Understanding **Electrocardiography**

Mary Boudreau Conover, RN, BSNed
Director of Education
Critical Care Conferences
Santa Cruz, California

With 689 illustrations

EIGHTH EDITION

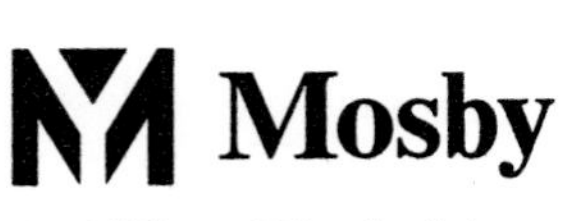

An Affiliate of Elsevier Science

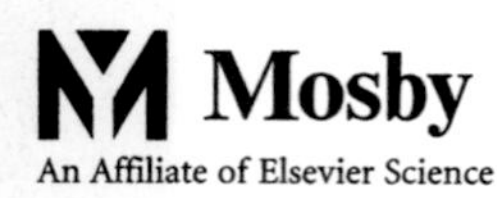

An Affiliate of Elsevier Science

11830 Westline Industrial Drive
St. Louis, Missouri 63146

UNDERSTANDING ELECTROCARDIOGRAPHY, EIGHTH EDITION
ISBN 0-323-01905-6

NOTICE

Nursing is an ever-changing field. Standard safety precautions must be followed, but as new research and clinical experience broaden our knowledge, changes in treatment and drug therapy may become necessary or appropriate. Readers are advised to check the most current product information provided by the manufacturer of each drug to be administered to verify the recommended dose, the method and duration of administration, and contraindications. It is the responsibility of the licensed health care provider, relying on experience and knowledge of the patient, to determine dosages and the best treatment for each individual patient. Neither the publisher nor the author assumes any liability for any injury and/or damage to persons or property arising from this publication.

Previous editions copyrighted 1972, 1976, 1980, 1984, 1988, 1992, 1996

Library of Congress Cataloging-in-Publication Data

Conover, Mary Boudreau
Understanding electrocardiography / Mary Boudreau Conover.—8th ed.
p.; cm
Includes bibliographical references and index.
ISBN 0-323-01905-6
1. Electrocardiography. I. Title.
[DNLM: 1. Electrocardiography. WG 140 C753u 2002]
RC683.5.E5 C65 2002
616.1′207547—dc21

2002029924

Vice President, Publishing Director: Sally Schrefer
Executive Publisher: Barbara Nelson Cullen
Acquisitions Editor: Sandra Clark Brown
Senior Developmental Editor: Cindi Anderson
Publishing Services Manager: Deborah L. Vogel
Project Manager: Deon Lee
Design Manager: Bill Drone
Background Cover Image: Gary and Vivian Chapman/Getty Images/The Image Bank

RT/QWV

Printed in the United States of America

Last digit is the print number: 9 8 7 6 5 4 3 2 1

To

Ara G. Tilkian, MD

In tribute to his excellence as a Cardiologist,
selfless concern for his patients,
innate sense of ethics, and wonderful sense of humor

Co-author, consultant, friend
"Thank you" never seems enough

Consulting Panel

Charles Antzelevitch, PhD, FACC
Executive Director and Director of Research
Gordon K. Moe Scholar
Masonic Medical Research Laboratory
Utica, New York
Professor of Pharmacology
SUNY Health Science Center at Syracuse
Syracuse, New York
Chapter 27, Brugada Syndrome

A. John Camm, MD, FRCP
Professor of Clinical Cardiology
Department of Cardiological Sciences
St. George's Hospital Medical School
London, England
Chapter 26, Torsades de Pointes in the Acquired Long QT Syndrome

Antonio Pelliccia, MD
Professor of Medicine
Institute of Sports Science
Medical Division
Italian National Olympic Committee
Rome, Italy
Chapter 20, The Athlete's ECG

Michael Sanguinetti, PhD
Professor, Department of Medicine
Division of Cardiology
Eccles Institute of Human Genetics
University of Utah
Salt Lake City, Utah
Chapter 25, Congenital Long QT Syndrome

Ara G. Tilkian, MD
Assistant Clinical Professor of Medicine
Division of Cardiology
University of California School of Medicine
Los Angeles, California
Director of Cardiology
Providence Holy Cross Medical Center
Mission Hills, California
Chapter 24, Acute Myocardial Infarction

Albert L. Waldo, MD
The Walter H. Pritchard Professor of Cardiology
Professor of Medicine
Professor of Biomedical Engineering
Case Western Reserve University
Adult Cardiac Electrophysiology Program
University Hospitals of Cleveland
Cleveland, Ohio
Chapter 9, Atrial Flutter

Hein J.J. Wellens, MD, PhD
Professor of Cardiology
University of Maastricht
Chairman, Department of Cardiology
University Hospital Maastricht
Maastricht, The Netherlands
Chapter 8, Atrial Fibrillation

Contributors

Mary G. Adams-Hamoda, RN, PhD
Assistant Professor
State University of New York at Buffalo
School of Nursing
Chapter 31, In-Hospital Cardiac Monitoring

John R. Buysman, PhD, BME
Product Ressearch Analyst
Customer Service Scientist
Medtronic Inc.
Minneapolis, Minnesota
Chapter 33, Electrical Stimulation Therapies
Chapter 34, Pacemaker Therapies for Bradyarrhythmias

Edward L. Conover, BSEE
Hughes Aircraft (retired)
Manager Electronic Design Automation
Santa Cruz, California
Chapter 32, Signal-Averaged ECG and Fast Fourier Transform Analysis

Michele M. Pelter, RN, PhD
Project Director
Department of Physiological Nursing
University of California, San Francisco
Chapter 31, In-Hospital Cardiac Monitoring

Preface

When combined with the patient's history, the electrocardiogram (ECG) is a superior diagnostic and prognostic tool. It also guides the clinician regarding referrals for permanent cures with radiofrequency ablation. Data accumulated from genetic research, activation mapping, entrainment techniques, radiofrequency ablation, and comparisons with surface ECGs have yielded an explosion of new information regarding mechanisms, risks, diagnosis, therapy, and cure, changing the way patients with arrhythmias and myocardial infarction are managed. These are the exciting possibilities that are offered in the eighth edition of this book.

The great physicist and Nobel prize recipient Richard P. Feynman once said that when people do not learn by understanding but rather by rote, "Their knowledge is so fragile!" The goal of this book is to impart an understanding of the ECG through comprehension of the mechanisms of cardiac rhythms and a systematic approach to ECG recognition. With these skills, clinical implications are appreciated, and better patient outcomes are ensured. This book has never been a "cookbook" approach to the ECG because of my belief that in emergency settings appropriate response is compromised when a background in the understanding of mechanisms is missing.

To facilitate your approach to understanding electrocardiography, the text is divided into four major sections:

I. Introduction to the 12-Lead Electrocardiogram
II. Arrhythmia Recognition
III. Abnormal 12-Lead Electrocardiograms
IV. Special Diagnostic and Therapeutic Procedures

As in the last edition, arrhythmias and ECG abnormalities are described according to ECG recognition, rhythm variations, mechanisms, causes, clinical implications, symptoms, pediatric considerations, bedside diagnosis, differential diagnosis, and treatment.

This edition includes new chapters on The Athlete's ECG, In-Hospital Cardiac Monitoring, Congenital Long QT Syndrome, and Brugada Syndrome.

Significant new information has been added to the chapters on Torsades de Pointes in the Acquired Long QT Syndrome, Atrial Fibrillation, Atrial Flutter, Acute Myocardial Infarction, and Pacemaker Therapies for Bradyarrhythmias.

As always, I hope that you enjoy learning from this book and learn to enjoy electrocardiography as I do. I have secured as my consulting panel the best and most current in the world in the field of electrocardiography and pacing techniques to ensure your confidence in the accuracy of each chapter; this has been my pledge through eight editions. It is my purpose to help you approach the ECG with confidence and eagerness born from understanding, especially in the emergency settings of tachycardia, profound bradycardia, and drug toxicity. Much good can be accomplished for our patients by an informed clinician and teacher. My sincere hope is that my readers will be both ... clinician and teacher.

Mary Conover

Acknowledgments

Mary G. Adams-Hamoda, RN, PhD, and Michele M. Pelter, RN, PhD Drs. Adams-Hamoda and Pelter wrote the chapter on In-Hospital Cardiac Monitoring, bringing this edition up to date on this important approach to excellent patient care.

Charles Antzelevitch, PhD, FACC Thank you, Dr. Antzelevitch, for your help on the genetics and electrophysiological mechanisms of Brugada syndrome. Your guidance and writings were indispensable to me in creating Chapter 27.

John R. Buysman, PhD, BME Dr. Buysman is a universally acknowledged scientist and expert in pacing technology. I would like to thank him for his considerable contribution to this and the last two editions of this book.

A. John Camm, MD, FRCP I am grateful to Dr. Camm for reviewing the chapter on Torsades de Pointes in the Acquired Long QT Syndrome. Dr. Camm is a universally acknowledged authority on the rapidly expanding list of drugs, new and old, cardiac and noncardiac, and their combinations capable of causing torsades de pointes. His advice on this and on the sections on mechanism, cellular electrophysiology, public health risks, and torsades de pointes in women is greatly appreciated.

Antonio Pelliccia, MD I am grateful to Dr. Pelliccia for reviewing the chapter on The Athlete's ECG. His responsibilities for the physiologic and medical evaluation of the athletes of the Italian national teams from which Olympic athletes are selected has made him a valued resource.

Michael Sanguinetti, PhD Chapter 25 could not have been written without the help of Dr. Sanguinetti, who guided me through the genetics of congenital long QT syndrome.

Ara G. Tilkian, MD I am grateful to Dr. Tilkian for his expert review and major contribution to the chapter on Acute Myocardial Infarction in this and the last four editions, involving considerable time and commitment.

Albert L. Waldo, MD Thank you, Dr. Waldo, for your advice regarding the new classification of atrial flutter.

Hein J.J. Wellens, MD, PhD Dr. Wellens needs no introduction to my readers. I would like to thank him for his review of the chapter on Atrial Fibrillation and for his participation in the formation of many of the chapters in this book over the last 25 years and six editions. His clinical expertise, research, publications, lectures, and genuine concern for good outcomes for cardiac patients everywhere has uniquely and indelibly influenced cardiology throughout the world. I am privileged to be associated with him.

Contents

PART I

Introduction to the 12-Lead Electrocardiogram

CHAPTER 1

The 12 Electrocardiogram Leads

The heart is an electrical field in which currents flow in repetitive patterns with each cardiac cycle, which consists of electrical systole (depolarization and repolarization) and electrical diastole (the resting phase). The arms and legs are linear extensions of this electrical field. Therefore the electrical activity of the heart can be detected at the extremities by placing electrodes of opposite polarity on the skin at opposite poles of the heart's electrical field.

A lead is composed of two electrodes of opposite polarity (bipolar) or one electrode and a reference point (unipolar). It is attached to an amplifier within an oscilloscope or strip recorder (Fig. 1-1). This instrument, the *electrocardiograph*, accurately records the electrical activity of the heart, being influenced by the direction and magnitude of current flow. The recording of the cardiac electrical cycle is called the *electrocardiogram (ECG)*.

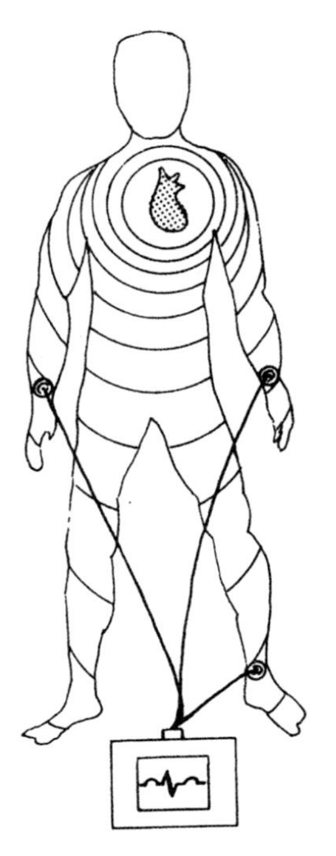

FIG. 1-1. The arms and legs are linear extensions of the electrical field of the heart. The current flow from each cardiac cycle is detected at the skin by electrodes, is amplified, and then displayed on an oscilloscope or written on a strip recorder.

There are 12 leads in the standard surface electrocardiogram, 3 bipolar and 9 unipolar. The only bipolar leads are on the limbs, and there are 3 unipolar limb leads as well; the remaining leads are on the chest (precordial). These leads record atrial activation (depolarization), ventricular activation (depolarization), and ventricular recovery (repolarization).

FRONTAL PLANE LEADS COMPARED WITH HORIZONTAL PLANE LEADS

Frontal plane leads are I, II, III, aV_R, aV_L, and aV_F. They are called *frontal plane leads* because they give information about current flow that is right, left, inferior, or superior.

Horizontal plane leads are the precordial leads V_1 to V_6. They give information about current flow on the horizontal plane (i.e., right, left, anterior, or posterior).

LIMB LEADS

Half of the limb leads are bipolar (I, II, and III) and half are unipolar (aV_R, aV_L, and aV_F).

Bipolar leads have two electrodes (positive [+] and negative [−]) about equidistant from the heart, with each contributing equally to the tracing. An imaginary line drawn between the two electrodes is the *axis of the lead*, illustrated in Fig. 1-2; all currents generated by the heart relate to the axis of each lead.

Unipolar leads have a positive electrode and an indifferent connection, which is achieved by connecting the electrodes from the three bipolar limb leads—I, II, and III—through resistances to a central terminal. The potential at

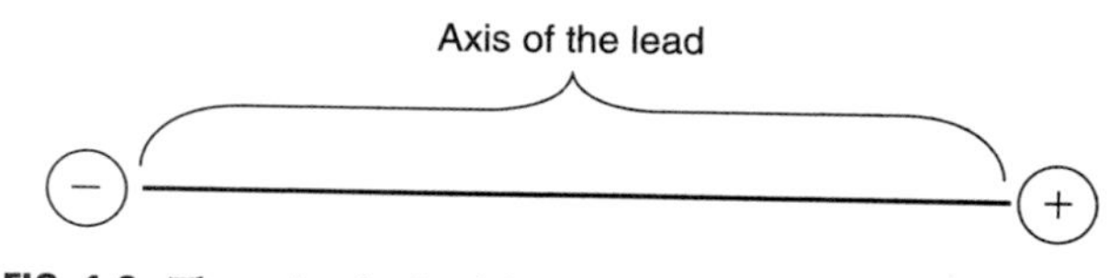

FIG. 1-2. The axis of a lead is an imaginary line drawn between the two electrodes of the bipolar lead or between the positive electrode and a reference point of the unipolar lead.

the central terminal, which represents the center of the electrical field of the heart, is almost zero, so the contribution to the tracing is made solely by the positive electrode. The axes of unipolar limb leads are from the positive electrode on the limbs (*R*, right arm; *L*, left arm; *F*, left leg) to the zero potential at the center of the electrical field, the heart.

EINTHOVEN'S TRIANGLE

Willem Einthoven, as a young scientist and professor of physiology at Leiden University in The Netherlands, first introduced the three bipolar limb leads (I, II, and III), whose axes form an inverted equilateral triangle (Fig. 1-3). The sum of voltages in any closed path such as Einthoven's triangle equals zero. However, because Einthoven reversed the positive and negative electrodes of lead II in his triangle, in the equation you would then subtract instead of add the voltage from lead II. That is, the voltages from lead I plus voltages from lead III, *minus* voltages from lead II, equals zero (I + III – II = 0).

The zero potential created by the vector sum of these voltages is the virtual ground used as a reference point for the unipolar leads; that reference point is in the center of the triangle.

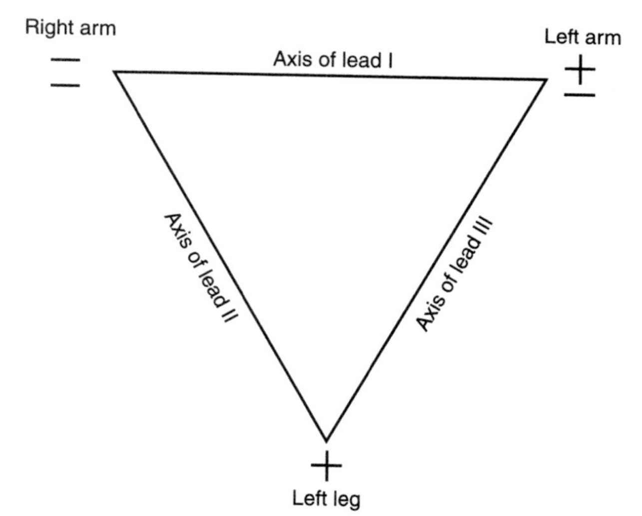

FIG. 1-3. Einthoven's triangle is formed by the axes of the three bipolar limb leads—I, II, and III. The diagram shows the placement of the positive and negative electrodes for each lead.

PLACEMENT OF ELECTRODES FOR EINTHOVEN'S TRIANGLE

Lead I

The negative electrode is placed on the right arm and the positive on the left arm. Thus the axis of lead I is from shoulder to shoulder.

Lead II

The negative electrode is placed on the right arm and the positive on the left leg. Thus the axis of lead II is from the right shoulder to the apex of the inverted triangle.

Note: Although the placement of an electrode on the left leg makes the triangle seem out of balance, it is nevertheless an equilateral triangle because all electrodes are about equidistant from the electrical field of the heart.

Lead III

The negative electrode is placed on the left arm and the positive on the left leg. Thus the axis of lead III is from the left shoulder to the apex of the triangle.

UNIPOLAR LIMB LEADS

The axes of the three unipolar limb leads—aV_R, aV_L, and aV_F—are illustrated in Fig. 1-4. Note that a positive electrode in the R, L, and F positions is compared with the zero potential at the center of the heart's electrical field (i.e., the center of Einthoven's triangle). The letter *a* stands for augmented, a term added when it was discovered that eliminating a negative electrode resulted in the amplitude of the recording being augmented by 50%. The letter *V* indicates a unipolar lead. The letters *R*, *L*, and *F* indicate where the positive electrode is placed; that is, right arm, left

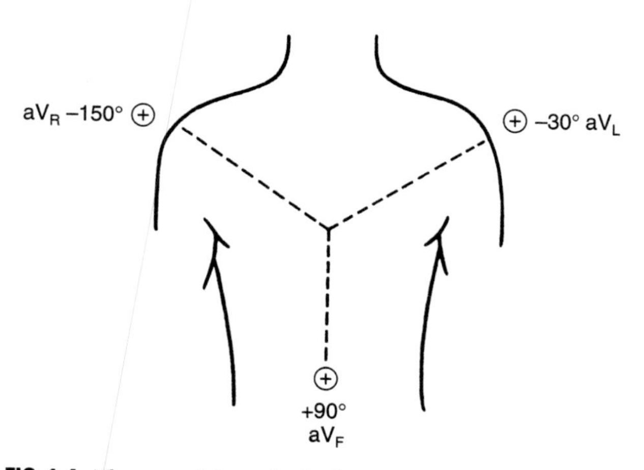

FIG. 1-4. The axes of the unipolar limb leads are from the positive electrode on each point of Einthoven's triangle to the center of the electrical field (the heart).

arm, and left leg. In some records these leads are simply designated R, L, and F instead of aV_R, aV_L, and aV_F.

PRECORDIAL LEADS

The axes of the precordial leads are illustrated in Fig. 1-5. This cross-section of the thorax demonstrates how valuable these leads are in recording anterior and posterior, right and left forces.

The placement of the precordial electrodes is shown in Fig. 1-6. As with the limb leads, the letter *V* indicates a unipolar lead. The numbers 1 to 6 are codes for locations on the precordium. To find the placement for the V_1 electrode place your fingers at the left sternal border just below the clavicle; you will feel the first rib. Below that is the first intercostal space. Slip your fingers down along the left sternal border over each rib, counting four intercostal spaces; place the electrode in the fourth intercostal space. Accustomed as one becomes to placing this electrode on the patient, it is still a good idea to count intercostal spaces; incorrect placement of this electrode may result in a slightly abnormal pattern. Additionally, position of the remaining chest electrodes would be affected. V_2 is located at the same interspace along the right sternal border. V_4 is at the midclavicular line, the fifth intercostal space. V_3 is halfway between V_2 and V_4. On the same level with V_4 are the two lateral chest leads, V_5 and V_6; they are placed in the anterior and midaxillary lines, respectively. Identify the placement for V_6 by first locating the fifth intercostal space at the sternal border and drawing a straight imaginary line across the chest to the midaxillary line.

Lead V_1 looks into the right ventricle, leads V_2 to V_3 span the interventricular septum, lead V_4 is over the cardiac apex, and leads V_5 and V_6 reflect the left lateral wall of the heart.

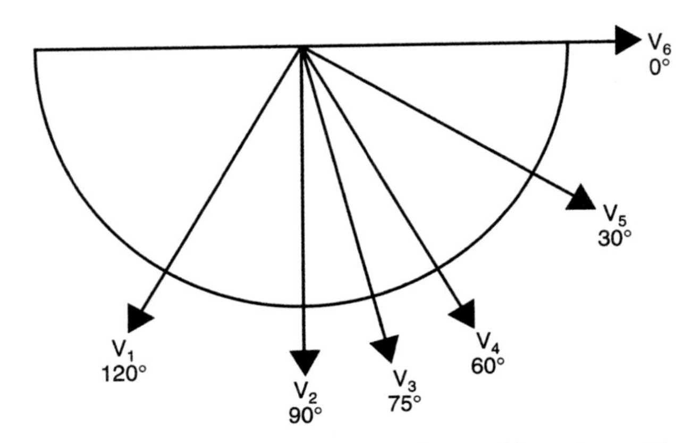

FIG. 1-5. The axes of the precordial leads extend from the positive electrode on the chest wall to the center of the heart's electrical field, which is the sum of Einthoven's triangle.

RIGHT CHEST LEADS

The right chest leads are V_{3R}, V_{4R}, V_{5R}, and V_{6R}. The positive electrodes for these leads are in the same position on the right side of the chest as their counterparts on the left side. Thus the positive electrode for V_{4R} is at the midclavicular line, fifth intercostal space, right chest; for V_{3R} it is halfway between V_{4R} and V_1 of the standard 12-lead ECG. The electrodes for V_{5R} and V_{6R} are on the same level with V_{4R}—in the anterior and midaxillary lines, respectively. The electrode position for V_{4R} is shown in Fig. 1-6. Lead V_{4R} is the most useful of the right chest leads in the emergency setting. It is used to evaluate risk in patients with acute inferior myocardial infarction (Chapter 25).

MCL LEADS

The MCL leads are bipolar precordial leads that simulate unipolar precordial leads. Although many critical care units now monitor with all 12 leads or at least have the facility for 7 leads, the MCL leads are still useful when only 2 electrodes and a ground are available.

Before 1960 the ECG sometimes contained three

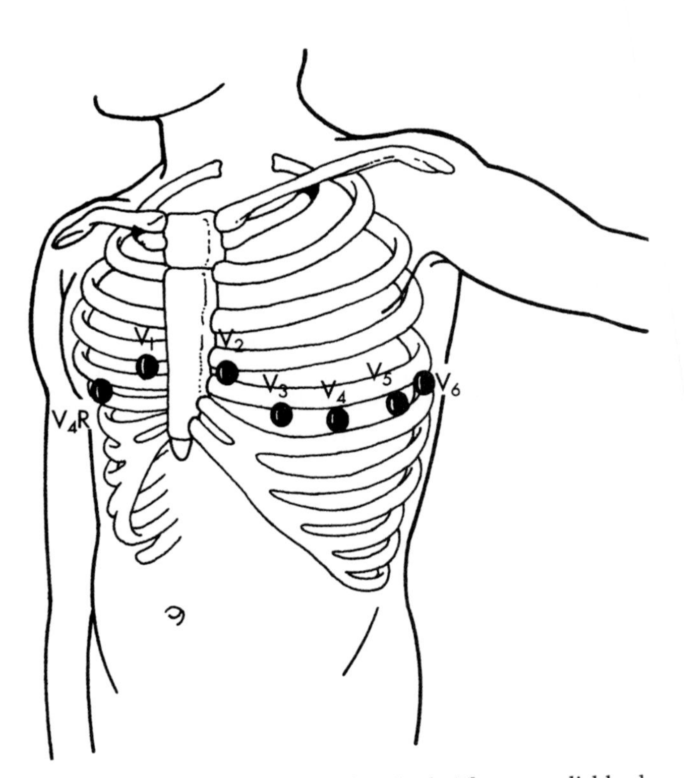

FIG. 1-6. Electrode sites for the chest leads. The precordial leads are on the left from V_1 on the right sternal border to V_6 at the left midaxillary line. One of the designated right chest leads is shown (V_{4R}), although V_1 is also a right chest lead. Please see text for exact placement of electrodes.

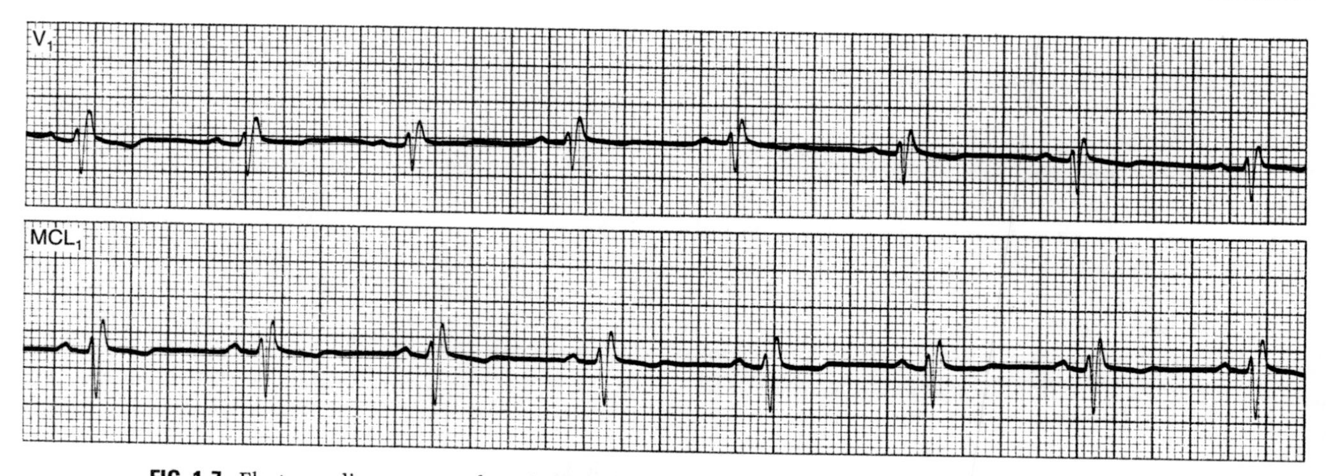

FIG. 1-7. Electrocardiogram complexes in V_1 and MCL_1 compared. The patterns in the two leads are virtually identical in this normal sinus rhythm with incomplete right bundle branch block, nicely illustrating the value of the bipolar set up for simulating a unipolar precordial lead.

bipolar chest leads with the positive electrode on the chest (C) and the negative electrode on an extremity (R [right arm], L [left arm], or F [left leg]). With the introduction of the coronary care units in 1962, there was only one monitoring lead available. Dr. Henry Marriott, in search of the best monitoring lead, modified the old bipolar CL lead, placing the positive electrode in the V_1 position and the negative electrode at the left shoulder under the left clavicle (modified CL in the V_1 position: MCL_1). This placement simulated the complex seen in the unipolar V_1 position. Since then, this bipolar lead has been used for monitoring in certain clinical settings when the unipolar lead, V_1, is not available. Fig. 1-7 illustrates the two recordings from the same patient, one of leads V_1 and the other of MCL_1. The two recordings are very similar and the diagnosis of right bundle branch block can be made from either lead. Any of the precordial leads can be simulated by this method. Think of the negative electrode at the left shoulder as an anchor (it doesn't change); turn the channel selection to one of the bipolar limb lead positions. Then take the negative electrode for that lead position and place it at the left shoulder. The positive electrode can be moved to the precordial position desired. Modern equipment with multiple monitoring leads eliminates the need for this useful lead.

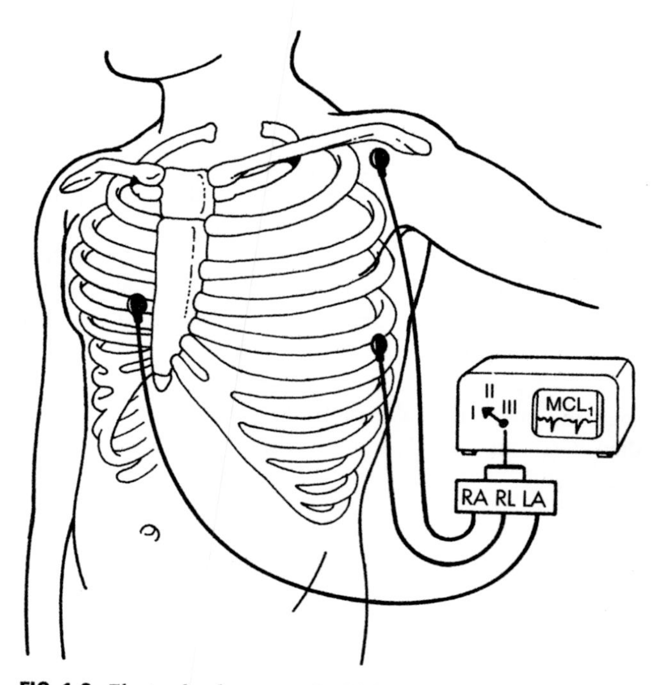

FIG. 1-8. Electrode placement for MCL_1 using the single-channel monitor with three lead-wire cables capable of recording only one bipolar lead.

Electrode Placement for MCL Leads

Single-channel monitor. When using the single-channel monitor you have three selections: lead I, II, or III. This is achieved simply by placing the electrodes in the inverted triangular position (both arms and the left leg). The ground is incorporated into the left leg lead wire; thus this lead is both positive and ground. Fig. 1-8 demonstrates the use of these three lead wires to obtain the MCL leads.

1. Place the electrodes in the positions illustrated in Fig. 1-9 (with one electrode in the V_1 position and another in the V_6 position; the third electrode is at the left shoulder).

2. Turn your lead selector to lead I, which means that the right arm cable is negative and the left arm cable is positive. Thus the right arm cable goes to the left shoulder electrode and the left arm cable to the V_1 position on the right sternal border; the third cable (RL) is attached to the electrode in the V_6 position.
3. You are now recording the bipolar lead, MCL_1, a simulation of the unipolar lead, V_1.
4. If you turn your lead selector to lead II, you will be recording the bipolar lead, MCL_6, a simulation of the unipolar lead, V_6.
5. To record a simulated V_2 or V_3 lead, simply move the electrode at the right sternal border to those positions.

Telemetry monitor. Many telemetry monitors have no selector dial for changing leads. In Fig. 1-9 the electrode positions for recording MCL_1 are illustrated. Should you wish to record a simulated V_2 or V_3, simply move the left arm electrode across the sternum to those positions.

PLACEMENT OF ELECTRODES FOR MULTICHANNEL MONITORING

Fig. 1-10 shows the correct placement for the electrodes of multichannel monitors with five lead-wire cables, negating the necessity for MCL_1 because V_1 will be available. Such an arrangement permits recording all the limb leads (I, II, III, aV_R, aV_L, aV_F) and one precordial lead. The precordial lead shown is V_1; however, it is possible to record other precordial leads by moving the C electrode to the desired position. Right chest leads may also be obtained by moving the C electrode to the V_{3R}, V_{4R}, V_{5R}, or V_{6R} positions.

SUMMARY

The standard ECG consists of 12 leads—6 frontal plane leads and 6 horizontal plane leads. There are only three bipolar leads—I, II, and III. The axes of these leads form an inverted equilateral triangle around the heart's electrical field. The sum of the potentials from these three bipolar leads offers a zero potential in the center of the triangle. All unipolar leads use this zero potential as a reference point. Thus the axis of all unipolar leads is from the positive electrode to the center of the triangle. There are three unipolar limb leads—aV_R, aV_L, and aV_F—and six precordial leads that form a curve from the right heart, across the septum, to the left ventricle (V_1 to V_6). The electrode for V_1 is located on the right chest at the sternal border; the electrode for V_6 is located at the left midaxillary line.

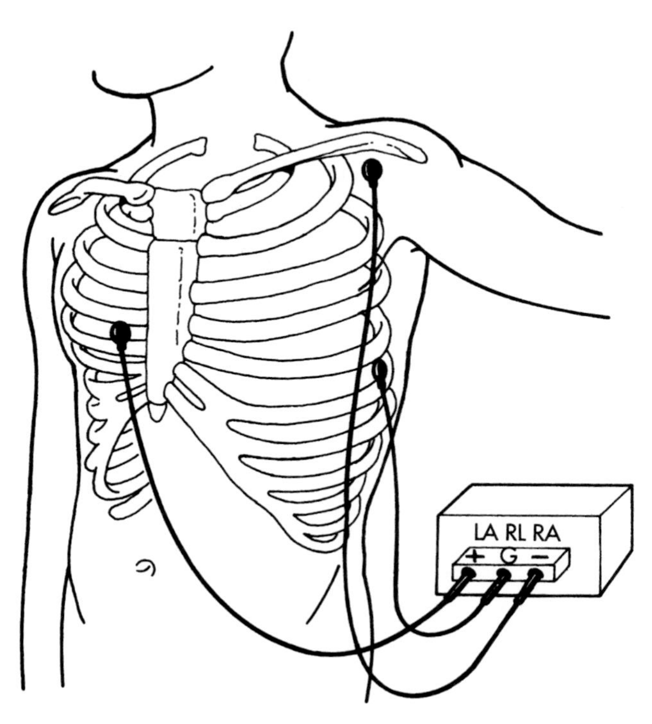

FIG. 1-9. Electrode placement for telemetry monitoring.

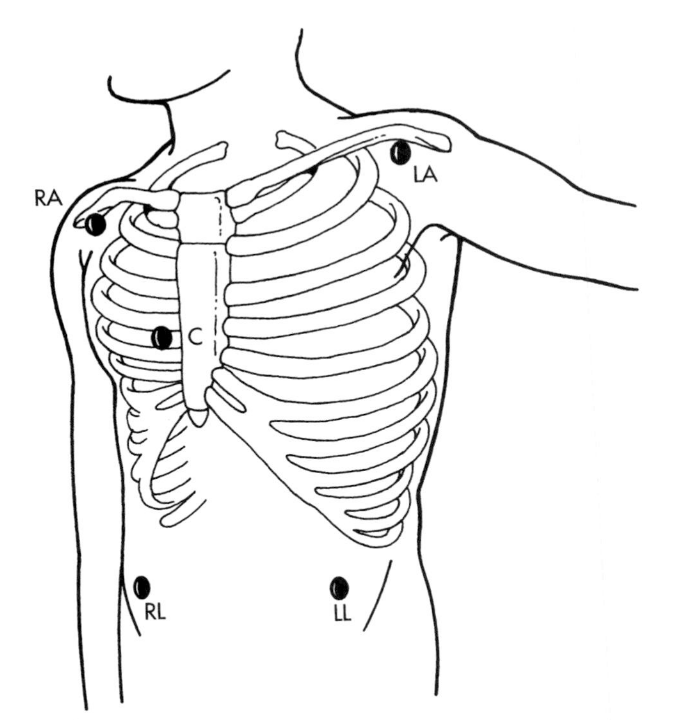

FIG. 1-10. Electrode placement for multichannel monitoring using five lead-wire cables capable of recording one or more limb leads and any one of the precordial leads, eliminating the necessity for MCL_1. (V_1 is shown here.)

CHAPTER 2

Normal Electrical Activation of the Heart

The normal activation of the heart is initiated by the sinus node, also called the sinoatrial (SA) node. The entire heart follows in an eloquently orchestrated sequence resulting in perfect pump function. Contributing to this perfection are the various geometrical structures of the cardiac fibers, the highly specific electrical properties of various cells, and their connections to each other.

Right and left atrial depolarization produces a P wave on the electrocardiogram (ECG). During and immediately after the inscription of the P wave the conduction system is activated (atrioventricular [AV] node, bundle of His, bundle branches, and Purkinje fibers). Activation of these structures is a silent event on the surface ECG, the impulses not being large enough to be transmitted to the skin.

As soon as the working ventricular muscle cells are activated, a ventricular complex (QRS) begins to be inscribed on the ECG. Ventricular depolarization proceeds from endocardium to epicardium starting with the interventricular septum.

The ST segment begins at the end of the QRS complex and ends at the beginning of the T wave; it should be isoelectric and slightly slanted up, although in athletes it can be elevated as much as 2 mm (see Chapter 20). The ST segment, along with the T wave, represents the different phases of ventricular repolarization.

The electrical cardiac cycle consists of three phases: depolarization, repolarization, and resting. The resting working atrial or ventricular cell is negatively charged to –90 mV. This negative charge is maintained until the cell is activated (depolarization).

A pacemaker cell does not have a resting phase; after the completion of the action potential, during electrical diastole, it begins the process of self-depolarization, known as the property of *automaticity*, which progresses until the cell reaches threshold potential and activates itself (SA nodal cells) or is activated by the SA nodal impulse (sinus rhythm) or another source (ectopic focus or artificial pacemaker).

DEPOLARIZATION

Depolarization is the process by which a resting cell becomes more positive. This process may be slow, as it is in pacemaker cells, or extremely rapid, as it is in atrial and ventricular myocardial cells. The cells of the sinus node, the normal pacemaker of the heart, depolarize relatively slowly, although it can hardly be thought of as slow when there is a sinus tachycardia. It is slow, however, compared to the explosive response of the myocardial cells when this sinus impulse reaches them. The rapid depolarization of a myocardial cell is accomplished by a sudden influx of sodium (Na^+) and calcium (Ca^{2+}) ions into the cell, driving it from its resting state of –90 mV to a positive charge that momentarily reaches 30 mV.

REPOLARIZATION

Repolarization is the process by which a depolarized cell is restored to its resting state. The repolarization process begins immediately after rapid depolarization; a complicated interaction of current flow first maintains the membrane at a *plateau* of approximately 0 mV and then rapidly restores the membrane to its resting state of –90 mV. The plateau permits a *refractory period* during which the cell cannot be activated again.

AUTOMATICITY

Automaticity is the ability of a cell to depolarize itself (slow depolarization), reach threshold potential, and produce a propagated action potential. Cardiac tissues that possess the property of normal automaticity are listed in Box 2-1. The sinus node normally paces the heart and the subsidiary pacemakers provide backup in the event that the sinus node fails (sinus arrest), is too slow (sinus bradycardia), or its impulse is blocked (sinoatrial [SA] block). Atrial and ventricular working myocardial cells do not depolarize spontaneously. As long as they remain healthy, their best feature is the ability to wait by maintaining their negative charge (i.e., they do not activate themselves, but await a stimulus from the sinus node or another pacing source).

BOX 2-1. Cardiac Tissues with Normal Automaticity

SINUS NODE

Parts of the atria (coronary sinus, inferior right atrium, Bachmann's bundle, the AV valves, and atrial fibers along the crista terminalis and interatrial septum)

AV nodal region

His-Purkinje system

AV, Atrioventricular.

ACTION POTENTIAL

The action potential is a graph of the electrical cardiac cycle of a single cell. It reflects the cellular events that take place during depolarization and repolarization. An appreciation for the normal action potential is necessary for an understanding of the effects of genetic mutations on the transfer of ions across the cell membranes in the chapters that deal with the congenital long QT syndrome (Chapter 26) and Brugada syndrome (Chapter 28).

One of the first things noticeable about the cardiac action potential is its long duration, which is necessary to prevent premature excitation. The different phases of the action potential are the result of multiple inward and outward ionic currents of Na^+, potassium (K^+), and Ca^{2+}. Some of the genes controlling these currents have been identified, facilitating our understanding of malfunctions (see Chapter 25).

The action potential of a ventricular myocardial cell is seen in Fig. 2-1, *A*. Note the phases of rapid depolarization (phase 0), initial repolarization (phase 1), the plateau (phase 2), rapid repolarization (phase 3), and quiescence (phase 4). The property of automaticity (phase 4 depolarization) can be seen in the second action potential (*B*); the slow rise of phase 4 to a more positive value reflects slow diastolic depolarization (automaticity). This cell is capable of of reaching threshold potential (–70 mV) without outside stimulus.

Phase 0

The ventricular cell is driven to threshold by the impulse from an outside source (normally the sinus node). Once at threshold, the cell depolarizes rapidly and inactivates immediately. A record of this event is seen in the graph of the ventricular action potential. It is the tall, swiftly drawn vertical line (phase 0), caused by the rapid influx of Na^+ via voltage-dependent sodium channels. (Notable exceptions are the sinus and AV nodes.) Slow and fast Ca^{2+} currents also make a contribution to this dramatic phase of the action potential. In most cardiac fibers the fast sodium channels open at approximately –65 mV, and are the main cause of the phase 0 spike, as well as determining conduction velocity. A second inward current is initiated during phase 0 in atrial, Purkinje, and nodal cells at about –60 to –50 mV when the T-type calcium channels briefly open. At approximately –40 mV the L-type (slow) calcium channels open with clustered bursts that continue during phase 2 in all cardiac cells.

Although the calcium current contributes little to phase 0 of the action potential, it plays a major role in triggering calcium release from its stores in the sarcoplasmic reticulum, permitting myocardial contraction to take place.

Phase 1

Phase 1 is the rapid, brief, and incomplete beginning of repolarization immediately following phase 0 that occurs because the fast sodium channels abruptly close and a transient outward potassium current is activated.

Phase 2

Phase 2 is the plateau or phase that depends on a delicate balance of inward and outward currents across the membrane to maintain an electrical equilibrium. The Ca^{2+} influx that was initiated during phase 0 continues but slowly declines as the slow Ca^{2+} channels inactivate. This, along with a rising K^+ permeability, ultimately repolarizes the cell. At least seven functionally distinct potassium currents have been described. It is these channels that are the target for drugs used to control arrhythmias (class III antiarrhythmic agents).

Phase 3

Phase 3 is the phase of late, rapid repolarization. This phase is initiated when the slow calcium channels close and is implemented by an exodus of potassium from the cell.

Phase 4

Phase 4 is electrical diastole when the heart rests, except for the pacemaker cells, especially the cells of the sinus

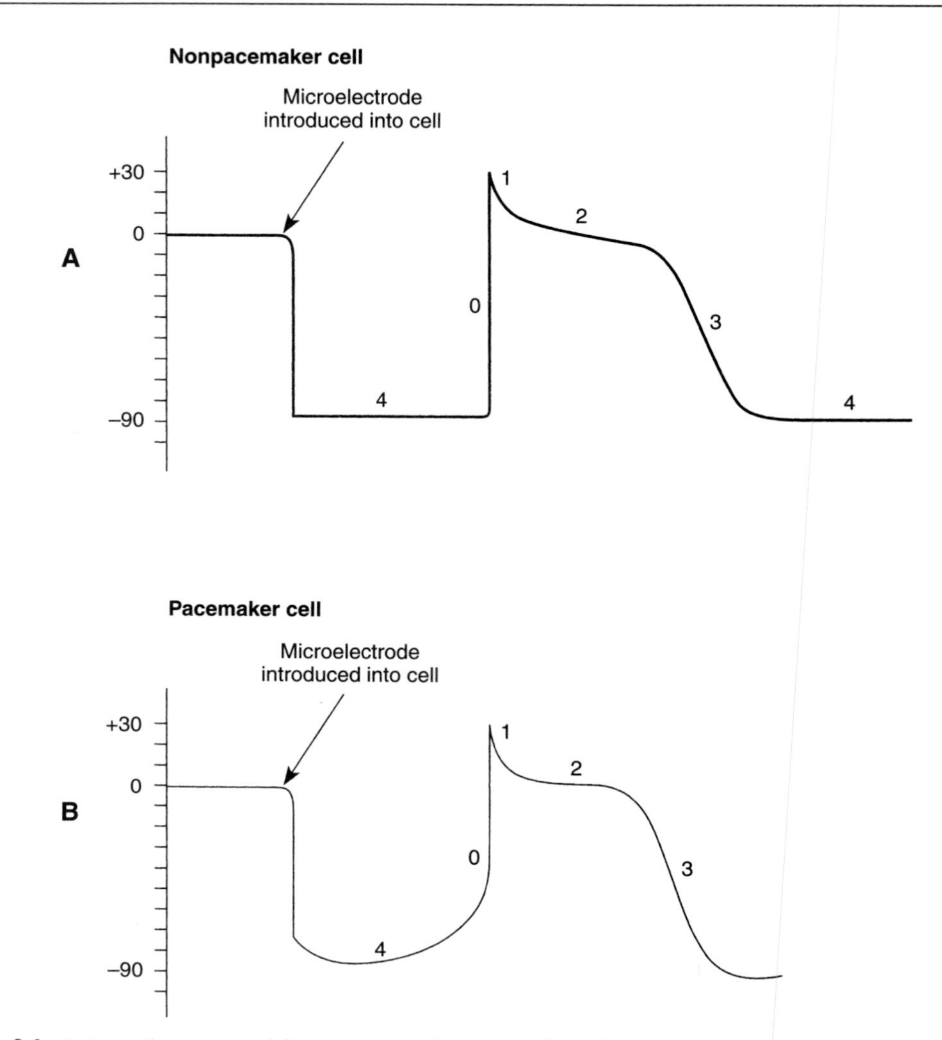

FIG. 2-1. **A**, An action potential from a ventricular myocardial cell. Phase 4 is flat, indicating lack of automaticity. **B**, An action potential from a pacemaker cell. In this case phase 4 slopes upward toward threshold potential, indicating the power of automaticity.

node; at the end of phase 3, pacemaker cells begin the process that is intended to bring them to threshold potential. In the normal heart only the sinus node reaches that threshold.

NORMAL PACEMAKER AND CONDUCTION SYSTEM OF THE HEART

The pacing and conduction system and the timing and form of the action potentials in different areas of the heart are illustrated in very diagrammatically in Fig. 2-2, *A* and *B*. In *A* note that the sinus or SA node and the AV node are both supplied by the vagus nerve. When the rate of the sinus node increases or decreases, so does AV conduction time. In *B*, note that the action potentials from the two nodes are similar in shape, a shape that permits only slow conduction—so that, although the rate of the sinus node can be rapid, conduction velocity through it is slow. Illustrated are the time sequence and shape of the normal action potentials from the sinus node that initiates the concatenation of action potentials of varying shapes and durations, to the ventricular epicardium. The ECG reflects the sequence of differences in electrical potentials and generated currents that exist between adjacent areas of the heart during the cardiac cycle. Note in Fig. 2-2, *B*, that the time

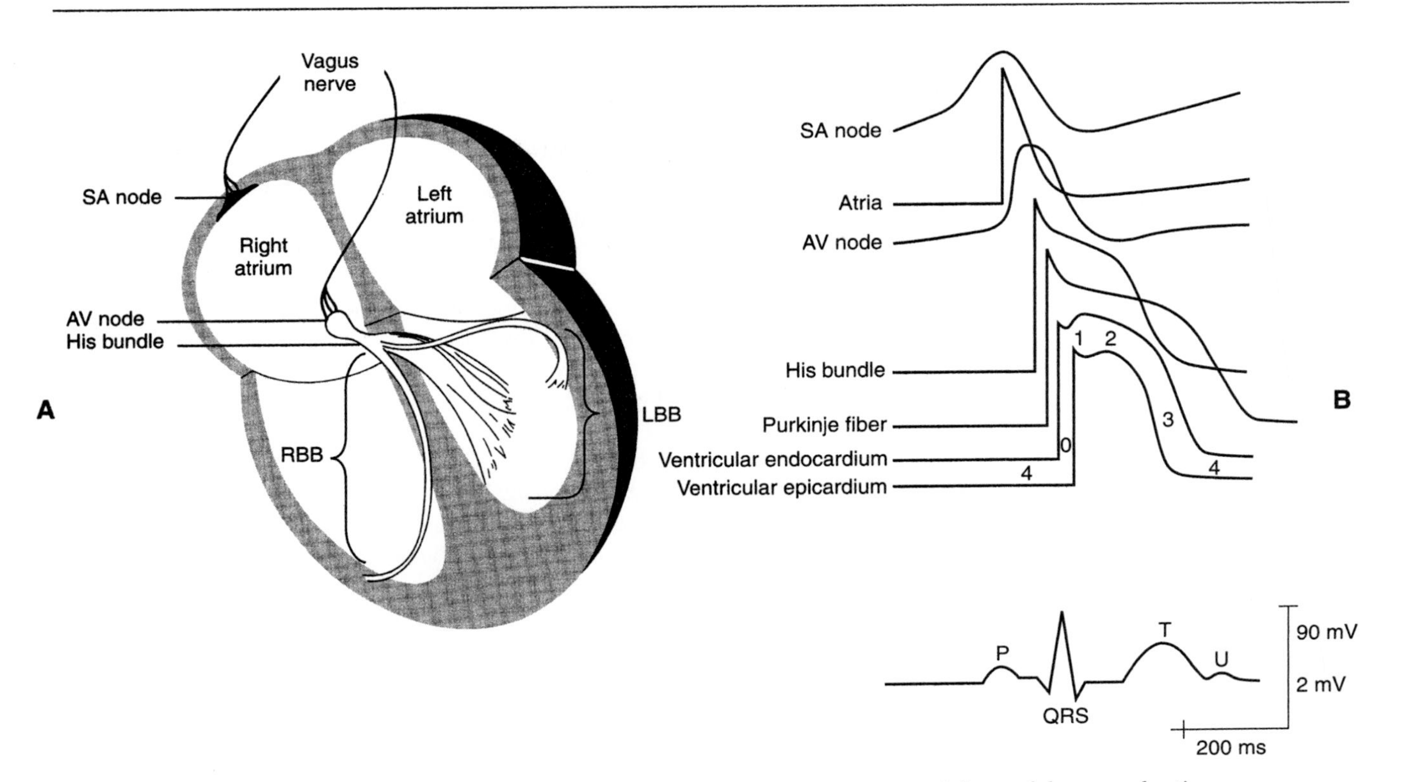

FIG. 2-2. **A,** The sinus node and conduction system. **B,** The time sequence and shape of the normal action potentials from the sinus node that initiates the concatenation of action potentials of varying shapes and durations to the ventricular epicardium. The ECG reflects the changing action potentials. *AV*, Atrioventricular; *LBB*, left bundle branch; *RBB*, right bundle branch; *SA*, sinoatrial.

lapse between ventricular endocardial and epicardial activation (phase 0 of the action potential) generates a current flow that creates the QRS complex. During phase 2, there is no difference in potential between those two areas of the heart, and the isoelectric ST segment appears on the ECG. During phase 3, the epicardium repolarizes first, creating a difference in potential between it and the endocardial cells, thus a current is generated, creating a positive T wave. Understanding this and how these currents relate to a lead axis (see Chapter 4) is the basis of understanding electrocardiography; the importance of fully grasping this before attempting to understand the mechanisms of arrhythmias and how they are reflected on the 12-lead ECG is often underestimated.

Sinus Node

The sinus node, located high in the right atrium near the superior vena cava, normally activates the atria at a rate consistent with the needs of the body. Thus atrial activation is from superior to inferior and from right to left. The impulse reaches the compact AV node via the fast AV nodal pathway before atrial activation is completed. It is then conducted down the bundle of His and into the ventricles via the bundle branches and the Purkinje fibers (the His-Purkinje system). Because the His-Purkinje system is a subendocardial structure, the impulse is delivered to the endocardium of both ventricles and activates them from endocardium to epicardium.

The AV Node, Its Atrial Pathways, and the His Bundle

The AV node, its atrial pathways, and the His bundle make up the conductive tissue of the AV junction (Fig. 2-3). They are located within the triangle of Koch, which is formed by the tricuspid annulus and the tendon of Todaro.

The compact AV node. The compact AV node is located just beneath the endocardium on the muscular septum that separates the right atrium from the left ventricle. It is

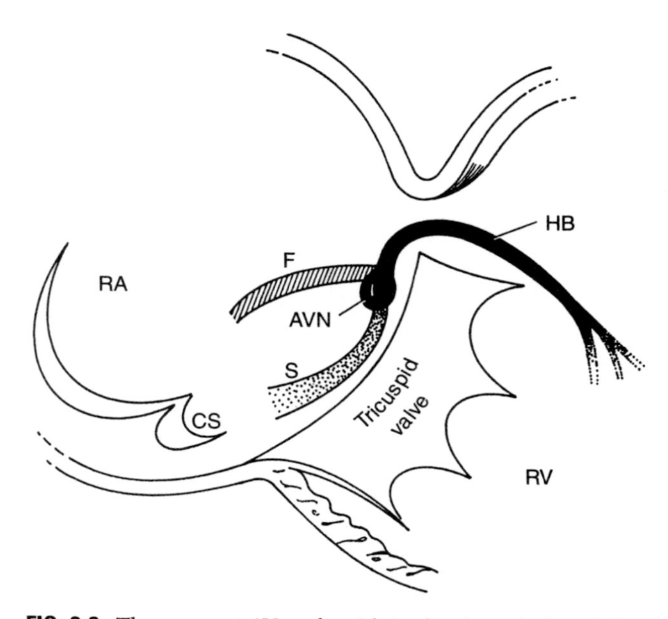

FIG. 2-3. The compact AV node with its fast (anterior) and slow (posterior) fibers. The slow pathway fibers extend from a broad area near the os of the coronary sinus and converge as a common pathway as they reach the compact AV node. The fast pathway fibers arise near the tendon of Todaro and enter the compact AV node superiorly. *RA*, Right atrium; *CS*, coronary sinus; *AVN*, atrioventricular node; *F*, fast pathway; *S*, slow pathway; *HB*, His bundle; *RV*, right ventricle. (Adapted from Keim S, Werner P, Jazayeri M et al: *Circulation* 86:919, 1992.)

directly above the insertion of the septal leaflet of the tricuspid valve and at the apex of the triangle of Koch. The compact node is isolated from the ventricular myocardial fibers by the annulus fibrosus and is usually far removed anteriorly from the coronary sinus.

Blood supply. In 90% of subjects the AV node receives its blood supply from the right coronary artery. In the remaining 10% the circumflex artery supplies the AV node.

Atrionodal pathways. Fig. 2-3 diagrammatically illustrates the parallel strands of fibers that emanate from the floor of the coronary sinus and are directed inferiorly along the tricuspid annulus toward the compact AV node. These strands are separated by fibrous tissue[1] and form a conduction pathway that is posterior and inferior to the compact node that has been called "slow." Another set of fibers are located anteriorly or superiorly along the compact AV node and exit into the atrial septum near Todaro's tendon, forming a conduction pathway that has been called "fast." Thus the fibers of the fast and slow pathways run along opposite edges of the compact AV node into the atrium in a fanlike fashion. Block in the slow pathway has no impact on the PR interval during sinus rhythm.[2]

His bundle. At the apex of the triangle of Koch, the compact AV node becomes the penetrating bundle of His, which crosses through while being encased in the insulating tissues of the central fibrous body (annulus fibrosus) and passes into the ventricular septum posterior to the membranous septum (see Fig. 2-3).[3] Normal cardiac conduction depends on the isolation of the atrial musculature from the ventricular musculature except at the point where the bundle of His penetrates the annulus. The His bundle has longitudinal strands of Purkinje-like cells with loosely arrayed mitochondria and few myofibrils.

Blood supply. The upper muscular ventricular septum, wherein the His bundle lies, receives its blood supply from branches of the left anterior and posterior descending coronary arteries.[4] The double blood supply makes this important link of the conduction system less vulnerable to ischemic damage.[5]

Right Bundle Branch

Fig. 2-4 illustrates the cordlike structure of the thin right bundle branch (RBB), explaining its vulnerability. It is supplied by the left anterior descending coronary artery. The RBB descends in its sheath to the bases of the papillary muscles, becoming a subendocardial structure in the middle and lower third of the ventricular septum. At its origin it is a direct continuation of the penetrating His bundle along the right side of the ventricular septum and remains unbranched until it reaches the apex of the right ventricle where it penetrates the right ventricular apex and sends a branch through the moderator band to the anterior papillary muscle of the tricuspid valve.

Terminal Purkinje fibers. The bundle branches terminate in a network of fibers on the endocardial surfaces of the ventricles that are very difficult to trace. The terminal Purkinje fibers tend to be concentrated at papillary muscles and to penetrate the subendocardium and myocardium.[5]

Left Bundle Branch

The left bundle branch (LBB) is illustrated in Fig. 2-5. It begins as a single structure and fans out into three divisions, originally described by Tawara in 1906.[6] This fan of conductive fibers streams down the left ventricular septum in a "virtual sheet"[7] forming large posterior, smaller anterior, and midseptal radiations. Thus there are three main interconnecting fascicles in the left ventricle rather than two. One supplies the anterior (superior) wall,

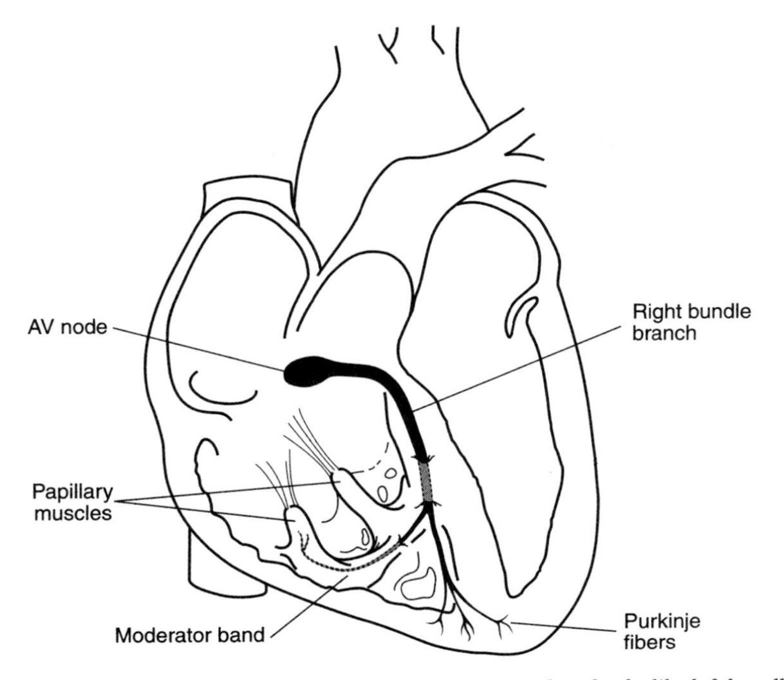

FIG. 2-4. Right bundle branch. Note its cordlike structure as opposed to the fanlike left bundle branch. *AV*, Atrioventricular.

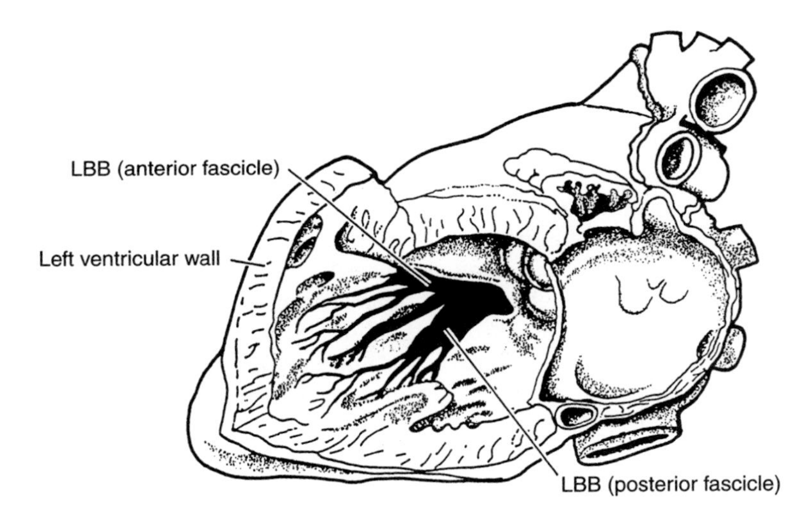

FIG. 2-5. Left bundle branch (*LBB*). Note the fanlike structure with its anterior and posterior fascicles and a medial fascicle in between.

another the posterior (inferior) wall, and a third the midseptum. The ECG pattern of left anterior hemiblock reflects LBB disease and is hardly ever confined solely to the anterior fascicle.

Blood supply. The posterior fascicle of the LBB receives its blood supply from both the left anterior descending and posterior descending coronary arteries. The anterior and medial fascicles of the LBB are supplied mainly by septal perforators from the left anterior descending coronary artery.

NORMAL ELECTROCARDIOGRAM

In Fig. 2-6 the normal ECG records atrial depolarization, represented by a small, rounded deflection called a *P*

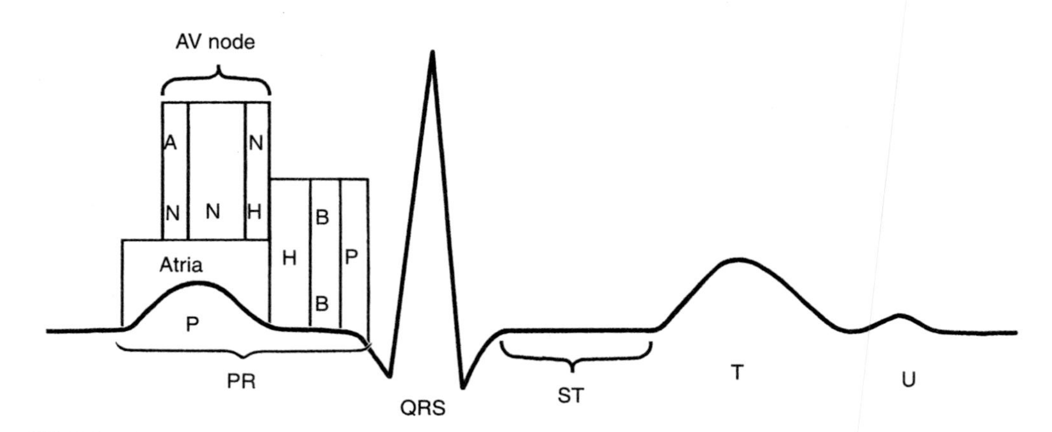

FIG. 2-6. The normal ECG: P wave, atrial depolarization; QRS, ventricular depolarization; ST segment and T wave, ventricular repolarization. The U wave is a small positive deflection. The PR interval reflects not only atrial depolarization but also the conduction time through the atrioventricular (*AV*) node, His bundle (*H*), bundle branches (*BB*), and Purkinje fibers (*P*). *AN*, Atrionodal; *N*, compact AV node; *NH*, nodal His.

wave; ventricular depolarization, represented by a swift, angular deflection called a *QRS complex*; and ventricular repolarization, called the *ST segment* and *T wave*. A *U wave* is a very small deflection that follows the T wave and has the same polarity. The PR interval represents atrial activation and the conduction time of the cardiac impulse as it passes down the AV node, His bundle, bundle branches, and Purkinje fibers.

STEP-BY-STEP ELECTRICAL ACTIVATION OF THE HEART (LEAD I)

The following sequence of illustrations and text demonstrates the step-by-step electrical activation of the heart and how each step is reflected on lead I of the ECG. The axis of lead I is depicted to show how the current flow relates to that lead axis. When current flows toward the positive electrode, the ECG stylus moves up; when current flows toward the negative electrode, the stylus moves down.

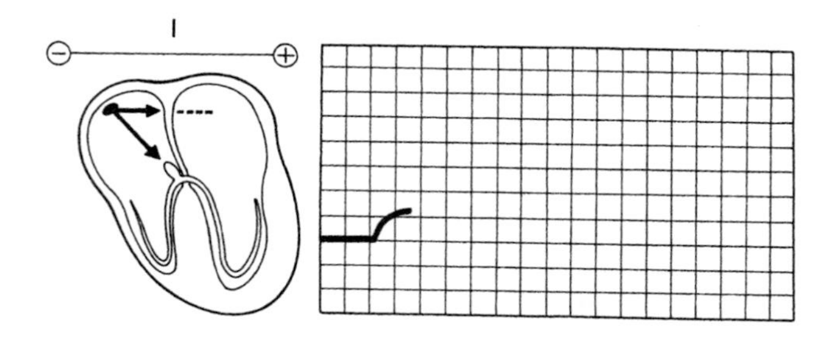

The first half of the *P wave* is inscribed in lead I when the sinus impulse activates the right atrium and reaches the AV node.

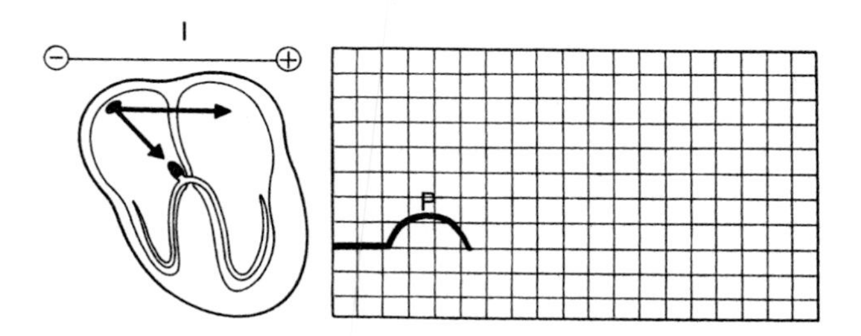

The left atrium and AV node have been activated by the time the P wave is completed. Note that the P wave represents both right and left atrial activation in sequence. Normally the P wave is smooth in contour, but if one or the other atrium is stretched or hypertrophied, the P wave can be distorted. At approximately the peak of the P wave the AV node is being activated. This is a "silent" event, not seen on the ECG because the currents involved are so small.

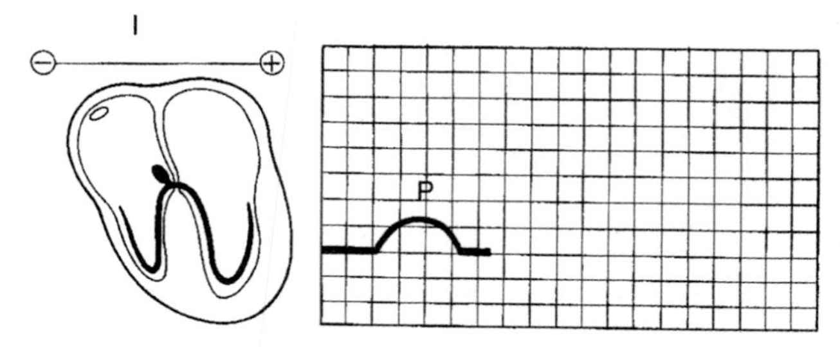

During the *PR segment* (end of the P wave to the beginning of the ventricular complex), the His-Purkinje system is being activated. This is another silent event, not seen on the surface ECG.

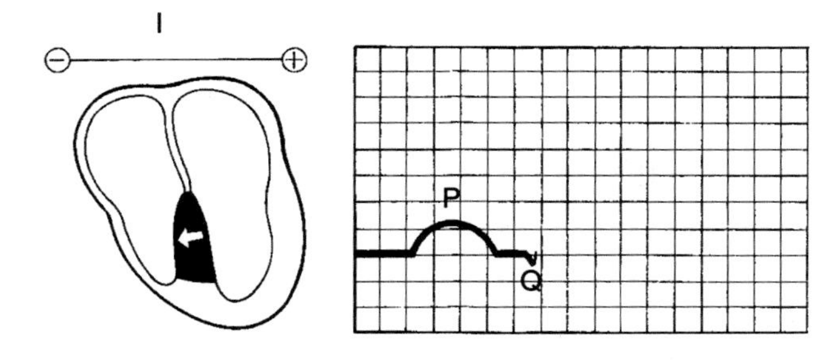

The middle of the interventricular septum from left to right is the first part of the ventricles to activate, followed immediately by opposing septal activation from the right to the left. Only the dominant left-to-right activation is shown. Note that this current moves toward the negative electrode of lead I and produces a small, narrow, negative deflection (*Q wave*). AV conduction, measured from the beginning of the P wave to the onset of the ventricular complex is called the *PR interval*, although in this case it is actually a "PQ" interval (this term is not used).

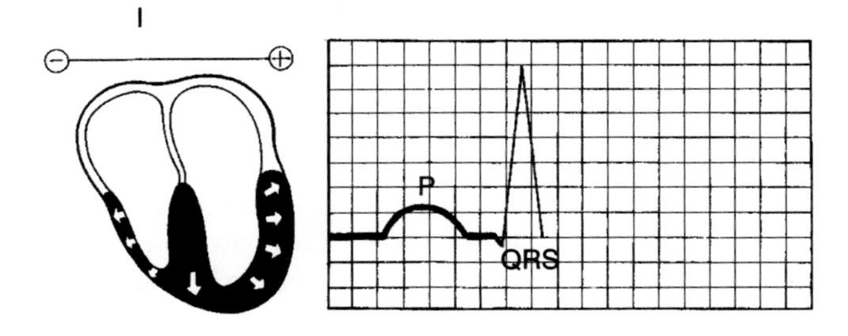

Immediately after the onset of septal activation, the impulse has activated the subendocardial walls of both ventricles, spreading from endocardium to epicardium. The larger left ventricular muscle mass dominates and produces a tall positive spike in lead I, the generic *QRS complex*. If the complex in this lead were to be described more accurately, it would be called a qR complex; that is, a small initial negative deflection (q) followed by a large positive one (R). In a significant number of individuals the complex in lead I is a qRs.

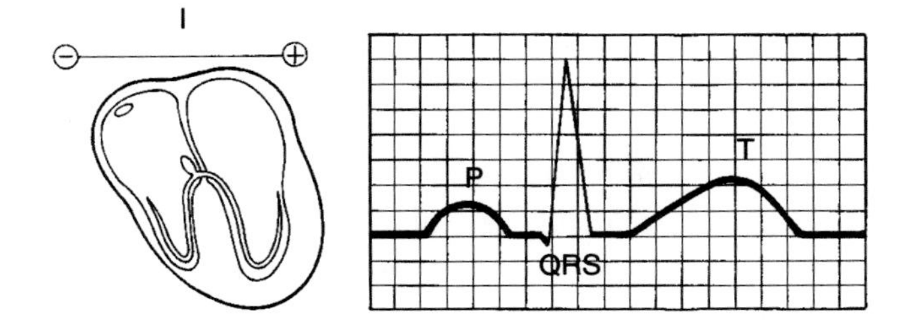

Electrical currents generated during repolarization of the ventricles are reflected in the *ST segment* and the *T wave*. The ST segment is the flat (isoelectric) portion following the QRS complex; it is followed by a slightly asymmetric curve (T wave). Having seen the normal ventricular complex in its step-by-step development in lead I, it would now be beneficial to evaluate the step-by-step progress of atrial and ventricular activation in all 12 leads.

The electrocardiogram is evaluated systematically:

1. Heart rate
2. Rhythm (regular or irregular)
3. P waves (position relative to the QRS; axis; amplitude; duration)
4. Intervals: PR, QRS, QT/QTc
5. QRS (axis; amplitude; morphology; Q waves)
6. ST segments (displacement)
7. T waves (polarity; shape; height)

These parameters will be discussed in subsequent chapters.

P WAVE

Duration

The duration of the P wave, which is not greater than 0.11 second in the normal heart, indicates the time it takes for the depolarization current to pass through the two atria. An increased width usually indicates left atrial abnormality or right atrial hypertrophy.

Height

In the limb leads the amplitude of the normal P wave is seldom more than 0.25 mV. In V_1 the positive component of the P wave is less than 0.15 mV, and the negative deflection usually less than 0.1 mV—or it should not take up more area than one small square on the graph. The atria are thin-walled structures. If the P wave is taller than this or, in V_1, deeper and wider, atrial enlargement is suspected and may indicate AV valvular problems, hypertension, cor pulmonale, or congenital heart disease. Increased P wave amplitude is seen occasionally in the athlete.

Polarity

The polarity of the P wave in leads I, II, aV_F, and V_4 to V_6 (Fig. 2-7) is normally positive because the P vector travels in a leftward, inferior direction toward the positive electrode of these leads.

In leads III, aV_L, and V_1 to V_3 (Fig. 2-8) the P wave may be upright, diphasic, flat, or inverted, depending on the position of the heart in the chest and on the orientation of the atrial vector to the positive terminals. The P wave may be diphasic in leads V_1 and V_2 because the activation of the

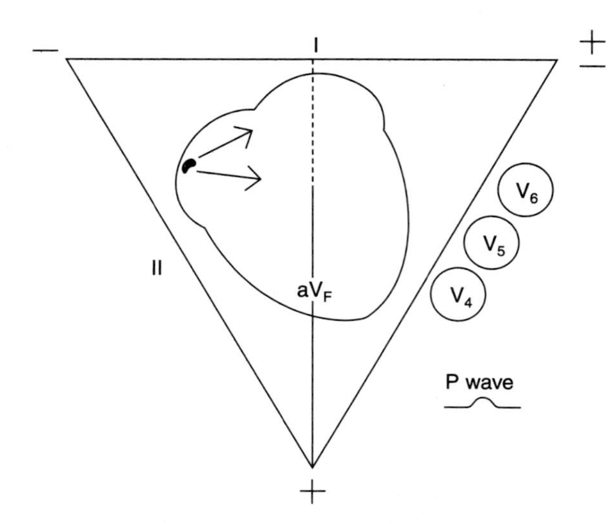

FIG. 2-7. The P vectors related to the axes of leads I, II, aV_F, and V_4 to V_6. The P wave is positive in these leads.

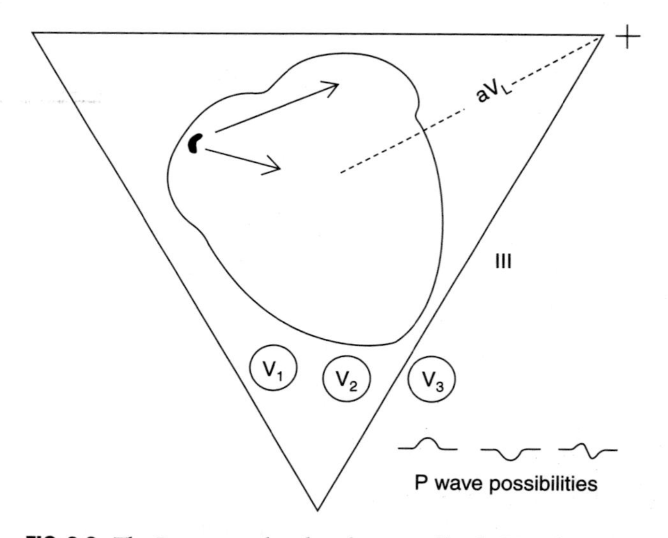

FIG. 2-8. The P vectors related to the axes of leads III and V_1 to V_3. The P wave may normally be positive, negative, or biphasic.

right atrium (anterior P vector) and the activation of the left atrium (posterior P vector) are recorded sequentially. In cases of left atrial enlargement, the second half of the P wave is significantly negative in lead V_1.

In lead aV_R the normal P wave is negative because the P vector travels away from the positive electrode of that lead (Fig. 2-9).

Axis

The normal P axis is about +60 degrees (range 0 to 75 degrees) in the frontal plane.

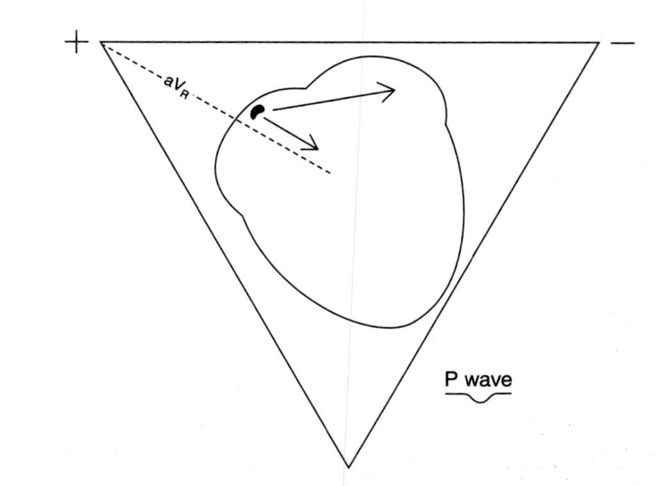

FIG. 2-9. The P vectors related to the axes of lead aV_R. The normal P wave is always negative in this lead.

Shape

Minor notching or slurring of the P wave is normal. Definite notching with a peak-to-peak interval of more than 0.04 second is usually considered abnormal.

Otherwise, a notched P wave that is upright in leads I, II, and V_4 to V_6 indicates left atrial abnormality. A tall, peaked P wave in the inferior leads and sometimes in lead V_1 is called *P-pulmonale* and is probably caused by the increased sympathetic stimulation and the low position of the diaphragm associated with diffuse lung disease. The increased sympathetic stimulation causes increased P amplitude, and low position of the diaphragm causes the P axis to be rightward.

Clinical Significance of P Wave Abnormalities

1. Increased width and notching: left atrial abnormality or right atrial hypertrophy
2. Increased amplitude: possible atrial enlargement and AV valvular problems, hypertension, cor pulmonale, or congenital heart disease
3. Diphasic with negative component excessively deep (–1.0 mm) and wide (0.04 second) in V_1: left atrial enlargement
4. Peaking that is taller in I than III: right atrial overload
5. Absent P waves: sinoatrial block, atrial standstill, junctional rhythm with hidden P waves
6. Inverted P wave in lead II, III, aV_F: ectopic atrial beat from low in the atrium, retrograde activation from junctional beats, or an AV reentry mechanism

Summary of the Normal P Wave

1. Not broader than 0.11 second in limb leads
2. Not taller than 2.5 mm in limb leads or 1.5 mm in V_1 (may be taller in athletes)

3. Upright in leads I, II, aV_F, and V_4 to V_6
4. Inverted in aV_R
5. May be positive, negative, or diphasic in leads III, aV_L, and V_1 to V_3, but the negative component in V_1 should not be excessively broad or deep
6. Smooth; not notched or peaked (may be notched in athletes)
7. Frontal plane axis between 0 degrees to + 75 degrees

NORMAL QRS COMPLEX IN THE LIMB LEADS

Figs. 2-10 and 2-11 illustrate the step-by-step evolution of the QRS complex in the limb leads (bipolar and unipolar). Numbers are used instead of letters to illustrate how each instantaneous event is reflected in a particular lead. For example, in this particular drawing, initial forces (septal) to the right is to the negative side of the lead I axis, producing a normal little q wave in that lead. The numbers correspond to the numbered currents in the heart. The long arrow represents the electrical axis of the heart (see Chapter 4). It is easy to see that the axis of the heart determines the complexes drawn in these two figures. For example, a more vertical orientation would not only produce little q waves in lead I, but in II, III, and aV_F as well, a pattern seen in more than half of normal adults.

These figures again illustrate that when the current is flowing toward a positive electrode, a positive deflection is recorded. The deflection is most positive when the current is parallel with the lead axis. When current flow is perpendicular to the lead axis, it is isoelectric (neither positive nor negative).

QRS COMPLEXES IN THE PRECORDIAL LEADS

The precordial chest leads give valuable information about anterior and posterior forces and, because of their proximity to the surface of the heart, are helpful in localizing pathologic changes in the myocardium. The six standard positive precordial electrodes form one fourth of a circle around the heart, beginning on the right side of the sternum, continuing over the right ventricle, across the interventricular septum, and ending on the left lateral chest wall over the left ventricle (Fig. 2-12). From V_1 to V_6 the positive electrode gets closer and closer to current flow in the thick-walled left ventricle, and the R wave (positive component) becomes taller and taller. This normal *R wave progression* reflects intact anterior forces; if anterior forces are lost, so are the R waves. The R wave in V_6 may actually be smaller than that of V_5 because the V_6 electrode is farther from the heart.

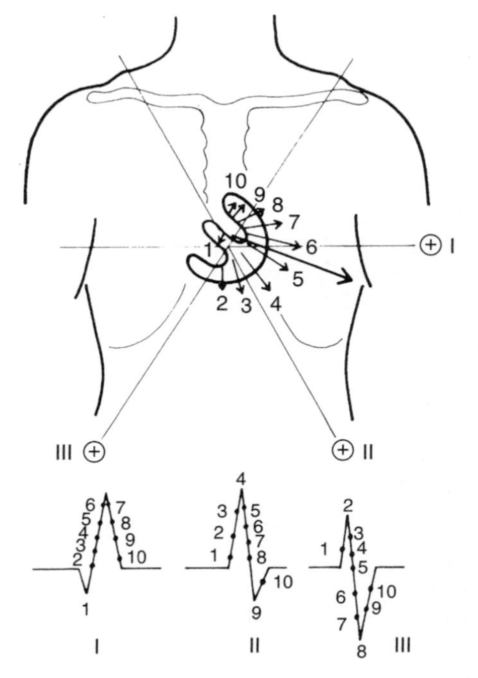

FIG. 2-10. Instant-to-instant cardiac vectors related to the bipolar limb leads. The numbers on the ventricular complexes correspond to the cardiac vectors. Septal activation is well-defined in lead I (vector 1).

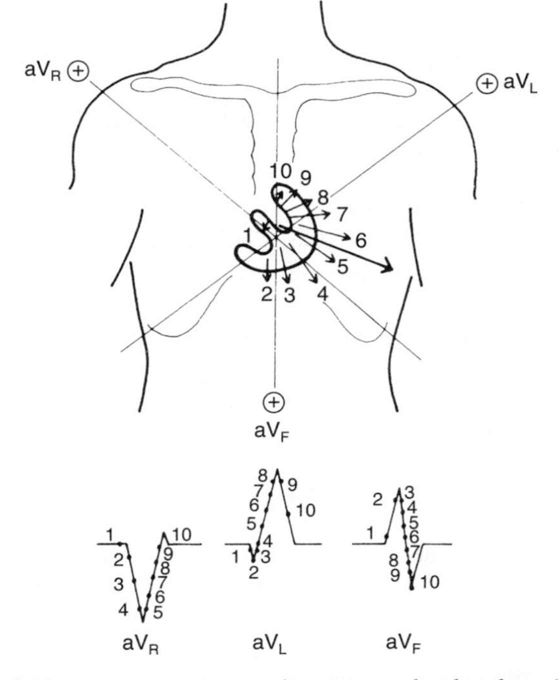

FIG. 2-11. Instant-to-instant cardiac vectors related to the unipolar limb leads. The numbers on the ventricular complexes correspond to the cardiac vectors.

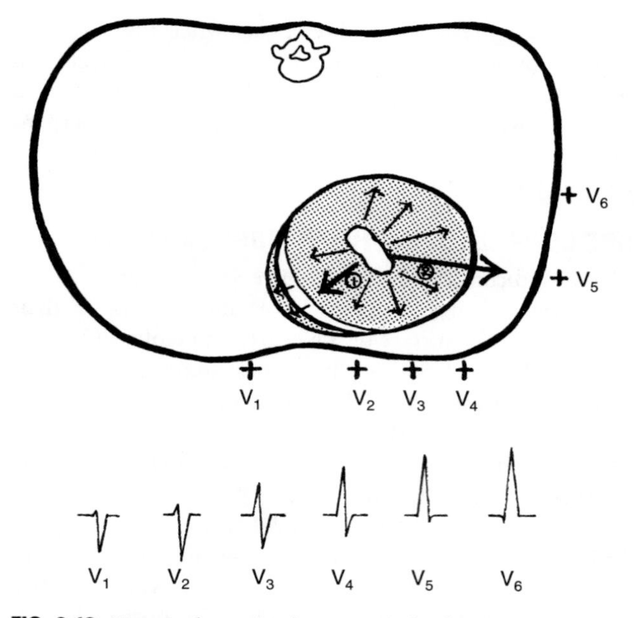

FIG. 2-12. Ventricular activation as seen in the precordial leads. Note the normal R wave progression.

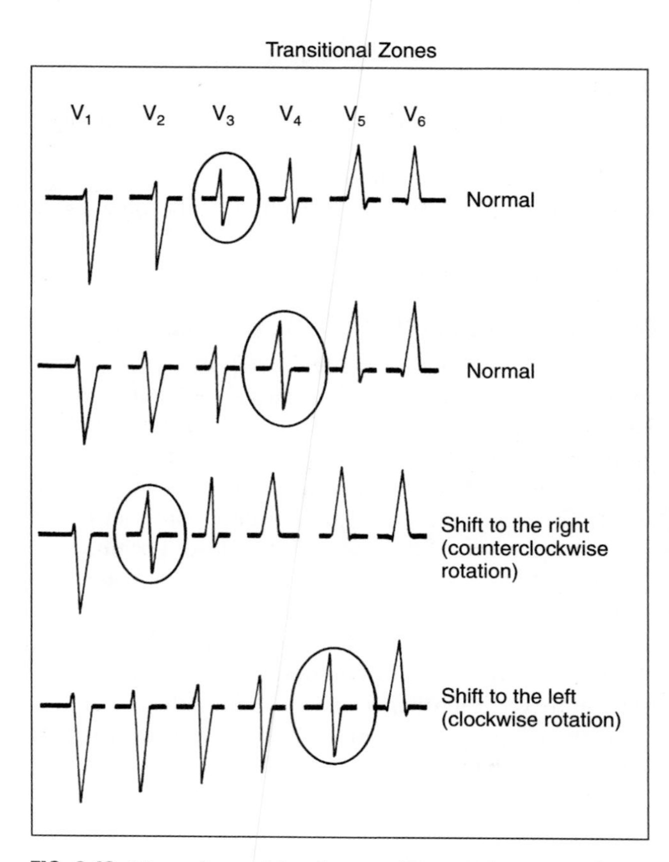

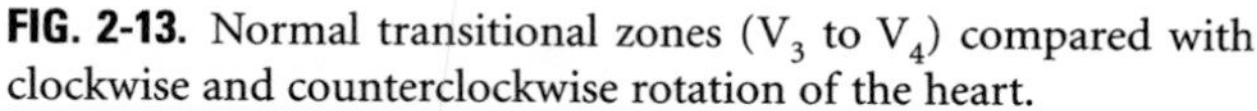

FIG. 2-13. Normal transitional zones (V_3 to V_4) compared with clockwise and counterclockwise rotation of the heart.

In V_1 the initial little r wave reflects both septal and right ventricular forces. However, when right ventricular activation is still just beginning, the dominant leftward force of the left ventricle produces a deep S wave. Thus a narrow rS complex is normal for V_1, although the little r wave may be normally absent. In V_6 normal septal activation can easily be detected. It is reflected by the small, narrow q wave (as seen in lead I).

Transitional Zone

The transitional zone—the isoelectric complex in the precordial leads—is produced by a horizontal electrical axis perpendicular to the lead axis. As the R wave becomes taller across the precordial leads, the S wave becomes smaller. Usually, between V_3 and V_4 the R and the S are equal. This equiphasic complex defines the *transitional zone.* If the transitional zone is to the left (toward V_6), there is clockwise rotation of the heart. If the shift is to the right (toward V_1), there is counterclockwise rotation of the heart.

A shift in the transitional zone to the left is one of the ECG signs of acute pulmonary embolism, right ventricular hypertrophy, and atrial septal defect. A shift to the right is seen in left ventricular hypertrophy. Fig. 2-13 illustrates the normal transitional zone compared with shifts to the right (counterclockwise rotation) and to the left (clockwise rotation).

EVALUATING THE QRS COMPLEX

Duration

In the adult the duration of the QRS complex is 0.05 to 0.10 second; in the newborn it is 0.04 to 0.05 second. It represents intraventricular conduction time.

Measurement

When measuring the QRS complex, be sure to take in any initial or terminal components (little q or s wave) and to look in more than one lead. Sometimes it is difficult to pinpoint the beginning of the complex. The duration of the QRS complex is measured from the moment the tracing leaves the baseline to the point at which it returns. In bundle branch block the duration is 0.12 second or more; in ventricular hypertrophy it is 0.10 to 0.11 second. In overt Wolff-Parkinson-White syndrome it is more than 0.10 second.

Best Leads for Measuring

The QRS complex may be narrower in one or two leads than it is in others. This is because either initial forces or terminal forces are perpendicular to that particular lead axis, causing the record to remain on, or return to, the isoelectric line. Wanderman et al[8] found a 5- to 20-ms delay in the onset of the QRS complex in one or two leads in almost half of more than 300 patients tested. Lead II was the lead that most frequently showed a delayed QRS onset and therefore would seem to be a poor choice for measuring the QRS duration. A right precordial lead (V_1 or V_2) was found to be most reliable for the actual QRS recording, and when this was combined with a simultaneous recording of a limb lead, the most accurate measurement was ensured. Fig. 2-14 illustrates the delay in onset of the QRS that is sometimes encountered. In this case the delay is in lead III. Note that the beginning of the QRS complex in lead II is slow, making it difficult to determine the precise point where it begins, unless the complex is recorded simultaneously with V_1.

Amplitude

QRS voltage varies with age, being greater in younger individuals, blacks, and in those with thin chest walls.

Upper Limit for the R Wave Amplitude

Lead I: 15 mm
aV_L: 10 mm
II, III, aV_F: 19 mm

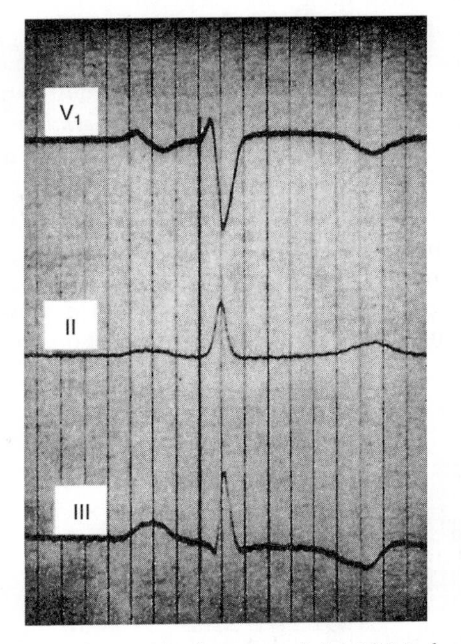

FIG. 2-14. Delay of 20 ms in the onset of the QRS in lead III as compared with V_1. (From Wanderman KL et al: *Circulation* 63:933, 1981.)

V_1: 6 mm but may normally be absent or, in young adults, higher
V_4: commonly tallest
V_5 and V_6: 25 mm; 30 mm in young adults

Lower Limit for the R Wave Amplitude

V_1 and V_6: 6 mm
V_2 and V_5: 8 mm
V_3 and V_4: 10 mm
I, II, III: 6 mm total value (positive + negative components)

Among the conditions causing low voltage are obesity, diffuse coronary disease, pericardial effusion, emphysema, myxedema, hemochromatosis, primary amyloidosis, and cardiac failure.

Upper Limit for the S Wave Amplitude

aV_R: 16 mm in younger individuals
III and aV_L: 9 mm
I, II, aV_F: 5 mm
V_1: 18 mm
V_2: 26 mm
V_3: 21 mm (occasionally up to 30 mm)

Lower Limit for the S Wave Amplitude in V_1

3 mm

Polarity

In the limb leads the polarity of the QRS depends on the QRS vectors in the frontal plane and their relationship to the axis of each lead. In the precordial leads the R wave increases in amplitude from the right to the left. In V_1 it may be absent.

Leads I, II, and V_3 to V_6: positive to equiphasic
Leads aV_L and aV_F: positive, negative, or equiphasic
Lead aV_R: negative

Shape

The term *QRS* may be used to refer in general to the ventricular complex, whatever its shape. It is a generic term not intended to describe the morphology of the complex. If it is necessary to describe precise deflections, uppercase and lowercase letters are used to indicate relative sizes of the components. All positive deflections are R or r waves. If there are two R (or r) waves in the same complex, the second is named R or r prime (R or r'). A negative component is either an uppercase or a lowercase Q or S; the Q is before the first R, and the S follows it. Fig. 2-15 illustrates a few possibilities. The normal shape of the QRS in the right precordial leads is rS. In

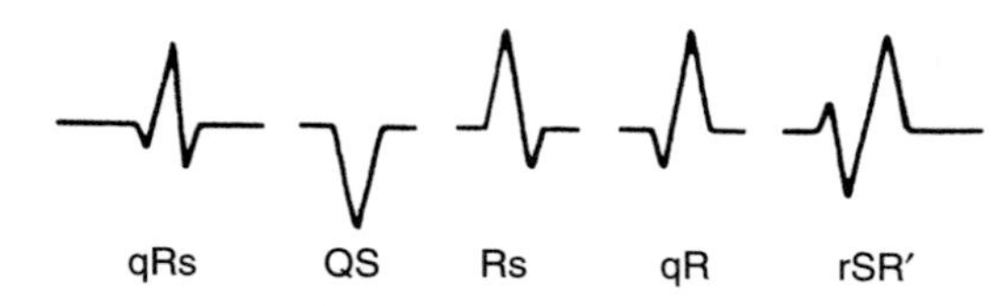

FIG. 2-15. QRS deflections described using uppercase and lowercase letters. R or r waves are always positive. A negative component is either a Q or an S. A Q is before an R wave, an S follows an R.

RBB block the shape of the QRS in V_1 is rSR' without myocardial infarction and qR or QR with myocardial infarction.

Pediatrics. In the normal child younger than 5 years of age a RSR' complex is sometimes seen in the right precordial leads, in which case the QRS duration is not more than 0.01 second longer than normal and the R' voltage in V_1 less than 15 mm in infants younger than 1 year and less than 10 mm in those older than 1 year of age.

NORMAL Q WAVE

A Q wave appears in a lead when initial ventricular forces are directed away from the positive electrode of that lead. Normal little q waves, reflecting the left-to-right forces of septal activation, are present in V_6 in more than 75% of normal individuals, and are sometimes seen in V_5 and V_4. The appearance of a normal q wave in the limb leads varies with the frontal plane QRS axis. A more vertical axis may produce normal q waves in leads II, III, and aV_F, occurring in more than half of normal adults. A more horizontal axis results in q waves in leads I and aV_L. When the transitional zone (p. 18) is to the right, more q waves are likely to be noted.

Duration of the Normal Q Wave

Limb leads (except III and aV_R) and left precordial leads: 0.03 second or less

Lead III: 0.04 second or less (rarely 0.05 second)

V_5 and V_6: 0.03 second or less

Amplitude of the Normal Q Wave

Limb lead (except III): less than 4 mm or less than 25% of the amplitude of the R wave; in lead I it is usually not over 1.5 mm except for individuals younger than 30 years of age

Lead III: may reach 5 mm

V_5 and V_6: less than 2 mm

In younger adults the amplitude of the q wave in the left precordial leads may be as deep as 3 mm, and in teenagers, 4 mm or more.

ST SEGMENT

The ST segment extends from the *J point* (at the end of the QRS) to the beginning of the T wave. The J point is identified in Fig. 2-16. The ST segment is part of the repolarization phase of the heart and is normally isoelectric, slanting slightly upward from the end of the QRS, into the T wave. To determine if the ST segment is displaced from the isoelectric line use the PR or the TP segment for reference, placing a straight edge from one PR segment to another. ST segment displacement will become apparent.

Normal ST Segment

Limb leads: isoelectric in approximately 75% of normal adults

Displacement in limb leads: up to 1 mm is normal, with ST elevation rather than depression being more common in inferior leads

ST elevation in precordial leads: seen in more than 90% of normal adults. More pronounced in youths and in athletes as part of the *early repolarization syndrome*. An elevation of more than 2 mm is uncommon in individuals more than 40 years of age

- Most common and marked in V_2 and V_3 (may reach 3 mm)
- Rarely more than 1 mm in V_4-V_6

ST depression in precordial leads: not depressed more than 0.5 mm in any lead; an abnormal finding

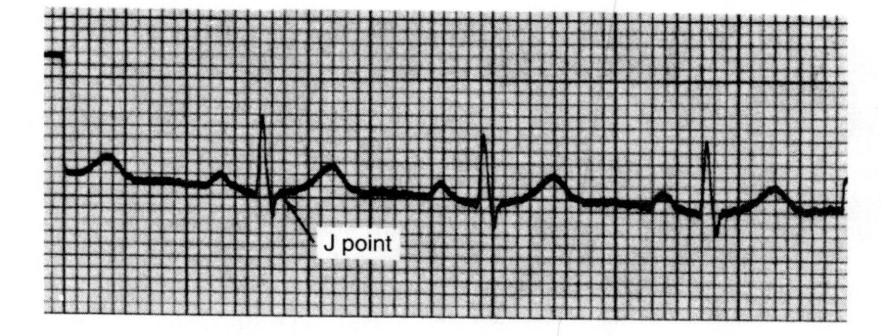

FIG. 2-16. The J point (*arrow*) defines the end of the QRS complex and the beginning of the ST segment.

Causes of Abnormal Deviation

1. Significant displacement: coronary artery disease
2. Marked elevation: acute myocardial infarction
3. Depression in eight leads with slight ST elevation in aV_R and V_1 reflects left main or three-vessel disease
4. Marked depression at rest: myocardial ischemia or subendocardial infarction
5. Depression during stress test: occult coronary artery disease
6. Digitalis: typical scooped-looking depression with QT shortening
7. Direct current cardioversion: may result in temporary elevation
8. 12-lead ST segment monitoring for displacement
   - Identifies transient periods of silent ischemia
   - Alerts to abrupt closure from spasm or thrombus postangioplasty
9. Location of culprit lesion
   - ST elevation in aV_L + V_2-V_5: proximal left anterior descending coronary artery before the first diagonal branch
   - ST elevation in aV_L + V_2 + isoelectric or depressed ST in V_3-V_5: first diagonal branch
   - ST elevation in aV_L + isoelectric or depressed ST in precordial leads: first obtuse marginal branch

Early Repolarization Syndrome

In the early repolarization syndrome the epicardial cells differ significantly from the endocardial cells in their repolarization process. This difference produces a small voltage gradient at the end of ventricular depolarization and the beginning of repolarization, causing a current to flow between the two myocardial layers. This is reflected in a small J wave, perceived as an ST segment elevation, almost always the rule in athletes (see Chapter 20) and adolescents.

Shape

The normal ST segment curves very slightly into the beginning of the T wave. In fact, an absolutely horizontal ST segment, which forms a sharp angle with the T wave, is highly suggestive of ischemia.

T WAVE

The T wave is the result of current generated during rapid repolarization of the heart.

Polarity

I, II, V_5, and V_6: Positive
aV_R: inverted
aV_F: usually positive, but may be flat or inverted if the QRS complex is less than 6 mm tall
III and aV_L: upright or inverted depending on T vector
V_1: negative in 50% of women; usually positive in men
V_2: usually positive, but in less than 10% may be inverted, diphasic, or flat
V_3: usually positive, but may be inverted, diphasic, or flat in youths
V_4: usually positive, rarely inverted, diphasic, or flat

Pediatric T Wave

Infants older than 48 hours should have inverted T waves in the right precordial leads, persisting throughout childhood. T wave inversion to V_4 is normal. As the child grows older there is a progressive change to an upright T wave across the precordial leads from left to right. Until 8 years of age an upright T wave in V_1 is considered to be a sign of right ventricular hypertrophy. Many children have and inverted T wave in V_1 until their late teens.

A *persistent juvenile pattern* is said to exist when the T wave is negative in two or more of the right precordial leads, V_1, V_2, and V_3 in the normal adult.

Amplitude

Limb leads: usually less than 6 mm; tallest in lead II and not less than 0.5 mm in leads I and II
Precordial leads: tallest in V_2 and V_3 and taller in men (about 6 mm, but may be as high as 12 mm in healthy men); in women, usually 3 to 4 mm and seldom more than 8 mm

Tall, pointed T waves reflect hyperkalemia or myocardial ischemia and are sometimes seen before the T wave inversion of myocardial infarction. T wave alternans may be seen in hypokalemia, hypocalcemia, hypomagnesemia, tachycardia, congestive heart disease, and pericardial disease.

Vulnerable Period

The vulnerable period is at the peak of the T wave, offset slightly toward the end of the T wave. During the recovery of cellular excitability there is a short period in which the heart is both refractory and excitable. A stimulus during this time is likely to be blocked by refractory tissue but conducted through excitable tissue, resulting in unidirectional conduction, intraventricular reentry, and ventricular tachycardia or fibrillation. The approximate location of the ventricular vulnerable period is shown in Fig. 2-17. The atrial vulnerable period is obscured by the QRS complex and has not been clearly defined.

Shape

The normal T wave is rounded and asymmetric. It usually ascends more slowly than it descends. A notched T wave is normal in children but may also be found in adults with pericarditis. Abnormal T wave shapes are seen in patients with long QT syndrome. The presence of "humps" near the apex or on the descending limb of upright T waves may suggest the presence of the long QT syndrome trait in symptomatic blood relatives with borderline QTc interval (see p. 370).

Whenever the depolarization process of the ventricles is abnormal, the repolarization process changes as well. Examples of such conditions are bundle branch block, digitalis therapy, quinidine therapy, ischemia (slow conduction), ventricular ectopic beats, and ventricular hypertrophy. T wave abnormalities are also sensitive indicators of a variety of conditions including hyperkalemia, hyperventilation, metabolic diseases, acid-base imbalance, and the presence of various drugs.

T waves in athletes may look abnormal, but are the normal physiologic signs of conditioning, in which case T waves can be tall, peaked, inverted, or isoelectric; such changes may normalize with exercise.[9] The athlete's ECG is covered in Chapter 20.

U WAVE

The U wave follows the T wave and is upright except in lead aV_R. It normally goes unnoticed because of its low voltage. Its mechanism is controversial. Some researchers believe that the U wave represents repolarization of Purkinje fibers; others believe it to be a reflection of a diastolic event. It becomes taller in hypokalemia and inverted in heart disease. Hypertension is the most common cause of a negative U wave. Transient U wave inversion can be caused by acute myocardial ischemia or a rise of blood pressure. Typically when associated with ischemia there is terminal U wave inversion (inversion after positive U-wave deflection). When associated with hypertension only the initial part of the U wave is negative.

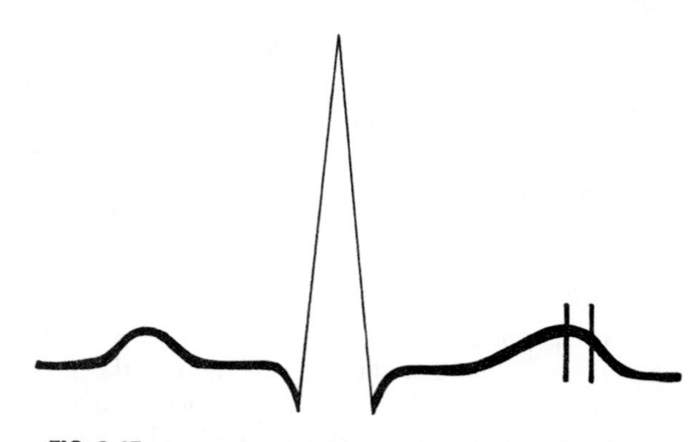

FIG. 2-17. Approximate location of the vulnerable period.

SUMMARY

The normal activation of the heart is initiated by the sinus node. In turn the atria depolarize and during this time the AV node is also depolarized; the P wave represents atrial depolarization. The bundle of His, bundle branches, and Purkinje fibers are then activated; this is not seen on the ECG. Ventricular depolarization begins and, with the interventricular septum, proceeds from endocardium to epicardium; the QRS complex represents ventricular depolarization. The ST segment is from the end of the QRS complex to the beginning of the T wave; it should be isoelectric and slightly slanted up. The T wave represents ventricular repolarization.

REFERENCES

1. Crick SJ, Wharton J, Sheppard MN et al: Innervation of the human cardiac conduction system. A quantitative immunohistochemical and histochemical study, *Circulation* 89:1697, 1994.
2. Keim S, Werner P, Jazayeri M et al: Localization of the fast and slow pathways in atrioventricular nodal reentrant tachycardia by intraoperative ice mapping, *Circulation* 86:919-925, 1992.
3. Ferguson TB Jr, Cox JL: Surgical treatment of arrhythmias. In Willerson JT, Cohn JN, editors: *Cardiovascular medicine*, New York, 1995, Churchill Livingstone, pp 1476-1494.
4. James TN: Anatomy of the conduction system of the heart. In Hurst JW, editor: *The heart*, New York, 1982, McGraw-Hill.
5. Waller BF, Gering LE, Branyas NA, Slack JD: Anatomy, histology, and pathology of the cardiac conduction system: Part II, *Clin Cardiol* 16:347, 1993.
6. Tawara S: *Das Reizleitungssystem des Saugetierherzens*, Jena, Gustav Fischer, 1906.
7. James TN: Anatomy of the conduction system of the heart. In Hurst JW, editor: *The heart*, ed 4, New York, 1978, McGraw-Hill.
8. Estes NAM III, Link MS, Homund M, Wang PJ: ECG findings in active patients. Differentiating the benign from the serious, *Phys Sports Med* 29(3):1-12, 2001.

PART II

Arrhythmia Recognition

CHAPTER 3

Mechanisms of Arrhythmias

An *arrhythmia* is an abnormal cardiac rhythm. It usually occurs when the normal sinus rhythm is interfered with by ectopic beats, ectopic rhythms, or compromised atrioventricular (AV) conduction. Sinus rhythms that are too fast or too slow or that fail also qualify as arrhythmias, even though sinus bradycardia, sometimes profound, is a normal occurrence during sleep and in athletes.

Two categories of arrhythmias and three basic tachycardia mechanisms have been described. The two categories of arrhythmias are abnormalities of conduction (block; reentry; or reflection, a type of reentry) and abnormalities of impulse initiation (early beats and tachycardia). The three tachycardia mechanisms are described in this chapter.[1]

ARRHYTHMIA OR DYSRHYTHMIA?

Both terms are acceptable. Marriott[2] has eloquently pointed out that the original meaning of the alpha privative often implied an "imperfection in" rather than the flat, negative absence of. Apart from original meanings, Marriott points out that the most important factor for retaining the term *arrhythmia* is "the sovereign role of usage," suggesting that both terms be accepted, "arrhythmia because it has tradition and no perceptible flaws, and dysrhythmia because it offers variety and satisfies spurious scholarship."

The determining factor may be Marriott's usage theory, for the term *dysrhythmia* has not caught on after more than two decades of pressure from militants. It hasn't even been considered as an option in the writings,[3-6] lectures, and scientific conversations of internationally known experts and world leaders in the field of cardiovascular medicine.

THREE BASIC TACHYCARDIA MECHANISMS

Three basic arrhythmogenic mechanisms are responsible for the initiation of tachyarrhythmias, all of which are caused by alterations in ionic currents that pass through the channels of the myocardial cell membrane. These mechanisms are altered automaticity, triggered activity, and reentry.[7]

Altered Automaticity

Altered automaticity is classified as either enhanced normal automaticity or abnormal automaticity, the first being relatively benign and the second being difficult to suppress.

Normal automaticity. Normal automaticity is the ability of a cardiac cell to *spontaneously* depolarize, reach threshold potential, and initiate a propagated action potential. Whether this property is normal, enhanced, or abnormal, spontaneous depolarization is the result of the development of a net inward ionic current during phase 4 of the action potential (slow diastolic depolarization); this current brings the cell to threshold potential and a propagated action potential is initiated. In all pacemaker cells except those of the sinus node this property is suppressed (overdrive suppression) because the impulse from the sinus node normally activates the remainder of the heart before subsidiary pacemakers can reach threshold potential on their own.

Normal automaticity is the physiologic response of the sinus node to the needs of the body—fast when running, slow when sleeping, and within the defined parameters of "normal" when slightly active or resting. The action potential of the sinus node is illustrated in Fig. 3-1. Note the hyperpolarization at the end of the action potential (most negative), the steep phase 4 leading to threshold potential, and a slow calcium channel action potential.

Enhanced normal automaticity. Enhanced normal automaticity is caused by a change in the magnitude of the ionic transmembrane currents responsible for normal automaticity of cardiac pacemaker cells. For example, the pacemaker cells of the His-Purkinje system may be functioning normally until a change is mediated by drugs, the autonomic nervous system, or hormones, causing a steepening of phase 4, resulting in extra beats or an increase of firing rate to about 100 beats/min (rarely more rapid). Such fibers are readily suppressed by overdrive pacing. Enhanced normal automaticity in a His-Purkinje cell is illustrated by the dotted line in Fig. 3-2, *A*.

Abnormal automaticity. Abnormal automaticity is caused by a disturbance of the ionic transmembrane currents of atrial or ventricular myocardial cells, resulting in the spontaneous firing of cardiac cells that, in health, did not have the capability of automaticity. Abnormal automaticity is also possible in pacemaker cells. For example, conditions such as ischemia, infarction, hypokalemia, hypocalcemia, or cardiomyopathy may cause a reduction in membrane potential. When the membrane potential is sharply reduced to a critical level (more positive than –60 mV) anywhere in the heart, spontaneous depolarization may occur. The tachycardia that results is not readily suppressed by overdrive pacing. Although the sinus node normally suppresses latent pacemaker activity, it may not have that power over fibers with abnormal automaticity. As a result, although a long sinus cycle may not elicit normal escape beats, areas of abnormal automaticity may easily surface when the rate of the sinus node drops below that of an ectopic focus. The action potential seen in cells with abnormal automaticity is compared with enhanced normal automaticity in Fig. 3-2, *A* and *B*.

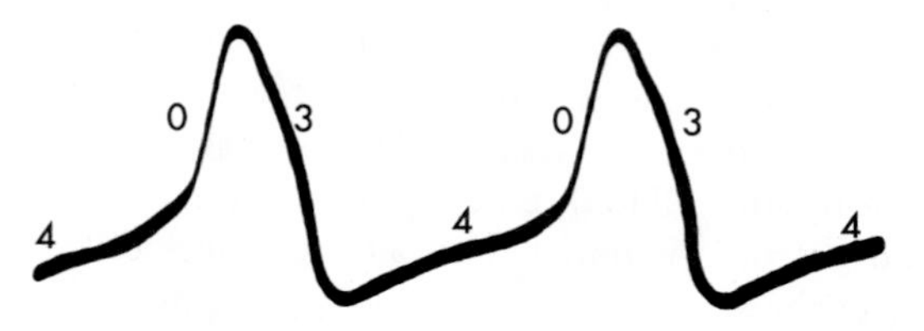

FIG. 3-1. Sinus node action potential. This is purely a slow calcium channel action potential (no fast sodium channels). Note the steepness of phase 4 depolarization and the deep negative (hyperpolarization) at the end of phase 3.

TRIGGERED ACTIVITY

Triggered activity occurs because of afterdepolarizations (i.e., oscillations of membrane potential before or after the completion of repolarization). When these oscillations depolarize the cell to threshold potential, they induce spontaneous action potentials (triggered activity) that are responsible for extrasystoles and tachycardia. Afterdepolarizations are divided into two subclasses: early and delayed, each with different causes and different mechanisms. Early afterdepolarizations are associated with slow rates and prolonged repolarization (long QT interval); delayed afterdepolarizations are associated with fast rates and conditions of calcium overload.

Early Afterdepolarizations

Early afterdepolarizations are oscillations of the membrane potential that interrupt or retard repolarization; they occur against a background of prolonged QT intervals and are exacerbated by bradycardia or pauses. Early afterdepolarizations are caused by congenital or acquired long QT syndrome (see Chapters 25 and 26) that either genetically or through QT prolonging drugs alters potassium or sodium currents during repolarization (phase 2 of the action potential), resulting in a life-threatening type of ventricular tachycardia called *torsades de pointes*. Fig. 3-3 illustrates an early afterdepolarization that occurs during phase 3; upon reaching threshold potential, it produces a propagated action potential *(dotted line)*—that is, a triggered beat.

Delayed Afterdepolarizations

Delayed afterdepolarizations are oscillations of the membrane potential after completion of the action poten-

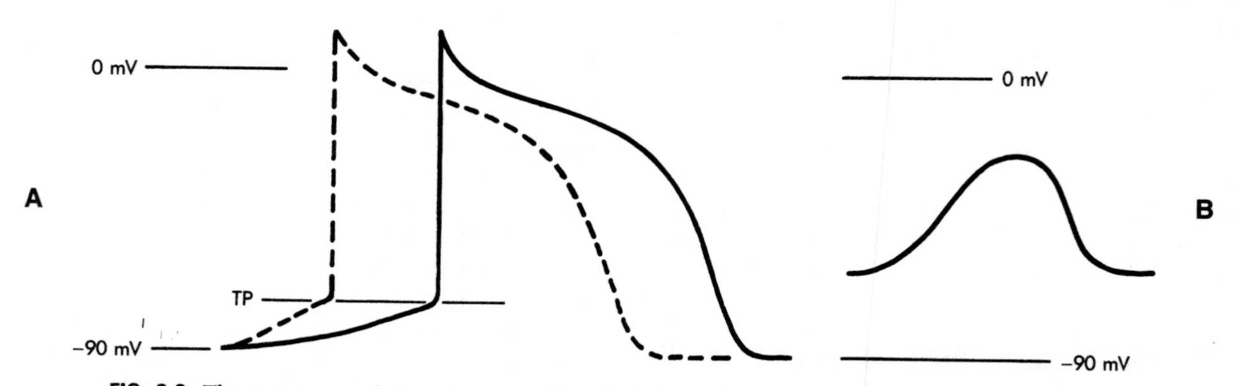

FIG. 3-2. The two types of altered automaticity. **A,** Enhanced normal automaticity is caused by catecholamines and occurs in pacemaker cells such as His-Purkinje cells. **B,** Abnormal automaticity is due to ischemia or injury and may occur anywhere in the heart. *TP,* Threshold potential.

tial (i.e., following full repolarization); they occur against a background of fast rates and conditions of calcium overload (digitalis toxicity and catecholamines). If the oscillation reaches threshold potential (*dotted line* in Fig. 3-4), it produces a propagated action potential (a triggered beat). Delayed afterdepolarizations are discussed more completely in Chapter 15.

REENTRY

Reentry is the arrhythmogenic mechanism by which a wave of excitation turns upon itself and reenters the tissue it had previously activated. The terms used to describe arrhythmias supported by reentry are *circus movement, reciprocal* or *echo beats, reciprocating tachycardia*, and, of course, *reentry* or *reentrant tachycardia.*

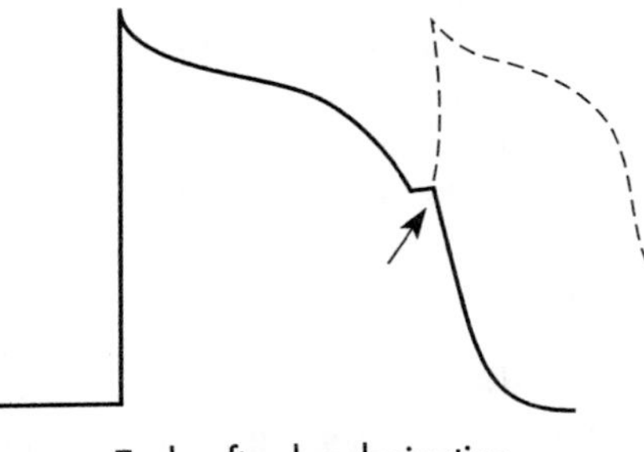

FIG. 3-3. An early afterdepolarization is shown distorting the action potential during phase 3. It reaches threshold potential and produces a triggered beat *(dotted line).*

Normally the cardiac impulse moves rapidly through the heart and is extinguished in its first pass because the entire heart becomes refractory and the impulse expires, having "no place to go."[13] Given the right conditions, it is possible for any part of the myocardium or conduction system to support reentry circuits. The right conditions are unidirectional conduction block, inexcitable tissue in the center of the reentry circuit, and excitable tissue ahead of the traveling impulse. All of these conditions are necessary so that the reentrant impulse is protected from extinction by collision with another impulse and has a place to go (excitable tissue in its advancing pathway). Thus reentry is dependent not only on slow conduction but also on the architecture of the myocardium through which the reentrant impulse circles.

Typically, reentrant tachycardia are *paroxysmal* and may be terminated with a critically timed, paced beat or, clinically in the case of paroxysmal supraventricular tachycardia (PSVT), with a vagal maneuver or a drug that slows or blocks AV nodal conduction, such as adenosine. In subsequent chapters you will become acquainted with reentry as the mechanism that sustains atrial flutter and atrial fibrillation and with PSVT because of its common causes (AV nodal reentry and AV reentry using the AV node and an accessory pathway) or its least common causes (sinoatrial [SA] reentry and intra-atrial reentry). Three types of

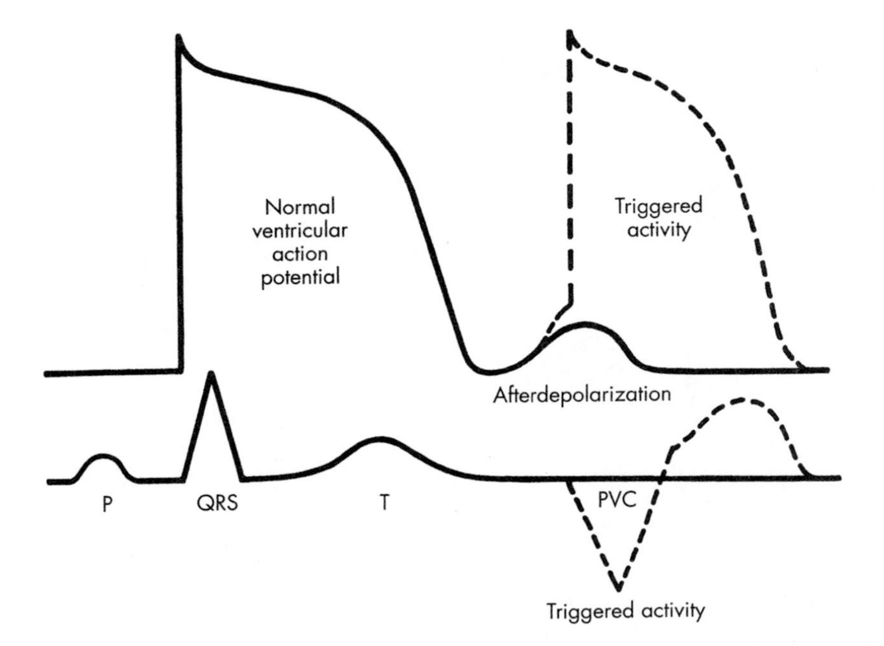

FIG. 3-4. A delayed afterdepolarization is shown following the action potential. It reaches threshold potential *(dotted line)* and produces a triggered beat. *PVC*, Premature ventricular complex.

reentry have been described: anatomic, functional, and anisotropic. Anatomic reentry can rotate or be terminated. Functional reentry can reproduce itself and result in fibrillation or it can convert into anatomic reentry by becoming captured in a fixed rotation around an orifice. Reentry in three dimensions has been described in cardiac muscle.

Anatomic Reentry

Anatomic reentry consists of an excitation wave that travels a fixed pathway as if it were a road. The classic example of anatomic reentry is that supporting the paroxysmal supraventricular tachycardia of Wolff-Parkinson-White syndrome, illustrated in Fig. 3-5. Other arrhythmias supported by anatomic reentry are atrial fibrillation, atrial flutter, and AV nodal reentry, discussed in Chapters 8, 9, and 11. In post–myocardial infarction patients the impulse may circulate around an anatomic obstacle such as an infarct scar.

The Mines model of reentry. The earliest and simplest model of reentry, introduced by Mines[8] in 1913, shows an impulse that circles a large anatomic obstacle (Fig. 3-6, *A*). The white part within the circle represents fibers that are nonrefractory. This "excitable gap" continues to move around the circle behind the refractory tissue (stippled area). The wave of excitation is thus propagated to produce a regular tachycardia.

The Lewis model. In 1920 Lewis[9] (Fig. 3-6, *B*) introduced a reentry loop whose pathway took in two anatomic obstacles (i.e., venae cavae). Such a large circuit could result in the impulse crossing at the isthmus to establish a smaller circuit and a faster tachycardia.

In the lower row of Fig. 3-6, *E*, *F*, and *G*, are also models of anatomical reentry. In Fig. 3-6, *E*, the impulse wave length is shortened. Such an impulse may circle an anatomic obstacle and produce a stable reentry circuit. In Fig. 3-6, *F*, there is an area of depressed conduction between the two anatomic boundaries, which allows for an excitable gap in the normal myocardium. In Fig. 3-6, *G*, note an area of prolonged refractoriness next to an anatomic obstacle; the depolarization wave encircles both in a pathway that may be long enough to create an excitable gap in the normal myocardium. Such a circuit may pivot at slightly different points, allowing for different cycle lengths; such a reentrant tachycardia could last for an extended time.[10]

Functional Reentry

Functional reentry does not require an anatomic structure to circle around; it depends on the local differ-

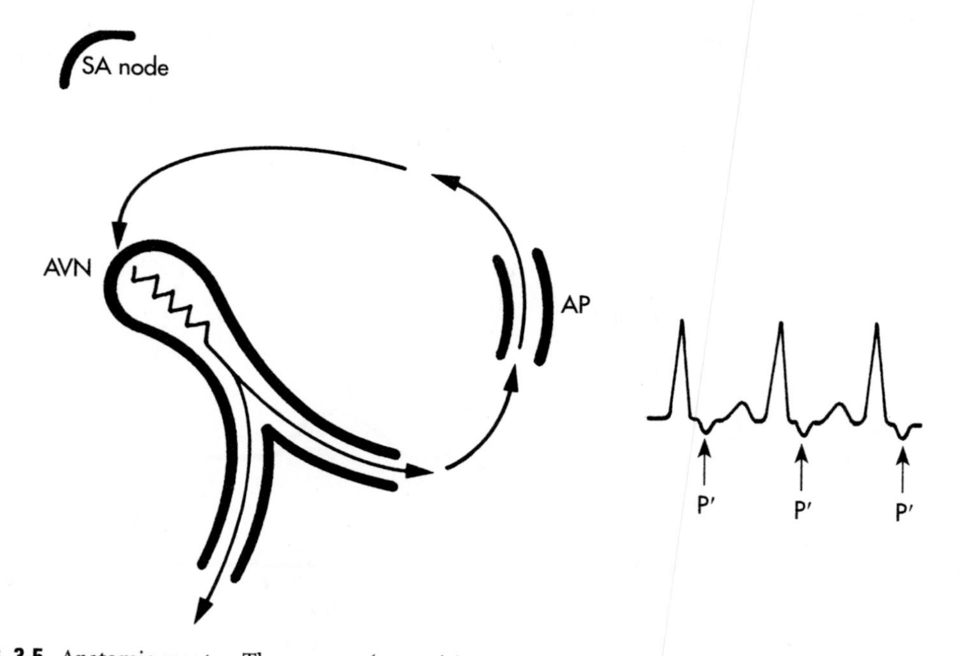

FIG. 3-5. Anatomic reentry. The current *(arrows)* is rotating through a fixed pathway, making a complete circle involving the atria, AV node *(AVN)*, ventricle, and accessory pathway *(AP)*, reactivating these structures with each passage. The *zig-zag line* in the AV node represents impulse slowing. This is the mechanism that supports the paroxysmal supraventricular tachycardia of Wolff-Parkinson-White syndrome. *APB*, Atrial premature beat.

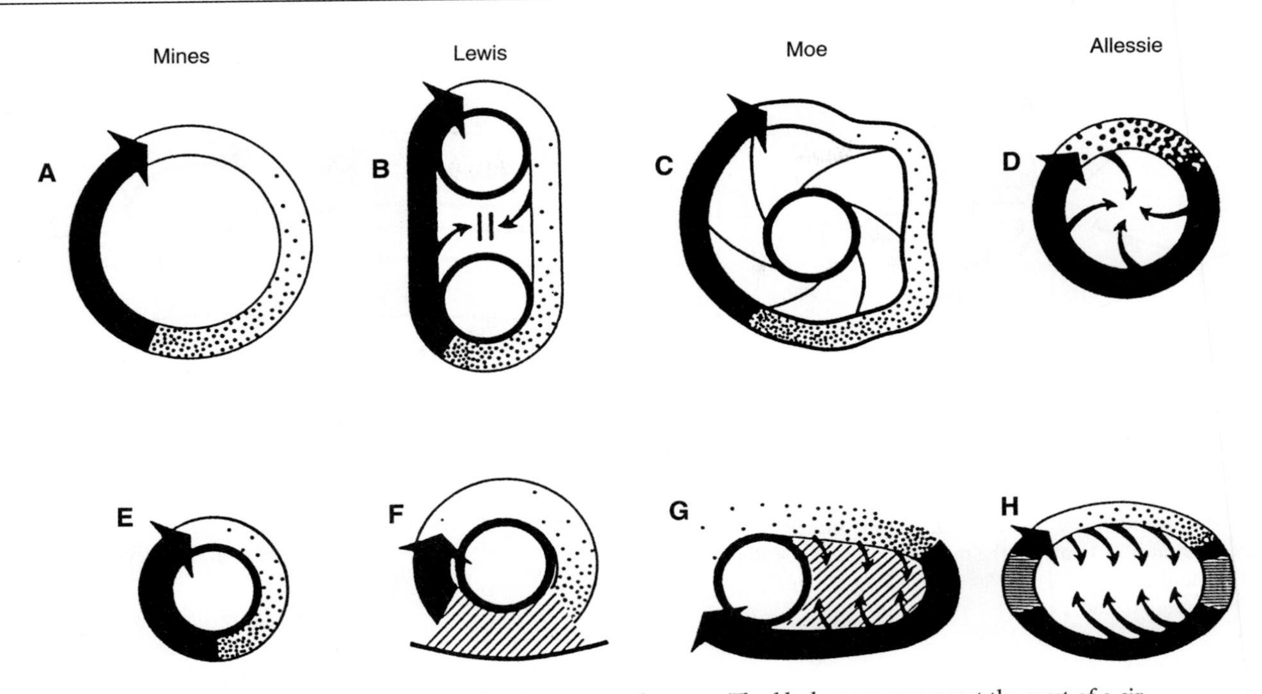

FIG. 3-6. Schematic representation of various types of reentry. The *black arrows* represent the crest of a circulating depolarization wave and the absolute refractory phase. The *stippled areas* indicate the refractory tail of the circuit. See text for description of **A** to **H**. (From Allessie MA, Rensma W, Brugada J et al: In Touboul P, Waldo AL, editors: *Atrial arrhythmias: current concepts and management*, St Louis, 1990, Mosby.)

ences in conduction velocity and is characterized by a "leading circle" (Moe and Allessie models in Fig. 3-6, *C* and *D*).

The *spiral* form of reentry was recorded in cardiac muscle for the first time in 1973 by Maurits Allessie and colleagues.[11] Before that time rotating waves had been described in excitable media by Selfridge[12] and by Balakhovsky.[13] Recently, colleagues in the laboratory of José Jalife[14] developed a video imaging technique that visualized spiral wave reentry (Fig. 3-7), demonstrating its behavior in isolated cardiac muscle[15-18] and its role in monomorphic and polymorphic tachycardia and fibrillation.[19-22] The spiral form of reentry is initiated by a "wavebreak" (i.e., a wave of electrical current that fails to propagate in its normal plane after meeting refractory tissue). The broken end of the wave curls, forms a vortex, and rotates permanently. Such a reentrant spiral suppresses normal pacemaker activity and may result in fibrillation. The spiral reentrant wave may drift, find an obstacle, and start rotating around it, thus converting to anatomical reentry (pinned, or anchored to the obstacle). By the same token, a classic reentry circuit (pinned to an obstacle) can leave the obstacle around which it was rotating and become functional.[23,24]

Anisotropic Reentry

Anisotropic reentry is a circuit that is determined by the difference in conduction velocities through the length of the fiber as opposed to across its width. *Isotropic* conduction would be uniform in all directions; *anisotropic* conduction would not. Slow conduction in at least part of the reentrant pathway, although not required for reentry to occur, facilitates the mechanism, allowing time for recovery of tissue in the path of the circulating wave front. One-

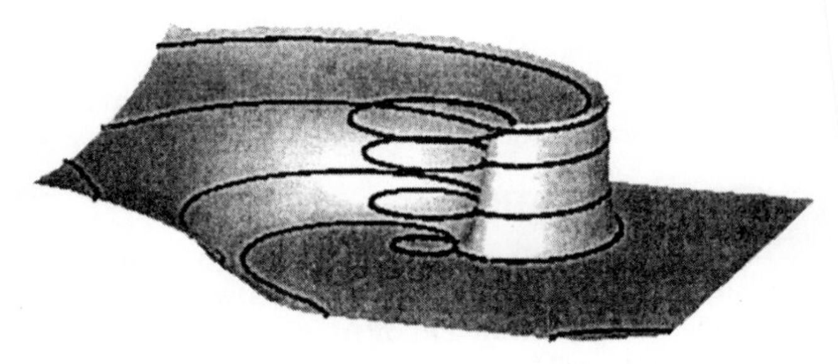

FIG. 3-7. A simulation of stationary spiral wave reentry at a given instant in time. (From Beaumont J, Jalife J: Rotors and spiral waves in two dimensions. In Zipes DP, Jalife J, editors: *Cardiac electrophysiology from cell to bedside*, ed 3, Philadelphia, 2000, WB Saunders, pp 327-335.)

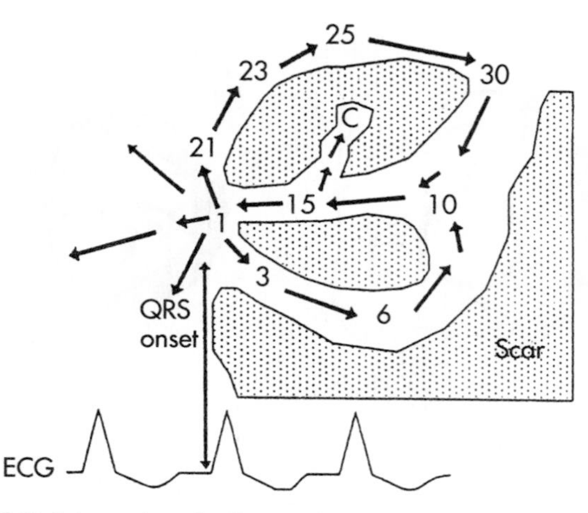

FIG. 3-8. Schematics of a figure-of-8 circuit through myocardial scar tissue late after a myocardial infarction. Sites 1 to 10 are the inner loop, sites 21 to 30 are the outer loop, and sites 10 to 20 are the common pathway. (From Stevenson WG, Khan H, Sager P et al: *Circulation* 88:1647, 1993.)

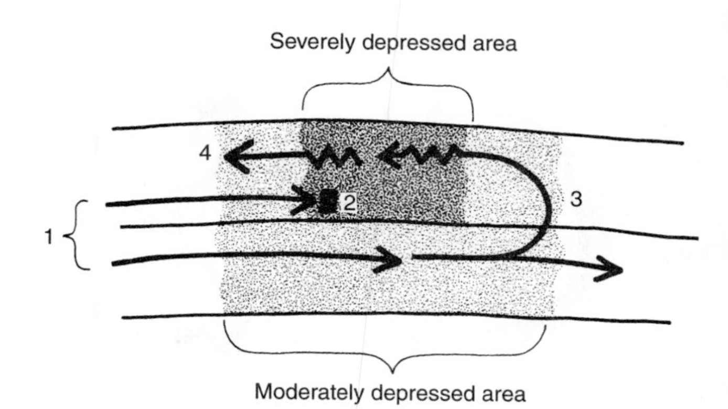

FIG. 3-9. Reflection, a type of reentry that occurs in depressed nonbranching Purkinje fibers. Impulse conduction *(1)* is blocked in a severely depressed segment *(2)* and is conducted slowly in a less severely depressed segment. It then returns to its origin *(3* and *4)* by traveling in a retrograde direction in the previously blocked segment.

way conduction (unidirectional block) is an essential component of the reentry circuit; otherwise, the impulse would be canceled out by opposing traffic. The anisotropic properties of cardiac muscle; that is, that conduction is faster lengthwise in the fiber than it is crossways, contribute to slow conduction and unidirectional block. An anisotropic reentry circuit is diagrammatically illustrated in Fig. 3-6, *H.* A figure-of-8 reentry circuit in a patient late after a myocardial infarction is shown in Fig. 3-8.

Reflection

Reflection is another form of reentry that occurs in parallel pathways of Purkinje fibers or myocardial tissue that have depressed segments. Fig. 3-9 illustrates a reflected impulse. When the cardiac impulse reaches the severely depressed segment, it is blocked there but transmitted slowly in a less severely depressed neighboring fiber. Upon reaching the end of the segment, the impulse activates the surrounding tissue and returns in the retrograde direction through the severely depressed segment.

CLINICAL APPLICATION

Electrocardiogram (ECG) differentiation among the mechanisms of reentry, altered automaticity, and triggered activity is at best difficult and often impossible because of the inability to reliably identify these mechanism in the electrophysiologic laboratory.[25] Occasionally, however, ECG clues suggest a particular mechanism.

Automaticity is suspected when the following occur: gradual acceleration or gradual emergence of an arrhythmia, long coupling or variable coupling intervals, and an arrhythmia that is introduced by a fusion beat. Automatic rhythms include parasystole, escape rhythms, nonparoxysmal junctional tachycardia, and accelerated idioventricular rhythms.

Triggered activity is more difficult to recognize but is suspected to be the mechanism of long-QT ventricular tachycardia (torsades de pointes) and the tachycardia of digitalis toxicity.

Reentry is suspected when the following occur: fixed coupling, abrupt termination of an arrhythmia by an extra beat, and, in the setting of prolonged conduction, the appearance of an ectopic rhythm. Verapamil has been shown to suppress arrhythmias thought to be caused by triggered activity.[26]

SUMMARY

Two categories of arrhythmias have been described: abnormalities of conduction caused by conduction block, reentry, or reflection and abnormalities of impulse initiation caused by altered automaticity (enhanced "normal" automaticity or "abnormal" automaticity), triggered activity, or reentry, which may be anatomic or functional. Enhanced normal automaticity is caused by a steepening of phase 4 in pacemaker cells; abnormal automaticity occurs in myocardial fibers (working or pacemaker) with abnormally reduced membrane potentials. Triggered activity is the result of afterdepolarizations; there are two types, early and delayed. Early afterdepolarizations are the result of prolonged QT intervals that may be congenital or acquired; delayed afterdepolarizations are the result of excess intracellular calcium, digitalis being a notable culprit. Anatomic reentry occurs in a set pathway as in the AV reciprocating circus movement tachycardia of Wolff-Parkinson-White syndrome or atrial flutter. Functional reentry is not pinned to an anatomic pathway.

REFERENCES

1. Peters NS, Cabo C, Wit AL: Arrhythmogenic mechanisms: automaticity, triggered activity, and reentry. In Zipes DP, Jalife J: *Cardiac electrophysiology from cell to bedside*, ed 3, Philadelphia, 2000, WB Saunders, pp 345-356.
2. Marriott HJL: Arrhythmia versus dysrhythmia, *Am J Cardiol* 53:628, 1984.
3. Arrhythmias and conduction disturbances; contents main heading, *Am J Cardiol* 89:A5, March 15, 2002.
4. Varma N, Stambler BS: Arrhythmia of the month, *J Cardiovasc Electrophysiol* 12:730, 2001.
5. Zipes DP, Jalife J: *Cardiac electrophysiology from cell to bedside*, ed 3, Philadelphia, 2000, WB Saunders, pp 447-481.
6. Kastor JA: *Arrhythmias*, ed 2, Philadelphia, 2000, WB Saunders.
7. Borchard U, Hafner D: [Ion channels and arrhythmias], *Z Kardiol* 89(Suppl 3):6, 2000.
8. Mines GR: On dynamic equilibrium in the heart, *J Physiol* (Lond) 46:349, 1913.
9. Lewis T: Observations upon flutter and fibrillation. IV. Impure flutter: theory of circus movement, *Heart* 7:293, 1920.
10. Allessie MA, Rensma W, Brugada J et al: Modes of atrial reentry. In Toboul P, Waldo AL, editors: *Atrial arrhythmias: current concepts and management*, St Louis, 1990, Mosby.
11. Allessie MA, Bonke FIM, Shopman FIG: Circus movement in rabbit atrial muscle as a mechanism of tachycardia, *Circ Res* 33:54, 1973.
12. Selfridge O: Studies of flutter and fibrillation, *Arch Inst Cardiol Mex* 58:177, 1948.
13. Balakhovsky IS: Several modes of excitation movement in the ideal excitable tissue, *Biophysics* 10:1175, 1965.
14. Beaumont J, Jalife J: Rotors and spiral waves in two dimensions. In Zipes DP, Jalife J, editors: *Cardiac electrophysiology from cell to bedside*, ed 3, Philadelphia, 2000, WB Saunders, pp 327-335.
15. Davidenko JM, Kent P, Chialvo DR et al: Sustained vortex-like weaves in normal isolated ventricular muscle, *Proc Natl Acad Sci U S A* 87:8785, 1990.
16. Davidenko JM, Kent P, Jalife J: Spiral waves in normal isolated ventricular muscle, *Physica D* 49:182, 1991.
17. Davidenko JM, Pertsov AM, Salomonsz R et al: Stationary and drifting spiral waves of excitation in isolated cardiac muscle, *Nature* 355:349, 1991.
18. Pertsov AM, Davidenko JM, Salomonsz R et al: Spiral waves of excitation underlie reentrant activity in isolated cardiac muscle, *Circ Res* 72:631, 1993.
19. Gray RA, Jalife J, Panfilov A et al: Nonstationary vortexlike reentrant activity as a mechanism of polymorphic ventricular tachycardia in the isolated rabbit heart, *Circulation* 91:2454, 1995.
20. Jalife J, Gray R: Drifting vortices of electrical waves underlie ventricular fibrillation in the rabbit heart, *Acta Physiol Scand* 157:123, 1996.
21. Asano Y, Davidenko JM, Baxter WT et al: Optical mapping of drug-induced polymorphic arrhythmias and torsade de pointes in the isolated heart, *Circulation* 91:2454, 1995.
22. Mandapati R, Asano Y, Davidenko JM et al: Effects of global ischemia on propagation during ventricular fibrillation in the isolated rabbit heart, *J Am Coll Cardiol* 330A(Suppl A):29, 1997.
23. Garfinkel A, Qu Z: Nonlinear dynamics of excitation and propagation in cardiac muscle. In Zipes DP, Jalife J, editors: *Cardiac electrophysiology from cell to bedside*, ed. 3, Philadelphia, 2000, WB Saunders, pp 315-320.
24. Krinsky V: Qualitative theory of reentry. In Zipes DP, Jalife J, editors: *Cardiac electrophysiology from cell to bedside*, ed 3, Philadelphia, 2000, WB Saunders, pp 320-327.
25. Saoudi N, Cosio F, Waldo A et al: Classification of atrial flutter and regular atrial tachycardia according to electrophysiologic mechanism and anatomic bases: a statement from a joint expert group from the Working Group of Arrhythmias of the European Society of Cardiology and the North American Society of Pacing and Electrophysiology, *J Cardiovasc Electrophysiol* 12:852, 2001.
26. Waldo AL, Wit AL: Mechanism of cardiac arrhythmias and conduction disturbances. In Fuster V, Alexander RW, King S et al, editors: *Hurst's the heart*, ed 10, New York, 2000, McGraw-Hill.

CHAPTER 4

Determination of the Electrical Axis

WHY IS AXIS DETERMINATION IMPORTANT?

The ability to determine the electrical axis of the heart is important for two main reasons. It is a necessary skill in the intelligent response to several cardiac emergencies, and it gives depth to understanding the 12-lead electrocardiogram (ECG) and monitoring leads.

Cardiac Emergencies

In the cardiac emergency of wide QRS tachycardia, rapid axis determination is helpful in many cases and diagnostic in some. This skill is a mandate for the speedy identification of patients with *hemiblock.* In the cardiac emergency of *broad QRS tachycardia,* axis determination can sometimes be diagnostic. Axis determination is also useful in the recognition of life-threatening *hyperkalemia.* An understanding of the QRS axis easily leads to an understanding of the P wave axis. Thus in paroxysmal supraventricular tachycardia, the ability to determine the P wave axis helps not only to determine the mechanism of the tachycardia, but also, in cases of *Wolff-Parkinson-White syndrome,* the location of an accessory pathway.

Understanding the 12-Lead ECG

An understanding of the 12-lead ECG and the nonstandard monitoring leads is not possible without a clear appreciation for the instant-to-instant electrical vectors of the heart and how they relate to each lead axis. This knowledge provides an important foundation in electrocardiography. After the axes of the six limb leads and the frontal plane electrical axis of the heart are understood, the student easily understands why the P wave or QRS complex is negative in one lead (aV_R for example) and positive in another (such as lead II).

METHODS OF AXIS DETERMINATION

Three methods for axis determination will be discussed: axis at a glance (for emergencies) and two other methods (the easy two-step method and the quadrant method). This will assist in providing the depth of understanding necessary for an appreciation of the normal ECG and how the mechanisms of arrhythmias and other abnormalities such as preexcitation, bundle branch block, hemiblock, acute myocardial infarction, and chamber enlargement are reflected on the ECG.

For completeness the *hexaxial figure* is also included in this chapter. It is an accurate, useful means of axis determination. However, I have found that although the student may understand the concept of the hexaxial figure in class, this understanding is generally not carried through to the pressured clinical setting. There is no doubt that visualizing the hexaxial wheel and plotting currents on it takes more time and requires a long-time familiarity. In the setting of cardiac emergencies, axis at a glance seems best.

INSTANT-TO-INSTANT ELECTRICAL ACTIVATION OF THE HEART

The impulse is delivered at the endocardial surface of the two ventricles almost simultaneously by the rapidly conducting His-Purkinje system. The impulse then travels from endocardium to epicardium; the numbers from 1 to 10 in Fig. 4-1 represent the sequence of impulse arrival at the epicardium. The whole process in the normal heart takes about 0.08 second or less.

VECTORS AND THE AXIS OF THE HEART

Vectors are quantities that have both a magnitude and direction. We use vectors many times in everyday life. For

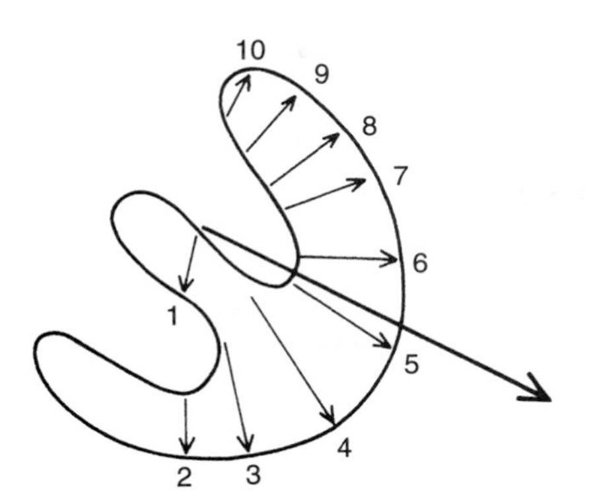

FIG. 4-1. Instant-to-instant currents *(1 to 10)* resulting from the orderly depolarization of the ventricular muscle mass. The prominent *arrow* between 5 and 6 represents the electrical axis of the heart.

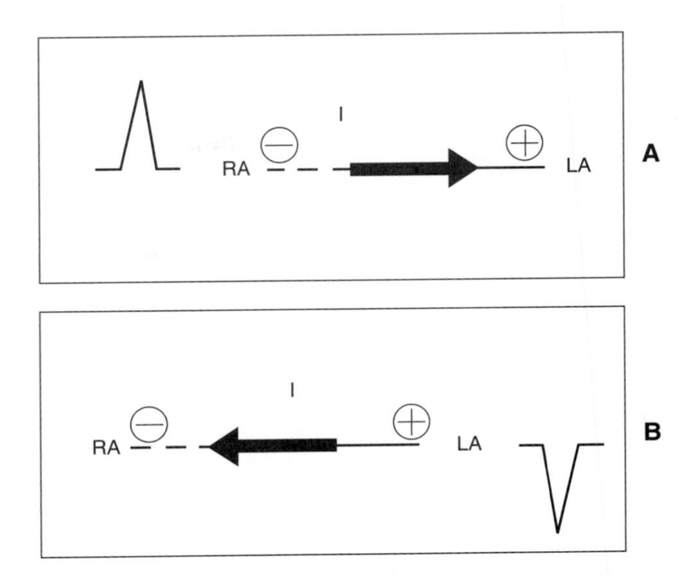

FIG. 4-2. Lead I is represented here (the *line* between the two electrodes). When current flow *(arrow)* is parallel to the axis of a lead (in this case, lead I) it results in, **A**, the tallest positive deflection or, **B**, the deepest negative deflection. *LA*, Left arm; *RA*, right arm.

example, if you live 10 miles southeast of the post office; that is a vector. The magnitude is 10 miles and its direction is southeast. The direction can also be expressed in degrees; in this case it would be 135 degrees. Vectors can also be added together to give a resultant vector. In adding vectors we simply travel along the first and then along the second and see where we end up. The process is not unlike the sailboat that sails northeast for 10 miles and then tacks to sail to the southeast for 10 miles. Our intrepid mariners will end up due east of the starting point because the northerly component of their travel exactly cancels the southerly component, leaving only the easterly component. Although the total distance traveled is 20 miles, the sailors end up only about 14 miles east of the starting point. This can be easily verified by using a ruler to make a scale drawing. As with ordinary addition, when many numbers can be added together to get a result, many vectors can be vector-added to get a resultant vector.

Current flow can be represented by a vector, with the amount of current being the magnitude and "downstream" being its direction. The small arrows in Fig. 4-1 represent the current flow vectors for the ventricles during electrical activation. If we add all of these vectors, the resultant vector, represented by the long, darker arrow, is called the *axis of the heart*. It may also be called the *QRS axis*. Just as the total effort of our sailors' Sunday afternoon sail was a 14-mile trip to the east, the total electrical effort of the heart is a current flow along its axis, represented by the long arrow in Fig. 4-1. Because we are primarily interested in the direction of current flow, I will refer to "currents" rather than vectors and to "axis" rather than "mean QRS vector."

CURRENT FLOW RELATED TO THE LEAD AXIS

The currents generated by the heart cause certain deflections on the ECG, according to how they relate to the lead axis.

1. When the main current flow of the heart is parallel to the lead axis, the resulting ECG complex is either the most positive or the most negative deflection of all, depending on whether it flows toward the positive or the negative electrode. This principle is illustrated in Fig. 4-2, where lead I is depicted; the negative electrode is on the right arm (RA), and the positive electrode is on the left arm (LA). The same principle is illustrated by two of the mean currents in Fig. 4-3. Two of the mean currents are superimposed on the lead axis (the line between the two electrodes), producing the tallest and deepest possible deflections, depending on which electrode is the target.
2. In Fig. 4-3, note the current that is perpendicular to the lead axis; it is neither positive nor negative and an isoelectric (equiphasic) deflection is written.

The remaining two mean currents drawn on the positive side of the lead axis are mostly positive, but become less so as the perpendicular orientation is approached.

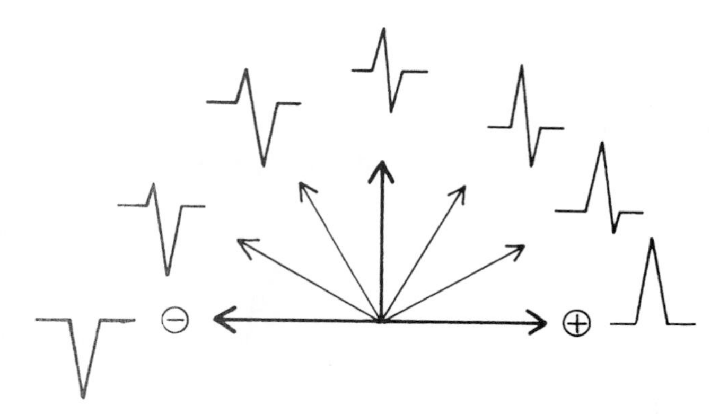

FIG. 4-3. Several electrical axes and their resultant ECG complex are represented. The *arrows* represent the electrical axes from seven different hearts. The lead axis is a straight line between the two electrodes. Take special note that a current perpendicular to the lead axis produces an equiphasic deflection and that a current parallel to the axis of the lead results in the tallest complex possible if the current flows toward the positive electrode and results in the deepest complex possible if the current flows toward the negative electrode.

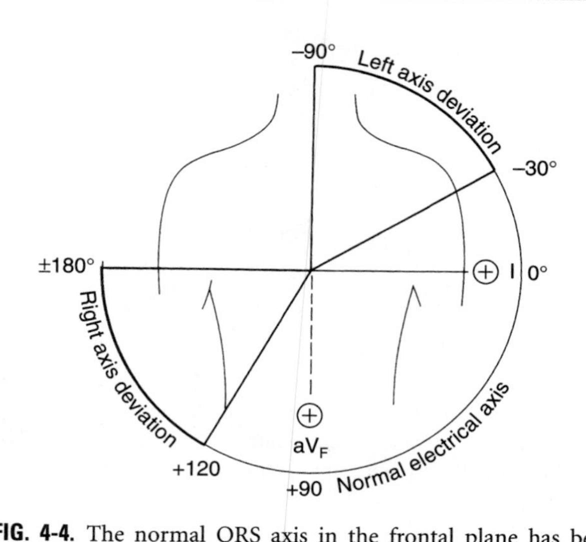

FIG. 4-4. The normal QRS axis in the frontal plane has been placed by various authors between −30 degrees and +120 degrees, depending on age, sex, and body build. See text for explanation.

Likewise, the remaining two mean currents between the perpendicular and parallel on the negative side of the lead axis are mostly negative, but become less so as they approach the perpendicular.

When studying this important illustration, keep in mind two facts: (1) Mean current parallel to a lead axis produces the deepest or tallest possible deflection. (2) Mean current perpendicular to a lead axis produces an isoelectric complex.

These concepts along with an understanding of the mechanisms of arrhythmias and cardiac disease, and where each lead axis is located are your keys to understanding the 12-lead ECG. If you are just beginning, the course will seem daunting. However, with these basic principles in hand, the need to memorize ECG patterns will be virtually nonexistent and your depth of understanding will be very rewarding clinically.

NORMAL QRS AXIS

The normal range of the QRS axis in the frontal plane is between −30 degrees and +105 degrees.[1] The definition of these boundaries varies among authors. Most seem to agree that the QRS axis should not be to the left of −30 degrees; however, opinions vary regarding the rightward boundary of the frontal plane QRS axis, placing it anywhere from +73 degrees to +120 degrees. The axis is left, of course, when it is beyond 0 degrees, but it is not an abnormal left axis deviation until it is beyond −30 degrees.

In 1960 Hiss et al[2] published findings in more than 67,000 asymptomatic individuals. Their findings indicate that the normal range of the QRS axis in the frontal plane is between +30 degrees and +75 degrees. These authors noted the influence of age as being significant in that there is a leftward shift of the axis in older individuals, but not into the abnormal range of beyond −30 degrees. Additionally, a thin person is likely to have a more vertical axis, and overweight individuals a more leftward axis, especially with aging. The difference in QRS axis between the sexes is insignificant, except from 40 to 50 years of age when women generally have less of a leftward axis shift than men (−53 degrees for women versus −37 degrees for men).[3,4]

Fig. 4-4 illustrates the outer boundaries of the normal QRS axis. In the clinical setting a change in the QRS axis is a reliable guide to a possible abnormality.

Pediatric QRS Axis[5]

Premature infant (less than 35 weeks' gestation): left and posterior
Full-term newborn: Right axis (up to +180 degrees)
1 week to 1 month: Right axis
1 month to 6 months: Right axis less than +120 degrees
6 months to 3 years: Usually less than +90 degrees

CAUSES OF AXIS DEVIATION

Left Axis Deviation

Anterior hemiblock
Q waves of inferior myocardial infarction
Ventricular pacing
Emphysema
Hyperkalemia (life-threatening)
Wolff-Parkinson-White syndrome (right-sided accessory pathway)
Tricuspid atresia
Injection of contrast into left coronary artery

Right Axis Deviation

Normal in children and tall thin adults
Right ventricular hypertrophy
Chronic lung disease even without pulmonary hypertension
Anterolateral myocardial infarction
Posterior hemiblock
Pulmonary embolus
Wolff-Parkinson-White syndrome (left-sided accessory pathway)
Atrial septal defect
Ventricular septal defect

Northwest Axis ("No Man's Land")

Emphysema
Hyperkalemia
Lead transposition
Ventricular pacing
Ventricular tachycardia

AXIS AT A GLANCE

In the emergency setting, knowing how to recognize an abnormal axis at a glance is most helpful. This is especially true when there is a broad QRS tachycardia or acute myocardial infarction.

Fig. 4-5 illustrates this useful shortcut to axis determination. Leads I and II are used as follows:

Normal axis: Leads I and II are upright (first three examples)
Left axis deviation: I is up; II is down
Right axis deviation: I is down; II is up
Northwest quadrant ("no man's land" or "indeterminate"): I and II are down

Note that when the complex in lead I is mainly positive and II is equiphasic, the axis is at –30 degrees. This is a borderline left axis deviation because if the complex in lead II were even a little more negative, it would be an abnormal left axis deviation.

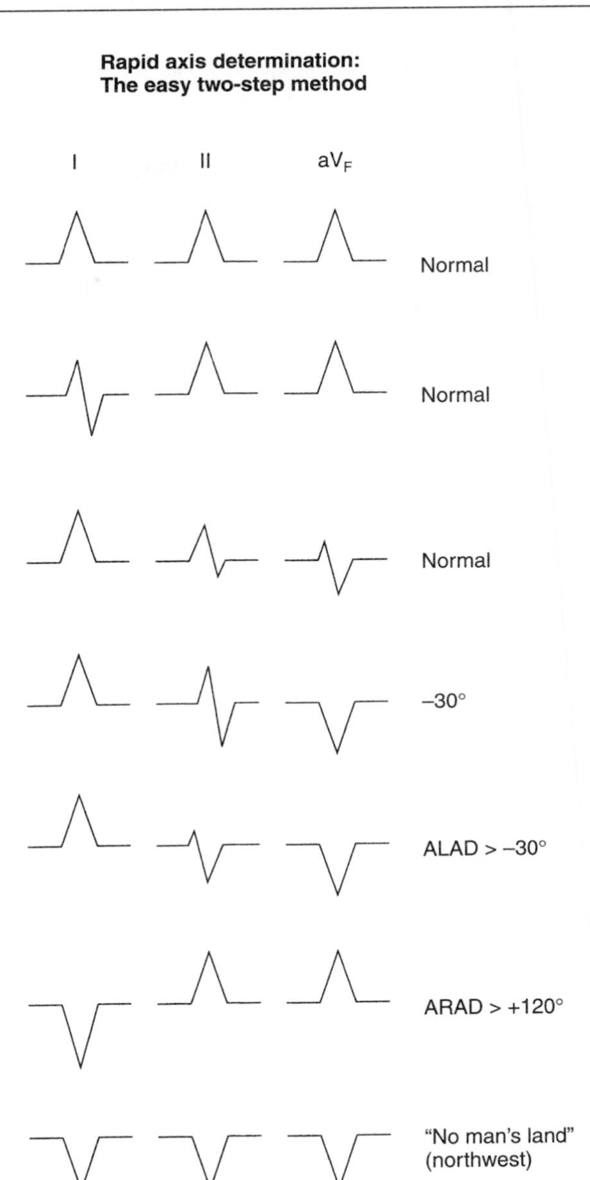

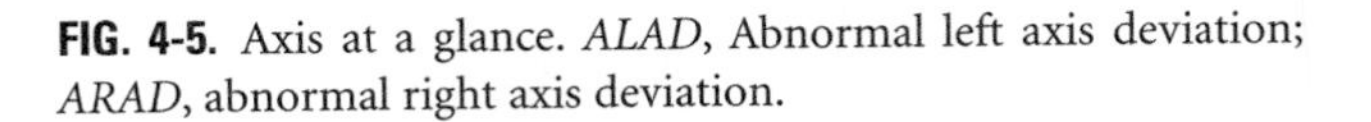

FIG. 4-5. Axis at a glance. *ALAD*, Abnormal left axis deviation; *ARAD*, abnormal right axis deviation.

EASY TWO-STEP METHOD OF AXIS DETERMINATION

When the Y shape of the three unipolar limb leads, aV_R, aV_L, and aV_F, is combined in a drawing with the inverted triangular shape formed by the three bipolar limb leads I,

II, and III, as seen in Fig. 4-6, each bipolar lead axis is perpendicular to a unipolar lead axis, providing an excellent frame of reference in which to determine the electrical axis of the heart.

For example, if the heart's electrical axis lies perpendicular to the lead axis of aV_R, it is also parallel to the lead axis of III. Thus when the equiphasic deflection is seen in one of these leads, a mostly positive or negative deflection is seen in the lead whose axis is perpendicular to it. Let us say that the equiphasic deflection is in lead aV_R (current flow is perpendicular to that lead axis). If the complex in lead III is positive, the QRS axis is to the right (toward the positive electrode); if the complex in lead III is negative, the QRS axis is to the left (toward the negative electrode). Thus you have the easy two-step method of axis determination.

1. Look for an equiphasic deflection; it tells you that current flow is perpendicular to that lead axis.
2. Now that the plane of current flow is known, look at the lead whose axis is parallel with the current flow to see whether current is flowing toward or away from its positive electrode. These principles will become clear when you follow the step-by-step exercises.

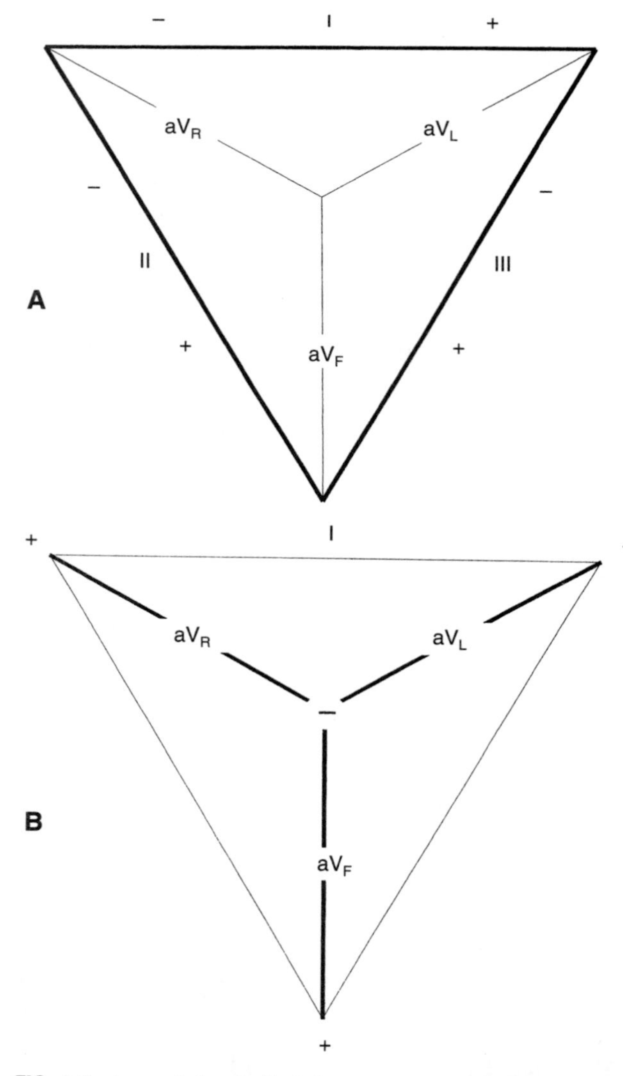

FIG. 4-6. Axes of the six limb leads. **A**, The inverted triangular shape is created by the axes of the three bipolar limb leads, I, II, and III. **B**, The Y shape is formed by the axes of the three unipolar limb leads, aV_R, aV_L, and aV_F. The center of the triangle is the zero reference point and the assigned negative for the unipolar leads.

EXERCISES FOR AXIS DETERMINATION

1. Place a piece of paper over all of the triangles on the right of the following exercises.
2. Draw your own triangle; then look for the equiphasic deflection in the frontal plane leads. If it is in a unipolar lead, draw that lead axis too, remembering that it will be perpendicular to a bipolar lead axis.
3. Draw a line indicating current flow, making the current flow line perpendicular to the axis of the lead where you found the equiphasic deflection.
4. Now evaluate the second lead of the easy two-step method. This will be the lead whose axis is parallel with the current flow. For example, if current flow is perpendicular to lead I, it will be parallel with lead aV_F.

Exercise 1: Normal Axis

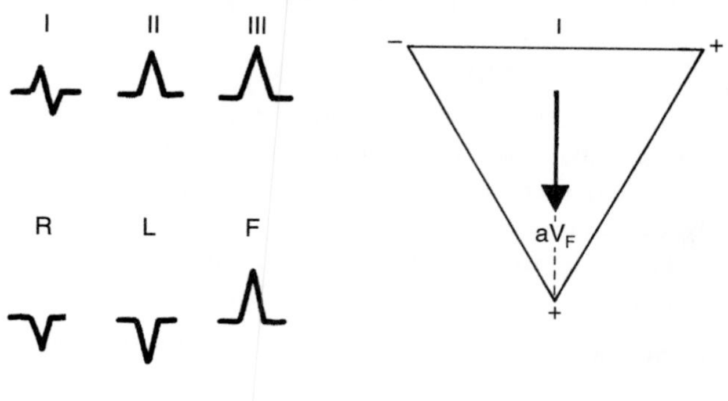

Step 1: Look for the equiphasic deflection. It is in lead I; therefore, current flow is perpendicular to that lead axis.

Step 2: Note that the lead axis of aV_F is also perpendicular to the lead axis of I.

Conclusion: Because the ECG complex in lead aV_F is positive, the mean current is flowing inferiorly toward the positive electrode of that lead. This is a normal axis.

Exercise 2: Normal Axis

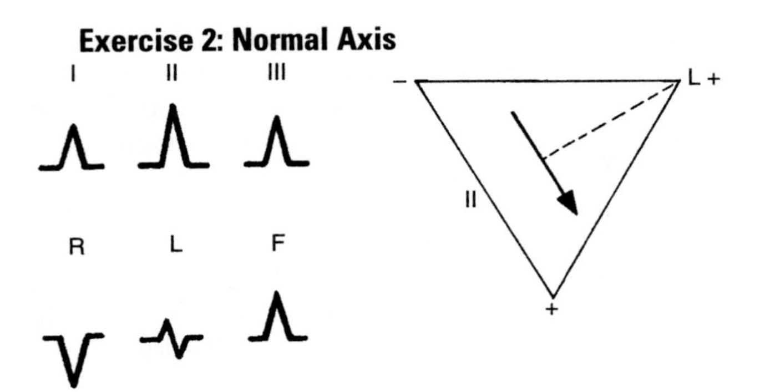

Step 1: Look for the equiphasic deflection. It is in lead aV_L; therefore, current flow is perpendicular to that lead axis.

Step 2: Note that the lead axis of aV_L is also perpendicular to the lead axis of II.

Conclusion: Because the ECG complex in lead II is positive, the mean current is flowing inferiorly toward the positive electrode of that lead. This is a normal axis.

Exercise 3: No Man's Land Axis

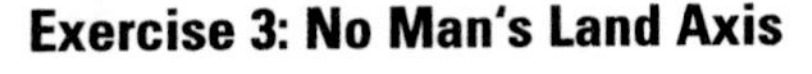

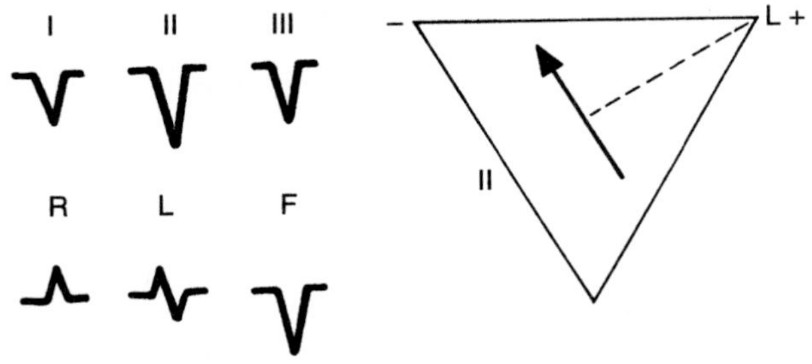

Step 1: Look for the equiphasic deflection. It is in lead aV_L (as it was in Exercise 2); therefore, current flow is perpendicular to that lead axis.

Step 2: Note that the lead axis of aV_L is also perpendicular to the lead axis of II.

Conclusion: Because the complex in lead II is negative (unlike that of Exercise 2), the mean current is flowing superiorly to the right and toward the negative electrode of lead II. This is commonly referred to as "no man's land," the northwest quadrant, or an indeterminate axis.

Exercise 4: Borderline Axis of –30 Degrees

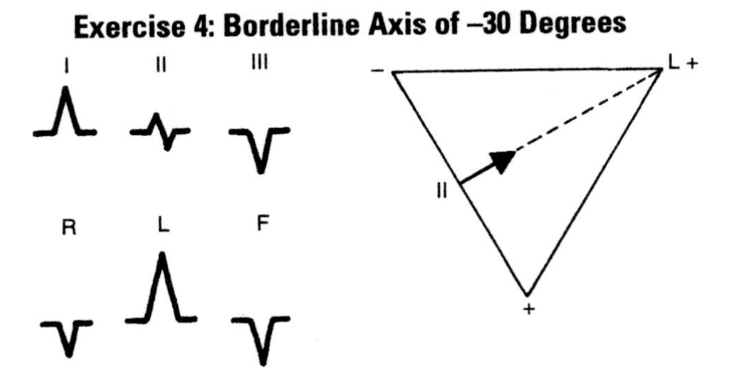

Step 1: Look for the equiphasic deflection. It is in lead II; therefore, current flow is perpendicular to that lead axis.

Step 2: Note that the lead axis of II is also perpendicular to the lead axis of aV_L.

Conclusion: Because the ECG complex in lead aV_L is positive, the mean current is flowing toward the positive electrode of that lead. This is a borderline axis (–30 degrees). If lead II were any more negative, the axis would be beyond –30 degrees, an abnormal left axis.

Exercise 5: Left Axis Deviation

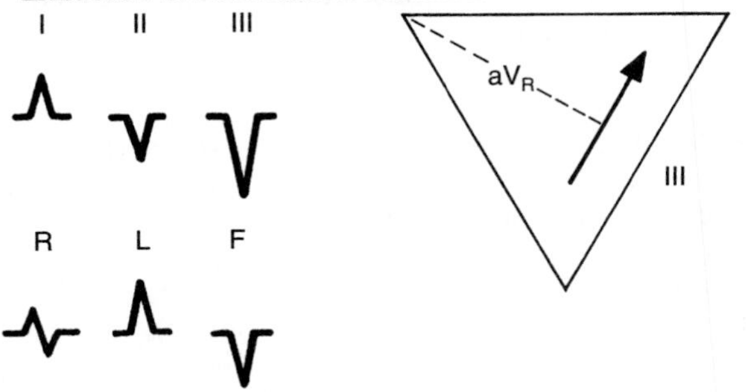

Step 1: Look for the equiphasic deflection. It is in lead aV_R; therefore, current flow is perpendicular to that lead axis.

Step 2: Note that the lead axis of aV_R is also perpendicular to the lead axis of III.

Conclusion: Because the ECG complex in lead III is negative, the mean current is flowing superiorly to the left and toward the negative electrode of lead III. This is an abnormal left axis (greater than –30 degrees).

Exercise 6: Right Axis Deviation

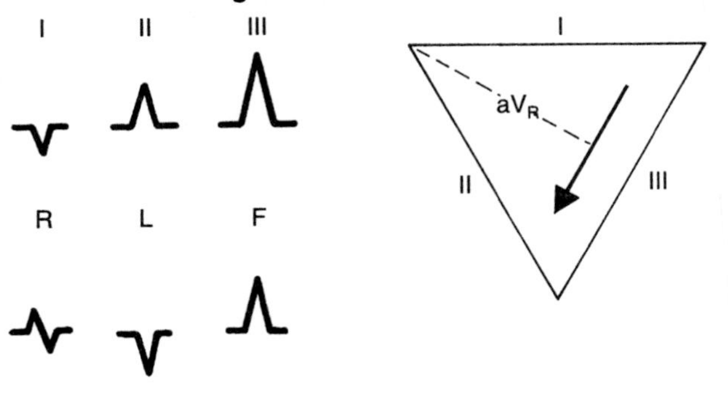

Step 1: Look for the equiphasic deflection. It is in lead aV_R; therefore, current flow is perpendicular to that lead axis.

Step 2: Note that the lead axis of aV_R is also perpendicular to the lead axis of III.

Conclusion: Because the complex in lead III is positive, the mean current is flowing inferiorly to the right and toward the positive electrode of lead III. This is an abnormal right axis deviation (greater than +120 degrees).

USE OF LEADS I AND aV_F IN AXIS DETERMINATION: THE QUADRANT METHOD

Note that in Fig. 4-7, *A*, the axes of leads I and aV_F divide the thorax into quadrants—normal, left, right, and northwest. The examples shown in Fig. 4-7, *B-E*, are meant to point out the advantages of this method and its single disadvantage; that is, the inability to determine whether a left axis is normal (less than –30 degrees) or abnormal (at or greater than –30 degrees).

In Fig. 4-7, *B*, note that the complex in lead I is mainly positive. Thus the axis must be to the left, between +90 degrees and –90 degrees.

If the complex in lead aV_F is also positive (Fig. 4-7, *C*), the axis is inferior and located in the normal quadrant (between 0 degrees and +90 degrees), since this is the quadrant that I and aV_F share when both are positive).

However, in the event of lead aV_F being negative (and lead I positive) (Fig. 4-7, *D*), the axis would be superior and somewhere in the left quadrant (between 0 degrees and –90 degrees). From this information alone it is not known whether the axis is left but normal (0 degrees to –30 degrees) or abnormal (–30 degrees to –90 degrees). To

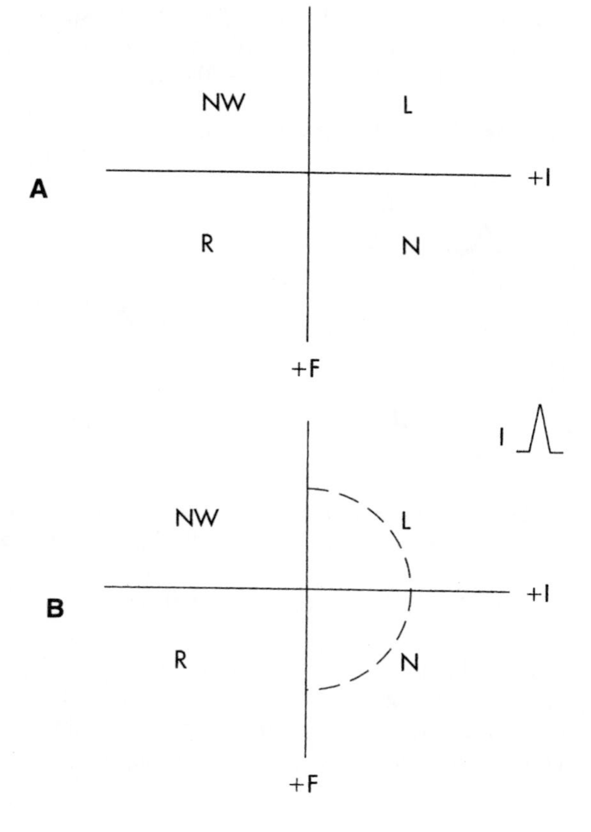

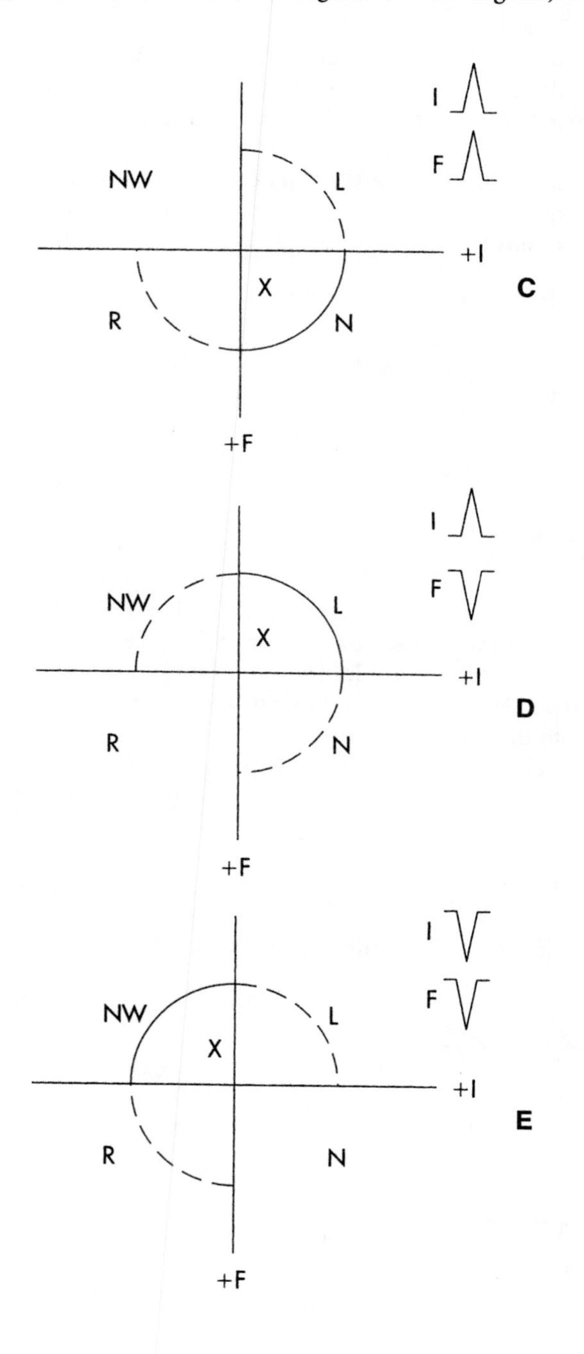

FIG. 4-7. A, The four quadrants of the thorax are defined by the axes of I and aV_F. B-D, The complexes in lead I are positive (the current flows toward the positive electrode). C, The complex in aV_F is positive (the current flows toward the positive electrode). *X* marks the normal *(N)* quadrant that both leads share. If the complex in lead I had been negative (and aV_F positive), the axis would have been in the right *(R)* quadrant. D, The complex in aV_F is negative (the current flows away from the positive electrode). *X* marks the left *(L)* quadrant that both leads share. In this case, without lead II a normal left axis cannot be distinguished from an abnormal left axis. E, The complexes in both leads are negative (current flows away from the positive electrodes). *X* marks the northwest *(NW)* quadrant that both leads share.

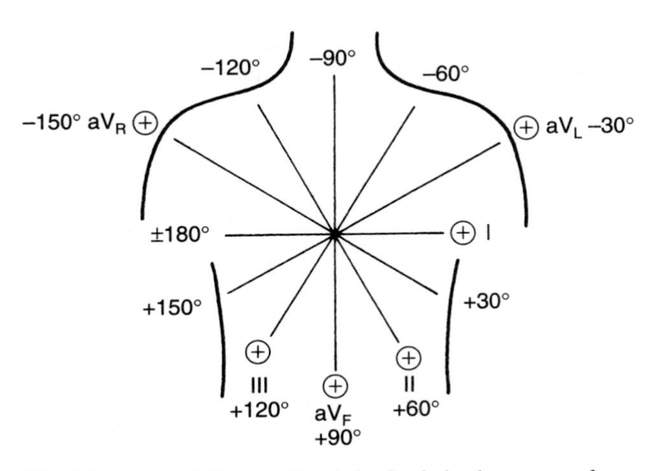

FIG. 4-8. Hexaxial figure. All of the limb lead axes are drawn through a central point. They are 30 degrees apart.

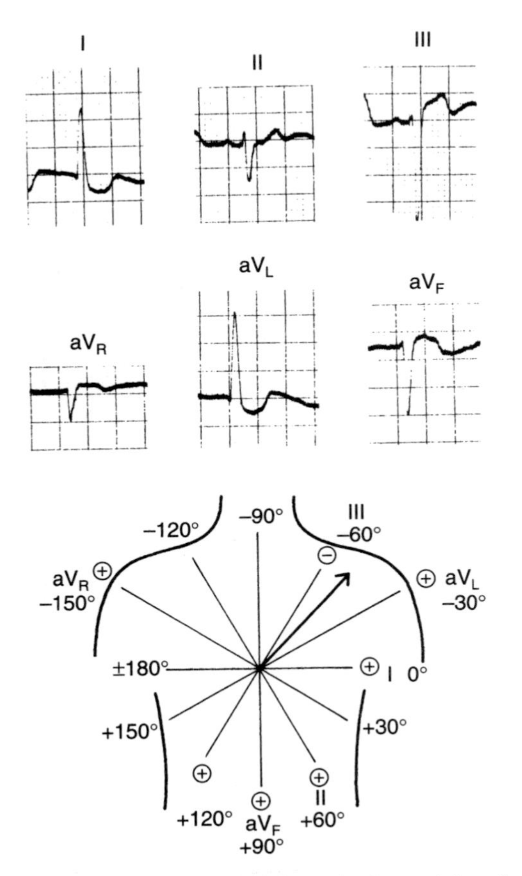

FIG. 4-9. The use of the hexaxial figure in determining electrical axis. Leads I and aV$_F$ reveal that the axis is in the left quadrant. Now look at the other two leads in this quadrant, III and aV$_L$. Lead III is more negative than lead aV$_L$ is positive; therefore the main current flow is closer to the axis of III than to that of aV$_L$, or at about −50 degrees, an abnormal left axis deviation.

obtain this information, lead II is needed (axis at a glance method). If the complex in II is mostly positive, the axis is left but normal; if equiphasic, the axis is −30 degrees (borderline); if negative, the axis is abnormal left.

As shown in Fig. 4-7, *E*, when the complex is negative in leads I and aV$_F$, the axis is in no man's land (northwest quadrant). In the setting of broad QRS tachycardia, such an axis is diagnostic of ventricular tachycardia.

HEXAXIAL FIGURE: A MORE PRECISE METHOD OF AXIS DETERMINATION

After becoming comfortable and adept at determining the electrical axis using axis at a glance, the easy two-step method, and the quadrant method, you may wish to refine

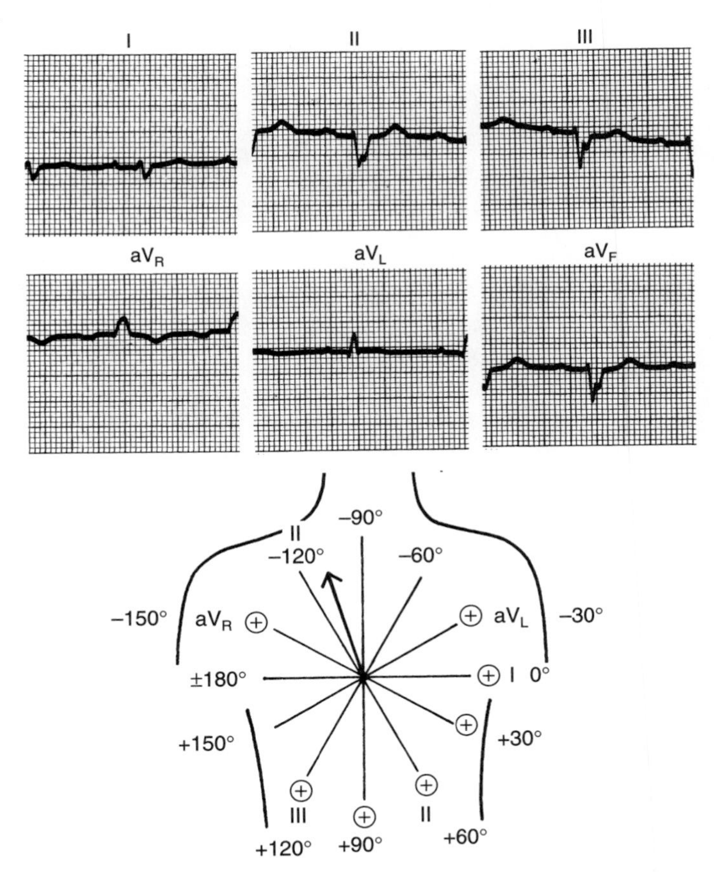

FIG. 4-10. Use of the hexaxial figure. In this illustration the axis is placed in "no man's land" (−90 degrees to ±180 degrees) because both I and aV$_F$ are negative. When the axis is in this quadrant, it is either extreme right or extreme left axis deviation. Now look at the other two leads within this quadrant (II and aV$_R$). The complex in lead II is clearly more negative than aV$_R$ is positive, placing the axis closer to II. However, if the main current were parallel to the axis of II, aV$_L$ would be equiphasic. Because this is not the case, aV$_L$ being positive, the axis is slightly to the right of −120 degrees, or −115 degrees.

your skill by learning to work with the hexaxial figure, which provides an excellent reference system for estimating the axis in degrees.

The hexaxial figure is drawn by shifting the axes of the six limb leads so that they all pass through the zero potential of the heart's electrical field (Fig. 4-8). There are 30-degree increments between lead axes. Figs. 4-9 and 4-10 describe the use of the hexaxial figure.

SUMMARY

The QRS axis may be quickly estimated by the polarity of the complexes in leads I and II; especially useful is the knowledge that the axis is normal if the complexes in leads I and II are upright. Leads I and aV_F may also be used to determine which quadrant (normal, left, right, or north-west) the axis is in. Other methods requiring more figuring are the easy two-step method and plotting current flow on the hexaxial figure.

REFERENCES

1. Chou TC, Knilans TK: *Electrocardiography in clinical practice adult and pediatric*, Philadelphia, 1996, WB Saunders, p. 6.
2. Hiss RG, Lamb LE, Allen MF: Electrocardiographic findings in 67,375 asymptomatic patients, *Am J Cardiol* 6:200, 1960.
3. Hakki AH, Anderson GJ, Ishandrisn AS et al: A simple method to determine the electrocardiographic frontal plane axis, *J Electrocardiol* 15:285, 1982.
4. MacFarlane PW, Lawrie TDV: *Comprehensive electrocardiology theory and practice in health and disease*, vol 3, Oxford, 1989, Pergamon Press.
5. Tipple M: Interpretation of electrocardiograms in infants and children, *Images Paediatr Cardiol* 1:3, 1999.

CHAPTER 5

Measurement of Heart Rate and Intervals

ECG PAPER

Time is measured on the horizontal plane. Each small square on the electrocardiogram (ECG) paper is 1 mm in length and represents 0.04 second. Each larger square, which is defined by the heavier lines, is 5 mm in length and represents 0.2 second in time when the paper speed is 25 mm/sec.

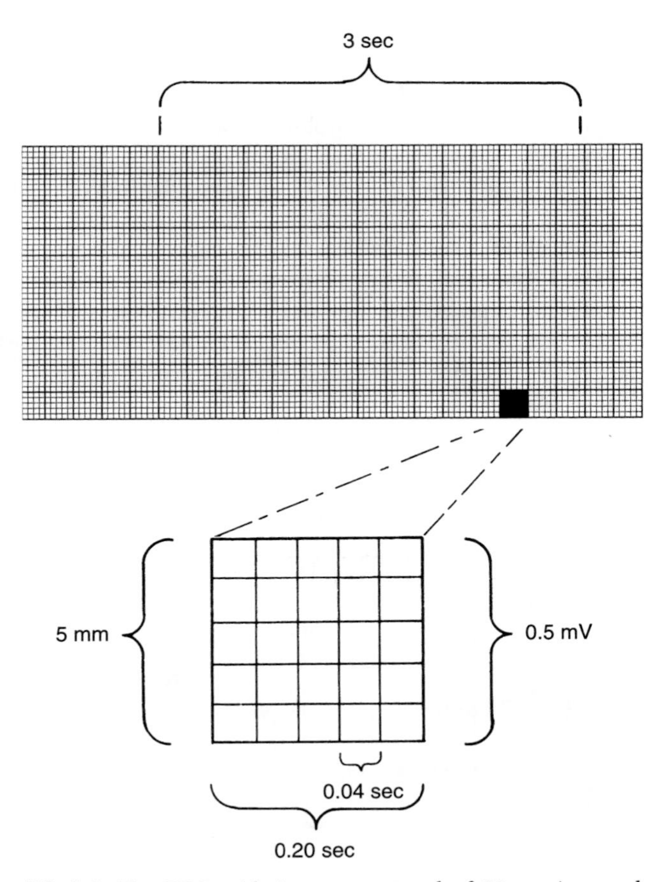

FIG. 5-1. The ECG grid. At a paper speed of 25 mm/sec, each small square represents 0.04 second and each large square, 0.20 second. In the standardized ECG, 5 mm equals 0.5 mV.

Amplitude (voltage) is measured on the vertical plane. All diagnostic 12-lead ECGs are standardized so that 1 mV is equal to 10 mm (two large squares).

The single vertical lines above the ECG grid are 3 inches apart and represent 3-second intervals (Fig. 5-1) when the paper speed is 25 mm/sec.

CALCULATION OF HEART RATE

Any of several methods can be used to calculate heart rate.

1. Count the number of cycles in a 6-second strip and multiply by 10. This method, which is fast and simple, can be used when the rhythm is either regular or irregular (Fig. 5-2).
2. Count the number of large squares between two R waves and divide into 300. This method is accurate only if the rhythm is regular (Fig. 5-3).
3. Measure the time interval in seconds between two R waves and divide into 60. For example, if the distance between the R waves of two consecutive beats is 0.60 second, the heart rate is 100 beats/min. This method is accurate only if the rhythm is regular.
4. For more rapid rhythms or to calculate a rapid atrial rate, count the number of small squares (0.04 second) between R waves or P waves and divide into 1500. This method is accurate only if the rhythm is regular.

PR INTERVAL

The PR interval (Fig. 5-4) is normally between 0.12 and 0.20 seconds. It represents the length of time it takes for the impulse to travel through the atria, across the atrioventricular (AV) node and bundle of His, and down the bundle branches and Purkinje fibers. It ends the moment the ventricular myocardium is activated. Thus the PR interval is measured from the very beginning of the P wave to the first ventricular deflection. Because the onset of the P wave and

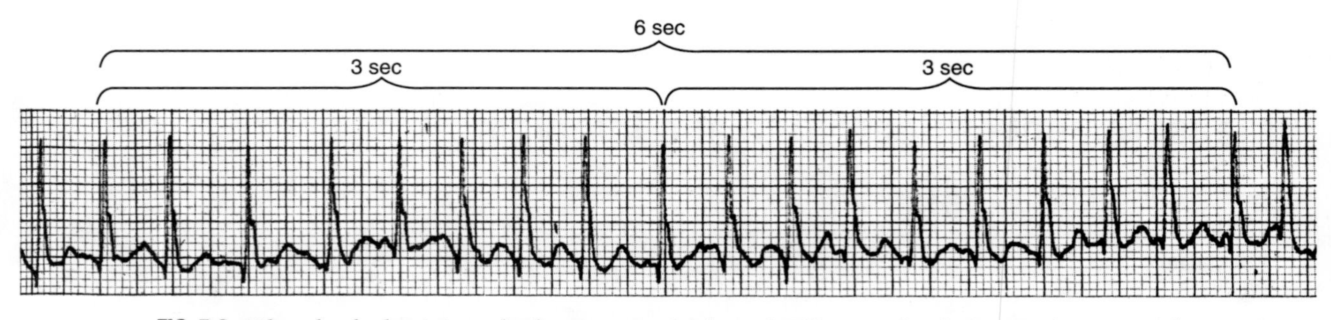

FIG. 5-2. When the rhythm is irregular, heart rate can be determined by counting the R waves in a 6-second strip and multiplying by 10. (Paper speed is 25 mm/sec.)

the onset of the QRS can be isoelectric (see Fig. 2-14), to be absolutely accurate the PR interval should be measured in the lead with the widest P and QRS. The onset of the P wave is the beginning of atrial activation, just as the onset of the QRS complex is the beginning of ventricular activation. The activation of the AV node and His-Purkinje system are silent events, not seen on the surface ECG.

The PR segment is part of the PR interval. It is that segment from the end of the P wave to the beginning of the QRS complex (Fig. 5-4). The PR segment is normally isoelectric but may be displaced in atrial infarction and in acute pericarditis. Normal displacement of the PR segment is usually the result of atrial repolarization and is more likely to be seen when the P waves are tall. Normally PR segment depression is less than 0.8 mm and PR segment elevation less than 0.5 mm.

Influence of Heart Rate

Because the sinus node and the AV node are both under the control of the vagus nerve, the PR interval varies with heart rate, becoming shorter during sinus tachycardia and longer during sinus bradycardia. The sinus node responds to the needs of the body. It increases its rate if more cardiac output is necessary. The AV node responds in kind by shortening its refractory period so that the quicker sinus rate will be able to reach the ventricles. This tandem functioning of the two nodes is noticeably absent when atrial tachycardia is caused by a rhythm outside the sinus node (an ectopic rhythm). Instead of shortening its refractory period in response to the tachycardia, the AV node lengthens this period so that at least the ventricles are somewhat protected from the unwelcome tachycardia.

Prolonged PR Interval

The PR interval may be prolonged because of AV block or hypothyroidism. However, a PR interval longer than the prescribed limits may be normal for a particular individual.

Shortened PR Interval

The PR interval may be shortened because of preexcitation syndromes, AV junctional rhythms, glycogen storage disease, or hypertension. However, a PR interval that is shorter than the prescribed limit may be normal for a particular individual.

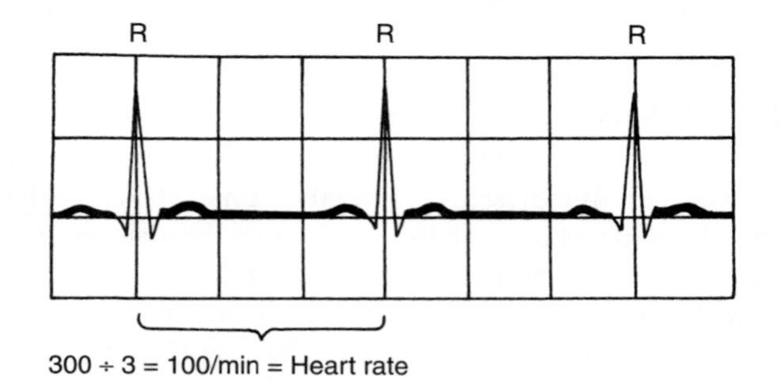

FIG. 5-3. When the rhythm is regular, heart rate can be determined at a glance.

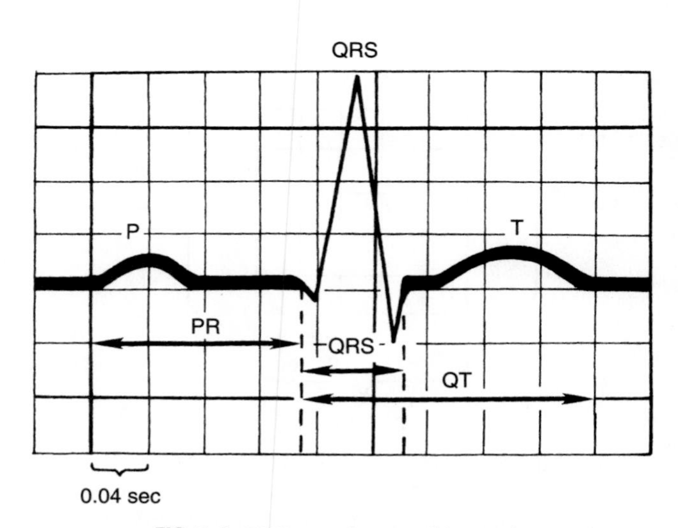

FIG. 5-4. ECG complexes and intervals.

QT INTERVAL

The QT interval is the distance from the beginning of the ventricular complex to the end of the T wave (Fig. 5-4). It represents the sum of depolarization and repolarization periods in the heart (refractory period of the ventricles). After myocardial infarction the longest QT interval is usually seen in leads V_2 to V_4.

The QT interval is significantly influenced by heart rate and autonomic tone; it also varies in males and females and with age. As the heart rate speeds up, the QT shortens; as the heart rate slows down, the QT lengthens. This response represents a fundamental physiologic phenomenon by which the heart is protected from stimulation before an adequate diastolic filling period can be achieved. QT prolongation reflects dispersion of repolarization within the myocardium, predisposing to a malignant polymorphous ventricular tachycardia known as torsades de pointes (see Chapters 25 and 26).

The QT interval may lengthen because of drugs, cardiac and noncardiac, and certain conditions. The QT interval may be prolonged by 10% to 15% in trained athletes (see Chapter 20).

For a complete list of cardiac and noncardiac drugs and the various conditions that can prolong the QT interval please refer to Chapter 27.

Measuring the QT Interval

The QT interval is measured in a lead in which the T wave is largest and its end best seen (Fig. 5-4). This may be leads V_2 and V_3. Measurement of the QT interval may be difficult when the T waves are flat, broad, or notched. A notched T wave could represent fusion of the T wave and the U wave. In such a case the duration of the QT interval cannot be exactly measured. The same problem exists when a P wave is superimposed on a T wave. Table 5-1 contains the longstanding Ashman and Hull correlation of cycle lengths and heart rate with normal QT intervals.

Corrected QT (QT_c)

Because the QT interval lengthens with tachycardia and shortens with bradycardia, it is corrected for heart rate. One of the ways to do that is to use Bazett's formula, which is based on the observation that the QT interval varies with the square root of the cycle length. (Divide the square root of the RR interval into the QT interval, measured in seconds.) However, a normal range for the QT_c remains

TABLE 5-1 Normal Q-T Intervals and the Upper Limits of the Normal

				Upper Limits of the Normal	
Cycle Lengths (sec)	Heart Rate (beats/min)	Men and Children (sec)	Women (sec)	Men and Children (sec)	Women (sec)
1.50	40	0.449	0.461	0.491	0.503
1.40	43	0.438	0.450	0.479	0.491
1.30	46	0.426	0.438	0.466	0.478
1.25	48	0.420	0.432	0.460	0.471
1.20	50	0.414	0.425	0.453	0.464
1.15	52	0.407	0.418	0.445	0.456
1.10	54.5	0.400	0.411	0.438	0.449
1.05	57	0.393	0.404	0.430	0.441
1.00	60	0.386	0.396	0.422	0.432
0.95	63	0.378	0.388	0.413	0.423
0.90	66.5	0.370	0.380	0.404	0.414
0.85	70.5	0.361	0.371	0.395	0.405
0.80	75	0.352	0.362	0.384	0.394
0.75	80	0.342	0.352	0.374	0.384
0.70	86	0.332	0.341	0.363	0.372
0.65	92.5	0.321	0.330	0.351	0.360
0.60	100	0.310	0.318	0.338	0.347
0.55	109	0.297	0.305	0.325	0.333
0.50	120	0.283	0.291	0.310	0.317
0.45	133	0.268	0.276	0.294	0.301
0.40	150	0.252	0.258	0.275	0.282
0.35	172	0.234	0.240	0.255	0.262

From Ashman R, Hull E: *Essentials of electrocardiography*, New York, 1941, Macmillan.

unsettled, a wide range being observed in normal subjects as in individuals with long QT syndrome.

"Rule of Thumb"

For decades, clinicians have been using a "rule of thumb" to quickly determine if a QT interval is normal. This undocumented rule states that at heart rates of 60 to 100 beats/min the normal QT does not exceed half the RR interval.[2] This shorthand rule was mathematically validated in 1998 by Phoon,[3] who plotted it against Bazett formula, the Framingham Heart Study's linear correction, and Fridericia's cube root prediction. The validated "rule of thumb" is essentially the same as the long-standing empirical one; the only change has been the heart rates at which it can be used. Thus *the normal QT_c is less than one half the RR interval when the HR is more than 70 beats/min.*

THE PEDIATRIC ECG

Before the pediatric ECG can be interpreted, the age of the child must be known, as must information about the indications for the testing, clinical diagnosis, medications, and electrolytes.

Interpretation of the neonatal ECG is the most challenging because of the rapid hemodynamic changes taking place causing the ECG to change rapidly during the first few weeks of life. At 3 years of age the child's ECG begins to resemble the adult's, although there remains significant, persistent differences.[4]

REFERENCES

1. Ashman R, Hull E: *Essentials of electrocardiography for the student and practitioner of medicine*, New York, 1941, Macmillan (appendix, table III).
2. Marriott HJL: *Practical electrocardiography*, Baltimore, 1983, Williams & Wilkins.
3. Phoon CKL: Mathematic validation of a shorthand rule for calculating QT_c, *Am J Cardiol* 82:400, 1998.
4. Tipple M: Interpretation of electrocardiogram in infants and children, *Images Paediatr Cardiol* 1:3-13, 1999.

CHAPTER 6

Arrhythmias Originating in the Sinus Node

The sinus node is located anteriorly at the junction of the right atrium and the superior vena cava in the superior part of the crista terminalis, a longitudinal band dividing the sinus venosum (venous portion of the right atrium) from the muscular right atrium (atrial appendage and pectinate muscles). The physiologic sinus node is thought to extend beyond its histologic boundaries to involve the crista terminalis. Fig. 6-1 shows a wax model of the human sinus node. The body of the sinus node blends with perinodal fibers, which in turn blend with atrial tissue (*1*, *2*, and *3* in the illustration).

SINUS P WAVE

The sinus node is a complex network with many dynamic points of impulse origin. The autonomic nervous system exerts exquisite control over the rate at which the sinus node paces the heart and the location of that pacing site within the node. Parasympathetic stimulation slows the rate of discharge and causes an inferior shift of impulse origin; sympathetic stimulation increases the rate of discharge and causes a superior shift of impulse origin, so that the shape of the sinus P wave may vary according to rate.[1] In the past this has been known as a *wandering pacemaker*.

SINUS NODE ACTION POTENTIAL

The action potential differs from that of atrial fibers in that it possesses the property of automaticity, has a less negative maximal diastolic potential, and therefore is depolarized mostly by a slow calcium current (rather than a fast sodium current), which in turn determines that, although

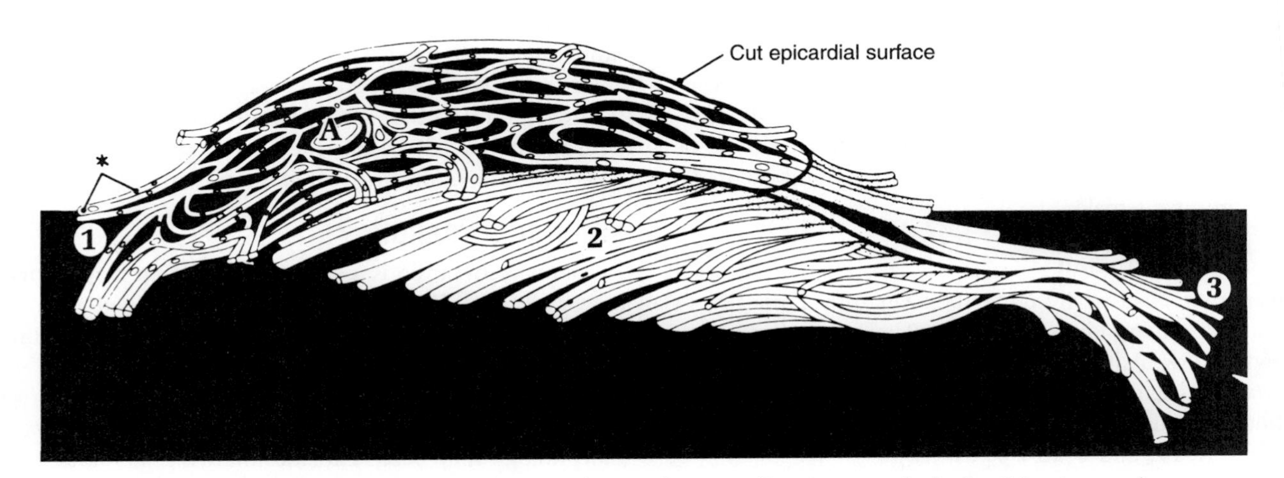

FIG. 6-1. A wax model of the human sinus node. *A* and surrounding tissue are the body of the sinus node; *1*, *2*, and *3* identify perinodal fibers. (From Truex RC. In Wellens HJJ, Lie KI, Janse MJ, editors: *The conduction system of the heart*, Hingham, Mass, 1976, Martinus Nijhoff.)

the sinus rate may be fast, conduction velocity through the sinus node itself is slow.

SINUS NODE ARRHYTHMIAS

Arrhythmias that originate in the sinus node are designated as such because the rate is too fast (sinus tachycardia) or too slow (sinus bradycardia); the sinus rhythm slows and accelerates with respirations (sinus arrhythmia); a sinus node impulse either does not form within the sinus node (sinus arrest), fails to exit from the sinus node (sinoatrial [SA] block), or repeatedly circulates through the sinus node (SA nodal reentry tachycardia); and inappropriate responses to the autonomic nervous system with episodes of atrial tachyarrhythmias (sick sinus syndrome [SSS]).

Such arrhythmias are not necessarily abnormal. For example, sinus tachycardia, when appropriate, is a physiologic response to the needs of the body (e.g., prompted by exercise, emotions, fever), sinus bradycardia is common in athletes and during sleep, and sinus arrhythmia is associated with the vagal effect of respirations and is common in children and athletes. When these arrhythmias are symptomatic or inappropriate, they are abnormal; SSS is exactly what its name implies.

NORMAL SINUS RHYTHM

Normal sinus rhythm is recognized because of sinus P waves normally conducted to and through the ventricles (normal PR; normal QRS), and a heart rate of 60 to 100 beats/min, a rate that has been generally agreed on for many years. However, in clinical practice most clinicians are alert to possible problems when the adult heart rate is faster than 90 beats/min and are not concerned unless the heart rate drops to less than 50 beats/min in a symptomatic patient. Faster rates are normal in infants and young children; and slower rates are seen in athletes and many healthy adults. In a Cleveland Clinic[2] study, 536 consecutive healthy subjects were studied. From this study came the recommendation that the normal sinus rate should be defined at 44 to 84 beats/min for males and 50 to 90 beats/min for females.

ECG Recognition

Heart rate: Historically, 60 to 100 beats/min. Clinically, 44 to 84 beats/min in males; 50 to 90 beats/min in females.
Rhythm: Regular or slightly irregular with respirations.
P waves: Usually all the same shape.
Mandatory normal polarities:

- I, II, aV_F and V_3 to V_6: positive
- aV_R: negative
- III, aV_L, V_1 and V_2: positive, negative, or biphasic

P wave axis: +15 degrees to +75 degrees.
PP interval: Minor variations are normal, but not usually more than 0.16 second difference between the longest and shortest intervals.
PR interval, QRS complex, and QT interval: Although the term *normal sinus rhythm* should logically refer to the P waves (rate, rhythm, and morphology), tradition requires us to limit that title to rhythms in which all measurements are normal. It is possible, of course, for the sinus rhythm to be normal and the other measurements to be abnormal (i.e., normal sinus rhythm with prolonged PR interval, bundle branch block, long QT syndrome).

Mechanism

The autonomic nervous system controls the discharge rate of the sinus node and the conduction velocity of the atrioventricular (AV) node. The two nodes work together; when the rate of the sinus node decreases, so does AV conduction velocity. When the rate of the sinus node increases, so does conduction velocity. Steady vagal stimulation (sinus slowing) dominates steady sympathetic stimulation (sinus acceleration).

Fig. 6-2 is a normal sinus rhythm (rate 62 beats/min) from a 48-year-old woman. Note the normal frontal plane QRS axis (+60 degrees), normal PR interval (0.13 second), normal QRS duration (0.08 second), and normal corrected QT (QTc) intervals (0.44). In the precordial leads one looks for R wave progression (reflecting normal anterior forces), septal activation (tiny q in leads I, V_5, and V_6), and a transitional zone (see Chapter 2) somewhere between V_3 and V_4.

Pediatrics

The younger the age, the faster the rate of the normal sinus rhythm. A rate of 200 beats/min may be the upper limit of normal for a 1-month-old infant but would be abnormal in an older child. Normal heart rate in the newborn varies from 110 to 200 beats/min; variability decreases with age. In the first week of life the average rate is less than 140 beats/min; in the first year, it is less than 120 beats/min.

SINUS TACHYCARDIA

Sinus tachycardia is a sinus rhythm at an inappropriately rapid rate. Traditionally, that rate is defined as more than 100 beats/min, as seen in Fig. 6-3. However, most clinicians would be suspicious of a resting heart rate of 90 beats/min or more.

In this figure the subtle but apparent changes in P wave morphology may be due to the following: (1) a shift of pacemaker site within the SA node, (2) a change in the exit pathway from the node so that a different part of the atrium becomes the first to be activated, or (3) to the initiation of the impulse from a pacemaker cell outside of the

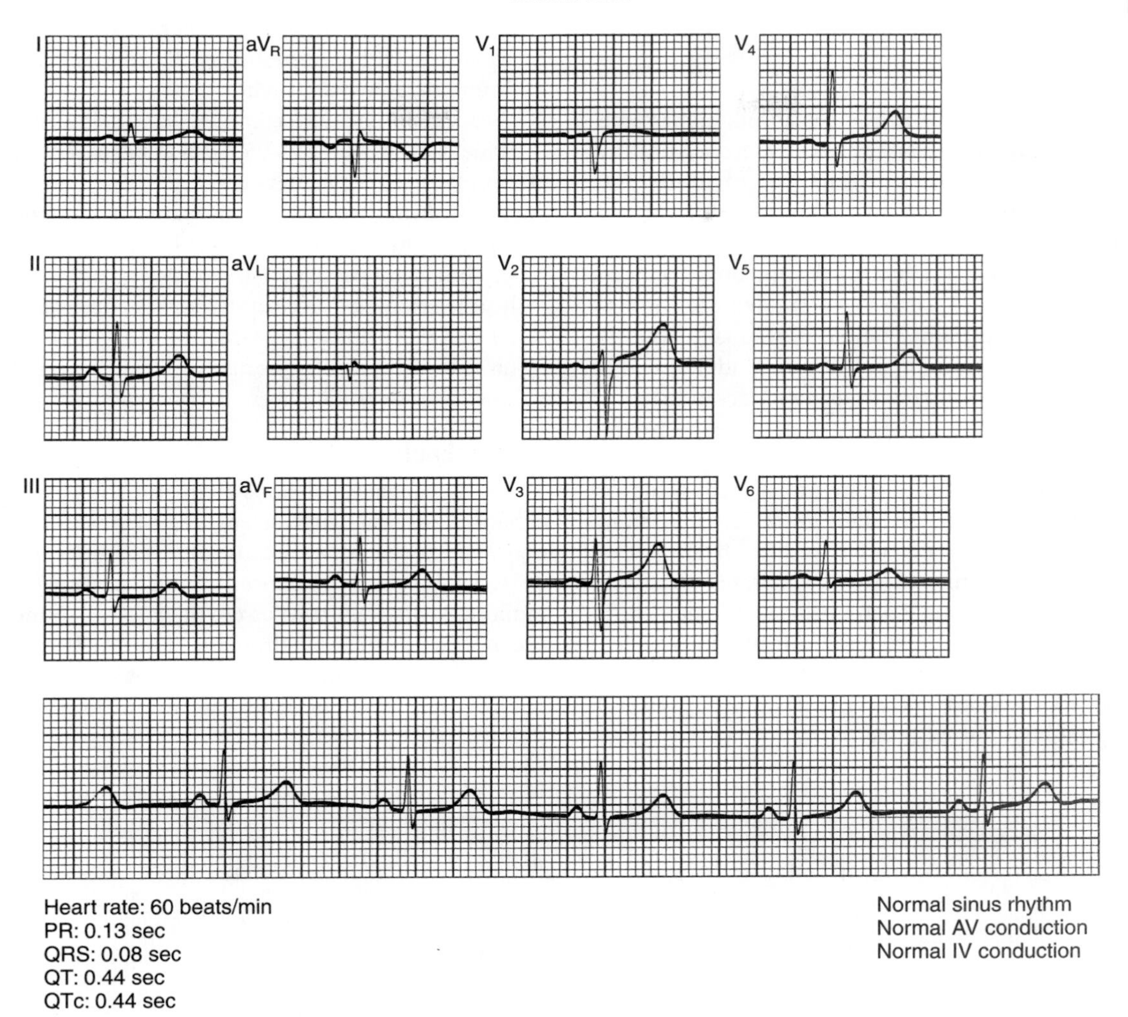

FIG. 6-2. Normal sinus rhythm. All measurements are normal (PR: 0.13 second; QRS: 0.08 second; QTc: 0.44 second; QRS axis: +60); heart rate is 62 beats/min.

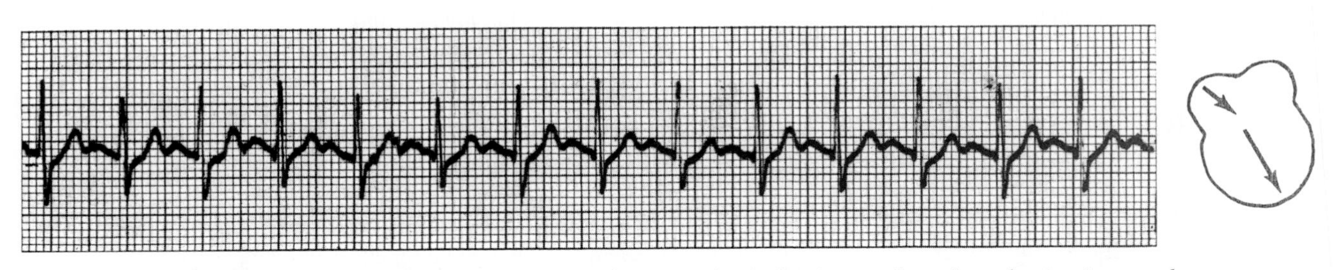

FIG. 6-3. Sinus tachycardia of 140 beats/min. The pacemaker is the sinus node, and conduction is normal. The undulating heights of the QRS complexes are caused by respirations. Note the subtle changes in the shape of the P wave morphology. See text for explanation.

SA node, which can occur under normal physiologic conditions.[3]

ECG Recognition

Heart rate: Ranges from 100 to 180 beats/min; higher with exertion. During strenuous physical exercise, healthy young adults may register a heart rate of nearly 200 beats/min, which decreases with age to less than 140 beats/min.[4]

Rhythm: Sinus tachycardia has an abrupt onset only in unusual circumstances, such as the sudden cessation of parasympathetic restraint. Rather, it gradually accelerates to a rapid, regular rhythm and then gradually decelerates when the physiologic needs no longer exist.

P waves: P waves are usually identical in shape to the P waves of slower, normal sinus rhythm. However, as already mentioned, with the tachycardia it is possible for the pacing site within the sinus node itself to shift, causing the shape of the P wave to differ from that of a slower sinus rhythm.[5-7] Fig. 6-4 illustrates variations in the shape of the sinus P wave because of microshifts of the focus within the SA node during sinus tachycardia.

PR interval: As the sinus rate accelerates, the PR interval shortens slightly. This is because the AV node is under the same autonomic nervous system control as the sinus node, and acceleration of the rate of sinus firing is accompanied by shortening of AV conduction.

PP intervals: May vary slightly.

QRS complex: The QRS complex during sinus tachycardia is identical in shape to the QRS at normal rates.

QT interval: The QT interval shortens.

Distinguishing features: (1) P waves are in front of the QRS; be careful not to mistake the T for the P. (2) This rhythm is not paroxysmal, rather the heart rate gradually accelerates and decelerates and is consistent with the needs of the body. (3) A rate of over 100 beats/min is quickly recognized because of less than three large squares between R waves.

Mechanism

The mechanism of sinus tachycardia is physiologically enhanced automaticity (steepening of phase 4 of the SA nodal action potential) because of sympathetic stimulation or vagal block. *Instantaneous sinus tachycardia* can be induced by an event such as the unexpected sound of gunfire at close range. This dramatic response is mediated by the sudden cessation of parasympathetic restraint on the sinus node, with sympathetic stimulation developing slightly later.[8]

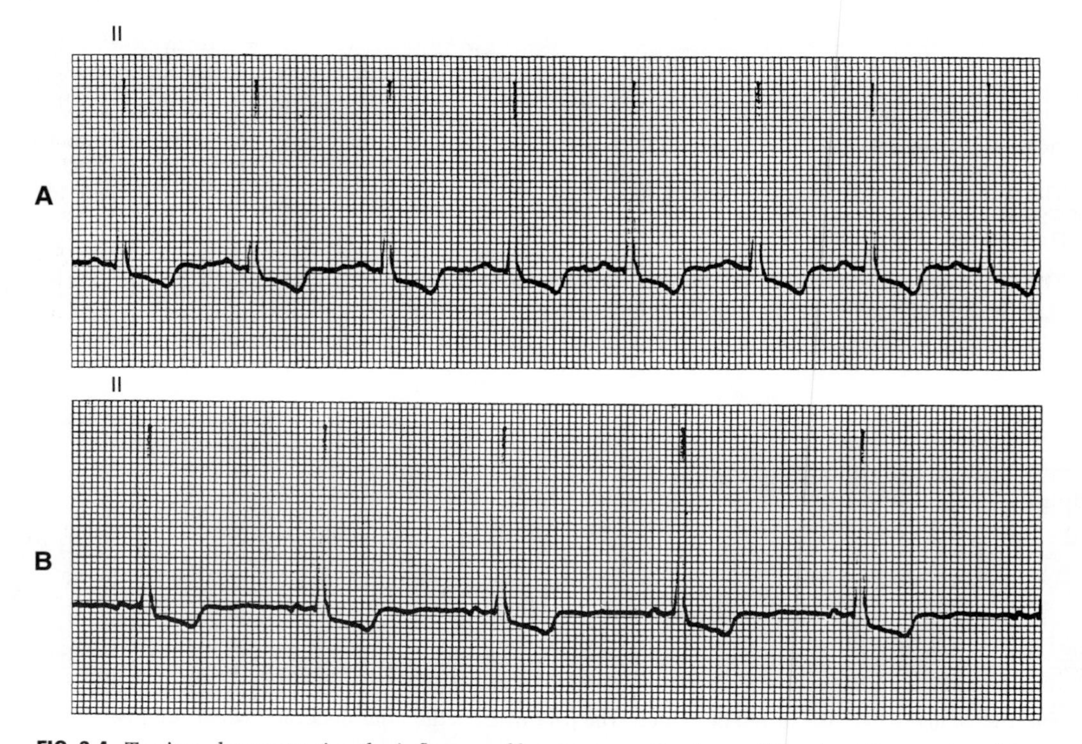

FIG. 6-4. Tracings demonstrating the influence of heart rate on the shape of the sinus P wave. **A** and **B** are from the same patient.

Causes

The physiologic causes of sinus tachycardia include fever, inflammation, congestive heart failure, cardiogenic shock, acute pulmonary embolism, acute myocardial infarction and its extension, sympathetic stimulation, atropine, thyrotoxicosis, alcohol, nicotine, and caffeine.

Clinical Implications

In the setting of mitral stenosis or severe ischemia, sinus tachycardia may precipitate other arrhythmias. Inappropriate sinus tachycardia may be related to a primary sinus node abnormality.[9]

Pediatrics

In an infant sinus tachycardia is a rate greater than 200 beats/min; in a child it is between 140 and 200 beats/min.

Bedside Diagnosis

- Regular pulse
- Normal neck vein pulsation
- Constant systolic blood pressure
- Constant intensity of the first heart sound

Differential Diagnosis

- Paroxysmal supraventricular tachycardia (PSVT)

In sinus tachycardia the heart rate gradually accelerates and gradually decelerates; in PSVT the rapid rate begins and ends abruptly between one beat and the next.

Response to carotid sinus massage. The sinus rate gradually and temporarily slows in response to vagal maneuvers, whereas PSVT abruptly terminates.

These two effects are caused by a slowing of the sinus rate in the case of sinus tachycardia and block of AV conduction in the case of PSVT.

Treatment

Sinus tachycardia itself is not treated. If the tachycardia is inappropriate or if the patient is symptomatic, the cause is identified and treated (e.g., hypovolemia or fever). In certain cases relief may be found in eliminating obvious causes such as tobacco, alcohol, or caffeine. An unsuspected cause may be the sympathomimetic agents in nose drops.

INAPPROPRIATE SINUS TACHYCARDIA

Inappropriate sinus tachycardia is a form of focal atrial tachycardia originating along the superior aspect of the crista terminalis in the "sinus node region" at rates above physiologic range, without relation to metabolic or physiologic demands.[10] It is characterized by an increased resting heart rate accompanied by an exaggerated response to exercise or stress[11]; it is chronic and nonparoxysmal. Most patients are female (90%).[12]

ECG Recognition

Heart rate: More than 100 beats/min at rest or with minimal exertion; the individual is symptomatic.

P waves: Positive in leads I, II, and aVF (identical to sinus rhythm).

PR, QRS, and QT intervals: Normal unless associated with conduction or repolarization abnormalities.

Mechanism

The mechanism of inappropriate sinus tachycardia is not known. Theories include autonomic dysfunction, abnormal SA nodal automaticity, and atrial focus near the node.[11] The discharge site of the tachycardia moves down the crista terminalis with changing autonomic tone.[10]

Symptoms

Symptoms include palpitations, presyncope, and exercise intolerance disproportionate with the degree of tachycardia. Symptoms may be severe, debilitating, and incessant.

Differential Diagnosis

The diagnosis is made after excluding physiologic sinus tachycardia, right atrial tachycardia, or sinus node reentry.

SINUS BRADYCARDIA

Sinus bradycardia is the slow beating of the sinus node at rates of less than 60 beats/min. However, clinicians would not be alarmed at a heart rate of less than this in a patient with hemodynamic stability. The sinus rate in Fig. 6-5, *A*, is 35 beats/min in an active healthy 53-year-old male athlete. Although not seen in this short tracing, he also had sinus arrhythmia, often associated with sinus bradycardia, especially in athletes. Fig. 6-5, *B*, is from the same athlete after a strenuous swim. His heart rate is 60 beats/min.

ECG Recognition

Heart rate: The heart rate is less than 60 beats/min in the adult, although a resting heart rate in the range of 35 to 50 beats/min in an athletic person is not abnormal.

Rhythm: Regular unless associated with sinus arrhythmia.

P waves: P waves are usually identical in shape to the P waves of normal sinus rhythm, or there may be a slight change in morphologic features.

PR interval: Normal.

QRS complex: The QRS complex during sinus bradycardia is identical in shape to the QRS at normal rates.

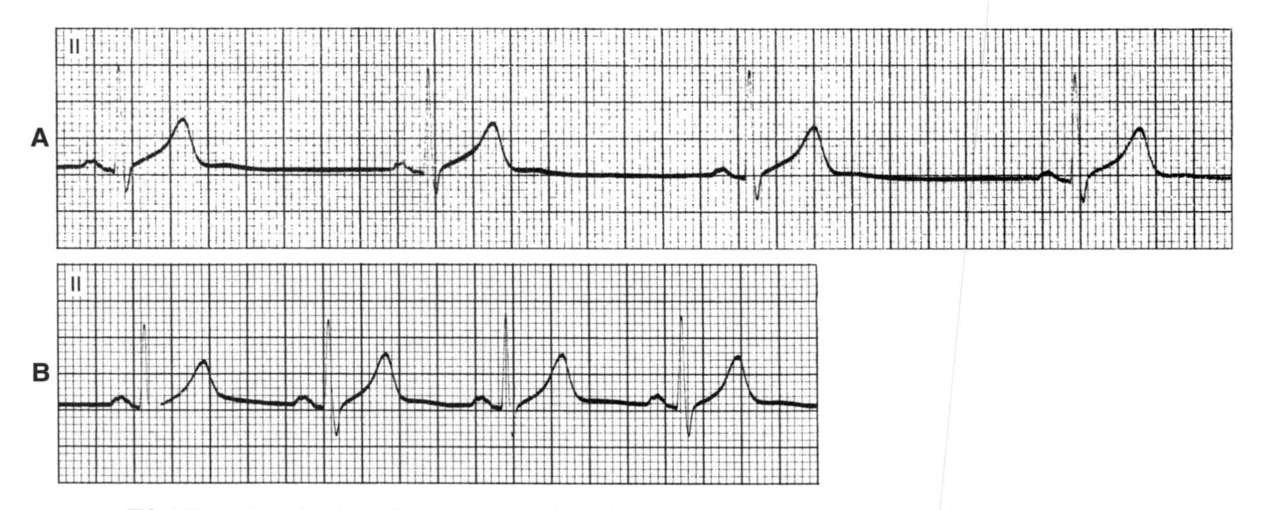

FIG. 6-5. A, Sinus bradycardia (35 beats/min) in a healthy 53-year-old male athlete, who was active but not exercising at the time of the tracing. The pacemaker is the sinus node. AV and intraventricular conduction are normal (normal PR; normal QRS). **B**, Normal sinus rhythm of 60 beats/min in the same individual, but this time after strenuous exercise trying to keep pace with a 27-year-old Olympic swimmer. (Tracings courtesy Coach Joel Wilson, Santa Cruz Masters Swimming, Santa Cruz, Calif.)

QT interval: The QT interval lengthens with bradycardia.

Distinguishing features: (1) The heart rate and the uniform shape of the P waves. (2) May coexist with sinus arrhythmia. (3) A rate of less than 60 beats/min is quickly recognized because of more than five large squares between R waves.

Mechanism

Sinus bradycardia may be caused by excessive vagal tone, decreased sympathetic tone, physiologic conditioning (athletes), anatomic changes (idiopathic degeneration of the SA node in the elderly), or increased intracranial pressure.

In most people vagal activity exerts a strong influence on the circadian variation in sinus rate that occurs during the normal sleep-wake cycle. Vagal activity also establishes a set point for mean sinus rate during inactivity. During sleep, enhanced vagal activity can result in sinus rates of less than 40 beats/min. In fact, one of the ways sinus nodal disease is recognized is by the reduction of such circadian variation. Transient sinus bradycardia occurs with the Valsalva maneuver, carotid sinus massage, or vomiting.

Causes

Among the causes of sinus bradycardia are sleep, an athletic heart, increased vagal tone, decreased sympathetic tone, meningitis, increased intracranial pressure, cervical or mediastinal tumor, hypoxia, myxedema, hypothermia, fibrodegenerative changes, gram-negative sepsis, mental depression, eye surgery, coronary arteriography, vomiting and vasovagal syncope, hyperkalemia, hypothyroidism, Cheyne-Stokes respiration (during the apneic phase), and organic heart disease.

Commonly used drugs causing sinus bradycardia include the following:

- Beta blockers
- Some calcium channel blockers (e.g., verapamil, diltiazem)
- Clonidine (Catapres)
- Digitalis
- Class IA antiarrhythmic drugs

Clinical Implications

Sinus bradycardia is a relatively benign condition; the rate in healthy individual who are not athletes is usually higher than 40 to 50 beats/min, but may be as low as 35 beats/min during sleep. Absence during sleep suggests sinus nodal disease. Syncope is considered an indication of severity, and is defined as a transient loss of consciousness with inability to maintain postural tone.[13]

Sinus bradycardia in myocardial infarction. In acute myocardial infarction, especially of the inferior wall, sinus bradycardia is common (25% to 40%)[14] and may be beneficial by producing a longer diastole and increased ventricular filling time. Sinus bradycardia without hypotension is associated with an equal or lower mortality rate than if the heart rate had been faster,[15] although ventricular ectopy may be more frequent during the bradycardia that occurs in the very early phase of myocardial infarction. When the sinus bradycardia is profound and associated with hypotension in the setting of acute myocardial infarction, the prognosis is poor, especially if the deteriorating hemodynamic situation is not corrected rapidly. Sinus bradycardia may occur during reperfusion with thrombolytic agents. If it occurs after resuscitation from cardiac arrest, it is associated with a poor prognosis.[16]

Pediatrics

Sinus bradycardia is rare in normal, healthy children. It may be seen in hypothyroidism, hypothermia, hypopituitarism, obstructive jaundice, and typhoid fever. Transient sinus bradycardia may be seen in normal premature infants. Reflex sinus bradycardia occurs because of increased intracranial pressure or increased systemic blood pressure and, occasionally, during cardiac catheterization.

Neonates can tolerate ventricular rates of 55 beats/min or greater if the heart is normal and 65 beats/min when associated with congenital heart disease. In addition, in the neonatal period rates are similar, asleep or awake.[17]

Bedside Diagnosis

Response to vagal block. Vagal block, such as with atropine, causes the normal sinus node to increase its rate, usually by more than 50% above baseline but not in excess of 120 beats/min. In fact, one of the signs of intrinsic sinus nodal dysfunction is that the heart rate does not exceed 90 beats/min after vagal block with 2 to 4 mg/kg of intravenous atropine.[17]

Treatment

Sinus bradycardia is not treated unless the patient is symptomatic; then atropine 0.04 mg/kg body weight is given. A temporary pacemaker may be indicated if the heart rate does not accelerate. A permanent pacemaker may be needed for patients with congestive heart failure or patients in whom the arrhythmia is chronic and associated with low cardiac output, or when the bradycardia is associated with sinus node dysfunction. This is because heart rate cannot be reliably and safely increased with drugs on a long-term basis.[18]

SINUS ARRHYTHMIA

Sinus arrhythmia is the variation in heart rate by more than 0.16 second. Respiratory sinus arrhythmia is the more common type, in which the heart rate is synchronized with breathing, slowing with expiration and accelerating with inspiration. In Fig. 6-6 the effect of respirations on the normal sinus rhythm in two 4-year-old children is shown.

ECG Recognition

Heart rate: More likely seen when the heart rate is slow and tends to become regular with faster rates or atropine. In the classic form of sinus arrhythmia the heart rate slows with expiration and accelerates with inspiration. The slow phase may be less than 60 beats/min in the adult and much less in athletes.

Rhythm: Irregular because of acceleration and deceleration of the heart rate.

P waves: Normal sinus P waves.

PP interval: Sinus arrhythmia is present when the difference between the shortest PP interval and the longest PP interval is greater than 0.16 second. Respiratory sinus arrhythmia is quite pronounced in children (Fig. 6-6). In 6-6, *A*, the difference between the longest and shortest PP interval is 0.26 second. The rate, taken over a full minute, is normal at approximately 75 beats/min.

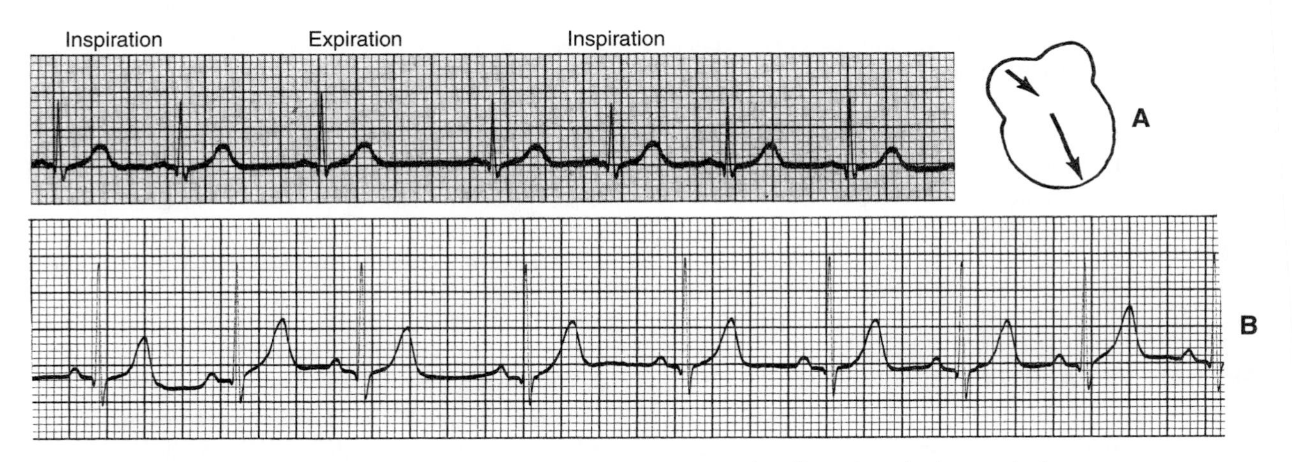

FIG. 6-6. Sinus arrhythmia in two 4-year-olds (**A** and **B**); note the effect of respiration on the heart rate.

PR interval: The PR interval may change slightly as the heart rate changes.

QRS complex: The QRS complex is not affected by the sinus arrhythmia.

QT interval: The QT interval changes with heart rate, becoming longer during the slow phase of this rhythm.

Distinguishing features: (1)The heart rate varies by more than 0.16 second, the rate increasing with inspiration and slowing with expiration. (2) P waves, PR interval, and QRS are normal.

Mechanism

The probable mechanism for respiratory sinus arrhythmia is a change in vagal tone arising from pulmonary and systemic reflex vascular mechanisms during respirations. Direct recordings from the sinus node have shown that sinus arrhythmia is associated not only with changes in sinus cycle length but also with changes in SA conduction time.[17]

Causes

Youth and athleticism are the main causes of respiratory sinus arrhythmia in the normal heart. Other causes are aging, postprandial hypotension, diabetes, and alcoholic cardiomyopathy.

Clinical Implications

Respiratory sinus arrhythmia is most pronounced in the young and becomes less and less marked as a child becomes older; it is a normal occurrence.

Nonrespiratory sinus arrhythmia is more often caused by cardiac disease or aging. It is common after acute inferior myocardial infarction and when there is an increase in intracranial pressure.

Symptoms

Symptoms are uncommon. However, excessively long pauses may result in dizziness or in some cases syncope, if not accompanied by an escape rhythm.

Pediatrics

Sinus arrhythmia is rare in the young infant but common in children and adolescents.

Treatment

Sinus arrhythmia is not treated unless the bradycardia phase of the arrhythmia is marked, causing symptoms.

HEART RATE VARIABILITY

Heart rate variability (HRV) refers to the different durations of individual normal cardiac cycles and is a tool for assessing cardiac autonomic status.

ECG Recognition

The evaluation of HRV is accomplished by extensive use of statistical methods, including time domain, frequency domain, and nonlinear analysis that classify the variations of normal-to-normal cardiac cycles.

Mechanism

In the healthy heart the sinus rhythm is not absolutely regular. Factors that cause heart rate variability include normal physical activity,[19] exercise, mental stress, respiration, blood pressure regulation, thermoregulation, actions of the renin-angiotensin system, some medications, and circadian rhythms. The effect of respirations on sinus rhythm is known to be an autonomic mechanism—a balance between sympathetic and parasympathetic tone. Normally during sleep parasympathetic activity predominates, although in patients with anterior myocardial infarcts this may be suppressed by the relatively high sympathetic activity.[20]

Clinical Implications

Thus far the analysis of HRV has been useful in risk stratification after acute myocardial infarction and in the early diagnosis of diabetic neuropathy.

Postinfarction risk. Decreased 24-hour HRV is a powerful risk predictor of postinfarction mortality.

Diabetic neuropathy. Clinical manifestation of diabetic neuropathy indicates a 5-year mortality rate of approximately 50%. This condition is a complication of diabetes mellitus in which there is widespread neuronal degeneration of small nerve fibers of the autonomic nervous system. Assessment of HRV helps to detect early subclinical autonomic dysfunction.[21]

Treatment

HRV is prognostic and elicits appropriate interventions.

TWO TYPES OF SA BLOCK

SA block is the failure of a sinus impulse to exit from the sinus node and activate the atria. There are two types of SA block: type I (SA Wenckebach) and type II. Both types are recognized because of dropped P waves. They are differentiated because type I SA block has the signs of Wenckebach and type II SA block has fixed PP intervals with the pause being an exact multiple. The two types of SA block are discussed separately.

Pediatrics

Second-degree SA block may be seen in infants (especially newborns) and children without heart disease. In adolescents it is usually caused by increased vagal tone.

Clinical Implications

SA block is usually a transient condition. Asymptomatic pauses of more than 2 seconds have been noted in ambulatory patients, trained athletes, and healthy young people and do not necessarily carry a poor prognosis. Transient SA block may be caused by digitalis toxicity and some antiarrhythmic agents. It is seen in patients with acute myocardial infarction and acute myocarditis.

SA Wenckebach, when associated with other arrhythmias, may be part of SSS.

SA WENCKEBACH (TYPE I SA BLOCK)

SA Wenckebach is the progressive lengthening of SA conduction until P wave conduction fails for one beat and the sequence begins again. This results in group beating, shortening PP intervals, and pauses that are less than twice the shortest cycle (Dr. Marriott's "footsteps of Wenckebach"). In the case of SA Wenckebach visualize conduction between the sinus node and the atrial fibers surrounding it. The sinus discharge is not seen on the surface electrocardiogram (ECG); it is the atrial activation that produces the P wave. It is possible for the sinus node to discharge and not produce a P wave. SA Wenckebach is diagnosed because of its "footsteps." Fig. 6-7 shows two instances of SA Wenckebach, one with a 4:3 conduction ratio and the other with a 3:2 conduction ratio. In Fig. 6-7, *A*, there are four discharges from the sinus node with three of them being conducted to produce three P waves in each group; in Fig. 6-7, *B*, there are three sinus node impulses with two being conducted, hence two P waves in each group. The best way to illustrate this mechanism is with a laddergram. There are four tiers in this particular laddergram. The top tier accommodates sinus node impulses and SA conduction; note that SA conduction time lengthens until one sinus impulse is not conducted.

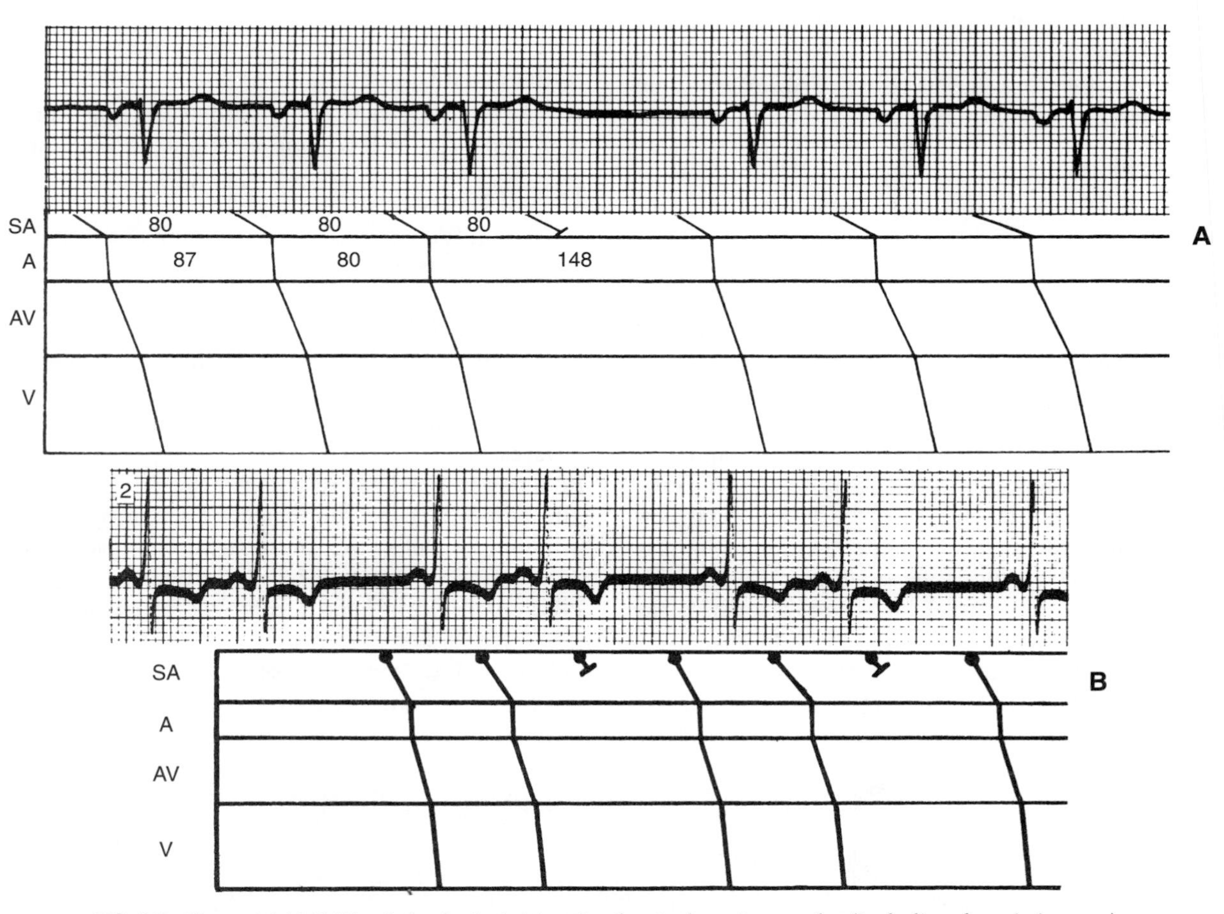

FIG. 6-7. Sinoatrial (*SA*) Wenckebach. **A,** A 4:3 ratio; that is, four sinus cycles (including the missing one) for three P waves. **B,** A 3:2 ratio (i.e., three sinus cycles for two P waves). *A*, Atrial; *AV*, atrioventricular; *V*, ventricular.

ECG Recognition

Heart rate: There may be bradycardia because of the pauses.
Rhythm: Group beating (usually groups of two or three).
P waves: Normal sinus P waves.
PP interval: Shortens until there is a pause, and then the sequence begins again (shortening PP intervals and a pause).
The pause: Less than twice the shortest cycle. Although a P wave is missing, the pause will not be twice the shortest cycle because SA conduction is lengthening with every sinus beat, placing the P waves later in the cycle than they would normally appear. However, SA conduction time for the P wave following the pause is at its shortest, causing this P wave to be earlier than the others.
PR interval: Normal and fixed unless there is an associated AV conduction problem.
QRS complex: Normal unless associated with an intraventricular conduction problem.
Distinguishing features: The diagnosis of SA Wenckebach is made because of normal P waves, group beating, shortening PP intervals (except when there are only two P waves in the group), and pauses that are less than twice the shortest cycle.

Mechanism

The Wenckebach conduction phenomenon (lengthening conduction time until there is a nonconducted beat) can be found anywhere there are slow-response action potentials, normally in the two nodes and abnormally in ischemic tissue anywhere in the heart. Thus the mechanism of SA Wenckebach is easily explained because of the type of tissue involved. Sinus nodal cells are quite similar to AV nodal cells; both have slow-response action potentials, slow conduction, and similar conduction problems. Although the sinus node is capable of beating very rapidly, the conduction of an impulse through this tissue is at least as slow as conduction through the AV node. SA exit block may result from drugs (e.g., quinidine, procainamide, digitalis), acute myocarditis, myocardial infarction, fibrosis of the atrium, or excessive vagal stimulation.[18]

In SA Wenckebach there is not the tell-tale lengthening of the PR interval seen in AV Wenckebach (see Chapter 16). The firing of the sinus node and the conduction time from that focus to the atrial tissue are concealed (not seen on the ECG). Therefore the problem is diagnosed by the tracks that it leaves on the ECG (its "footsteps").

Causes

Causes of SA Wenckebach are drugs such as digitalis, quinidine, and procainamide; acute myocarditis; myocardial infarction; fibrosis of the atrium; and excessive vagal stimulation.

Clinical Implications

SA Wenckebach is usually transient in trained athletes and healthy young people. When it is associated with other arrhythmias it may be part of SSS.

Pediatrics

SA Wenckebach is seen in infants and children without heart disease. In adolescents it is usually caused by increased vagal tone.

Treatment

SA Wenckebach is not treated unless the pauses are symptomatic; then it is managed as a sinus bradycardia.

TYPE II SA BLOCK

Type II SA block is the regular firing of the sinus node with periodic failure of conduction.

ECG Recognition

Heart rate: Pauses in the sinus rhythm may cause bradycardia.
Rhythm: Regular before and after the pauses.
P waves: Normal sinus P waves.
PP interval: Fixed before and after the pauses.
The pause: Can be multiplied by an integer (a whole number). Unlike SA Wenckebach, a P wave is dropped without increments in SA conduction.
PR interval: Normal and fixed unless there is an associated AV conduction problem.
QRS complex: Normal unless associated with an intraventricular conduction problem.

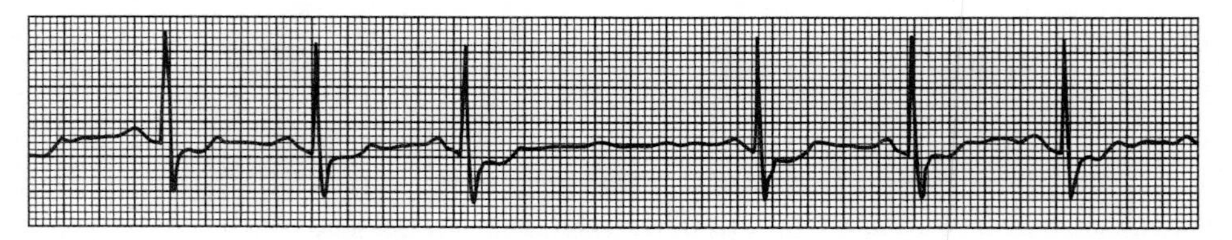

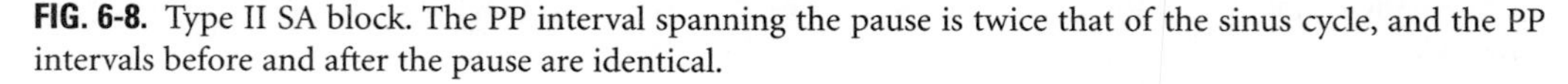

FIG. 6-8. Type II SA block. The PP interval spanning the pause is twice that of the sinus cycle, and the PP intervals before and after the pause are identical.

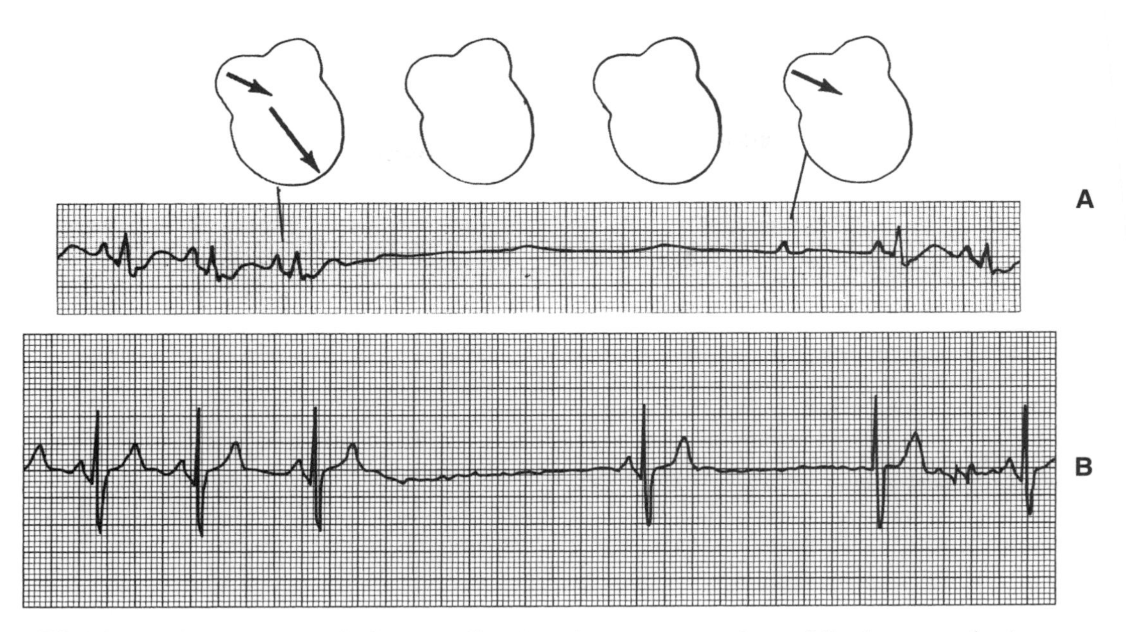

FIG. 6-9. **A** and **B**, Sinus arrest. (**B** from Angeli SJ: Superior vena cava syndrome following pacemaker insertion post atrial septal defect repair, *Am Heart J* 120(2):433, 1990.)

Distinguishing features: The diagnosis of type II SA block is made because of dropped P waves against a background of fixed PP intervals and pauses that are multiples of the uninterrupted sinus rhythm, as seen in Fig. 6-8.

SINUS ARREST OR SINUS PAUSE

Sinus arrest or sinus pause is a failure of impulse formation in the sinus node, an event that is impossible to determine with certainty on the surface ECG. One can, however, be suspicious of this condition if the PP intervals of the basic cycle cannot be "walked out" across the pause, ending on a P wave. Fig. 6-9 shows two examples of sinus arrest. In Fig. 6-9, *A*, during a long sinus pause there is an absence of an appropriate escape junctional beat. When another P wave appears, AV conduction is a problem. The long pause without relief from the junction is a manifestation of SSS. In Fig. 6-9, *B*, the second pause is interrupted by a junctional escape beat and all P waves are conducted. Fig. 6-10 shows SA block or sinus arrest compounded by other problems (SSS). The main dramatic concern for this patient was the long pauses unrelieved by a junctional escape beat. The pauses were due not only to the SA block, but also to AV Wenckebach and nonconducted premature atrial complexes, profound overdrive suppression, and failure of a junctional escape mechanism . . . a sick sinus

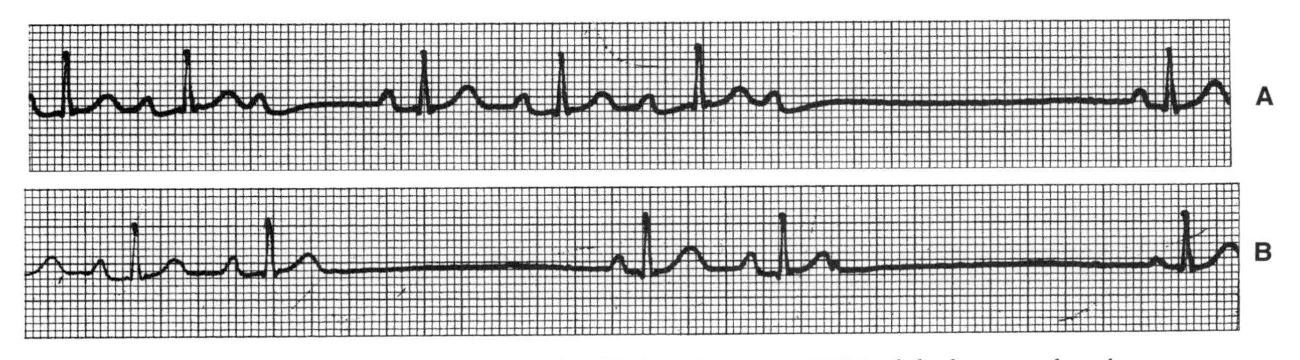

FIG. 6-10. Sick sinus syndrome consisting of SA block or sinus arrest, AV Wenckebach, nonconducted premature atrial complex, and profound overdrive suppression. The sinus arrest is seen in the long pauses. **A**, There are shortening PP intervals in the center, indicating incremental SA conduction time. The nonconducted premature atrial complex (distorting the T wave) initiates the last pause in **B**.

node. Note in Fig. 6-10, *A*, the small increments in PR intervals until there is a dropped beat (AV Wenckebach); in Fig. 6-10, *B*, a nonconducted premature atrial beat is seen just before the last pause.

ECG Recognition

Heart rate: May be marked bradycardia because of long pauses.

Rhythm: Regular with pauses that have no numeric relationship to the basic cycle length.

P waves: There may be normal sinus P waves along with atrial escape beats.

PP interval: May be fixed before and after the pauses.

The pause: Not a multiple of a whole number. That is, the basic PP interval cannot be "walked out" across the pause and end on a P wave.

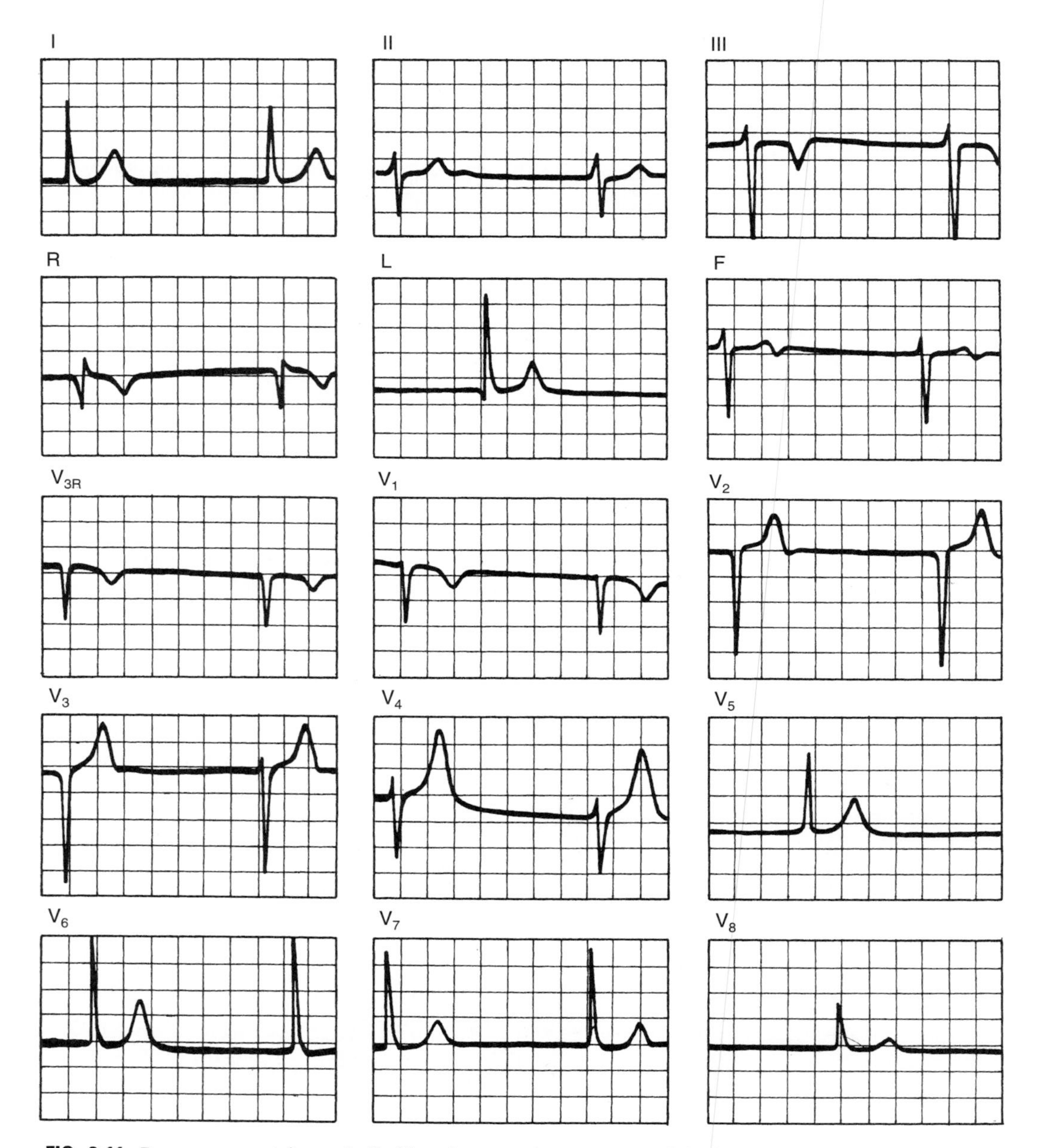

FIG. 6-11. Permanent atrial standstill. The absence of P waves in all leads is evident, including a right precordial lead (V_{3R}) and extreme left precordial leads V_7 and V_8. (Courtesy Dr. James Wolliscroft, Ann Arbor, Mich.)

PR interval: Normal and fixed unless there is an associated AV conduction problem.

QRS complex: Normal unless associated with an intraventricular conduction problem.

Distinguishing features: The diagnosis of sinus arrest is made because of a pause (or pauses) in a sinus rhythm that is not a multiple of a whole number.

Treatment

SA block is not treated unless the pauses are symptomatic and complicated by other arrhythmias (SSS); then, a pacemaker may be indicated.

PERMANENT ATRIAL STANDSTILL

Permanent atrial standstill is the inability of the atria to respond to stimuli. It is an infrequently recognized arrhythmia and has been diagnosed in three clinical settings: long-standing progressive cardiac disease, neuromuscular disease, and patients with vertigo or syncope. Not only were P waves absent in all leads of the surface ECG (Fig. 6-11) and in the atrial electrogram (not shown), but also the A waves were absent in the jugular venous pulse and right atrial pressure tracings (not shown).

ECG Recognition

P waves: Absent in all leads, including right precordial leads and extreme left precordial leads.

QRS complex: Junctional or ventricular escape beats.

Distinguishing features: The diagnosis of permanent atrial standstill is made because the ECG and atrial electrogram have absent P waves, and pressure tracings from the jugular venous pulse and right atrium have absent A waves.

Mechanism

The atria are immobile on fluoroscopy and cannot be stimulated electrically, so it is possible that the sinus node may actually be firing but the atria are incapable of responding.

SINUS NODE REENTRY TACHYCARDIA

Sinus node reentry or SA nodal reentry tachycardia is a proposed uncommon cause of PSVT sustained by a reentry circuit through or in the vicinity of the sinus node. It is recognized because of its paroxysmal nature, the shape of the P waves (sinus), and its termination with use of vagal maneuvers, adenosine, or a premature beat (Fig. 6-12). It should be noted that a reentry circuit limited to the sinus node has never been demonstrated and is questionable.[10,22]

ECG Recognition

Precise identification of reentrant sinus tachycardia is elusive.

Heart rate: 100 to 160 beats/min (average, 130 beats/min).

Rhythm: PSVT.

P waves: The P waves of the paroxysmal tachycardia are in front of the QRS complex and identical or similar in shape to the normal sinus beats.

PR interval: Normal and fixed; during the paroxysm of tachycardia the PR shortens slightly along with the cycle length.

QRS complex: Normal unless associated with an intraventricular conduction problem.

AV conduction: AV block may be present, especially AV Wenckebach; the PSVT is not affected.

Distinguishing features: Paroxysmal narrow QRS tachycardia in which the P waves immediately precede the QRS, are upright in lead II, and are the same shape as the normal sinus beats. Vagal maneuvers usually slow or terminate the tachycardia.

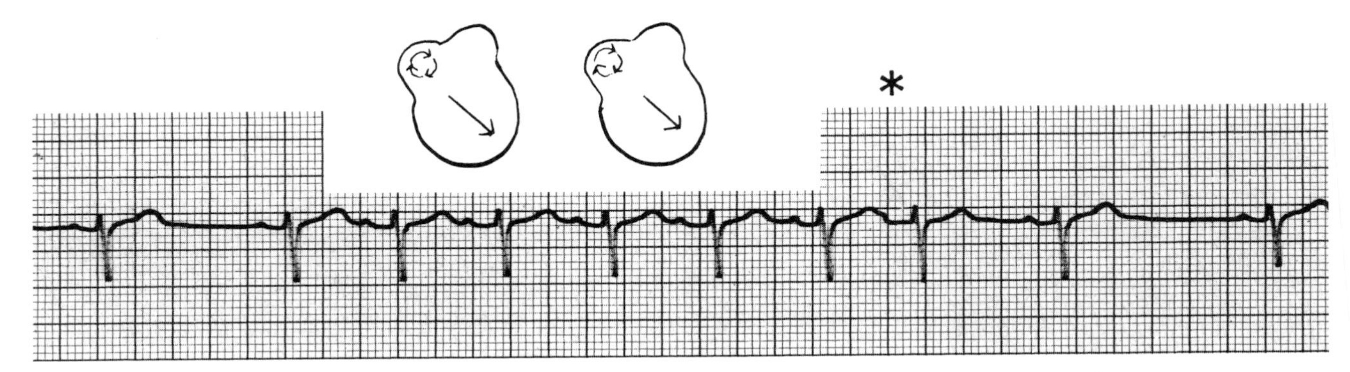

FIG. 6-12. Paroxysmal supraventricular tachycardia presumably resulting from SA or sinus node reentry. The tachycardia is terminated by a single premature atrial complex (in the T wave with the *asterisk*).

Mechanism

The reentry circuit supporting this arrhythmia is not known. It may be isolated to the sinus node itself (sinus node reentry), it may involve perinodal fibers (SA nodal reentry), or it may circulate around a portion of the crista terminalis.

Clinical Implications

Reentry in the region of the SA node usually occurs in patients with organic heart disease.[23]

Pediatrics

SA nodal reentry tachycardia has been reported in infants, particularly after surgery for congenital heart disease. Although it is a relatively slow tachycardia, it can cause hemodynamic compromise. It is managed acutely with adenosine.[24]

Differential Diagnosis

SA or sinus node reentry tachycardia may easily be mistaken for sinus tachycardia because it is hemodynamically tolerated and has a heart rate similar to that of sinus tachycardia and because the P waves are the same shape as normal sinus P waves. It differs from sinus tachycardia in that it may be abruptly terminated with a vagal maneuver, whereas sinus tachycardia slows gradually. SA or sinus node reentry may also be mistaken for a marked sinus arrhythmia; however, SA or sinus node reentry tachycardia does not fluctuate with respirations.

Treatment

SA nodal reentry tachycardia may be terminated by a vagal maneuver or adenosine. The diagnosis is made during electrophysiologic study as is radiofrequency ablation of a critical part of the reentry pathway.

SINUS NODE DYSFUNCTION

Sick sinus syndrome (SSS) includes disorders of impulse generation and conduction, failure of escape pacemakers, and a susceptibility to paroxysmal or chronic atrial tachyarrhythmias. When bradycardia is associated with recurrent episodes of supraventricular tachycardia, including atrial fibrillation, it is called *bradycardia-tachycardia syndrome* and has important therapeutic implications.

ECG Recognition

Rate: Too fast, too slow, or alternating.

Rhythm: Irregular.

P waves: Sinus, atrial, or absent (atrial fibrillation).

Distinguishing features: In SSS any of the following may be present or alternate with each other, and are associated with syncope:

1. Isolated marked sinus bradycardia in the absence of significant vagal tone
2. Inappropriate sinus node response to exercise or stress
3. Sudden prolonged sinus pauses, especially after premature atrial beats of following a bout of atrial tachycardia
4. Chronic atrial tachyarrhythmias, especially atrial fibrillation associated with a slow ventricular response (unrelated to drugs)
5. Bradycardia that alternates with tachycardia, usually paroxysmal atrial fibrillation or flutter (bradycardia-tachycardia syndrome; Fig. 6-13)
6. Persistent profound sinus bradycardia and episodic sinus pauses that are due to sinus arrest or SA block and are frequently accompanied by episodic atrial fibrillation, atrial flutter, and atrial tachycardia

The bradycardia-tachycardia syndrome often precedes the development of chronic atrial fibrillation and is a common manifestation of SSS. The tachycardia phase is often paroxysmal atrial fibrillation or flutter but may be atrial ectopic or junctional. Often in the transition between the tachycardia and the bradycardia there are long pauses caused by overdrive suppression of the sinus node or the escape atrial pacemaker.

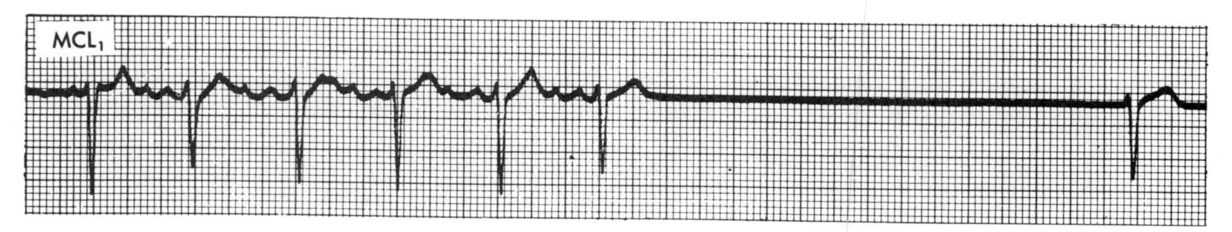

FIG. 6-13. Sick sinus syndrome caused by bradycardia-tachycardia. (From Marriott HJL, Conover M: *Advanced concepts in arrhythmias*, St Louis, 1983, Mosby.)

Causes

Disease of SA nodal fibers may cause dysfunction of impulse formation, propagation, or recovery from overdrive suppression. Disease of the atria may affect the sinus node in addition to generating atrial tachyarrhythmias. In adult patients, about 40% with SSS have coronary atherosclerosis. Approximately 5% to 10% have idiopathic cardiomyopathy. It is, however, not certain if the SSS is caused by the cardiac disease. SSS is frequently intermittent and unpredictable and may occur in the absence of other cardiac disease. The sinus node itself may be partially or totally destroyed. There may be discontinuity between the SA node and atrial tissue; the nervous system surrounding the SA node or the atrial wall may be altered because of inflammatory or degenerative processes.[18]

Drugs most often implicated as an extracardiac factor include cardiac glycosides, sympatholytic antihypertensive agents, beta blockers, calcium channel blockers, and membrane-active antiarrhythmic agents. Marked hypervagotonia, sometimes combined with certain drugs, may be implicated in some cases of SSS.

Symptoms

The major complaint of individuals with SSS is usually fatigue or lightheadedness and dyspnea on exertion, although they may be asymptomatic or symptomatic only with exertion.

Syncope and presyncope usually occur after termination of atrial fibrillation or other tachyarrhythmias. Fatigue is usually caused by insufficient cardiac output when physical demands are increased.

Pediatrics

SSS is seen in children during the postoperative period, usually after extensive intra-atrial surgery (especially surgery for transposition of the great vessels). The rhythms seen are profound sinus bradycardia, periods of sinus arrest, atrial or junctional rhythms, atrial flutter, and rarely atrial fibrillation. The focus may switch from one to another, especially during the immediate postoperative period.

Treatment

Treatment is determined by the patient's symptoms and ECG findings. Important therapeutic considerations include the following[25,26]:

1. Thromboembolism (anticoagulation and preservation of organized atrial activation)
2. Symptoms of exertional intolerance (chronotropic support when indicated)
3. Survival (enhanced by physiologic pacing therapy along with appropriate pharmacologic interventions)

When symptoms of dizziness and syncope are related to bradyarrhythmia in patients with SSS, permanent cardiac pacemaker therapy is usually indicated. In some patients theophylline may suppress sinus pauses, sinus bradycardia, and associated symptoms.[27]

HYPERSENSITIVE CAROTID SINUS SYNDROME

Carotid sinus hypersensitivity is ventricular asystole of more than 3 seconds during even mild carotid sinus stimulation.

ECG Characteristics

A sinus pause of more than 3 seconds coupled with failure of junctional or ventricular escape beats.

Mechanism

Hypersensitive carotid sinus syndrome is a circulatory vagal reflex. Atherosclerosis of the carotid sinus region of the carotid artery causes excessive sensitivity of the baroreceptors located in the arterial wall of the carotid sinus. In cases of hypersensitivity, even mild pressure on the carotid sinus causes a strong baroreceptor reflex, releasing acetylcholine, which inhibits sinus node automaticity and AV conduction. The reflex may be powerful enough to stop the heart for 5 to 10 seconds.[28]

Causes

- Atherosclerotic process in the carotid sinus region of the carotid artery

SUMMARY

The arrhythmias originating in the sinus node that are physiologic are sinus tachycardia (a response to exercise, emotions, fever, among others), sinus bradycardia (common in athletes and during sleep), and sinus arrhythmia (associated with the vagal effect of respirations). When these arrhythmias are symptomatic or inappropriate, they are abnormal. Sinus nodal disease may manifest itself as SA block, sinus arrest, or SSS.

REFERENCES

1. Olgin JE: Sinus tachycardia and sinus node reentry. In Zipes DP, Jalife J, editors: *Cardiac electrophysiology from cell to bedside*, ed 3, Philadelphia, 2000, WB Saunders, pp 459-468.
2. Yang XS, Beck GJ, Wilkoff BL: Redefining normal sinus heart rate, *J Am Coll Cardiol* 749-1:193A, 1995.
3. Schuessler RB, Boineau JP, Saffitz JE et al: Cellular mechanisms of sinoatrial activity. In Zipes DP, Jalife J, editors: *Cardiac elec-*

trophysiology from cell to bedside, ed 3, Philadelphia, 2000, WB Saunders, p 193.

4. Weisfeldt ML, Lakatta EG, Gerstenblith G: Aging and the heart. In Braunwald E, editor: *Heart disease*, ed 4, Philadelphia, 1992, WB Saunders.
5. Boineau JP, Schuessler RB, Roeske WR et al: The quantitative relation between sites of atrial impulse origin and cycle length, *Am J Physiol* 245:H781, 1983.
6. Gomes JA, Winters SL: The origins of the sinus node pacemaker complex in man: demonstration of dominant and subsidiary foci, *J Am Coll Cardiol* 9:45, 1987.
7. Schuessler RB, Boineau JP, Saffitz JE et al: Cellular mechanisms of sinoatrial activity. In Zipes DP, Jalife J, editors: *Cardiac electrophysiology from cell to bedside*, ed 3, Philadelphia, 2000, WB Saunders, pp 187-195.
8. Braunwald E, Sonnenblick EH, Ross J: Mechanisms of cardiac contraction and relaxation. In Braunwald E, editor: *Heart disease*, ed 4, Philadelphia, 1992, WB Saunders.
9. Morillo CA, Klein GJ, Thakur RK et al: Mechanism of "inappropriate" sinus tachycardia; role of sympathovagal balance, *Circulation* 90:873, 1994.
10. Saoudi N, Cosio F, Waldo A et al: Classification of atrial flutter and regular atrial tachycardia according to electrophysiologic mechanism and anatomic bases: a statement from a joint expert group from the Working Group of Arrhythmias of the European Society of Cardiology and the North American Society of Pacing and Electrophysiology, *J Cardiovasc Electrophysiol* 12:852, 2001.
11. Ren JF, Marchlinski FE, Callans DJ, Zado ES: Echocardiographic lesion characteristics associated with successful ablation of inappropriate sinus tachycardia. *J Cardiovasc Electrophysiol* 12:814, 2001.
12. Tielman RG, De Langen CDJ, Van Gelder JC et al: Verapamil reduces tachycardia-induced electrical remodeling of the atria. *Circulation* 95:1945, 1997.
13. Alboni P, Menozzi C, Brignole M et al: An abnormal neural reflex plays a role in causing syncope in sinus bradycardia, *J Am Coll Cardiol* 22:1130, 1993.
14. Pasternak RC, Braunwald E, Sobel BE: Acute myocardial infarction. In Braunwald E, editor: *Heart disease*, ed 4, Philadelphia, 1992, WB Saunders.
15. Corr P, Gillis R: Autonomic neural influences on the dysrhythmias resulting from myocardial infarction, *Circ Res* 43:1, 1978.
16. Juma Z, Castellanos A, Myerburg RJ: Prognostic significance of the electrocardiogram in patients with coronary heart disease. In Wellens HJJ, Kulbertus HE, editors: *What's new in electrocardiography?* The Hague, 1981, Martinus Nijhoff.
17. Reiffel JA: Clinical electrophysiology of the sinus node in man. In Mazgalev T, Dreifus LS, Michelson EL, editors: *Electrophysiology of the sinoatrial and atrioventricular nodes*, New York, 1988, Alan R Liss.
18. Zipes DP: Specific arrhythmias: diagnosis and treatment. In Braunwald E, editor: *Heart disease*, ed 4, Philadelphia 1992, WB Saunders.
19. Ito H, Nozaki M, Maruyama T et al: Shift work modifies the circadian patterns of heart rate variability in nurses. *Int J Cardiol* 79:231, 2001.
20. Stein PK, Bosner MS, Kleiger RE, Conger BM: Heart rate variability: a measure of cardiac autonomic tone, *Am Heart J* 127:1376, 1994.
21. Malik M: Heart rate variability. In Zipes DP, Jalife J, editors: *Cardiac electrophysiology from cell to bedside*, ed 3, Philadelphia, 2000, WB Saunders, pp 753-766.
22. Kirchhof CJHJ, Bonke Fi M, Allessie MA: Sinus node reentry: fact or fiction? In Brugada P, Wellens HJJ, editors: *Cardiac arrhythmias. Where to go from here?* Mount Kisco, NY, 1987, Futura Publishing, p 53.
23. Chou TCC, Knilans TK: *Electrocardiography in clinical practice adult and pediatric*, ed 4, Philadelphia, 2000, WB Saunders, p 326.
24. Blaufox AD, Numan M, Knick BJ, Saul JP: Sinoatrial node reentriant tachycardia in infants with congenital heart disease. *Am J Cardiol* 88:1050, 2001.
25. Benditt DG, Sakaguchi S, Goldstein MA et al: Sinus node dysfunction: pathophysiology, clinical features, evaluation, and treatment. In Zipes DP, Jalife J, editors: *Cardiac electrophysiology from cell to bedside*, ed 2, Philadelphia, 1995, WB Saunders.
26. Tchou P, Chung MK: Sick sinus syndrome and hypersensitive carotid sinus syndrome. In Zipes DP, Jalife J, editors: *Cardiac electrophysiology from cell to bedside*, ed 3, Philadelphia, 2000, WB Saunders, pp 862-871.
27. Kastor JA: *Arrhythmias*, ed 2, Philadelphia, 2000, WB Saunders, p 578.
28. Guyton AC, Hall JE: *Textbook of medical physiology*, ed 10, Philadelphia, 2000, WB Saunders, p 13.

CHAPTER 7

Premature Atrial Complexes and Atrial Tachycardia

PREMATURE ATRIAL COMPLEXES

A premature atrial complex (PAC) is an ectopic impulse from an atrial focus outside of the sinus node; it emerges earlier than the next expected sinus beat. An ectopic P′ wave is called a *P′ (P prime) wave*; it is recognized because it has a different shape from that of the sinus P wave unless the ectopic focus is near the sinus node, in which case the shape can be identical or similar to that of the sinus P wave. Fig. 7-1 illustrates the sinus node and the resulting sinus P wave compared with an atrial ectopic focus and the resulting P′.

"Walking Out" the Rhythm

Irregularities, premature beats, and the presence or absence of atrioventricular (AV) dissociation are evaluated by using a caliper or a piece of paper and a sharp

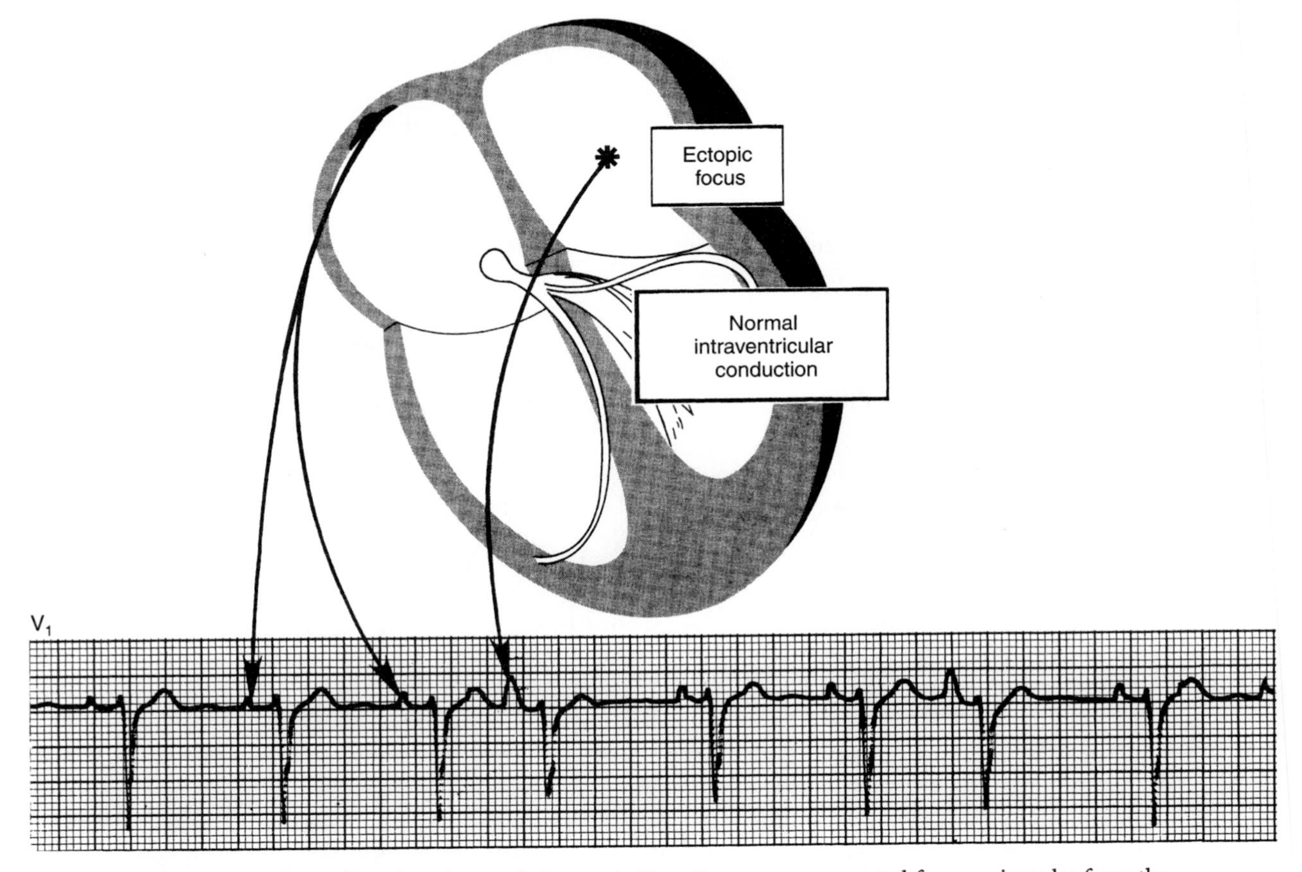

FIG. 7-1. Two PACs (fourth and seventh P waves). Sinus P waves are generated from an impulse from the sinus node and have a uniform shape in a single lead. In addition to being premature, PACs are generated from a focus outside of the sinus node and are shaped differently.

pencil to mark off ("walk out") the P waves or QRS complexes.

Although the two premature atrial complexes in Fig. 7-1 are immediately apparent by simply looking at the tracing (fourth and seventh beats), this tracing can be used for practice. Mark off the first three P waves, and you will find that the PP intervals are identical and that the PAC is easily found. If you continue to walk out the sinus rhythm across the PAC, you will find that the sinus P wave after the PAC falls earlier than expected. This is because of the early discharge and resetting of the sinus node by the PAC. This shortened pause is referred to as a *noncompensatory pause* (i.e., less than a full compensatory pause).

It is important to understand that "walking out" a rhythm is an exercise that is not used in isolation.

Full Compensatory Pause

A *full compensatory* pause is discussed in Chapter 12. Briefly, it occurs when a premature ventricular beat does not disturb the regular sinus rhythm, but the P wave that occurs during or immediately after the premature beat is not conducted, creating a pause. The P waves are all on time when the PP intervals are walked out across the premature beat.

ECG Recognition

Heart rate: That of the underlying sinus rhythm.

Rhythm: Irregular because of the PACs.

P wave shape: The PAC usually has a different shape from that of the sinus P wave: different focus, different shape.

P wave location: Premature; may be hidden in the T wave.

PP interval: Irregular because of the PAC.

P′R interval: May be the same as the PR interval but is usually prolonged because of the prematurity of the P′ wave. The P′ wave may be nonconducted (followed by a pause).

QRS complex: Normal unless there is an intraventricular conduction problem. The PAC may or may not be followed by a QRS.

Distinguishing features: A PAC is diagnosed because of a premature beat with a narrow QRS (a supraventricular complex) preceded by a P′ wave, or because of a pause preceded by a distorted T wave (hidden nonconducted PAC).

AV conduction after a PAC: Atrioventricular conduction after a PAC depends on the prematurity of the P′ wave and the health of the AV node, bundle of His, and bundle branches. The possibilities for AV conduction of a PAC are the following:

1. Normal conduction (narrow QRS)
2. Nonconduction resulting in no QRS and a sudden pause; the block could be anywhere in the AV node or even in the His-Purkinje system
3. Aberrant ventricular conduction (broad QRS because of bundle branch block [BBB]); the BBB is functional and is the result of the sudden shortening of the cycle length rather than to any disease in the bundle branches
4. Conducted down only one AV nodal pathway (there are two) to set up a reentry circuit within the AV node; this is the most common mechanism of symptomatic paroxysmal supraventricular tachycardia (PSVT) (discussed in Chapter 11)
5. Conducted down the AV node and up an accessory pathway to establish a circus movement tachycardia (see Chapter 11); this is the second most common cause of symptomatic PSVT

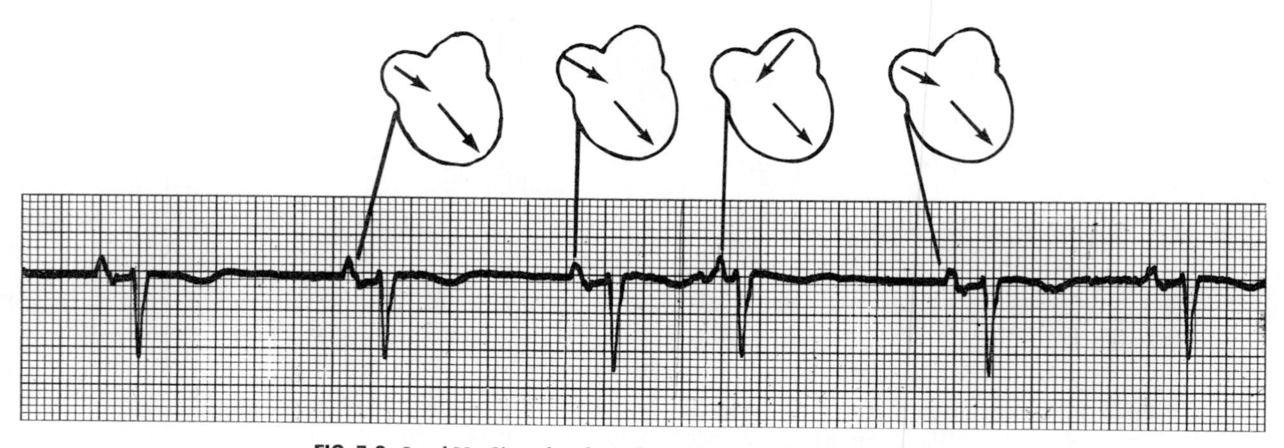

FIG. 7-2. Lead V_1. Sinus bradycardia with a PAC (the fourth P wave).

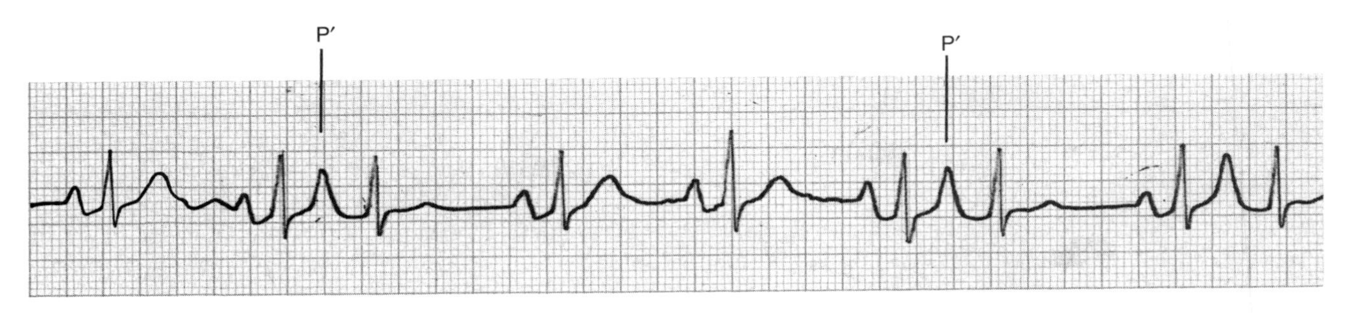

FIG. 7-3. PACs hidden in T waves (lead II). Notice how the T waves before the premature beats are distorted by the hidden P′ waves compared with the two sinus-conducted beats in the middle of the tracing.

Overdrive Suppression

Overdrive suppression is a property belonging to pacemaker cells in which their cycle length may be lengthened if they are depolarized from an outside source. For example, the sinus node normally exerts overdrive suppression on all subsidiary pacemakers. Conversely, a PAC may exert overdrive suppression on the sinus node.

In Fig. 7-1 you walked out the sinus rhythm and noted that the PAC had reset the sinus node, causing the pause following the PAC to be less than compensatory.

Fig. 7-2 shows a PAC in a patient with sinus bradycardia of 48 beats/min. The PAC is the fourth P wave in the tracing. It occurs early, before the next expected sinus P wave. It is also shaped differently, being a little narrower and more pointed than the sinus P waves. The QRS configuration is the same as for the sinus-conducted beats, proving that the stimulus originated above the branching portion of the bundle of His (supraventricular).

The two PACs in Fig. 7-3 are followed by a less than full compensatory pause as would be expected. Sometimes, however, the PAC suppresses the sinus node (overdrive

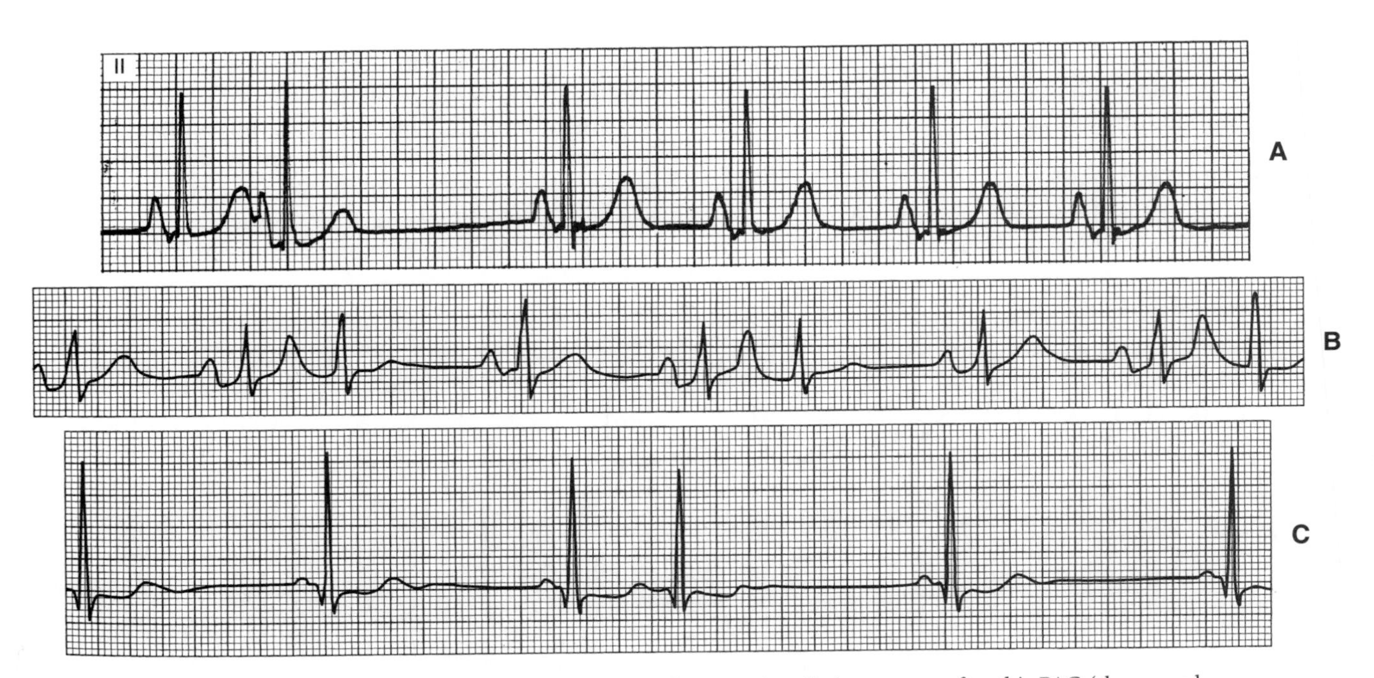

FIG. 7-4. Overdrive suppression (lead II). **A,** Note the exceptionally long pause after this PAC (the second P wave). **B,** Atrial trigeminy. There is a PAC every third beat. The overdrive suppression is exerted on the sinus node by the PAC, causing the P′P interval to be longer than the PP interval. **C,** There is a PAC in the third T wave. The suppressant effect it has on the sinus node can be seen.

suppression), and the sinus P wave that follows the PAC is delayed (Fig. 7-4). This may result in a pause that is equal to, less than, or more than a full compensatory pause.

Rhythm Variations

PACs are sometimes difficult to detect because they conceal themselves in T waves or masquerade as profound bradycardia when bigeminal and not conducted.

PACs That Hide in T Waves

The PACs in Fig. 7-3 are hidden in the preceding T waves. This is a common hiding place for PACs, although they can be easily spotted as follows:

1. By noting the irregular rhythm and the narrow QRS, indicating a supraventricular mechanism
2. By comparing the shape of the T waves preceding the early QRS; the taller, peaked T waves are distorted by PACs. Three of them are found in this tracing

Bigeminal PACs

Whenever the cardiac rhythm occurs in groups of two beats, it is called bigeminal. One of the causes of such a rhythm is a PAC following every sinus beat. In Fig. 7-5 you will note bigeminal PACs; it is immediately recognized as a supraventricular rhythm because all QRS complexes are narrow. If you compare the shape of the end of the T wave preceding the pause with the shape of the one following the pause, you will easily find the PACs.

Nonconducted PACs

When the PAC falls in the T wave, it may not be conducted. Fig. 7-6 illustrates the nonconducted PAC and its mechanism. The block is usually due to refractoriness in the AV node or bundle of His. The nonconducted PAC in Fig. 7-6 is not difficult to see, but in Fig. 7-7 it is more subtle. An abrupt pause is always a striking occurrence on the ECG. When this is encountered, examine the T wave preceding the pause carefully, comparing its shape with other T waves. The PAC can usually be found easily in this manner.

Bigeminal Nonconducted PACs

Bigeminal nonconducted PACs can masquerade as sudden, inappropriate, profound sinus bradycardia and may be mistaken for sick sinus syndrome (SSS) because the sudden bradycardia is associated with syncope or presyncope. It should be suspected when the bradycardia is of sudden onset. In Fig. 7-8 there are two sinus conducted beats at the beginning of the tracing. The first PAC is in the third T wave, and it is conducted normally, after which there is a nonconducted P′ wave in every T wave (bigeminal nonconducted PACs). The failure of the PACs to conduct to the ventricles, plus some degree of overdrive suppression, causes the heart rate to suddenly plunge from about 80 beats/min to less than 48 to 50 beats/min. This sudden change in cardiac output often results in loss of consciousness. In locating the P′ waves and making the diagnosis, it is helpful to remember that bigeminal nonconducted PACs are a far more common cause of sudden bradycardia than sinoatrial (SA) block and that in such a case the T waves do not necessarily look abnormal, but they are different in shape from the T waves before the first PAC and they are slightly different in shape from one another. If there is a PAC in every T wave, it distorts the T wave a little differently each time because the P′ is not part of the T wave mechanism. Note in Fig. 7-8 that not only are

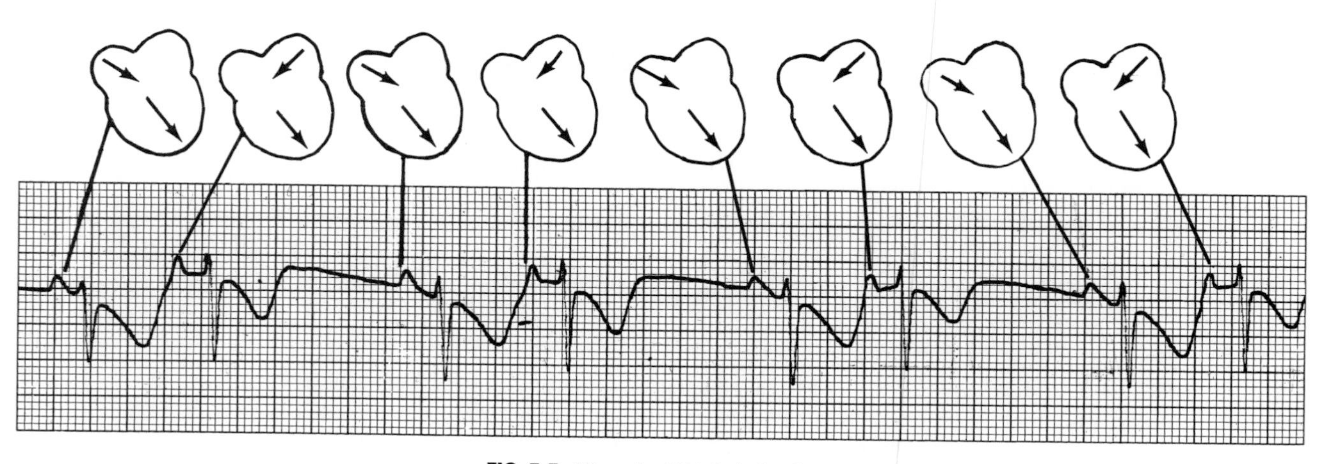

FIG. 7-5. Bigeminal PACs in lead V_1.

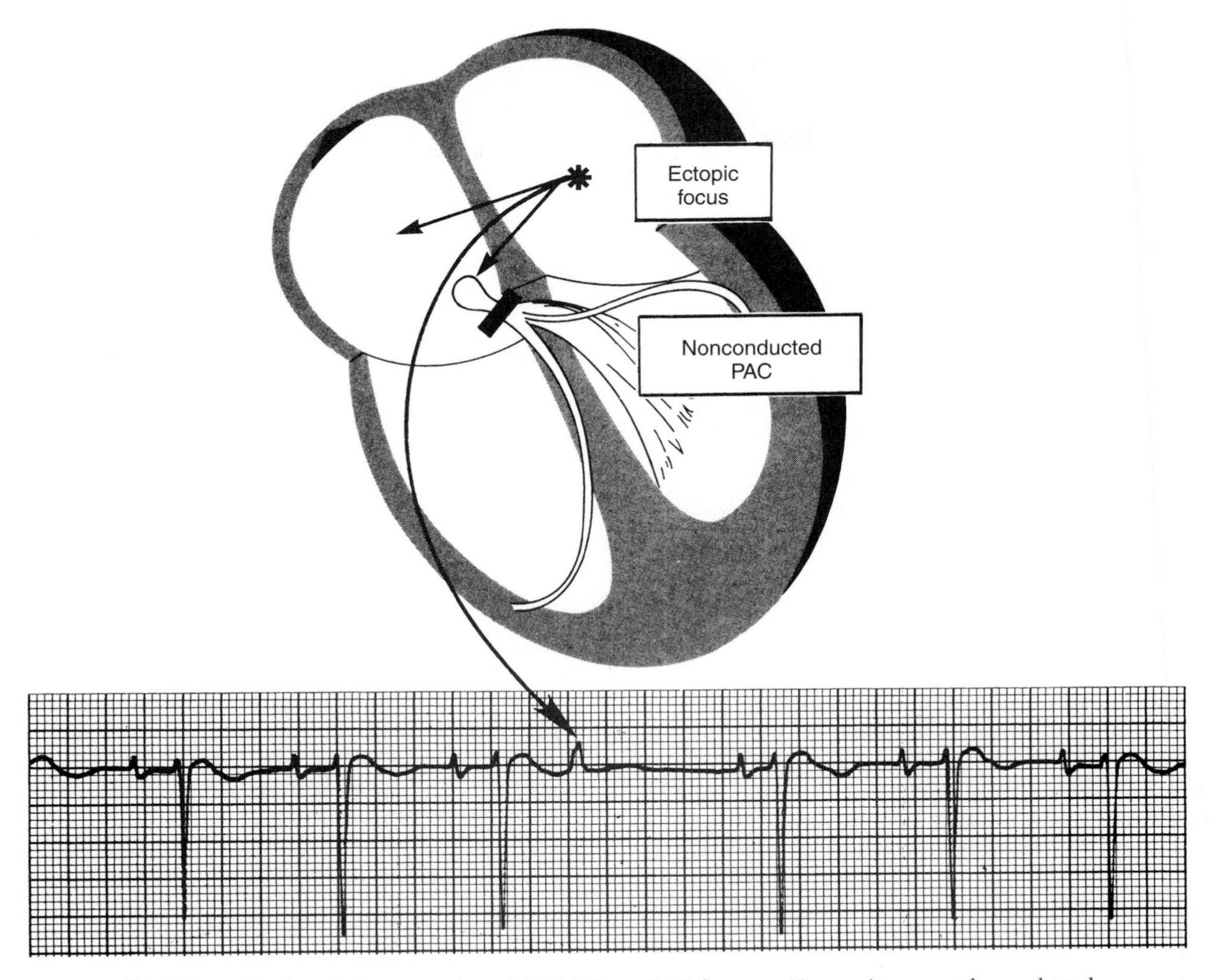

FIG. 7-6. Mechanism of the nonconducted PAC. When a PAC fires on a T wave, it may not be conducted because the AV node, bundle of His, or bundle branches are still refractory.

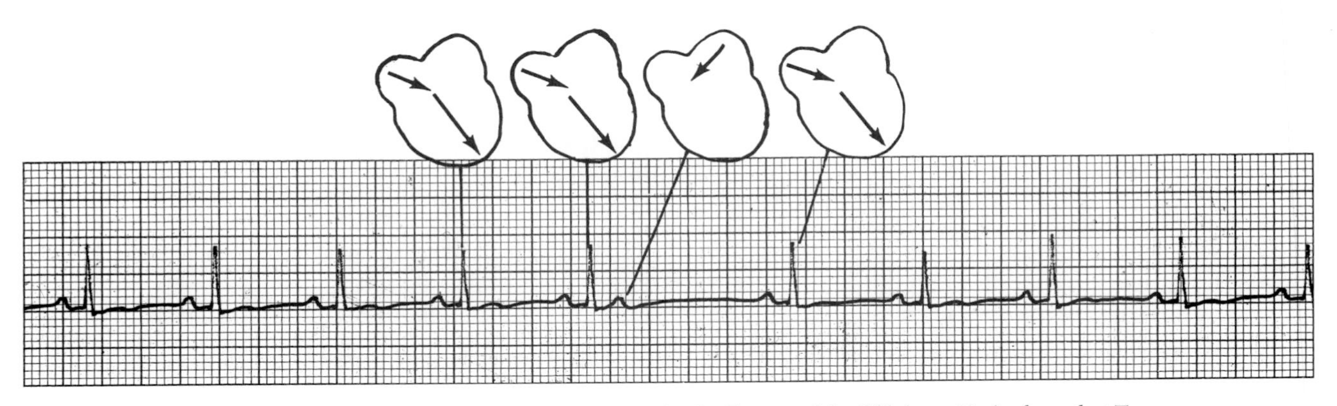

FIG. 7-7. Nonconducted PAC; lead II. There is a PAC in the T wave of the fifth beat. Notice how that T wave is different from the others, a sign of a hidden P′.

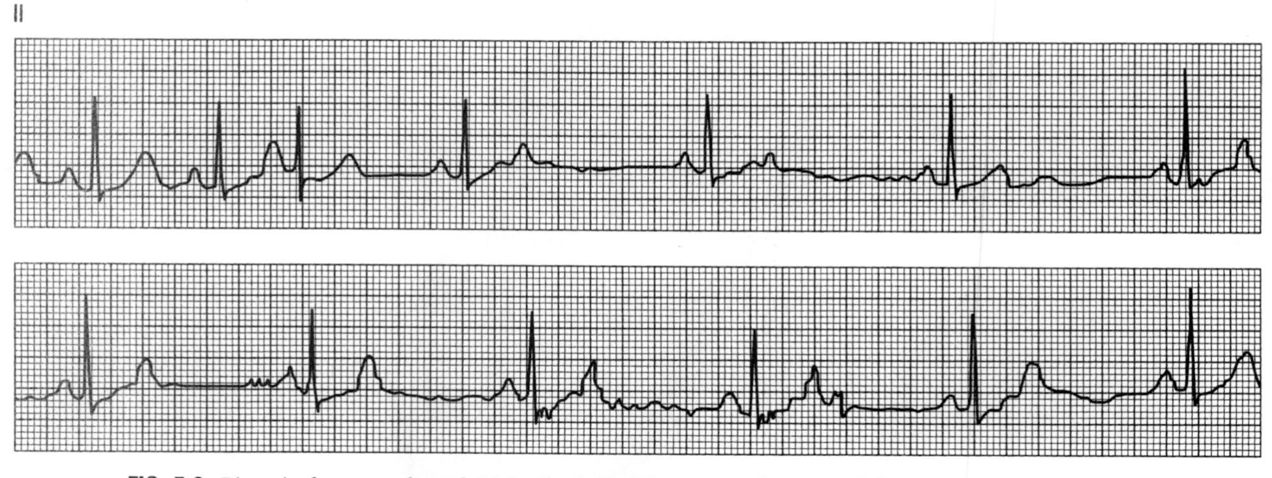

FIG. 7-8. Bigeminal nonconducted PACs (lead II). The nonconduction of the PAC in every other beat causes an abrupt, symptomatic bradycardia (continuous tracing). The PACs are easily found because they distort the T waves differently each time. There is considerable artifact in the middle of the bottom tracing.

the T waves before the pauses different from the two normal T waves at the beginning of the tracing, but they are also different from each other.

Fig. 7-9 provides another example of bigeminal nonconducted PACs. In Fig. 7-9, *A*, there is one nonconducted PAC. It is a sharp spike distorting the sixth T wave. In Fig. 7-9, *B*, P′ waves can be seen distorting every T wave.

Fig. 7-10 demonstrates a sinus tachycardia with two nonconducted PACs. Note that the PACs cause an irregular shape of the T waves preceding the pauses. We have spent some time on the nonconducted PAC because it is often misdiagnosed. The diagnosis is straightforward (1) if you know what to expect (nonconducted PACs are more common than what they simulate [sinus pauses]); and (2) if you know what to look for (distorted T waves when compared).

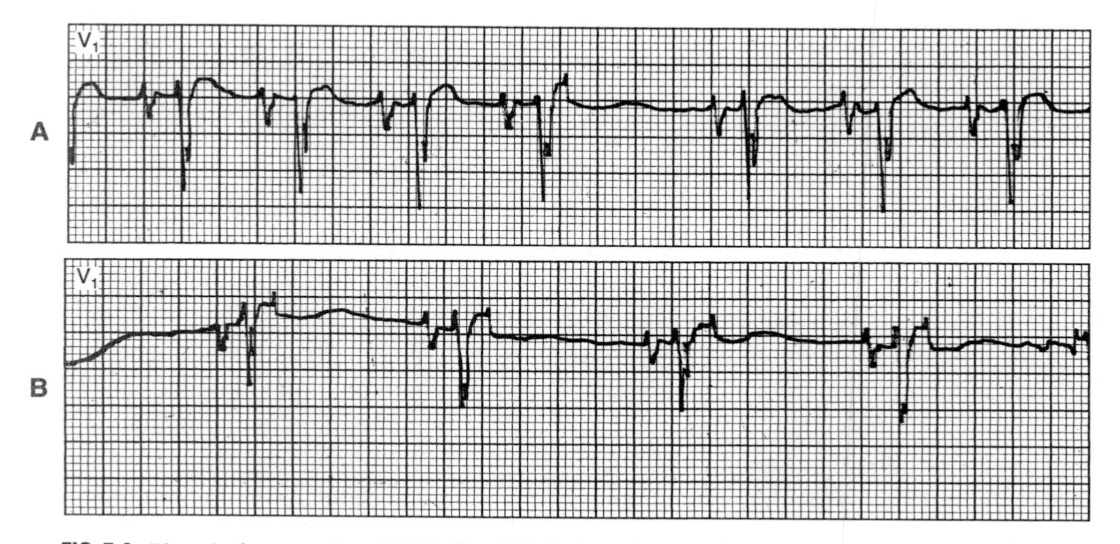

FIG. 7-9. Bigeminal nonconducted PACs (lead V_1). Both tracings are from the same patient. **A,** A PAC is distorting the sixth T wave. **B,** Same patient, moments later. Every T has a PAC in it (nonconducted), resulting in a heart rate of 52 beats/min. Nonconducted PACs are more common than the conditions that they mimic—sinoatrial block and sinus arrest.

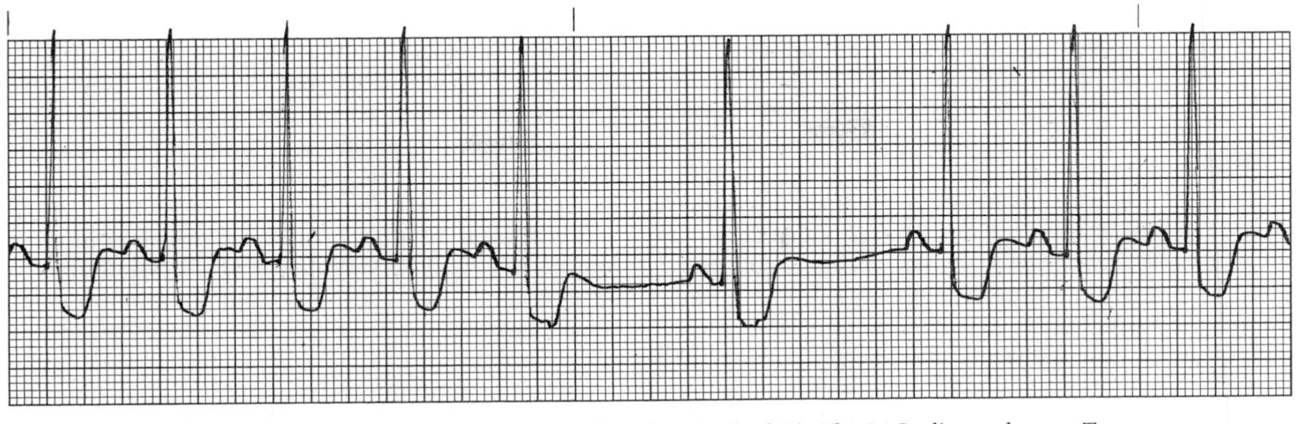

FIG. 7-10. Sinus tachycardia with two nonconducted PACs (lead II). The PACs distort the two T waves before the pauses; this is recognized when the T waves are compared.

Mechanism

The electrophysiologic mechanism for PACs is abnormal automaticity or delayed afterdepolarization. The mechanism determining the shape of the P′ wave is the location of the ectopic focus in the atria and its position in the cardiac cycle (i.e., whether it occurs on a T wave or not). If the focus is in the vicinity of the sinus node (as it is in the atrial tachycardia of digitalis toxicity), the resultant P′ wave closely resembles the normal sinus P wave. If the ectopic focus is low in the atrium toward the septum, there will be a negative P′ wave in leads II, III, and aV_F because the P′ vector moves away from the positive electrode of those leads. An ectopic focus in the left atrial appendage would result in a negative P′ wave in lead I because the current would be moving toward the right shoulder and the position of the negative electrode for lead I. By the same token, a PAC arising from the right free wall of the atrium would produce a positive P wave in lead I.

Causes

In normal individuals PACs may be the result of various stimuli, such as strong emotion (catecholamines), tobacco, alcohol, and caffeine to name a few. Premature atrial complexes are also associated with myocardial ischemia, infection, a variety of medications, low potassium or low magnesium blood levels, and hypoxia.

Clinical Implications

1. With critical timing a PAC may precipitate PSVT, atrial flutter, or atrial fibrillation.
2. In acute myocardial infarction (MI), PACs may result from catecholamines secondary to apprehension and pain or may warn of congestive heart failure and electrolyte imbalance.
3. PACs may be seen when mitral stenosis or atrial septal defect causes dilated or hypertrophied atria.

Most individuals with PACs do not have organic heart disease. However the incidence of PACs is increased in patients with organic heart disease, especially when there is atrial disease or enlargement, mitral stenosis, or cor pulmonale.

Symptoms

The patient is often unaware of the presence of isolated PACs. When PACs are not conducted, some may feel their heart "skips a beat." However, the sudden onset of the bradycardia of bigeminal nonconducted PACs may be profound enough to cause presyncope or syncope, even in an otherwise healthy heart.

Pediatrics

PACs are common in healthy children, even in newborn infants, and require no treatment. However, PACs may also be associated with structural heart disease.

Differential Diagnosis

Sinus bradycardia or SA block. Bigeminal nonconducted PACs with the P′ waves buried in T waves can be mistaken for profound sinus bradycardia or SA block. When P′ waves distort T waves, they do so a little differently each time so that the T waves will not be uniform, nor will they look like the T waves in the patient's normal sinus rhythm if this is available.

Atrial tachycardia with 2:1 block and ventriculophasic PP intervals. This particular tachycardia is seen in digitalis toxicity and can be mistaken for bigeminal nonconducted PACs. In atrial tachycardia with 2:1 block that is due to digitalis toxicity there is often a shorter PP interval in the cycle that contains the QRS (ventriculophasic PP intervals), causing it to resemble bigeminal nonconducted PACs. The differential diagnosis is made because of the clinical setting and by comparing the shapes of the P waves and P′ waves.

Treatment

PACs are not treated, although the cause is investigated, especially if the patient is aware of and bothered by an irregular heart beat caused by the PACs. Some simple measures in treatment would be to improve electrolyte intake, eliminate sources of caffeine from the diet, and stop smoking. If the PACs are the result of apprehension and pain (acute MI), reassurance and morphine may cause them to disappear. If they are the cause of hypoxia (especially in smokers), oxygen may be effective.

In the setting of Wolff-Parkinson-White (WPW) syndrome, these precautions along with instructions about performing a vagal maneuver would be especially important because it is usually a PAC that initiates one of the two common arrhythmias associated with WPW syndrome (i.e., paroxysmal supraventricular tachycardia). WPW syndrome is covered in Chapter 21.

FOCAL ATRIAL TACHYCARDIA

Focal atrial tachycardia is a regular atrial rhythm at a constant rate of 100 beats/min or more with a focus that is often located on the crista terminalis or in the pulmonary veins. It is characterized by atrial activation starting rhythmically at a small focus and spreading centrifugally from there.[1]

ECG Recognition

Atrial rate: Typically 130 to 240 beats/min, but may range from 100 to 300 beats/min.

Atrial rhythm: When associated with AV block, the atrial rhythm is irregular in approximately 50% of cases.[2]

P′ waves: Usually there is a clearly defined isoelectric baseline between P′ waves in all leads. Shape of the P waves depends on location of the focus. If it is high on the crista terminalis the P′ waves will closely resemble sinus P waves; such is the case in the atrial tachycardia of digitalis toxicity. If the rate is rapid or conduction within the atria is compromised, there may be no isoelectric baseline between P′ waves, causing the rhythm to resemble atrial flutter on the ECG in spite of its focal origin.

AV conduction: Block is often present; during AV block the atrial rate is not influenced.

Effect of vagal maneuvers: Atrial tachycardia continues unabated, although the maneuvers do, of course, cause AV block.

Mechanism

The mechanism of focal atrial tachycardia can be enhanced automaticity, triggered activity, or microreentry (i.e., very small reentrant circuits). From such a focus the electrical activation spreads centrifugally to both atria. The sudden onset of atrial tachycardia would suggest a microreentry mechanism.

Focal atrial tachycardia with prolonged or incessant episodes of a rapid atrial rhythm in which the rate becomes faster ("warm up") after onset and slows down ("cool down") before termination suggests enhanced automaticity as the mechanism.[3]

The appearance of nonparoxysmal atrial tachycardia is itself a sign of digitalis toxicity, in which case the mechanism is triggered activity caused by elevated intracellular calcium and early afterdepolarizations.

Causes

- Digitalis toxicity
- Intra-atrial disease

Clinical Implications

- Persistent type results in progressive cardiac dilation and congestive heart failure, which are potentially reversible with ablation of the focus
- More common when right ventricular dysfunction accompanies inferior wall MI

Pediatrics

In neonates and infants atrial tachycardia is often mistaken for atrial flutter. It is, however, more persistent than atrial flutter and may be associated with atrial septal defect. If drug therapy is successful in slowing the ventricular rate but not that of the atria, the atria dilate, the arrhythmia is exacerbated, and congestive heart failure results.[4]

Differential Diagnosis

Sinus tachycardia. A rapidly firing focus high on the crista terminalis cannot be differentiated from inappropriate sinus tachycardia or SA nodal reentry tachycardia on the surface electrocardiogram (ECG), and only with difficulty by endocardial mapping.[5]

Atrial tachycardia of digitalis toxicity. In the atrial tachycardia caused by digitalis toxicity the mechanism is triggered activity (delayed afterdepolarizations), in which case the P′R interval lengthens and the atrial rate increases gradually as the digitalis is continued and ranges from 130 to 250 beats/min. Atrial tachycardia with block associated with digitalis toxicity is illustrated in Fig. 7-11. For further discussion and examples, please refer to Chapter 15.

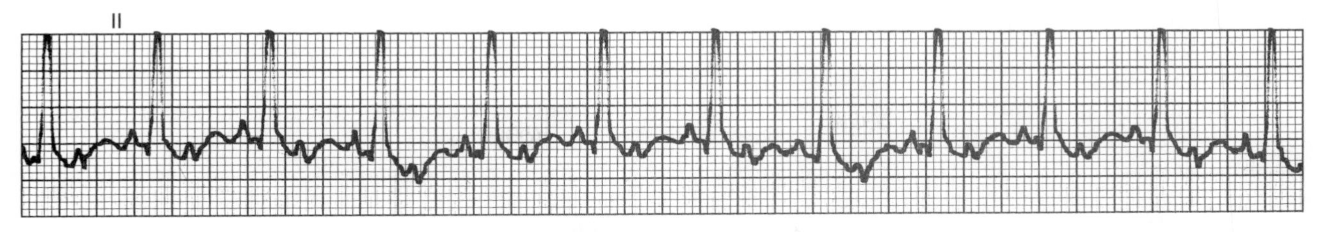

FIG. 7-11. Atrial tachycardia 200 beats/min with a 2:1 block.

INCESSANT ATRIAL TACHYCARDIA

In its incessant form, atrial tachycardia is present more than half the day and can result in dilated cardiomyopathy if untreated (tachycardiomyopathy). Incessant atrial tachycardia in a patient with dilated cardiomyopathy is seen in Fig. 7-12. The left ventricular dysfunction is reversible after cure by radiofrequency ablation.[3,6]

ECG Recognition

Atrial rate: About 130 to 180 beats/min.

Rhythm: Usually regular; can be started and stopped with atrial stimulation. Spontaneous termination can be sudden, or it can be preceded by progressive slowing or long-short cycles.[2]

P′ waves: The polarity of the P′ wave is determined by the site of the ectopic focus in the atria.

P′R interval: Normal or prolonged because of digitalis, in which case there may be a gradual prolongation of the PR interval as the heart rate increases. AV dissociation may be present as a result of digitalis toxicity.

QRS complexes: Normal, unless associated with BBB.

AV conduction: Ratio may be 1:1, or there may be atrial tachycardia with block (2:1 ratio, Wenckebach [Mobitz type I]), depending on the atrial rate.

Clinical Implications

Atrial tachycardia is a relatively uncommon arrhythmia and an infrequent cause of symptomatic supraventricular

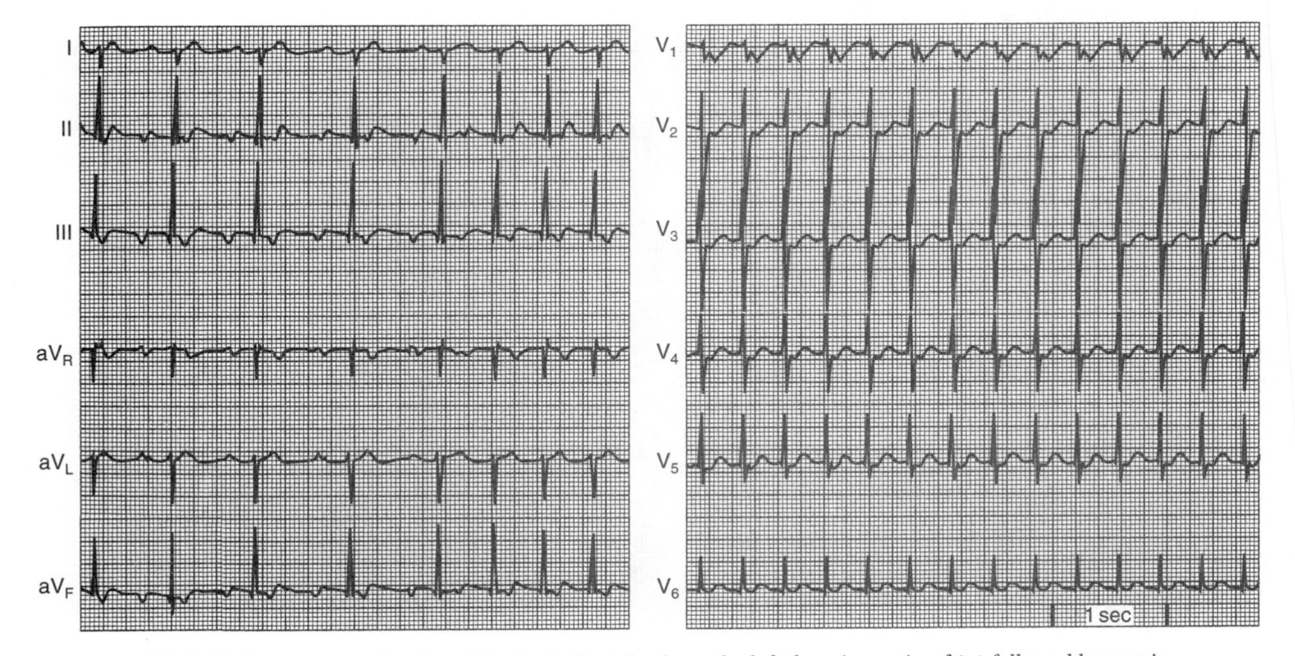

FIG. 7-12. Incessant atrial tachycardia. In the limb leads on the left there is a ratio of 2:1 followed by a ratio 1:1 AV conduction. This patient has been continuously in tachycardia for 12 years and came to medical attention with dilated cardiomyopathy. (From Wellens HJJ: In Willerson JT, Cohn JN, editors: *Cardiovascular medicine*, New York, 1995, Churchill Livingstone.)

tachycardia (SVT). Over a period of 17 years the Wellens group in the Netherlands examined 1834 patients with ECG documentation of SVT; 7% of these patients had atrial tachycardia, and one fourth of those cases were of the incessant form. Of patients with incessant atrial tachycardia, 40% came to medical attention with dilated cardiomyopathy.[6] Because incessant long-term atrial tachycardia is especially difficult to control pharmacologically, it can result in progressive cardiac dilation and congestive heart failure. These debilitating conditions are potentially reversible after the arrhythmia focus is ablated or the tachycardia controlled.[7]

In cases of atrial tachycardia with block the signs, symptoms, and prognosis are usually related to the cardiovascular status. Most of the time atrial tachycardia with block occurs in patients who have heart disease (coronary artery disease or cor pulmonale) or in patients who are taking digitalis (a sign of intoxication), in which case hypokalemia can precipitate the atrial tachycardia.[2] Patients who have inferior wall MI that is accompanied by right ventricular dysfunction are more prone to have atrial rhythms than are patients who have preserved right ventricular function.[8]

Bedside Diagnosis[2]

First heart sound. Varying intensity with varying AV block.

Jugular venous pulse. Auscultation reveals an excessive number of A waves.

Carotid sinus massage. Causes an increase in the degree of AV block and a stepwise slowing of the ventricular rate without termination of the atrial tachycardia.

Warning. In cases of suspected or confirmed digitalis toxicity carotid sinus massage should not be performed (or it is performed with extreme caution by an experienced physician); serious ventricular arrhythmias can result.

Differential Diagnosis

The differential diagnosis is *lesion macroreentrant atrial tachycardia* (Fig. 7-13) that, because of its mechanism and the ability to entrain and ablate it, is covered under Atrial Macroreentrant Mechanisms on pp. 104-107.

Treatment

In the incessant form of atrial tachycardia the focus of impulse formation is ablated with radiofrequency energy.

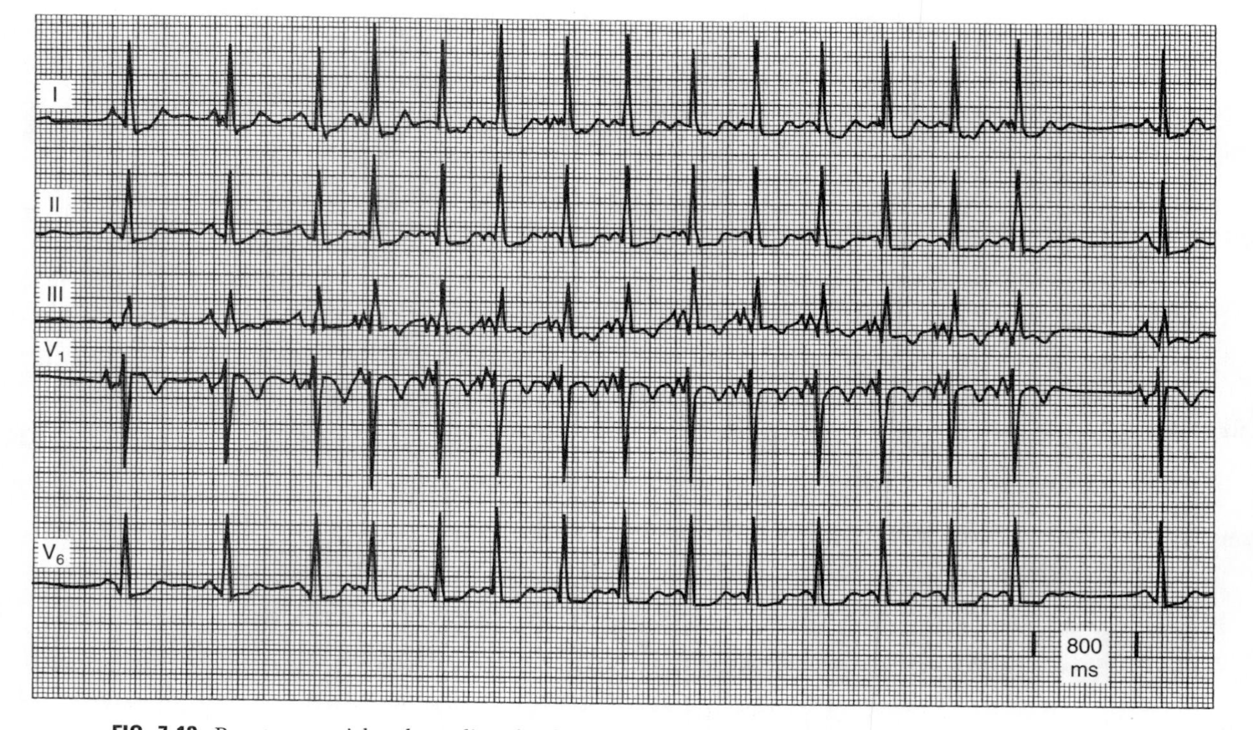

FIG. 7-13. Reentrant atrial tachycardia. The first three beats are preceded by a sinus P wave. The atrial tachycardia begins with the fourth cycle; the configuration of the P waves changes with that beat. (From Wellens HJJ: In Willerson JT, Cohn JN, editors: *Cardiovascular medicine*, New York, 1995, Churchill Livingstone.)

In cases such as this, it is very common for drug therapy to fail.

When atrial tachycardia develops in a patient taking digitalis, the assumption is made that the arrhythmia is due to digitalis toxicity; failure to discontinue the drug can result in death. The mortality rate in such a clinical situation has been shown to be 100%.[8] The patient should be confined to bed, the digitalis withheld, potassium chloride administered orally or intravenously if serum potassium level is not elevated; the patient's condition should be monitored continuously (ECG and hemodynamics), and the patient protected from sympathetic stimulation (complete bed rest) because catecholamines can aggravate the triggered activity responsible for this arrhythmia. If phenytoin is used, a ventricular pacing lead should be in place and the rhythm monitored. Because of its cost, digitalis antibody is usually reserved for patients who are hemodynamically compromised.[10]

MULTIFOCAL (CHAOTIC) ATRIAL TACHYCARDIA

Multifocal or chaotic atrial tachycardia is the rapid firing of atrial foci from more than two locations. It is characterized by multiple shapes of P waves and an irregular rhythm. It occurs relatively infrequently (0.36% of patients admitted to the hospital)[11] and usually in critically ill, elderly patients. Multifocal atrial tachycardia can be seen in Fig. 7-14. In this tracing of lead II at least three different shapes of P waves can be identified.

ECG Recognition

Rhythm: Irregular.

P waves: Three or more different morphologic appearances in a single ECG lead.

PP intervals: Varying; isoelectric PP segment.

PR intervals: Varying.

QRS complexes: Normal unless an intraventricular conduction problem exists.

AV conduction: Usually all P′ waves are conducted to the ventricles.

Distinguishing features: Multifocal atrial tachycardia is recognized because of its rapid rate and several P′ shapes, often in a patient with chronic pulmonary disease.

Mechanism

The mechanism for multifocal atrial tachycardia is thought to be triggered activity because the arrhythmia responds to calcium channel blockers such as verapamil and magnesium sulfate and because the clinical conditions associated with this arrhythmia have in common the cellular potential for triggered activity.

Clinical Implications and Causes

Multifocal atrial tachycardia is a difficult clinical problem, seen primarily in the elderly and generally associated with acute cardiorespiratory illness or chronic obstructive pulmonary disease. Less commonly, pulmonary infections or pulmonary embolism may be present. Multifocal atrial tachycardia is the result not only of the pathophysiologic features of severe pulmonary disease but also of the treatment. For example, right atrial enlargement, hypercapnia, hypoxia, acidosis, adrenergic stimulation, and drugs used for the treatment of pulmonary disease, such as isoproterenol and aminophylline, are all proarrhythmic. When the diagnosis of multifocal atrial tachycardia is first made, the clinical setting is often that of congestive heart failure. Diabetes, a common condition in patients with this arrhythmia, is present in 24% of patients.[11,12]

Pediatrics

The majority of children with multifocal atrial tachycardia (MAT) are healthy infants less than 1 year of age; a few may exhibit mild to life-threatening cardiorespiratory disease. Less often, multifocal atrial tachycardia accompanies structural heart disease. Mild ventricular dysfunction may be observed in the presence of MAT, but symptoms are few and resolution is generally complete. Response to antiarrhythmic agents is mixed, and cardioversion is of no

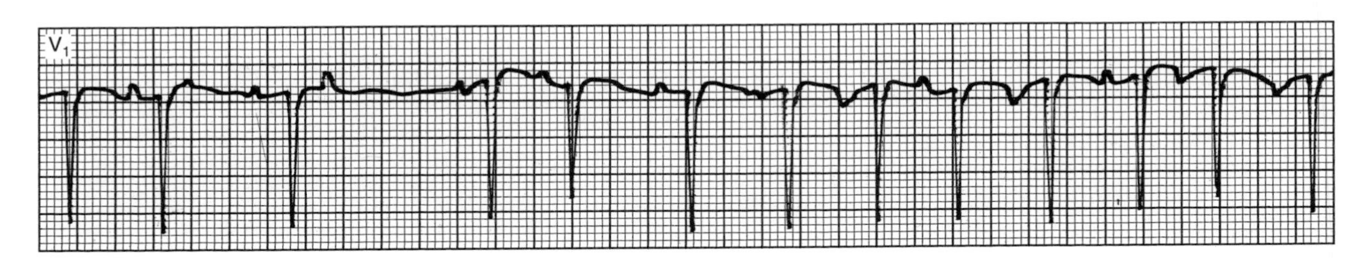

FIG. 7-14. Multifocal atrial tachycardia (lead V_1). Notice the different shapes of the P′ waves.

avail. Finally, long-term cardiovascular and developmental outcome depends principally on underlying condition; for otherwise healthy children, it is excellent.[13]

Treatment

Therapy is supportive and directed at correcting the predisposing cardiac, pulmonary, metabolic, and infectious conditions that have caused the arrhythmia. Because multifocal atrial tachycardia is commonly a secondary phenomenon; antiarrhythmic drugs are often ineffective and their role is unclear.[12] The tachycardia may be suppressed by potassium and magnesium, improvement in oxygenation, ventilation, and the treatment of congestive heart failure. Metoprolol, magnesium, and verapamil have been evaluated in a few treatment studies, and may have a role in the treatment of multifocal atrial tachycardia.[14]

SUMMARY

The PAC is early in the cycle and abnormal in configuration. This early atrial beat may either reset the sinus node or it may suppress the next expected sinus beat (overdrive suppression). PACs are usually of no clinical significance, but may cause AV nodal reentry tachycardia or atrial fibrillation in some cases. They are associated with atrial disease and atrial dilatation, mitral stenosis, or cor pulmonale.

Atrial tachycardias are regular rhythms of more than 100 beats/min with a focal origin outside of the sinus node or a reentry circuit. Focal atrial tachycardia may be the result of enhanced automaticity, triggered activity, or microreentry. It is possible to ablate the focus with radiofrequency energy.

REFERENCES

1. Saoudi N, Cosio F, Waldo A et al: Classification of atrial flutter and regular atrial tachycardia according to electrophysiologic mechanism and anatomic bases: a statement from a joint expert group from the Working Group of Arrhythmias of the European Society of Cardiology and the North American Society of Pacing and Electrophysiology, *J Cardiovasc Electrophysiol* 12:852, 2001.
2. Zipes DP: Specific arrhythmias: diagnosis and treatment. In Braunwald E, editor: *Heart disease*, ed 4, Philadelphia, 1992, WB Saunders.
3. Lesh MD: Radiofrequency catheter ablation of atrial tachycardia and flutter. In Zipes DP, Jalife J, editors: *Cardiac electrophysiology from cell to bedside*, ed 2, Philadelphia, 1992, WB Saunders.
4. Wren C: Treatment of tachycardia in infants and children, *Indian Pediatrics* 36:1091-1096, 1999.
5. Kalman JM, Olgin JE, Karch MR et al: "Cristal tachycardias." Origin of right atrial tachycardias from the crista terminalis identified by intracardiac echocardiography, *J Am Coll Cardiol* 31:451-459, 1998.
6. Wellens HJJ, Rodriquez LM, Smeets JLRM et al: Tachycardiomyopathy in patients with supraventricular tachycardia with emphasis on atrial fibrillation. In Olsson SB, Allessie MA, Campbell RWF, editors: *Atrial fibrillation: mechanisms and therapeutic strategies*, Armonk, NY, 1994, Futura.
7. Wellens HJJ: Atrial tachycardia: how important is the mechanism? *Circulation* 90:1576, 1994.
8. Rechavia E, Strasberg B, Mager A et al: The incidence of atrial arrhythmias during inferior wall myocardial infarction with and without right ventricular involvement, *Am Heart J* 124:387, 1992.
9. Driefus LS, McKnight EH, Katz M et al: Digitalis intolerance, *Geriatrics* 18:494, 1963.
10. Wellens HJJ, Conover M: *The ECG in emergency decision making*, St Louis, 1992, Mosby.
11. Kastor JA: Multifocal atrial tachycardia, *N Engl J Med* 322:1713, 1990.
12. McCord J, Borzak S: Multifocal atrial tachycardia, *Chest* 113:203, 1998.
13. Bradley DJ, Fischbach PS, Law IH et al: The clinical course of multifocal atrial tachycardia in infants and children, *J Am Coll Cardiol* 38:401, 2001.
14. Scher DL, Arsura EL: Multifocal atrial tachycardia: mechanisms, clinical correlates, and treatment, *Am Heart J* 118:574, 1990.

CHAPTER 8
Atrial Fibrillation

Atrial fibrillation is the fragmented and rapid electrical activity resulting from multiple, simultaneous reentrant waves within the atria. The normal response of the ventricles to this rampant atrial activity is irregular and rapid (approximately 140 to 150 beats/min). The major risks are stroke and death. Current therapy seeks prevention of thromboemboli, control of ventricular response, and restoration and maintenance of sinus rhythm. Atrial fibrillation has been referred to as "a growth industry for the 21st century."[1] Internationally, a remarkable effort is being made to develop a safe and reproducible cure.

CLASSIFICATION AND TERMS

In clinical practice atrial fibrillation is generally classified into paroxysmal, persistent, and permanent. These terms can be qualified by adding an adjective that describes the arrhythmia further, such as paroxysmal lone atrial fibrillation or persistent hypertensive atrial fibrillation.

Paroxysmal atrial fibrillation begins abruptly and converts to sinus rhythm spontaneously within minutes or hours; frequency, duration, and severity of symptoms vary among individuals. *Persistent atrial fibrillation* requires intervention for conversion to sinus rhythm. *Permanent atrial fibrillation* cannot be cardioverted, or if cardioverted, sinus rhythm is not maintained.

Other designations are *acute or first onset* atrial fibrillation; *chronic*, which may be permanent or recurrent (paroxysmal or persistent); *silent* atrial fibrillation is not subjectively noticed; the terms *slow* and fast refer to the ventricular response, rather than to the atrial fibrillatory rate; *controlled* is the term generally used to indicate what the physician judges to be an "ideal" long-term rate for this arrhythmia and this individual.

ECG CHARACTERISTICS

Ventricular rate: Usually 100 to 160 beats/min in the untreated patient with normal atrioventricular (AV) conduction; the rate is determined by the refractory period of the AV node and its conduction velocity, plus concealed conduction (p. 77).

Ventricular rhythm: Irregular unless complicated by complete AV block, digitalis toxicity, or conversion to atrial

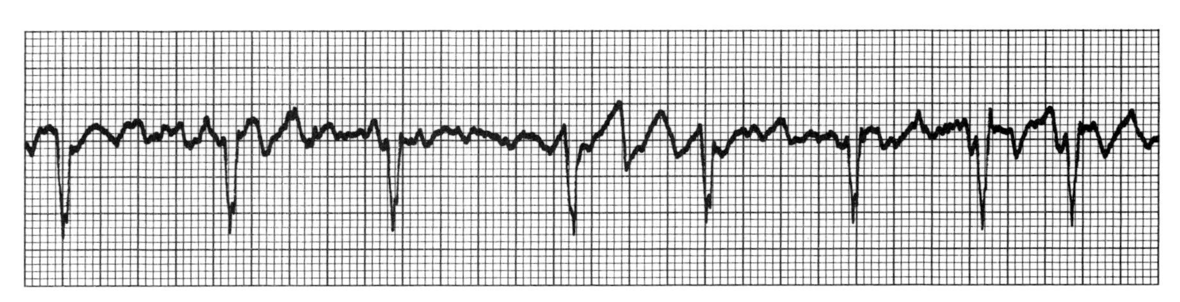

FIG. 8-1. Marked coarse atrial fibrillation. The irregular rhythm indicates intact AV conduction.

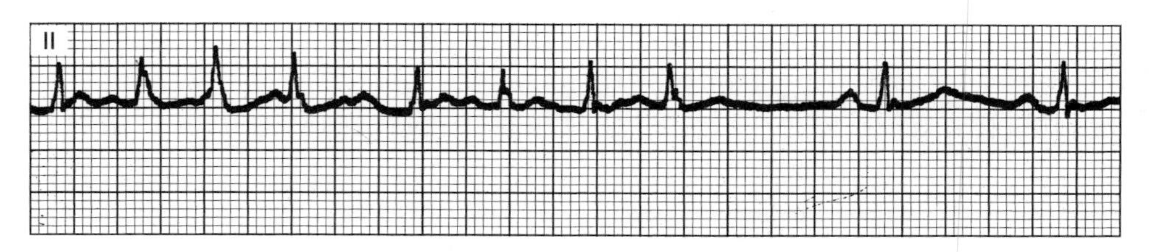

FIG. 8-2. Coarse paroxysmal atrial fibrillation and its conversion to sinus rhythm.

flutter with fixed 1:1 or 2:1 conduction; very rapid rates may appear to be regular.

P waves: Absent.

Fibrillatory (f) waves: The fibrillatory line may be *coarse or fine*, depending on the amplitude of the atrial waves. When the amplitude of the f waves in lead V_1 is 0.1 mV or more, they are described as coarse. Figs. 8-1 and 8-2 are examples of coarse atrial fibrillation. The termination of a run of paroxysmal atrial fibrillation is seen in Fig. 8-2.

Kirchhof et al[2] report a transition from coarse to fine f waves after carotid sinus massage and immediately before spontaneously converting to sinus rhythm. It is known that alterations in vagal tone can influence the atrial fibrillatory process by changing the atrial refractory period.

QRS complex: Narrow unless complicated by bundle branch block or Wolff-Parkinson-White (WPW) syndrome.

Distinguishing features: Acute atrial fibrillation is notable because of an absence of P waves and its rapid rate, irregular rhythm, and variable hemodynamic symptoms.

Summary of Ventricular Responses

Possible ventricular responses to atrial fibrillation are as follows:

- Irregular rhythm at a rate of 100 to 160 beats/min when AV conduction is normal and no AV blocking drugs are being used. The QRS may be narrow or broad with a bundle branch block (BBB) pattern. Such a rhythm is sometimes called "irregularly irregular" to distinguish it from group beating.
- Irregular rhythm at a rate of 280 to 300 or more with broad QRS complexes (WPW syndrome). The QRS is broad with a ventricular ectopic morphology (pp. 178 and 182).
- Regular rhythm, indicating digitalis toxicity, AV block, or conversion to atrial flutter. The QRS may be narrow or broad with a RBBB pattern. Of course, the rhythm would also be regular if there was conversion to normal sinus rhythm.
- Group beating, indicating digitalis toxicity or conversion to atrial flutter with Wenckebach conduction. The QRS may be narrow or broad with a BBB pattern.

THE ECG: HOW TO BEGIN

Although atrial fibrillation is a common and so called "basic" arrhythmia, its recognition on the electrocardiogram (ECG) is often missed because the clinician is expecting the ventricular rhythm to always be irregular. In cases of atrial fibrillation complicated by AV block or digitalis toxicity, the ventricular rhythm may be perfectly regular or there may be group beating. Additionally, when the rate is rapid, the rhythm at first glance may appear to be regular. To avoid these pitfalls, always define atrial activity first and know what drugs the patient is taking. Do not be tempted to address AV conduction and the ventricular rhythm before this is done. When the atrial rhythm is ignored, the wrong diagnosis, or, at best, an incomplete one is the result. So, in Fig. 8-3, first evaluate the longer lead II tracing at the bottom in the following sequence:

1. **Are there P waves?**

If so, are they sinus P waves or ectopic (atrial tachycardia, atrial flutter)?

If not:

2. **Is there AV conduction?** (i.e., a grossly irregular ventricular rhythm)

If yes, what is the ventricular rate, QRS width, QRS axis, and QTc?

If not, what is the ventricular rhythm (junctional, narrow QRS; ventricular, broad QRS)? (Answers are found in the legend for Fig 8-3.)

Fig. 8-4 is a 12-lead ECG from a woman with paroxysmal atrial fibrillation. The patient was on propranolol for rate control. This episode lasted for 12 hours. Follow steps 1 and 2 above to evaluate the rhythm.

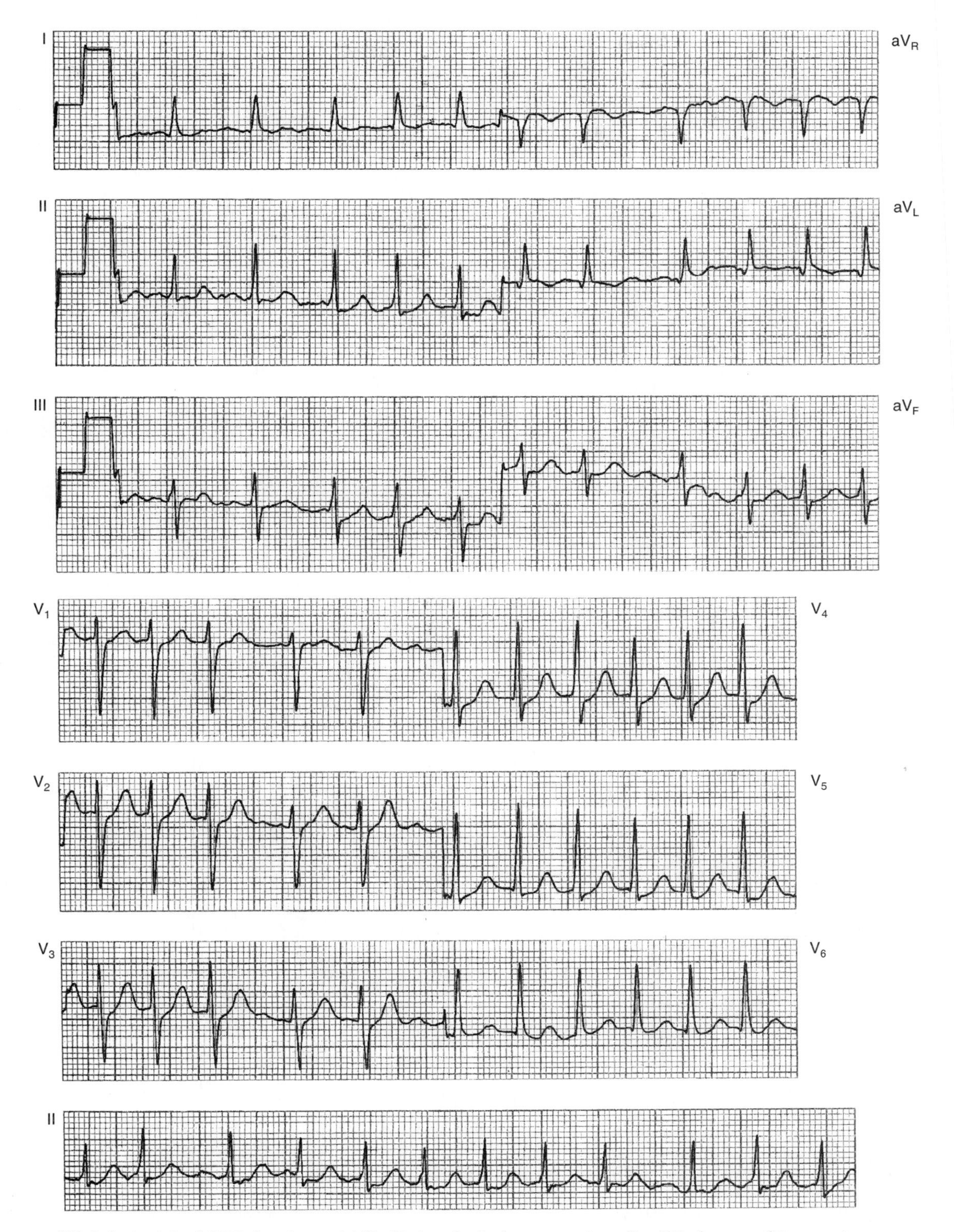

FIG. 8-3. A 12-lead ECG showing atrial fibrillation. In the longer tracing of lead II, absence of P waves, intact AV conduction, and the fine fibrillatory line are noted. In V_1 the QRS is normal (no bundle branch block). Leads I and II show a normal axis. The grossly irregular ventricular response at a rate of approximately 140 beats/min indicates intact AV conduction.

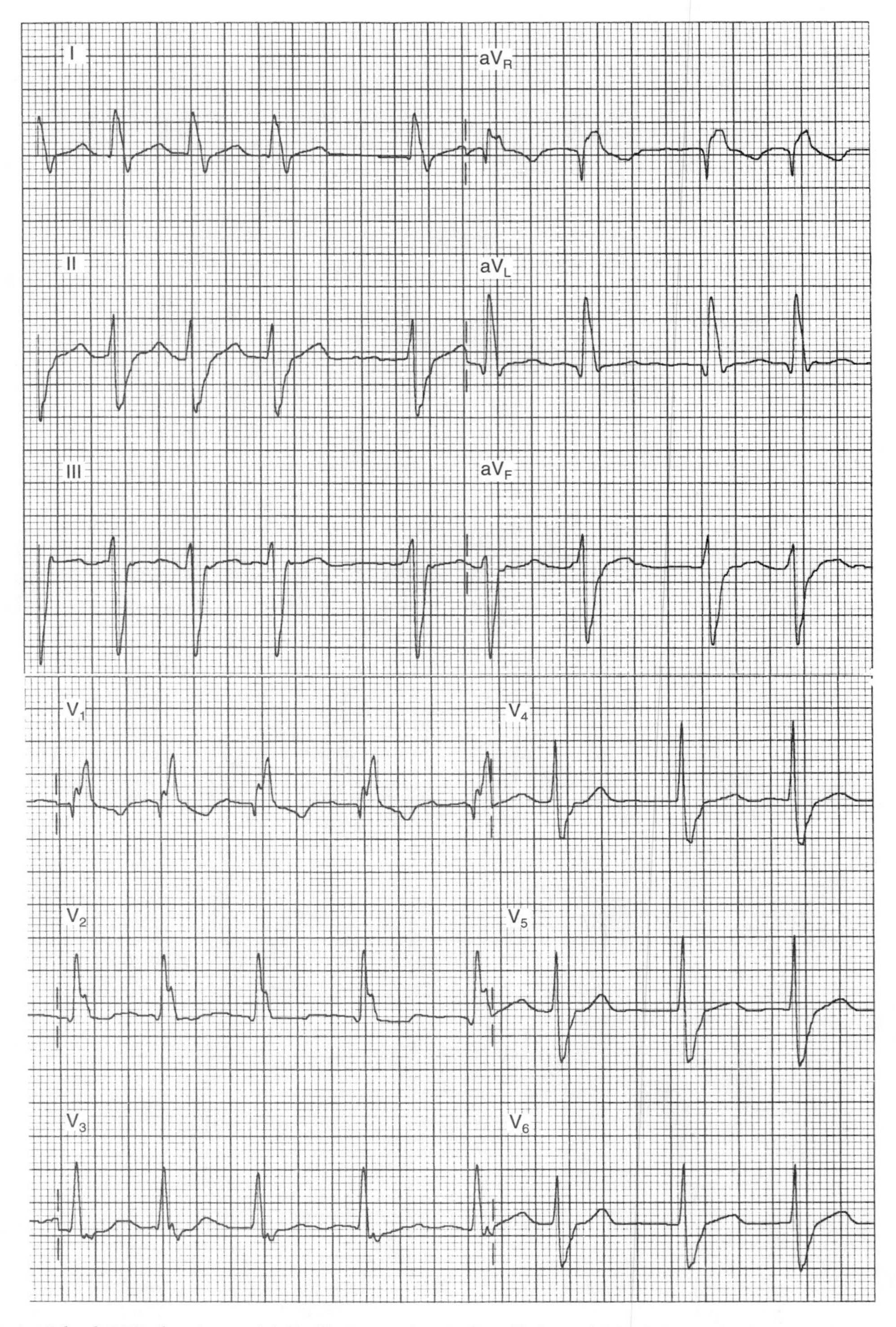

FIG. 8-4. A 12-lead ECG showing atrial fibrillation and right bundle branch block (RBBB). Absence of P waves and a fine fibrillatory line are noted. Leads I and II show left axis deviation. The grossly irregular ventricular response at approximately 102 beats/min indicates intact AV conduction.

TROUBLESHOOTING THE ECG IN ATRIAL FIBRILLATION

Important clue: The ventricular rhythm in uncomplicated atrial fibrillation is never regular or in fixed groups.

A. Conversion to a regular rhythm

May indicate	ECG
1. Conversion to sinus rhythm	P waves precede every QRS; rate normal or a little slow because of the rate control drug already aboard
2. Conversion to atrial flutter with 1:1 or 2:1 conduction	Ventricular rate increases to 150 to 220 beats/min; saw-tooth pattern will be difficult to see
3. Digitalis toxic rhythm (junctional tachycardia or fascicular ventricular tachycardia [VT])	No P waves; narrow QRS (junctional; 70-140 beats/min) or right BBB pattern (fascicular VT; 90-160 beats/min)
4. Digitalis toxic junctional tachycardia with 2:1 Wenckebach exit block	No P waves; narrow QRS (unless BBB); group beating; rate <70 beats/min
5. Complete AV block (possibly caused by rate-control drugs)	No P waves; narrow QRS (unless BBB); rate approximately 60 beats/min

B. Conversion to a rhythm with group beating (irregular, but in fixed groups; groups indicate Wenckebach conduction)

May indicate	ECG
1. Digitalis toxic junctional tachycardia with 3:2 Wenckebach exit block	No P waves; narrow QRS (unless BBB); group beating; rate <95 beats/min
2. Digitalis toxic fascicular VT with Wenckebach exit block (rare)	No P waves; RBBB pattern; group beating
3. Atrial flutter with Wenckebach AV conduction (3:2 or 4:3 ratios)	Saw-tooth pattern; fixed groups of two (3:2 conduction) or three (4:3 conduction); narrow QRS (unless BBB)

MECHANISMS

Normal Cardiac Cycle Reviewed

The normal cardiac cycle as reflected on the ECG is briefly reviewed here. Normally, the atria are activated by impulses generated by the sinus node at a rate in keeping with the physiologic needs of the body. This sinus rate is complemented by adjustments in AV nodal conduction velocity and action potential duration (refractory period). In tandem with the acceleration and slowing of the rate of the sinus node, conduction velocity in the AV node also accelerates and slows. The cardiac refractory period shortens with tachycardia and lengthens with bradycardia, all adjustments intended for the well-ordered and safe operation of the pump.

The two atria are activated (depolarized) by the sinus impulse, resulting in a *P wave.* They contract, expelling their blood pool into the ventricles. When the atrial excitation wave reaches the AV node, there is a delay before activation of the ventricles occurs *(PR interval).* Ventricular depolarization *(QRS complex)* is followed by ventricular contraction. The heart repolarizes *(T wave)*, relaxes, and the cycle repeats.

Cardiac Cycle During Atrial Fibrillation

When the atria are fibrillating, they are no longer activated in an orderly fashion, but rather with very rapid, fragmented, electrical activity; they do not pump and *P waves are absent.* The normal ventricular response to this abnormal erratic atrial activity is a *rapid, irregular ventricular rhythm*, rate and rhythm being influenced by concealed conduction, AV nodal refractory period, and AV nodal conduction velocity.

Abnormal Ventricular Response to Atrial Fibrillation

A ventricular rate or rhythm that is abnormal for atrial fibrillation may be caused by AV block (pathologic or iatrogenic) or digoxin-induced emergence of junctional or ventricular pacemakers. These conditions would result in an abnormal ventricular rhythm that may be slow and regular or irregular, fast and regular, or in fixed groups (see section on Troubleshooting the ECG in Atrial Fibrillation). Fig. 8-5 is an example of profound bradycardia because of AV block in a patient with atrial fibrillation.

Concealed Conduction

Concealed conduction is the propagation of electrical activity into or from the AV node and His bundle (anterogradely or retrogradely) that is not seen on the surface ECG because it never reaches its target chambers (ventricles or atria). Electrical activity in the bundle of His cannot be detected by the surface ECG; rather, it is assumed because of its results. For example, during normal sinus rhythm P waves are followed by QRS complexes with fixed PR intervals. We can assume AV conduction through the His-Purkinje system, although such conduction is not actually seen on the surface ECG.

Anterograde concealed conduction usually begins in the atria, but does not reach the ventricles. Here again, we recognize it because of its effect on subsequent events. During acute atrial fibrillation without AV nodal conduc-

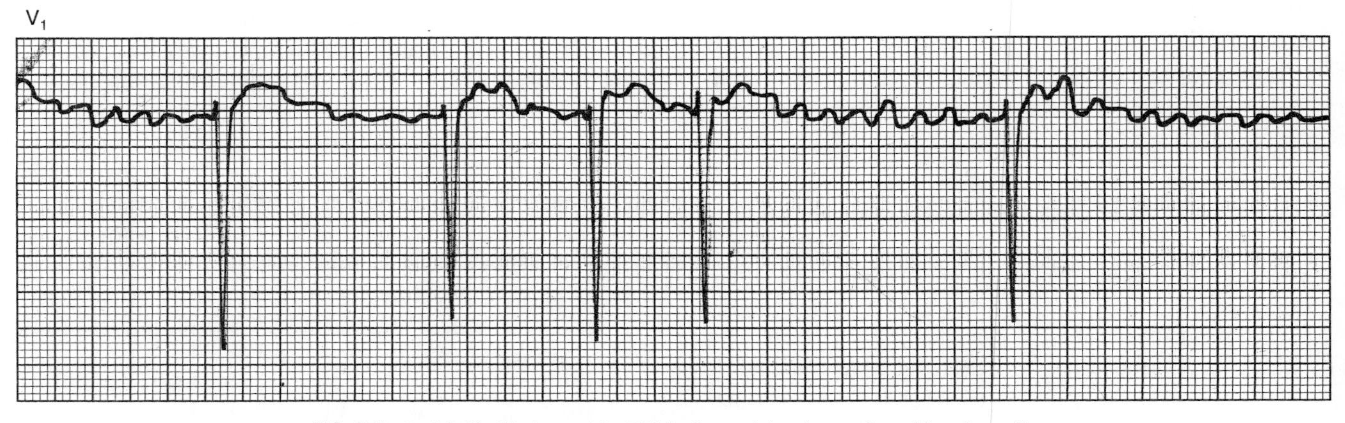

FIG. 8-5. Atrial fibrillation with AV block resulting in profound bradycardia.

tion-blocking drugs, the rate at which the ventricles respond is slower than their capability and the capability of the AV junction to conduct. Thus we assume concealed conduction into the AV node from the erratic atrial activity, leaving the node refractory for longer than its native time. Additionally, if the ventricles were activated as soon as the AV nodal refractory period was completed, the rhythm would be fairly regular. It is concealed conduction that contributes to the irregular RR intervals in atrial fibrillation and the relatively tolerable heart rate of 140 to 150 beats/min.

Retrograde concealed conduction follows ventricular depolarization, but does not reach the atria. It is recognized because of its effect of lengthening the next PR interval, such as would occur with an interpolated premature ventricular complex (PVC) (p. 142). In the case of atrial fibrillation, retrograde concealed conduction is possible, but, of course, cannot be precisely identified on the surface ECG because of the absence of PR intervals. It can be suggested, however, by a long pause after a PVC.

Intra-atrial Reentry

The mechanism that sustains atrial fibrillation is multiple reentrant wavelets, first submitted by Moe in 1962.[3] Fig. 8-6 illustrates atrial activity during atrial fibrillation in which the atria are activated by multiple reentrant wavelets that continuously change in size and direction. Multiple waves are generated from a larger circuit and die out at the AV ring, collide with other waves to become wavelets, or meet with refractory tissue and reverse direction by 180 degrees or a full 360 degrees to form a short-lived, closed local circuit and an irregular and fractionated type of intraatrial reentry.[4]

Konings et al[5] have identified the following types of atrial fibrillation based on mapping studies in 25 patients with WPW syndrome undergoing surgery for interruption of their accessory pathway or pathways.

Type I. Activation of the right atrium by broad wave fronts propagating uniformly and without significant conduction delay (40% of patients)

Type II. One or two nonuniformly conducting wavelets, with a higher degree of conduction delay and intraatrial block than seen in type I (32% of patients)

Type III. Activation of the right atrium by three or more highly fragmented wavelets that frequently change direction of propagation because of numerous arcs of functional conduction block (28% of patients)

Triggering Mechanisms

Premature atrial complexes (PACs). Paroxysmal atrial fibrillation is usually (95%) triggered by one or more rapidly firing atrial ectopic foci clustered at the ostium or within the first centimeters of the atrial muscle sleeves into the pulmonary veins.[6-9] In a few cases the initiating foci are localized in the right atrium.[10] Other locations for initiation of atrial fibrillation are the crista terminalis, superior vena cava, ostium of the coronary sinus, interatrial septum, ligament of Marshall, or left atrial posterior free wall.[11]

Paroxysmal supraventricular tachycardia (PSVT). During PSVT the atrial stretch caused by the atria contracting against closed AV valves may create the unstable milieu necessary to support atrial fibrillation.

Autonomic nervous system. A correlation between vagal stimulation and paroxysmal atrial fibrillation has been reported by Coumel.[12,13]

Vagal stimulation causes a shortening of the effective refractory period and an increased dispersion of refractoriness in atrial myocardium, both of which are proarrhythmic for atrial fibrillation. The part played by the autonomic nervous system can be suspected from the clinical history;

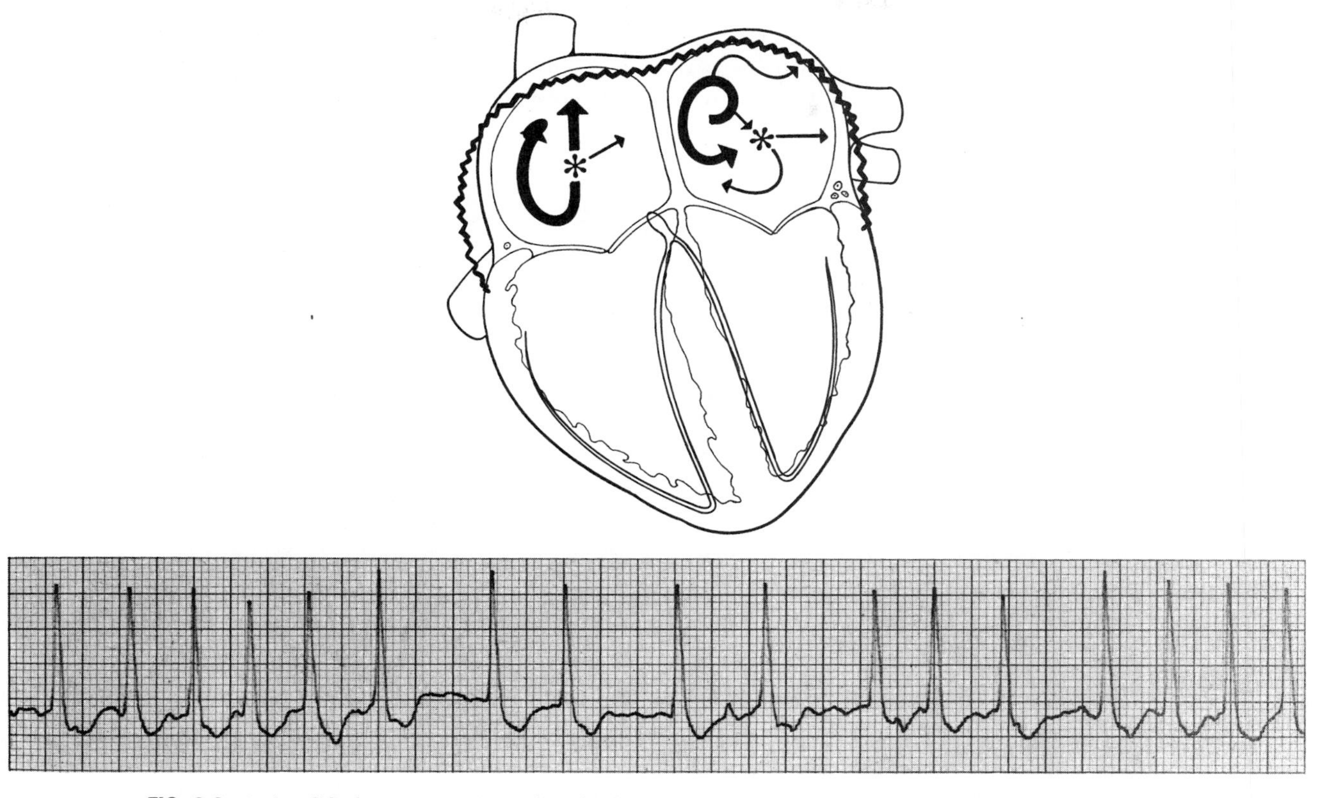

FIG. 8-6. A simplified representation of multiple reentry currents during atrial fibrillation. The tracing shows the irregular ventricular response erratic atrial activity.

notable are whether the arrhythmia was triggered during exercise or at rest, night or day, and the heart rate up to 10 minutes before the attacks.[14]

PATHOPHYSIOLOGY

Electrical and structural changes inflicted even by short-term atrial fibrillation are reflected by an increase in postconversion ectopics and eventual tachycardia-mediated cardiomyopathy. Hypercoagulability and changes in the autonomic nervous system are additional by-products of atrial fibrillation.

Electrical Remodeling

The electrophysiologic changes that occur in atrial tissue secondary to atrial fibrillation are called *electrical remodeling*. Specifically, they are progressive and are characterized by significant shortening of the atrial effective refractory period and inability of atrial cells to adapt to heart rate.[15-17] Among other factors, calcium overload, modulated ionic pumps, and angiotensin II are implicated in the perpetuation of atrial fibrillation and facilitate its reinduction.[18]

Calcium overload. Wijffels et al[19] were the first to describe electrical remodeling. It was later shown that the rapid atrial rates of atrial fibrillation cause an intracellular calcium overload,[20] and possibly mitochondrial swelling and lysis of the cristae.

Modulated ion pumps. It is known that with the onset of atrial fibrillation there is a reduction in at least three of the potassium currents involved in the repolarization process.[21] Barbey et al[22] further showed that the energy demands of atrial fibrillation can rapidly modulate two ion pumps that are crucial for the regulation of membrane potential. Even a small change in pump current alters the action potential duration and could explain the tendency of atrial fibrillation to become self-perpetuating and the extreme vulnerability of patients following a bout of paroxysmal atrial fibrillation to experience the arrhythmia repeatedly.

Angiotensin II. Studies have implicated angiotensin II in atrial remodeling. In the future, it may be that blockage of this enzyme will have a role in preventing shortening of the atrial effective refractory period during atrial fibrillation.[23-25]

Structural Remodeling

Structural abnormalities after conversion from chronic atrial fibrillation to sinus rhythm were found to persist longer in the canine model than electrophysiologic abnormalities and to be more of a factor in the recurrence of atrial fibrillation.[26,27]

Even to the untrained eye, Fig. 8-7 reveals the striking difference between the myocardial structure of goat atrial

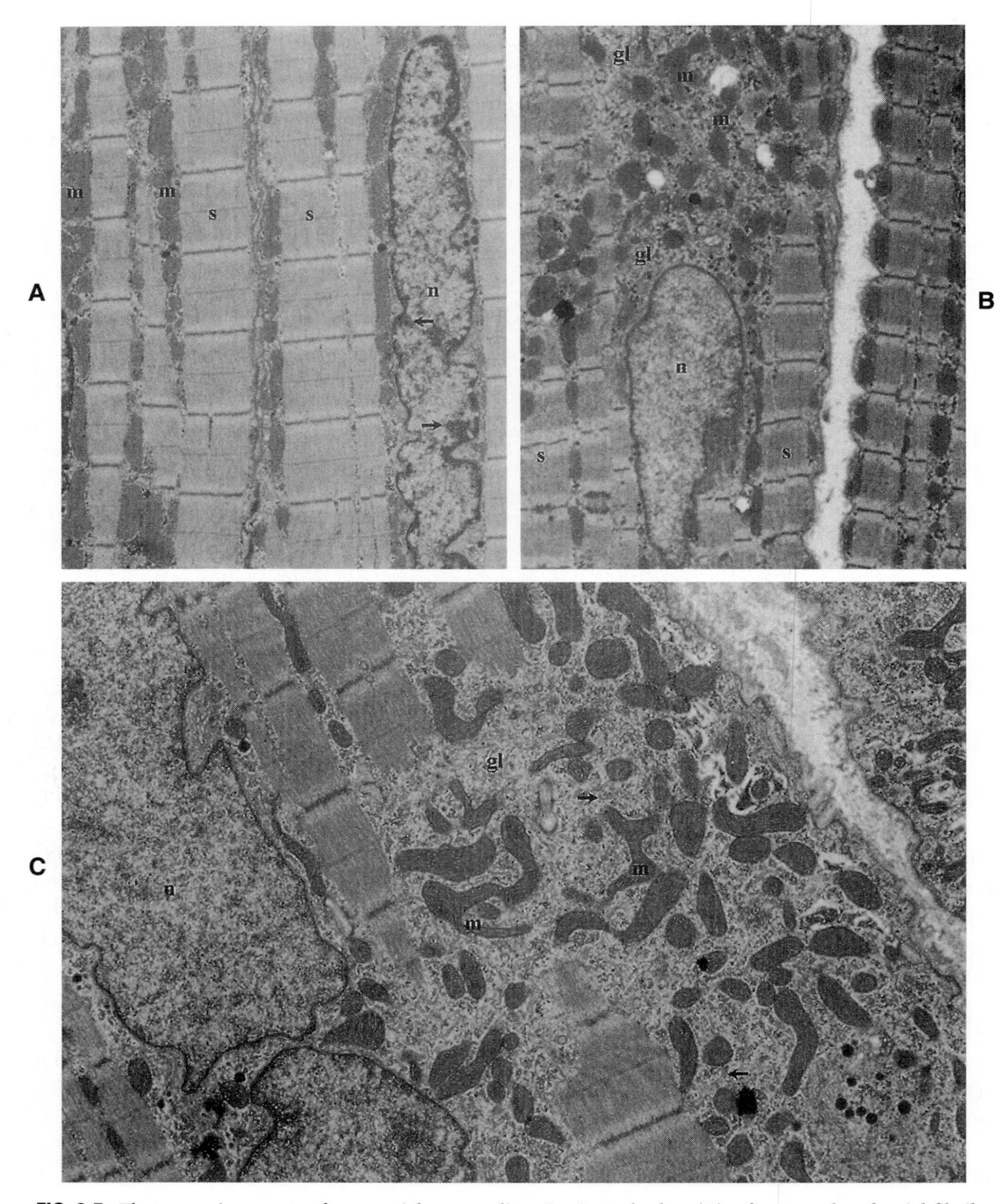

FIG. 8-7. Electron microscopy of goat atrial myocardium in sinus rhythm (**A**), after 4 weeks of atrial fibrillation (**B**), and after 16 weeks of atrial fibrillation (**C**). *Arrows* in **A** point to clustered heterochromatin; *arrows* in **C** point to remnants of sarcoplasmic reticulum. *s*, Sarcomeres; *m*, mitochondria; *n*, nucleus; *gl*, glycogen. See text for explanation. (From Thijssen VLJL, Ausma J, Liu GS et al: Structural changes of atrial myocardium during chronic atrial fibrillation, *Cardiovasc Pathol* 9:17-28, 2000.)

myocardium in sinus rhythm *(A)* compared to that after 4 weeks *(B)* and 16 weeks *(C)* of sustained atrial fibrillation, providing a strong case in favor of efforts to attempt conversion to sinus rhythm. Thijssen et al[28] describe the electron microscope findings in Fig. 8-7 as follows:

In *A*, while in sinus rhythm, the sarcomeres are regularly structured and surrounded by rows of mitochondria *(m)*. In the nucleus *(n)*, clustered heterochromatin *(arrows)* is visible at the nuclear membrane.

In *B*, after 4 weeks of atrial fibrillation, myolysis has occurred in the vicinity of the nucleus; glycogen *(gl)* is present in the myolytic area, the mitochondria are misshapen, and heterochromatin is evenly distributed throughout the nucleoplasm instead of being clustered at the nuclear membrane.

In *C*, after 16 weeks of atrial fibrillation, a myolytic area with glycogen accumulation, abnormally shaped mitochondria, and remnants of sarcoplasmic reticulum *(arrows)* can be seen; the chromatin has been dispersed in the nucleus.[28]

The Maastricht group[29] found that during chronic atrial fibrillation structural remodeling develops progressively; after 8 weeks about 40% of the atrial myocytes were affected. Other studies[30] have shown structural remodeling of the left atrial appendage in the form of dilation, stretching, reduction in pectinate muscle volume, and endocardial fibroelastosis.

Tachycardia-Related Cardiomyopathy

Poor control of the ventricular rate during atrial fibrillation ranks next to stroke as a risk to survival.[31] In addition to the structural changes sustained by the atria, a fast ventricular response during atrial fibrillation may cause extensive structural and functional damage to the ventricles resulting in cardiomyopathy.[32,33] Thus, although a patient may begin his or her history of atrial fibrillation as "lone atrial fibrillation," the damage from an uncontrolled ventricular response can soon change that classification. After the ventricular rate has been controlled, a significant number of patients show marked improvement in the ejection fraction to a value higher than 45% after ablation.[34]

Tachycardia-related ventricular dysfunction is related to the duration and rate of the tachycardia, with initial changes at rates as low as 100 beats/min.[35] Patients with a fast ventricular response to atrial fibrillation have been shown to have decreased left ventricular ejection fraction, increased end-systolic and end-diastolic volumes, and increased pulmonary artery pressures.[36]

Increase in PACs

In the canine model of atrial fibrillation, Everett et al[26] observed increases in spontaneous PAC frequency, vulnerability to induced atrial fibrillation, and gross and multiple ultrastructural anatomical changes (discussed previously).

Hypercoagulable State of Chronic Atrial Fibrillation

Three contributing factors to the persistent hypercoagulable state of chronic atrial fibrillation leading to the increased risk of thromboembolic complications in patients with chronic atrial fibrillation have been suggested. These include the following:

1. Structural remodeling in the left atrial appendage[30]
2. Blood flow stasis in the left atrial appendage
3. Elevation in lipoprotein(a)[37]

Autonomic Nervous System

In addition to the structural and electrophysiologic atrial changes that occur with the prolonged rapid rates of atrial fibrillation, a toll is also exacted from the autonomic nervous system in the form of a heterogeneous increase in atrial sympathetic innervation.[38]

CAUSES OF ATRIAL FIBRILLATION

Normal Aging Process

The normal age-related fibrotic changes in the myocardium predispose to delayed and inhomogeneous conduction, the prerequisites for atrial fibrillation. These changes begin by the third decade of life and continue into old age, with 1% of the myocardium being replaced each year by fibrous tissue when we are older than 50 years of age.[39] This eventually leads to decreased ventricular compliance, atrial dilation, and, in some individuals, a predisposition to atrial fibrillation.[40] Other nonacute factors that may be present along with the aging process to create a favorable milieu for atrial fibrillation are valvular and congenital heart disease, particularly mitral stenosis (left atrial stretch) and left ventricular hypertrophy (resulting from longstanding hypertension or hypertrophic cardiomyopathy).

Acute Causes

Exclusion of treatable underlying disease is part of the fabric of managing patients with atrial fibrillation. The acute problems that may predispose the patient to the development of atrial fibrillation are as follows[41]:

Myocardial

Infarction and ischemia
Myocarditis
Congestive heart failure
Cardiac surgery
Irritation (intracardiac catheters, pericarditis)

Pulmonary disease
- Bronchopneumonia
- Pulmonary embolus
- Chronic airflow limitation
- Carcinoma of the bronchus

Endocrine disease
- Thyrotoxicosis
- Pheochromocytoma

Metabolic disturbance and toxins
- Electrolyte imbalance
- Alcohol intake, chronic or acute, moderate to heavy
- "Recreational" drug use

Lone Atrial Fibrillation

Lone atrial fibrillation is a condition that exists in the apparent absence of identifiable causes. However, a study comparing 28 patients with lone atrial fibrillation with 14 control patients with WPW syndrome demonstrated the presence of diastolic left heart dysfunction (significantly increased early-diastolic and end-diastolic left ventricular pressure) in the patients with so-called "lone" atrial fibrillation.[42] Falk points out that lone atrial fibrillation is not really atrial fibrillation with a structurally normal heart; instead, it is atrial fibrillation with a heart that is echocardiographically normal but electrophysiologically abnormal. Although patients with lone atrial fibrillation are at a low risk for thromboembolism, the clinician should be alert to the possibility of the patient developing tachycardia-mediated cardiomyopathy.[40]

SYMPTOMS

Paroxysmal atrial fibrillation is likely to be symptomatic and frequently presents with specific symptoms, whereas permanent atrial fibrillation is usually associated with less specific symptoms.

The symptoms associated with paroxysmal atrial fibrillation are palpitations, dyspnea, chest discomfort, fatigue, dizziness, and syncope, depending on many factors, especially the cardiac status. This form of atrial fibrillation is often associated with severe dyspnea because of the abrupt reduction in cardiac output resulting from the loss of atrial kick and the uncontrolled rapid ventricular response.

Silent Atrial Fibrillation

In at least one third of patients, no obvious symptoms or noticeable degradation of quality of life are observed. This asymptomatic, or silent, atrial fibrillation is diagnosed incidentally during routine physical examinations or preoperative assessments.[31]

Cardiac Output

Atrial fibrillation usually is tolerated well after the heart rate is controlled. However, some patients show new or exacerbated symptoms of congestive heart failure because of the reduction in cardiac output associated with the arrhythmia. In patients with normal or hypertrophic left ventricles (i.e., relatively small ventricular volumes) the loss of the atrial contribution to diastolic filling ("atrial kick") may result in a 25% to 30% reduction in cardiac output, whereas with moderate to severe compromises in left ventricular function, atrial kick contributes less to ventricular filling and cardiac output. In such patients cardiac output may decrease by only 5% to 15%.

Angina

The exacerbation of angina in some patients is due to increased oxygen demand, which results from the increased heart rate.

Polyuria

In patients with paroxysmal atrial fibrillation, as in paroxysmal supraventricular tachycardia, the tachycardia may be associated with polyuria, which may be profound enough to cause hypovolemic hypotension in the period after return to sinus rhythm. Oral fluid intake and electrolyte replacement are usually enough to correct this symptom.

BEDSIDE DIAGNOSIS

Physical findings include a slight variation in the intensity of the first heart sound, absence of A waves in the jugular venous pulse, and a grossly irregular pulse. Often, with fast ventricular rates, a significant pulse deficit appears, during which the auscultated or palpated apical rate is faster than the rate palpated at the wrist (pulse deficit) because each contraction is not sufficiently strong to open the aortic valve or to transmit an arterial pressure wave through the peripheral artery.

Pulse Deficit

When comparing the apical and radial pulses there is often a discrepancy called a pulse deficit. The irregular ventricular rhythm creates different ventricular filling volumes with each cycle, which in turn result in a variation in stroke volumes. Thus the beats after the shorter cycles are not strong enough to open the aortic valve or to transmit an arterial pressure wave that can be felt at the radial pulse, but they can be heard with the stethoscope at the apex.[43] Because of this, the heart rate is best evaluated by listening for a full minute with your stethoscope at the apex. The ECG monitor measures for a few seconds and multiplies, giving you a false reading.

PHYSICAL ASSESSMENT

Physical assessment includes the following:

- Checking for thromboemboli (peripheral, coronary, pulmonary, or cerebral)
- Looking for signs of decreased cardiac output such as hypotension, a pulse deficit, signs of heart failure, and decreased cerebral oxygen supply (presyncope or syncope)

CLINICAL IMPLICATIONS

Atrial fibrillation is associated with the following clinical implications:

- A 10% to 20% reduction in cardiac output resulting from the loss of active atrial transport and the irregularity of the ventricular rhythm
- A substantial excess morbidity, decreased life expectancy,[44] and a significantly impaired quality of life. In fact, quality of life is reported to be as impaired in patients with paroxysmal atrial fibrillation as in patients with significant structural heart disease[45,46]
- A risk of thromboembolism that varies with the underlying disease[40]

Because of these facts and because after it is initiated this arrhythmia tends to recur, the primary therapeutic goal for patients with atrial fibrillation is restoration and maintenance of sinus rhythm. Once maintained, sinus rhythm increases left ventricular ejection fraction, cardiac output, and exercise capacity, while restoring physiologic rate control and improving the quality of life.

Predisposing Conditions

- Aging
- Coronary artery disease
- Congestive heart failure
- Mitral or aortic valvular disease
- Symptomatic hypertension

Fibrotic changes in the atria normally associated with aging predispose to delayed and inhomogeneous conduction, conditions that support the mechanisms of atrial fibrillation.[40]

PEDIATRICS

Atrial fibrillation in a child with a structurally normal heart is extremely rare. In children with WPW syndrome, atrial fibrillation is a possibility. If the refractory period of the accessory pathway is short, the risk of sudden death is the same as for the adult with this condition. When seen in an infant or child, atrial fibrillation is often associated with a structural heart abnormality, particularly after surgical repair of congenital heart disease.[47]

COMPLICATIONS

The major complication of atrial fibrillation is of course thromboemboli. Other situations promoting atrial fibrillation are WPW syndrome, myocardial infarction (MI), and cardiac surgery.

Stroke

Stroke is a potentially devastating complication of atrial fibrillation, with stroke rates increasing with age.[48] During atrial fibrillation, thrombi may form inside the left atrial appendage. When the thrombus embolizes, it may lodge in the brain, causing a "stroke," which often leaves the patient suddenly and severely disabled.

Numerous randomized controlled trials of warfarin have conclusively demonstrated that long-term, well-controlled anticoagulation therapy can safely reduce the risk of stroke by approximately 68% per year in patients with nonvalvular atrial fibrillation, and even more in patients with valvular atrial fibrillation.[49] Because the risk of hemorrhage increases with the intensity of anticoagulation, the international normalized ratio (INR) is maintained between 2.0 and 3.0. At lower levels anticoagulation is less effective and at higher levels the risk of hemorrhage rises rapidly (INR > 4.0 to 5.0).[50,51]

WPW Syndrome

Atrial fibrillation with conduction over an accessory pathway seriously complicates the occurrence of atrial fibrillation. This is the case when the accessory pathway has a short anterograde refractory period. The life-threatening character of this arrhythmia is recognized because of a broad QRS tachycardia and a very fast irregular rhythm (Fig. 8-8). It is the second most common arrhythmia in patients with WPW syndrome. Without knowledgeable emergency intervention, this rapid rhythm may deteriorate into ventricular fibrillation. The mechanism, ECG recognition, emergency treatment, and cure of this life-threatening arrhythmia are covered in Chapter 21.

Atrial Fibrillation in Acute MI

Atrial fibrillation after the first 24 hours. Atrial fibrillation occurs in approximately 20% of cases after the first 24 hours of the onset of MI as a result of either pericarditis or heart failure and carries with it a worse prognosis than patients who were admitted with the arrhythmia already present.[52]

In the elderly. Atrial fibrillation is a common complication of acute MI in elderly patients and independently

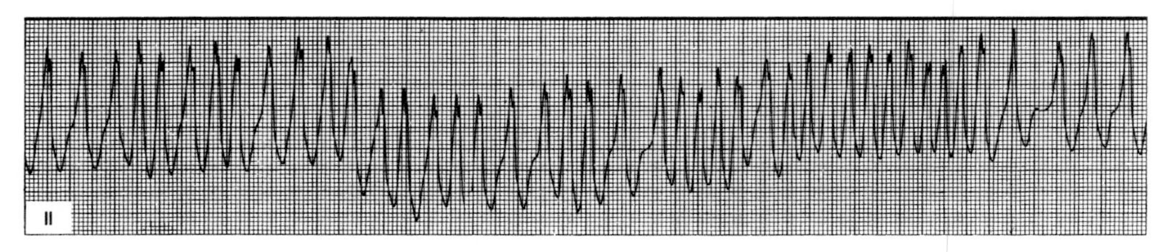

FIG. 8-8. Atrial fibrillation with conduction over an accessory pathway with a short refractory period. Note the diagnostic features of this arrhythmia: fast ventricular rate greater than 300 beats/min; broad QRS; irregular rhythm. (From Goldberger AL, Goldberger E: *Clinical electrocardiography*, ed 5, St Louis, 1994, Mosby.)

influences mortality, particularly when it develops during hospitalization. Rathore et al[53] evaluated 106,780 patients who were 65 years old or more and being treated for acute MI and found that medical therapies are currently being underused in the treatment of female, black, and poor patients.

In the emergency department. It is common for patients with atrial fibrillation to present in the emergency department with chest pain and ST segment depression. However, such symptoms have limited power in predicting the presence of MI. ECG evidence of ST segment elevation or depression of more than 2 mm appears to be a reliable discriminator of which patient presenting in the emergency department with a diagnosis of atrial fibrillation is at risk for MI (sensitivity of 100% and a specificity of 99%).[54]

Possible mechanisms of atrial fibrillation in MI. Atrial fibrillation in the early hours after the infarction is rare and is thought to be the result of impaired left atrial perfusion secondary to coexistent occlusion of the proximal left circumflex artery and the AV nodal artery.[52]

In patients with inferior and right ventricular MI one of the possible mechanisms related to atrial fibrillation is an increase in right atrial pressure associated with atrial distention.[55]

In patients with acute Q wave anterior infarction, one possible mechanism is the increase in atrial pressure resulting from hemodynamic changes caused by more extensive myocardial damage.[56]

Atrial Fibrillation after Cardiac Surgery

Atrial fibrillation is a common arrhythmia after cardiac surgery; it occurs in at least 25% to 30% of patients after coronary artery bypass grafting and in 60% of patients after valvular surgery, usually appearing on the second or third postoperative day. Additionally, postdischarge recurrences of atrial fibrillation are frequent during the first postoperative month.

The main independent predictor of postoperative atrial fibrillation is reported to be cardiopulmonary bypass with cardioplegic arrest.[57,58]

Conversion to Class IC Atrial Flutter

Fig. 8-9 is a rhythm strip showing atrial flutter in a patient who was admitted in atrial fibrillation and later converted to atrial flutter. It is known that atrial fibrillation may convert to or recur as atrial flutter in some patients who are taking class IC antiarrhythmic drugs, such as flecainide (Tambocor), propafenone (Rythmol), or amiodarone (Cordarone).[59] This patient was taking only propranolol for rate control.

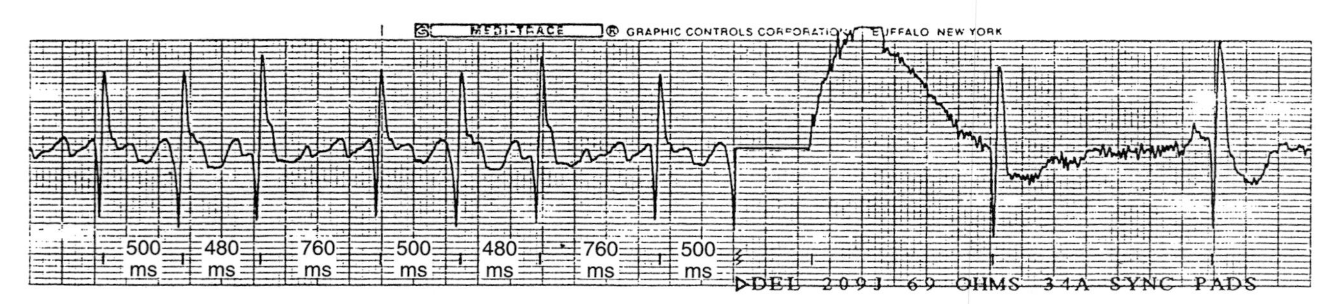

FIG. 8-9. Lead II showing atrial flutter with 4:3 Wenckebach conduction. The patient was admitted with atrial fibrillation with propranolol for rate control. The rhythm subsequently converted to atrial flutter with Wenckebach conduction (note the group beating). You will note that because the atrial flutter was not recognized, 209 J was used for cardioversion.

Mechanism. In addition to suppressing excitability, class IC antiarrhythmic drugs depress conduction velocity and cause rate-dependent prolongation of the atrial refractory period, the combination of which causes atrial fibrillatory wavelengths to prolong, setting the stage for the development of the right atrial macroreentrant circuit that causes atrial flutter[60] (illustrated and discussed in Chapter 9). It may do this by preventing the formation of the little wavelets that peel off from the larger "mother" wave during atrial fibrillation (Fig. 8-6), causing the smaller wavelets to decrease in number while increasing in size,[59] or widening the temporal excitable gap.[61] Either scenario may result in the well-known single macroreentrant circuit of atrial flutter.

On the other hand, class IC drugs and amiodarone may also terminate or prevent atrial fibrillation by blocking conduction within the atria, thereby preventing reentry circuits from developing.

When atrial fibrillation converts to atrial flutter, the atrial rate slows to 300 beats/min or less and becomes organized. Concealed conduction is no longer as prominent in determining AV conduction and the ventricular rate can increase depending on the AV conduction ratio (e.g., 2:1; 1:1; Wenckeback).

Warning. Drugs that keep the ventricular rate under control during atrial fibrillation may become less effective during atrial flutter because of the absence of concealed conduction. Thus a ventricular rate of 80 beats/min during atrial fibrillation may suddenly accelerate to 150 beats/min during atrial flutter.

Digitalis Toxicity

The ECG signs of digitalis toxicity in patients with atrial fibrillation include regularization or group beating of the ventricular rhythm. When not recognized and treated, the mortality rate with such rhythms is 100%. The mechanism, ECG recognition, clinical implications, and emergency treatment of digitalis toxicity are illustrated and discussed in detail in Chapter 15.

TREATMENT

Delay in converting atrial fibrillation to sinus rhythm results in damage to the atria (atrial remodeling) and affects the patient's future exposure to this arrhythmia, possibly accelerating the progression to permanent atrial fibrillation. On the other hand, speedy conversion to sinus rhythm may slow down this debilitating process. Dittrich et al[62] report that the longer the duration of atrial fibrillation before conversion, the higher the recurrence rate.

The acute treatment of atrial fibrillation includes control of rate, prevention of thromboembolism, restoration and maintenance of sinus rhythm, and treatment of underlying cardiac disease.

Antiarrhythmic agents terminate atrial fibrillation either by slowing conduction or by lengthening the atrial refractory period. The risks and benefits of each treatment modality are assessed according to the individual patient's circumstances. Unlike other arrhythmias, there is still no uniformly highly successful therapy for treating atrial fibrillation and the response to treatment seems to vary among patients. However, significant advances are being made using nonpharmacologic approaches to cure this troublesome arrhythmia.

Rate Control

Patients with hemodynamic instability require urgent direct current (DC) cardioversion. In patients who are stable, intravenous calcium antagonists or beta blockers slow the heart rate by 25% within 3 to 7 minutes of administration, relieving symptoms.[63] This being said, another consideration may enter into the decision regarding drug choice for ventricular rate control. It is that of the cellular effect of the drug on the atria itself. Duytschaever et al[64] have concluded from studies on goats with paroxysmal atrial fibrillation, that *verapamil has a proarrhythmic effect* on atrial fibrillation because it shortens the atrial cycle length and atrial refractory period, causing the paroxysm to last longer, and lessening the chances for spontaneous conversion and the efficacy of chemical cardioversion. In their goat model, verapamil exerted a marked proarrhythmic effect converting paroxysmal atrial fibrillation (type I) into sustained atrial fibrillation (type III).

Why not digoxin? Digitalis, even after intravenous administration, will take several hours to take effect. Then, even after reaching the desired blood level, it may not be enough to control the ventricular rate during exercise because increased sympathetic tone and reduced vagal tone overcome its effects.[65,66]

Although the effects of digoxin on the course of atrial fibrillation are controversial,[67,68] its potential proarrhythmic effects are specific and there are clinical indications that digoxin may cause a recurrence of atrial fibrillation.[69]

It is precisely the desired therapeutic effects of digoxin (inotropy and AV block) that turn against it in the treatment of atrial fibrillation. The inotropic effect of digoxin is achieved by an increase of intracellular calcium; AV block is accomplished by its parasympathetic effect. Likewise, atrial fibrillation itself causes intracellular calcium overload and shortening of the atrial action potential duration by its parasympathetic effect.[70,71] Thus the damaging electrical remodeling of myocardial cells seen in atrial fibrillation are compounded by the effects of digoxin,[72] potentially increasing the difficulty of converting to and maintaining sinus rhythm.

Other disadvantages of digoxin are its narrow therapeutic window and the possibility of toxic effects preceding the desired therapeutic effect, especially in the elderly.[73] The significant disadvantages just listed have led some to conclude that emergency use of intravenous digoxin for ventricular rate control in atrial fibrillation or atrial flutter is rarely indicated, even after decades of use for this purpose.[74] However, when left ventricular function is impaired, digoxin remains the drug of choice for rate control.

Warning. Digoxin, as with calcium channel blockers, is not given for atrial fibrillation in patients with accessory pathways (WPW syndrome). In 30% of patients digoxin shortens the refractory period of the accessory pathway, causing the ventricular rate to accelerate.[75,76]

Conversion to Sinus Rhythm

Persistent atrial fibrillation requires cardioversion to restore sinus rhythm.

Paroxysmal atrial fibrillation converts to sinus rhythm spontaneously without intervention. However, because it may take hours to do this, early pharmacologic conversion may be desirable (because of the inevitability of electrical and structural remodeling, even after short atrial fibrillation times). Table 8-1 supplies information about the class I and III agents used for acute cardioversion of paroxysmal atrial fibrillation. The Vaughn Williams classification of antiarrhythmic agents is displayed in Box 8-1.

BOX 8-1. Vaughn Williams Classification of Antiarrhythmic Agents

CLASS IA (QUINIDINE, PROCAINAMIDE, DISOPYRAMIDE, AMIODARONE, IMIPRAMINE)
Sodium channel blockade (moderate)
Decreases conduction velocity
Prolongs repolarization (QT interval)

CLASS IB (LIDOCAINE, MEXILETINE, TOCAINIDE, PHENYTOIN)
Sodium channel blockade (mild)
Decreases conduction velocity
Shortens repolarization

CLASS IC (FLECAINIDE, ENCAINIDE, PROPAFENONE)
Sodium channel blockade (marked)
Decreases conduction velocity

CLASS II (PROPRANOLOL, ESMOLOL, SOTALOL, AMIODARONE)
Beta adrenergic blockade

CLASS III (BRETYLIUM, SOTALOL, AMIODARONE)
Potassium channel blockade
Prolongs repolarization

CLASS IV (VERAPAMIL, DILTIAZEM, AMIODARONE)
Calcium channel blockade

Carotid Sinus Massage

Alterations in vagal tone can influence the atrial fibrillatory process by changing the atrial refractory period. Kirchhof et al[2] observed in a patient with paroxysmal atrial fibrillation that carotid sinus massage changed the fibrillatory line from coarse to fine, upon which the arrhythmia converted to sinus rhythm. They concluded that before other interventions, carotid sinus massage is worth a try.

Maintenance of Sinus Rhythm

After sinus rhythm is restored, drug choices are made on an individual basis and always with the approval of a cardiologist. Roy et al[77] found amiodarone to be more effective than sotalol or propafenone for the prevention of recurrences of atrial fibrillation.

Fig. 8-10 presents one approach to maintaining sinus rhythm. In permanent atrial fibrillation the drugs listed are of course for rate control and their choice is guided by the clinical setting (Box 8-2). In *structurally normal hearts,*

BOX 8-2. Approach to Ventricular Rate Control in Permanent Atrial Fibrillation

I. **Heart rate goal**
   A. Resting (apical) heart rate ≤80 beats/min
   B. Ambulatory ECG: ambulatory heart rate ≤90 beats/min for all hours (mean hourly heart rate)
   C. If exercise testing is available, exercise duration and time-to-target heart rate are considered; peak heart rate 20% less than age-predicted
II. **Recommended sequence of drug selection for rate control**
   A. No structural heart disease
      1. Diltiazem, mibefradil, or verapamil
      2. Beta blockers
   B. Ischemic heart disease, LVEF ≥40%
      1. Beta blockers
      2. Diltiazem, mibefradil, or verapamil
   C. LV dysfunction, LVEF <40%, and/or clinical heart failure
      1. Digoxin
      2. Mibefradil

From Pratt CM: Impact of managed care on the treatment of atrial fibrillation, *Am J Cardiol* 81(5A):30C-34C, 1998.

ECG, Electrocardiogram; *LVEF,* left ventricular ejection fraction.

TABLE 8-1 Agents for Acute Cardioversion

	Dosing	Maintenance	Peak Concentration	Steady State	Half-life	Rate of Elimination	Active Metabolite	Comments
Quinidine sulfate	PO: 300-600 mg single oral dosing	200-400 mg every 6 hr (20 mg/kg/day)	1-3 hr	1-1.5 days	Elimination in 6-7 hr	Hepatic (50%-90%), renal (10%-30%)	3-OH-quinidine, 2-O-quinidine	GI effects (diarrhea); drug interactions (digoxin, warfarin, fl-blockers, amiodarone, cimetidine)
Procainamide	IV: 5-15 mg/kg at 0.2-0.4 mg/kg/min over 10-15 min (maximum: 1000 mg)	IV: 2-6 mg/min	PO: 1-2 hr IV: 15-60 min	12 hr	3-4 hr	Hepatic (40%-70%); renal (30%-60%)	N-acetyl-procainamide	GI effect (nausea) IV: hypotension
Flecainide	PO: 50-150 mg 3 times/day; IV: (not available in the United States) 2 mg/kg over 10 min (bolus)	PO: 100-200 mg/day in divided doses	PO: 3 hr	PO: 2-3 days	16-20 hr	Hepatic (70%); renal (25%)	Meta-O-de alkylated flecainide; meta-O-dealkylated lactam of flecainide	IV: hypotension, proarrhythmia
Propafenone	PO: 150-300 mg 3 times/day; IV: (not available in the United States) 2 mg/kg over 10 min (bolus)	PO: 450-900 mg/day in 3 divided doses	PO: 2-3 hr	PO: 1-1.5 days	2-10 hr (10-30 hr for poor metabolizers)	Hepatic (90%)	5-OH-propafenone	GI effects, proarrhythmia
Amiodarone	IV: 150 mg over 10-30 min	IV: 1 mg/min (6 hr, 0.5 mg/min	1-3 hr	NA	Acute 3-21 hr	Hepatic	Mono-N-desethylami-odarone; Bis-N-desethylami-odarone	IV: hypotension, bradycardia Drug interactions: warfarin, digoxin, procainamide, quinidine, flecainide, flecainide, phenytoin
Ibutilide	IV: 1 mg over 30 min; may repeat once 10 min after initial infusion is complete if arrhythmia persists (<60 lb, 0.1 mL/kg)	NA	Rapidly distributed, effect within 1 hour	NA	6 hr	Renal (82%)	Hydroxy-ibultide	Proarrhythmia

From Kowey PR, Marinchak RA, Rials SJ et al: Acute treatment of atrial fibrillation, *Am J Cardiol* 81:16C-22C, 1998, p. 19C.
PO, By mouth; *GI*, gastrointestinal; *IV*, intravaneous; *NA*, not applicable.

class IC antiarrhythmic drugs are least proarrhythmic and least organ toxic. Other considerations are class III drugs.[78-80] In *hypertrophied hearts*, the risk of torsade de pointes with class III and IA agents is enhanced. In hearts damaged by *ischemia, fibrosis*, or *infiltration*, class I agents are associated with an enhanced risk of arrhythmias.[81]

External Electrical Cardioversion for Atrial Fibrillation

More than 25 years ago Warner et al[82] submitted that the severity of the cardiac dysfunction caused by the delivery of electrical energy to the heart is related to the magnitude of the current. Although external electrical cardioversion has been deemed safe and effective for terminating atrial fibrillation, it takes its own significant toll on the heart, causing membrane damage similar to ischemic injury.[83,84]

Electrical cardioversion inhibits membrane activity of Na, K-ATPase, the enzyme that establishes and maintains cellular transmembrane sodium and potassium gradients and plays a crucial role in the regulation of cardiac contractility and excitability, as well as being the site for digitalis binding. Its inhibition could result in the disruption of ionic balance in ventricular myocardial cells.[85] Ionic imbalance in turn creates a hot bed for ectopic activity and a suitably unstable milieu for atrial fibrillation. New drugs for the conversion of atrial fibrillation should relieve the necessity to inflict this type of membrane damage on a heart already compromised by the arrhythmia.

Biphasic Defibrillation

Studies have demonstrated a superior efficacy of biphasic waveforms as compared with monophasic waveforms for transthoracic ventricular defibrillation and cardioversion of atrial fibrillation in humans,[86,87] particularly in patients with high transthoracic impedance. Biphasic shocks have been shown to defibrillate with nearly 68% less current than conventional monophasic waveforms[88,89] and have demonstrated improved outcomes and reduction in postshock dysfunction, cellular injury, recovery time, and skin burns.[90-94]

Surgery

Given the random multiple-reentrant wavelets that sustain atrial fibrillation, Cox et al[95] demonstrated that surgical atrial compartmentalization can cure atrial fibrillation. *The Cox maze procedure* involves critically applied linear incisions in both atria and bilateral atrial appendectomy.[96,97] The scars created by the incisions plus the reduced mass of atrial tissue created by the amputation of the atrial appendages, prevents the formation of the critical number of reentry wavelets (more than 3) necessary for stable atrial fibrillation. The maze procedure was first performed in 1987. Since then many patients have undergone the operation for the treatment of atrial fibrillation. The

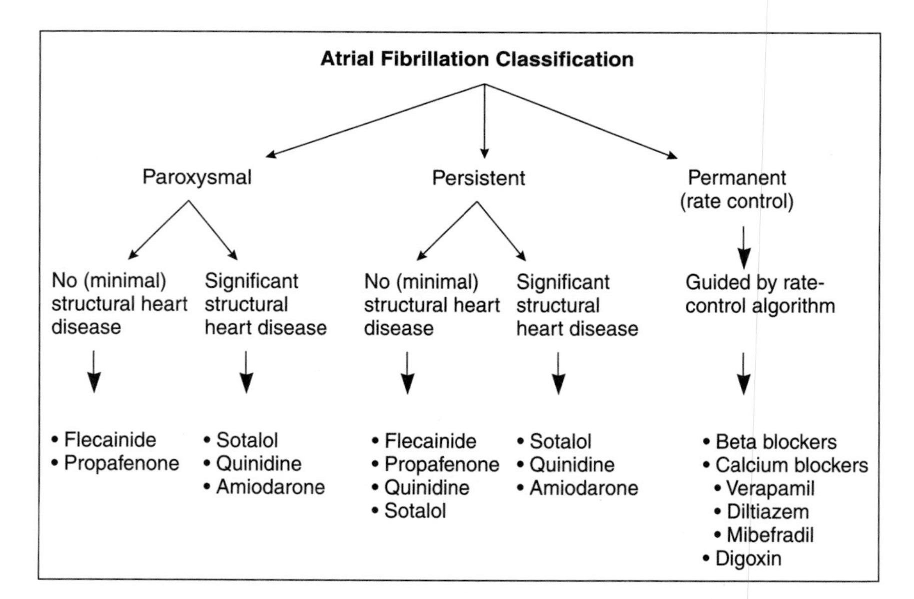

FIG. 8-10. Selection of antiarrhythmic therapy. This algorithm focuses on preferred choices; other antiarrhythmic drugs are occasionally selected. (From Pratt CM: Impact of managed care on the treatment of atrial fibrillation, *Am J Cardiol* 81[5A]:30C-34C, 1998.)

initial open heart operation performed through a median sternotomy has been modified (Maze-III procedure) so that it can be done by minimally invasive techniques without the use of cardiopulmonary bypass.[98] The Mayo Clinic experience with the maze procedure reports 90% of patients operated for atrial fibrillation are restored to sinus rhythm, thereby abolishing symptoms and reducing risks of thromboembolism and anticoagulant-associated hemorrhage.[99]

Disadvantages of the Cox maze procedure are long procedure time, impaired atrial function, and postoperative bleeding.

Catheter Techniques

Transcutaneous catheter techniques using radiofrequency energy to replicate the maze procedure have been proposed.[100-102] Although moderately successful in preventing atrial fibrillation, this approach carries with it the possibility of serious complications, such as cerebrovascular accidents resulting from thromboembolism from the burned myocardium, cardiac tamponade, impaired atrial contractility because of loss of atrial myocardial mass, loss of atrial rhythm, regional delays in atrial activation, and splinting of the atria by scarring.[103] Technical difficulties with this technique include catheter instability, accessibility of a continuous line with the atria, and a mapping technique to validate that the radiofrequency lesion is unbroken.

A more successful catheter technique is that used to ablate the right atrial isthmus in patients who developed fibrillation secondary to atrial flutter.[39]

Focal Radiofrequency Ablation

Catheter mapping in patients with paroxysmal atrial fibrillation has revealed atrial foci that can trigger the onset of the arrhythmia. Ablation of foci originating from the pulmonary veins has been reported first by Haïssaguerre[104] and then replicated by that group and others.[8,105-109] Preliminary reports have demonstrated that mapping and radiofrequency ablation of pulmonary vein ectopy initiating atrial fibrillation is feasible using new mapping techniques.[108,110,111] Ablatable foci may also be present in the right atrium and within the muscle fibers around the superior vena cava.[112] Although such procedures are still in their infancy, they do hold hope for a safe and reproducible cure.

Risks. Multiple radiofrequency applications inside the ostia of the pulmonary veins can lead to severe pulmonary venous stenosis and a venoocclusive pulmonary syndrome,[113-115] especially when a distal ablation site has been targeted (as opposed to the ostium). Reported incidence of stenosis ranges from as high as 42% in one group[8] to as low as 2.7% in another.[116] The resultant pulmonary venous occlusion can be severe.

Other possible serious complications include thromboembolism, air embolism, hemopericardium, and possible damage to adjacent structures, such as bronchioles, the right pulmonary artery, and lung tissue, and eventual recurrence of the atrial fibrillation.

Circumferential Radiofrequency Ablation of Pulmonary Vein Orifices

Ablation of the earliest site initiating atrial fibrillation is dependent on successful mapping and identification of the precise target. When this focus is elusive, complete electrical isolation of the pulmonary veins with multiple radiofrequency lesions has been used as an alternative technique.[117]

One disadvantage of this approach is the time required to make circular lesions with the catheters currently in use.[39]

SUMMARY

Atrial fibrillation in its uncomplicated form is recognized on the ECG because of absence of P waves, narrow QRS complexes, and an irregular ventricular response. The failure of the atria to pump results in a drop in cardiac output up to 20%, a tendency to develop thromboembolism, and an increased mortality rate. Atrial fibrillation may be paroxysmal, persistent, or permanent. Treatment of the persistent or permanent atrial types includes antithrombotic therapy, ventricular rate control, and attempts to convert to normal sinus rhythm.

Abnormal ventricular responses to atrial fibrillation are those that are too fast and too broad (WPW syndrome), regular (AV block or drug toxicity), or in groups (drug toxicity).

REFERENCES

1. Alpert JS: Atrial fibrillation: a growth industry in the 21st century, *Eur Heart J* 21:1207, 2000.
2. Kirchhof CJ, Gorgels AP, Wellens HJ: Carotid sinus massage as a diagnostic and therapeutic tool for atrial flutter-fibrillation, *Pacing Clin Electrophysiol* 21:1319, 1998.
3. Moe GK: On the multiple wavelet hypothesis of atrial fibrillation, *Arch Int Pharmacodyn Ther* 140:183, 1962.
4. Allessie MA, Lammers WJEP, Bonke FIM, Hollen J: Experimental evaluation of Moe's multiple wavelet hypothesis of atrial fibrillation. In Zipes DP, Jalife J, editors: *Cardiac arrhythmias*, New York, 1985, Grune & Stratton, pp 265-276.
5. Konings KTS, Kirchhof CJHJ, Smeets JRLM et al: High density mapping of electrically induced atrial fibrillation in man, *Circulation* 89:1665, 1994.
6. Nathan H, Eliakim M: The junction between the left atrium and the pulmonary veins: an anatomic study of human hearts, *Circulation* 34:412-422, 1966.

7. Jaïs P, Haïssaguerre M, Shah DC et al: A focal source of atrial fibrillation treated by discrete radiofrequency ablation, *Circulation* 95:572, 1997.
8. Chen SA, Chen YC, Yeh HI et al: Electrophysiology and arrhythmogenic activity of single cardiomyocytes from canine superior vena cava, *Circulation* 105:2679-2685, 2002.
9. Jaïs P, Shah DC, Haïssaguerre M et al: Atrial fibrillation: role of arrhythmogenic foci, *J Interv Card Electrophysiol* 1:29, 2000.
10. Haïssaguerre M, Marcus FI, Fischer B et al: Atrial fibrillation: report of three cases, *J Cardiovasc Electrophysiol* 5:743, 1994.
11. Chen SA; Tai CT; Tsai CF et al: Radiofrequency catheter ablation of atrial fibrillation initiated by spontaneous ectopic beats, *Curr Cardiol Rep* 2:322, 2000.
12. Coumel P, Attuel P, Leclercq JF: Arrhythmies auriculaires d'origine vagale ou catécholergique: effects comparé du traitment bêta-bloquer et phénomènes d'échappement. *Arch Mal Coeur Vaiss* 75:373, 1982.
13. Schauerte P, Scherlag BJ, Pitha J et al: Catheter ablation of cardiac autonomic nerves for prevention of vagal atrial fibrillation. *Circulation* 102:2774, 2000.
14. Coumel P: Clinical approach to paroxysmal atrial fibrillation, *Clin Cardiol* 13:209, 1990.
15. Allessie M, Konings K, Wijffels M: Electrophysiological mechanism of atrial fibrillation. In DiMarco JP, Prystowsky EN, editors: *Atrial arrhythmias: state of the art*, Armonk, NY, Futura Publishing, 1995, pp. 155-161.
16. Daoud EG, Bogun F, Goyal R et al: Effect of atrial fibrillation on atrial refractoriness in humans, *Circulation* 94:1600, 1996.
17. Osaka T, Itoh A, Kodama I: Action potential remodeling in the human right atrium with chronic lone atrial fibrillation, *Pacing Clin Electrophysiol* 23:960, 2000.
18. Goette A, Honeycutt C, Langberg JJ: Electrical remodeling in atrial fibrillation: time course and mechanisms, *Circulation* 94:2968, 1996.
19. Wijffels MCEF, Kirchoff CJHJ, Dorland R, Allessie MA: Atrial fibrillation begets atrial fibrillation: a study in awake chronically instrumented goats, *Circulation* 92:1954, 1995.
20. Yue L, Feng J, Gaspo R et al: Ionic remodeling underlying action potential changes in a canine model of atrial fibrillation, *Circ Res* 81:512, 1997.
21. Brandt MC, Priebe L, Bohle T et al: The ultrarapid and the transient outward K(+) current in human atrial fibrillation. Their possible role in postoperative atrial fibrillation, *J Mol Cell Cardiol* 32:1885, 2000.
22. Barbey O, Pierre S, Duran MJ et al: Specific up-regulation of mitochondrial F0F1-ATPase activity after short episodes of atrial fibrillation in sheep, *J Cardiovasc Electrophysiol* 11:432, 2000.
23. Nakashima H, Kumagai K, Urata H et al: Angiotensin II antagonist prevents electrical remodeling in atrial fibrillation, *Circulation* 101:2612, 2000.
24. Goette A, Arndt M, Rocken C et al: Regulation of angiotensin II receptor subtypes during atrial fibrillation in humans, *Circulation* 101:2678, 2000.
25. Goette A, Staack T, Rocken C et al: Regulation of angiotensin II receptor subtypes during atrial fibrillation, *J Am Coll Cardiol* 35:1669, 2000.
26. Everett TH 4th, Li H, Mangrum JM et al: Electrical, morphological, and ultrastructural remodeling and reverse remodeling in a canine model of chronic atrial fibrillation, *Circulation* 102:1454, 2000.
27. Hobbs WJ, Fynn S, Todd DM et al: Reversal of atrial electrical remodeling after cardioversion of persistent atrial fibrillation in humans, *Circulation* 101:1145, 2000.
28. Thijssen VLJL, Ausma J, Liu GS et al: Structural changes of atrial myocardium during chronic atrial fibrillation, *Cardiovasc Pathol* 9:17, 2000.
29. Ausma J, Coumans WA, Duimel H et al: Atrial high energy phosphate content and mitochondrial enzyme activity during chronic atrial fibrillation, *Cardiovasc Res* 47:788, 2000.
30. Shirani J, Alaeddini J: Structural remodeling of the left atrial appendage in patients with chronic non-valvular atrial fibrillation: implications for thrombus formation, systemic embolism, and assessment by transesophageal echocardiography, *Cardiovasc Pathol* 9:95, 2000.
31. Savelieva I, Camm AJ: Clinical relevance of silent atrial fibrillation: prevalence, prognosis, quality of life, and management, *J Interv Card Electrophysiol* 4:369, 2000.
32. Fenelon G, Wijns W, Andries E, Brugada P: Tachycardiomyopathy: mechanisms and clinical implications, *Pacing Clin Electrophysiol* 19:95, 1996.
33. Shingane JS, Wood MA, Jensen DN et al: Tachycardia-induced cardiomyopathy: a review of animal models and clinical studies, *J Am Coll Cardiol* 29:709, 1997.
34. Redfield MM, Kay GN, Jenkins LS et al: Tachycardia-related cardiomyopathy: a common cause of ventricular dysfunction in patients with atrial fibrillation referred for atrioventricular ablation, *Mayo Clin Proc* 75:790, 2000.
35. Van Gelder IC, Crijns JH, Blanksma PK: Time course of hemodynamic changes and improvement of exercise tolerance after cardioversion of chronic atrial fibrillation unassociated with cardiac valve disease, *Am J Cardiol* 72:560, 1993.
36. Schumacher B, L¸deritz B: Rate issues in atrial fibrillation: consequences of tachycardia and therapy for rate control, *Am J Cardiol* 82:29N, 1998.
37. Igarashi Y, Kasai H, Yamashita F et al: Lipoprotein(a), left atrial appendage function and thromboembolic risk in patients with chronic nonvalvular atrial fibrillation, *Jpn Circ J* 64:93, 2000.
38. Jayachandran JV, Sih HJ, Winkle W et al: Atrial fibrillation produced by prolonged rapid atrial pacing is associated with heterogeneous changes in atrial sympathetic innervation, *Circulation* 101:1185, 2000.
39. Wellens HJJ: Pulmonary vein ablation in atrial fibrillation. Hype or Hope? *Circulation* 102:2562, 2000.
40. Falk RH: Etiology and complications of atrial fibrillation: insights from pathology studies, *Am J Cardiol* 182:10N, 998.
41. Waktare JEP, Camm AJ: Acute treatment of atrial fibrillation: why and when to maintain sinus rhythm, *Am J Cardiol* 81:3C, 1998.
42. Jaïs P, Peng JT, Shah DC et al: Left ventricular diastolic dysfunction in patients with so-called lone atrial fibrillation, *J Cardiovasc Electrophysiol* 11:623, 2000.
43. Zipes DP: Specific arrhythmias: diagnosis and treatment. In Braunwald E, editor: *Heart disease*, ed 4, Philadelphia, 1992, WB Saunders.
44. Benjamin EJ, Wolf PA, D'Agostino RB et al: Impact of atrial fibrillation on the risk of death. The Framingham heart study, *Circulation* 98:946, 1998.
45. Dorian P, Jung W, Newman D et al: The impairment of health-related quality of life in patients with intermittent atrial fibrillation: implications for the assessment of investigational therapy, *J Am Coll Cardiol* 36:1303, 2000.
46. Paquette M, Roy D, Talajic M et al: Role of health-related quality of life in intermittent atrial fibrillation, *Am J Cardiol* 86:764, 2000.
47. Zachary CH, Cyran SE: Spontaneous-onset atrial fibrillation in a toddler with review of mechanisms and etiologies, *Clin Pediatr* 39:453, 2000.

48. Frost L, Engholm G, Johnsen S et al: Incident stroke after discharge from the hospital with a diagnosis of atrial fibrillation, *Am J Med* 108:36, 2000.
49. Bungard TJ, Ghali WA, Teo KK et al: Why do patients with atrial fibrillation not receive warfarin? *Arch Intern Med* 160:41, 2000.
50. Hylek EM, Skates SJ, Sheehan MA, Singer DE: An analysis of the lowest effective intensity of prophylactic anticoagulation for patients with nonrheumatic atrial fibrillation, *N Engl J Med* 335:540, 1996.
51. Singer DE: Anticoagulation to prevent stroke in atrial fibrillation and its implications for managed care, *Am J Cardiol* 81:35C, 1998.
52. Hod H, Lew AS, Keltai M et al: Early atrial fibrillation during evolving myocardial infarction: a consequence of impaired left atrial perfusion, *Circulation* 75:146, 1987.
53. Rathore SS, Berger AK, Weinfurt KP et al: Acute myocardial infarction complicated by atrial fibrillation in the elderly: prevalence and outcomes, *Circulation* 101:969, 2000.
54. Zimetbaum PJ, Josephson ME, McDonald MJ et al: Incidence and predictors of myocardial infarction among patients with atrial fibrillation, *J Am Coll Cardiol* 36:1223, 2000.
55. Sugiura T, Iwasaka T, Takahashi N et al: Atrial fibrillation in inferior wall Q-wave acute myocardial infarction, *Am J Cardiol* 67:1135, 1991.
56. Sugiura T, Iwasaka T, Takahashi N et al: Factors assocated with atrial fibrillation in Q-wave acute myocardial infarction, *Am Heart J* 121:1409, 1991.
57. Ascione R, Caputo M, Calori G et al: Predictors of atrial fibrillation after conventional and beating heart coronary surgery: a prospective, randomized study, *Circulation* 102:1530, 2000.
58. Hogue CW Jr, Hyder ML: Atrial fibrillation after cardiac operation: risks mechanisms, and treatment, *Ann Thorac Surg* 69:300, 2000.
59. Nabar A, Rodriquez LM, Timmermans C et al: Radiofrequency ablation of "class IC atrial flutter" in patients with resistant atrial fibrillation, *Am J Cardiol* 83:785, 1999.
60. Cryns HJGM: Clinical manifestations of use-and reverse-use dependence. In Crijns HJGM, editor: *Changes of intracardiac conduction induced by antiarrhythmic drugs: importance of use- and reverse use-dependence.* The Netherlands, 1993, Groningen Knoop, pp. 38-105.
61. Wijffels MC, Dorland R, Mast F, Allessie MA: Widening of the excitable gap during pharmacological cardioversion of atrial fibrillation in the goat: effects of cibenzoline, hydroquinidine, flecainide, and d-sotalol, *Circulation* 102:260, 2000.
62. Dittrich HC, Erickson JS, Schneiderman T et al: Echocardiographic and clinical predictors for outcome of elective cardioversion of atrial fibrillation, *Am J Cardiol* 63:193, 1989.
63. Naccarelli GV, Dell'Orfano JT, Wolbrette DL et al: Cost-effective management of acute atrial fibrillation: role of rate control, spontaneous conversion, medical and direct current cardioversion, transesophageal echocardiography, and antiembolic therapy, *Am J Cardiol* 85(10 Suppl 1):36D, 2000.
64. Duytschaever MF, Garratt CJ, Allessie MA: Profibrillatory effects of verapamil but not of digoxin in the goat model of atrial fibrillation, *J Cardiovasc Electrophysiol* 11:1375, 2000.
65. The Digitalis in Acute Atrial Fibrillation (DAAF) Trial Group Investigators: Intravenous digoxin in acute atrial fibrillation: results of a randomized, placebo-controlled multicentre trial in 239 patients. The Digitalis in Acute Atrial Fibrillation (DAAF) Trial Group, *Eur Heart J* 18:649, 1997.
66. Falk RH, Knowlton AA, Bernard SA et al: Digoxin for converting recent-onset atrial fibrillation to sinus rhythm: a randomized, double-blinded trial, *Ann Intern Med* 106:503, 1987.
67. Weiner P, Bassan MM, Jarchovsky J et al: Clinical course of acute atrial fibrillation treated with rapid digitalization, *Am Heart J* 105:223, 1983.
68. Rawles JM, Metcalfe MJ, Jennings K: Time of occurrence, duration and ventricular rate of paroxysmal atrial fibrillation: the effect of digoxin, *Br Heart J* 63:225, 1990.
69. Twileman RG, Van Gelder IC, Crijns HJ et al: Early recurrences of atrial fibrillation after electrical cardioversion: a result of fibrillation-induced electrical remodeling of the atria? *J Am Coll Cardiol* 31:167, 1998.
70. Hordof AJ, Spotnitz A, Mary RL et al: The cellular electrophysiologic effects of digitalis on human atrial fibers, *Circulation* 57:2223, 1978.
71. Roden DM: Mechanisms and management of proarrhythmia, *Am J Cardiol* 82:491, 1998.
72. Coumel P: Autonomic influences in atrial tachyarrhythmias, *J Cardiovasc Electrophysiol* 7:999, 1996.
73. Blazing MA, Morris JJ Jr: Atrial fibrillation: conventional wisdom reappraised, *Heart Dis Stroke* 1(2):79, 1992.
74. Ewy GA: Urgent parenteral digoxin: a requiem, *J Am Coll Cardiol* 15:1248, 1990.
75. Wellens HJJ, Durrer D: Effects of digitalis on atrioventricular conduction and circus movement tachycardia in patients with Wolff-Parkinson-White syndrome, *Circulation* 47:1229, 1973.
76. Shettigar UR: Management of rapid ventricular rate in acute atrial fibrillation, *Int J Clin Pharmacol Ther* 32:240, 1994.
77. Roy D, Talajic M, Dorian P et al: Amiodarone to prevent recurrence of atrial fibrillation. Canadian Trial of Atrial Fibrillation Investigators, *N Engl J Med* 342:913, 2000.
78. Page RL, Abrol R: Azimilide dihydrochloride: a new class III antiarrhythmic agent, *Expert Opin Investig Drugs* 9:2705, 2000.
79. Pritchett EL, Page RL, Connolly SJ et al: Antiarrhythmic effects of azimilide in atrial fibrillation: efficacy and dose-response. Azimilide Supraventricular Arrhythmia Program 3 (SVA-3) Investigators, *J Am Coll Cardiol* 36:794, 2000.
80. Clemett D, Markham A: Azimilide, *Drugs* 59:271, 2000.
81. Reiffel JA: Drug choices in the treatment of atrial fibrillation, *Am J Cardiol* 85:12D, 2000.
82. Warner ED, Dahl CF, Ewy GA: Myocardial injury from transthoracic defibrillation countershock, *Arch Pathol* 99:55, 1975.
83. Xie J, Weil MH, Sun S et al: High-energy defibrillation increases the severity of postresuscitation myocardial dysfunction, *Circulation* 96:683, 1997.
84. Vikenes K, Omvik P, Farstad M, Nordrehaug JE: Cardiac biochemical markers after cardioversion of atrial fibrillation or atrial flutter, *Am Heart J* 140:690, 2000.
85. Maixent JM, Barbey O, Pierre S et al: Inhibition of Na,K-ATPase by external electrical cardioversion in a sheep model of atrial fibrillation, *J Cardiovasc Electrophysiol* 11:439, 2000.
86. Bardy GH, Ivey TD, Allen MD et al: A prospective randomized evaluation of biphasic versus monophasic waveform pulses on defibrillation efficacy in humans, *J Am Coll Cardiol* 14:728, 1989.
87. Saksena S, An H, Mehra R et al: Prospective comparison of biphasic and monophasic shocks for implantable cardioverter-defibrillators using endocardial leads, *Am J Cardiol* 70:304, 1992.
88. Mittal S, Ayati S, Stein KM et al: Transthoracic cardioversion of atrial fibrillation: comparison of rectilinear biphasic versus damped sine wave monophasic shocks, *Circulation* 101:1282, 2000.
89. Mittal S, Ayati S, Stein KM et al: Comparison of a novel rectilinear biphasic versus damped sine wave monophasic waveform for transthoracic ventricular defibrillation, *J Am Coll Cardiol* 34:1595, 1999.

90. Bardy GH, Marchlinski FE, Sharma AD, et al for the Transthoracic Investigators: Multicenter comparison of truncated biphasic shocks and standard damped sine wave monophasic shocks for transthoracic ventricular defibrillation, *Circulation* 94:2507-14, 1996.
91. Heere JM, Higgins SL, Epstein AE et al: A comparison of biphasic and monophasic shocks for external defibrillation of humans, *Circulation* 96(Suppl):I-173, 1999.
92. Augostini RS, Tchou PJ, Love C et al: Multicenter trial of a biphasic external defibrillation waveform, *PACE* 22:4(Part II):827, 1999.
93. Tang AS, Yabe S, Wharton JM et al: Ventricular defibrillation using biphasic waveforms: the importance of phasic duration, *J Am Coll Cardiol* 13:207, 1989.
94. Yamanouchi Y, Brewer JE, Mowrey KA et al: Sawtooth first phase biphasic defibrillation waveform: a comparison with standard waveform in clinical devices, *J Cardiovasc Electrophysiol* 8:517, 1997.
95. Cox JL, Boineau JP, Schuessler RB et al: Five-year experience with the maze procedure for atrial fibrillation, *Ann Thorac Surg* 56:814, 1993.
96. Cox JL, Boineau JP, Schuessler RB et al: Modification of the maze procedure for atrial fibrillation. I. Rationale and surgical results, *J Thorac Surg* 110:473, 1995.
97. Cox JL, Ad N, Palazzo T et al: The Maze-III procedure combined with valve surgery, *Semin Thorac Cardiovasc Surg* 12:53, 2000.
98. Cox JL, Ad N, Palazzo T et al: Current status of the Maze procedure for the treatment of atrial fibrillation, *Semin Thorac Cardiovasc Surg* 12:15, 2000.
99. Schaff HV, Dearani JA, Daly RC et al: Cox-Maze procedure for atrial fibrillation: Mayo Clinic experience, *Semin Thorac Cardiovasc Surg* 12:30, 2000.
100. Swartz JF, Pellersel G, Silvers J et al: A catheter-based curative approach to atrial fibrillation in humans, *Circulation* 90:I-335, 1994 (abstract).
101. Maloney JD, Milner L, Barold S et al: Two staged biatrial linear and focal ablation to restore sinus rhythm in patients with refractory chronic atrial fibrillation, *Pacing Clin Electrophysiol* 21:2527, 1998.
102. Haïssaguerre M, Jaïs P, Shah DC et al: Right and left atrial radiofrequency catheter therapy of paroxysmal atrial fibrillation, *J Cardiovasc Electrophysiol* 7:1132, 1996.
103. Thomas SP, Nicholson IA, Nunn GR et al: Effect of atrial radiofrequency ablation designed to cure atrial fibrillation on atrial mechanical function, *J Cardiovasc Electrophysiol* 11:77, 2000.
104. Haïssaguerre M, Shah DC, Jaïs P et al: Spontaneous initiation of atrial fibrillation by ectopic beats originating in the pulmonary veins, *N Engl J Med* 339:659, 1998.
105. Haïssaguerre M, Jaïs P, Shah DC et al: Catheter ablation of chronic atrial fibrillation targeting the reinitiating triggers, *J Cardiovasc Electrophysiol* 11:2, 2000.
106. Chen SA, Hsieh MH, Tai TC et al: Initiation of atrial fibrillation by ectopic beats originating from the pulmonary veins: electrophysiologic characteristics, pharmacologic responses, and effects of radiofrequency ablation, *Circulation* 100:1879-1886, 1999.
107. Chen SA, Tai CT, Tsai CF et al: Radiofrequency catheter ablation of atrial fibrillation initiated by pulmonary vein ectopic beats, *J Cardiovasc Electrophysiol* 11:218, 2000.
108. Michael Mangrum J, Haines DE et al: Elimination of atrial fibrillation initiated by pulmonary vein for computerized activation sequence mapping, *J Cardiovasc Electrophysiol* 11:1159, 2000.
109. Shah DC, Haissaguerre M, Jais P et al: Electrophysiologically guided ablation of the pulmonary veins for the curative treatment of atrial fibrillation, *Ann Med* 32:408, 2000.
110. Schneider MA, Ndrepepa G, Zrenner B et al: Noncontact mapping-guided catheter ablation of atrial fibrillation associated with left atrial ectopy, *J Cardiovasc Electrophysiol* 11(4):475, 2000.
111. Friedman PA, Grice S, Munger TM et al: EP images: from cell to bedside. Spot welding the trigger in focal atrial fibrillation ablation, *J Cardiovasc Electrophysiol* 11:1061, 2000.
112. Tsai CF, Tai CT, Hsieh MH et al: Initiation of atrial fibrillation by ectopic beats originating from the superior vena cava: electrophysiological characteristics and results of radiofrequency ablation, *Circulation* 102(1):67, 2000.
113. Robbins IM, Colvin EV, Doyle TP et al: Pulmonary vein stenosis after catheter ablation of atrial fibrillation, *Circulation* 98:1769, 1998.
114. Scanavacca MI, Kajita LJ, Vieira M, Sosa EA: Pulmonary vein stenosis after catheter ablation of atrial fibrillation, *J Cardiovasc Electrophysiol* 11:677, 2000.
115. Sohn RH, Schiller NB: Left upper pulmonary vein stenosis complicating catheter ablation of atrial fibrillation, *Circulation* 101:E154, 2000.
116. Jaïs P, Shah DC, Hocini M et al: Radiofrequency catheter ablation for atrial fibrillation. *J Cardiovasc Electrophysiol* 11:758, 2000 (editorial comment).
117. Pappone C, Fosanio S, Oreto G et al: Circumferential radiofrequency ablation of pulmonary vein ostia: a new anatomic approach for curing atrial fibrillation, *Circulation* 102:2619, 2000.

CHAPTER 9

Atrial Flutter

TERMINOLOGY

atrial flutter A rapid atrial rhythm sustained by a macroreentrant circuit

atrial tachycardia A single focus firing rapidly

entrainment The ability to capture the reentry circuit with atrial pacing

excitable gap A cyclic area of nonrefractory tissue within the pathway of a reentry circuit

F wave An atrial flutter wave composed of a P′ wave and a Ta wave (atrial repolarization)

flutter A continuously waving pattern on the ECG without isoelectric baseline in at least one lead, irrespective of the rate

macroreentry (intra-atrial) A current that circles around a large (several centimeters in diameter) normal or abnormal structure that may be fixed and/or functional

Atrial flutter is a rapid and remarkably regular form of atrial tachycardia that is sustained by a macroreentrant circuit almost always, but not exclusively, located in the right atrium; it is usually paroxysmal, lasting for seconds to hours and occasionally even days. Chronic atrial flutter is unusual because if the arrhythmia lasts for a prolonged period it usually converts to atrial fibrillation.[1]

Although atrial flutter was described in 1911[2] not much progress was made in defining its mechanisms or diagnosing and managing it until relatively recently. Mechanisms of all the tachycardias originating in the atria are now known because of the data accumulated from activation mapping, entrainment techniques, radiofrequency ablation, and comparisons with surface electrocardiograms (ECGs). In particular, there is a sophisticated understanding of the several mechanisms that are capable of initiating and supporting the macroreentry circuit of atrial flutter. Additionally, new diagnostic techniques have evolved as well as improvements in acute and long-term management.[3]

ECG FINDINGS IN GENERAL

Atrial flutter is characterized by uniformity in its rate, configuration, and beat-to-beat cycle length (Fig. 9-1). It

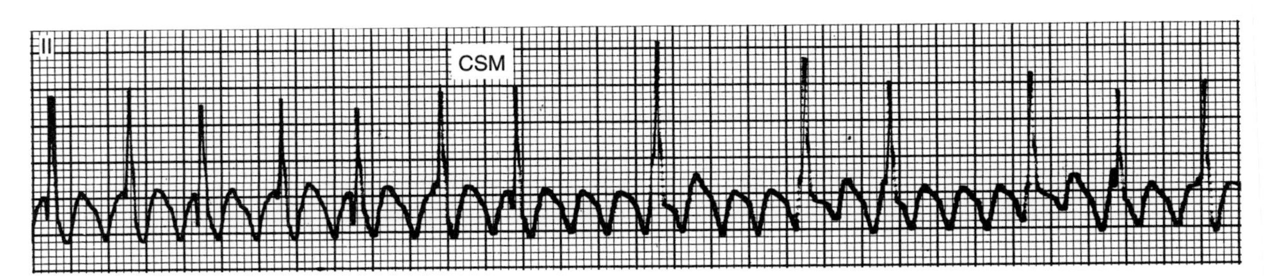

FIG. 9-1. Type I atrial flutter showing the typical sawtooth pattern with 2:1 conduction at the beginning of the tracing and 4:1 conduction because of carotid sinus massage *(CSM)*.

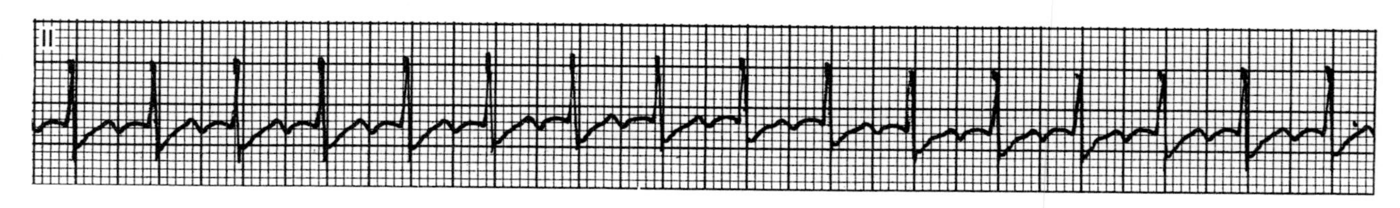

FIG. 9-2. Atrial flutter with 2:1 conduction.

can usually be recognized in the ECG by its sawtoothed flutter waves in leads II, III, aV_F, and by a typical pattern in lead V_1 sometimes resembling a child's drawing of little waves on water. It may however, also resemble atrial tachycardia on the ECG (isoelectric line separating P′ waves) and still be supported by the mechanism associated with a sawtooth pattern.

Ventricular Rate

Depends on atrioventricular (AV) conduction ratio; usually 150 to 170 beats/min because of a 2:1 AV conduction ratio, as shown in Fig. 9-2. In this rate range flutter should be considered, although other tachycardias may also have a rate in that range.

Atrial Rhythm

Regular sawtooth pattern is the usual in atrial flutter, although its absence does not negate the possibility that the macroreentrant mechanism is present. Electrophysiologists have found that "neither rate nor lack of isoelectric baseline is specific for any tachycardia mechanism."[3]

Ventricular Rhythm

Regular if there is a fixed conduction ratio or AV dissociation; group beating if there is Wenckebach conduction, a common conduction pattern in atrial flutter (Fig. 9-3); and irregular if there is variable AV conduction.

Usual AV Conduction Ratio

Conduction ratios are usually even (e.g., 2:1, 4:1, 6:1). With a normal AV node there is usually a physiologic AV block with 2:1 conduction or Wenckebach. As demonstrated in Fig. 9-4, Wenckebach conduction often causes group beating. It has been proposed that atrial impulses that appear to be completely blocked actually penetrate into different levels of the AV node (concealed conduction),[4] with 2:1 conduction at the level of the proximal AV node and Wenckebach conduction of the beats that reach the distal level of the AV node.

In 1996 Page et al[5] presented data supporting a mechanism other than two levels of AV nodal block to explain the 2:1 and 4:1 conduction in atrial flutter. These investigators demonstrated that heightened vagal tone

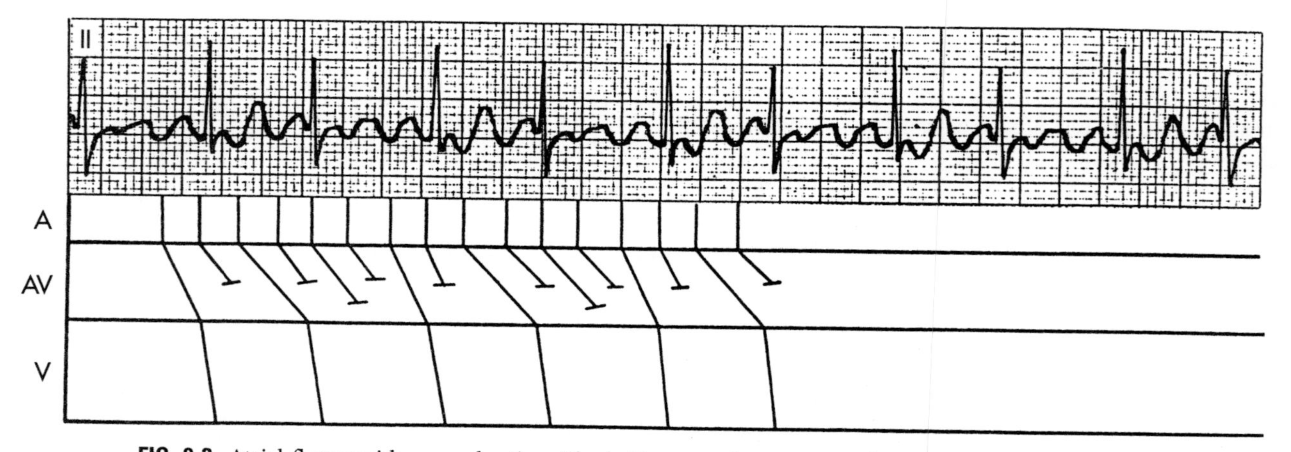

FIG. 9-3. Atrial flutter with group beating. The laddergram demonstrates the mechanism. The atrial tier *(A)* shows a regular atrial rhythm. There are two levels in the AV tier. In the upper level there is 2:1 conduction. In the lower atrioventricular node there is 3:2 Wenckebach conduction. This results in group beating.

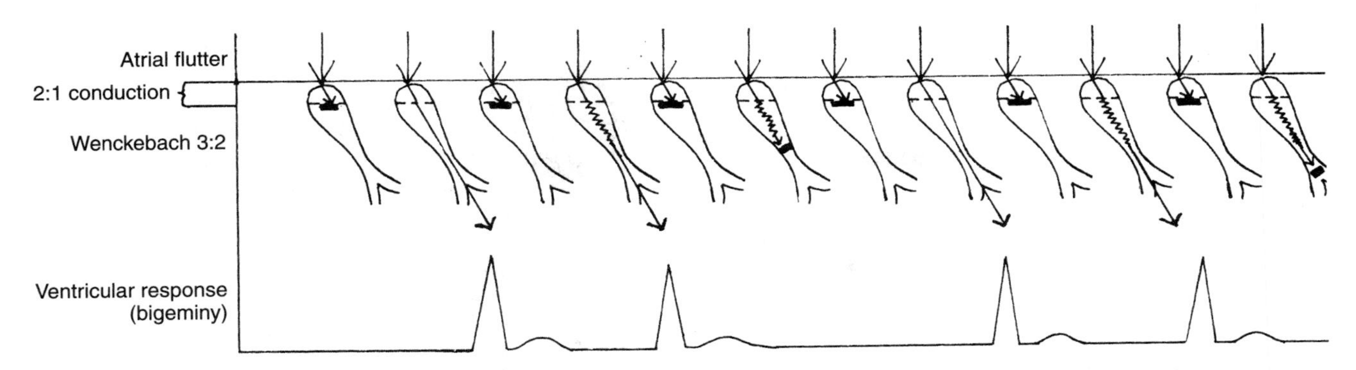

FIG. 9-4. A common mechanism for AV conduction during atrial flutter: 2:1 conduction at the top of the AV node and Wenckebach conduction (3:2) at the lower AV node. Atrial flutter is represented by the regularly spaced vertical arrows at the top. At the top of the AV node 2:1 conduction is shown (only every other beat gets through to the lower AV node) from where they are conducted to the ventricles with a 3:2 Wenckebach ratio; that is, for every three beats, only two are conducted to the ventricles, causing the typical group beating.

could substantially prolong the effective refractory period of the AV node, resulting in block of two consecutive atrial impulses. The second blocked beat would then increase the AV nodal effective refractory period enough to prevent the next beat from conducting, producing 4:1 conduction.

Other AV Conduction Ratios

- Higher degrees of AV block, as seen in Fig. 9-5, can occur with AV nodal disease, increased vagal tone, or when drugs that cause AV block are in use.
- A 1:1 conduction ratio may be seen in patients with preexcitation syndromes such as Wolff-Parkinson-White and Lown-Ganong-Levine syndromes, during exertion, or in those taking catecholamines or sympathomimetic amines. Atrial flutter in a patient with an accessory pathway, even with 2:1 conduction, is indistinguishable from ventricular tachycardia, as shown in Fig. 9-6. In this situation, the patient is usually seriously compromised hemodynamically and requires immediate electrical cardioversion.
- In patients taking class I antiarrhythmic agents (especially class 1C), the atrial rate may slow to as little as 180 to 200 beats/min. With the slower atrial rate, 1:1 AV conduction is more likely; such a case is illustrated in Fig. 9-7.

F-R Relationship

As you have seen, the relationship between the F wave (or the P′ wave) and the R wave that follows should be fixed *if the ventricular rhythm is regular*. This F-R relationship alternates *if there is group beating*, a normal AV nodal response to atrial flutter. However, if the F-R relationship is not fixed, despite a regular ventricular rhythm,

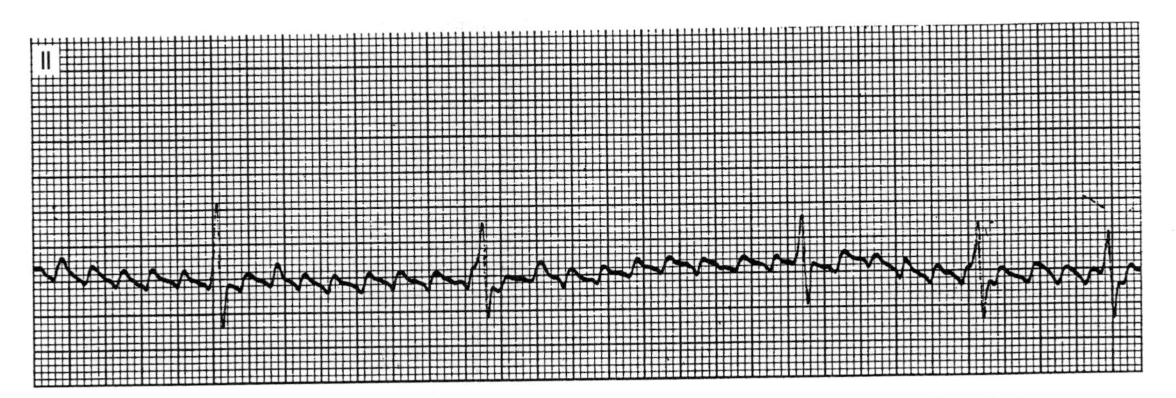

FIG. 9-5. Atrial flutter with high-grade and variable AV block. The atrial rate is 345 beats/min.

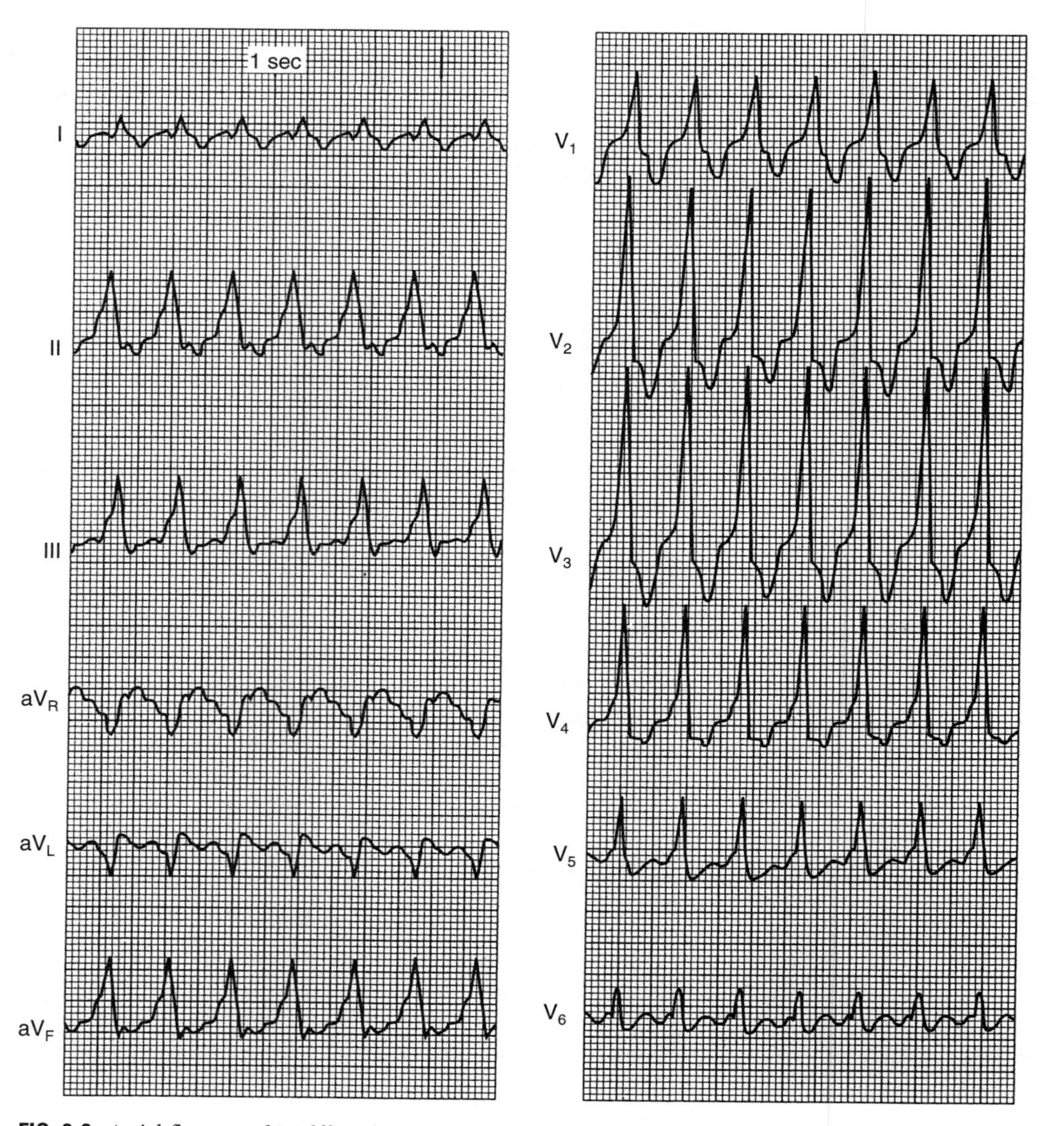

FIG. 9-6. Atrial flutter and Wolff-Parkinson-White syndrome. The conduction ratio is 2:1 over a left-sided accessory pathway. The QRS is broad because the atrial impulses are entering the ventricles via a rapidly conducting pathway rather than via the AV node. (From Wellens HJJ, Conover M: *The ECG in emergency decision making*, Philadelphia, 1992, WB Saunders.)

there is AV dissociation, which is the result of complete AV block or an accelerated idiojunctional or idioventricular rhythm. Fig. 9-8 shows the onset of atrial flutter, along with the development of an accelerated idioventricular rhythm. The atria are in flutter, and the ventricles are under the control of a ventricular focus. The AV dissociation can be nicely seen in changing F-R relationships in this figure.

Fig. 9-9 is another example of the onset of atrial flutter; this time it begins with a wandering atrial pacemaker. There are four different P′ wave shapes before the onset of the atrial flutter. If you walk out the R waves, you will find three of them are a little early. These are *capture beats* (C); the first has a PR interval of 0.30 second.

Response to Carotid Sinus Massage

Carotid sinus massage is a strong vagal maneuver that causes temporary slowing of the ventricular rate because

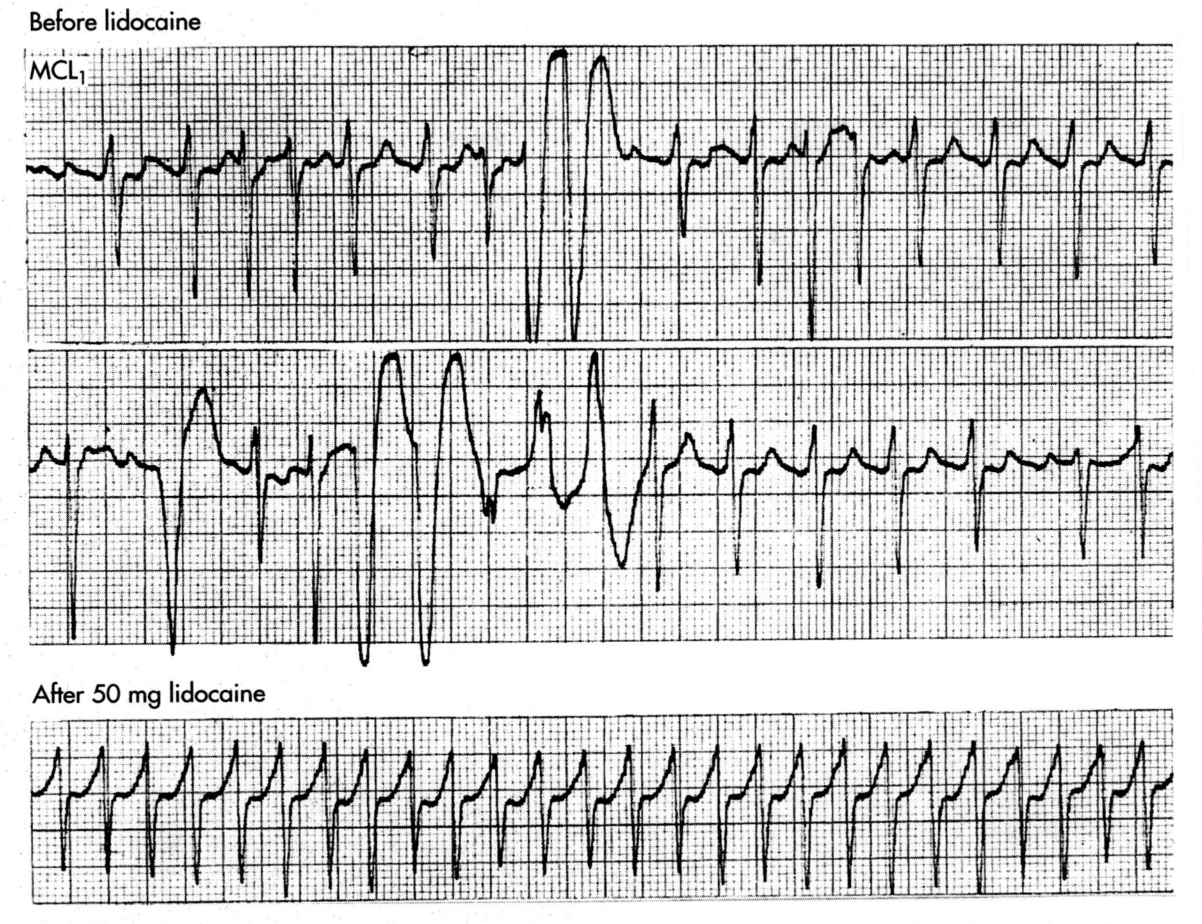

FIG. 9-7. The upper two strips are continuous and show atrial flutter at a rate of 285 beats/min with varying AV conduction interrupted by multiform anomalous beats. The *bottom strip* was recorded after administration of 50 mg of lidocaine. The atrial rate has decreased to 265 beats/min, with an alarming acceleration of the ventricular rate because of 1:1 conduction. (Courtesy H.J.L. Marriott, MD, Tampa, Fla.)

of AV block, as shown in Fig. 9-10. It is especially helpful in revealing an underlying atrial flutter that is not apparent when associated with physiologic (aberrancy) or pathologic left bundle branch block. A more complete discussion of carotid sinus massage can be found on pp. 132-133.

MECHANISMS

Numerous studies from electrophysiologic laboratories have shown that atrial mechanisms do not always correlate with the traditional ECG patterns that have been classified by the atrial rate and the shape of the P′ waves, dividing them strictly into "atrial flutter" or "atrial tachycardia." We now know that there is a crossover of atrial rates and P′ wave morphologies within the traditional classification of atrial tachycardia and atrial flutter. This has spawned mechanistic terms that cover all abnormal tachycardias originating in the atria outside of the sinus node that have a regular rhythm at a constant rate of 100 beats/min or more.[3] Included in this list are focal atrial tachycardia (see Chapter 7), inappropriate sinus tachycardia (see Chapter 6), and macroreentrant atrial flutter. The macroreentrant pathways of atrial flutter have been further described from the left anterior oblique fluoroscopic view as counterclockwise, clockwise, lesion, lower loop, double wave reentry, right atrial free-wall macroreentry without atriotomy, left atrial macro-

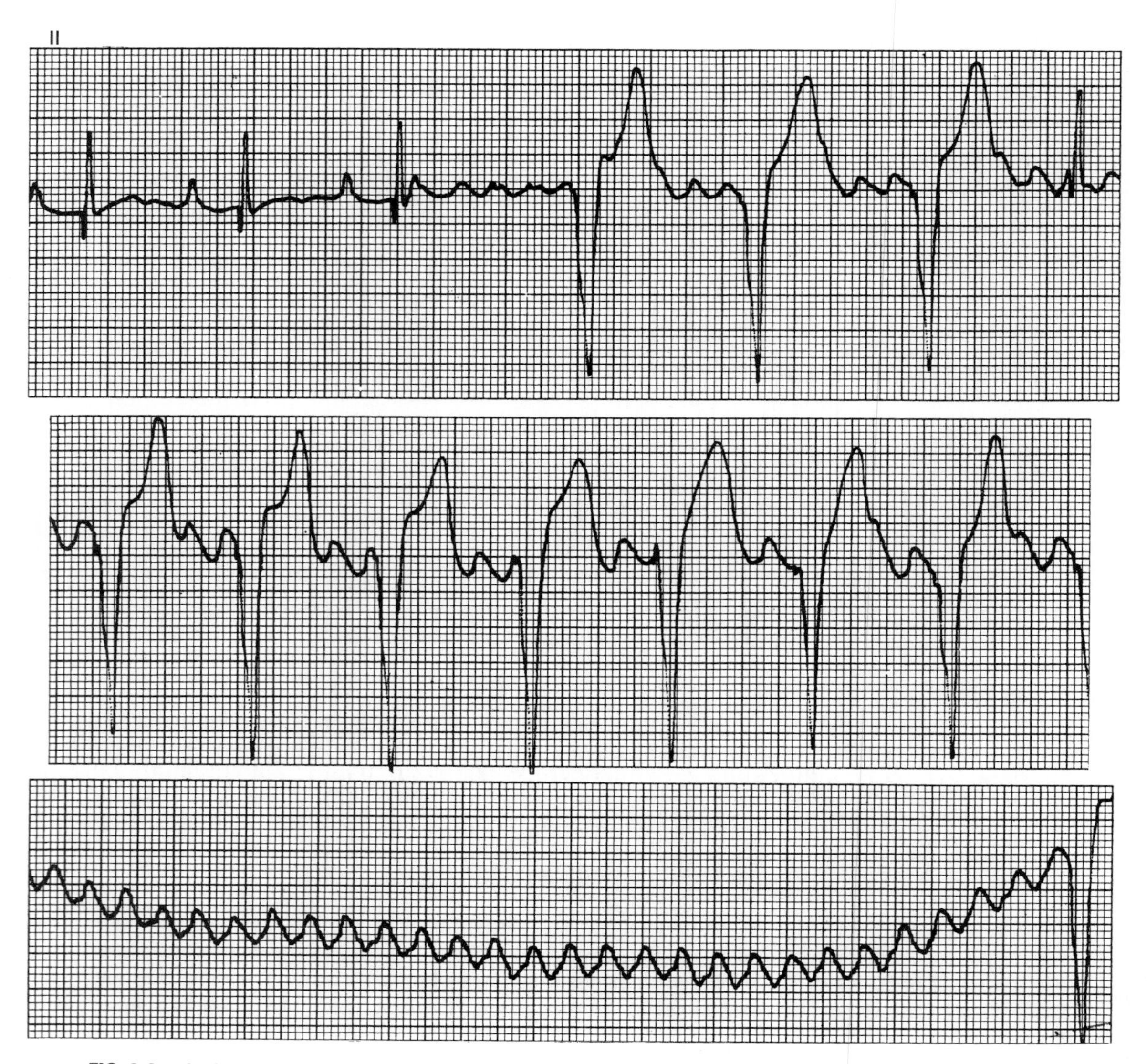

FIG. 9-8. The beginning of the tracing shows sinus rhythm with a prolonged PR interval. A premature atrial complex fires in the ST segment of the third complex, resulting in atrial flutter. An accelerated idioventricular rhythm interrupts a pause and beats at a rate of 63 beats/min, "warming up" to 85 beats/min in the middle tracing, where the signs of atrial flutter with AV dissociation are nicely seen. Note the changing F-R relationship. When the ventricular rhythm is regular the F-R relationship will be fixed if there is AV conduction. In the *bottom tracing* from the same patient, the idioventricular rhythm failed, presumably because of a bolus of lidocaine. One can observe the rigid regularity of atrial flutter and appreciate its morphology.

reentry, and atypical. In this chapter, the classification will be simplified.

RIGHT ATRIAL ANATOMIC STRUCTURES

Fig. 9-11 illustrates the atrial structures important in forming a protected pathway for the macroreentrant circuit of atrial flutter.

Crista Terminalis

This is a terminal crest of the right atrium, a ridge on the internal surface of the right atrium located laterally to the orifices of the superior and inferior venae cavae. It corresponds to a groove on the external surface of the heart called the sulcus terminalis. The portion of the atrium behind the crista is smooth; it developed from the embry-

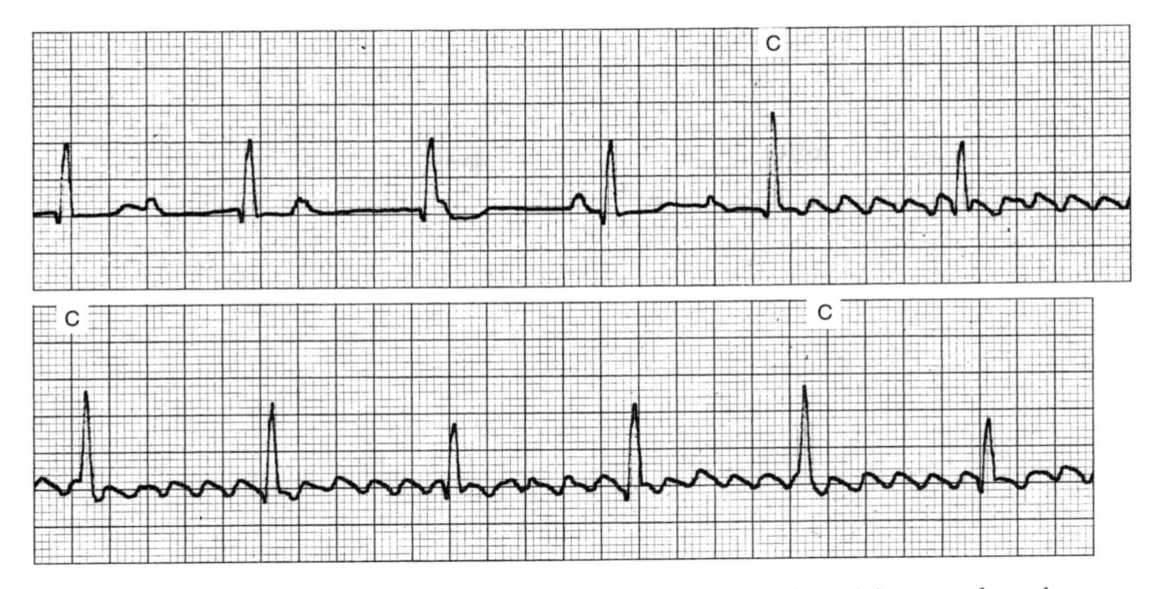

FIG. 9-9. The onset of atrial flutter with AV dissociation and three capture beats *(C)*. See text for explanation. (Strips are not continuous.)

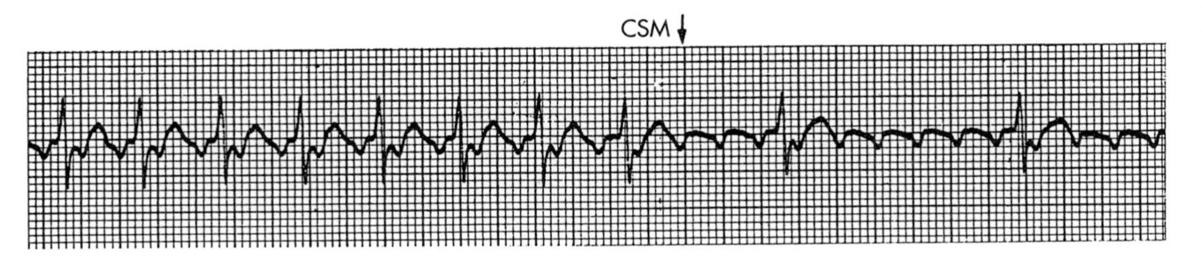

FIG. 9-10. Atrial flutter with 2:1 atrioventricular conduction that changes to 4:1 and 6:1 because of carotid sinus massage *(CSM)*. (From Marriott HJL, Conover M: *Advanced concepts in arrhythmias*, ed 3, St Louis, 1998, Mosby.)

onic structure, the sinus venosus. The portion of the atrium in front of the crista is trabeculated, having developed from the primitive atrium.

Eustachian Valve

Valve of the inferior vena cava; it forms its inferior lip.

Eustachian Ridge

With the eustachian valve, forms a barrier to conduction between the inferior vena cava and the coronary sinus.

Coronary Sinus

The terminal portion of the great cardiac vein, which empties into the right atrium. The orifice of the coronary sinus opens between the orifice of the inferior vena cava and the tricuspid annulus. It is guarded by a fold that is often perforated like a piece of lace and is known as the *valve of the coronary sinus.*

Fossa Ovalis

A depression on the right interatrial septum representing the remains of the fetal *foramen ovale*. The fossa ovalis does not participate in the macroreentrant circuit of atrial flutter,[6] but is included here for its landmark value. When dissecting a cadaver heart, a forceps passed up the inferior vena cava will be arrested by the crescentic upper margin of the fossa ovalis. But in about 25% of cases it will pass onward through a valve-like slit in the septum (foramen ovale) into the left atrium. This is the course much of the blood took until birth.

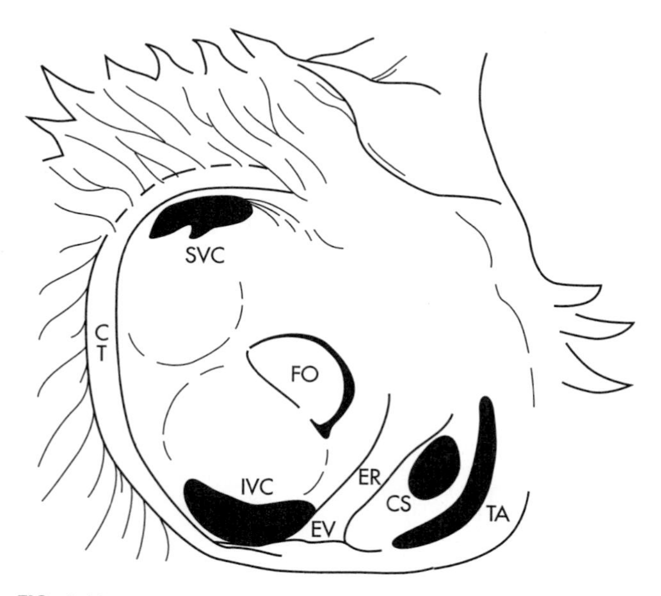

FIG. 9-11. Pertinent anatomic landmarks in the right atrium. The eustachian ridge *(ER)* is between the inferior vena cava and the tricuspid annulus *(TA)*. Refer to text for description. *CS*, Coronary sinus; *CT*, crista terminalis; *FO*, fossa ovalis; *IVC*, inferior vena cava; *SVC*, superior vena cava; *EV*, eustachian valve.

Tricuspid Annulus

A fibrous ring surrounding the orifice of the tricuspid valve. Such a ring surrounds each of the four orifices guarded by a valve. The aortic ring is the strongest and is like a cuff. Without the rings, the orifices would stretch and the valves be rendered incompetent.

VARIATIONS

The main varieties of atrial flutter are listed below and summarized in Table 9-1.[7] Keep in mind that if the patient is taking Class IA or IC antiarrhythmic drugs, or amiodarone, the rate of atrial flutter may be as low as 180 beats/min.

- **Typical atrial flutter:** 240 to 350 beats/min; negative P′ waves in leads II, III, aV_F
- **Reverse typical atrial flutter:** 240 to 350 beats/min; positive or negative P′ waves in II, III, aV_F
- **Lesion macroreentrant atrial flutter:** rate varies; flutter wave morphology varies with lesion location
- **Left atrial macroreentrant atrial flutter:** rate and flutter wave morphology vary
- **Atypical atrial flutter:** rate varies; flutter wave morphology varies with reentry circuit location

TYPICAL ATRIAL FLUTTER

Typical atrial flutter is seen in patients with or without heart disease and can be entrained and cured by radiofrequency ablation.[8] It occurs in two forms according to the direction of rotation of its macroreentrant circuit: up the septum and down the right atrial free wall (typical) or down the septum and up the right atrial free wall (reverse typical).

ECG Recognition

Atrial rate: Ranges from 240 to 350 beats/min. The rate may be as slow as 180 to 200 beats/min with class IA, IC antiarrhythmic drugs, or amiodarone, or because of right atrial enlargement.
Atrial rhythm: Regular.
P′ wave axis: Superior.
The 12-lead ECG in Fig. 9-12 demonstrates the typical form of the flutter waves:
Leads II, III, and aV_F (the inferior leads): P′ wave negative; sawtooth pattern.

TABLE 9-1 Classification of Atrial Flutter

Type	Mechanism	P′ Wave Axis	P′ Waves II, III, aV_F	Atrial Rate
Typical	Macroreentry	Superior	Negative	240-350 beats/min Slower with class IA, class IC, or amiodarone
Reverse typical	Macroreentry	Usually inferior; may be superior	Positive or negative	240-350 beats/min Slower with class IA, class IC, or amiodarone
Lesion	Macroreentry	Varies with lesion location	Varies	Varies
Left atrial	Macroreentry	Varies	Varies	Varies
Atypical	Macroreentry	Varies with reentry circuit location	Varies	Varies

Note: A superior P′ wave axis will have negative P′ waves and positive Ta waves forming the sawtooth pattern in leads II, III, and aV_F. An inferior P′ wave axis will have positive P′ waves and negative Ta waves forming a sawtooth pattern in those leads.

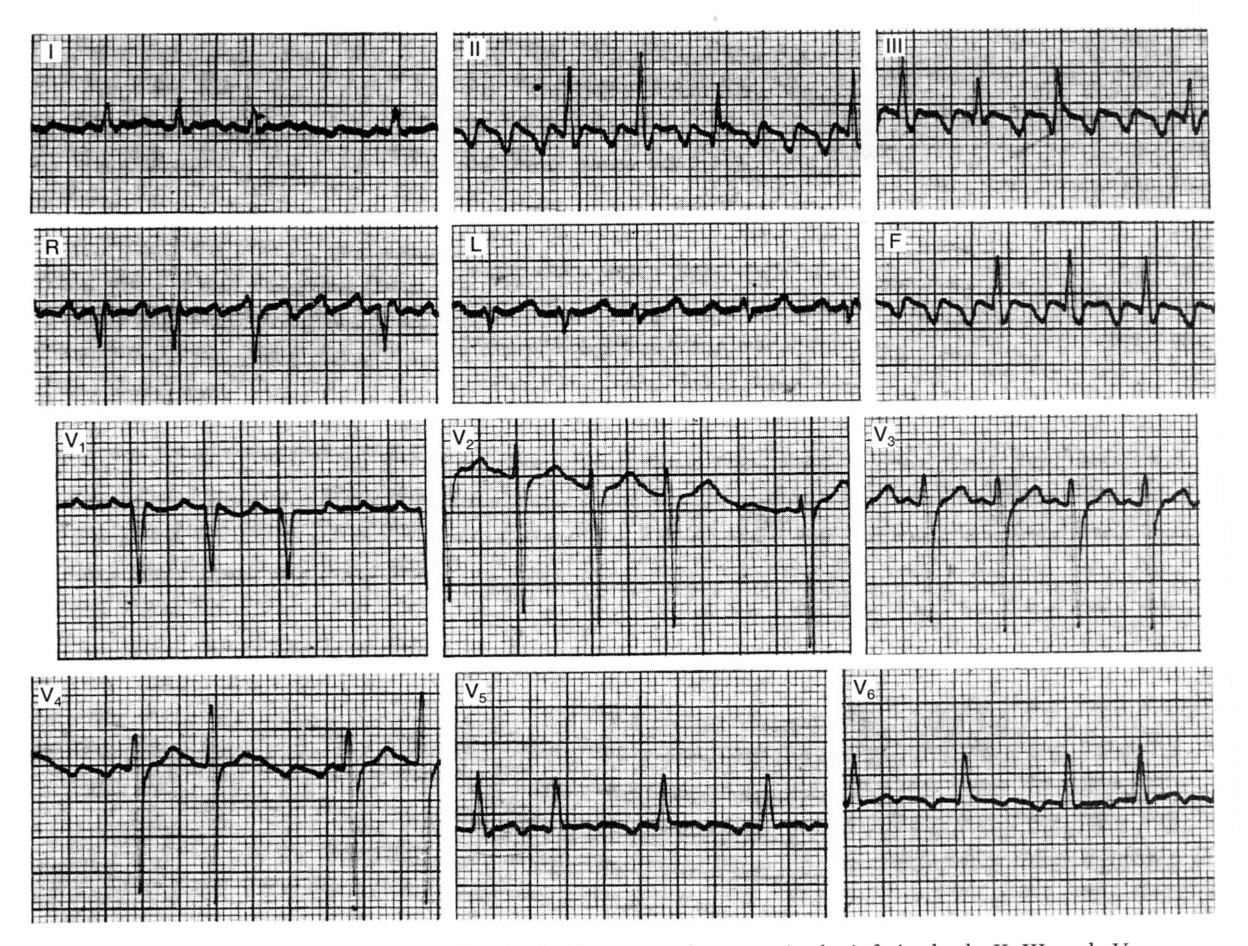

FIG. 9-12. Typical atrial flutter in all 12 leads. The sawtooth pattern in the inferior leads, II, III, and aV_F with negative P′ waves and the little positive peaks in lead V_1 are evident. Typically, in lead I the flutter waves are not seen, but in this case resemble atrial fibrillation, especially because of the varying conduction ratio.

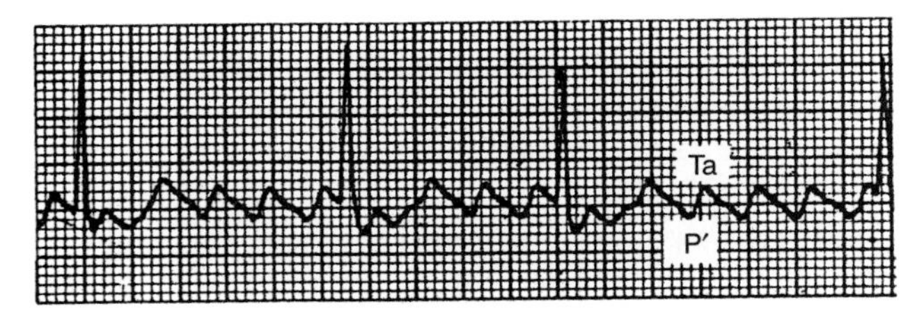

FIG. 9-13. The P′ and Ta wave in typical atrial flutter.

Lead V_1: P′ wave positive and separated by an isoelectric line.

Lead I: P′ wave isoelectric or looking like atrial fibrillation.

The Genesis of Flutter Waves

Although atrial flutter is generated by a macroreentry circuit in the right atrium, the P′ wave polarity on the ECG is determined primarily by the sequence of activation in the left atrium, activating it in an inferior/superior direction.

As noted in Fig. 9-13, in typical atrial flutter when the activation current travels away from the diaphragmatic surface of the heart, the F waves in the inferior leads (II, III, aV_F) are composed of a negative component (the P′ wave) and a positive component (the Ta wave), producing a very distinctive sawtooth pattern with slight variations among patients. Fig. 9-12 has shown that lead I is not helpful in recognizing atrial flutter. Atrial activity is often not seen or resembles atrial fibrillation. This is because the P′ wave axis is perpendicular to the axis of lead I and therefore atrial activity is isoelectric in that lead. This also demonstrates Einthoven's equation (II = I + III). The ECG pattern of the F waves is similar in both forms of typical atrial flutter in the inferior leads (i.e., "sawtooth"), although the P′ wave may be positive and the Ta wave negative in clockwise rotation.

The Macroreentrant Circuit

When seen in the left anterior oblique fluoroscopic view, the rotation of the macroreentrant circuit of typical atrial flutter is counterclockwise (up the septum and down the right atrial free wall), barriers to conduction playing an important role in the establishment and maintenance of the circuit. They provide a protected pathway for the wave front and prevent stray currents from traversing the smooth-walled posterior right atrium and terminating the mechanism by introducing refractory tissue.[6]

Fig. 9-14 demonstrates the pathway sustaining this most common form of atrial flutter as constructed from activation and entrainment mapping during electrophysiologic studies.

1. Note in Fig. 9-14 the line drawn on the left next to the *crista terminalis* (CT); here the broad inferiorly directed wave front is confined by the line of conduction block formed by the crista terminalis and the *eustachian valve and ridge* (EV, ER), which together form a line of conduction block between the *inferior vena cava* (IVC) and the *coronary sinus* (CS).
2. The wave front then proceeds through an isthmus of slow conduction between the *tricuspid annulus* (TA) and the eustachian valve and ridge. Together, the posterior and anterior barriers form a continuous protected pathway for the macroreentrant circuit. It is this so called *IVC-tricuspid isthmus* that is ablated with radiofrequency energy, curing the patient of typical atrial flutter.
3. The wave front then continues its loop, ascending the septum between the coronary sinus ostium and the septal tricuspid annulus.
4. The upper link in the circuit is not well-defined, but probably includes the roof of the right atrium anterior to the orifice of the orifice of the superior vena cava. It is also possible for the activation front to cross the top of the crista terminalis or lower.[9] From this point it completes its rotation anterior to the supero/medial portion of the crista terminalis.

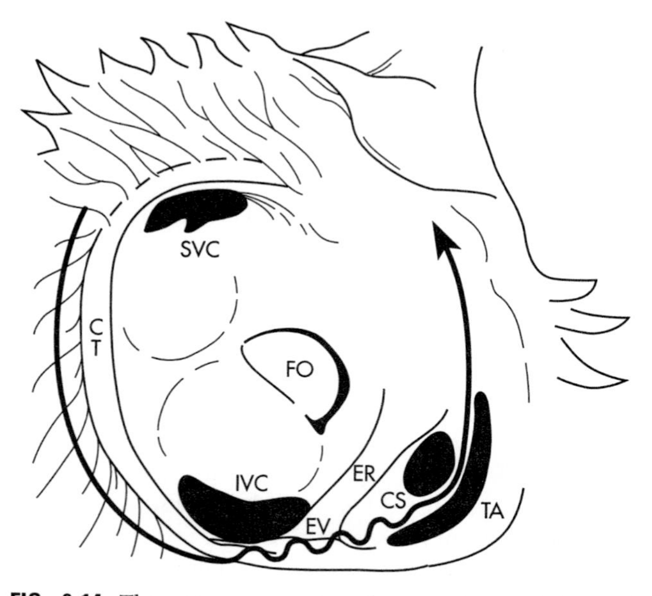

FIG. 9-14. The macroreentrant path taken by typical atrial flutter: up the septum and down the right atrial free wall. This is a counterclockwise direction when seen in the left anterior oblique fluoroscopic view. *SVC*, Superior vena cava; *CT*, crista terminalis; *IVC*, inferior vena cava; *CS*, coronary sinus; *TA*, tricuspid annulus; *FO*, fossa ovalis; *ER*, eustachian ridge; *EV*, eustachian valve.

Note that the macroreentrant wave front does not bridge the barrier of the crista terminalis at any point. This is because of a functional rather than a fixed conduction block across the crista terminalis.[9] The cycle length of this circuit is dependent on atrial size, underlying disease, and the presence of antiarrhythmic drugs.[6]

Radiofrequency Ablation—The Isthmus of Slow Conduction

One critical element of both forms of the typical atrial flutter reentrant circuit is a narrow isthmus of slow conduction that can be interrupted by a lesion created by radiofrequency energy, eliminating the possibility of such a reentrant circuit being initiated or sustained, and providing a cure.

There is a posterior isthmus and a septal isthmus that can be interrupted. The posterior isthmus is in the low posterior right atrium between the inferior vena cava and the tricuspid annulus. The septal isthmus, from the tricuspid annulus to the posteroapical margin of the coronary sinus ostium is the narrower of the two possible ablation sites, illustrated in Fig. 9-15 by Warren Jackman's group.[10]

In patients who do not have conduction in the narrow space between the coronary sinus ostium and the eustachi-

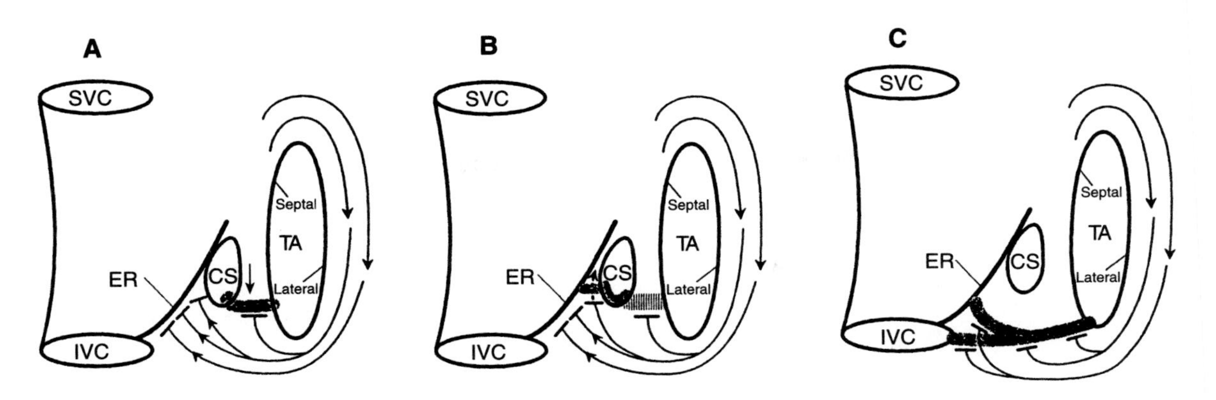

FIG. 9-15. Schematics of the right atrium in the right anterior oblique projection illustrate the three approaches used for ablation of counterclockwise typical atrial flutter. **A,** Ablation *(wide gray line)* across the septal isthmus from the tricuspid annulus *(TA)* to the posteroapical margin of the coronary sinus *(CS)* ostium. **B,** The ablation line can be extended along the posterior margin of the coronary sinus ostium and to the eustachian ridge *(ER)* in patients who have conduction through this space *(dashed arrow)*. **C,** Ablation line across the posterior isthmus from the tricuspid annulus to the inferior vena cava *(IVC)* or the eustachian valve and ridge. (From Nakagawa H, Lazzara R, Khastgir T et al: Role of the tricuspid annulus and the eustachian valve/ridge on atrial flutter. Relevance to catheter ablation of the septal isthmus and a new technique for rapid identification of ablation success, *Circulation* 94:407, 1996.)

an ridge, the ablation line illustrated in Fig. 9-15, *A*, should produce a complete arc of conduction block extending from the tricuspid annulus to the coronary sinus ostium and to the inferior vena cava and eliminate both forms of typical atrial flutter.

In patients who do have conduction in the narrow space between the coronary sinus ostium and the eustachian ridge (*dashed arrow*), the ablation line is extended along the posterior margin of the coronary sinus ostium and to the eustachian ridge (Fig. 9-15, *B*). Fig. 9-15, *C*, shows the longer ablation line across the posterior isthmus from the tricuspid annulus to the inferior vena cava or to the eustachian ridge.

REVERSE TYPICAL ATRIAL FLUTTER

This less common type of macroreentrant atrial flutter, as with the more common typical form, is seen in patients with or without heart disease and do not require a scar from prior atriotomy.[11] Both can be cured by radiofrequency ablation.[8]

ECG Recognition

Atrial rate: Ranges from 240 to 350 beats/min. The rate may be slower (in right atrial enlargement, for example).

Atrial rhythm: Regular.

P′ wave axis: Usually inferior, but may be superior.

Flutter Waves

ECG recognition

Leads II, III, and aV$_F$: The F waves of reverse typical atrial flutter in the inferior leads are usually composed of a positive component (the P′ wave) and a negative component (the Ta wave) in the inferior leads because the direction of the reentry circuit is reversed from that of typical atrial flutter. However, it is possible for the P′ waves to have a superior axis so that the sawtooth flutter waves may be identical to those of the more common counterclockwise form of atrial flutter.[12] Reversed typical atrial flutter is seen in Fig. 9-16.

Lead V$_1$: The P′ waves may be negative or may mimic the positive P′ wave of the more common counterclockwise mechanism.[8] Fig. 9-17, *A*, is an atrial flutter with 2:1 conduction and an atrial rate of 280 beats/min. Note the negative P′ waves in lead V$_1$.

Mechanism

Fig. 9-17, *B*, demonstrates the pathway of the reverse and rare (10%) form of typical atrial flutter. Its circuit is anatomically identical to that of the counterclockwise rotation, but travels in the opposite direction (down the septum and up the right atrial free wall). In the left anterior oblique fluoroscopic view this is a clockwise direction. Both share similar right atrial conduction disturbances and normal left atrial conduction times.[13]

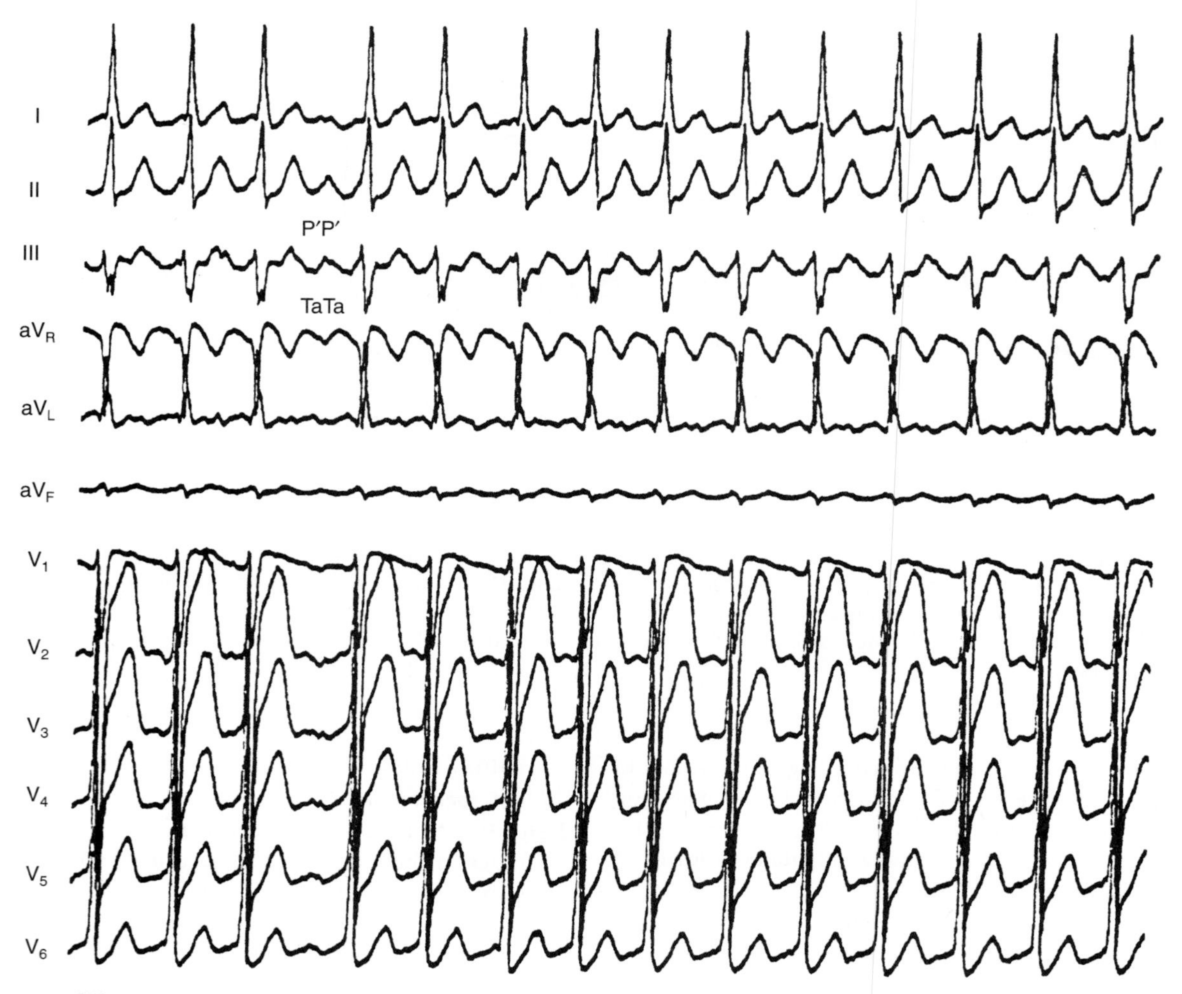

FIG. 9-16. Twelve-lead ECG of reversed typical atrial flutter. There is less agreement regarding the ECG features of reverse right atrial rotation in typical atrial flutter. In the majority of cases the atrial flutter waves are described as predominantly positive in the inferior leads and negative in lead V_1. (From Saoudi N, Cosio F, Waldo A et al: Classification of atrial flutter and regular atrial tachycardia according to electrophysiologic mechanism and anatomic bases: a statement from a joint expert group from the Working Group of Arrhythmias of the European Society of Cardiology and the North American Society of Pacing and Electrophysiology, *J Cardiovasc Electrophysiol* 12:852, 2001.)

Treatment

Radiofrequency ablation as described for the counterclockwise macroreentrant circuit is a cure.

LESION MACROREENTRANT ATRIAL FLUTTER

Intraatrial reentrant flutter is a well-described complication in as many as 25% of patients after repair of complex congenital heart disease, leaving a scar in the right atrium, although the lesion is not limited to being scar tissue.[7]

ECG Recognition

Atrial complexes may be low voltage and not the typical sawtooth pattern. Fig. 9-18, *A*, is an example of this. The 12-lead ECG from a patient with an intraatrial scar from a past atrial septal defect repair shows an atrial rate of 240 caused by a macroreentrant circuit, yet without the sawtooth pattern.

The morphology of the atrial waves in right atrial free wall atriotomy tachycardia range from typical sawtooth to distinct P′ waves separated by an isoelectric line, the same

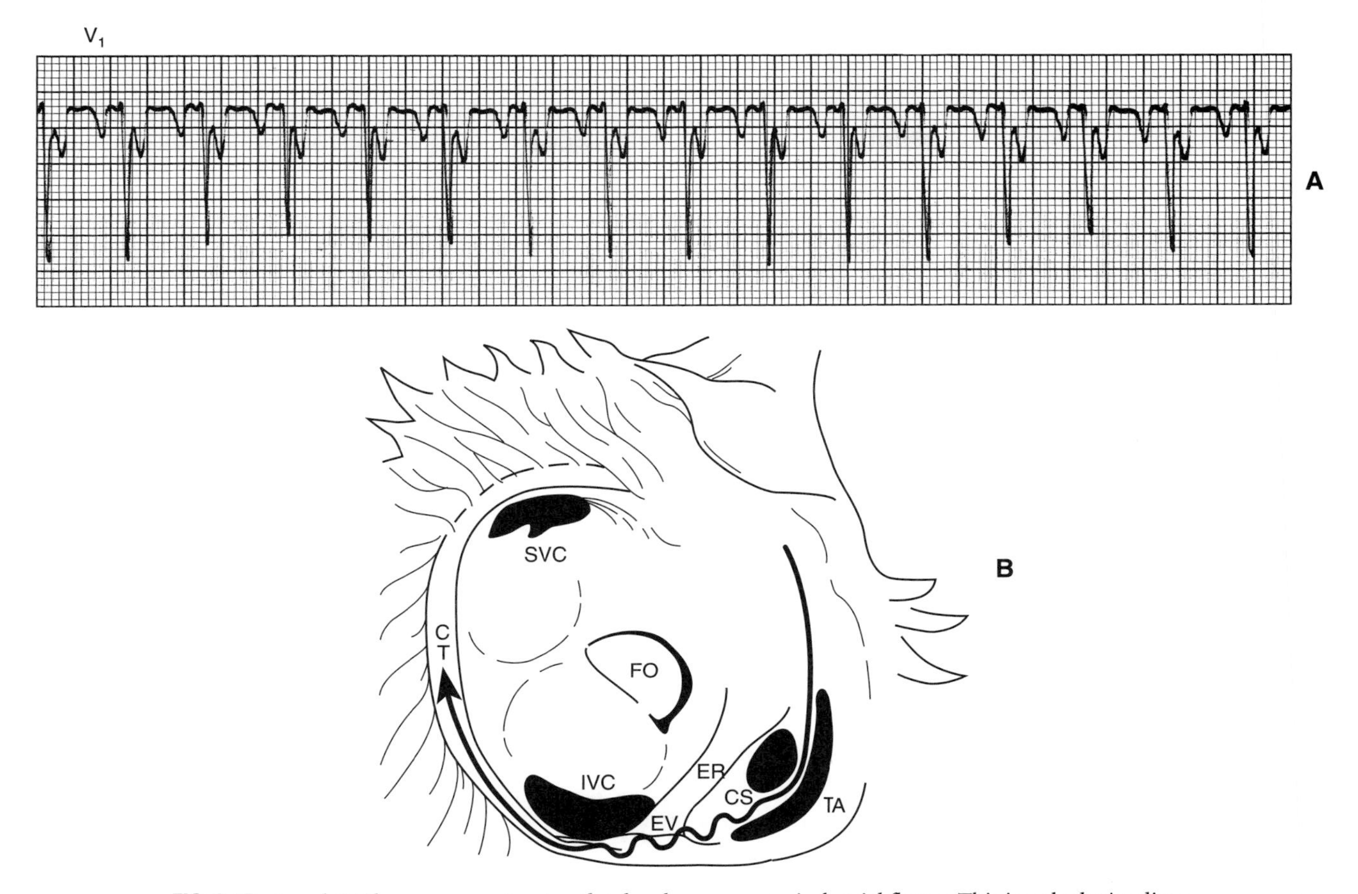

FIG. 9-17. **A** and **B**, The macroreentrant path taken by reverse typical atrial flutter. This is a clockwise direction when seen in the left anterior oblique fluoroscopic view. The route is the same as that of typical atrial flutter just described, but in the opposite direction: down the septum and up the right atrial free wall. *SVC*, Superior vena cava; *CT*, crista terminalis; *IVC*, inferior vena cava; *CS*, coronary sinus; *TA*, tricuspid annulus; *FO*, fossa ovalis; *ER*, eustachian ridge; *EV*, eustachian valve.

as the typical pattern of focal atrial tachycardia. After this type of macroreentry circuit is ablated with radiofrequency energy, another may be unmasked.

Mechanism

Lesion macroreentrant circuits are diverse and different from those of typical atrial flutter.[14] However, because of the atrial rate and the possibility for radiofrequency ablation, it is classified as type I. The scar from the patient whose ECG was seen in Fig. 9-18, *A*, is shown in *B* extending obliquely from the right atrial appendage to the low right atrium. When the incision scar is in the lateral right atrial wall electrophysiologists identify the arrhythmia as *right atrial free wall atriotomy tachycardia*. It is commonly supported by a reentry circuit around the scar.

The onset of lesion macroreentrant atrial flutter is almost always preceded by transitional atrial fibrillation, during which time the macroreentrant circuit necessary to support atrial flutter develops.[15]

Causes

Lesion macroreentry defines a circuit around a central obstacle such as an atriotomy scar, septal prosthetic patch, suture line, a scar from the right atrial radiofrequency ablation line for atrial fibrillation, or atrial fibrosis. The superior and inferior vena cava may also provide a central obstacle to circulate around. In any patient with a previous atriotomy, there is a high degree of suspicion regarding a macroreentrant circuit around the incision scar. Complex and multiple reentrant circuits are noted after the following:

1. Placement of an intra-atrial baffle for transposition of the great vessels (Mustard, Senning)
2. Fontan procedure in a dilated right atrium
3. Maze surgery for atrial fibrillation

Long-Term Treatment

Such circuits are difficult to manage with antiarrhythmic drug therapy, but can be successfully ablated with radiofrequency energy. The reentrant circuit shown in

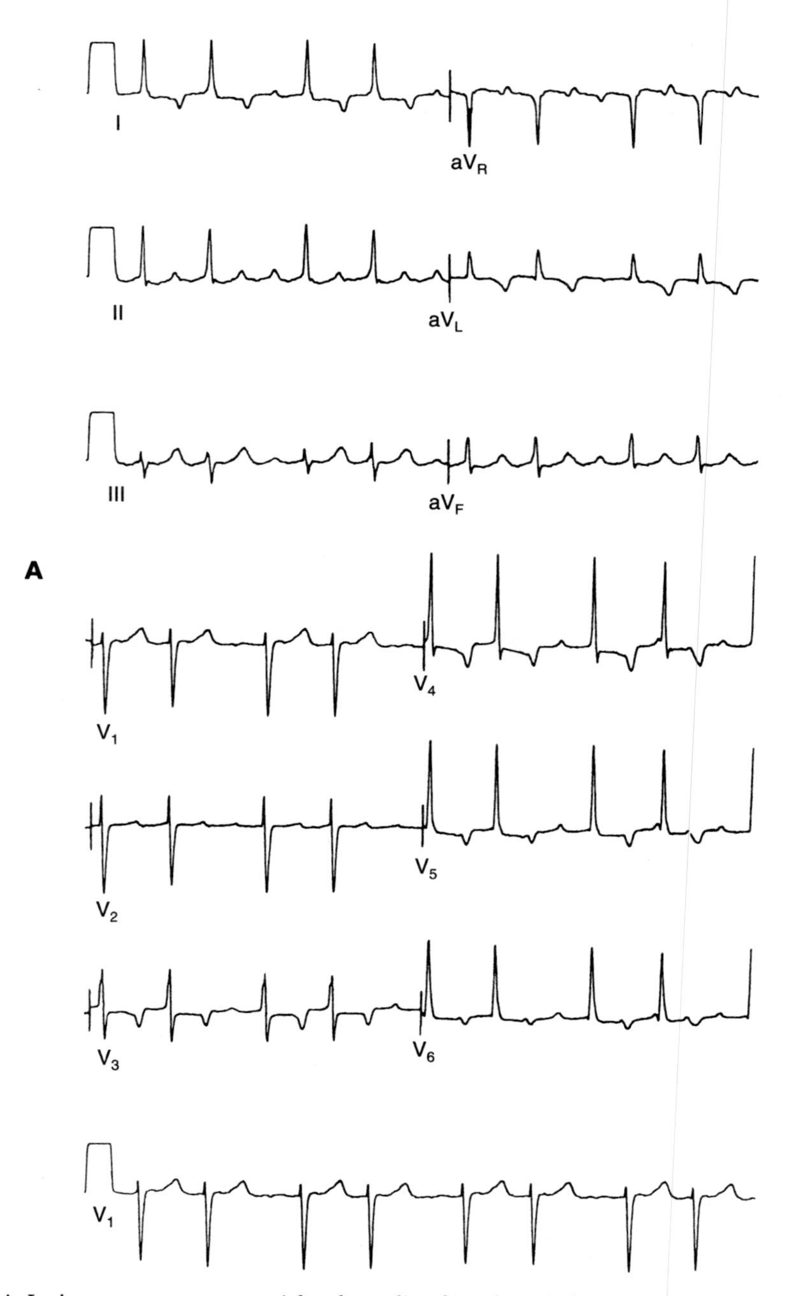

FIG. 9-18. **A**, Lesion macroreentrant atrial tachycardia of 240 beats/min. P waves are positive in lead I and in the inferior leads. The P waves are negative in aV_R and negative or isoelectric in leads V_1 and aV_L. (**B** from Lesh MD, Van Hare GF, Epstein LM et al: Radiofrequency catheter ablation of atrial arrhythmias: results and mechanisms, *Circulation* 89:1074, 1994.)

Continued

Fig. 9-18, *B*, was terminated promptly with ablation and could not be reinduced. Note the position of the catheter at the site of successful ablation.

An essential electrophysiologic substrate is an isthmus of myocardium between the atriotomy and the atriopulmonary connection. Interruption of conduction through this isthmus terminates the atrial flutter in this model and suggests a technique for ablation of atrial flutter in patients who have undergone a classic Fontan operation.[16]

Prevention

It has been shown that if atriotomy incisions are altered slightly to coincide with nonconductive atrial borders such as the inferior or superior vena cava, pulmonary veins, and the tricuspid annulus, the incidence of incisional reentrant tachycardia may be substantially reduced.[17] For example, Henglein et al,[18] to avoid incisional atrial flutter, successfully performed the atriotomy incision for atrial septal defect perpendicular to the terminal groove and extending towards the tricuspid annulus, placing some cryothermal lesions between the end of the incision and the annulus.

LEFT ATRIAL MACROREENTRANT TACHYCARDIA

It is possible for a stable macroreentrant circuit to originate in the left atrium. A reentry circuit can be established around the pulmonary veins, within the inferior posterior left atrium, or even around the mitral valve ring.[7]

ECG Recognition

P′ waves may be discrete with an isoelectric line between them or that of reverse typical atrial flutter with a positive P′ wave and negative Ta wave forming the flutter wave morphology. The diagnosis cannot, however, be made from the surface ECG, instead requiring recordings from the right atrium, coronary sinus esophagus, and right pulmonary artery.[3]

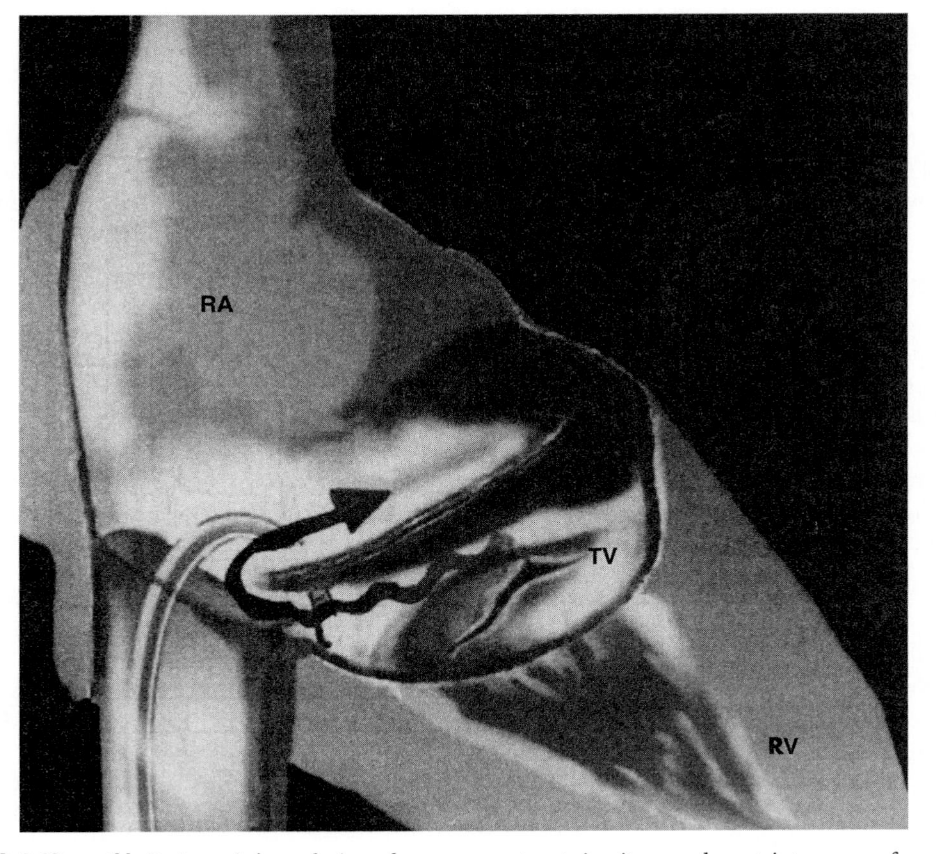

FIG. 9-18, cont'd. B, An artist's rendering of a macroreentrant circuit around an atriotomy scar from an old surgery for atrial septal defect. Also shown are the presumed reentry circuit (note its slow arm inferior to the scar) and the radiofrequency catheter poised for successful ablation of the circuit. *RA*, Right atrium; *RV*, right ventricle; *TV*, tricuspid valve.

ATYPICAL ATRIAL FLUTTER

Atypical atrial flutter is a rare form of rapid macroreentrant tachycardia that is difficult to characterize because of its instability.

ECG Recognition

Atypical atrial flutter rates may be in the usual range or much faster. The flutter wave morphology and axis depend on where the reentry circuit is located.

Mechanism

The rhythm of atypical atrial flutter is unstable because reentry circuits may vary in size and location. It is possible for a macroreentrant circuit in the right atrium to be the mechanism of this tachycardia.

Acute Treatment

Difficult to terminate.

Long-Term Treatment

Radiofrequency ablation of atypical atrial flutter is difficult to achieve. However, most patients are still candidates for electrophysiologic studies.[19,20] In one study of 75 consecutive patients undergoing catheter ablation of typical atrial flutter, additional atypical types were found in 11 patients. In 3 of the 11, the circuit was confined to the right atrial free wall and was successfully ablated with a linear lesion directed at the lateral right atria.[21]

TYPE I AND TYPE II CLASSIFICATION

The classification of atrial flutter as type I and type II is still widely used. Type I atrial flutter encompasses typical and reverse typical atrial flutter on the basis of rate, stability, morphology, and entrainment. Type II atrial flutter is defined on the basis of an atrial rate of more than 340 beats/min, with the most rapid having been documented at 433 beats/min.[1] In Fig. 9-19 the rate of the atrial flutter is 380 beats/min. The mechanism of type II atrial flutter is not known because it is an unstable rhythm and has not been entrained. It is more easily diagnosed from the atrial electrogram than from the surface ECG.[1] The short cycle lengths of type II atrial flutter produce fibrillatory conduction and an ECG pattern of atrial fibrillation.[15] Fig. 9-20 is an example of atrial flutter that looks like atrial fibrillation on the surface ECG. At times it is difficult to make the diagnosis of atrial flutter from the ECG alone. The atrial electrogram clearly demonstrates the mechanism to be that of atrial flutter with an atrial rate of approximately 340 beats/min.

CLINICAL IMPLICATIONS

It is estimated that there are 200,000 cases of new onset atrial flutter in the United States per year.[22] Atrial flutter is commonly associated with atrial fibrillation and may alternate in the same patient. Among other supraventricular tachycardias (SVTs), atrial flutter is common during the first week after open heart surgery, and especially common after repair of congenital cardiac lesions (e.g., Mustard, Senning, Fontan procedures). It is also associated with right atrial dilatation.

Postoperative

Acute or transient atrial flutter is one of the atrial tachyarrhythmias that is a typical complication after open heart surgery. SVT occurs in 30% of patients, one third of whom have atrial flutter that may convert to atrial fibrillation and back again, especially immediately after the surgery.[23] In this clinical setting, atrial flutter is probably caused by the diffuse sterile pericarditis and atrial inflammation associated with the surgical procedure.[24]

Post–Myocardial Infarction

Atrial flutter may also be seen during the acute phase of myocardial infarction and in patients with pulmonary embolism with or without preexisting cardiac disease.[25]

Chronic atrial flutter is rare and is most often seen in

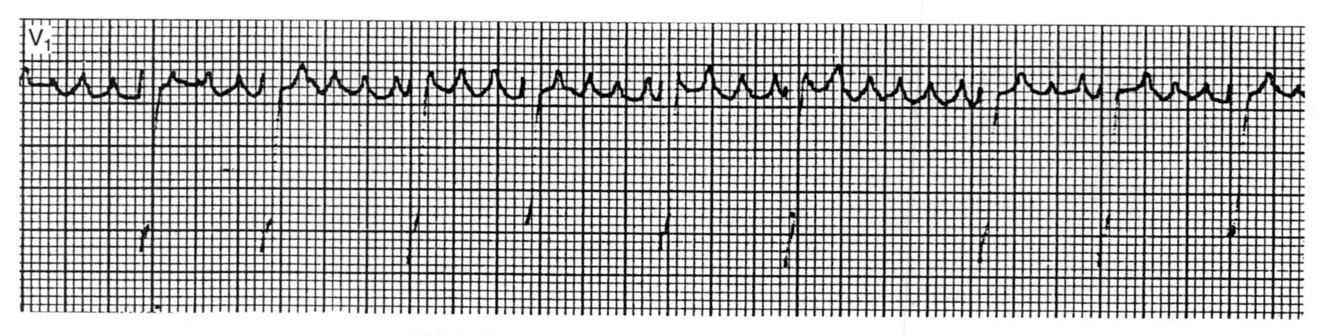

FIG. 9-19. Atrial flutter with a rate of 428 beats/min.

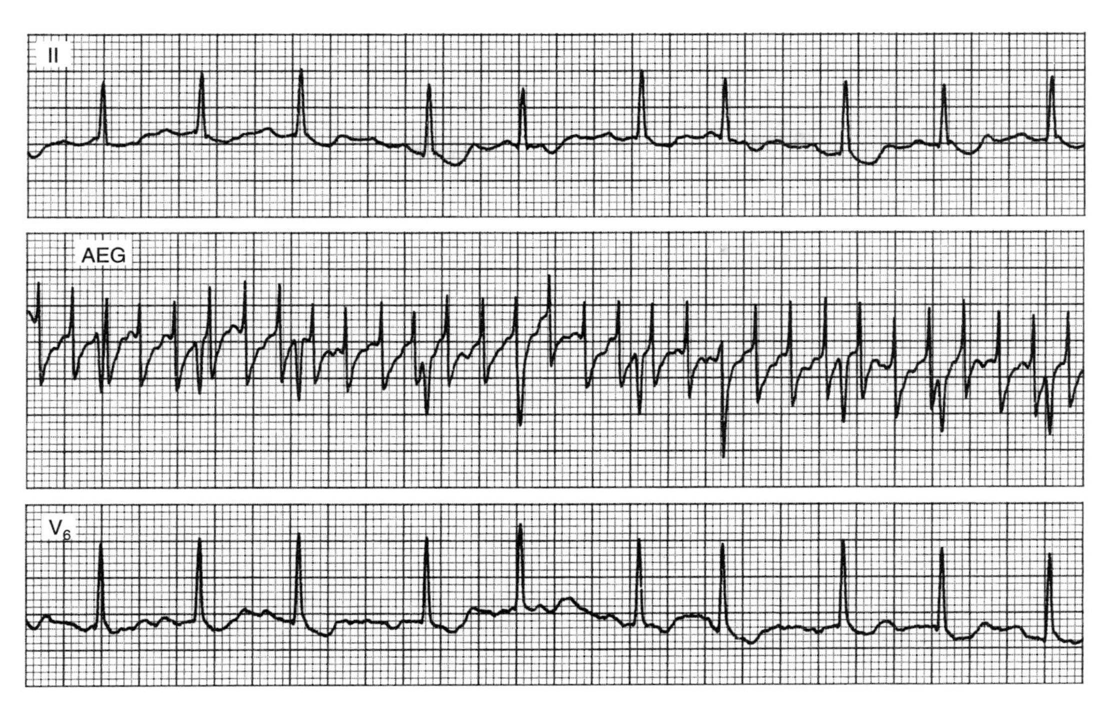

FIG. 9-20. Atrial flutter with variable conduction to the ventricles. The atrial electrogram *(AEG)* demonstrates that the diagnosis of atrial flutter is sometimes difficult with the electrocardiogram alone. In the AEG the regular biphasic deflections represent atrial activation and the mainly negative deflections represent ventricular activation. The regular biphasic spikes represent the atrial rhythm; the negative spikes represent the ventricular rhythm. This regular atrial activity is not recorded on the surface leads II and V_6. (Tracings courtesy Susan Quaal, PhD, Salt Lake City, Utah.)

persons older than 40 years of age and is commonly associated with organic heart disease, making termination and prevention of the arrhythmia important.[26]

Wolff-Parkinson-White Syndrome

Patients with accessory pathways who develop atrial flutter are particularly at risk because of the high rate of ventricular response, sometimes 1:1.

PEDIATRICS

Atrial flutter occurs in two distinct pediatric groups: the fetus and newborn and the older infant, child, or adolescent. In the newborn in most cases the arrhythmia is associated with normal cardiac structure. Atrial rates are usually between 400 and 500 beats/min with sawtooth flutter waves and 2:1 conduction (Fig. 9-21).[27] In the fetus atrial flutter can be diagnosed by fetal echocardiography. Hydrops fetalis may be secondary to intrauterine atrial flutter, and aggressive treatment is called for. In the newborn it can be treated by transesophageal overdrive pacing or external synchronized cardioversion. Once treated, in some it may never return. Most infants outgrow this arrhythmia by 12 to 18 months of age.[28-30]

In the older infant, child, or adolescent, atrial flutter often develops after surgical repair of congenital heart disease, such as atrial septal defect and tetralogy of Fallot. In most cases, the isthmus of slow conduction between the tricuspid annulus and the inferior vena cava is part of the reentrant circuit. Thus after repair of a congenital heart defect, the atrial flutter isthmus is evaluated.[30] Some patients have cardiomyopathy. Only 8% of this age group has structurally normal hearts.[31]

BEDSIDE DIAGNOSIS

Neck Veins

Rapid, rippling flutter waves may be seen in the jugular venous pulse if the conduction ratio is 4:1; with a 2:1 ratio, there is little chance of seeing this.

Heart Sounds

The first heart sound has a constant intensity if the AV relationship remains constant. It is possible on occasion to

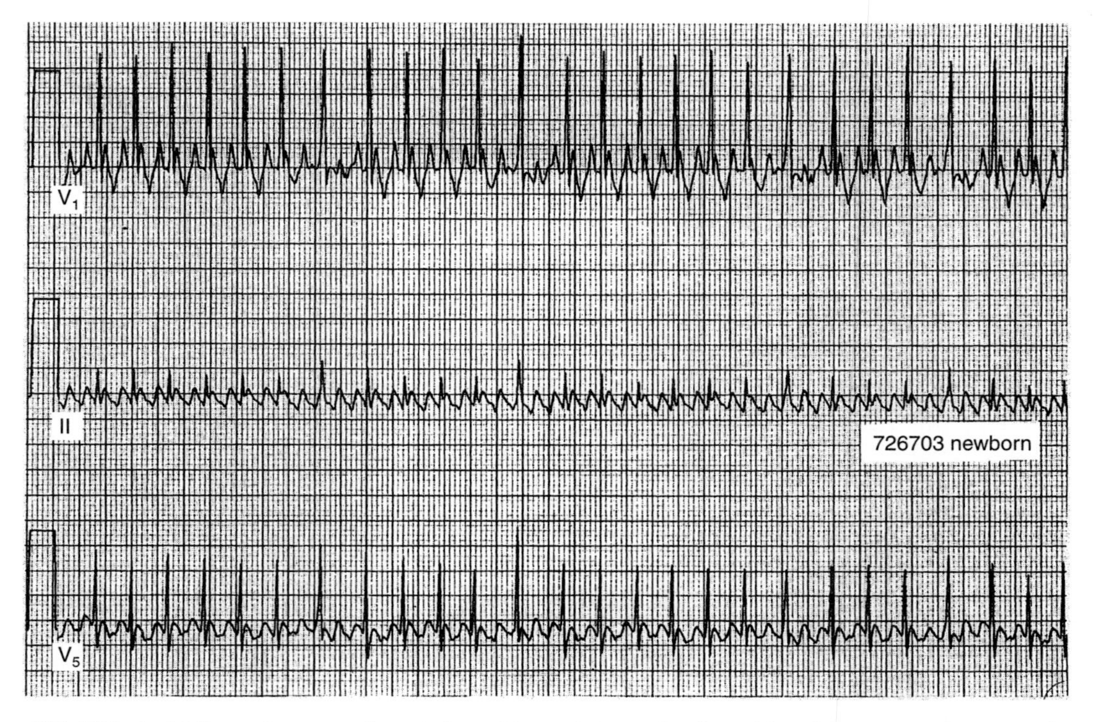

FIG. 9-21. Atrial flutter from a newborn infant of 30 weeks' gestational age. Note the presence of a sawtooth pattern seen in leads V_1, II, and V_5. The atrial rate is approximately 400 beats/min, and there is variable but predominantly 2:1 AV conduction. The infant received synchronized cardioversion for the presenting arrhythmia and was noted to develop orthodromic AV reentrant tachycardia using a concealed left-sided accessory AV connection. (From Chou TC, Knilans TK: *Electrocardiography in clinical practice: adult and pediatric*, ed 4, Philadelphia, 1996, WB Saunders.)

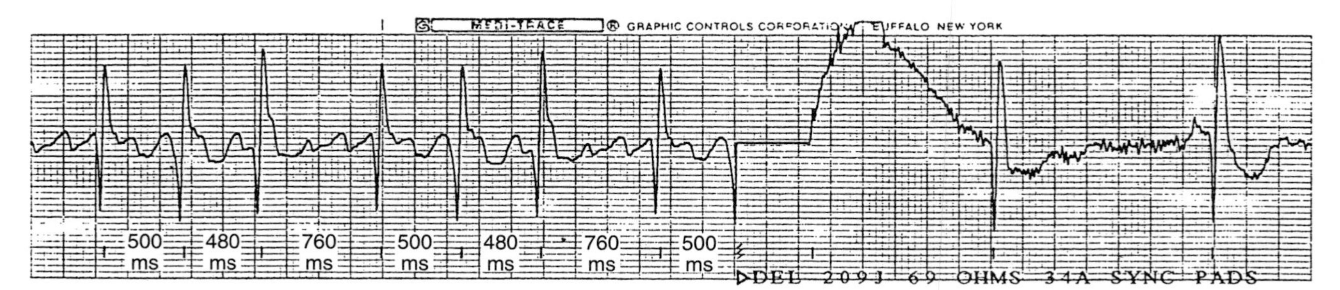

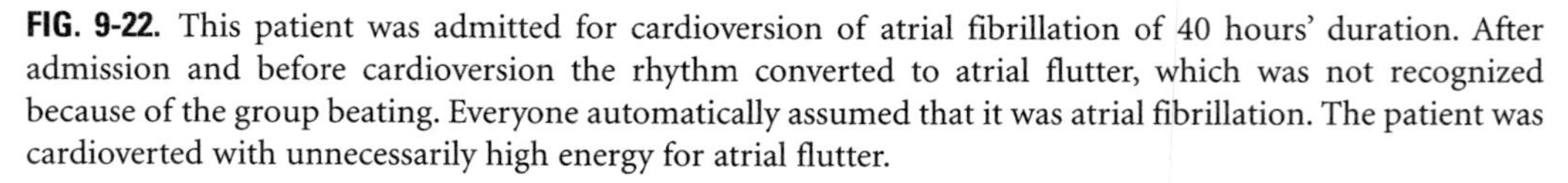

FIG. 9-22. This patient was admitted for cardioversion of atrial fibrillation of 40 hours' duration. After admission and before cardioversion the rhythm converted to atrial flutter, which was not recognized because of the group beating. Everyone automatically assumed that it was atrial fibrillation. The patient was cardioverted with unnecessarily high energy for atrial flutter.

hear the rapid sounds of the atrial contractions at the 4:1 ratio, but there is little chance of this at the 2:1 ratio.

Pulse

In atrial flutter with a fixed conduction ratio the pulse will be regular. If there is a variable conduction ratio, the irregularity of the ventricular rhythm will exactly mimic that of atrial fibrillation.

Class IC Atrial Flutter

An important in-hospital scenario is the patient who is admitted for elective direct current (DC) cardioversion of atrial fibrillation and converts to class IC atrial flutter[32] before the DC cardioversion. If the atrial flutter is not recognized, an unnecessarily high level of energy will be used for the conversion, as shown in Fig. 9-22 in which 209 J were used to convert this atrial flutter with Wenckebach conduction. This unnecessarily high level of electrical energy delivered to the myocardium is not without its price (see p. 88).

EMERGENCY TREATMENT

Acute treatment of atrial flutter depends on the clinical setting and the type of flutter (atypical atrial flutter is difficult to terminate). In typical (type I) atrial flutter restoration of sinus rhythm is accomplished by one of the following[2]:

1. Antiarrhythmic drug therapy
2. Direct current cardioversion
3. Rapid atrial pacing to interrupt the atrial flutter

In cases of chronic obstructive pulmonary disease or if the patient has taken a meal recently, rapid atrial pacing or antiarrhythmic drugs to slow the ventricular response are preferred to DC cardioversion, which requires an anesthetic. In postoperative patients who have an epicardial wire, rapid atrial pacing is performed to convert the atrial flutter.

SUMMARY

Atrial flutter is a rapid, regular form of atrial tachycardia that is sustained by a macroreentrant circuit; it is usually paroxysmal, lasting for from seconds to hours and occasionally even days. The well-known classification of atrial flutter into type I and type II has given way to a classification of typical, reverse typical, lesion, left atrial macroreentrant, and atypical.

REFERENCES

1. Waldo AL: Atrial flutter: mechanisms, clinical features, and management. In Zipes DP, Jalife J, editors: *Cardiac electrophysiology from cell to bedside*, ed 2, Philadelphia, 1995, WB Saunders.
2. Jolly WA, Ritchie WJ: Auricular flutter and fibrillation, *Heart* 2:177, 1911.
3. Saoudi N, Cosio F, Waldo A et al: Classification of atrial flutter and regular atrial tachycardia according to electrophysiologic mechanism and anatomic bases: a statement from a joint expert group from the Working Group of Arrhythmias of the European Society of Cardiology and the North American Society of Pacing and Electrophysiology, *J Cardiovasc Electrophysiol* 12(7):85, 2001.
4. Langendorf R: Concealed A-V conduction: the effect of blocked impulses on the formation and conduction of subsequent impulses, *Am Heart J* 35:542, 1948.
5. Page RL, Wharton JM, Prystowsky EN: Effect of continuous vagal enhancement on concealed conduction and refractoriness within the atrioventricular node, *Am J Cardiol* 77:260, 1996.
6. Kalman JM, Olgin JE, Saxon LA et al: Activation and entrainment mapping defines the tricuspid annulus as the anterior barrier in typical atrial flutter, *Circulation* 94:398, 1996.
7. Waldo AL: Personal communication, 17 Oct 2001.
8. Feld G: Catheter ablation for atrial flutter, Session ACC96-327; and Morady F, Borggrefe M, Epstein L et al: Changing concepts in treatment of supraventricular tachycardia, Session ACC96-327, *Am Coll Cardiol* 45th Annual Scientific Sessions, Orlando, Fla, March 24-27, 1996.
9. Matsuo K, Uno K, Khrestian CM et al: Conduction left-to-right and right-to-left across the crista terminalis, *Am J Physiol Heart Circ Physiol* 280:H1683, 2001.
10. Nakagawa H, Lazzara R, Khastgir T et al: Role of the tricuspid annulus and the eustachian valve/ridge on atrial flutter. Relevance to catheter ablation of the septal isthmus and a new technique for rapid identification of ablation success, *Circulation* 94:407, 1996.
11. Lesh MD, Kalman JM: To fumble flutter or tackle “tach?” Toward updated classifiers for atrial tachyarrhythmias, *J Cardiovasc Electrophys* 7:460, 1996.
12. Lesh MD: Personal communication, 13 August, 1996.
13. Aziz AA, Saoudi N, Nair M et al: Intra and interatrial conduction abnormalities in atrial flutter. A comparison between clockwise and counterclockwise right atrial rotation, *J Am Coll Cardiol* 27(Suppl A):189-A, 1996.
14. Triedman JK, Jenkins KJ, Colan SD et al: High-density transcatheter mapping shows diverse mechanisms for atrial reentrant tachycardia after congenital heart surgery, *J Am Coll Cardiol* 27(Suppl A), 768:189A, 1996.
15. Waldo AL, Cooper TB: Spontaneous onset of type I atrial flutter in patients, *J Am Coll Cardiol* 28:707, 1996.
16. Gandhi SK, Bromberg BI, Schuessler RB et al: Characterization and surgical ablation of atrial flutter after the classic Fontan repair, *Ann Thorac Surg* 61:1666, 1996.
17. Baker BM, Lindsay BD, Bromberg BI et al: Catheter ablation of clinical intraatrial reentrant tachycardias resulting from previous atrial surgery: localizing and transecting the critical isthmus, *J Am Coll Cardiol* 28:411, 1996.
18. Henglein D, Cauchemez B, Bloch G: Simultaneous surgical treatment of atrial septal defect and atrial flutter using a simple modification of the atrial incision, *Cardiol Young* 9:197, 1999.
19. Kirkorian G, Moncada E, Defeo M et al: Radiofrequency ablation of atrial tissue is also effective in atypical atrial flutter, *Circulation* 90:1802, 1994 (abstract).
20. Satake S, Okishiga K, Azegami K et al: Radiofrequency catheter ablation of uncommon type atrial flutter, *Circulation* 90:3201, 1994 (abstract).
21. Kall J, Rubenstein D, Kopp D et al: Characterization and catheter ablation of right atrial free wall atypical atrial flutter, *Circulation* 94(8 Suppl):3949, 1996.
22. Uribe W, Vidaillet H, Granada J et al: Incidence and cause of death among patients with atrial flutter in the general population, Circulation 94(8 Suppl):2269, 1996.
23. Waldo AL, MacLean WAH: *Diagnosis and treatment of arrhythmias following open-heart surgery: emphasis on the use of epicardial wire electrodes*, New York, 1980, Futura Publishing.
24. Pagè PL, Plumb VJ, Okumura K et al: A new animal model of atrial flutter, *J Am Coll Cardiol* 8:872, 1986.
25. Brugada P, Gorgels AP, Wellens HJJ: The electrocardiogram in pulmonary embolism. In Wellens HJJ, Kulbertus HE editors: *What's new in electrocardiography*? The Hague, 1981, Martinus Nijhoff, pp. 366-380.
26. Wellens HJJ: Atrial flutter: progress but no final answer, *J Am Coll Cardiol* 17:1235, 1991.

27. Porter CJ: Premature atrial contractions and atrial tachyarrhythmias. In Gillette PC, Garson A Jr, editors: *Pediatric arrhythmias: electrophysiology and pacing*, Philadelphia, 1990, WB Saunders, pp 328-359.
28. Dunnigan A, Benson DW Jr, Benditt DG: Atrial flutter in infancy: diagnosis, clinical features, and treatment, *Pediatrics* 75:725, 1985.
29. Gillette PC, Zeigler VL, Case CL: Pediatric arrhythmias: Are they different? In Zipes DP, Jalife J, editors: *Cardiac electrophysiology from cell to bedside*, ed 2, Philadelphia, 1995, WB Saunders, pp 1265-1268.
30. Chan DP, Van Hare GF, Mackall JA et al: Importance of atrial flutter isthmus in postoperative intra-atrial reentrant tachycardia, *Circulation* 102:1283, 2000.
31. Chou TC: *Electrocardiography in clinical practice: adult and pediatric*, Philadelphia, 1996, WB Saunders.
32. Nabar A, Rodriquez LM, Timmermans C et al: Radiofrequency ablation of "class IC atrial flutter" in patients with resistant atrial fibrillation, *Am J Cardiol* 83:785, 1999.

CHAPTER **10**

Junctional Beats and Rhythms

TERMINOLOGY

nonparoxysmal Of gradual onset and termination

accelerated junctional rhythm When the junctional rate is more than 60 beats/min and less than 100 beats/min. The term implies retrograde conduction to the atria (i.e., atrioventricular [AV] dissociation is not present)

accelerated idiojunctional rhythm "Idio-" added to the word junctional implies independent beating of the ventricles (AV dissociation) under the control of the junctional focus; the atria are beating to another stimulus (sinus or atrial)

junctional tachycardia The term *junctional tachycardia*, in its strict sense, is used when the junctional rate is 100 beats/min or more. Junctional tachycardias with rates of less than 100 beats/min are, strictly speaking, *accelerated idiojunctional rhythms*. Whether the rate is 70 beats/min, 99.8 beats/min, or 100 beats/min, the mechanism is the same; therefore, it seems less cumbersome to simply refer to any junctional rhythm with a rate greater than 60 beats/min as junctional tachycardia. This term makes dialogue easier and acknowledges that any rate more than 60 beats/min is too fast to qualify as junctional escape

retrograde conduction This term implies that a junctional or ventricular focus is conducted up the AV node to activate the atria inferiorly to superiorly. Whether retrograde conduction to the atria occurs depends on the physiologic properties of the individual AV node and the effect of drugs on AV nodal conduction. When retrograde conduction does occur, the retrograde P′ wave that results is negative in the inferior leads (II, III, and aV_F) and isoelectric in lead I because the current proceeds from an inferior position to the top of the heart (away from the positive electrodes of the inferior leads). Because the AV node is located more or less equidistant between the right and left atria, the mean current proceeds straight up, crossing the axis of lead I at right angles and resulting in an isoelectric P′ wave. The location of the P′ wave relative to the QRS, of course, depends on the speed of retrograde AV nodal conduction

AV dissociation AV dissociation is the independent beating of atria and ventricles (see Chapter 18). If retrograde conduction from a junctional or ventricular pacemaker is blocked, the atria are under the control of the sinus node or an atrial ectopic focus and the ventricles are under the control of the junctional or ventricular focus

ATRIOVENTRICULAR JUNCTION

The atrioventricular (AV) junction consists of the AV node and the bundle of His down to where it begins to branch. The different regions of the AV junction are divided according to the various cell types: atrionodal (AN), nodal (N), nodal-His (NH), and His bundle. Fig. 10-1 is an artist's conception of the divisions of the AV junction.

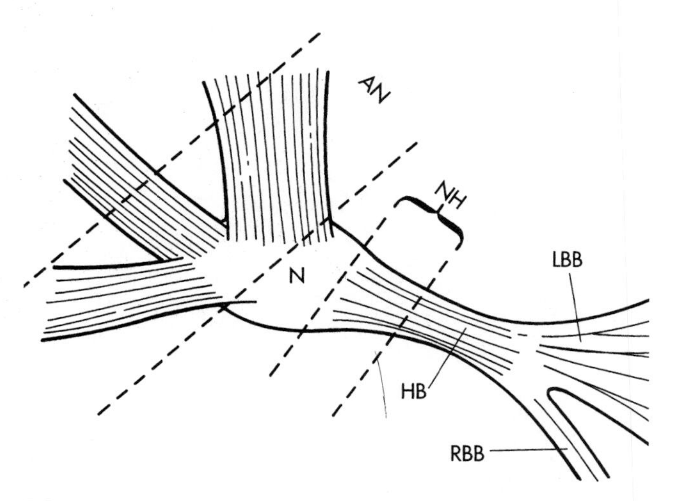

FIG. 10-1. The divisions of the AV junction. *AN*, Atrionodal; *N*, compact AV node; *NH*, nodal-His; *HB*, His bundle; *LBB*, left bundle branch; *RBB*, right bundle branch.

AN Region

The AN region is a transitional zone where the atrial fibers gradually merge with the compact AV node. The best-known AV nodal fibers are found posteriorly (the slow pathway) and anteriorly (the fast pathway). These pathways are responsible for the maintenance of the AV nodal reentry mechanism, one of the most common causes of paroxysmal supraventricular tachycardia (see Chapter 11).

N Region

The N region is the compact AV node, especially the midnodal region. It is noted for the virtual absence of junctional beats along with an increase in the electrical resistance at the coupling of the cells. In the N region the normal and rate-related conduction delay occurs. A simplified drawing of the "fast" (f) and "slow" (s) atrial fibers emanating from the compact AV node can be seen in Fig. 10-2.

NH Region

The NH region is the merging of fibers from the lower AV node with those of the His bundle. Some investigators have defined this region as the primary focus for the junctional escape rhythm.

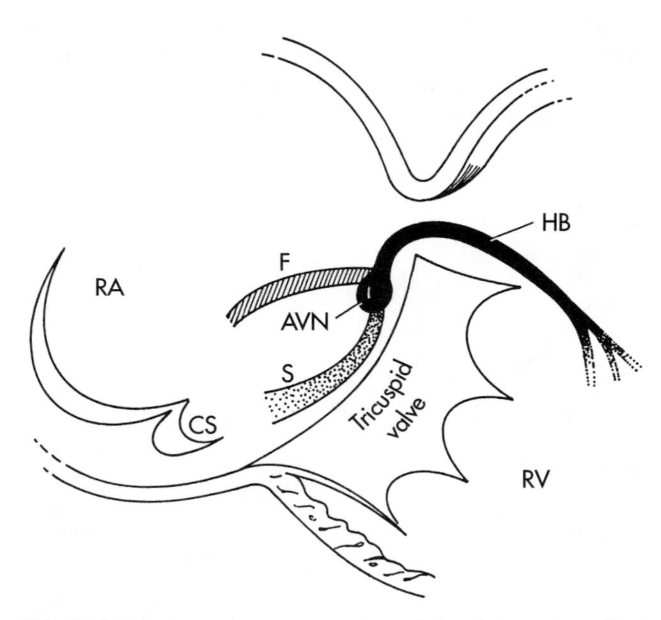

FIG. 10-2. A schematic representation of the right atrium *(RA)* and right ventricle *(RV)* opened to reveal the compact atrioventricular node *(AVN)* and its atrial fibers. The fast fibers *(F)* are superior; the slow fibers *(S)* are inferior, arising near the os of the coronary sinus *(CS)*. *HB*, His bundle. (Adapted from Kiem S, Werner P, Jazayeri M et al: *Circulation* 86:919, 1992.)

PREMATURE JUNCTIONAL COMPLEX

A premature junctional complex (PJC) originates in the AV junction, usually in the NH region. It discharges before the next expected sinus impulse and activates the ventricles through the His bundle and bundle branches in the normal manner. In fact, it is recognized because its shape does not differ from that of the normal sinus-conducted beat. There may be retrograde conduction to the atria from this focus. This depends on the ability of the AV node to conduct in a retrograde fashion. For example, in cases of digitalis toxicity, there is some degree of AV block, impairing conduction in both directions across the AV node.

If retrograde conduction does take place, the resulting P′ wave is negative in the inferior leads II, III, and aV_F. The location of the retrograde P′ wave relative to the QRS depends on the speed of conduction up into the atria compared with the conduction speed down to the ventricles. Thus the P′ wave may occur before, during, or after the QRS. Fig. 10-3 illustrates the possibilities for P′ wave location in PJCs. It is also possible for a junctional focus to discharge and fail to conduct anterogradely or retrogradely. Such an occurrence is called a *concealed junctional extrasystole*; it is recognized because of the effect it has on the subsequent cycle. For example, there may be unexplained lengthening of the PR interval, as seen in Fig. 10-4, or an unexplained type II AV block.

ECG Recognition

Heart rate: That of the underlying rhythm.
Rhythm: Irregular because of the PJC.
P′ wave: If a P′ wave occurs, it is negative in leads II, III, and aV_F and may occur before, during, or after the QRS.
P′R interval: If the P′ wave occurs before the QRS, the P′R interval is less than 0.12 second.
QRS complex: Normal in shape and duration unless there is an intraventricular conduction abnormality.

Treatment

PJCs are not usually treated. If they initiate a more serious arrhythmia (for example, ventricular tachycardia [VT]), therapy is directed at the VT.[1]

JUNCTIONAL TACHYCARDIA

Junctional tachycardia is a narrow QRS tachycardia with gradual onset and termination that originates within AV junctional fibers (AV node-His bundle).

ECG Recognition

Heart rate: Ranges from 70 to 140 beats/min (may be seen between 60 beats/min and 70 beats/min if there is sinus bradycardia or sinoatrial [SA] block). As with atrial

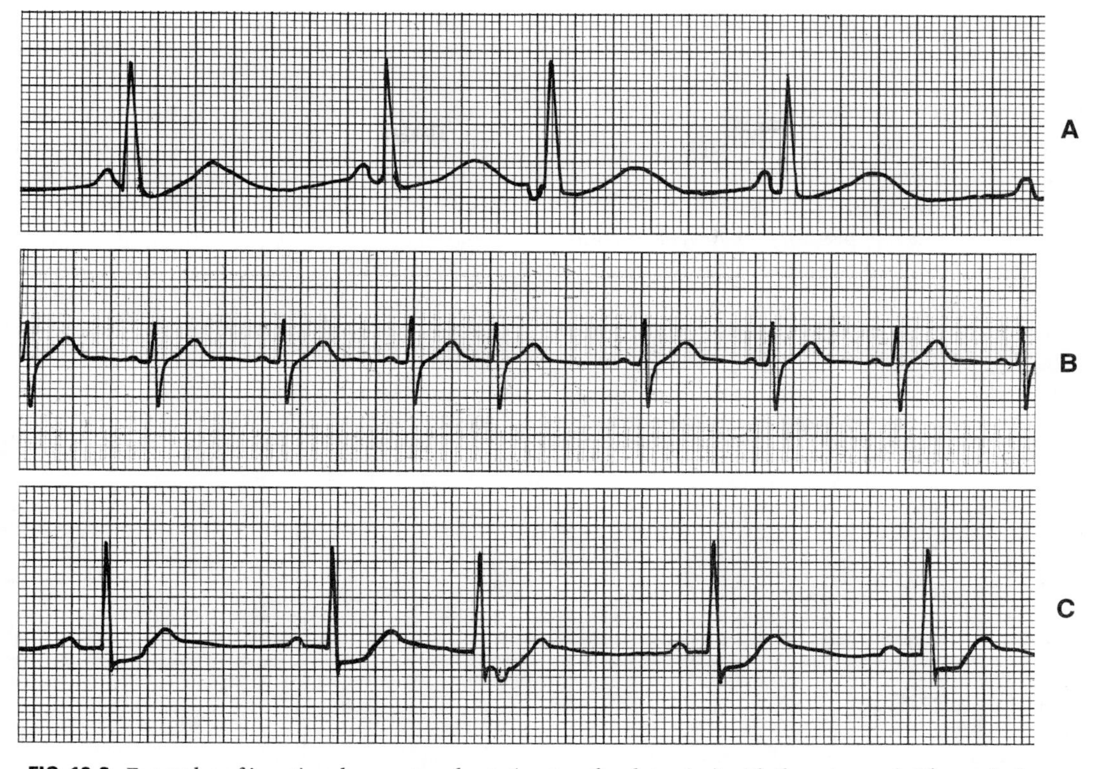

FIG. 10-3. Examples of junctional premature beats (*center of each tracing*) with the retrograde P′ wave before (**A**), during (**B**), and after (**C**) the QRS.

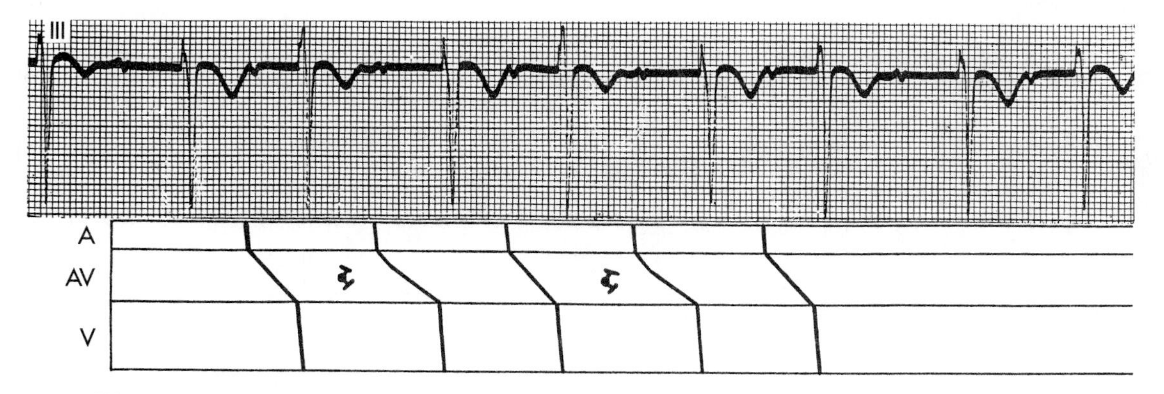

FIG. 10-4. Concealed junctional extrasystoles (shown in the atrioventricular *[AV]* tier of the laddergram) produce alternating PR and RR intervals. The mechanism is suspected because of the unexplained PR lengthening. (It is obviously not a Wenckebach period because there are no dropped beats.) *A*, Atrial; *V*, ventricular. (From Marriott HJL, Conover M: *Advanced concepts in arrhythmias*, ed 2, St Louis, 1992, Mosby.)

tachycardia resulting from digitalis toxicity, the rate of the junctional tachycardia gradually increases as more digitalis is given.[1]

Rhythm: Nonparoxysmal; appears to be regular but may slowly increase its rate.

P waves: Retrograde P′ waves before, during, or after the QRS. If there is AV dissociation (junctional tachycardia with retrograde AV block), there will be normal sinus P waves.

P′R interval: Less than 0.12 second if the P′ wave occurs before the QRS.

QRS complex: Normal in duration and shape.

Response to carotid sinus massage: No response. (This is not a reentry mechanism as with that of paroxysmal supraventricular tachycardia.)

AV dissociation: The atria and the ventricles usually beat independently in the presence of junctional tachycardia. The ventricles are under the control of the junctional focus, and the atria are in sinus rhythm or their own ectopic rhythm. It is even possible to have a second junctional focus controlling the atria.

There is AV dissociation in all of the tracings in Fig. 10-5. For further discussion of AV dissociation, see Chapter 18. Fig. 10-6, *A* and *B*, are examples of junctional tachycardia of 110 and 75 beats/min, respectively, both without AV dissociation. Note the retrograde conduction to the atria immediately after the QRS complexes in both tracings (negative P′ wave in lead II).

Distinguishing features: The distinguishing feature of a junctional rhythm is a QRS complex that is supraventricular in shape and has a regular rhythm with a rate of 70 to 140 beats/min. AV dissociation may be present.

Mechanism

Because the ectopic focus of junctional tachycardia is pacemaker tissue, it is possible for the mechanism to be enhanced normal automaticity in the His bundle; of course, abnormal automaticity or triggered activity is also a possibility.

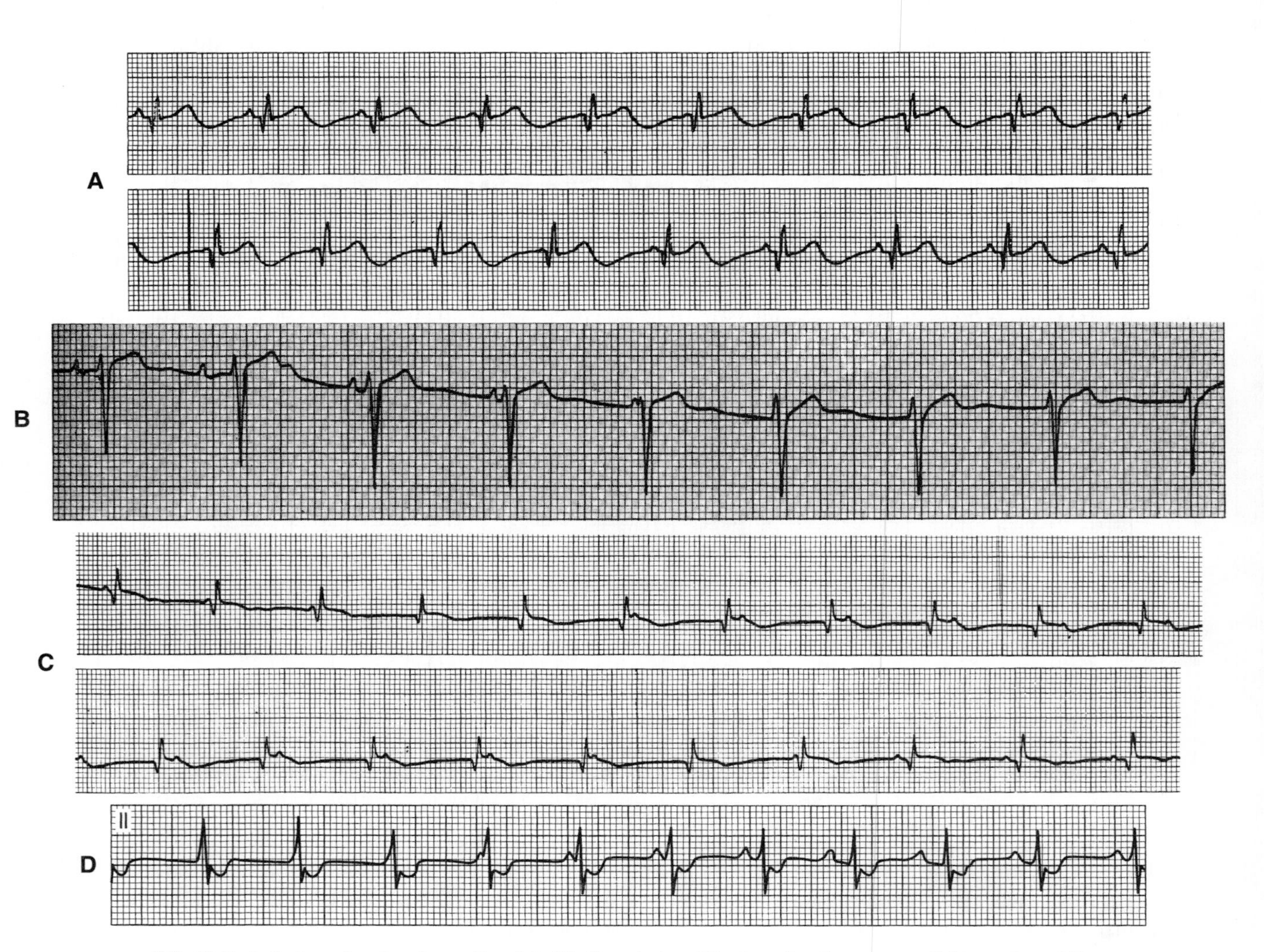

FIG. 10-5. **A-D**, Junctional tachycardia with AV dissociation. The junctional rates are all lower than 100 beats/min but too fast for the atrioventricular junction. **D** is from a 16-year-old boy who attempted suicide with an overdose of digitalis. (**D** courtesy William P. Nelson, MD.)

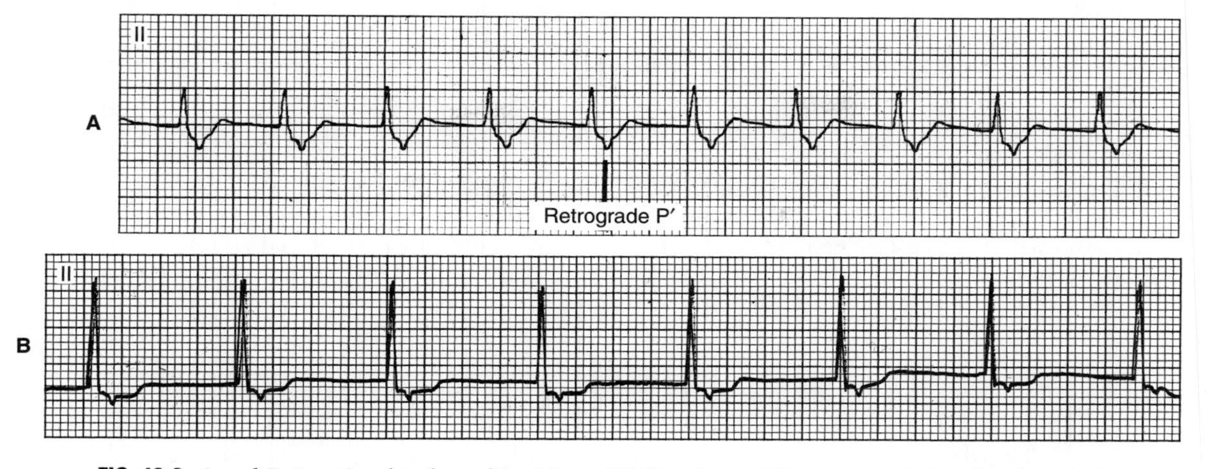

FIG. 10-6. **A** and **B**, Junctional tachycardia without AV dissociation. The rates are 110 and 75 beats/min, respectively. The retrograde P′ waves immediately follow the QRS waves.

Causes

Probably the most important cause of nonparoxysmal junctional tachycardia is digitalis toxicity[2]; in such cases, the mortality rate can be very high when the condition is not treated properly.

Other causes include the following:

- Inferior myocardial infarction
- Myocarditis, often a result of acute rheumatic fever
- After open heart surgery
- Idiopathic

Pediatrics

Junctional ectopic tachycardia in children occurs most frequently after operative repair of congenital heart defects. The mechanism is thought to involve direct trauma to the AV node and His bundle resulting in an ectopic focus. Cardiovascular function in the postoperative patient can be significantly compromised because heart rates may exceed 200 to 300 beats/min, leaving inadequate time for ventricular filling, and because of the lack of synchrony between the atria and the ventricles.[3]

Bedside Diagnosis

The physical signs of nonparoxysmal AV junctional tachycardia, as in other arrhythmias, are determined by the ventricular rate, the atrial rate, the relationship of the P wave to the QRS complex, ventricular function, and the absence or presence of underlying heart disease.[1]

First heart sound: Varies in intensity if AV dissociation is present; is of constant intensity if AV dissociation is not present (i.e., there is retrograde conduction to the atria).

Jugular venous pulse: Irregular cannon a waves appear if AV dissociation is present (in the absence of coexisting atrial fibrillation).

Treatment

If the junctional tachycardia is due to digitalis toxicity, it is usually sufficient to discontinue the drug. However, if there is hemodynamic compromise, digitalis antibody may be lifesaving.

JUNCTIONAL ESCAPE BEATS AND RHYTHMS

Junctional escape beats and rhythms are protective mechanisms that are normally prevented from pacing the heart because they are discharged by the sinus rhythm. Junctional cells have an inherent rate of 35 to 60 beats/min. When they are not discharged in a timely fashion by the impulse from the sinus node, they reach threshold and discharge themselves. Thus AV junctional cells can normally assume the passive role of pacemaker only when the sinus node defaults; for example, in marked sinus bradycardia and SA block, during the pause caused by a nonconducted premature atrial complex (PAC), or when there is AV block.

ECG Recognition

Heart rate: Bradycardia (35 to 60 beats/min).

Rhythm: Regular for junctional escape rhythms, although at its onset the rate increases ("warm-up" phenomena characteristic of automatic fibers).

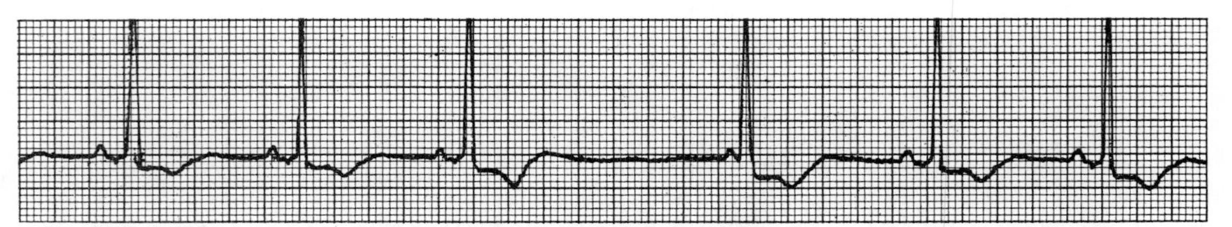

FIG. 10-7. Junctional escape beat after a pause created by a nonconducted PAC (distorting the third T wave). The premature atrial complex is not conducted because it is very early; a pause results and is terminated by a junctional escape beat (fourth complex). The sinus P wave immediately in front of the escape beat is too close to have been conducted.

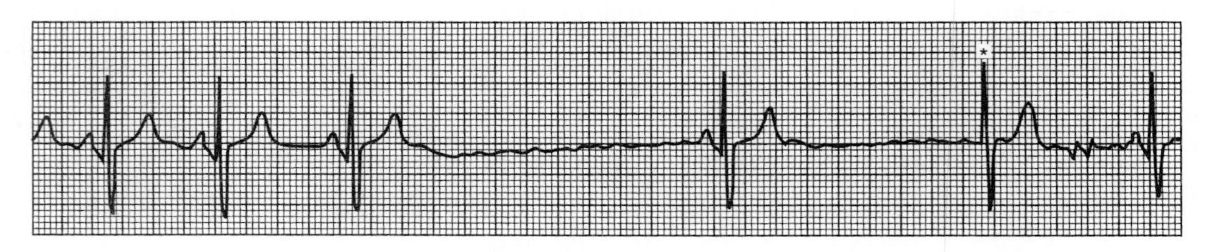

FIG. 10-8. Sinoatrial block and sinus arrest with a 2.4-second pause. A junctional escape beat (*) terminates the second pause. This beat resembles the sinus-conducted ones, missing only the initial q wave. There is artifact in the tracing after the junctional escape beat. This patient had presyncope as a result of these pauses. (From Angeli SJ: *Am Heart J* 120:433, 1990.)

P′ waves: May or may not be linked to the junctional complex.

QRS complex: Normal or the same shape as the sinus conducted beats.

Junctional escape beats and rhythms are recognized because of an underlying bradycardia or pauses that are terminated by the appearance of a normal QRS complex with or without a retrograde P′ wave. In Fig. 10-7, for example, there is a PAC distorting the third T wave (making it deeper and bigger), followed by overdrive suppression of the sinus node. Thus the next sinus beat is delayed, causing the junctional focus to "escape." Although there is a sinus P wave in front of the fourth QRS it does not conduct to the ventricles (the PR is too short). Note that the junctional escape beat is identical in shape to the sinus conducted beats.

In Fig. 10-8 the pause is caused by SA block or sinus arrest. After 2.4 seconds, a sinus P wave appears and is conducted to the ventricles and is followed by another pause, terminated with a junctional escape beat, apparently without retrograde ventriculoatrial conduction.

In Fig. 10-9 there is an underlying sinus arrhythmia and sinus tachycardia dominated by a junctional escape rhythm of 57 beats/min. Only one of the sinus P waves conducts to the ventricles. When this happens it is called a "capture" beat *(C)*.

Fig. 10-10 is a junctional escape rhythm of 60 beats/min without AV dissociation. The retrograde P′ waves is immediately in front of the QRS with a very short P′R interval

Treatment

Frequently no treatment is necessary. At times, consideration may be given to increasing the rate of the sinus node to improve cardiac output by restoring AV synchrony.[1]

SUMMARY

Junctional beats and rhythms are recognized because the QRS is narrow and the P wave either is not associated with the QRS (AV dissociation) or is retrograde (negative in leads II, III, and aV_F). When the rate of a junctional rhythm exceeds that expected of a junctional focus (approximately 60 beats/min), this is an abnormal acceleration and the cause should be identified and treated. Junctional rates up to 140 beats/min may be seen with digitalis toxicity. When the junctional rhythm is less than 60 beats/min, it is a protective escape mechanism, usually in the setting of sinus bradycardia or complete AV nodal block.

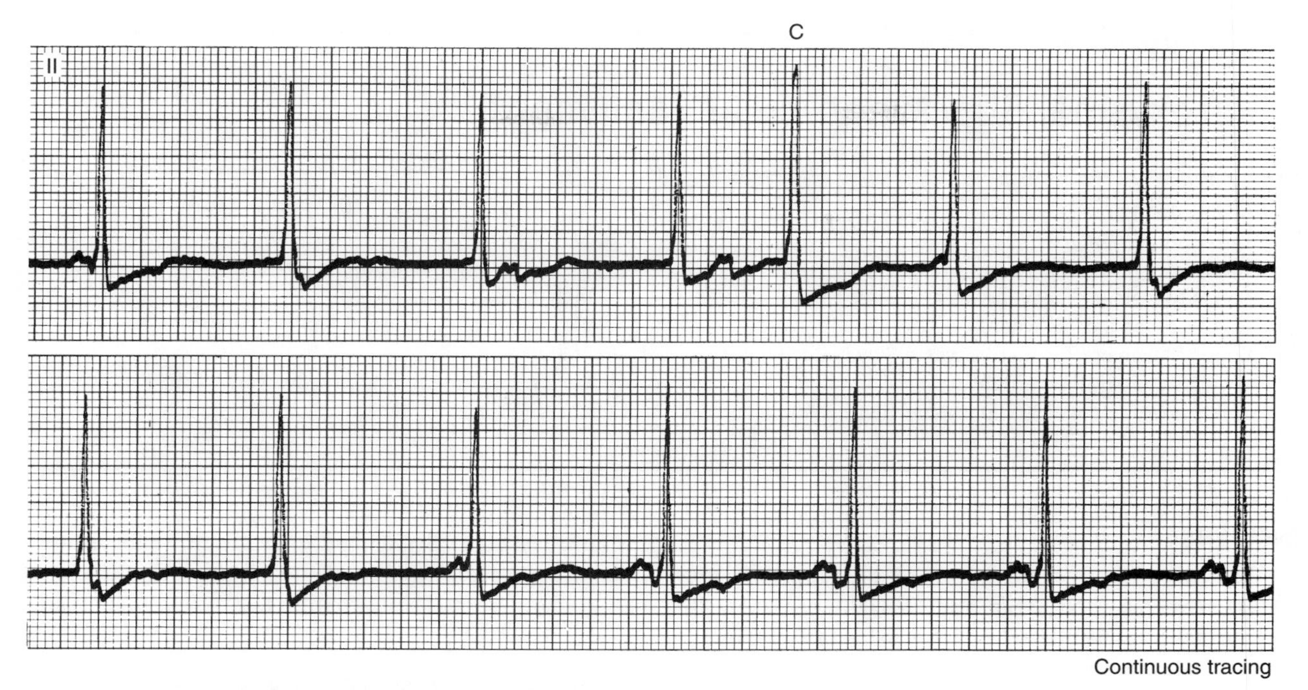

FIG. 10-9. Sinus arrhythmia and sinus bradycardia dominated by a junctional escape rhythm. There is one capture (conducted; *C*) beat.

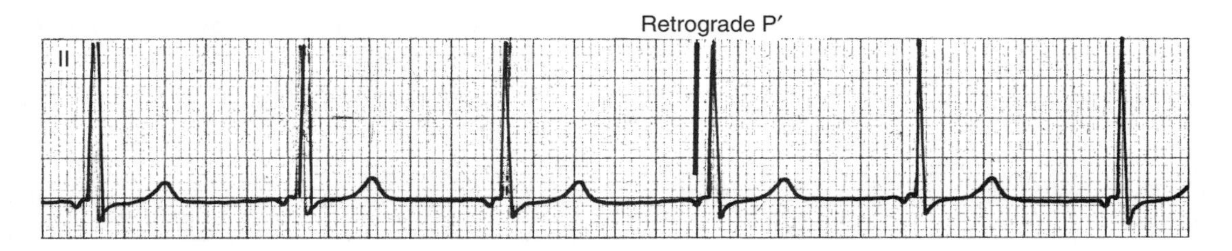

FIG. 10-10. Junctional escape rhythm with retrograde conduction to the atria. Atrial activation takes place slightly before ventricular activation.

REFERENCES

1. Zipes DP: Specific arrhythmias: Diagnosis and treatment. In Braunwald E, editor: *Heart disease*, ed 4, Philadelphia, 1992, WB Saunders.
2. Naccarelli GV, Shih HT, Jalal S: Sinus node reentry and atrial tachycardias. In Zipes DP, Jalife J, editors: *Cardiac electrophysiology from cell to bedside*, ed 2, Philadelphia, 1995, WB Saunders.
3. Michael JG, Wilson WR Jr, Tobias JD: Amiodarone in the treatment of junctional ectopic tachycardia after cardiac surgery in children: Report of two cases and review of the literature, *Am J Ther* 6:223, 1999.

CHAPTER **11**

Paroxysmal Supraventricular Tachycardia

INCIDENCE

According to one study[1] there are approximately 89,000 new cases per year and 570,000 persons with paroxysmal supraventricular tachycardia (PSVT) in the United States, with the two most common mechanisms being atrioventricular nodal reentry tachycardia (AVNRT) and circus movement tachycardia (CMT) using the atrioventricular (AV) node anterogradely and an accessory pathway retrogradely (Wolff-Parkinson-White syndrome [WPW], see Chapter 21). Of cases of symptomatic PSVT, in one study AVNRT accounted for 50% of cases and CMT for 40%.[2]

In another institution[3] out of 1,500 consecutive patients with symptomatic tachycardia, 987 (65.8%) had CMT. The second most common mechanism was AVNRT, found in 321 (21.4%) of patients. The less common arrhythmias were atrial flutter in 109 (7.2%), atrial tachycardia in 13 (1.7%), and ventricular tachycardia (VT) in 37 (2.4%).

TERMINOLOGY

orthodromic In the same direction as the normal current through the AV node; "-dromic" refers to conduction

antidromic In the opposite direction of the normal current through the AV node

reciprocating The return of an impulse to its place of origin; for example, in AV reciprocating tachycardia the supraventricular impulse enters the ventricles via one AV pathway and then returns to the atria via another pathway

circus movement A reentry circuit; commonly used to refer to the AV reentry circuit using an accessory pathway and the AV node

paroxysmal Begins and ends abruptly; for example, a rapid rhythm of sudden onset that changes from normal sinus rhythm to a tachycardia in one beat

ATRIOVENTRICULAR NODAL REENTRY TACHYCARDIA

AVNRT is a PSVT caused by a reentry circuit using multiple pathways into the AV node. Recent studies by the Zipes group[4] demonstrated multiple preferential AV nodal input pathways.

Location of the Fast and Slow Atrioventricular Nodal Pathways

It has been suggested[3] that the fibers of the fast and slow pathways run along opposite edges of the compact AV node into the atrium in a fanlike fashion. Fig. 11-1, *A*, shows the compact AV node and two of its atrial input fibers. The fast fibers are located superiorly along the compact node and exit into the atrial septum near the tendon of Todaro. The slow fibers arise near the coronary sinus os and are directed inferiorly along the tricuspid annulus toward the compact AV node. Block in the slow pathway has no impact on the PR interval during sinus rhythm.

Mechanism of the Common Form of AVNRT

The reentrant circuit of the common form of AVNRT ("slow/fast") uses the slowly conducting pathway anterogradely and the more rapidly conducting pathway retrogradely.

Fig. 11-1, *B-D*, takes you step-by-step through the sequence of events that result in PSVT caused by the common form of AVNRT.

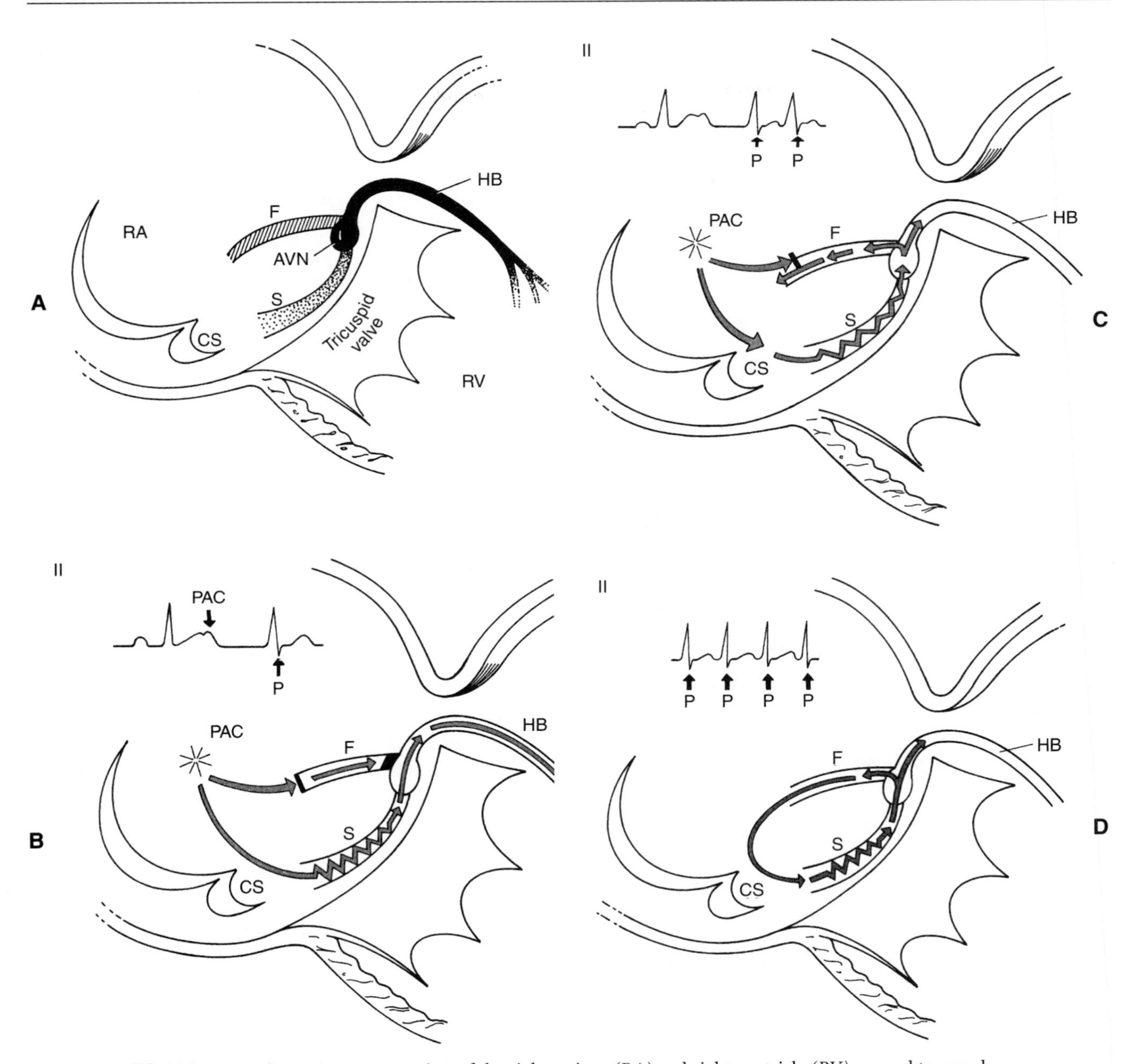

FIG. 11-1. **A,** A schematic representation of the right atrium *(RA)* and right ventricle *(RV)* opened to reveal the compact atrioventricular node *(AVN)* and two of its atrial input fibers. The fast fibers *(F)* are superior; the slow fibers *(S)* are inferior, arising near the os of the coronary sinus *(CS)*. **B-D,** Events that lead to PSVT caused by AVNRT. *HB,* His bundle; *PAC,* premature atrial complex. (Adapted from Kiem S, Werner P, Jazayeri M et al: *Circulation* 86:919, 1992.)

In Fig. 11-1, *B*, note that the reentry circuit is initiated by an early premature atrial complex (PAC) that is blocked in the fast pathway at its interface with the AV node.[4] It, however, does pass down the slow pathway. The delay in slow pathway conduction to the compact AV node results in a prolonged P′R interval of about 0.38 second. Note the distance between the PAC and the next QRS.

Fig. 11-1, *C*, shows that within the AV node the impulse travels in two directions *simultaneously*—down to activate the ventricles and up to the atrium via the fast pathway. This

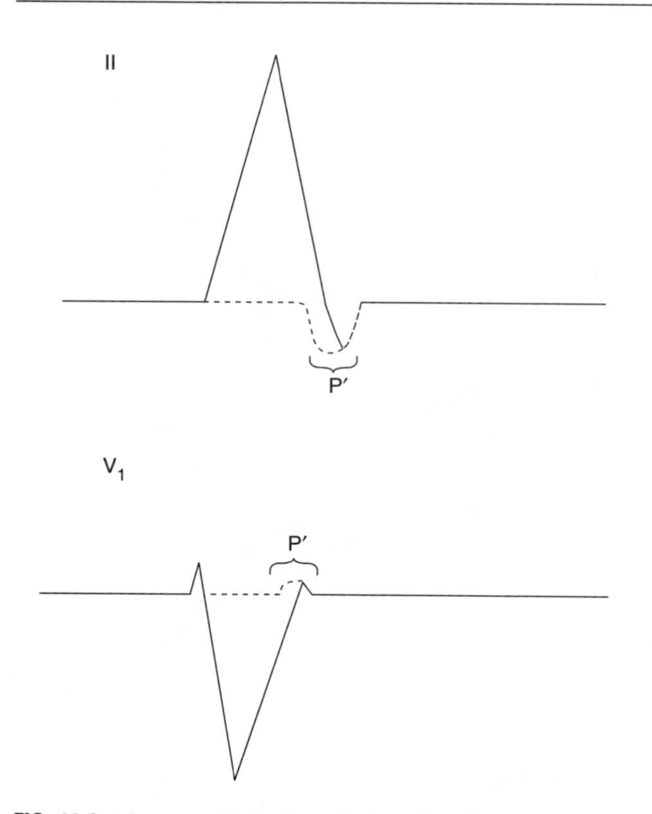

FIG. 11-2. The partially hidden P′ wave *(dotted line)* in leads II and V_1 during AVNRT. The end of the P′ wave looks like an S wave in lead II or an r′ wave in lead V_1.

part of the mechanism is important to understand and remember because it supports the differential diagnosis between AVNRT and CMT using an accessory pathway. From the fast pathway the impulse rapidly returns to the slow pathway through the atrial tissue located at the base of Koch's triangle.

In Fig. 11-1, *D*, the AV nodal reentry circuit is in full swing and can be terminated by lengthening the refractory period in the AV node (vagal maneuver). Note that the P′ wave is within or distorting the end of the QRS looking like an S wave in the inferior leads and an r′ in V_1 (not shown).

The common form of AV nodal reentry is established as a result of (1) an early PAC blocked in the fast pathway (2) conducted down the slow pathway to the AV node (3) where it simultaneously activates upper and lower chambers, placing the P′ wave within the QRS.[5] Fig. 11-2 shows how the partially hidden retrograde P′ wave can distort the QRS and give us the diagnostic clue in leads II and V_1. When atrial activation lags slightly behind ventricular activation, the end of the retrograde P′ wave can be seen protruding from the end of the QRS. Because it is only partially seen, it resembles part of the QRS (i.e., a pseudo–s wave in the inferior leads and a pseudo–r′ wave in lead V_1).

Although the mechanism of AVNRT is not difficult to understand and in the drawings it is clear why the P′ waves are completely or partially hidden, in clinical practice the differential diagnosis between this and CMT can be difficult. However, the more understanding you have of the mechanism, the easier it is to spot the end of the small P′ wave.

Fig. 11-3, *A* and *B*, show the two electrocardiogram (ECG) patterns seen in the common form of AVNRT.

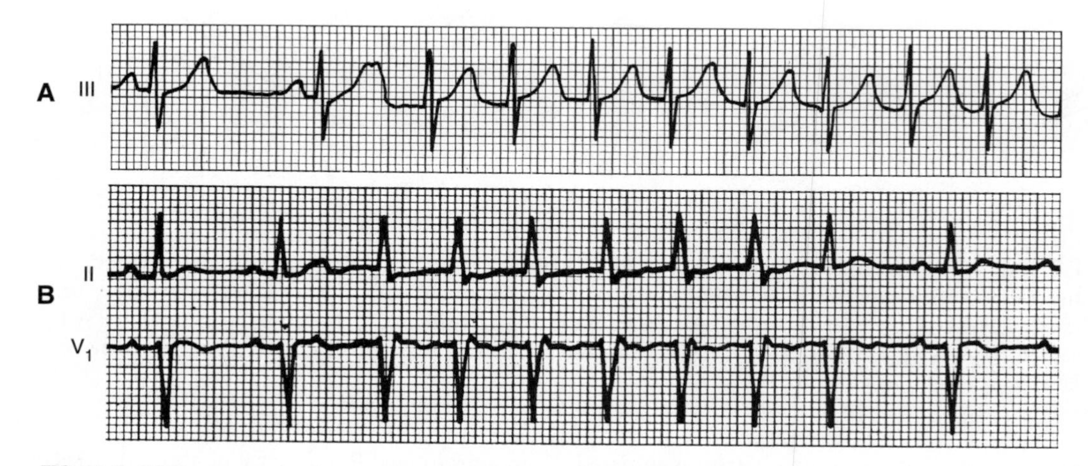

FIG. 11-3. ECG patterns in the two most common forms of AVNRT. At the onset of these tachycardias are premature atrial complexes (second T wave of both tracings). Each P′ is followed by a critically prolonged P′R interval (0.36 second in both cases.) **A**, During this tachycardia the P′ wave is completely hidden within the QRS. The QRS of the tachycardia is identical to that of the sinus beat. **B**, During this tachycardia the P′ wave is distorting the end of the QRS. Compare the QRS of the tachycardia with that of the sinus beat: you will note that the P′ wave looks like an S wave in lead II and like r′ in lead V_1.

Examine the tracings for the ECG signs that confirm the diagnosis. Keep in mind that this mechanism is the cause of approximately half of symptomatic PSVT. Without an understanding of the statistics and the mechanism the examiner would be looking *in front of* the QRS for the P wave instead of looking for a distorted terminal QRS, as would be seen in AVNRT or for a P′ wave immediately after the QRS, as would be seen in CMT.

The following properties of the AV node make it particularly vulnerable for dissociation of the atrial-nodal pathways and the establishment of a reentry circuit:

- The possibility for retrograde conduction through the AV node exists in many individuals. In most cases the impulse is conducted up the fast AV nodal fibers to the atria. In fact, half of all ventricular rhythms are conducted retrogradely into the atria.
- There are multiple AV nodal input pathways capable of conduction in both directions with differing conduction velocities and refractory periods.[4]

ECG Recognition

Heart rate: 150 to 250 beats/min.

Rhythm: May be regular or irregular because of varying conduction through the AV node.

Initiating P′R interval: Approximately 0.38 second because of anterograde conduction down the slow AV nodal fibers.

Location of the P′ waves: Buried within the QRS and not seen at all or distorting the end of the QRS, looking like terminal QRS forces.

Polarity of the P′ waves: Negative in leads II, III, and aV_F. This is because atrial activation originates inferiorly in the right atrium. Therefore if the P′ wave can be seen in the inferior leads, it will appear in the QRS as a *pseudo–s wave*. It will not be seen in lead I because in this lead it is isoelectric as a result of the atrial impulse originating at the AV node and traveling more or less straight up (perpendicular to the axis of lead I). If the P′ wave can be seen in lead V_1, it will look like an r′ wave (described by Wellens as a "pseudo right bundle branch block [RBBB] pattern").

QRS complex: Normal if the P′ is completely hidden, as it is in Fig. 11-3, *A*. However, the QRS is often distorted by the P′ wave, causing a pseudo–s wave in the inferior leads or a pseudo-r′ in lead V_1, as seen in Fig. 11-3, *B*.[6] QRS alternans (alternating heights of the R wave or depths of the S wave) are rare in AVNRT.

Conduction ratio: The conduction ratio is usually 1:1; that is, every time the ventricles are activated, so are the atria.

Aberrant ventricular conduction: Uncommon. This is because in the common form of AVNRT the impulse reaches the ventricles by way of the slow atrial-nodal pathway, giving the bundle branches time to repolarize. Aberrant ventricular conduction is discussed in Chapter 14.

Distinguishing features: AV nodal reentry tachycardia is recognized because of a paroxysmal, narrow QRS tachycardia that is either identical in shape to the normal sinus-conducted beats in all leads (hidden P′ waves) or distorted by the P′ wave (pseudo–s wave in leads II, III, and aV_F or pseudo-r′ in lead V_1).

Uncommon Forms of AVNRT

In the uncommon forms of AVNRT (fast/slow and slow/slow) the reentry circuit passes in the opposite direction to that just described. The fast/slow type passes down the fast AV nodal approach pathway and back up to the atria via the slow pathway. There is also a slow/slow type of AVNRT in that both arms of the reentry circuit use slow pathways; anterograde conduction is over an intermediate pathway and retrograde conduction up to the atria is over the slow pathway.[4] In both of the uncommon forms of AVNRT the AV nodal reentry impulse is delayed in its return to the atria, placing the retrograde P′ wave at a distance behind the QRS instead of being buried within it as in the more common form. In the fast/slow form of AVNRT the P′ wave is closer to the next QRS causing the rhythm to resemble that of junctional tachycardia. In the slow/slow form of AVNRT the P′ wave is between two QRS complexes.

Clinical Implications

AVNRT is usually benign and self-limiting or easily terminated by a vagal maneuver. Prolonged runs of PSVT may result in atrial fibrillation or atrial flutter.

Patient education. The patient should understand that PSVT is usually initiated by a PAC. Therefore the preventable arrhythmogenic practices in a patient's lifestyle should be eliminated or controlled (such as too much caffeine, cigarette smoking, stress, or poor nutrition). Additionally, show your patient several vagal maneuvers with instructions to terminate the tachycardia as soon as it is perceived. Often one vagal maneuver will terminate the tachycardia and another will not; show your patient at least three. It has been my experience that some patients "freeze" and hold their breath during their palpitations, hoping it will "go away," even after having been told how to perform a vagal maneuver. Getting a return demonstration from your patient may help him or her to act.

Emergency Treatment

Emergency treatment for AVNRT and CMT is exactly the same as that of PSVT; long-term treatment differs. Please turn to p. 130 for a discussion of emergency response to PSVT.

Treatment with Radiofrequency Ablation

In a significant number of cases, AVNRT can be recurrent and symptomatic. For such patients radiofrequency ablation has been shown to be safer than pharmacologic treatment. These patients are candidates for selective ablation or modification of the slow posterior pathway with radiofrequency energy and should be referred to centers skilled in this procedure.

In ablating the posterior slow pathway there is some risk (1%) of causing complete AV block. Great care is taken and the amount of radiofrequency energy used is sometimes not enough to completely ablate the pathway; a repeat procedure on another day is often necessary.

The results of the North American Society for Pacing and Electrophysiology (NASPE) prospective Voluntary Registry have been reported.[7] Of the 3,357 patients entered, 1,197 patients underwent AV nodal modification for AVNRT, which was successful in 96.1%; the only significant complication was development of AV block (1%).

CIRCUS MOVEMENT TACHYCARDIA (ATRIOVENTRICULAR RECIPROCATING TACHYCARDIA)

CMT is a PSVT that is the most common arrhythmia in individuals with WPW syndrome (see Chapter 21). It is caused by a reentry circuit using the normal atrial-nodal pathways for entrance into the ventricles and an accessory pathway for return to the atria. Thus, although there may be a delta wave and a QRS of 0.10 second or more in duration while in sinus rhythm, during PSVT the QRS will not have a delta wave and will be narrow, unless there is physiologic (aberrant) or pathologic BBB. Because anterograde conduction proceeds normally down the AV node, this type of CMT is called *orthodromic*. There are two less common forms of CMT, *incessant CMT* and *antidromic CMT*, which are discussed in more detail in Chapter 21.

Location of the Accessory Pathways

Accessory pathways may be located at almost any point around the annulus fibrosus, although the two most common locations are the left free wall (58%) and the posterior septum (24%). The ECG can be very helpful in determining the location of the accessory pathway, as is explained on p. 277.

Mechanism of Orthodromic CMT

Preexcitation syndromes such as WPW syndrome are of interest because they often result in PSVT or in atrial fibrillation with a ventricular response so rapid that it may deteriorate into ventricular fibrillation. Preexcitation exists when all or part of the ventricular muscle is activated by a P wave earlier than would occur if the current had proceeded through a normal route. The next three illustrations take you step by step through the sequence of events that results in PSVT caused by orthodromic CMT.

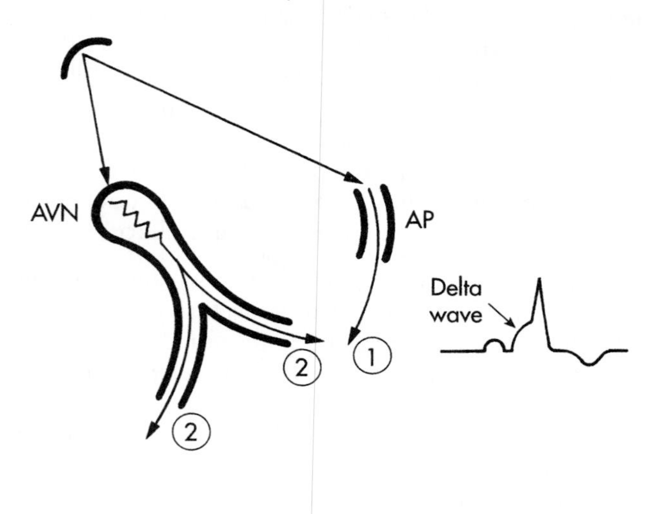

Note that in overt WPW syndrome there is preexcitation. The normal sinus rhythm is conducted first down the accessory pathway (AP) closely followed by conduction down the normal route (AVN). This results in (1) a delta wave and (2) a fusion beat because the delta force fuses with the normal activation wavefront. This delta force is traveling outside the conduction system and it is therefore slower than the normal initial forces. This is reflected on the ECG by a slow beginning to the QRS called a *delta wave*. The fusion beat is of course dependent on how fast the sinus impulse passes down the accessory pathway and arrives in the ventricle compared to how rapidly the AV node can deposit its impulse into the ventricles. If intra-atrial conduction or AV nodal conduction is a little slow, or if accessory pathway conduction is very fast, it is possible for the entire QRS to be the result of the delta force (no fusion). Additionally, the polarity of the delta wave changes with the location of the accessory pathway.

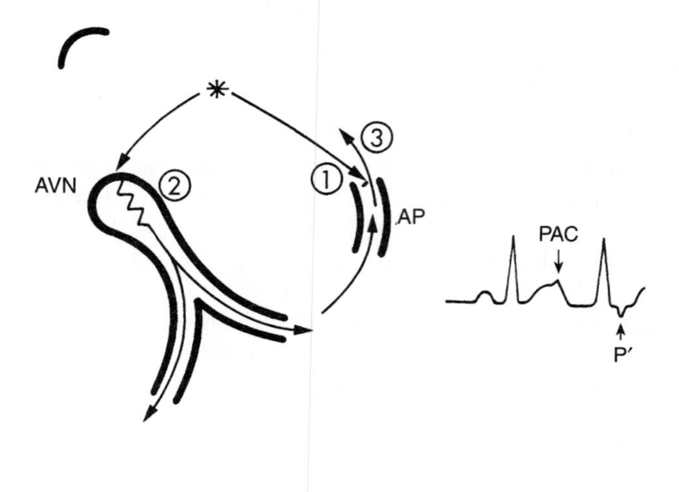

Note the PAC hiding in the T wave of the ECG. Now, note the mechanism that follows the PAC (*). (1) The impulse is blocked in the AP, but (2) it is conducted normally down the AV node (AVN) to produce a narrow QRS (no delta wave). This leaves the AP nonrefractory and free to conduct the ventricular impulse up to *reenter* the atrium (3). Now the stage is set for the next picture, the reentry circuit.

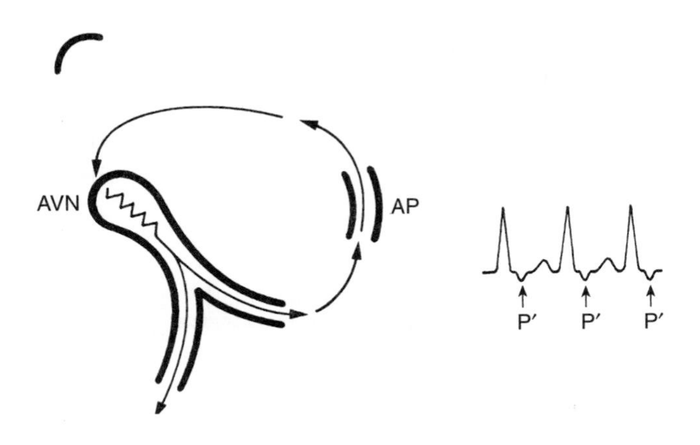

The impulse passes retrogradely up the accessory pathway, activates the atria, and reenters the AV node, the ventricles, the accessory pathway, back to the atria, and round and round in this sequence. Note that the P′ wave is separate from and immediately following the QRS.

To become proficient in differentiating this PSVT from that of AVNRT, the most essential point to note is that the reentry circuit of CMT activates the ventricles and atria in sequence, not simultaneously as in AVNRT. Although the P′ wave is small, the ECG pattern is distinctive in CMT, with the P′ wave separate from and immediately following the QRS, as seen in all three leads in Fig. 11-4. Study this figure for a moment before going on until the mechanism is quite clear. Then compare it with the mechanism of AVNRT on pp. 120-121. It is apparent that although to the uninformed observer the two types of PSVT seem to be identical, that they are in fact very different: AVNRT with the P′ buried and distorting the QRS and CMT with the P′ separate from the QRS 100% of the time.

In the common form of CMT, conduction up the accessory pathway is rapid, placing the P′ wave close to the preceding QRS. Other forms of CMT are illustrated and discussed on pp. 287-291.

ECG Recognition

Heart rate: 170 to 250 beats/min, often ≥200 beats/min (tends to be faster than AVNRT).

Rhythm: Regular but may be irregular because of changing conduction through the AV node.

Initiating P′R interval: Not prolonged as it is in AVNRT (p. 121), because anterograde conduction uses the fast atrial-nodal pathway.

Location of the P′ waves: Always immediately after and separate from the QRS.

Polarity of the P′ waves: The polarity of the P′ wave depends on the atrial location of the accessory pathway because atrial activation during CMT proceeds from the ventricle through the atrial insertion to activate the atria. For example, with left-sided accessory pathways atrial activation is from left to right (toward the negative electrode of lead I); thus the P′ wave is negative in lead I. With right-sided pathways it is positive in that lead.

QRS complex: Normal unless there is aberrant ventricular conduction (see Chapter 14).

Conduction ratio: Always 1:1.

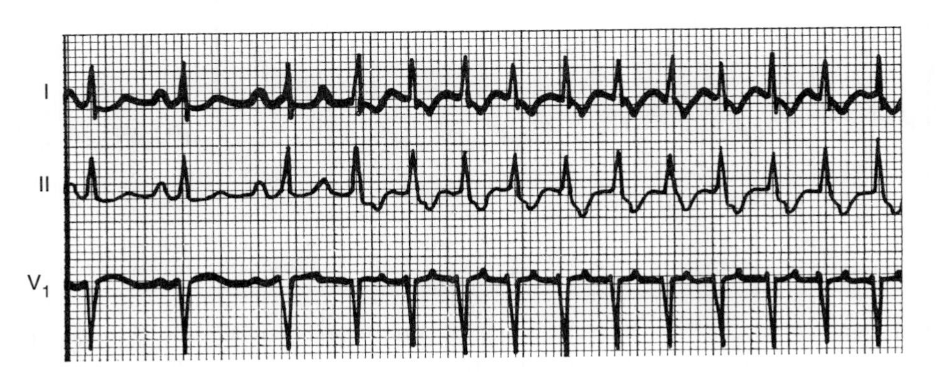

FIG. 11-4. Orthodromic circus movement tachycardia. The initiating PAC is distorting the third T wave. Note that the initiating P′R interval is normal. (In AVNRT it would be prolonged.) During the tachycardia the P′ waves are nicely seen in all three leads.

Aberrant ventricular conduction: Common. Fig. 11-5 shows an RBBB aberration in a patient with a right-sided accessory pathway.

Heart rate during aberrancy: When the accessory pathway is on the same side as the BBB, the heart rate is slower during the aberrancy than it is without, as shown in Fig. 11-5. When this is seen, it is diagnostic. The mechanism is demonstrated in Fig. 11-6. If at the onset of PSVT there were left bundle branch block (LBBB) aberrancy because of the sudden rate acceleration in an individual with a left-sided accessory pathway, the impulse entering the ventricles via the AV node would not be able to travel directly to the ventricular insertion of the left-sided pathway, but would have to take a detour through the right bundle branch and interventricular septum (*broken lines* in Fig. 11-6). When the aberrancy is no longer present the pathway of the impulse would be shorter (i.e., down the AV node, left bundle branch to the accessory pathway). Thus the RR intervals would be shorter. This is demonstrated in the ECG seen in Fig. 11-5.

QRS alternans: QRS alternans (alternating heights of R peaks or depths of S nadirs) is frequently present and is helpful in the diagnosis of CMT when it persists after the first 5 to 6 seconds.[2]

QRS alternans is remarkable in all leads except V_4 of Fig. 11-7. This is a phenomenon that is present 25% to 30% of the time during CMT but is rarely seen in AVNRT. QRS alternans may be seen with and without aberrant ventricular conduction and is seen especially

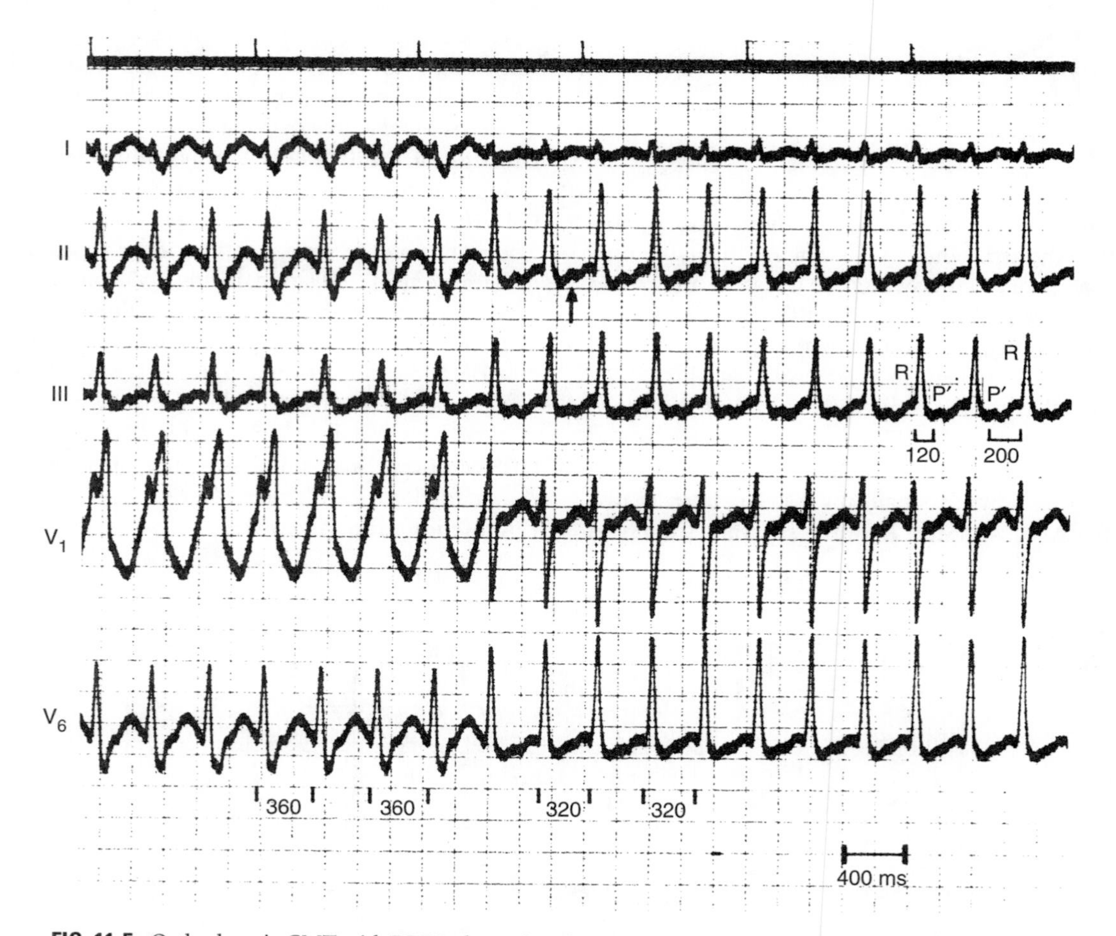

FIG. 11-5. Orthodromic CMT with RBBB aberration that resolves after seven beats. In this tracing there are four signs that support or are diagnostic of CMT: (1) the aberration itself, (2) the slower heart rate during aberration, (3) the QRS alternans, and (4) a P′ wave separate from and after the QRS *(arrow)*. (Courtesy Hein J.J. Wellens, MD, Maastricht, The Netherlands.)

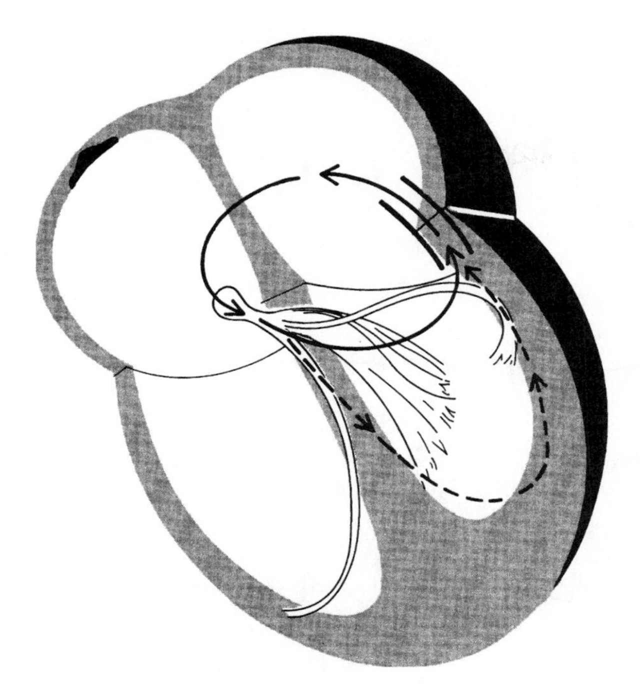

FIG. 11-6. The mechanism for the phenomenon of a slower heart rate during aberrancy than without aberrancy. Note that in the presence of a functional block in the left bundle branch, after entering the ventricles through the AV node and bundle of His, the impulse must take the long way around *(broken line)* to complete the reentry loop back into the atria via the left-sided accessory pathway. Without the block the route is shorter *(solid lines)*. Of course, if the accessory pathway were on the right side and the aberration that of LBBB, there would be no change in heart rate with or without aberration. This phenomenon occurs only when the accessory pathway is on the same side as the aberration (i.e., RBBB and right-sided accessory pathway or LBBB and left-sided accessory pathway).

in RBBB aberration, but not if there is preexisting BBB. QRS alternans may also be seen in VT but not usually in more than four leads. The presence or absence of this sign is evaluated only after the first 5 to 6 seconds of the tachycardia because AVNRT may also have QRS alternans at its onset.

Distinguishing features: CMT is recognized because of a paroxysmal narrow QRS tachycardia with a P′ wave separate from and after the QRS. CMT is frequently associated with QRS alternans and aberrant ventricular conduction.

CMT Initiated by a Premature Ventricular Complex

When PSVT is initiated by a premature ventricular complex (PVC), the mechanism is usually CMT. The ventricular impulse easily enters the atria via the rapidly conducting accessory pathway, whereas retrograde penetration of the AV node occurs more slowly than it would through the accessory pathway, if it occurs at all. Having activated the atria, the impulse passes down the AV node to the ventricles and a reentry circuit is established with the two AV structures (node and accessory pathway) being out of synchronization with each other. This lack of synchronization perpetuates the reentry circuit in all forms of reentry.

ECG Signs Negating the Possibility of CMT

AV dissociation: Because the atria and ventricles are activated in sequence during CMT, AV dissociation is not possible.

Second- or third-degree AV block: Because second- or third-degree AV block eliminates the ventricles from the reentry circuit, neither condition is possible in CMT.

No visible P waves: Absence of P waves during the tachycardia after all leads have been carefully searched implies simultaneous activation of atria and ventricles and rules out CMT.

Differential Diagnosis

Table 11-1 is a summary of the ECG differences between CMT and AVNRT. The distinction between the two mechanisms is made because of the position of the P′ wave in the cardiac cycle. In AVNRT the P′ wave is buried

TABLE 11-1 Differential Diagnosis in Paroxysmal Supraventricular Tachycardia

ECG Sign	AV Nodal Reentry Tachycardia	Circus Movement Tachycardia
QRS alternans	Rare	Common
Initial P′R interval	Prolonged	Normal
P′ wave location	Hidden in the QRS or may look like terminal QRS forces	Always separate; follows the QRS
P′ polarity	Negative in inferior leads (pseudo–S wave); positive in lead V_1 (pseudo-r′); isoelectric in lead I	Varies with accessory pathway location
Aberrancy	Rare	Common
AV conduction	Usually 1:1	Always 1:1

ECG, Electrocardiogram; *AV*, atrioventricular.

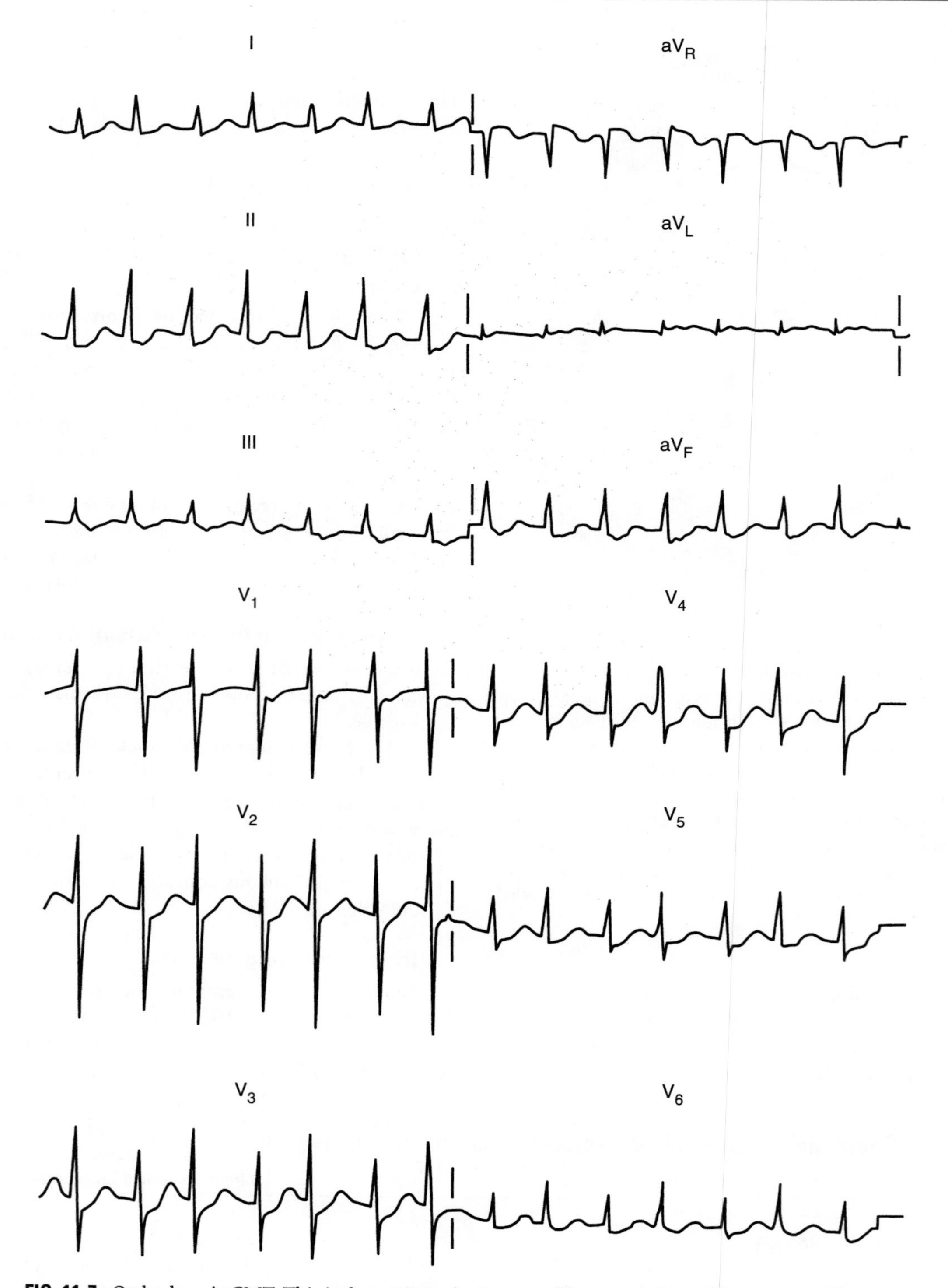

FIG. 11-7. Orthodromic CMT. This is the tracing of a 41-year-old woman who had been symptomatic for 5 years. Note the QRS alternans and the small P′ wave immediately after the QRS, best seen in leads III, aV_F, and V_1. A nursing diagnosis was made because of this emergency tracing, and the patient was referred to a physician for successful ablation of her accessory pathway with radiofrequency energy. (Courtesy Teresita Harrison, RN, Calgary, Alberta, Canada.)

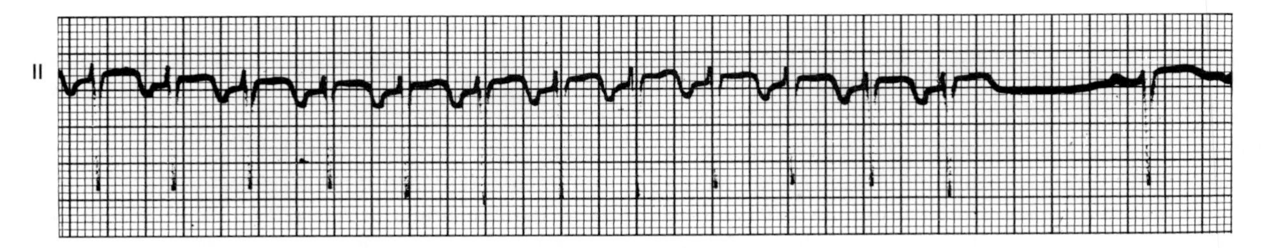

FIG. 11-8. CMT using a slowly conducting accessory pathway ("permanent CMT"). This condition is recognized because of the persistent nature of the tachycardia (more than 12 hr/day) and the ECG (RP longer than PR). A slowly conducting accessory pathway is inserted into the coronary sinus os, accounting for the negative P′ wave in lead II. In this tracing there are two sinus beats in the middle of the strip.

within the QRS; in CMT, the P′ wave is separate from the QRS. In addition, QRS alternans and aberrant ventricular conduction are more common in CMT than in AVNRT; a slowing of the rate during aberration as compared with the rate without aberration is diagnostic of CMT, and when a PVC initiates PSVT, the mechanism is usually CMT.

Clinical Implications

A patient who is symptomatic with CMT is in danger of developing atrial fibrillation, in which case the ventricular response is more than 200 beats/min and often as fast as 300 beats/min. Thus it is important for clinicians who evaluate ECGs to be skilled in the recognition of CMT.

Emergency Treatment

Emergency treatment for AVNRT and CMT is the same as that of PSVT. Please refer to p. 130 for this discussion.

Treatment (Cure) with Radiofrequency Ablation

Long-term treatment for symptomatic CMT is transvenous radiofrequency ablation of the accessory pathway; this cures the patient of PSVT and eliminates the threat of sudden death should atrial fibrillation develop (see Chapter 21).

Of the 3,357 patients entered in the NASPE prospective Voluntary Registry,[7] accessory pathway ablation was performed in 654 patients and was successful in 94%. Major complications included cardiac tamponade (7 patients), acute myocardial infarction (1 patient), femoral artery pseudoaneurysm (1 patient), AV block (1 patient), pneumothorax (1 patient), and pericarditis (2 patients).

CIRCUS MOVEMENT TACHYCARDIA WITH A SLOWLY CONDUCTING ACCESSORY PATHWAY

When CMT is supported by a slowly conducting accessory pathway, the RP interval is longer than the PR interval and the tachycardia usually occupies more than 12 hours of the patient's day. "Permanent," "incessant," and "persistent" are all terms given to this relatively rare and extremely debilitating type of CMT. The persistent nature of this tachycardia leads to atrial damage and congestive heart failure. The reentry circuit consists of conduction into the ventricles via the AV node (thus the narrow QRS) and retrograde conduction to the atria via a slowly conducting accessory pathway, placing the P′ wave well beyond the QRS (RP > PR). Remember that during CMT using a rapidly conducting accessory pathway the P′ wave is located close to but separate from the preceding QRS (RP < PR). Fig. 11-8 shows a permanent CMT. Such a tachycardia can be cured with radiofrequency ablation of the slowly conducting accessory pathway, after which the tachycardia related cardiomyopathy resolves considerably. In one study the ejection fraction in patients with tachycardiomyopathy was 28% and rose to 51% after ablation.[8]

ECG Features

Rate: 130 to 200 beats/min.
QRS complex: Narrow.
Rhythm: Regular.
P waves: Retrograde. The accessory pathway is located posterior-septally. Thus the P′ waves are equiphasic or flat in leads I and V_1 and negative in leads II and III and leads V_2 through V_6.
Main diagnostic features: Orthodromic CMT with a slowly conducting accessory pathway is most recognizable because of it resembles a junctional tachycardia with retrograde Ps in front of the QRS and because it alternates with brief periods of sinus rhythm. It is present more than 12 hours/day.

Mechanism

The unusual form of orthodromic CMT just described is supported by a reentry circuit using the AV node in an anterograde direction and using a slowly conducting accessory pathway in a retrograde direction. The slow conduction from the ventricle to the atria over the accessory pathway produces a long RP interval, so the retrograde P′ wave—along with the QRS that follows it—resembles a junctional beat (negative P′ in inferior leads immediately preceding a QRS complex). The pathway in most cases is inserted into the ostium of the coronary sinus, although left-sided pathways with slow conduction have also been identified.[12] Because of a response similar to that of the AV node to drugs and vagal maneuvers, the slowly conducting accessory pathway is thought to have nodal-like tissue.

Symptoms

Patients may be unaware of the tachycardia, having lived with it as a prevailing condition. It is often not diagnosed until their early teenage years when they seek medical attention because of symptoms of congestive heart failure resulting from their tachycardia-induced dilated cardiomyopathy.

Treatment

Antiarrhythmic drugs are usually ineffective in treating orthodromic CMT with a slowly conducting accessory pathway.

Transvenous radiofrequency catheter ablation of the accessory pathway offers a complete cure and a dramatic cessation of the tachycardia. In many patients there is a dramatic improvement of ventricular function after the ablation of the accessory pathway.[13,14]

EMERGENCY RESPONSE TO PAROXYSMAL SUPRAVENTRICULAR TACHYCARDIA

Hemodynamically Stable Patient

- **Record** the tachycardia in at least five leads (I, II, III, V_1, and V_6).
- **Terminate** the tachycardia.[9]
  1. Vagal maneuver; if unsuccessful:
  2. Adenosine 6 mg intravenous (IV), rapidly; if it is unsuccessful, the dosage is increased to 12 mg. This may be repeated once; if unsuccessful:
  3. Procainamide 10 mg/kg body weight IV over 5 minutes; if unsuccessful:
  4. Electrical cardioversion
- **Record** the sinus rhythm in the same leads.
- **Stabilize** the patient and take a history.
- **Diagnose** by close examination of the tracings with and without the tachycardia.
- **Refer** for radiofrequency ablation if CMT or refractory AVNRT is diagnosed.

Hemodynamically Unstable Patient

If the patient is hemodynamically unstable, record the rhythm in at least five leads and terminate the tachycardia with synchronized direct-current cardioversion. After the patient is stabilized, the ECG tracings should be carefully examined and a differential diagnosis made. This symptomatic patient should be referred for evaluation to a center experienced in the use of radiofrequency ablation.

Rationale of Emergency Response

Why multiple lead recordings? In PSVT, unlike VT, it is not necessary to make the differential diagnosis before terminating the tachycardia because emergency treatment is the same for the two common forms of PSVT. In hemodynamically stable patients the primary consideration is to record the tachycardia in as many leads as possible. Obtaining a record in at least five leads (I, II, III, V_1, and V_6) is considered a minimal requirement. For patients with PSVT this is extremely important because such patients have often had symptoms of palpitations and even presyncope for many years without seeking medical attention. The PSVT may be a fleeting experience for the patient, so the opportunity to record it is fortunate and the responsibility to do so should be taken very seriously.

Such tachycardias in patients with WPW syndrome may be harbingers of a more life-threatening arrhythmia. If delta waves are not present during sinus rhythm, as would be the case with latent or concealed WPW syndrome, short of invasive studies, the diagnosis can only be made during the tachycardia by observing the presence and position of P′ waves. Therefore the responsibility of the emergency department, critical care unit, or telemetry unit personnel to record the tachycardia in multiple leads cannot be overemphasized. Even if the admitting professional is not skilled in making the differential diagnosis of PSVT, a strict protocol should be followed so that the cardiologist has the opportunity to evaluate the tachycardia in enough leads to make the diagnosis and proper recommendations.

When the symptomatic patient is evaluated by cardiac catheterization, arrhythmias that are not clinically significant can be elicited by the intracardiac catheter. It is of great help to the examining physician to have a record of the clinical arrhythmia, another compelling reason to record multiple leads during the tachycardia.

Interrupting the Reentry Circuit. Treatment of the hemodynamically stable patient is initially aimed at lengthening the refractory period in the AV node with the vagal maneuver, adenosine, or verapamil. If this fails, procainamide is used. It blocks the retrograde fast atrial-nodal pathway and thus terminates AVNRT; it also blocks an accessory pathway

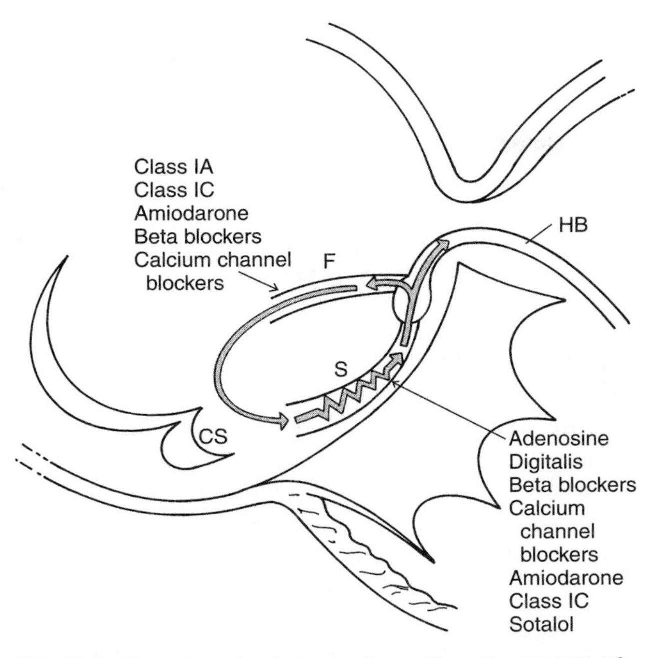

FIG. 11-9. Sites of antiarrhythmic drug effects in AVNRT. The common form of AV nodal reentry is depicted, in which anterograde conduction is via the slow atrial-nodal pathway and retrograde conduction is via the fast atrial-nodal pathway. Although the main action of calcium channel blockers is along the slow atrial-nodal pathway, on occasion the retrograde fast atrial-nodal pathway is remarkably suppressed. Class IA is quinidine, procainamide, and disopyramide; class IC is flecainide propafenone and encainide.

should it be part of the reentry circuit and thus terminates CMT. The action of some of the antiarrhythmic drugs on the slow and fast pathways of the AV node and on the accessory pathway is illustrated in Figs. 11-9 and 11-10. If the tachycardia continues after these three approaches, electrical cardioversion is indicated.

Vagal Maneuver

After the tachycardia has been recorded, a vagal maneuver can be used to terminate it. The mechanism of the vagal maneuver and the different types are described later in this chapter. If carotid sinus massage fails to terminate the tachycardia, it may be that the rhythm has been established for so long that the sympathetic nervous system is dominating.

Adenosine (Adenocard)

Adenosine blocks the AV node and has the advantage of an extremely short half-life (0.6 to 10 seconds). Because of its short half-life, correct administration procedure is critical. The drug must be delivered quickly to the heart by very rapid IV push followed by a saline flush in the antecubital fossa or another vein close to the heart. The arm is then raised and the vein milked down to the axilla to ensure as rapid a delivery as possible.

Unlike verapamil, adenosine does not usually cause a fall in blood pressure. Adenosine is also given as a central IV bolus for termination of PSVT.

Adenosine is not used in the differential diagnosis of

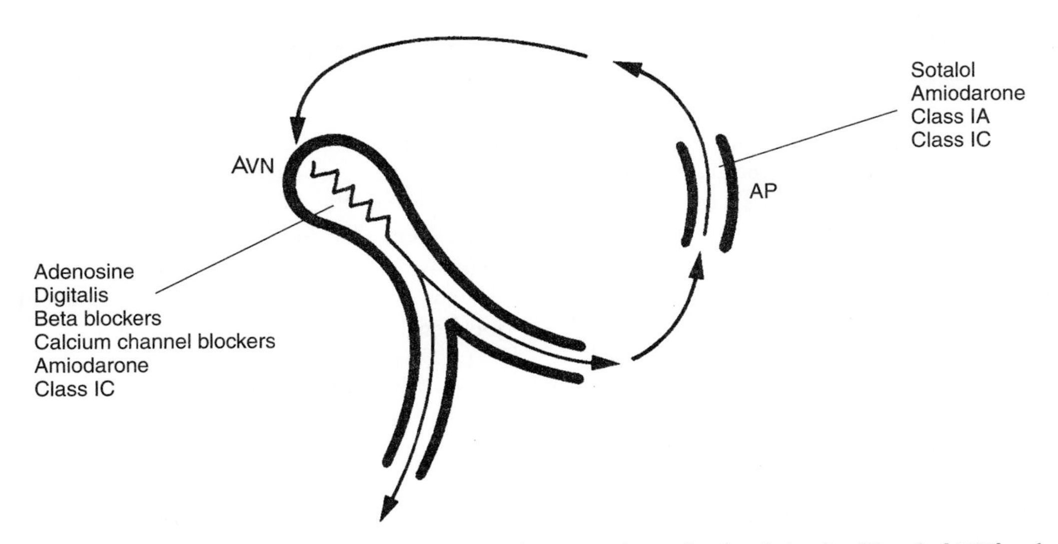

FIG. 11-10. Site of drug action in orthodromic CMT (anterograde conduction down the AV node *[AVN]* and retrograde conduction up the accessory pathway *[AP]*). Calcium channel blockers act primarily on the AV nodal component of the circuit, whereas class I drugs exert a more pronounced effect on the retrograde component (the accessory pathway). (From Akhtar M, Tchou P, Jazayeri M: *Circulation* 80[Suppl 4]:31, 1989.)

broad QRS tachycardia or in the "diagnosis of SVT" because of two important pitfalls. First, although noted for its blocking action on the AV node, adenosine is also capable of terminating certain types of VT ("adenosine-sensitive VT")[16] and incapable of terminating certain types of SVT (atrial fibrillation or atrial flutter with accessory pathways). Thus an idiopathic VT (adenosine-sensitive) would be assumed to be SVT, unless, of course, the informed practitioner was aware of this action of adenosine and suspected this type of VT from the QRS morphologic appearance, QRS axis, and history (see p. 159). Second, atrial fibrillation or atrial flutter with an accessory pathway may be misdiagnosed (VT). Both cases can be cured by radiofrequency ablation, and misdiagnosis deprives such patients of a correct diagnosis, referral, and cure.

Adverse effects. Adverse effects include flushing, dyspnea, headache, cough, chest pain, sinus bradycardia, atrial fibrillation, ventricular arrhythmias, and various degrees of AV block. The atrial fibrillation may develop because adenosine shortens the refractory period of atrial fibers. Because of the short half-life, the adverse effects are transient and well-tolerated.

Verapamil

If verapamil is used instead of adenosine, it is given IV 10 mg over 3 minutes. If the patient is taking a beta blocker or is hypotensive, the dose is reduced to 5 mg.[9]

Procainamide (Pronestyl)

Procainamide has the advantages of lengthening the refractory period in retrograde fast atrial-nodal pathways, which interrupts AVNRT, and lengthening the refractory period in accessory pathways, which interrupts CMT.

Cardioversion

If vagal maneuvers, including carotid sinus massage (performed by the physician), and drugs have not converted the PSVT to sinus rhythm, electrical cardioversion should now be used. As little as 10 J is frequently effective; 100 J is almost always successful.

Recording the Sinus Rhythm

After converting the patient to sinus rhythm, a 12-lead ECG is taken. At the very least, the sinus rhythm should be recorded in the same leads that recorded the tachycardia (I, II, III, V_1, and V_6). The purpose of this is not only to look for delta waves or other abnormalities during sinus rhythm, but also that P′ waves can be more easily located by comparing the shape of the ST segment during sinus rhythm with that during the tachycardia. The P′ wave will not necessarily be seen clearly in all leads, so comparison with the shape of the J point (the point where the QRS ends and the ST segment begins), ST segment, and T wave is very helpful in locating a P′ in hiding.

Taking a History

The history may reveal the occurrence of previous incidences of tachycardia. The patient should be queried about polyuria associated with the tachycardia. Such a finding is present in 20% to 50% of patients with physical signs of PSVT.

MECHANISM AND METHODS OF VAGAL STIMULATION

Stimulation of the vagal nerve causes a release of acetylcholine, which in turn lengthens the refractory period of the AV node and thus terminates PSVT; the maneuver, however, may also have no effect on the tachycardia. The reentry circuits responsible for both CMT and AVNRT use the AV node as one arm of the reentry circuit, or a microreentry circuit is confined to the compact AV node and its atrial pathways. The AV block produced by the vagal maneuver upsets the delicate balance between anterograde and retrograde currents supporting the reentry circuit. Of course, because the AV and sinus nodes are closely related and are both supplied by the vagus nerve, automaticity of the sinus node is also suppressed. With strong vagal stimulation the sinus node may cease to beat.

Vagal Maneuvers

Coughing is an excellent prehospital vagal maneuver. The patient may also be instructed to lie on the floor with legs elevated against the wall or perform Valsalva's maneuver, such as blowing against a closed glottis, gagging, or squatting. In the hospital setting, carotid sinus massage (described in the next section) and immersion of the face in cold water (the dive reflex) are excellent and strong vagal maneuvers. **Caution:** Never use eyeball pressure. Such a maneuver is extremely dangerous: it may cause retinal detachment. It is unpleasant for the patient and usually ineffective.

Carotid Sinus Massage

The carotid sinus is located at the bifurcation of the carotid artery at the angle of the jaw (not in the neck). The location of the carotid body is illustrated in Fig. 11-11. In the hands of the informed physician carotid sinus stimulation is an excellent diagnostic and therapeutic vagotonic maneuver. Massage of this area creates an elevation of blood pressure in the carotid sinus so that there will be reflex slowing of AV conduction.

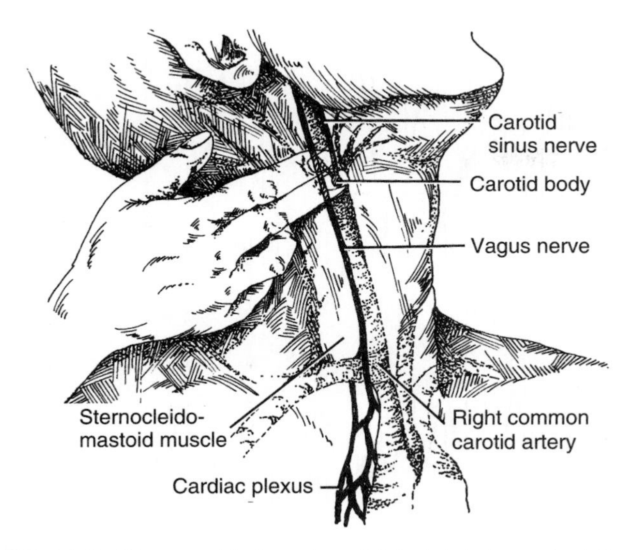

FIG. 11-11. The carotid sinus (carotid body) is located at the bifurcation of the carotid artery at the angle of the jaw.

Carotid sinus massage may be either diagnostic or therapeutic. It is diagnostic when it causes a transient block in AV conduction and unmasks atrial flutter (Fig. 11-12, *A*) or atrial tachycardia or when it causes temporary sinus slowing during sinus tachycardia. It is therapeutic when it terminates the tachycardia (Fig. 11-12, *B*). The abrupt termination of the tachycardia means only that the AV node was part of the reentry circuit; the decision regarding mechanism must still be made by closely examining the ECG during the tachycardia and noting the position and polarity of the P′ waves.

Effect of Carotid Sinus Massage on Supraventricular Tachycardia[10]

Sinus tachycardia: Gradual and temporary slowing of the heart rate.

Atrial tachycardia: When, because of reentry, there is cessation of the tachycardia or the maneuver has no effect.

Atrial fibrillation or persistent atrial tachycardia (also called "incessant" atrial tachycardia): Temporary slowing of the ventricular rate, AV block, or the maneuver has no effect.

Atrial flutter: Temporary slowing of ventricular rate, AV block, conversion into atrial fibrillation, or the maneuver has no effect.

PSVT: Termination of the tachycardia or no effect.

CAUTION

1. Do not use carotid sinus massage on patients with a history of transient ischemic attacks, the findings of carotid artery stenosis on palpation, or carotid bruits.
2. Do not apply pressure for longer than 5 seconds.
3. Do not use carotid sinus massage on patients older than 65 years of age; sinus pauses of 3 to 7 seconds have been reported under such circumstances. With aging there is a normal development of the parasympathetic nervous system, which is exacerbated by carotid sinus massage.

Procedure

1. After listening for carotid bruits, place the patient in a supine position with a small pillow or your arm under the patient's shoulders to extend the neck.
2. Turn the patient's head away from the side to be massaged.
3. Locate the bifurcation of the carotid artery just below the angle of the jaw (Fig. 11-11).
4. If the patient is not hypersensitive (begin with slight pressure), press the carotid sinus against the lateral processes of the cervical vertebrae with a massaging action for no more than 5 seconds.
5. Monitor the effect of carotid sinus massage on the ECG; if an ECG monitor is not available, listen to the heart with the stethoscope as you massage the carotid sinus.

SYMPTOMS OF PAROXYSMAL SUPRAVENTRICULAR TACHYCARDIA

Symptoms include feelings of palpitations, nervousness, polyuria, anxiety, angina, heart failure, syncope, or shock, depending on the duration and rate of the tachycardia and whether there is structural heart disease.

Syncope may be caused by the tachycardia itself (fall in cardiac output and reduced cerebral circulation) or by the overdrive suppression after the termination of the tachycardia (automaticity of the sinus node is suppressed by the tachycardia.) The prognosis for patients without heart disease is usually good.

PHYSICAL SIGNS OF PAROXYSMAL SUPRAVENTRICULAR TACHYCARDIA

The Neck Veins

"Frog sign." Even before the ECG electrodes are applied, observation of the neck veins often helps to rapidly distinguish between SVT and VT. During PSVT the atria contract against closed AV valves, causing a reflux of blood up the jugular veins. This results in a rapid, regular expansion of the neck veins resembling the rhythmic puffing motion of a frog. Wellens refers to this physical finding as the "frog sign." The patient usually reports a history of pal-

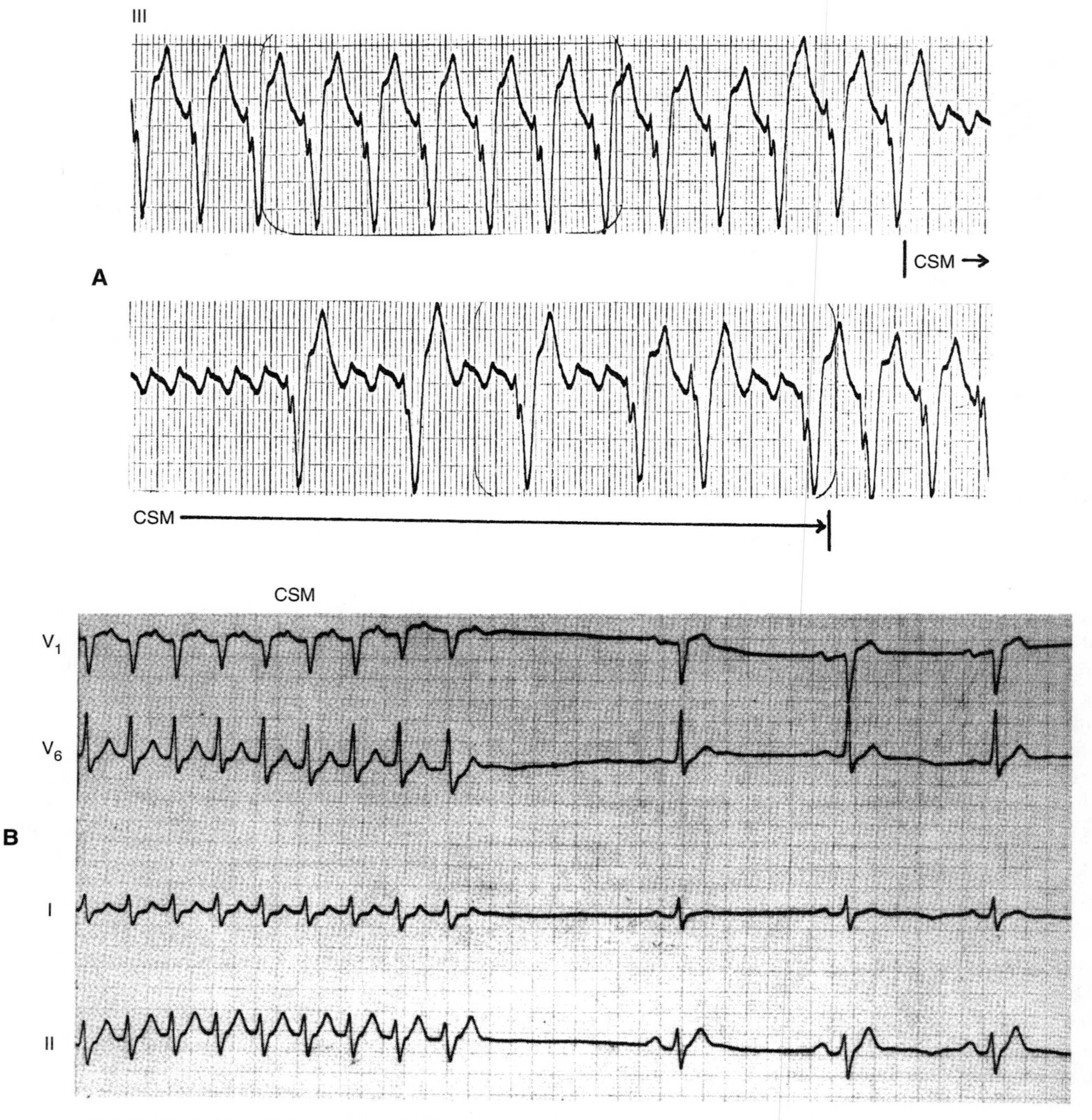

FIG. 11-12. **A**, Carotid sinus massage *(CSM)* causes AV block and reveals the underlying atrial flutter. **B**, The AV block caused by carotid sinus massage in this patient terminated circus movement tachycardia. During the tachycardia, the P′ waves can be seen in lead V_1, following and separate from the QRS. (**A**, From Stein E: *The electrocardiogram*, Philadelphia, 1976, WB Saunders. **B**, Courtesy Hein J.J. Wellens, MD, Maastricht, The Netherlands.)

pitations and seeks medical attention when the palpitations are associated with lightheadedness, shortness of breath, or anxiety. When questioned, the patient or family may have noticed the frog sign.

Other tachycardias. The pulsations in the neck veins often reveal the mechanism of other tachycardias as well.[10] Sinus tachycardia and atrial tachycardia are the only two SVTs that do not result in abnormal pulsations in the neck veins. In atrial flutter there are flutter waves, and in atrial fibrillation, irregular pulsations in the neck veins. In VT with AV dissociation these pulsations are irregular because of the occasional simultaneous beating of atria and ventricles.

Pulse, Blood Pressure, and Heart Sounds

In all types of regular SVT, the pulse is regular and the blood pressure and the loudness of the first heart sound constant. On the other hand, these parameters vary when there are changing RR intervals and AV conduction varies, as in atrial fibrillation and atrial flutter with variable conduction ratios. The jugular venous pressure may be elevated, but the waveform generally remains constant.[11]

Polyuria

In a significant number of patients (20% to 50%) PSVT is associated with polyuria. This response typically occurs with heart rates greater than 120 beats per minute and a duration of 10 to 30 minutes. Polyuria has also been noted during episodes of atrial fibrillation, atrial flutter, and VT. Factors responsible are changes in atrial rhythm and pressure, resulting in the release of the atrial natriuretic factor, a hormone that causes diuresis and may also play a role in the posttachycardia, hypovolemic hypotension sometimes associated with PSVT.[12]

Syncope

The syncope that frequently occurs in upright PSVT is thought to be caused by a particular hemodynamic response to the stress of tachycardia and does not imply a more malignant or rapid tachycardia. The sequence is thought to be as follows[13]:

1. Paroxysmal supraventricular tachycardia causes a short diastolic filling time and ineffective timing of atrial and ventricular contraction, reducing left ventricular filling.
2. An increase in sympathetic tone occurs at the onset of the tachycardia.
3. The upright position also causes reduced left ventricular volume and increased sympathetic tone.
4. This in turn may precipitate inappropriate stimulation of left ventricular stretch receptors, causing an inadequate hemodynamic response to the tachycardia and syncope. The mechanism is similar to that postulated for vasovagal syncope.
5. During the tachycardia, syncope can occur because the rapid ventricular rate fails to provide adequate cerebral circulation; after the tachyarrhythmia, syncope can occur because of overdrive suppression of the sinus node by the tachycardia.

PEDIATRICS: PSVT IN THE FETUS AND NEONATE

CMT is the most common arrhythmia in the neonate and accounts for most of the PSVTs that occur in infants. WPW syndrome is overt in 50% of cases and concealed in the other half (see Chapter 23).[14] AV nodal reentry tachycardia is also a significant cause of PSVT in the pediatric population.

Heart rate: The usual rate of SVT in an infant is 300 beats/min.

Mechanisms: The two common mechanisms for SVT in the fetus are intraatrial reentry and atrioventricular reentry using an accessory pathway.

Diagnosis: During random fetal heart rate monitoring the tachycardia is noted; rarely, the mother reports a decrease in fetal movements. The mechanism is diagnosed by visualizing on echocardiography the atrial and ventricular contractions or the movement of the AV valves, or both. For example, if the atrial contractions outnumber the ventricular ones, intraatrial reentry is diagnosed. Because of the AV block, it is assumed that the AV junction is not part of the reentry circuit. This type of PSVT is present in many fetuses. However, should there be a 1:1 relationship between the atria and the ventricle, an AV reciprocating tachycardia is assumed. This, of course, produces a faster ventricular rate than the SVT with AV block.

Symptoms and Clinical Implications

Fetus. In the fetus, the heart rate associated with PSVT is not well-tolerated and results in hydrops fetalis in just a few hours.

Newborn babies. In the newborn, PSVT is usually associated with signs of congestive heart failure.

Infants up to 1 year of age. In infants up to the age of 1 year a rate of 300 beats/min is generally well-tolerated for several hours.

Older children. In older children and adolescents, palpitations are the leading symptom of PSVT, but these children may also experience chest pain, fatigue, lightheadedness, and syncope.[15] Persistent or "incessant" tachycardia often results in a secondary form of dilated cardiomyopathy, the so-called *tachymyopathy*.[16] Persistent forms of SVT are atrial reentrant tachycardias after surgical correction of congenital heart disease (p. 107) and orthodromic CMT using a slowly conducting accessory pathway (p. 129).

Treatment

AVNRT. In children radiofrequency catheter ablation has been increasingly used to cure AVNRT.[15] In this procedure the slow pathway is modified using low temperature and low energy. This approach can be performed successfully with a low incidence of recurrence in the pediatric patient.[17]

CMT. Although 30% of the children with overt WPW syndrome lose the delta wave in the first year of life, 50% of them no longer have their CMT after that time. However, the PSVT returns by the time they are 20 years of age. Until then, no treatment is required.[14]

SUMMARY

The most common type of PSVT is AV-nodal reentry tachycardia, followed by AV reentry tachycardia (circus movement) using an accessory pathway. A smaller group (10%) consists of paroxysmal atrial flutter or fibrillation and focal atrial tachycardia. Symptoms are usually mild in people with otherwise normal hearts and include palpitations, polyuria, and an uneasy feeling in the chest. Some describe precordial pain, weakness, dizziness, nausea, vomiting, and syncope. Whenever possible, obtain a 12-lead ECG during an episode of PSVT. Otherwise a Holter ECG or an event recorder may be helpful. Termination of PSVT and conversion to sinus rhythm can usually be accomplished by vagal maneuvers; if these do not terminate the PSVT, intravenous adenosine is used. These measures block the AV node; if this is unsuccessful, IV procainamide will block an accessory pathway and a retrograde fast AV nodal pathway. If the tachycardia persists after this, cardioversion is attempted. Further diagnostic procedures prove or rule out structural heart disease. Therapeutic options are chosen according to the mechanism of the PSVT and the patient's symptoms. A better understanding of PSVT mechanisms, which has developed over the past 20 years, has led to dramatic improvements in therapy.

A cure for both AVNRT and CMT can be achieved by use of catheter-mediated radiofrequency ablation in 95% to nearly 100% of cases.

REFERENCES

1. Orejarena LA, Vidaillet H Jr, DeStefano F et al: Paroxysmal supraventricular tachycardia in the general population, *J Am Coll Cardiol* 31:150, 1998.
2. Josephson ME, Wellens HJJ: Differential diagnosis of supraventricular tachycardia, *Cardiol Clin* 8:411, 1990.
3. Iturralde Torres P, Colin Lizalde L, Guevara Valdivia M et al: [Experience in 1,500 patients undergoing radiofrequency ablation in the treatment of tachycardias], *Arch Inst Cardiol Mex* 70:349, 2000.
4. Wu J, Wu J, Olgin J et al: Mechanisms underlying the reentrant circuit of atrioventricular nodal reentrant tachycardia in isolated canine atrioventricular nodal preparation using optical mapping, *Circ Res* 88:1189, 2001.
5. Keim S, Werner P, Jazayeri M et al: Localization of the fast and slow pathways in atrioventricular nodal reentrant tachycardia by intraoperative ice mapping, *Circulation* 86:919, 1992.
6. Farré J, Wellens HJJ: The value of the electrocardiogram in diagnosing site of origin and mechanism of supraventricular tachycardia. In Wellens HJJ, Kulbertus JE, editors: *What's new in electrocardiography*, The Hague, 1981, Martinus Nijhoff.
7. Scheinman MM, Huang S: The 1998 NASPE prospective catheter ablation registry, *Pacing Clin Electrophysiol* 23(6):1020, 2000.
8. Aguinaga L, Primo J, Anguera I et al: Long-term follow-up in patients with the permanent form of junctional reciprocating tachycardia treated with radiofrequency ablation, *Pacing Clin Electrophysiol* 21(11 Pt 1):2073, 1998.
9. Wellens HJJ, Conover M: *The ECG in emergency decision making*, Philadelphia, 1992, WB Saunders.
10. Wellens HJJ, Brugada P, Bär F: Diagnosis and treatment of the regular tachycardia with a narrow QRS complex. In Kulbertus HE, editor: *Medical management of cardiac arrhythmias*, Edinburgh, 1986, Churchill Livingstone.
11. Zipes DP: Specific arrhythmias: diagnosis and treatment. In Braunwald E editor: *Heart disease*, ed 4, Philadelphia 1992, WB Saunders.
12. Kojima S, Fujii T, Ohe T et al: Physiologic changes during supraventricular tachycardia and release of atrial natruretic peptide, *Am J Cardiol* 62:576, 1988.
13. Leitch JW, Klein GJ, Yee R et al: Syncope associated with supraventricular tachycardia; an expression of tachycardia rate or vasomotor response? *Circulation* 85:1064, 1992.
14. Gillette PC, Zeigler VL, Case CL: Pediatric arrhythmias: Are they different? In Zipes DP, Jalife J, editors: *Cardiac electrophysiology from cell to bedside*, ed 2, Philadelphia, 1995, WB Saunders.
15. Ro PS, Rhodes LA: Atrioventricular node reentry tachycardia in pediatric patients, *Prog Pediatr Cardiol* 13:3, 2001.
16. Paul T, Bertram H, Kriebel T et al: [Supraventricular tachycardia in infants, children and adolescents: Diagnosis, drug and interventional therapy], *Z Kardiol* 89:546, 2000.
17. Rhodes LA, Wieand TS, Vetter VL: Low temperature and low energy radiofrequency modification of atrioventricular nodal slow pathways in pediatric patients, *Pacing Clin Electrophysiol* 22:1071, 1999.

CHAPTER 12

Premature Ventricular Complexes

A premature ventricular complex (PVC) is a single or pair of ventricular ectopic beats that occurs before the expected sinus-conducted QRS. Other terms used are ventricular premature beat or ventricular premature complex. A PVC is recognized on the electrocardiogram (ECG) because of its prematurity and its shape.

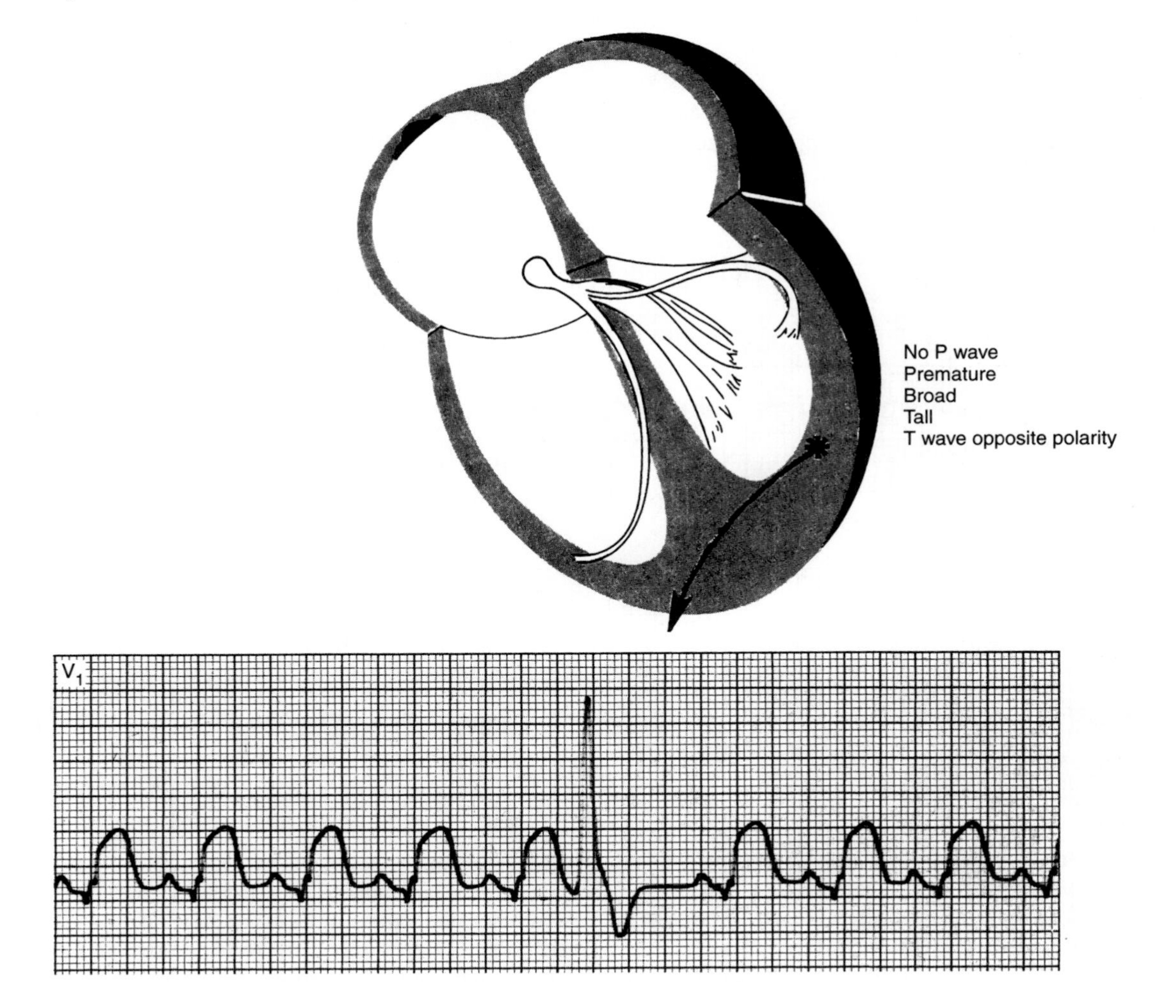

FIG. 12-1. A premature ventricular complex is initially suspected because of its prematurity, width, and full compensatory pause. The diagnosis is confirmed because of the monophasic R wave in V_1 (see Chapter 14).

ECG RECOGNITION

Heart rate: Underlying rate may be normal or abnormal. PVCs are more likely to appear during bradycardia, when there is more time for them to emerge.

Rhythm: Irregular because of the PVC.

P wave: The PVC does not have a related P wave unless there is retrograde conduction, and then the P′ wave follows the PVC and is buried in its T wave. The PVC may be preceded by a sinus P wave (end-diastolic PVC), in which case the resultant beat may be part sinus conducted and part ventricular ectopic (end-diastolic fusion beat) or all ventricular ectopic.

PP intervals: Can be "walked out" across the PVC approximately 50% of the time (atrioventricular [AV] dissociation).

QRS complex: That of the PVC is broad, usually more than 0.12 second, premature, and has increased amplitude. There is a differential diagnosis between the PVC and a supraventricular beat conducted with physiologic bundle branch block (BBB) (aberration). The shape of the QRS can be of help in distinguishing (see Chapter 14).

Full compensatory pause: Present approximately 50% of the time (discussed and illustrated on p. 146).

T wave: The T wave of the PVC is large and opposite in polarity to the terminal QRS.

Distinguishing features: A PVC is usually recognized because it is broad and premature and has an increased amplitude and a T wave of opposite polarity to the QRS. Fig. 12-1 illustrates a single PVC in a patient with acute myocardial infarction. The prematurity of the PVCs in Fig. 12-2 is not quite so obvious.

VARIATIONS

PVCs may occur at any time during the cardiac cycle from one, two, or many foci and may occur in certain shapes and sets. The many different types of PVC are illustrated in the following section.

The "Ugly PVC"

Clinical implications may be derived from the shape of the PVC. The "ugly PVC" is broad (0.16 second) with a notch of 0.04 second and has been shown to indicate a dilated and globally hypokinetic left ventricle in a nonspecifically diseased heart, whereas the smooth, narrower PVC reflects normal heart size and normal or near-normal systolic function, despite the presence of underlying

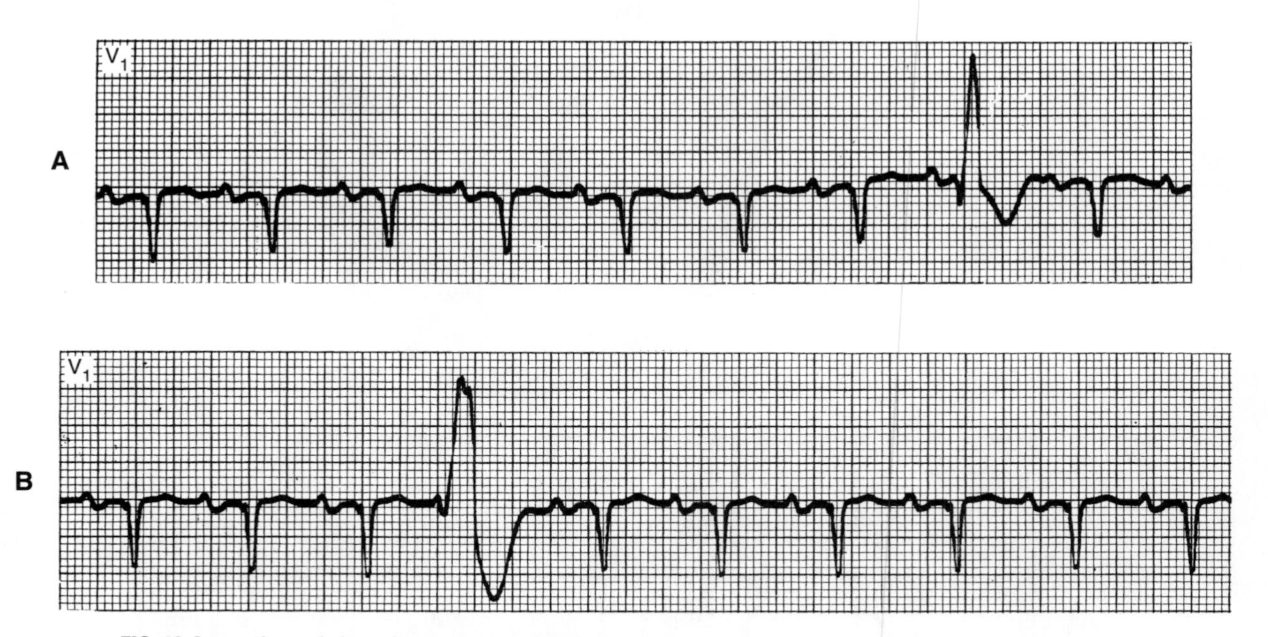

FIG. 12-2. **A**, The end-diastolic PVC. Note that this PVC is premature by only 0.08 second and occurs at the end of diastole, after the P wave but before the normal ventricular response is expected. Both the ectopic focus and the normally conducted beat activate the ventricles simultaneously (a fusion beat). **B**, Tracing from the same patient. This end-diastolic PVC is too early to be a fusion beat (i.e., the ventricles have already been completely activated by the ectopic focus). The sinus P wave can be seen distorting the beginning of the PVC, but its shape is purely that of the PVC. The PVC in **A** is narrower than the one in **B** (the hallmark of a fusion beat).

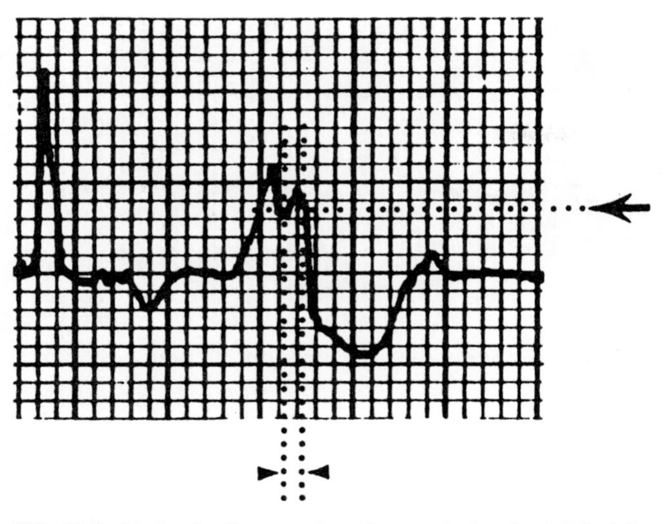

FIG. 12-3. Method of measuring the notch in the PVC. (1) Draw a horizontal line at the level of the lowest point in the notch (its nadir). (2) Make vertical lines at the two peaks. (From Moulton KP, Medcalf T, Lazzara R: *Circulation* 81:1245, 1990.)

disease.[1] Fig. 12-3 demonstrates the method of measuring ugliness (i.e., the notch). In Fig. 12-4, ugly PVCs are compared with smooth PVCs and the clinical implications are explained.

Unifocal PVCs

Unifocal PVCs are illustrated in Fig. 12-5. They are identical in form to each other because they originate from the same focus. Every time the ectopic focus fires, currents pass through the ventricular myocardium, taking the same route as before so that the complex is identical in shape each time, as long as the ECG lead remains the same.

Multifocal PVCs

Multifocal PVCs or ventricular extrasystoles are generated from different foci; other terms are *multiform* or *polymorphic.* Note in Fig. 12-6 that the ventricular extrasystoles have four different shapes.

Bigeminy, Trigeminy, Quadrigeminy, and Pairs

A bigeminal rhythm consists of pairs. In ventricular bigeminy, every other beat is a PVC. Note in Fig. 12-7 that

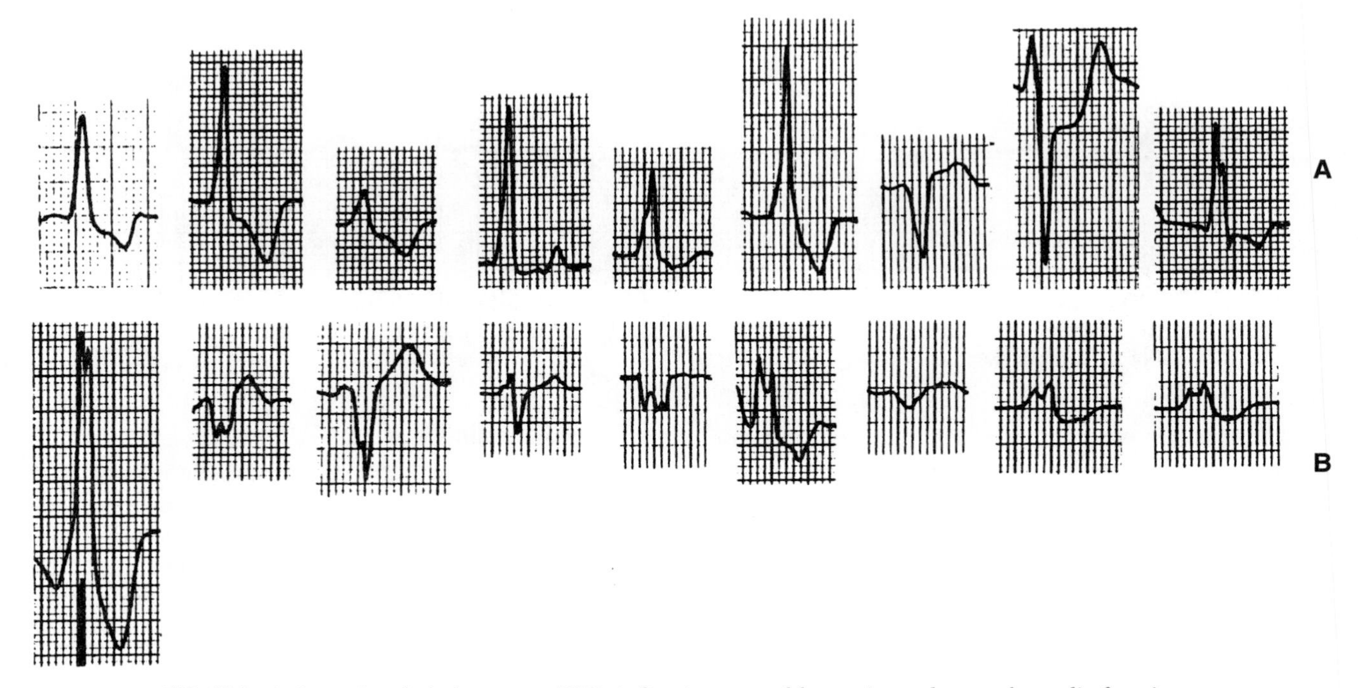

FIG. 12-4. **A**, Smooth, relatively narrow PVCs indicating normal heart size and normal systolic function, despite presence of underlying disease. **B**, "Ugly PVCs" are broad (more than 0.16 second) with a notch of 0.04 second or more, indicating a dilated and globally hypokinetic left ventricle in a nonspecifically diseased heart. (From Moulton KP, Medcalf T, Lazzara R: *Circulation* 81:1245, 1990.)

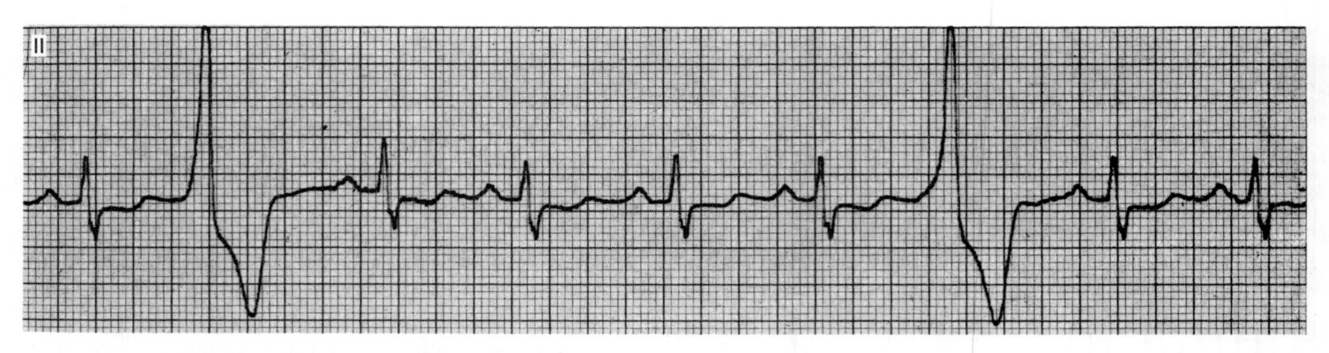

FIG. 12-5. Unifocal PVCs originate in the same focus, take the same route of conduction, and are identical in shape.

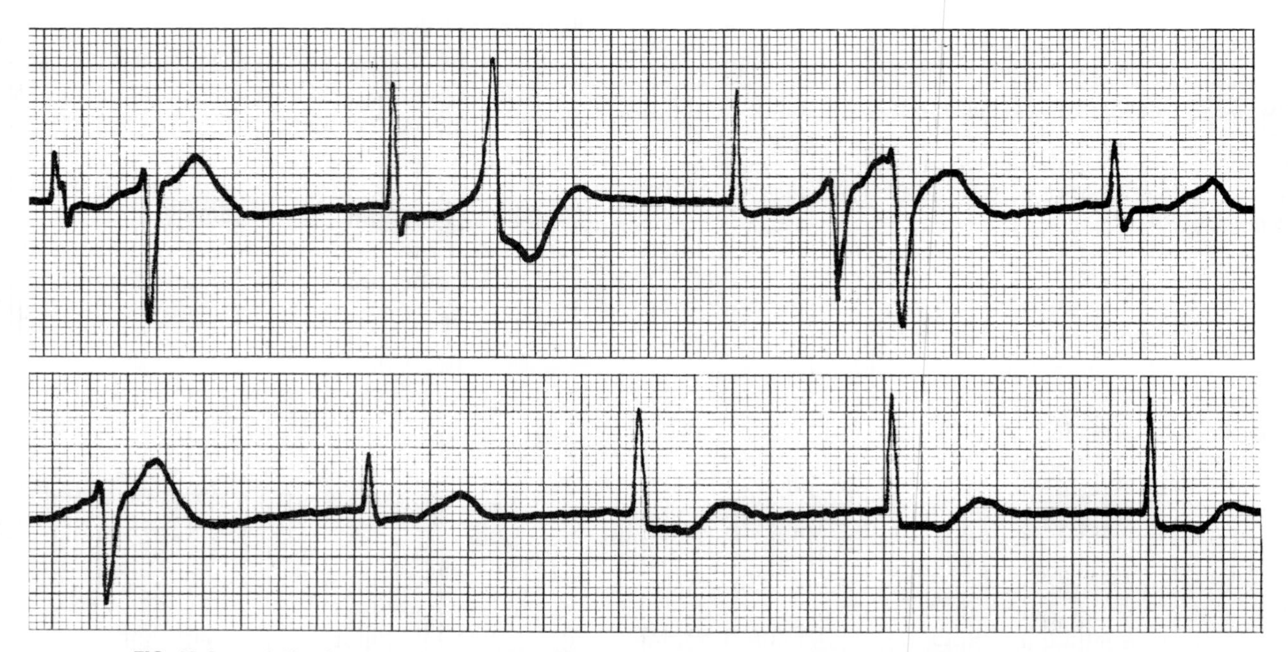

FIG. 12-6. Multifocal ventricular extrasystoles in a patient with digitalis toxicity. The underlying rhythm is atrial fibrillation with complete heart block and a junctional escape rhythm of 44 beats/min, as seen at the end of the bottom tracing.

each PVC is also precisely coupled to the preceding normal complex. The most common cause of this precise coupling is coronary artery disease. In that case the mechanism is reentry resulting from slow conduction in one area of the myocardium; ventricular bigeminy is sometimes seen in digitalis toxicity, in which case the mechanism is probably triggered activity. A trigeminal rhythm is made up of groups of three (Fig. 12-8, *A*). Fig. 12-8, *B*, is an example of quadrigeminy. Fig. 12-9 illustrates PVCs that occur in pairs or back to back. When there are three or more ventricular ectopic beats, the rhythm is called *ventricular tachycardia.*

End-Diastolic PVCs

PVCs that occur at the end of diastole may be only slightly premature, and they may be fusion beats. The end-diastolic PVC occurs late in the cardiac cycle before the ventricles can be activated or partially activated by the sinus beat. In Fig. 12-10, *A*, there is a P wave immediately preceding but unrelated to an end-diastolic PVC. The PR interval preceding the end-diastolic PVC may be shorter than the dominant one. In Fig. 12-10, *B*, the end-diastolic PVC is a fusion beat because it was late enough to permit the sinus impulse entrance into the ventricles at the same time as ectopic activation. An end-diastolic PVC may be

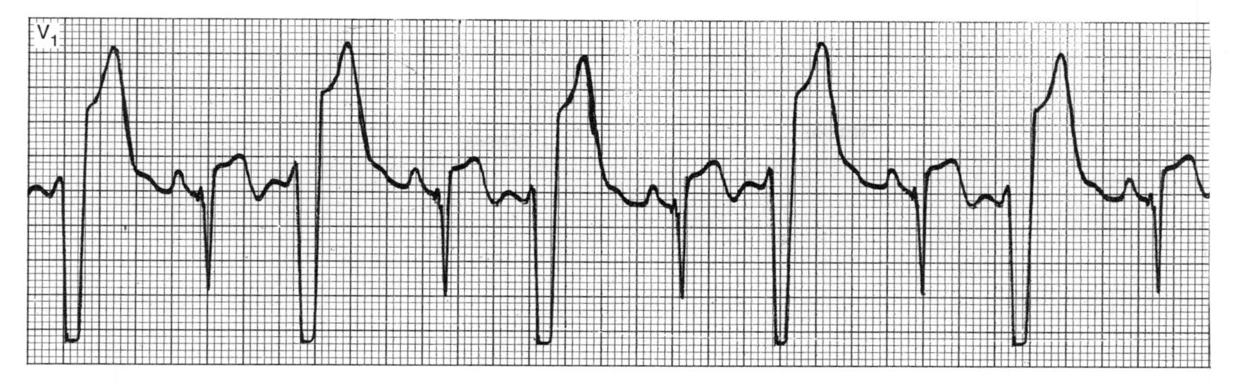

FIG. 12-7. Ventricular bigeminy with fixed coupling. Fixed coupling means that the interval between the sinus beat and the PVC is the same each time, implying a cause-and-effect relationship.

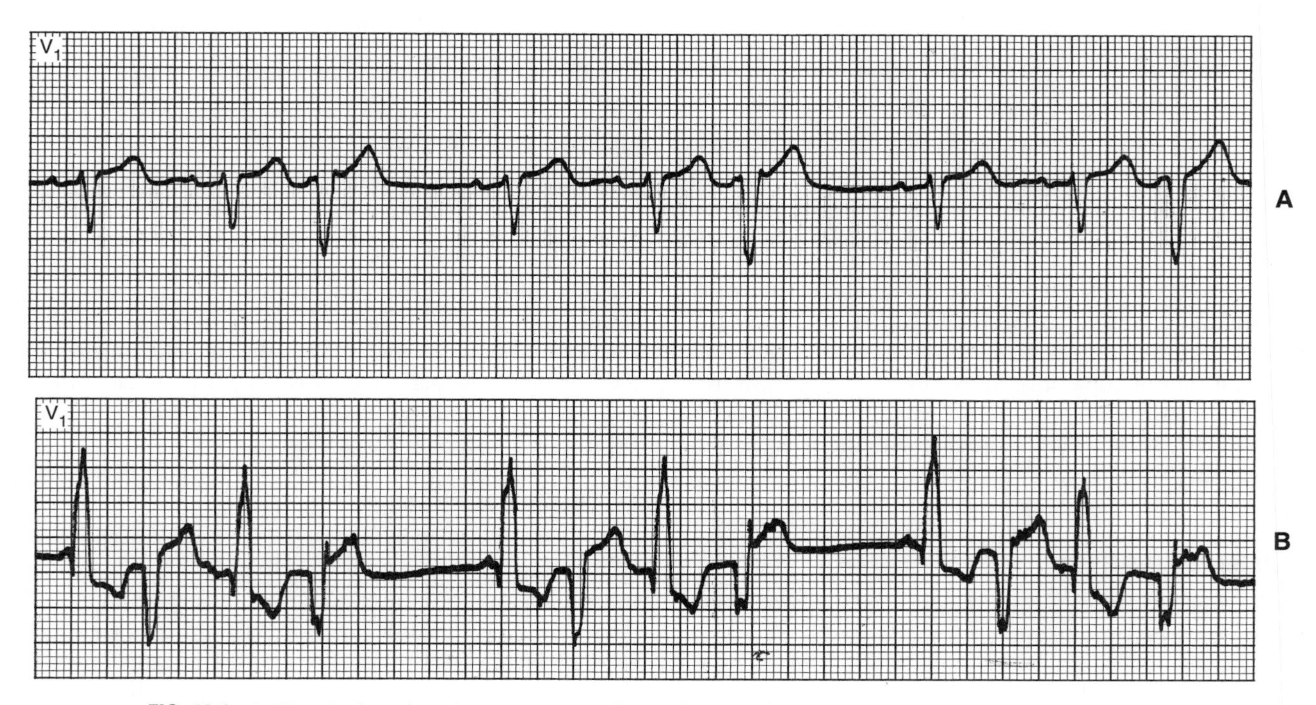

FIG. 12-8. **A**, Ventricular trigeminy—two normal complexes and one PVC. **B**, Ventricular quadrigeminy—groups of four.

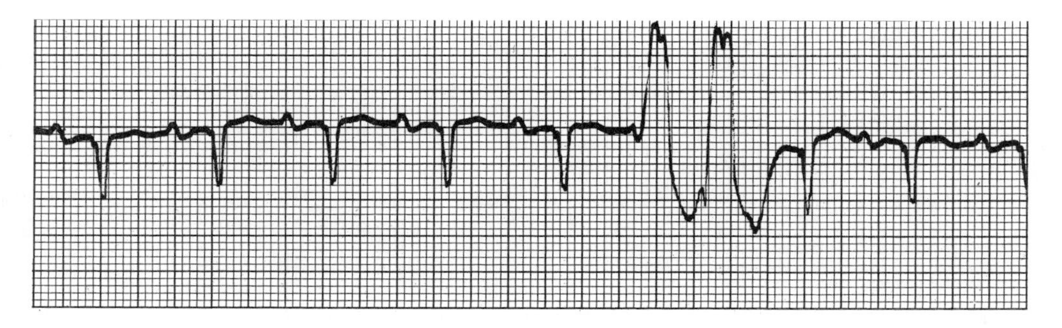

FIG. 12-9. Paired or "back-to-back" PVCs.

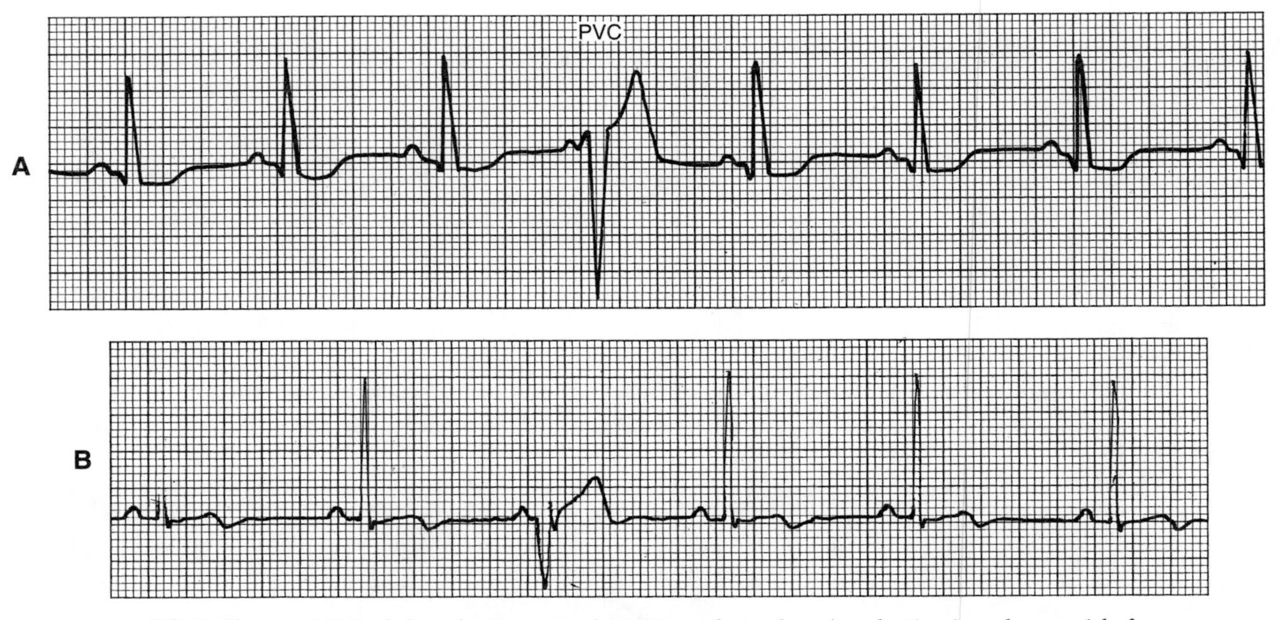

FIG. 12-10. A and B, End-diastolic PVCs. B, The PVC is a fusion beat (conduction into the ventricle from both the sinus beat and the ventricular ectopic focus).

the occasional manifestation of an accelerated idioventricular rhythm trying to surface or, if such PVCs occur frequently, in the setting of acute myocardial infarction they may be a sign of congestive heart failure. It is known that enhanced automaticity may result when myocardial fibers are stretched. Such would be the case with the elevated left-ventricular end-diastolic pressure that results from heart failure.

Interpolated PVCs

An interpolated PVC is a premature ectopic beat sandwiched between two normal sinus-conducted beats; therefore, it does not have a full compensatory pause. In fact, there is no pause at all in the sinus rhythm and ventricular response. Many times there is retrograde concealed conduction into the fast pathway of the AV node, causing the P wave after the PVC to be conducted into the ventricles via the slow AV nodal pathway. Thus the PR interval after the PVC is often longer than normal. Such is the case in Fig. 12-11: the sinus rate is 65 beats/min. Notice the long PR interval of the sinus beat after the PVC.

Fascicular PVCs

PVCs originating in the fascicles of the intraventricular conduction system are narrower than other PVCs and have morphologic appearances identical to left or right BBB aberration. The relative narrowness (approximately 0.13 second) of the QRS results because the impulse is within the intraventricular conduction system rather than in ventricular myocardium where conduction is slower.

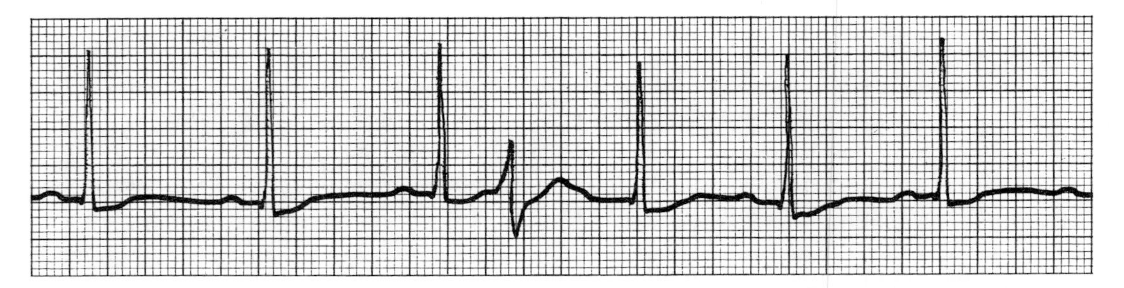

FIG. 12-11. Interpolated PVC. There is a PVC between the third and fourth QRS. The PR interval after the PVC is longer than the others. (The P wave can be found distorting the T wave of the ectopic beat.)

Anterior fascicular beats have right axis deviation (Fig. 12-12), posterior fascicular beats, and left axis deviation (Fig. 12-13); both have a right BBB configuration in lead V_1 and a relatively narrow QRS (less than 0.14 second). Axis deviation occurs whenever there is an ectopic focus in the fascicles of the left bundle branch or when there is a block in one of these fascicles. The right BBB pattern occurs because the impulse originates within the left ventricular fascicles and the right ventricle is the last to be activated. The complexes are narrower than other ventricular ectopic beats because they originate within the conduction system and the impulse is therefore delivered to both ventricles very rapidly.

R-on-T Phenomenon

As early as 1928 Louis Katz[2] emphasized the danger of PVCs falling on the T wave. The term *R-on-T phenomenon* was used by Wiggers[3] in 1940 and Smirk[4] in 1949, who found that many patients showed the R-on-T phenomenon and that they were subject to lethal ventricular tachycardia and sudden death. The term indicates that an R wave (PVC) has occurred at the peak of the T wave—the vulnerable period of the ECG when not all of the ventricular myocardium has fully repolarized. In the setting of acute myocardial infarction it is of course possible for the vulnerable period to extend throughout most of the cardiac cycle because of the heterogeneity of repolarization and conduction velocity in injured and ischemic tissue. Thus late-coupled PVCs are at least as likely to initiate ventricular tachycardia.[5]

The appearance of a PVC on the T wave is prevalent during the first 24 hours after the onset of symptoms of myocardial infarction, especially during thrombolysis and particularly if nonreperfused. This type of PVC decreases in frequency rapidly with time, and in the thrombolytic era the ventricular tachycardia produced tends to be a self-limited monomorphic type that seldom causes symptoms.[6]

Fig. 12-14 shows emergency department tracings from a patient in the prethrombolytic era. The patient had shortly before sustained an inferior wall myocardial infarction. At the slower heart rate (Fig. 12-14, *A*) the R on T did not result in ventricular tachycardia or fibrillation. However, Fig. 12-14, *B*, shows the increase in heart rate and the pause before the R on T resulted in ventricular fibrillation (VF). The increase in sympathetic drive (increased heart rate) and the pause in rhythm are factors that have been identified as two main determinants of sudden death in a study of 45 Holter monitor tapes of VF recorded during ambulatory monitoring.[7,8]

Rule of Bigeminy

The rule of bigeminy refers to the situation in which the PVC only occurs when in the setting of relatively long cycles.[9] This is illustrated in Fig. 12-15. In Fig. 12-15, *A* and *B*, there were no PVCs until a long cycle appeared, after which there was a PVC after every normal beat. In Fig. 12-15, *C*, the pause after one PVC perpetuated a bigeminal rhythm until the pause after the fourth PVC shortened, terminating the bigeminal rhythm. The implication is that the long cycle causes a longer refractory period and perhaps

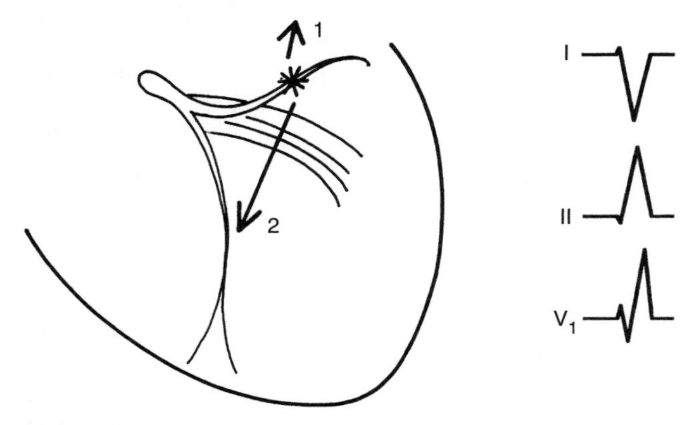

FIG. 12-12. An anterior fascicular beat and its ECG complexes. The QRS is relatively narrow (less than 0.14 second) because of an origin within the conduction system. There is right axis deviation and a right bundle branch block pattern. The indicated 1-2 conduction sequence explains the right axis deviation and the QRS shape in the limb leads.

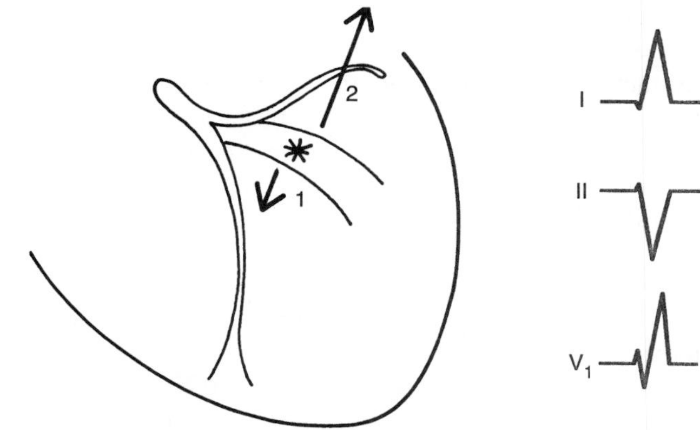

FIG. 12-13. A posterior fascicular beat and its ECG complexes. The QRS is relatively narrow (less than 0.14 second) because of an origin within the conduction system. There is left axis deviation and a right bundle branch block pattern. The indicated 1-2 conduction sequence explains the left axis deviation and the QRS shape in the limb leads.

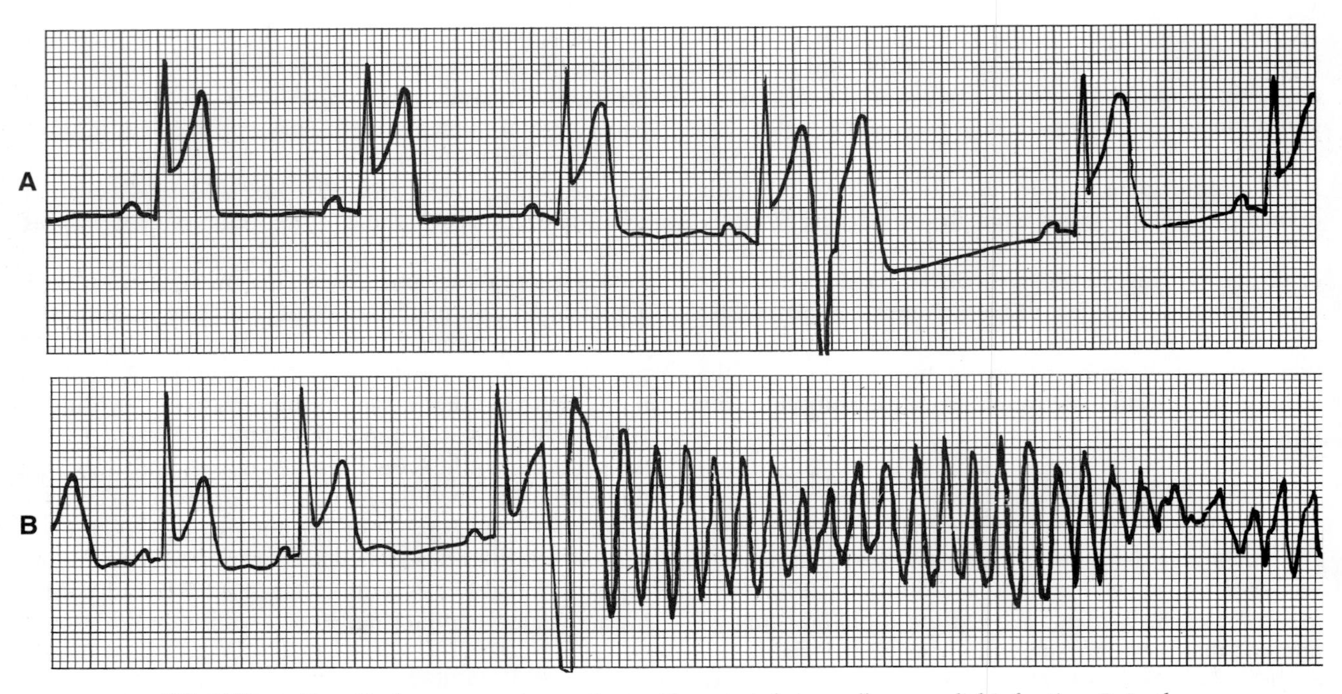

FIG. 12-14. **A**, R-on-T phenomenon in a patient with acute inferior wall myocardial infarction. **B**, In the same patient, R on T later causes ventricular fibrillation.

inhomogeneity of refractoriness. Thus the bigeminal rhythm perpetuates itself, since there is usually a pause after every PVC.

MECHANISMS

A PVC may be the result of enhanced normal automaticity in the His-Purkinje system (catecholamines); abnormal automaticity anywhere in the ventricles (ischemia, electrolyte imbalance, or injury); reentry through slowly conducting tissue within the ventricles (ischemia or injury); or triggered activity occurring within the His-Purkinje system (digitalis excess or catecholamines) or within the ventricular myocardium (e.g., class 1A, 1C drugs).

R on T

The mechanism of the R-on-T phenomenon is thought to be early afterdepolarizations. In fact, early afterdepolarization and phase 2 reentry (p. 142) are the only mechanism capable of producing an extrasystole that arises during the T wave; an extrasystole caused by the more common forms of reentry would come after the T wave, and one caused by a delayed afterdepolarization tends to appear in early or mid-diastole.[10]

One of the characteristics of this mechanism is a short coupling interval; ectopic firing occurs at the beginning of phase 3 of the action potential. This would coincide with the apex of the T wave, the vulnerable period of the ECG. Simultaneously present during the T wave are dispersions of repolarization, excitability, and the possibility for slow conduction. A stimulus applied in such an environment can provoke fibrillation. The R-on-T phenomenon is clearly a cause for concern when it appears in adults with a history of ischemic heart disease or Brugada syndrome (Chapter 27). However, the early emphasis on the R on T as a potentially lethal arrhythmia was placed during the prefibrinolytic era. In the postthrombolytic era the occurrence of R on T is an early rare feature of acute myocardial infarction and does not trigger severe ventricular tachycardia.[6]

Broad QRS

The excessive width of the PVC is due to ventricular activation that begins outside the conduction system and therefore does not have the advantage of speedy, organized delivery to the myocardium. A width of 0.14 second or more is one of the distinguishing features of the ventricular ectopic beat or rhythm. Exceptions are ventricular fascicular beats (see p. 142) and fusion beats (see Chapter 19). PVCs may also appear to be narrow in certain leads when initial or terminal forces are isoelectric; this is easily recognized by looking at the

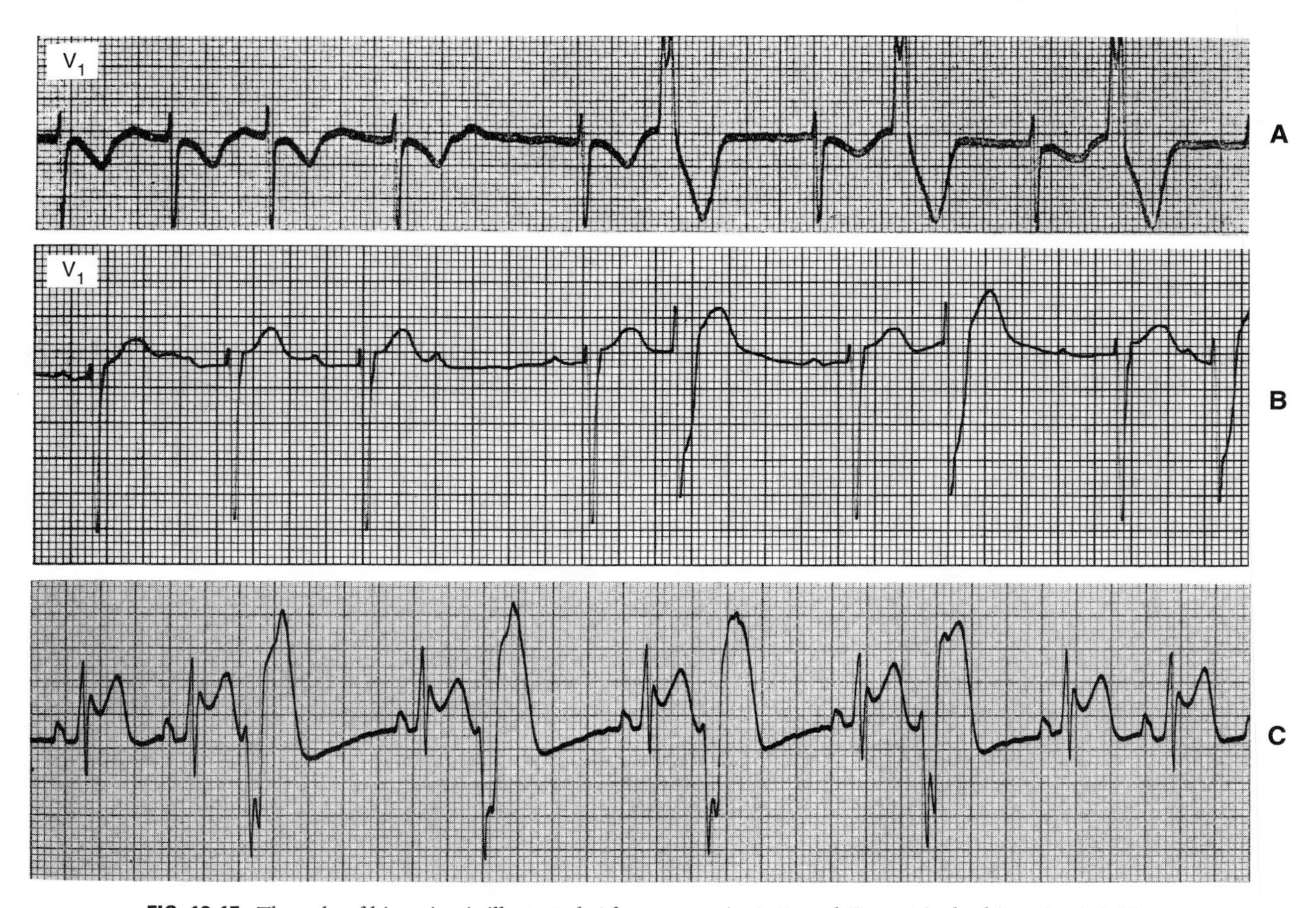

FIG. 12-15. The rule of bigeminy is illustrated. After a pause in **A**, **B**, and **C**, ventricular bigeminy is initiated. The underlying rhythm in **A** is atrial fibrillation (note absence of P waves); in **B** the underlying rhythm is AV Wenckebach. In **C** a PVC creates a pause that initiates ventricular bigeminy. At the end of this tracing the sinus rate increases, shortening the pause and eliminating the ventricular bigeminy.

questionable beat in other leads (in which the PVC is broad).

QRS Shape

The shape of the QRS can be diagnostic of ventricular ectopy. To make this judgment, lead V_1 must be available; sometimes leads V_2 and V_6 are also necessary. If V1 is positive, look for a monophasic or biphasic complex to indicate a PVC; two peaks with the first peak higher is also diagnostic for a PVC. If the complex in V_1 is negative, any one of the following signs indicates ventricular ectopy: R wave broader than 0.03 second, a slurred S downstroke, delayed S nadir in V_1 or V_2, or q in V_6.

Increased Amplitude

The greater amplitude of the PVC is caused by a stronger vector, not a stronger beat. Normally the right and left ventricles are activated simultaneously from endocardium to epicardium, with the currents activating the right ventricle being canceled out by the stronger ones in the left ventricle. With a ventricular ectopic beat the sequence of activation is such that most currents are traveling in one direction (e.g., from the left to the right ventricle) without the canceling-out effect of the normal activation sequence. The resultant stronger vector is reflected in the ECG tracing by a complex of higher amplitude than that of the dominant sinus rhythm.

The bigger vector of the PVC does not mean that the premature muscle contraction is stronger than normal. On the contrary, it is weaker because it occurs early, not allowing for complete ventricular filling, and because the contraction resulting from a PVC is not uniform. In fact, it is the conducted sinus beat after the PVC that is stronger than other sinus beats. This is because the pause after the PVC allows for more ventricular filling.

T Wave of Opposite Polarity

Whenever the process of depolarization is abnormal, as it is with a PVC or BBB, the repolarization sequence produces a T wave that is opposite in polarity to the terminal part of the QRS. This is called a *secondary T wave change* and is expected in these conditions. The normal repolarization process produces a T wave that is the same polarity as the QRS. After a PVC the repolarization process is reversed, producing a T wave that is opposite in polarity to the QRS.

The Full Compensatory Pause

A full compensatory pause is the pause that follows a PVC and is caused by nonconduction of a normal sinus beat. The sinus beat fails to conduct to the ventricles because the PVC has left them refractory. Thus a full compensatory pause is found only when the sinus rhythm is uninterrupted by the PVC and when one sinus P wave is not conducted. True full compensatory pauses are seen after

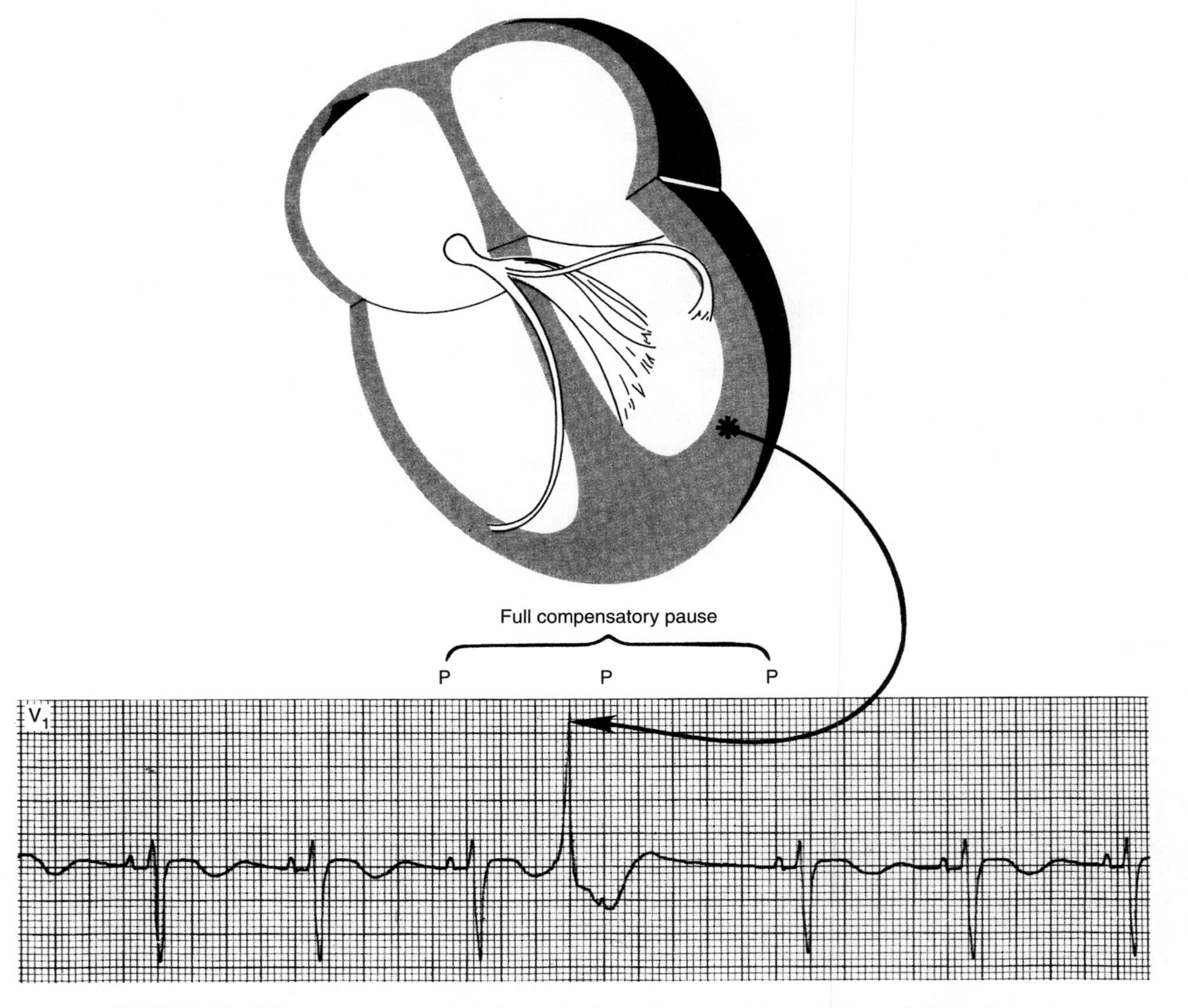

FIG. 12-16. The full compensatory pause is the result of an uninterrupted sinus rhythm and a sinus P wave that is not conducted to the ventricles. The sinus P wave that is not conducted in this tracing is seen in the T wave of the PVC; note that it is right on time with the other PP intervals.

only about half of the PVCs (the ones with retrograde block to the atria); the other half have retrograde conduction to the atria, which resets the sinus rhythm and negates the possibility for a true full compensatory pause. In Fig. 12-16 the sinus rhythm can be "walked out" across the PVC. The sinus P wave can actually be seen within the T wave of the PVC. To measure for the presence of a full compensatory pause, place a piece of paper under the tracing and mark precisely three P waves. Then move the paper so that the first mark is on the conducted beat before the PVC; the third mark should fall exactly on the P wave after the pause. A caliper can also be used to walk out the sinus rhythm; the P waves will be on time, despite the interruption by the PVC; one P wave is not conducted, causing the "pause."

Although a noncompensatory pause indicates atrial involvement, a full compensatory pause does not prove ventricular ectopy. This is because a premature atrial complex (PAC) may be followed by such a pause if the PAC discharges the sinus node and instead of resetting it depresses it. This phenomenon is called "overdrive suppression"; the next expected discharge from the sinus node is delayed. Of course, such a depression may also result in a longer pause than expected.

Thus a full compensatory pause is not a diagnostic clue for PVCs unless the nonconducted sinus P wave can be seen; a PAC may be followed by a compensatory, noncompensatory, or more than compensatory pause.

The atrial involvement mentioned above may occur because a PVC has retrograde conduction to the atria. This could produce any kind of a pause—full (chance), less than full, or more than full. Thus it is that the full compensatory pause is a "broken reed" (H. J. L. Marriott, MD). You can count on it as a diagnostic sign of a PVC *only* if the nonconducted sinus P wave can actually be seen (as in Fig. 12-16).

In Fig. 12-17 there is retrograde conduction to the atria, causing the sinus node to be discharged early and the next sinus P wave to be early. Thus although this is a PVC, there is not a full compensatory pause. More weight is placed on the morphologic appearance of the PVC in lead V_1 than on the presence of a full compensatory pause. For example, the broad beat in Fig. 12-18 is followed by a full compensatory pause. However, the sinus P wave occurring during the broad beat cannot be seen, placing the accuracy of such a pause in doubt. The monophasic R wave in V_1 plus the excessive width of the QRS (0.16 second) and its prematurity identify it as a PVC.

Overdrive Suppression

Overdrive suppression is a property belonging to all pacemaker cells by which their premature discharge causes their cycle to lengthen. For example, the sinus node sometimes is delayed in reaching threshold potential if it is discharged early by retrograde conduction to the atria or by any other early beat (e.g., PAC). This can be seen in the length of the P′P interval (the distance from the ectopic P to the next sinus P). This distance is longer than the PP intervals of the dominant rhythm.

CAUSES

PVCs are aggravated by ischemia, increased sympathetic activity, and tachycardia or bradycardia. Other

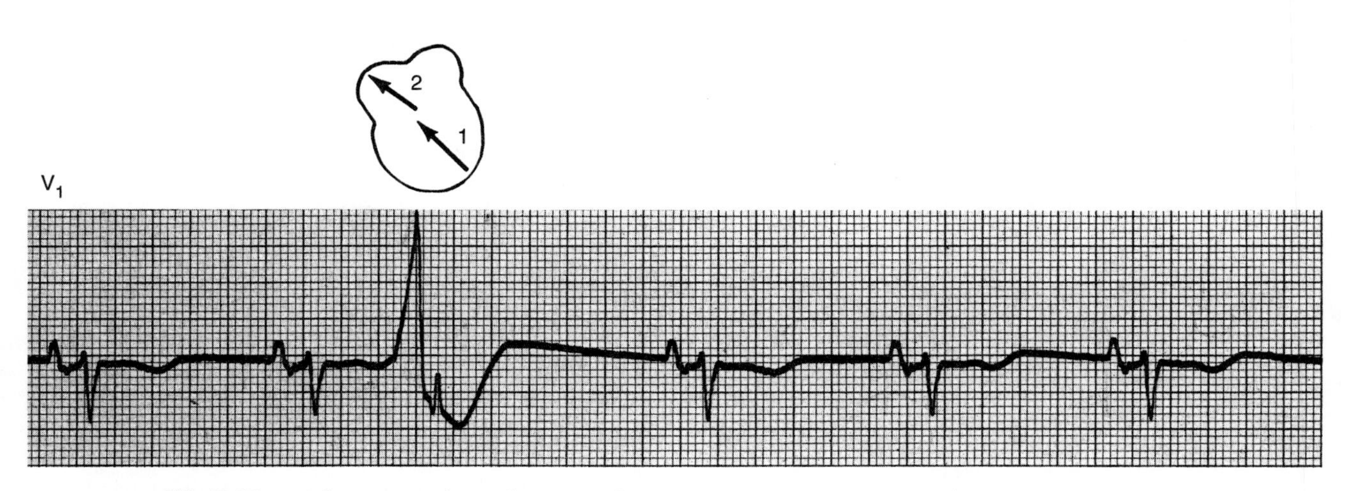

FIG. 12-17. PVC has retrograde conduction to the atria. Note that the retrograde P′ wave is distorting the T of the PVC. When you attempt to "walk out" this rhythm, the retrograde P′ is premature and disturbs the regular beating of the sinus node. In this case it suppresses the sinus node, causing the next expected sinus beat to be later than expected (overdrive suppression).

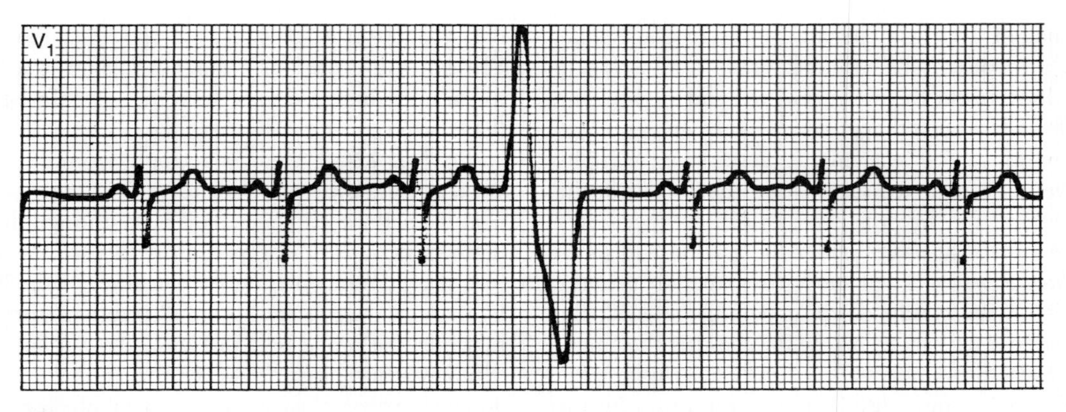

FIG. 12-18. An apparently full compensatory pause follows this PVC. However, the nonconducted sinus P wave cannot be seen, leaving some doubt. The morphologic appearance of the broad complex in V_1 identifies it as a PVC (monophasic R).

causes include the following: fever, volume depletion, infection, drug excesses of all types, hypokalemia, hypercalcemia, and excess or even moderate alcohol intake in certain individuals.

CLINICAL IMPLICATIONS

PVCs are a common occurrence, even without heart disease, and increase in number with age. The incidence of PVCs is greater with acute myocardial infarction and ventricular scarring resulting from infarction, hypertrophy, or infection, and may be aggravated by ischemia, increased sympathetic activity, and increased or reduced heart rate.[11] Other causes include fever, volume depletion, infection, drug excesses of all types, hypokalemia, hypercalcemia, and excess or even moderate alcohol intake in certain individuals.[12]

Symptomatic Patient with No Structural Heart Disease

In this setting PVCs are considered benign and are not treated; they have no impact on longevity nor do they require restricted activity. A symptomatic patient is reassured.[13]

Apparently Healthy Individuals

PVCs and complex ventricular arrhythmias may be markers of heart disease but have not been shown to play a role in sudden death, nor has antiarrhythmic therapy been shown to reduce the incidence of sudden death in such patients.[13]

Acute Myocardial Infarction

In the prethrombolytic era, the presence of PVCs after myocardial infarction identified a patient at greater risk for sudden cardiac death. In the thrombolytic era, a twofold increase in the number of PVCs is among the ECG signs of reperfusion and occurs before other reperfusion arrhythmias. For a list of ECG signs of reperfusion see p. 363.

Although PVCs of any type have not been shown to be prognostically helpful in the setting of acute myocardial infarction, frequent or complex (multiform, couplets, R on T) PVCs have been regarded as "malignant" or likely to result in VF.

In half of the patients with myocardial infarction who have these types of PVCs, VF does not develop, and of those patients in whom VF does develop, approximately half had not manifested such PVCs before the VF.

PVCs Associated with Left Ventricular Hypertrophy

Echocardiographically determined left ventricular hypertrophy is associated with increased risk for ventricular arrhythmias. When frequent (more than 30 PVCs per hour) or complex (multiform, couplets, R on T) they are associated with higher mortality.[14]

PVCs in Athletes

When PVCs in an athlete are associated with structural and functional heart adaptations, as demonstrated by echocardiography, the PVCs are not simply a physiologic phenomenon. Rather, the individual may be at high risk for lethal arrhythmias according to a study by Claessens et al[15] who tested 52 well-trained triathletes and compared the number of PVCs during a maximal exercise test with those of 22 control subjects. There were more PVCs among the athletes than among the control group. An increased risk of PVCs in the triathlon group was found to be associated with cardiac hypertrophy, increased diastolic reserve, duration of the exercise, existence of an aortic insufficiency jet, and some specific ECG findings.

PEDIATRICS

PVCs are seen in term infants on the first day of life and are commonly seen in pediatric patients and are considered benign in a structurally normal heart.[16]

BEDSIDE DIAGNOSIS

Compensatory pause: Follows the premature beat; it is longer than normal and does not change the timing of the basic rhythm.

Heart sounds: Often decreased intensity; the first heart sound can be sharp and snapping, and the second heart sound can be abnormally split, depending on the origin of the ventricular complex.

Peripheral pulse: Decreased or absent. The signs of AV dissociation are present about half the time.

DIFFERENTIAL DIAGNOSIS

The differential diagnosis is aberrant ventricular conduction, that is, physiologic BBB caused by activation of the ventricles by a PAC when one of the bundle branches is still refractory and cannot conduct. The differential diagnosis between aberration and ectopy is covered in Chapter 14.

TREATMENT

It has been found that the combination of amiodarone and beta blockade can safely be administered to patients at high risk for arrhythmic death.[17,18] Although ventricular arrhythmias in patients with left ventricular systolic dysfunction can be suppressed by class I antiarrhythmic drugs (blocking sodium channels), a study confined to patients who had sustained a prior myocardial infarction showed that these same drugs produced an increased mortality in most, if not all, subsets of patients with ischemic heart disease. The unexpected and dramatic results of the Cardiac Arrhythmia Suppression Trials first became available in 1989.[19,20] It is now suspected that all class I antiarrhythmic drugs may increase mortality in patients with prior myocardial infarction and in those with cardiac arrest or atrial fibrillation because the drugs themselves have proarrhythmic effects.[18] Thus prophylactic use of lidocaine is no longer routinely indicated for patients with acute myocardial infarction, and it is rarely indicated for patients without symptomatic arrhythmias or sustained VT or VF.[21,22]

SUMMARY

A PVC is noticed first because of its prematurity, excessive width, increased amplitude, and T wave of opposite polarity. If the sinus rhythm can be seen to be uninterrupted by the premature beat (full compensatory pause), this is a helpful sign in identifying a PVC. The morphologic appearance of the premature beat is often diagnostic.

REFERENCES

1. Moulton KP, Medcalf T, Lazzara R: Premature ventricular complex morphology: a marker for left ventricular structure and function, *Circulation* 81:1245, 1990.
2. Katz LN: The significance of the T wave in the electrogram and the electrocardiogram, *Physiol Rev* 8:447, 1928.
3. Wiggers CJA: The mechanism and nature of ventricular fibrillation, *Am Heart J* 20:399, 1940.
4. Smirk FH: R waves interrupting T waves, *Br Heart J* 11:23, 1949.
5. Rukbin AM, Morganroth J, Kowey PR: Ventricular premature depolarizations. In Podrid PJ, Kowey PR, editors: *Cardiac arrhythmia: mechanisms, diagnosis, and management*, Philadelphia, 1995, Williams & Wilkins.
6. Chiladakis JA, Karapanos G, Davlouros P et al: Significance of R-on-T phenomenon in early ventricular tachyarrhythmia susceptibility after acute myocardial infarction in the thrombolytic era, *Am J Cardiol* 85:289, 2000.
7. Coumel P, Leclerck J, Qimmerman M, Funck-Brentano J: Antiarrhythmic therapy: noninvasive guided strategy versusempirical or invasive strategies. In Brugada P, Wellens HJJ, editors: *Cardiac arrhythmias: where to go from here?* Mount Kisco, NY, 1987, Futura.
8. Leclerck JF, Coumel P, Maisonblanch P et al: Mechanisms determining sudden death: a cooperative study of 69 cases recorded during the Holter method, *Arch Mal Coeur Vaiss* 79:1420, 1986.
9. Langendorf R, Pick A, Winternitz M: Mechanisms of intermittent bigeminy. I. Appearance of ectopic beats dependent upon the length of the ventricular cycle: the "rule of bigeminy," *Circulation* 11:422, 1955.
10. Campbell RWF, Murray A, Julian DG: Ventricular arrhythmias in the first 12 hours of acute myocardial infarction, *Br Heart J* 46:351, 1981.
11. Bigger JT Jr: Definition of benign versus malignant ventricular arrhythmias: targets for treatment, *Am J Cardiol* 52:47C, 1983.
12. Naccarelli GV, Willerson JT, Blomquist CG: Recognition and physiologic treatment of cardiac arrhythmias and conduction disturbances. In Willerson JT, Choh JN, editors: *Cardiovascular medicine*, New York, 1995, Churchill Livingstone.
13. Zipes DP: Specific arrhythmias: diagnosis and treatment. In Braunwald E, editor: *Heart disease*, ed 4, Philadelphia, 1992, WB Saunders.
14. Bikkina M, Larson MG, Levy D: Asymptomatic ventricular arrhythmias and mortality risk in subjects with left ventricular hypertrophy, *J Am Coll Cardiol* 22:1111, 1993.
15. Claessens P, Claessens C, Claessens M et al: Ventricular premature beats in triathletes: still a physiological phenomenon? *Cardiology* 92:28, 1999.
16. Chou TC, Knilans TK: *Electrocardiography in clinical practice adult and pediatric*, ed 4, Philadelphia, 1996, WB Saunders.
17. Ogunyankin KO, Singh BN: Mortality reduction by antiadrenergic modulation of arrhythmogenic substrate: significance of combining beta blockers and amiodarone, *Am J Cardiol* 84:76R, 1999.

18. Yap YG, Camm AJ: Lessons from antiarrhythmic trials involving class III antiarrhythmic drugs, *Am J Cardiol* 84:83R, 1999.
19. Echt DS, Liebson PR, Mitchell LB et al: Mortality and morbidity in patients receiving encainide, flecainide or placebo: the Cardiac Arrhythmia Suppression Trial, *N Engl J Med* 324:781, 1991.
20. The Cardiac Arrhythmia Suppression Trial II Investigators: Effect of the anti-arrhythmic agent moricizine on survival after myocardial infarction, *N Engl J Med* 327:227, 1992.
21. Singh BN: Do anti-arrhythmic drugs work? Some reflections on the implications of the Cardiac Arrhythmia Suppression Trial, *Clin Cardiol* 13:725, 1990.
22. Singh BN: Routine prophylactic lidocaine administration in acute myocardial infarction: an idea whose time is all but gone? *Circulation* 86:1033, 1992.

CHAPTER **13**

Monomorphic Ventricular Rhythms

VENTRICULAR TACHYCARDIA

Ventricular tachycardia (VT) consists of at least three consecutive ventricular complexes with a rate of more than 100 beats/min. The focus is distal to the branching portion of the His bundle. Monomorphic VT is usually regular and has a uniform beat-to-beat QRS morphologic appearance.

ECG Recognition

Heart rate: 100 beats/min or more.
Rhythm: Regular.
P waves: Dissociated or retrograde.
QRS complex: Broad.
Distinguishing features: Monomorphic VT has a uniform beat-to-beat appearance and is identified as ventricular in origin because of its morphology (see Chapter 14) and the physical and electrocardiographic (ECG) signs of atrioventricular (AV) dissociation or ECG recognition of retrograde conduction to the atria. Figs. 13-1 and 13-2 show nonsustained and sustained monomorphic VT. Note the uniform beat-to-beat appearance of the broad ventricular complexes. In Fig. 13-1, 2:1 retrograde conduction to the atria is seen, is present in 50% of VTs, and is diagnostic of VT. In Fig. 13-2 the monophasic R wave in V_1 is diagnostic of VT.

Evaluation of QRS morphology. Evaluation of the QRS morphologic appearance is helpful in differentiating VT from SVT with aberrant ventricular conduction and in

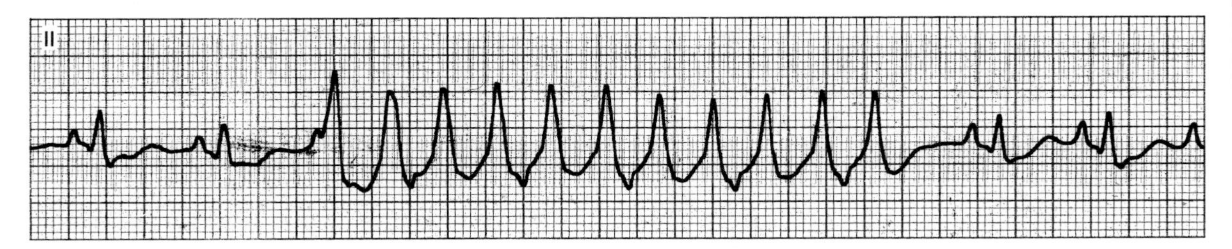

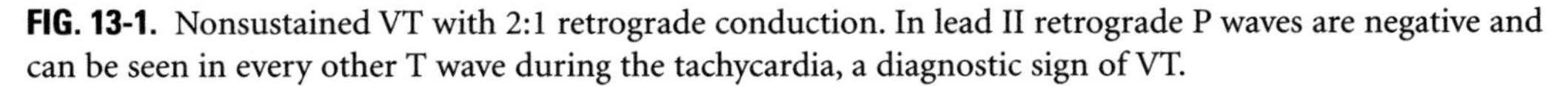

FIG. 13-1. Nonsustained VT with 2:1 retrograde conduction. In lead II retrograde P waves are negative and can be seen in every other T wave during the tachycardia, a diagnostic sign of VT.

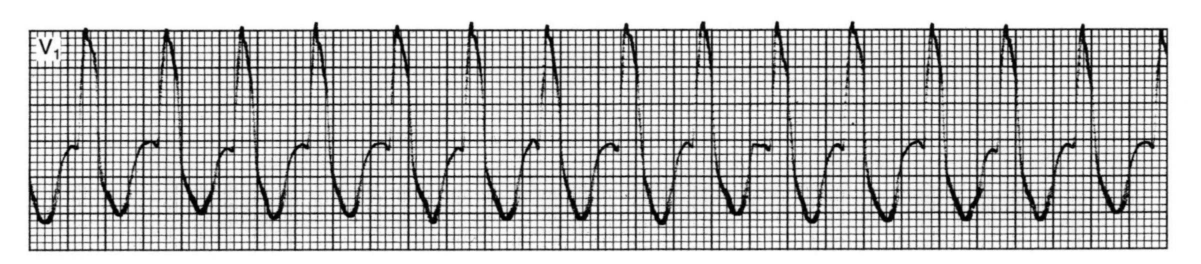

FIG. 13-2. Sustained VT. In lead V_1 the monophasic R wave is diagnostic of VT.

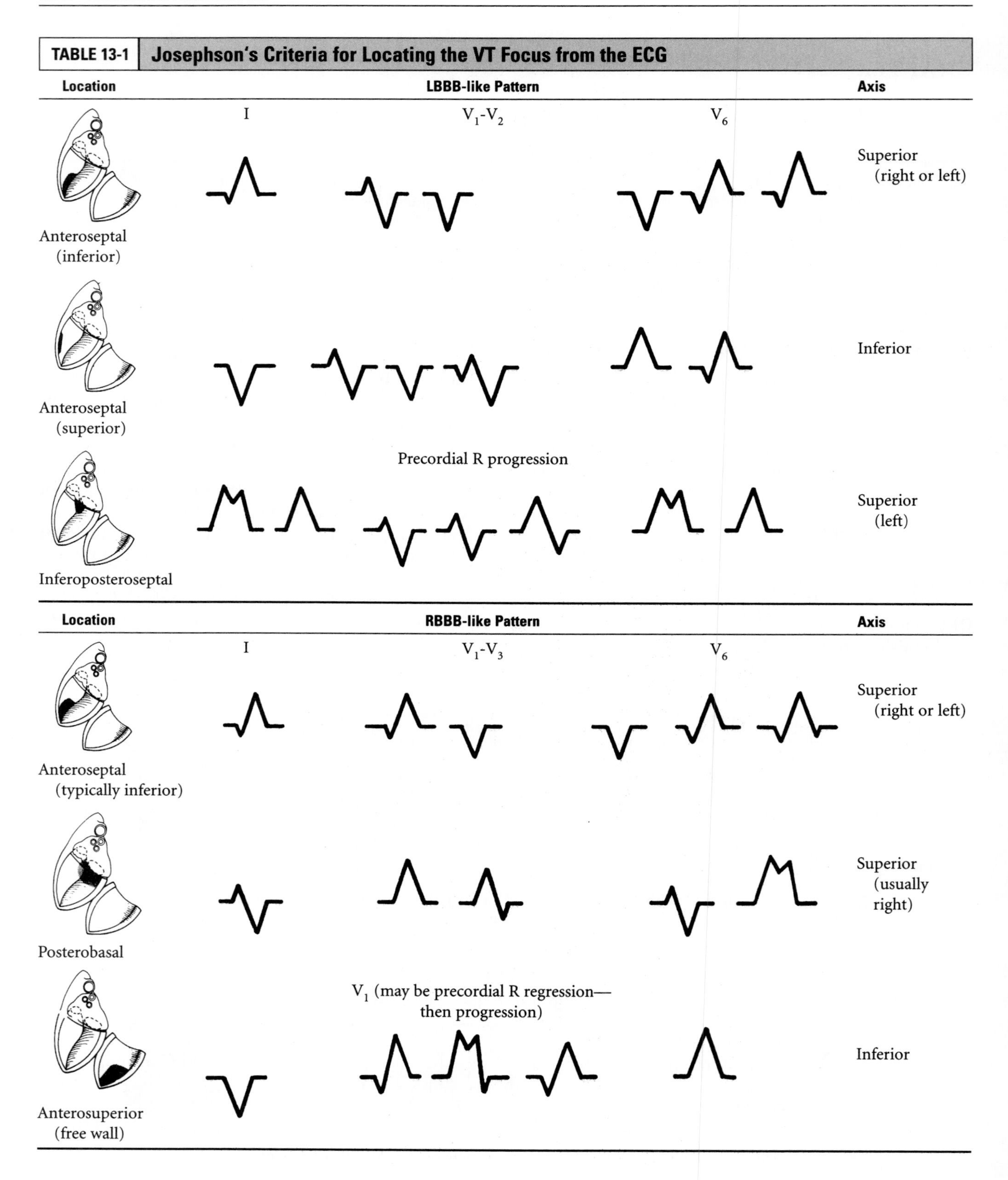

TABLE 13-1 Josephson's Criteria for Locating the VT Focus from the ECG

Location	LBBB-like Pattern: I	LBBB-like Pattern: V_1-V_2	LBBB-like Pattern: V_6	Axis
Anteroseptal (inferior)				Superior (right or left)
Anteroseptal (superior)				Inferior
Inferoposteroseptal		Precordial R progression		Superior (left)

Location	RBBB-like Pattern: I	RBBB-like Pattern: V_1-V_3	RBBB-like Pattern: V_6	Axis
Anteroseptal (typically inferior)				Superior (right or left)
Posterobasal				Superior (usually right)
Anterosuperior (free wall)		V_1 (may be precordial R regression—then progression)		Inferior

determining the location of the ventricular focus. However, when applying morphologic rules, it is important to also consider information from the history and physical examination.

Locating the VT focus. Josephson et al[1] have correlated the 12-lead ECG with endocardial pacing sites and known sites of origin of VT. Table 13-1 offers a useful method to localize the origin of VT. This method is especially accurate when the complex is mainly negative in V_1 (the so-called *left bundle branch block [LBBB] pattern*). The ECG is useful in distinguishing apical from basal and inferior from superior ventricular ectopic foci. In general, the following apply:

Apical location: A q wave in leads I, V_2, and V_6 (present in all three leads).
Basal location: An R wave in leads I, V_2, and V_6.
Posterobasal location: Positive precordial concordance.
Superior location: Inferior axis (normal or right).
Inferior location: Superior axis (left or northwest).

VT that looks like SVT with aberration. As you will see, some VTs have the QRS width and morphologic appearance of SVT with aberration on the ECG—for example, idiopathic VT, bundle branch reentrant VT, and fascicular VT.

SVT that looks like VT. Some SVTs are identical in QRS morphologic appearance to VT—that is, the SVTs that use an accessory pathway for entry into the ventricles, covered in Chapter 21.

Use of Precordial Leads in Locating VT Focus in Myocardial Infarction

Table 13-2 defines the different patterns of R wave progression during VT in patients with myocardial infarction (MI).[2]

Anterior wall MI. A V_1-negative pattern with left axis deviation and no late R wave progression means an *inferoapical septal focus.* An inferior axis (normal or right) means an *anterosuperior apical septal focus.*

A V_1-positive pattern with right axis deviation and dominant or abrupt loss of R wave progression means an *anteroapical septal focus.*

Inferior MI. A V_1-negative pattern with left axis deviation and a growing R wave progression means an *inferobasal septal focus.*

A V_1-positive pattern with a superior axis and reverse (early or late) R wave progression means an *inferobasal free wall focus.*

A V_1-negative pattern with an inferior right axis deviation and reverse (late) R wave progression means a *mid-posterior septal focus.*

Mechanisms and Causes

Sustained monomorphic VT is most commonly seen in adults with prior MI or chronic coronary artery disease. It is also seen in patients with dilated cardiomyopathy, arrhythmogenic right ventricular dysplasia, and in those with no apparent structural heart disease (idiopathic VT). Typically the patient with sustained VT has a history of MI with extensive muscle necrosis and an ejection fraction of less than 40%, marked wall motion abnormality, aneurysm (70%), and acute complications within the first 48 hours after the infarction (80%). These complications include bundle branch block (in anterior wall MI), congestive heart failure, primary ventricular fibrillation (VF), and hypotension.

Reentry. Most instances of monomorphic VT associated with coronary artery disease, MI, and dilated cardiomyopathy arise as a result of a stable reentrant circuit with an area of slow conduction within the circuit.[3]

Among the VTs that do originate from the right ventricle or use right ventricular structures as part of their circuit are idiopathic VT, bundle branch reentrant VT, the VT of arrhythmogenic right ventricular dysplasia, and the VT of Brugada syndrome.

Abnormal automaticity. In the postinfarction period the ischemia itself results in fibers with low membrane potentials that cause abnormal automaticity and slow conduction. Abnormal automaticity can occur in any ischemic fibers, even those that did not have the capability of automaticity in health.

Triggered activity. A less common mechanism of monomorphic VT is triggered activity in the form of delayed afterdepolarizations. When digitalis intoxication or excessive catecholamines are factors, triggered activity caused by delayed afterdepolarizations with foci in the His-Purkinje system is the suspected mechanism (see Chapter 15). Ischemia can cause afterdepolarizations and triggered activity in experimental preparations, but reentry is the commonly accepted mechanism of VT that follows MI. When class IA drugs are being used, triggered activity caused by long QT intervals and early afterdepolarizations may cause polymorphic VT (see Chapter 26).

Pediatrics

VT is rare in children. When it does occur, the QRS duration is longer than normal for the patient's age, but is narrow compared to VT in adults.[4] When VT occurs in children with a normal heart, the prognosis is good.[5] Common causes are cardiomyopathy or myocarditis.[6] Other causes include long QT syndrome, arrhythmogenic right ventricular dysplasia, and coronary artery anomalies.

TABLE 13-2 Type of Precordial R Wave Progression Pattern Seen in VT, Helping to Localize the Focus

Pattern	V_1	V_2	V_3	V_4	V_5	V_6
Increasing						
None or late						
Regression/growth (not QS)						
Regression/growth (QS)						
Dominant						
Abrupt loss						
Late reverse						
Early reverse						

From Miller JM et al: Relationship between the 12-lead electrocardiogram during ventricular tachycardia and endocardial site of origin in patients with coronary artery disease, *Circulation* 77:759, 1988.

Surgery for tetralogy of Fallot or more complex congenital defects carries with it a risk of ventricular arrhythmias and sudden death, especially if repair was late and the results were not optimal. Prognosis is better when VT occurs during the first year of life compared with beyond the first year of life. The clinical profile is more favorable for patients with presumed right VT (VT resolution in 76%, symptoms in 25% of patients) compared with patients with presumed left VT (VT resolution in 37%, symptoms in 67% of patients).[5]

Bedside Diagnosis

1. Irregular cannon A waves in the jugular pulse
2. Varying intensity of the first heart sound
3. Beat-to-beat changes in systolic blood pressure
4. ECG signs of AV dissociation

Any one of the preceding clues indicates AV dissociation, although the absence of clues does not rule out VT, nor does it rule out AV dissociation. For example, in atrial fibrillation with VT there is AV dissociation without its usual physical or ECG signs.

Jugular pulse. During AV dissociation the atria and the ventricles are beating independently; this beating occasionally coincides, so that the atria contract against closed AV valves, causing a reflux of blood up the jugular veins. Such irregular, unpredictable expansions in the pulsation of the jugular pulse are called *cannon A waves.*

Varying intensity of the first heart sound. The first heart sound is caused by the closing of the AV valves. During sinus rhythm it has a fixed intensity because the position of the leaflets of the AV valves is the same for every ventricular systole. During AV dissociation this position differs from beat to beat, causing a varying intensity of the first heart sound. Other conditions in which this would occur are complete heart block, AV Wenckebach, and atrial fibrillation.

Changes in systolic blood pressure. AV dissociation can be identified at the bedside by using the sphygmomanometer and blood pressure cuff. During AV dissociation there are beat-to-beat changes in systolic blood pressure because the lapse of time between atrial and ventricular contraction is different with each cycle, resulting in varying ventricular filling times.

ECG signs of atrioventricular dissociation. AV dissociation is often missed on the surface ECG. In one study[7] involving 150 patients with wide QRS tachycardia, AV dissociation was present in 67 patients (45%) but could be detected by the surface ECG in only 38 of those patients. The greatest danger is that the clinician may mistake T waves for P waves, a mistake that leads to an incorrect diagnosis and possibly lethal consequences. During the broad QRS tachycardia P waves can best be found by looking for a distortion in one cycle that cannot be found in another. Examples of this process are provided in Chapter 14.

Looks like VT, rhythm irregular, rate more than 200 beats/min? The irregular rhythm is a cue to give **procainamide;** do not give verapamil or digitalis.[8] In such a case atrial fibrillation with conduction over an accessory pathway is highly suspect, and blocking the AV node with verapamil or digitalis is of no help and may cause the rate to accelerate and VF to develop. If procainamide does not slow this rhythm, perform cardioversion immediately. The patient is referred to a center experienced in the treatment of patients with Wolff-Parkinson-White syndrome.

When in doubt. If the patient's condition is relatively stable, vagal maneuvers can be tried at any time (carotid sinus massage or Valsalva's maneuver). If these are unsuccessful, adenosine may be used. The effect is transient and should not make VT worse.[9]

ARRHYTHMOGENIC RIGHT VENTRICULAR CARDIOMYOPATHY

Arrhythmogenic right ventricular cardiomyopathy[10] (ARVC) or dysplasia is a myocardial disorder that is familial in more than 50% of cases and is characterized by fibrofatty replacement of the right ventricular myocardium.

ECG Recognition

The ECG is an initial diagnostic test that is useful but not sensitive; a normal ECG does not exclude the possibility of ARVC. The most frequent ECG abnormalities include the following.[10]

T waves: Inverted in V_1 through V_4.

QRS morphology during sinus rhythm:

- Incomplete or complete right bundle branch block (RBBB) pattern reflecting conduction delays through the right ventricle.
- Epsilon wave (a notch in the terminal portion of the QRS in V_1 reflecting delayed right ventricular activation). Fig. 13-3 is an example of the epsilon wave followed by a saddle back pattern of ST segment, another ECG sign seen in ARVC.

QRS duration: Prolonged to greater than 0.11 second in leads V_1 and V_2 as compared to the shorter QRS duration in V_6, as illustrated in Fig. 13-4.

QRS morphology of premature ventricular complexes (PVCs) or during VT: V_1-negative pattern with a superior axis (left or northwest). Fig. 13-5 is a Holter recording that begins with a PVC with a V_1-negative pattern (three PVCs had preceded the one seen). The short run

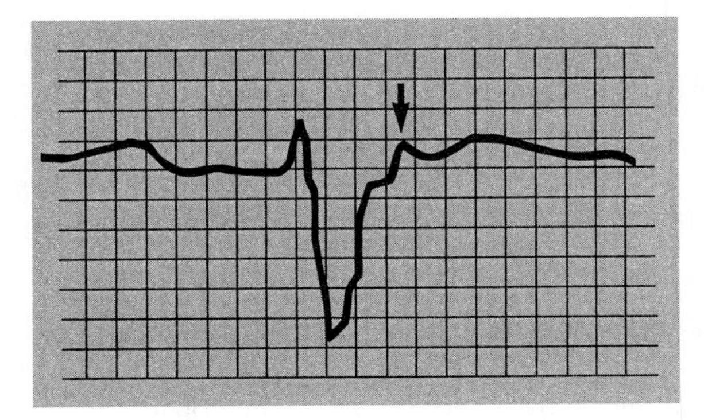

FIG. 13-3. Epsilon wave *(arrow)* in lead V_1, which is highly specific for arrhythmogenic right ventricular cardiomyopathy. (Courtesy Andrea Natale, MD, Department of Cardiology, Cleveland Clinic Foundation.)

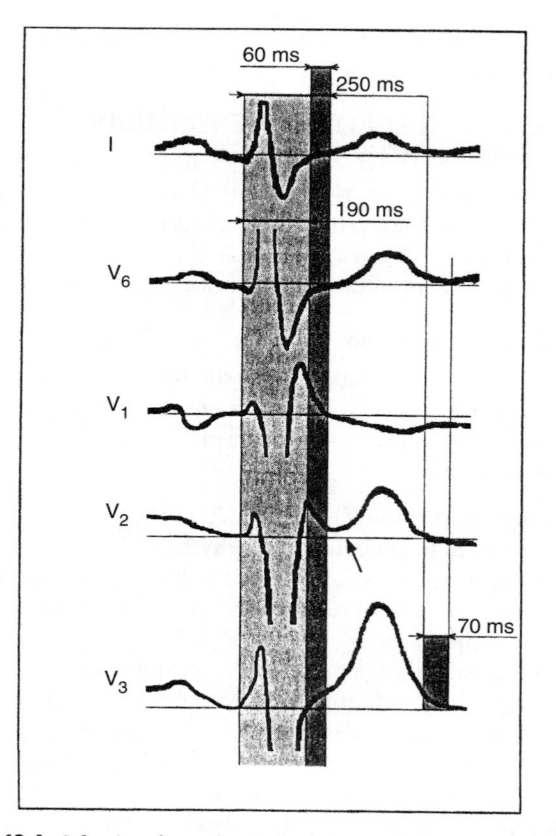

FIG. 13-4. Selection from the 12-lead ECG of a 56-year-old man who had the histologic diagnosis of arrhythmogenic right ventricular cardiomyopathy that could be suspected by the analysis of the ECG, showing an rSR' pattern in right ventricular precordial leads with a QRS complex of 250 ms in V_1 or V_2 as compared with 190 ms in lead V_6, suggesting the pattern of parietal block superimposed on a complete RBBB. Note the saddle-back pattern of the ST segment in lead V_2 *(arrow)* frequently seen in patients with arrhythmogenic right ventricular dysplasia. (From Fontaine G, Tonet J, Frank R: Ventricular tachycardia in arrhythmogenic right ventricular dysplasia. In Zipes DP, Jalife J, editors: *Cardiac electrophysiology from cell to bedside,* Philadelphia, 2000, WB Saunders.)

of VT at approximately 295 beats/min quickly deteriorates into VF, resulting in a sudden arrhythmic death during sleep.

Pathophysiology

The degenerative process begins with a genetic predisposition to fatty infiltration of the right ventricular myocardium from which it eventually degenerates into a fibrofatty form that over time involves both ventricles. In its terminal stage it is clinically indistinguishable from dilated cardiomyopathy.

Symptoms

Ventricular tachycardia and sudden death mostly in young adult males and athletes are the most common manifestations of arrhythmogenic right ventricular dysplasia. Often, there are a variety of symptoms related to episodes of VT, such as palpitations, dizzy spells, blurred vision, syncope, malaise, or abrupt extreme weakness in an individual who is apparently in good health.

Treatment

Treatment is controversial with options that include antiarrhythmic drugs, radiofrequency ablation, or an implantable cardioverter-defibrillator.[11] Cardiac transplantation may ultimately be an option in cases of progressive biventricular failure.

IDIOPATHIC VT

Idiopathic VT[12] is a generic term indicating that the arrhythmia originates in hearts without structural disease. Nearly 80% of cases originate from the right ventricle, usually the right ventricular outflow tract (RVOT); approximately 10% originate in the left ventricular outflow tract (LVOT).

Symptoms

Palpitations, dizziness, presyncope, and syncope

Prognosis

The prognosis of RVOT tachycardia is excellent with radiofrequency ablation of the arrhythmogenic focus.

Emergency Response

Wilber et al[13] recommend that idiopathic VT be managed like other VTs. Unless the physician is an expert electrophysiologist, verapamil is contraindicated for all wide-QRS tachycardias. Adenosine can be used and is effective for some of the right ventricular outflow tract VTs.

Long-Term Treatment

The decision to treat idiopathic VT is dependent on symptoms. If symptomatic, then radiofrequency catheter ablation of the focus may be indicated. Fig. 13-6 shows ablation sites in the right ventricular outflow tract. Adenosine-sensitive VT appears to arise from relatively discrete sites predominantly located in the free wall of the pulmonary infundibulum. The localized nature of this tachycardia renders it amenable to cure by catheter ablation techniques.[13] Pacing is performed in the right ventricular outflow tract, and the complexes are analyzed with respect to R/S ratio and fine notching in each lead until the paced complexes match the spontaneous QRS patterns during tachycardia. This site becomes the site of ablation. Fig. 13-7

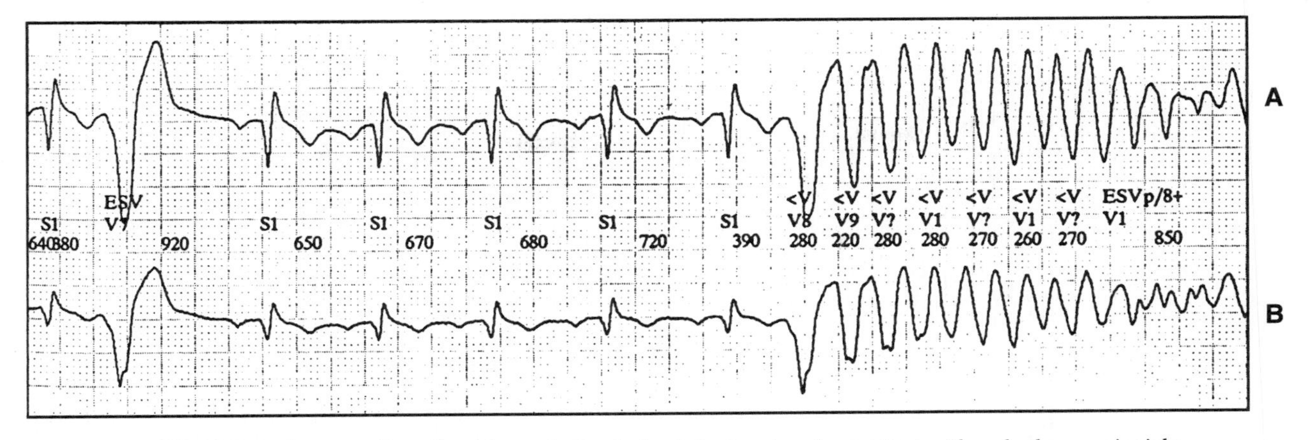

FIG. 13-5. Holter recording of sudden arrhythmic death during sleep in a patient with arrhythmogenic right ventricular cardiomyopathy. Ventricular fibrillation is preceded by four extrasystoles (only one shown here at the beginning of the tracing) and a short run of very rapid VT degenerating into ventricular fibrillation. (From Fontaine G, Tonet J, Frank R: Ventricular tachycardia in arrhythmogenic right ventricular dysplasia. In Zipes DP, Jalife J, editors: *Cardiac electrophysiology from cell to bedside,* Philadelphia, 2000, WB Saunders.)

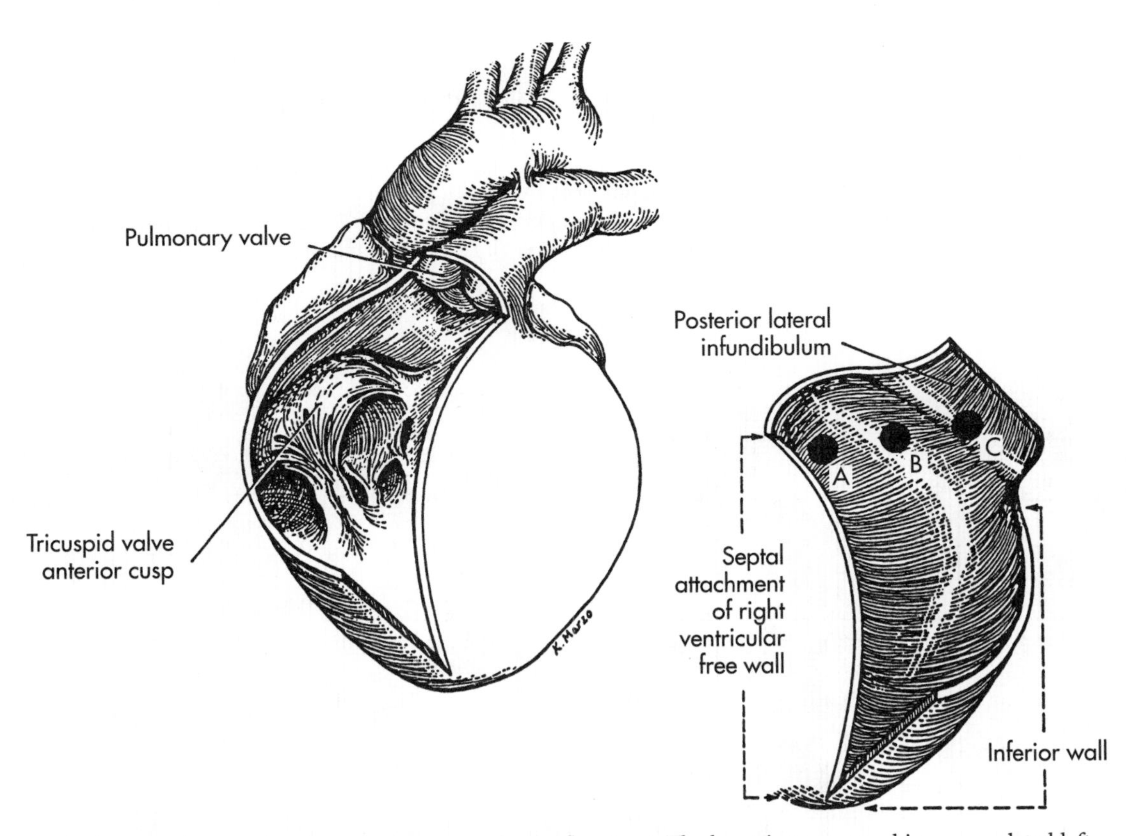

FIG. 13-6. Ablation sites in the right ventricular outflow tract. The heart is represented in an angulated left anterior oblique projection. The right ventricle is opened with the endocardial surface of the free wall depicted on the segment to the right. *A, B,* and *C* represent the sites in the right ventricular outflow tract that, during pace mapping, produced QRS complexes identical to the VT. Radiofrequency ablation was successfully performed at these sites in seven patients. (Redrawn from Wilbur DJ, Baerman J, Olshansky B et al: *Circulation* 87:126, 1993.)

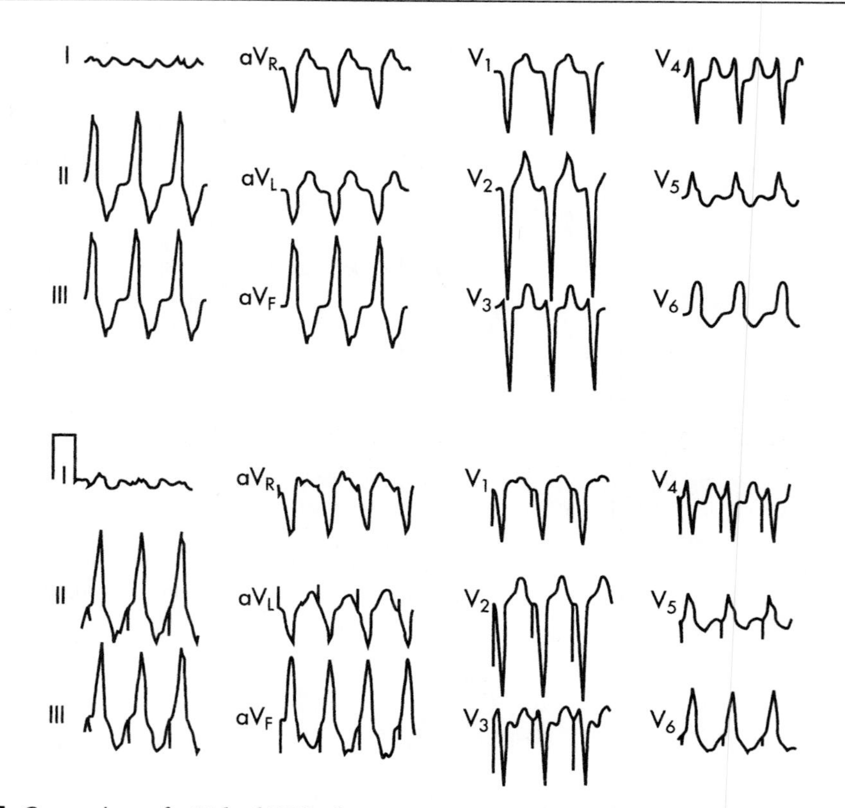

FIG. 13-7. Comparison of a 12-lead ECG of spontaneous VT and a pace map at the successful ablation site in the posteroseptal region of the left ventricle. The very close match of both R/S ratio and fine notching in all leads is evident. (From Coggins DL, Lee RJ, Sweeney J et al: *J Am Coll Cardiol* 23:1333, 1994.)

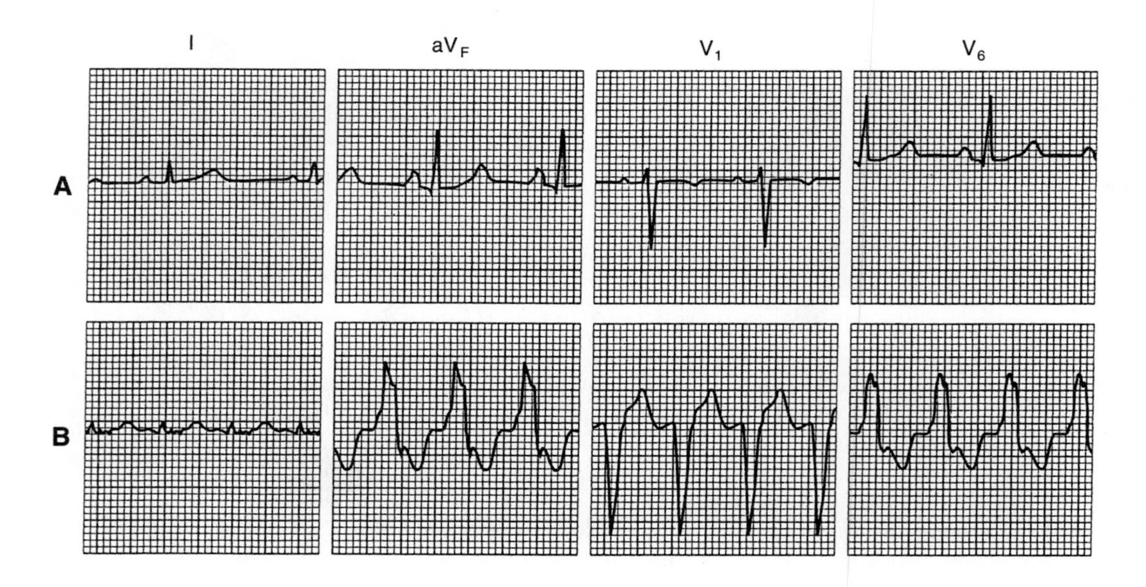

FIG. 13-8. **A,** Sinus rhythm. Relatively narrow QRS, the LBBB pattern in V_1 and V_6, and the inferior axis (aV_F positive) are evident. **B,** Idiopathic right VT at a rate of 145 beats/min (focus in the right ventricular outflow tract). (From Bhadha K, Marchlinski FE, Iskandrian AS: *Am Heart J* 126:1194, 1993.)

shows a representative pacing map from a successful ablation site.[14]

ADENOSINE-SENSITIVE RVOT TACHYCARDIA

Most of the idiopathic VTs with a focus in the RVOT are one of two forms of adenosine-sensitive VT: *nonsustained, repetitive monomorphic VT,* characterized by frequent PVCs, ventricular couplets, and salvos of nonsustained VTs interrupted by brief periods of sinus rhythm; and *paroxysmal exercise-induced sustained VT*, the mechanism of which may be triggered activity.[15]

ECG Characteristics

- Left bundle branch–like pattern in V_1
- Inferior axis (right or normal quadrants)

In Fig. 13-8, *A* and *B*, the ECG characteristics of RVOT idiopathic VT are compared to the patient's sinus rhythm.

Mechanism

Most forms of RVOT tachycardia are adenosine-sensitive and catecholamine-mediated triggered activity in response to delayed afterdepolarizations.

Differential Diagnosis

In the absence of coronary artery disease the following are considered in the differential diagnosis:

- Arrhythmogenic right ventricular cardiomyopathy
- Postsurgical repair of congenital heart disease
- Atriofascicular and nodofascicular reentry
- Bundle branch reentrant VT
- SVT with aberrant ventricular conduction

ADENOSINE-SENSITIVE LVOT TACHYCARDIA

Approximately 10% of adenosine-sensitive idiopathic VTs originate in the left ventricular outflow tract. The ECG

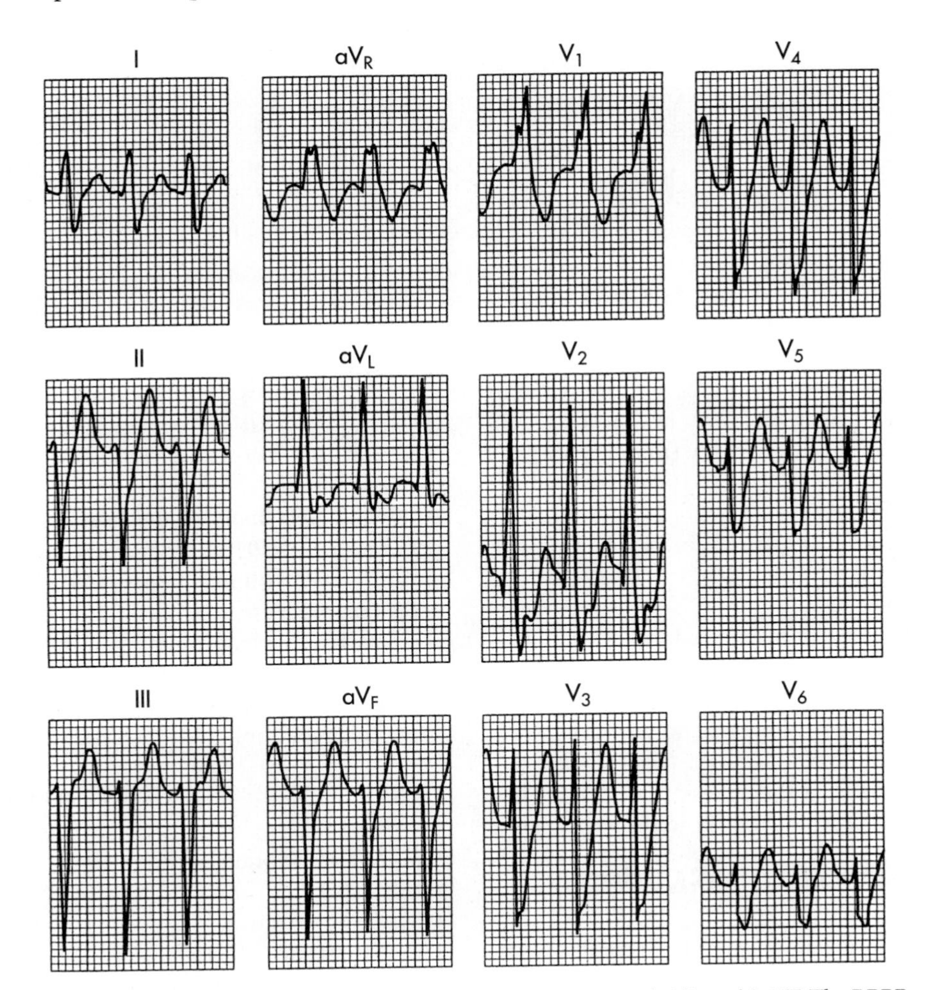

FIG. 13-9. An emergency department tracing from a 27-year-old man with idiopathic VT. The RBBB pattern in V_1 and superior axis are evident. (Courtesy Ara Tilkian, MD, Van Nuys, Calif.)

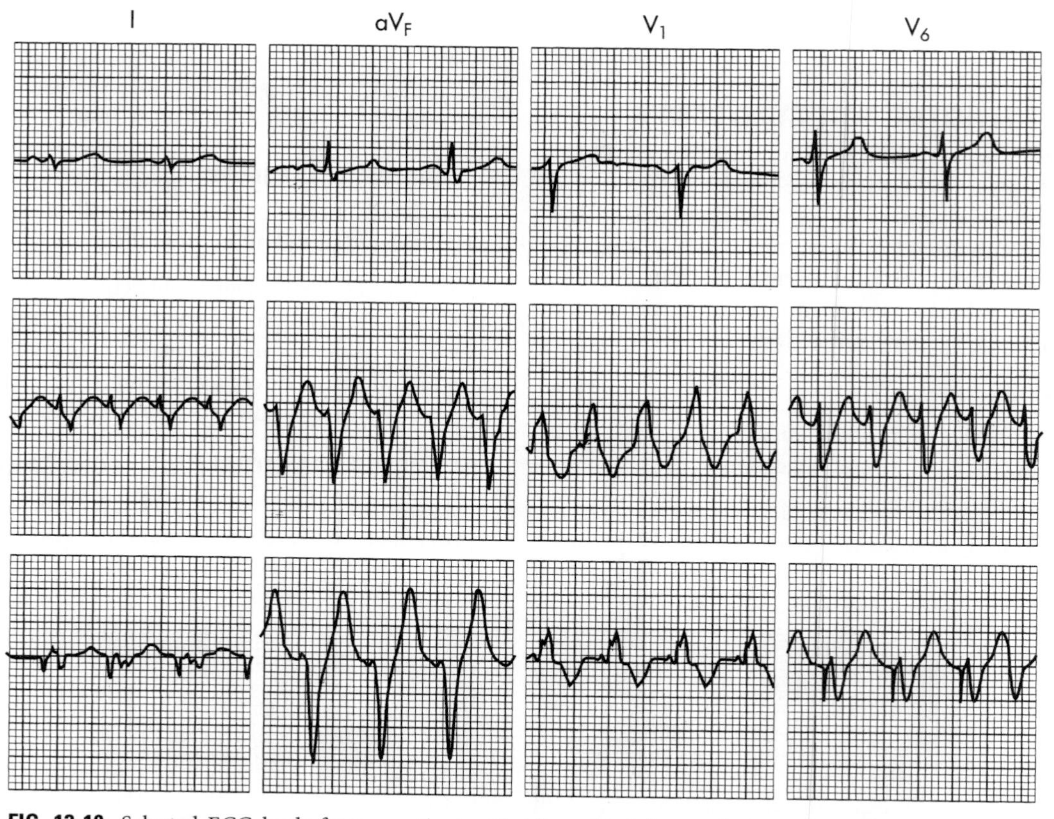

FIG. 13-10. Selected ECG leads from a patient with idiopathic left ventricular tachycardia. *Top,* baseline ECG; *middle,* idiopathic LV tachycardia;. *bottom,* ventricular pacing from the LV. (From Bhadha K, Marchlinski FE, Iskandrian AS: *Am Heart J* 126:1194, 1993.)

characteristics are seen in Fig. 13-9. The bottom panel in Fig. 13-10 shows the pacing site that produced a QRS pattern most like the clinical experience (middle panel).

ECG Characteristics

- Right bundle branch–like pattern in V_1; left bundle branch–like pattern is also possible, in which case the transition zone would be in V_2.
- QRS axis is superior (left or no-man's-land).

Mechanism

The sensitivity of LVOT tachycardia to adenosine, verapamil, and vagal maneuvers suggest a triggered mechanism. The focus is usually in the superior basal region of the left interventricular septum, inferior to the aortic valve.

VERAPAMIL-SENSITIVE INTRAFASCICULAR IDIOPATHIC VT

Verapamil-sensitive intrafascicular tachycardia is the most common form of idiopathic left VT and is usually seen in individuals between the ages of 15 and 40 years (range, 7-65 years). Approximately 60% to 80% of the afflicted individuals are men. When the tachycardia is incessant it may cause reversible tachycardia related cardiomyopathy.

Posterior fascicle of the left bundle branch. In most patients (90% to 95%) the focus is near the posterior fascicle of the left bundle branch near the inferoapical left ventricular septum.

Anterior fascicle of the left bundle branch. In the remainder of patients the focus is near the anterior fascicle of the left bundle branch near the anterosuperior left ventricular septum.

ECG Characteristics of Posterior Fascicular Location

- Right bundle branch–like pattern
- Left axis
- May be incessant
- QRS duration 0.14 second or less
- RS interval (R to nadir of the S) is 0.06 to 0.08 second in precordial leads

ECG Characteristics of Anterior Fascicular Location

- Right bundle branch–like pattern
- Right axis
- QRS duration 0.14 second or less
- RS interval 0.06 to 0.08 second in precordial leads

Mechanism

Occurs at rest but may also be activated by catecholamines during exercise, after exercise, or during emotional distress. The mechanism is thought to be a relatively focal reentry circuit.

Differential Diagnosis

Fascicular VT may also result from advanced digitalis toxicity and is covered in Chapter 15. The morphology of digitalis-toxic VT is identical to that of fascicular VT; the clinical picture differs.

AUTOMATIC (PROPRANOLOL-SENSITIVE) IDIOPATHIC VT

Automatic propranolol-sensitive idiopathic VT occurs most often in individuals who are younger than 50 years of age. The focus of the tachycardia can be in either ventricle.

ECG Characteristics

- Monomorphic or polymorphic
- Often precipitated by exercise

Mechanism

The mechanism is thought to be adrenergically mediated automaticity because it can be induced by catecholamines and terminated by beta blockade.

BUNDLE BRANCH REENTRANT VT

Sustained bundle branch reentrant VT[16,17] (BBR-VT) is a highly malignant form of monomorphic VT. It is important to recognize BBR-VT because it can be cured with radiofrequency ablation although the structural heart disease, usually dilated cardiomyopathy, associated with this type of VT remains.

ECG Recognition During Sinus Rhythm

PR interval: Prolonged.
QRS pattern: Incomplete LBBB pattern consistent with

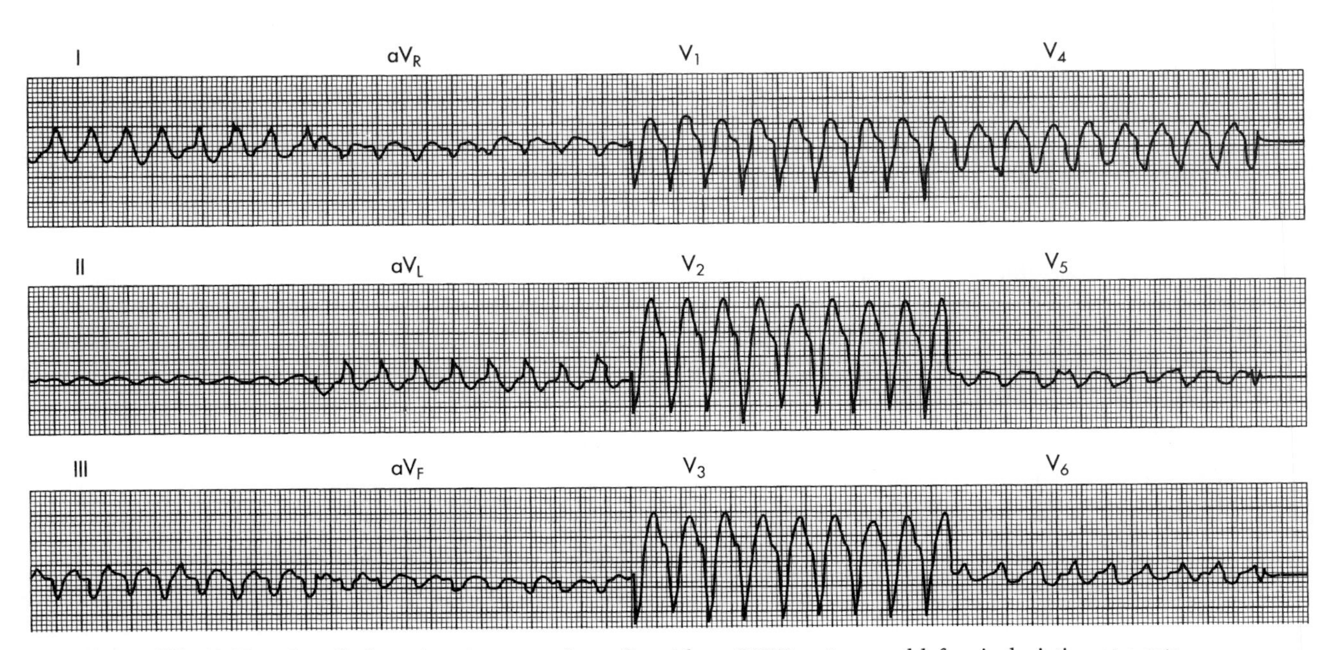

FIG. 13-11. A bundle branch reentrant tachycardia with an LBBB pattern and left axis deviation at a rate of 215 beats/min. Because ventricular activation occurs by way of the right bundle branch, the QRS is relatively narrow and its configuration suggests supraventricular tachycardia with LBBB aberrant ventricular conduction. (From Blanck Z, Sra J, Dhala A et al. In Zipes DP, Jalife J, editors: *Cardiac electrophysiology from cell to bedside,* ed 2, Philadelphia, 1995, WB Saunders.)

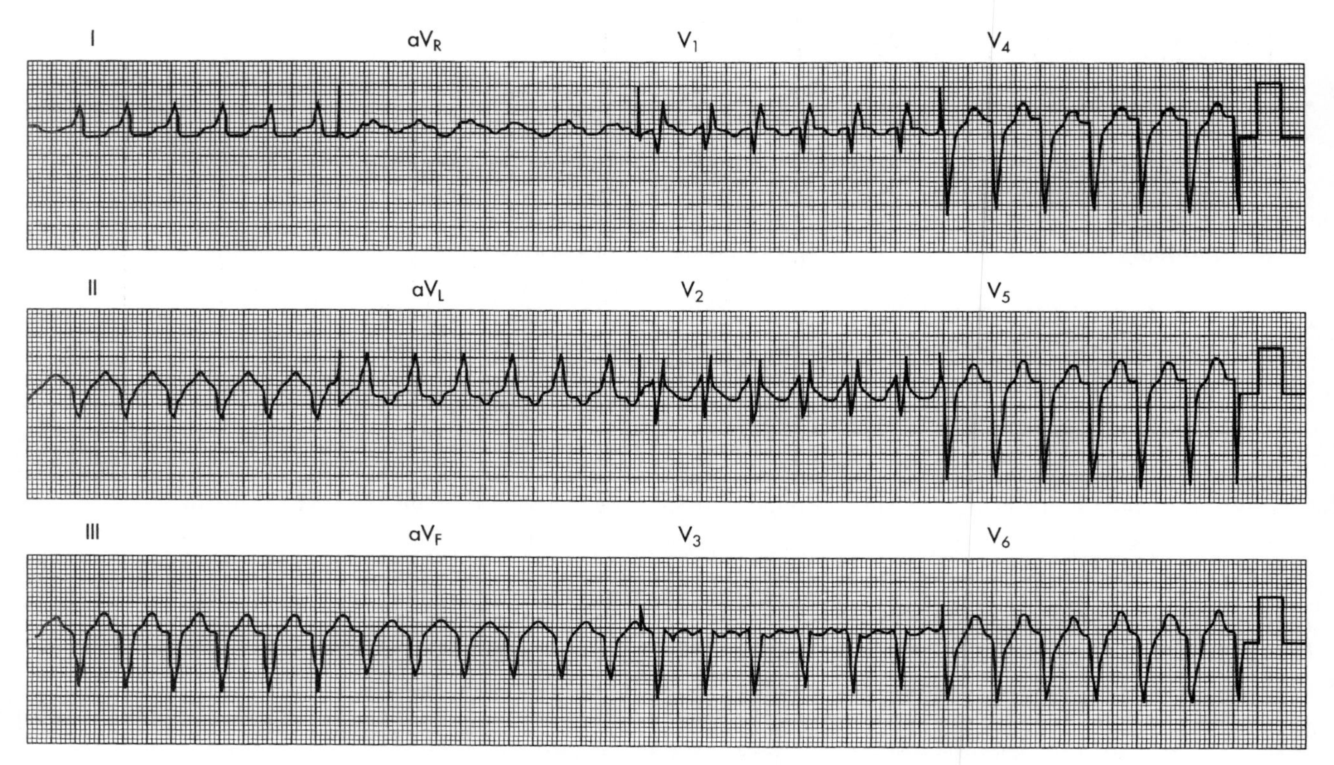

FIG. 13-12. A bundle branch reentrant tachycardia with an RBBB pattern and left axis deviation at a rate of 150 beats/min. Because ventricular activation occurs by way of the left bundle branch, the QRS is relatively narrow and its configuration suggests supraventricular tachycardia with RBBB aberrant ventricular conduction. (From Blanck Z, Sra J, Dhala A et al. In Zipes DP, Jalife J, editors: *Cardiac electrophysiology from cell to bedside,* ed 2, Philadelphia, 1995, WB Saunders.)

His-Purkinje system disease; a complete LBBB pattern or a complete RBBB pattern, although rare, is a possibility. Thus the patterns of BBR-VT mimic those of SVT with aberration, another one of the VTs that look like SVT. Others are idiopathic VT and fascicular VT. Note that the broad QRS complexes in Fig. 13-11 have the morphology of LBBB, and those in Fig. 13-12 have the morphology of RBBB. In this case the mechanism is being sustained by a reentry loop within the His-Purkinje system.

Note: When not in VT there is either sinus rhythm or atrial fibrillation.

ECG Recognition During BBR-VT with LBBB Pattern

- QRS morphology identical to that of sinus rhythm (LBBB)
- AV dissociation
- A very prolonged QRS duration (0.16 second or more)
- Frontal plane axis normal or leftward

ECG Recognition During BBR-VT with RBBB Pattern

- QRS morphology identical to that of sinus rhythm (RBBB)
- AV dissociation
- Frontal plane axis normal, left, or right depending on which left bundle branch fascicle (anterior or posterior) is used for anterograde conduction in the reentrant circuit

Mechanisms

The presence of conduction abnormalities in the His-Purkinje system is a prerequisite for sustained BBR-VT.

Conduction delay in the left bundle branch. The mechanisms of two forms of BBR-VT are illustrated in Fig. 13-13. Note the well-defined macroreentry circuit in which the His bundle, the right and left bundle branches, and transseptal ventricular muscle conduction are the components of the reentrant circuit. An absolute prerequisite for such a reentry loop is conduction delay in the His-Purkinje system, usually the left bundle branch; note the slow

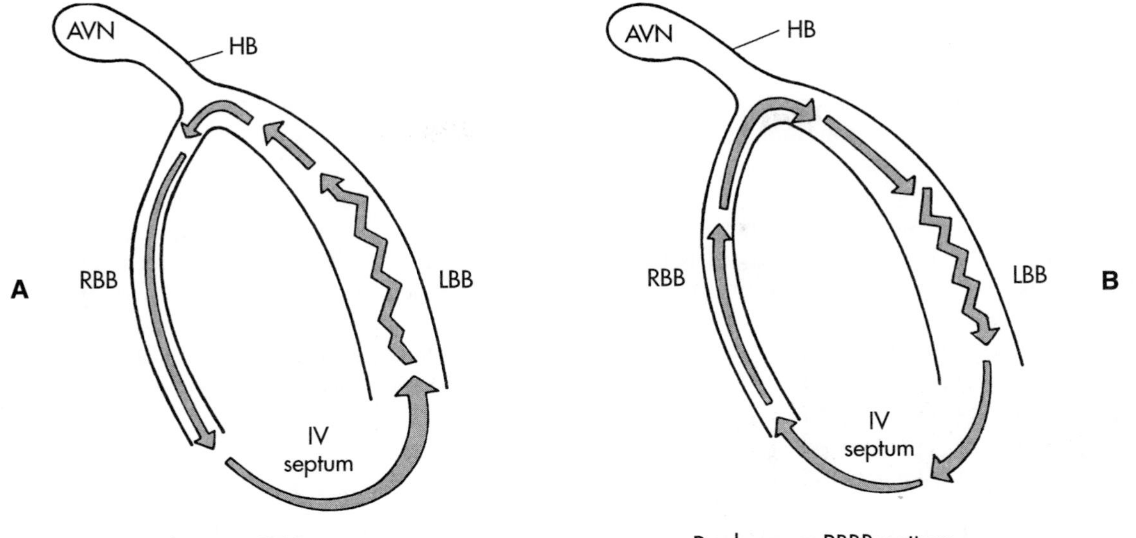

FIG. 13-13. The mechanism of bundle branch reentry VT is schematically depicted. **A,** Its most common form, with anterograde conduction in the right bundle branch *(RBB)* to produce an LBBB pattern; the required delay of conduction is evident in the ascending limb of the circuit. **B,** The least common form, with anterograde conduction in the LBBB to produce an RBBB pattern. *LBB,* Left bundle branch; *AVN,* atrioventricular node; *HB,* His bundle.

conduction depicted within that bundle.

It is also possible for the ECG pattern of LBBB to be caused by complete block rather than conduction delay. In such a case, slow retrograde conduction through the compromised left bundle branch may also support the bundle branch reentrant circuit.

Most common. The more common form of BBR-VT is seen in Fig. 13-13, *A*. When the anterograde arm of the reentrant loop is down the right bundle branch, the left ventricle is activated last, producing an LBBB pattern on the ECG, as seen in Fig. 13-11.

Least common. A less common form of BBR-VT is seen in Fig. 13-13, *B*. When the anterograde arm of the reentrant loop is down the right bundle branch, the left ventricle is activated last, producing an RBBB pattern on the ECG, as seen in Fig. 13-12.

Conduction delay in the right bundle branch. Cases of BBR-VT with a conduction delay in the right bundle branch are rare but may be more common in patients with valvular heart disease.

Causes

BBR-VT usually occurs in individuals with significant structural heart disease such as dilated cardiomyopathy of unknown origin (45%) and idiopathic cardiomyopathy (41%). Other underlying conditions are dilated ischemic cardiomyopathy and nonspecific intraventricular conduction abnormalities. BBR-VT may also occur in the setting of dilated ventricles resulting from coronary artery disease or significant valvular heart disease such as aortic or mitral regurgitation.

Symptoms

BBR-VT frequently becomes evident with syncope, palpitations, or sudden cardiac death.

Differential Diagnosis

Because the BBR-VT may resemble *myocardial reentrant VT*, *SVT with aberrancy*, and *atriofascicular reentry (Mahaim fiber)*, electrophysiologic studies are necessary for the detailed analysis of the activation sequence of the His bundle and bundle branches.

Emergency Treatment

For the patient in unstable condition, treatment consists of cardioversion; for the patient in stable condition, treatment consists of procainamide or lidocaine.

Long-Term Treatment (Cure)

If electrophysiologic studies establish that the mechanism of the VT is bundle branch reentry, as is often the case in dilated cardiomyopathy, catheter ablation of the right bundle branch eliminates the possibility of reentry and is a permanent cure of the reentrant tachycardia and the treatment of choice.[18] Because of the availability of such a cure, recognition of this condition through electrophysiologic studies avoids therapy with the implantable cardioverter-defibrillator or antiarrhythmic drugs. However, in almost 25% of such patients another form of VT (within the myocardium itself) emerges, requiring additional treatment with antiarrhythmic drugs. If, after ablation, atrial pacing reveals AV block or if the HV interval is 100 ms or more, a permanent pacemaker is implanted.[16]

Prognosis

The prognosis is generally poor, and some patients with the combination of BBR-VT and dilated cardiomyopathy may be considered for cardiac transplantation.

CLASS IC VT[8]

Class IC drugs include flecainide, encainide, indecainide, recainam, and propafenone. An adverse drug effect would be suspected if a sustained VT emerged after starting or increasing the dosage of the drug. The drug dose does not have to be toxic but merely large enough to slow conduction velocity sufficiently to facilitate circulation of the impulse within the reentry circuit. Induction of VT by a class IC drug

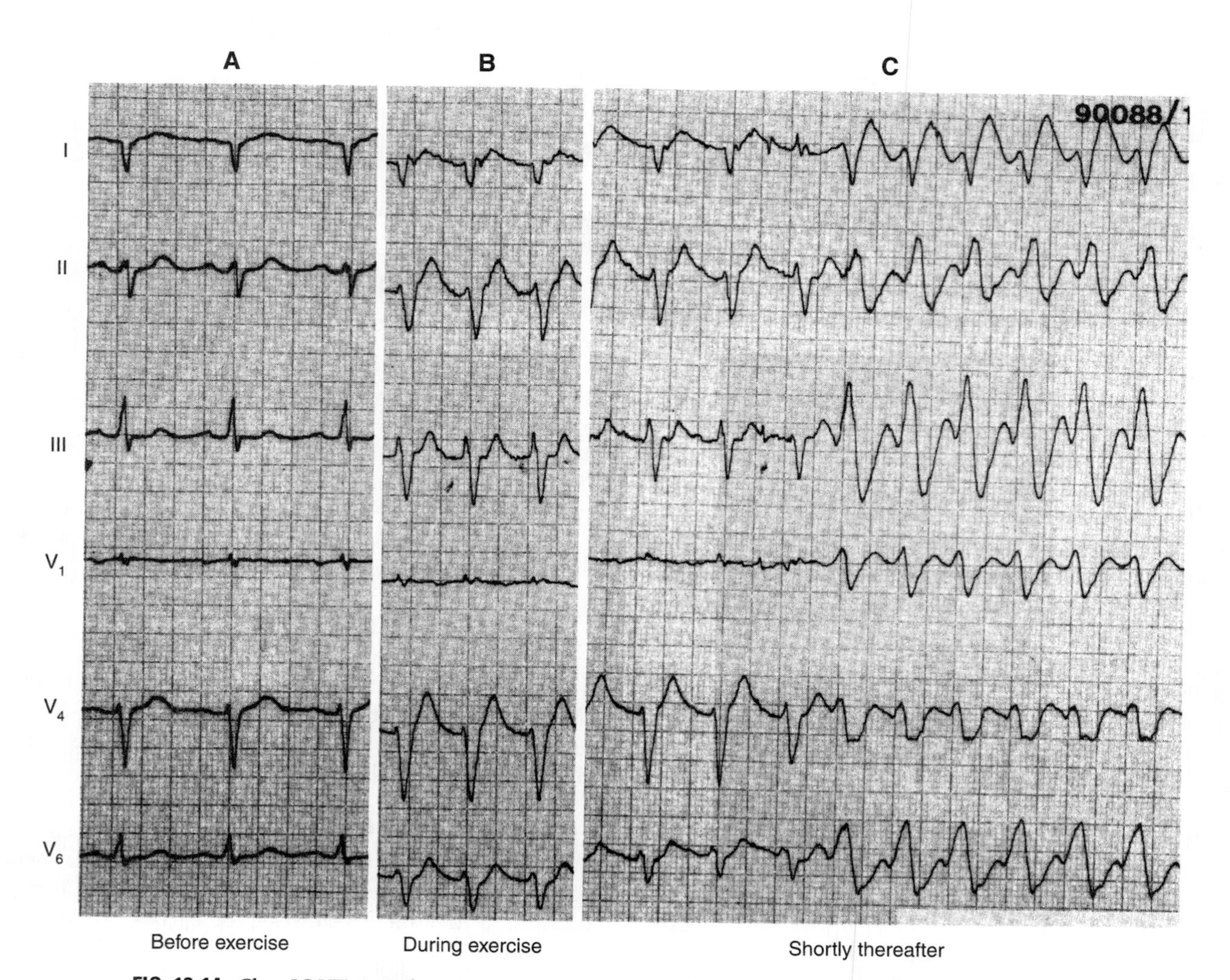

FIG. 13-14. Class IC VT. **A,** Before exercise, the heart rate is 80 beats/min, and the QRS is 100 ms in duration. **B,** During exercise, the heart rate is 130 beats/min, and the QRS is 160 ms; there is axis deviation. **C,** Shortly thereafter, a VT begins with a rate of 150 beats/min. (From Wellens HJJ, Conover M: *The ECG in emergency decision making,* Philadelphia, 1992, WB Saunders.)

is promoted by a fast heart rate as seen in Fig. 13-14. This is because class IC drugs are "use-dependent" (i.e., their action becomes more marked as the heart rate increases).

ECG Recognition

- Spontaneous onset after starting the drug or increasing the dose
- Sustained or persistent nature
- Extremely wide QRS complexes

Mechanism

The slow conduction within the ventricles induced by class IC or IA drugs is enough to sustain a reentry circuit.

Emergency Treatment of Class IC VT

- Often cannot be terminated by cardioversion or programmed ventricular stimulation
- Stop the offending drug
- If hemodynamically impaired, inotropic support with isoproterenol or epinephrine is given to counteract the slowing of conduction
- If the VT persists, the atrium is paced at the rate of the VT using an AV interval optimal for ventricular filling

VENTRICULAR FIBRILLATION

VF[19] is a severe derangement of the electrical rhythm of the heart, associated with hemodynamic collapse.

ECG Recognition

Electrical activation in the ventricles is fractionated, resulting in an ECG of irregular undulations without clear-cut ventricular complexes. Fig. 13-15, *A*, shows a VT of 110 beats/min that slows to below 100 beats/min and then deteriorates into VF. In Fig. 13-15, *B*, a supraventricular rhythm at 150 beats/min is interrupted with a short run of VT at 300 beats/min followed by VF. As already noted Fig. 13-5 the VT preceding VF may be 300 beats/min, a rhythm that is sometimes called *ventricular flutter.*

Mechanisms

VF is usually preceded by VT and appears to be sustained by wandering reentry wavelets of activation that may represent incomplete rotations of a spiraling pattern. In many cases the wavelets change from cycle to cycle, but in some cases appear somewhat repeatable.

Causes

The most common setting for the development of VF is coronary artery disease with and without acute MI. Other structural cardiac diseases include cardiomyopathy, valvular heart disease, congenital heart disease, and myocarditis. Functional causes include autonomic imbalance, electrolyte imbalance, and drug toxicity (torsades de pointes). Other causes are genetic mutations (Brugada syndrome and long QT syndromes), Wolff-Parkinson-White syndrome, and myocardial scar (surgical and structural heart disease).

Prognosis

The recurrence of VF is highly dependent on the circumstance of the first event. For example, the recurrence rate is less than 2% when cardiac arrest occurs during acute

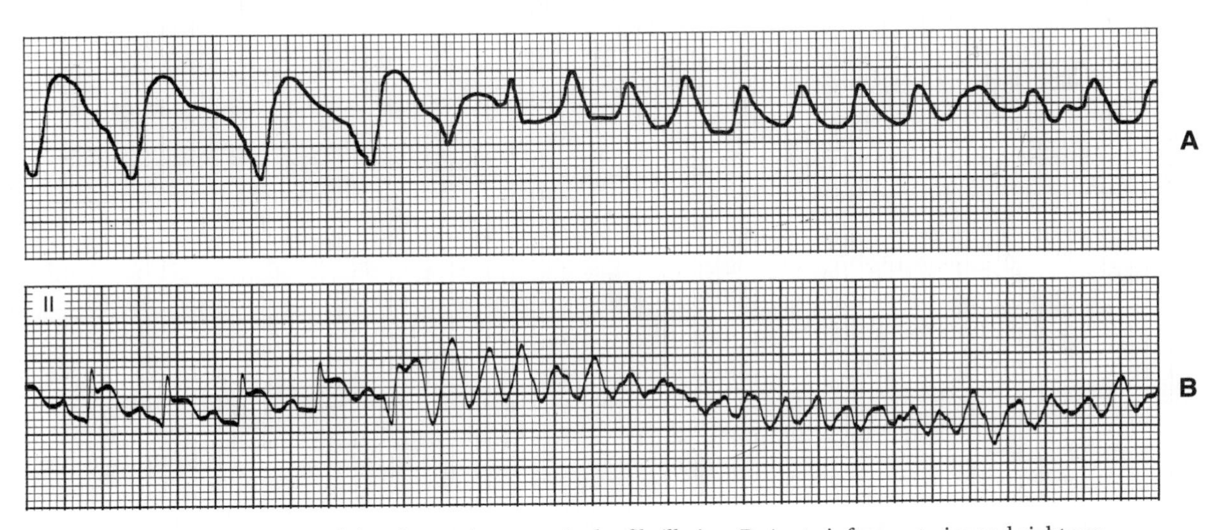

FIG. 13-15. **A,** A "slow VT" deteriorates into ventricular fibrillation. **B,** Acute inferoposterior and right ventricular myocardial infarction in sinus tachycardia deteriorating into a few ventricular beats at 300/min and ventricular fibrillation.

MI, whereas the recurrence rate is 30% or more at 1 year when cardiac arrest is associated with chronic ischemic heart disease without acute MI.

Risk factors associated with the recurrence of ventricular fibrillation include hypertension, hyperlipidemia, cigarette smoking, obesity, impaired glucose tolerance, left ventricular hypertrophy, digitalis use, and prior MI.

Symptoms

During ventricular flutter, a rhythm that commonly precedes VF, the patient may be hypotensive or unconscious. VF itself may have no warning. The patient loses consciousness and is cyanotic, blood pressure and pulse cannot be obtained, and heart sounds are absent. In response to the lack of oxygen to the brain there are seizures, apnea, and finally death if the fibrillation is not terminated.

Emergency Response

The reader is urged to become familiar with the article, Guidelines 2000 for cardiopulmonary resuscitation and emergency cardiovascular care (*Circulation* 102[8 Suppl], 2000).

1. Open the airway and deliver a few quick breaths. Cardiopulmonary resuscitation (CPR) is used only until the defibrillator is readied.
2. Defibrillate
3. Manage airway and ventilation
4. Administer intravenous medications

When CPR, defibrillation, and definitive treatment are delayed more than 8 to 10 minutes after collapse, the "chain of survival" is broken.

If the patient is not being monitored at the time of collapse, blind defibrillation is seldom necessary thanks to the universal availability of quick-look paddles. If it's bradycardia, do not defibrillate. If it's VF or if you're not sure, administer ***immediate*** electrical shock.

ACCELERATED IDIOVENTRICULAR RHYTHM

An *accelerated idioventricular rhythm* (AIVR) consists of three or more successive ventricular beats with a rate between 60 and 110 beats/min that begin with a long coupling interval. Because its rate is so similar to that of the sinus node, there are fusion beats at its beginning and end (Figs. 13-16 and 13-17) or even throughout its duration as the two pacemakers (sinus and ventricular) compete for dominance. In Fig. 13-18 find the fusion beats; to do this, you must identify two nonfusion complexes and compare with the others. They are the pure sinus conducted impulse, like the deepest one in the top tracing and the pure ventricular ectopic impulse, like the tallest one in the bottom tracing.

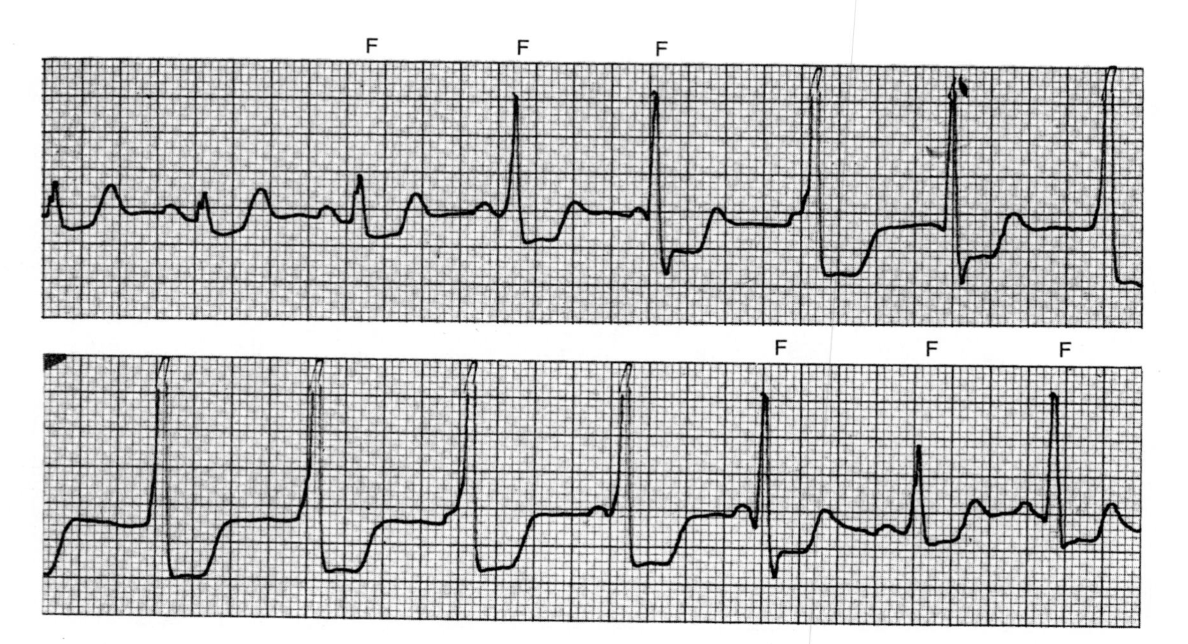

FIG. 13-16. AIVR. Note the fusion *(F)* beats at the onset of the tachycardia and at the end of this continuous tracing. The rate of the tachycardia is approximately that of the sinus rhythm, which explains the fusion beats at the onset and at the end.

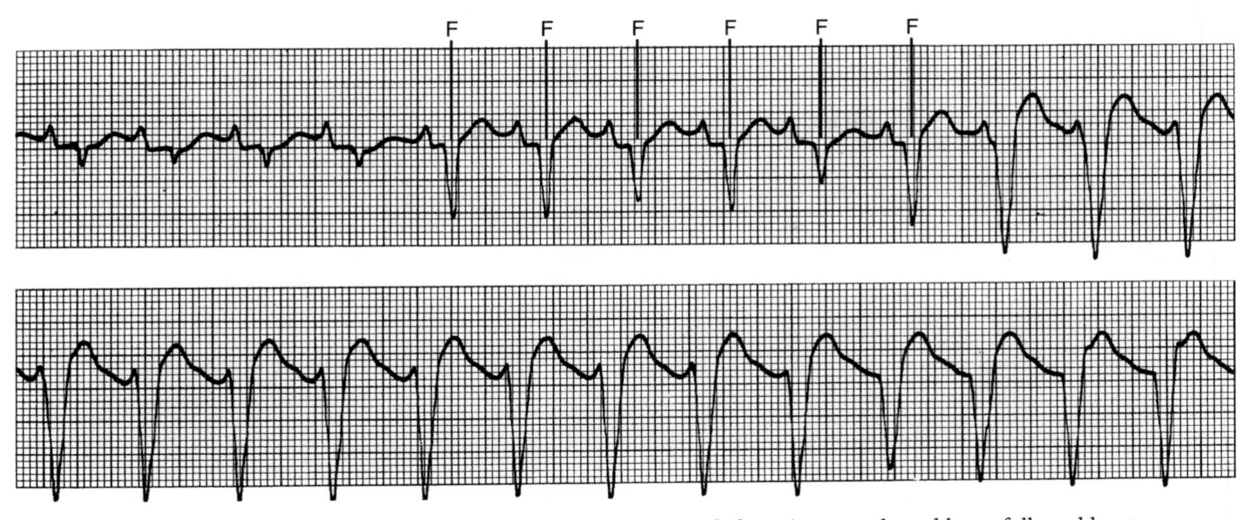

FIG. 13-17. AIVR (continuous tracing). The tracing begins with four sinus-conducted beats followed by at least six fusion beats (*F*) at the onset of the AIVR.

In AIVR the ventricular rhythm achieves dominance when it accelerates or when the sinus node slows its rate. Sinus rhythm dominates when the sinus rhythm increases its rate or the ventricular rhythm decreases its rate. The fusion beats, of course, are proof of the ventricular origin of the ectopic rhythm.

ECG Recognition

Sometimes an AIVR is unmasked because of a pause. For example, in Fig. 13-19 the AIVR emerges during the pause following a nonconducted premature atrial complex (PAC) and the initiation of atrial flutter. The bottom tracing is the result of the administration of lidocaine for the AIVR.

Rhythm: Transient and intermittent; lasting for three or more successive beats to 1 minute; may be regular or irregular.

Rate: Faster than the intrinsic escape rate of the ventricles (30 to 40 beats/min) but usually slower than VT; usually between 60 and 110 beats/min.

Onset: Gradual (nonparoxysmal), beginning with a long coupling interval, often with a ventricular fusion beat.

Termination: Gradual, often ending in ventricular fusion beats.

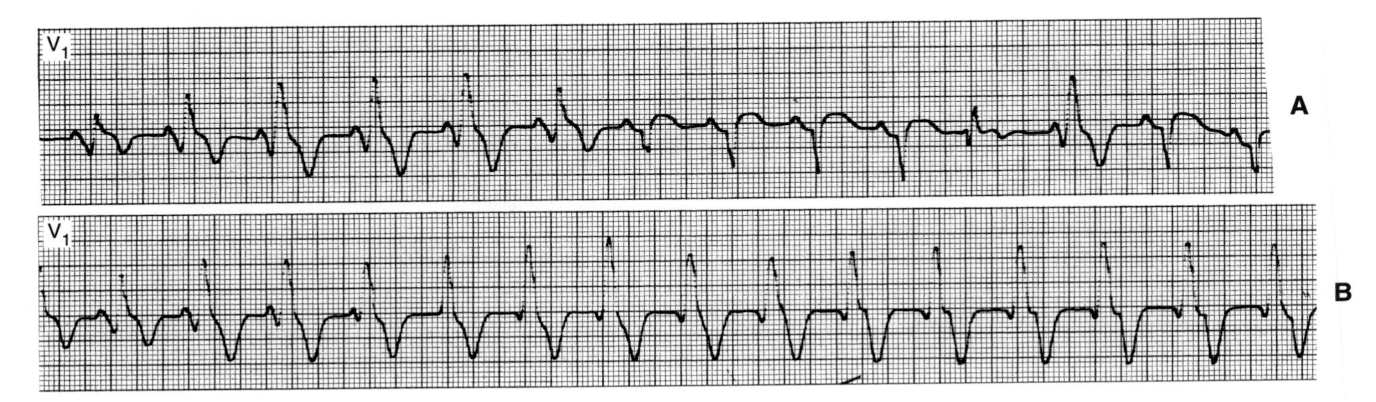

FIG. 13-18. **A,** An AIVR composed mostly of fusion beats. The last complex (the only one that is not fusion) has a PR interval of 0.16 second, slightly longer than the two similar-looking beats. **B,** The tracing shows the dominance of the AIVR with a rate of 96 beats/min.

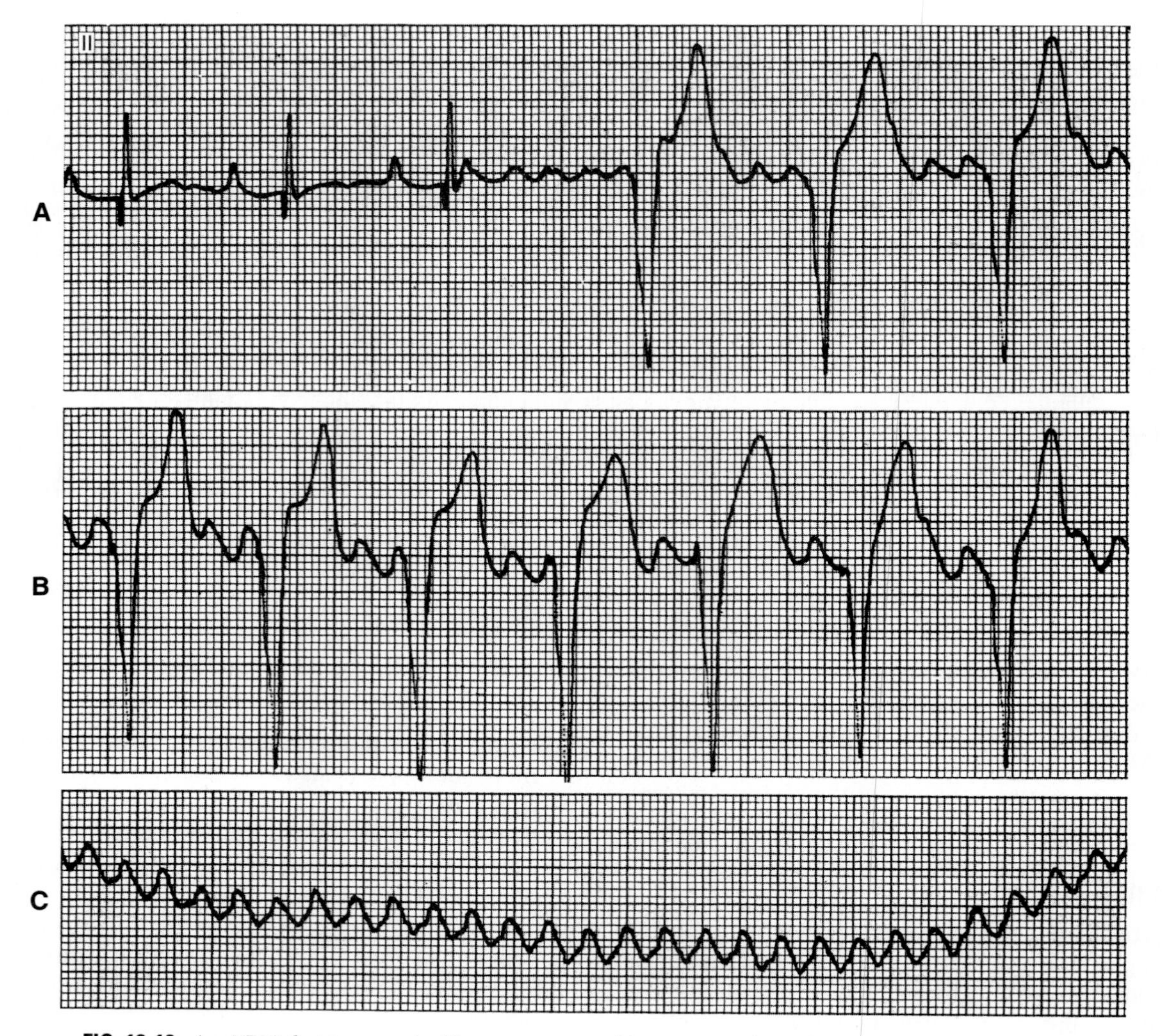

FIG. 13-19. An AIVR that is unmasked by a pause caused by a PAC and atrial flutter. **A,** There is first-degree AV block that is complicated by the appearance of a very early PAC (in the third ST segment). Atrial flutter ensues, compounding the AV block. An AIVR emerges because of the pause. Its initial rate is 64 beats/min, and it "warms up" to 78 beats/min (**B**). **C,** When lidocaine was given, the AIVR was completely suppressed, leaving the patient with nothing but atrial flutter and complete AV block.

Atrioventricular dissociation: Common, often isorhythmic (sinus and ventricular rhythms maintain the same rate).

AIVR Identifies Area of Reperfusion

The ECG is also of help in identifying the area of reperfusion in that the QRS configuration and the axis of the AIVR may identify or at least in rule out the occluded vessel:

Left anterior descending coronary artery: Multiple QRS configurations during the AIVR and a relatively narrow QRS.

Circumflex: Ruled out when lead V_1 is negative.

Right coronary artery: Ruled out when the electrical axis is inferior (between 0 and 180 degrees).[20]

ECG Recognition of AIVR *Not* Related to Reperfusion

The AIVR that occurs during the first 24 hours of infarction but after the reperfusion phase should be distinguished from that which occurs during reperfusion. The former is recognized because it begins with a short coupling interval, as shown in Fig. 13-20. Obviously then, because the onset is more premature, it does not begin with

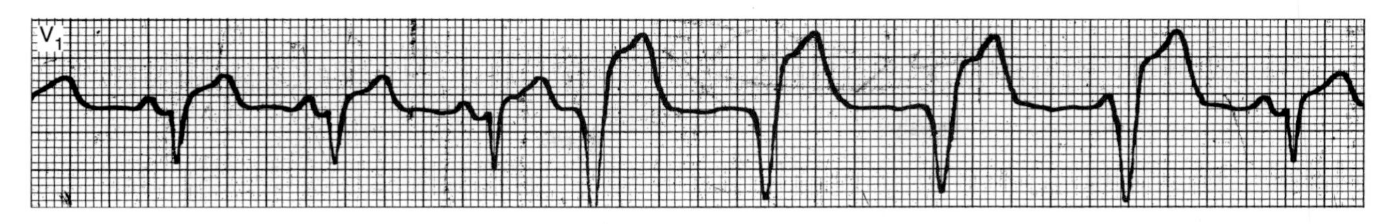

FIG. 13-20. AIVR not caused by reperfusion. Note the short initial coupling interval and the negative complex in V_1.

fusion beats, as does the reperfusion-related AIVR, although it may end with them. This type of AIVR is sometimes called "slow VT."[20]

Clinical Implications

The AIVR is usually benign (even when multiform) and of short duration (lasting seconds to a minute), is well-tolerated in hemodynamic terms, and does not seriously affect the clinical course or prognosis. It is usually associated with heart disease of some type, especially *acute myocardial infarction* (occurring at the moment of reperfusion) or digitalis toxicity, and can also be seen in cocaine intoxication and normal hearts of adults and children.

The AIVR indicates both reperfusion (spontaneous or following thrombolytic therapy) and myocardial necrosis. Approximately 50% of patients with reperfusion after MI have this arrhythmia. It has a high specificity (>80%) for reperfusion; that is, its presence strongly favors reperfusion. However, the sensitivity is only moderate (50% or less); that is, its absence does not preclude reperfusion. In addition, there is an equal distribution of AIVR in inferior and anterior MI, and the appearance of AIVR does not depend on infarct size.[20,21] Thus when coronary angiography is not available, this sign may be helpful in recognizing reperfusion.[8] Other ECG signs of reperfusion are normalization of the ST segment, development of terminal T wave inversion, and a twofold increase in PVCs.[22]

Mechanisms

The mechanism of the AIVR is not known. Its ECG characteristics are suggestive of altered automaticity.[23,24]

Treatment

Reperfusion arrhythmia. An AIVR requires no treatment other than the care of the underlying problem. Reperfusion arrhythmias have not been associated with an increased incidence of ventricular fibrillation or in-hospital mortality.[24]

Digitalis toxicity. When digitalis is the cause, the drug should be discontinued.

Hemodynamic symptoms. When associated with hemodynamic impairment, the sinus rate may be increased with

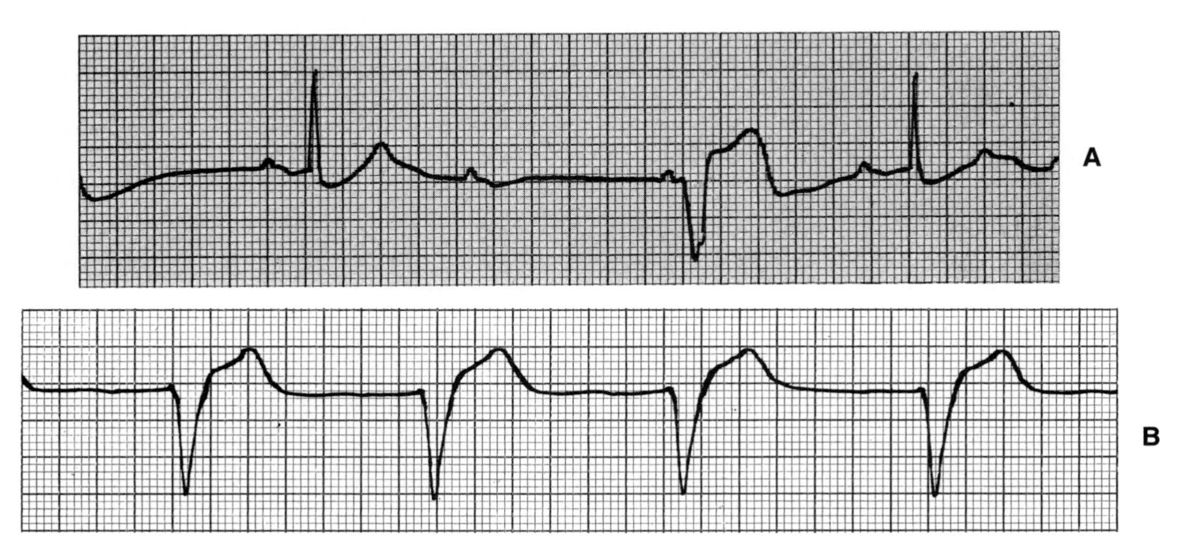

FIG. 13-21. A, Ventricular escape (the second ventricular complex). **B,** A ventricular escape rhythm with an appropriately slow rate (45 beats/min) and no evidence of atrial activity.

atropine or atrial pacing. This is usually sufficient to suppress the AIVR. Such hemodynamic symptoms are caused either by the atrioventricular dissociation (loss of "atrial kick") or by the ventricular rate being too fast.[19,24]

VENTRICULAR ESCAPE

If the ventricles are not being activated from the sinus node, an atrial or junctional pacemaker usually "escapes" and paces the ventricles. If both of these also fail, a slow ventricular focus will take over. Fig. 13-21, *A*, illustrates a single ventricular escape beat. There is AV block in which not every sinus P wave results in a ventricular complex, nor are there junctional escape beats to terminate the long pause. In Fig. 13-21, *B*, the ventricular rate is 45 beats/min and the QRS complexes are broad, giving evidence of a pacemaker that is low in the conductive system. No P waves are apparent. They may be seen in another lead, or they may be truly absent; if absent, there is atrial standstill with a slow ventricular escape rhythm.

REFERENCES

1. Josephson ME, Horowitz LN, Waxman HL: Sustained ventricular tachycardia: role of the 12 lead electrocardiogram in localizing site of origin, *Circulation* 64:257, 1981.
2. Miller JM, Marchlinski FE, Buxton AE et al: Relationship between the 12-lead electrocardiogram during ventricular tachycardia and endocardial site of origin in patients with coronary artery disease, *Circulation* 77:759, 1988.
3. Richardson AW, Callans DJ, Josephson ME: Electrophysiology of postinfarction ventricular tachycardia: a paradigm of stable reentry, *J Cardiovasc Electrophysiol* 10:1288, 1999.
4. Chou TC, Knilans TK: *Electrocardiography in clinical practice adult and pediatric,* ed 4, Philadelphia, 1996, WB Saunders.
5. Pfammatter JP, Paul T: Idiopathic ventricular tachycardia in infancy and childhood: a multicenter study on clinical profile and outcome. Working Group on Dysrhythmias and Electrophysiology of the Association for European Pediatric Cardiology, *J Am Coll Cardiol* 33:2067, 1999.
6. Davis AM, Gow RM, McCrindle BW et al: Clinical spectrum, therapeutic management, and follow-up of ventricular tachycardia in infants and young children, *Am Heart J* 131:186, 1996.
7. Josephson ME, Gottlieb CD: Ventricular tachycardias associated with coronary artery disease. In Zipes DP, Jalife J, editors: *Cardiac electrophysiology,* Philadelphia, 1990, WB Saunders.
8. Wellens HJJ, Conover M: *The ECG in emergency decision making,* Philadelphia, 1992, WB Saunders.
9. Zipes DP: Personal communication, February 1995.
10. Mcrae AT III, Chung MK, Asher CR: Arrhythmogenic right ventricular cardiomyopathy: a cause of sudden death in young people, *Cleveland Clinic J Med* 69:459, 2001.
11. Pinski SL: The right ventricular tachycardias, *J Electrocardiol* 33(Suppl):103, 2000.
12. Lerman BB, Stein KM, Markowitz SM et al: Ventricular tachycardia in patients with structurally normal hearts. In Zipes DP, Jalife J, editors: *Cardiac electrophysiology from cell to bedside,* ed 3, Philadelphia, 2000, WB Saunders.
13. Wilber IDJ, Baerman J, Olshansky B et al: Adenosine-sensitive ventricular tachycardia: clinical characteristics and response to catheter ablation, *Circulation* 87:126, 1993.
14. Coggins DL, Lee RJ, Sweeney J et al: Radiofrequency catheter ablation as a cure for idiopathic tachycardia of both left and right ventricular origin, *J Am Coll Cardiol* 23:1333, 1994.
15. Lerman BB, Stein K, Engelstein ED et al: Mechanism of repetitive monomorphic ventricular tachycardia, *Circulation* 92:421, 1995.
16. Blanck Z, Sra J, Dhala A et al: Bundle branch reentry: mechanisms, diagnosis, and treatment. In Zipes DP, Jalife J, editors: *Cardiac electrophysiology from cell to bedside,* ed 3, Philadelphia, 2000, WB Saunders.
17. Oreto G, Smeets JL, Rodriguez LM et al: Wide complex tachycardia with atrioventricular dissociation and QRS morphology identical to that of sinus rhythm: a manifestation of bundle branch reentry, *Heart* 76:541, 1996.
18. Delacretaz E, Stevenson WG, Ellison KE et al: Mapping and radiofrequency catheter ablation of the three types of sustained monomorphic ventricular tachycardia in nonischemic heart disease, *J Cardiovasc Electrophysiol* 11:11, 2000.
19. Zipes DP: Specific arrhythmias: diagnosis and treatment. In Braunwald E, editor: *Heart disease,* ed 4, Philadelphia, 1992, WB Saunders.
20. Gorgels APM, Vos MA, Letsch IS et al: Usefulness of the accelerated idioventricular rhythm as a marker for myocardial necrosis and reperfusion during thrombolytic therapy in acute myocardial infarction, *Am J Cardiol* 61:231, 1988.
21. Goldberg S, Greenspon AJ, Urban PL et al: Reperfusion arrhythmia: a marker of restoration of anterograde flow during intracoronary thrombolysis for acute myocardial infarction, *Am Heart J* 105:26, 1983.
22. Doevendans PA, Gorgels AP, van der Zee R et al: Electrocardiographic diagnosis of reperfusion during thrombolytic therapy in acute myocardial infarction, *Am J Cardiol* 75:1206, 1995.
23. Wit AL, Janese MJ: Relationship of experimental delayed ventricular arrhythmias to clinical arrhythmias. In Wit AL, Janese MJ, editors: *The ventricular arrhythmias of ischemia and infarction: electrophysiological mechanisms,* New York, 1993, Futura.
24. Grimm W, Marchlinski FE: Accelerated idioventricular rhythm: bidirectional ventricular tachycardia. In Zipes DP, Jalife J, editors: *Cardiac electrophysiology from cell to bedside,* ed 3, Philadelphia, 2000, WB Saunders.

CHAPTER 14

Aberrant Ventricular Conduction

Aberrant ventricular conduction is the intermittent abnormal intraventricular conduction of a supraventricular impulse in the form of bundle branch block (BBB) or hemiblock. Pathologic BBB is of course also a form of aberrant ventricular conduction, as is preexcitation. However, the term is generally reserved for the transient physiologic condition.

ECG RECOGNITION

- Relatively narrow QRS, usually 0.14 second or less
- Right bundle branch block (RBBB) pattern in V_1 (rSR′ pattern)[1-4] or
- Left bundle branch block (LBBB) pattern in V_1 and V_2 (narrow r, swift S downstroke)[5]
- Occurs as a single beat preceded by a premature atrial complex (PAC), at the onset of paroxysmal supraventricular tachycardia (PSVT), or may be sustained during atrial flutter
- Single beat is often, but not necessarily, followed by a less than full compensatory pause

The tracings in Fig. 14-1, *A* and *B*, are examples of RBBB and LBBB aberration after PACs as seen in lead V_1. Note the classical rSR′ pattern of RBBB in *A* and the slick downstroke of the LBBB pattern in *B*. Even if V_1 had not been available,

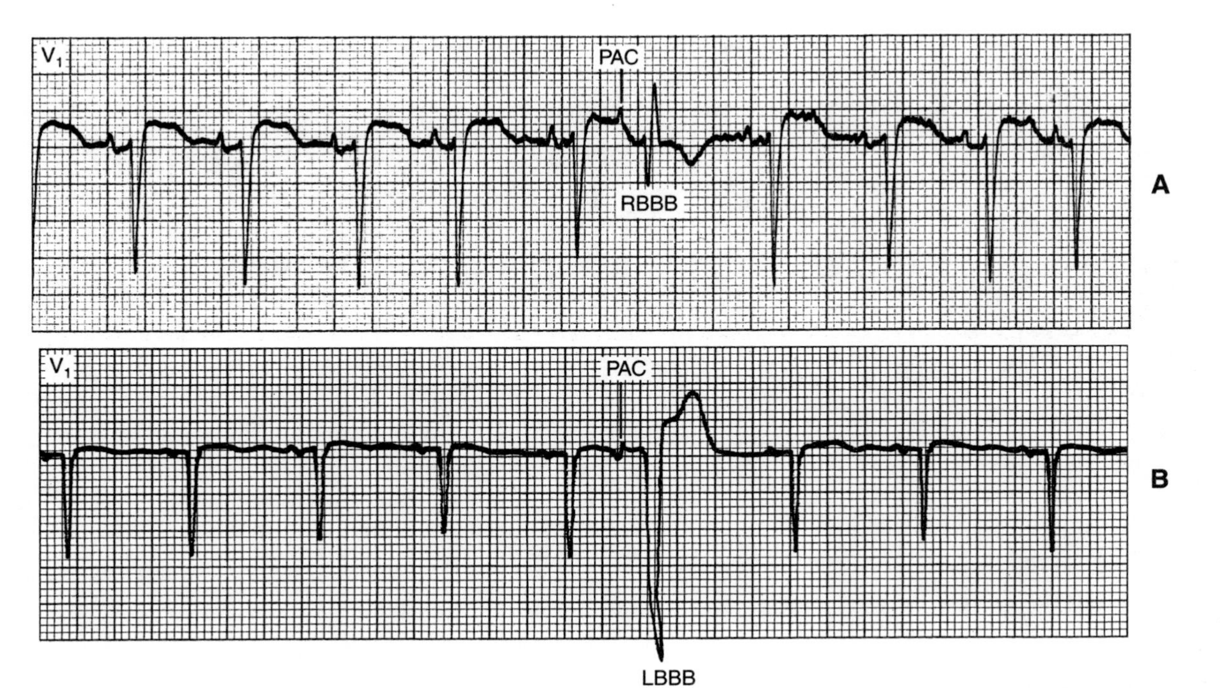

FIG. 14-1. Phase 3 aberration. In each tracing the PAC occurs early (in the T wave), finds one of the bundle branches still refractory, and is therefore conducted with RBBB in **A** and LBBB aberration in **B**.

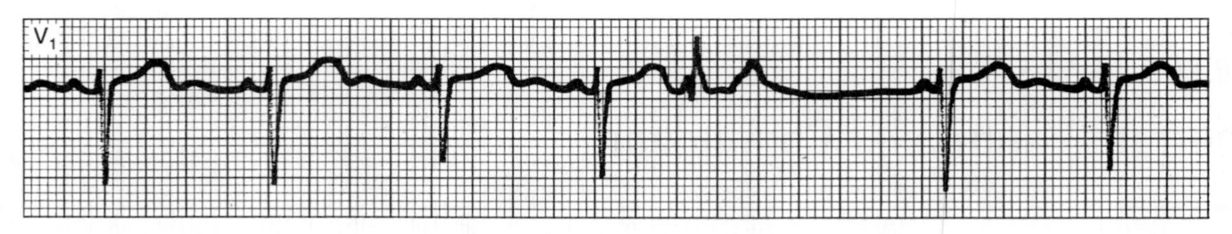

FIG. 14-2. PAC with RBBB aberration and overdrive suppression. An early PAC (in the fourth T wave) is conducted with RBBB aberrancy. Note the long pause after the aberrant beat, the result of overdrive suppression. The PAC has suppressed the sinus node, temporarily slowing its rate of discharge. The PR interval following the pause is slightly shorter because of a junctional escape beat.

the presence of the PACs would have been diagnostic. Both tracings also have less than full compensatory pauses, a strong indication of premature atrial activity. However, in the words of Dr. H.J.L. Marriott, the compensatory pause itself is a "broken reed" because it is possible for a premature ventricular complex (PVC) with retrograde conduction to the atria to have a less than full compensatory pause if the sinus node is discharged early. Additionally, a PAC may be followed by a full or more than full compensatory pause when there is overdrive suppression causing the next sinus P wave to be late, as shown in Fig. 14-2.

MECHANISMS

Aberrant ventricular conduction can be caused by phase 3 block and occasionally by phase 4 block or retrograde concealed conduction.

Phase 3 Block

Phase 3 block is also known as phase 3 aberration, functional BBB, or physiologic BBB because it does not require pathology. This is the type of aberrant ventricular conduction with which we are most familiar in the clinical setting.

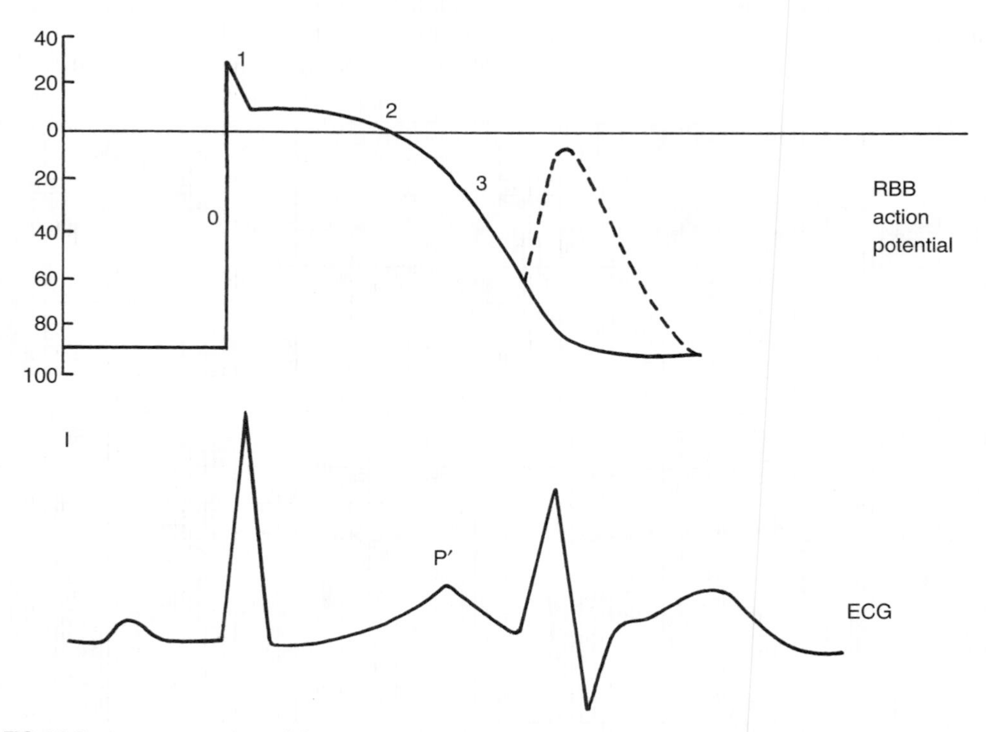

FIG. 14-3. A representation of the action potential from the right bundle branch *(RBB)* along with the concurrent ECG to demonstrate the mechanism of phase 3 block (aberration or functional BBB). A very early PAC *(P′)* occurs during phase 3 of the action potential when the right bundle branch is still repolarizing. The left bundle branch is free to conduct the impulse and does so with an RBBB pattern.

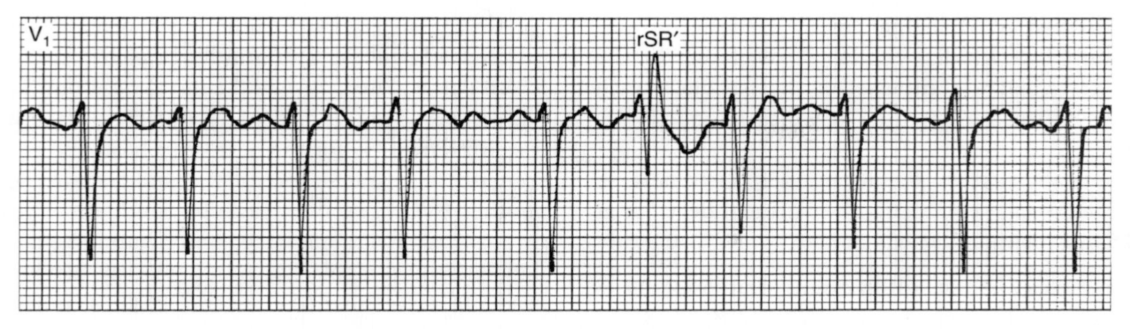

FIG. 14-4. Atrial fibrillation and RBBB *(rSR′)* aberration after a long-short sequence. The longer cycle presumably causes the refractory period of the next beat to lengthen. When this is followed by a short cycle, aberrant ventricular conduction results.

When stimulation occurs while one bundle branch is still refractory (phase 3 of the action potential), BBB is the result. Fig. 14-3 illustrates how the stimulus from an early PAC can be conducted with BBB if it reaches one of the bundle branches during phase 3 of the action potential. Because the right bundle branch repolarizes slightly later than the left bundle branch it is the more susceptible to block or at least to delay in conduction when confronted with an early impulse, although LBBB aberration is common in circus movement tachycardia (CMT) using an accessory pathway. In fact, aberration itself is more common in CMT than it is in atrioventricular (AV) nodal reentry tachycardia, as discussed in Chapter 11.

Phase 3 aberrations may also occur pathologically if the refractory period in the bundle branches is abnormally prolonged and the involved bundle is stimulated at a relatively rapid rate. Thus the term *tachycardia-dependent BBB* is sometimes used.

Phase 3 aberration is also likely to occur after a *long-short cycle sequence*, as shown in Fig. 14-4. The refractory period of the beat after the long cycle is prolonged, increasing the possibility of a PAC or early stimulation during atrial fibrillation, reaching a bundle branch during its refractory period. The fact that a long cycle causes a longer refractory period also comes into play in the initiation of torsades de pointes after a long-short sequence (p. 381)

Phase 4 Block

Phase 4 aberration is reflected on the electrocardiogram (ECG) by a BBB pattern after a long pause and preceded by atrial activity, as represented in Fig. 14-5. Because better conduction would be expected at the end of a long rest, this form of aberration is known as *paradoxical critical rate*. It is also sometimes referred to as *bradycardia-dependent BBB*, but this is unsatisfactory as an inclusive term because it is not always necessary to achieve a rate that merits the designation "bradycardia" to initiate the BBB.

Aberrant ventricular conduction caused by phase 4 block is infrequently seen and is usually not recognized as such because aberration after a long pause is unexpected. Phase 4 aberration is usually associated with organic heart disease and requires one or more of the following[6]:

1. The presence of slow diastolic depolarization (phase 4 depolarization), such as normally occurs in the bundle branches.
2. A decrease in excitability (shift in threshold poten-

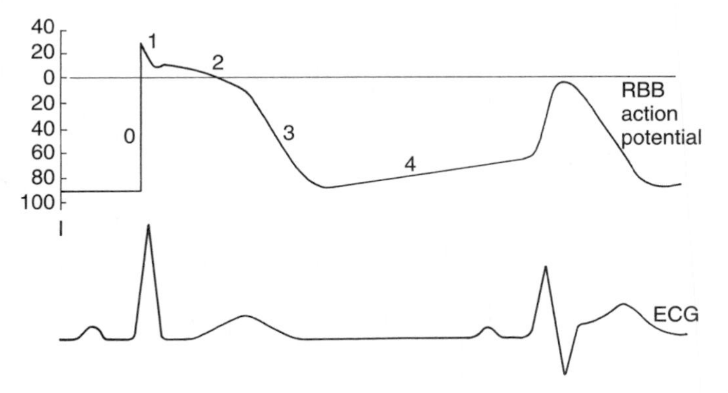

FIG. 14-5. A representation of the action potential from the right bundle branch *(RBB)* along with the concurrent ECG to demonstrate the mechanism of phase 4 aberration. After a long pause a sinus beat is surprisingly conducted, albeit with aberrant ventricular conduction. During phase 4 of the action potential all pacemaker cells are slowly depolarizing (as shown here), reducing their membrane potential. A stimulus at a reduced membrane potential may result in block if all conditions are favorable. See text for explanation.

tial toward zero) so that, in the presence of significant bradycardia, enough time elapses before the arrival of the impulse for the bundle branch fibers to reach a potential at which conduction is impaired.

3. A deterioration in membrane responsiveness so that significant conduction impairment develops at –75 mV instead of at –65 mV.

Two examples of phase 4 BBB can be seen in Fig. 14-6. In *A*, the longer sinus cycles end with LBBB; in *B*, the lengthened postextrasystolic cycles end with RBBB conduction.

Retrograde Concealed Conduction

Retrograde concealed conduction into one of the bundle branches is a very common mechanism for aberrant ventricular conduction.[7] Fig. 14-7 is an excellent example of aberrant ventricular conduction caused by retrograde concealed conduction in which RBBB aberration is initiated and terminated by a left ventricular premature beat. Note in the drawings below the tracings in Fig. 14-7 that a premature beat in the left ventricle activates the right bundle branch retrogradely and late so that the right bundle remains refractory for the next sinus beat (phase 3 aberration), although normal conduction proceeds down the left bundle branch, producing the RBBB pattern. By this time the distal right bundle branch has recovered and is again activated retrogradely, leaving it again refractory for the next sinus beat, and so on. This scenario is repeated for each ensuing sinus beat until another PVC breaks the cycle by conducting all the way up to the atria, allowing both bundle branches to depolarize and repolarize simultaneously. Note the retrograde P′ wave after the second PVC. A normal sinus rhythm follows.

CAUSES

The broad QRS in SVT may be caused by any one of the following conditions:

- Aberrant ventricular conduction during any supraventricular tachycardia (sinus tachycardia, atrial flutter, atrial fibrillation, AV nodal reentry tachycardia, orthodromic circus movement tachycardia, atrial tachycardia)
- Pathologic BBB
- Antidromic circus movement tachycardia
- AV nodal reentry tachycardia using a Mahaim fiber for anterograde conduction

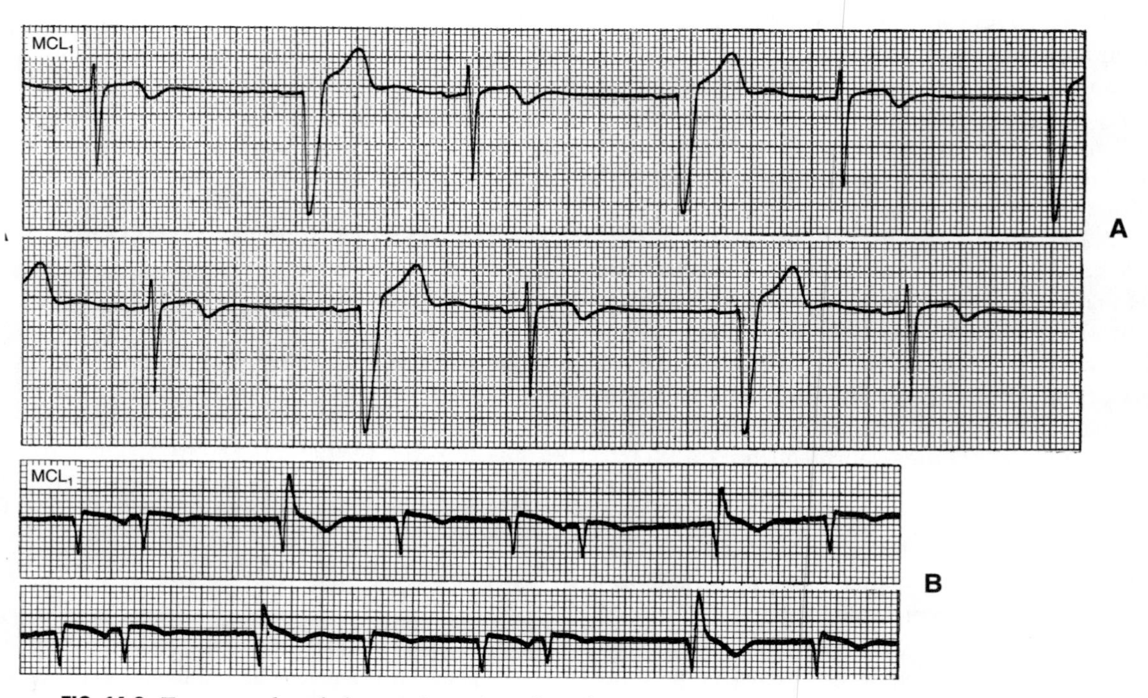

FIG. 14-6. Two examples of phase 4 aberration after a long pause. In **A** there is LBBB aberration and in **B** there is RBBB aberration. (Courtesy Henry J.L. Marriott, MD, Tampa, Fla.)

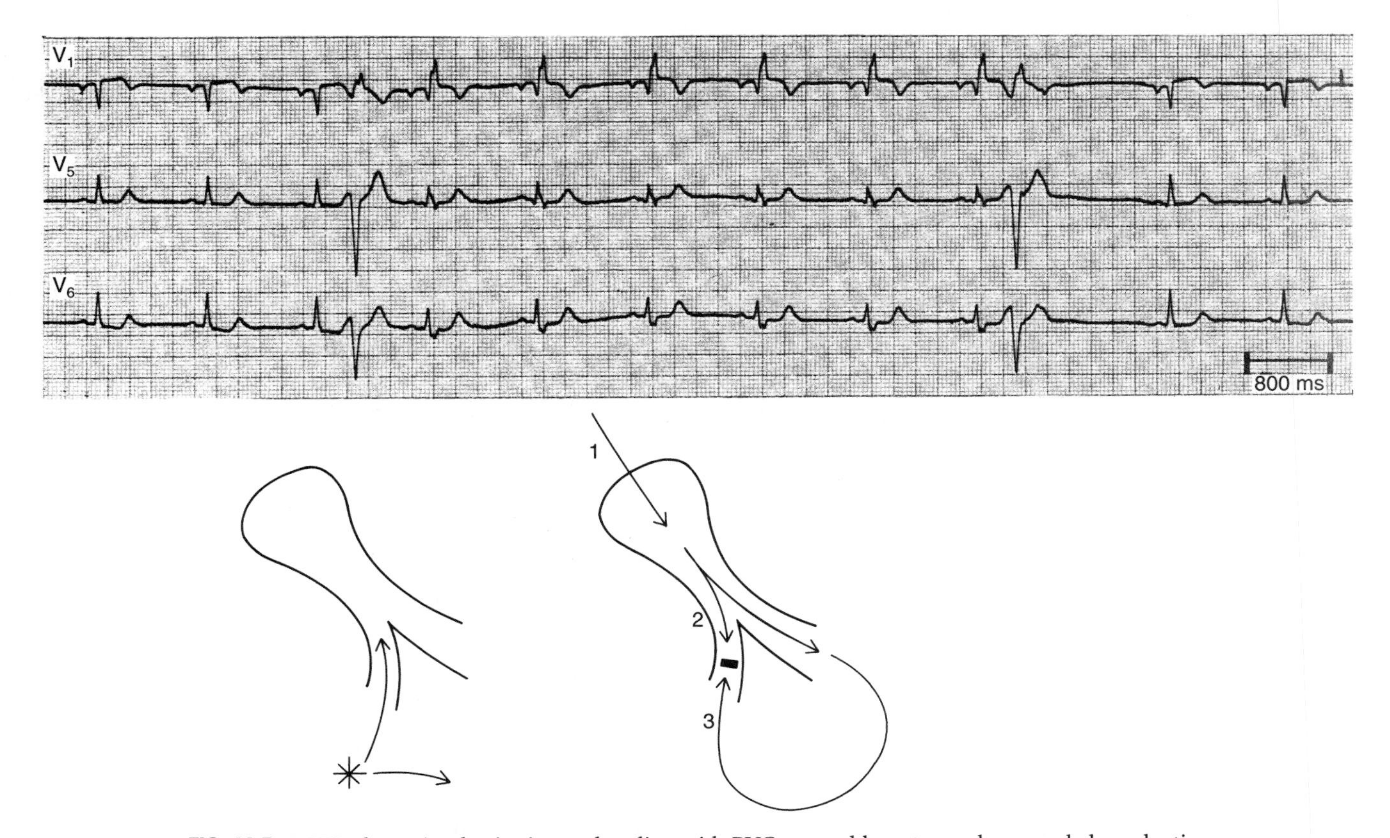

FIG. 14-7. RBBB aberration beginning and ending with PVCs caused by retrograde concealed conduction into the right bundle branch. The mechanism is illustrated: A PVC *(*)* is conducted retrogradely up the right bundle branch and not up the left. When the next sinus impulse *(1)* arrives at the bundle branches, it finds the right bundle still refractory *(2)* because of the retrograde invasion into it. Thus the sinus impulse is conducted with RBBB *(3)*. The retrograde conduction continues with each sinus beat because the right bundle branch, not having been activated, is open for retrograde conduction again and again, until the sequence is finally interrupted by another PVC. (Tracing courtesy Hein Wellens, MD, Maastricht, The Netherlands.)

CLINICAL IMPLICATIONS

Misdiagnosis of ventricular tachycardia (VT) may result in immediate hemodynamic collapse in the acute stage of therapy. If the patient survives, subsequent mismanagement may result in death. Not only is it important to recognize VT because of the dire consequences that result from mistreatment and subsequent mismanagement of such patients, but also it is important to recognize supraventricular tachycardia (SVT), especially when an accessory pathway is involved because of the possibility of atrial fibrillation with its life-threatening heart rate. Additionally, if a diagnosis of PSVT with a circus movement tachycardia using an accessory pathway is missed, the patient is denied a permanent cure.

Akhtar et al[8] analyzed the data obtained from 150 consecutive patients with broad QRS tachycardia and found that 122 patients had VT, 21 had SVT with aberration, and 7 had accessory pathway conduction. One of the findings of this study was that only 39 of the 122 patients with VT received a correct diagnosis in the acute setting. Reasons for this shocking discovery were unclear, but the following were suggested:

1. There is an erroneous perception that SVT with aberrancy is as common as VT.
2. In most patients who come to medical attention with wide-complex tachycardia and hemodynamic stability, the clinician wrongly assumes that VT is unlikely.
3. The emergency nature of the clinical setting moti-

vates the clinician to judge quickly rather than to thoroughly analyze the 12-lead ECG, take a history, and perform a physical examination. Certain findings on physical examination and on the ECG often swiftly provide a correct diagnosis.

BEDSIDE DIAGNOSIS

The patient is examined for the physical signs of PSVT or AV dissociation.

Physical Signs of PSVT

The neck veins. Even before the ECG electrodes are applied, observation of the neck veins often helps to rapidly distinguish between SVT and VT. During PSVT the atria contract against closed AV valves, causing a reflux of blood up the jugular veins. This results in a rapid, regular expansion of the neck veins resembling the rhythmic puffing motion of a frog. H.J.J. Wellens, MD, refers to this physical finding as the "frog sign." The patient usually reports a history of palpitations and seeks medical attention when the palpitations are associated with lightheadedness, shortness of breath, or anxiety. When questioned, the patient or family may have noticed the frog sign.

Other tachycardias. The pulsations in the neck veins often reveal the mechanism of other tachycardias as well.[9] Sinus tachycardia and atrial tachycardia are the only two SVTs that do not result in abnormal pulsations in the neck veins. In atrial flutter, there are flutter waves; in atrial fibrillation, there are irregular pulsations in the neck veins. In VT with AV dissociation these pulsations are irregular because of the occasional simultaneous beating of atria and ventricles.

Pulse, blood pressure, and heart sounds. In all types of regular SVT, the pulse is regular and the blood pressure and the loudness of the first heart sound constant. On the other hand, these parameters vary when there are changing RR intervals and AV conduction varies, as in atrial fibrillation and atrial flutter with variable conduction ratios. The jugular venous pressure may be elevated, but the waveform generally remains constant.[10]

Polyuria. In a significant number of patients (20% to 50%) PSVT is associated with polyuria. This response typically occurs with heart rates greater than 120 beats per minute and a duration of 10 to 30 minutes. Polyuria has also been noted during episodes of atrial fibrillation, atrial flutter, and VT. Factors responsible are changes in atrial rhythm and pressure, resulting in the release of the atrial natriuretic factor, a hormone that causes diuresis and may also play a role in the posttachycardia, hypovolemic hypotension sometimes associated with PSVT.[11]

Syncope. The syncope that frequently occurs in PSVT is thought to be caused by a particular hemodynamic response to the stress of tachycardia and does not imply a more malignant or rapid tachycardia. The sequence is thought to be as follows[12]:

1. PSVT causes a short diastolic filling time and ineffective timing of atrial and ventricular contraction, reducing left ventricular filling.
2. An increase in sympathetic tone occurs at the onset of the tachycardia.
3. The upright position also causes reduced left ventricular volume and increased sympathetic tone.
4. This in turn may precipitate inappropriate stimulation of left ventricular stretch receptors, causing an inadequate hemodynamic response to the tachycardia and syncope. The mechanism is similar to that postulated for vasovagal syncope.
5. During the tachycardia, syncope can occur because the rapid ventricular rate fails to provide adequate cerebral circulation; after the tachycardia, syncope can occur because of overdrive suppression of the sinus node by the tachycardia.

Physical Signs of VT (AV Dissociation)

The independent beating of atria and ventricles is present in approximately 50% of VTs and is therefore a reliable criterion for a correct diagnosis of VT. Look for these physical signs:

1. Irregular cannon A waves in the jugular pulse
2. Varying intensity of the first heart sound
3. Beat-to-beat changes in systolic blood pressure

Any one of the preceding clues indicates AV dissociation, although the absence of clues does not rule out VT, nor does it rule out AV dissociation. For example, in atrial fibrillation with VT there is AV dissociation without its usual physical or ECG signs. The possibility also exists for VT with retrograde conduction to the atria and for junctional tachycardia with retrograde block. Given the rarity of such rhythms, AV dissociation is still a valuable diagnostic clue for VT.

Jugular pulse. During AV dissociation the atria and the ventricles are beating independently; this beating occasionally coincides, so that the atria contract against closed AV valves. In the right heart, this causes a reflux of blood up the jugular veins. Such irregular, unpredictable expansions in the pulsation of the jugular pulse are called *cannon A waves.*

Varying intensity of the first heart sound. Listen at the apex or fourth left intercostal space for the closing of the mitral valve. During sinus rhythm it has a fixed intensity because the position of the leaflets of the AV valves is the same for every ventricular systole. During AV dissociation this position differs from beat to beat, causing a varying intensity of the first heart sound. Other conditions in which this would occur are complete heart block, AV Wenckebach, and atrial fibrillation.

Changes in systolic blood pressure. AV dissociation can be easily identified at the bedside by using the blood pressure recorder. During AV dissociation there are beat-to-beat changes in systolic blood pressure because the lapse of time between atrial and ventricular contraction is different with each cycle, resulting in varying ventricular filling times and beat-to-beat changes in systolic stroke volume into the aorta. Thus although the rhythm is regular, the systolic blood pressure differs from beat to beat.

DIFFERENTIAL DIAGNOSIS

The challenge of the differential diagnosis in broad QRS tachycardia is met with an understanding of the patient's history, the ECG and physical signs of PSVT and VT just discussed, and the morphologic distinction between the QRS of SVT with aberrant ventricular conduction and VT.

Value of the Patient's History

When the history can be obtained, QRS morphology provides greater than 90% accuracy.[13] In the setting of broad QRS tachycardia this information is not always available, which limits the value of QRS morphology in the differential diagnosis between VT and SVT.[8]

One study[14] found that a history of structural heart disease suggested VT in 112 (95%) of 118 patients, and a history of myocardial infarction (MI) was associated with a high incidence of VT as the mechanism of wide-complex tachycardia in 87 (98%) of 89 patients.

QRS Morphology

The QRS morphology is judged by different rules according to its polarity in V_1. This is because it is being compared to RBBB or LBBB patterns. RBBB is positive in V_1, and LBBB is negative in V_1, thus the V_1-positive and V_1-negative classification. It must be emphasized that in applying the morphologic criteria, especially in V_1-positive tachycardias, an understanding of the clinical setting (drugs being taken, history of MI, cardiomyopathy, presence of heart disease) is critical.

V_1-Positive Broad QRS Tachycardia

Fig. 14-8 illustrates the patterns seen in V_1 during broad QRS tachycardia when the QRS is upright in that lead, comparing the morphology of VT with that of SVT with aberration. Fig. 14-9 further demonstrates the patterns seen in V_1 during VT.[1-4]

The triphasic pattern. An RBBB (rSR′ in V_1 and qRs in V_6) pattern (Fig. 14-10) occurs more often in SVT than in VT. In V_1 during the tachycardia the small r wave reflects septal activation from left to right, the S wave reflects left ventricular activation, and the terminal R wave reflects late activation of the right ventricle caused by the physiologic block in the right bundle branch.

Note: Certain types of VT may also have this triphasic pattern in V_1 and the relatively narrow QRS (i.e., fascicular VT, left ventricular idiopathic VT, and bundle branch reentry VT).

BOX 14-1. Differential Diagnosis When V_1 Is Mainly Positive

MORPHOLOGIC SIGNS OF VT

- A monophasic R in V_1
- Biphasic complex in V_1
- Tall initial rabbit ear sign in V_1 (Rr′)
- R:S ratio in V_6 <1 when the QRS axis is left
- QRS >0.14 second

MORPHOLOGIC SIGNS OF SVT

- Triphasic RBBB pattern in V_1 (rSR′)
- Triphasic RBBB pattern in V_6 (qRs) ONLY if V_1 is positive
- QRS of 0.14 second or less

BOX 14-2. Differential Diagnosis When V_1 Is Mainly Negative

MORPHOLOGIC SIGNS OF VT

- Broad R (>0.03 second V_1 or V_2)
- Slurred S downstroke (V_1 or V_2)
- Delayed S nadir (>0.06 second V_1 or V_2)
- Any Q in V_6
- Right axis deviation
- QRS >0.16 second

MORPHOLOGIC SIGNS OF SVT

- Narrow initial r wave in V_1 or V_2
- Slick, quick S downstroke in V_1 or V_2
- Early S nadir in V_1 or V_2
- No Q in V_6

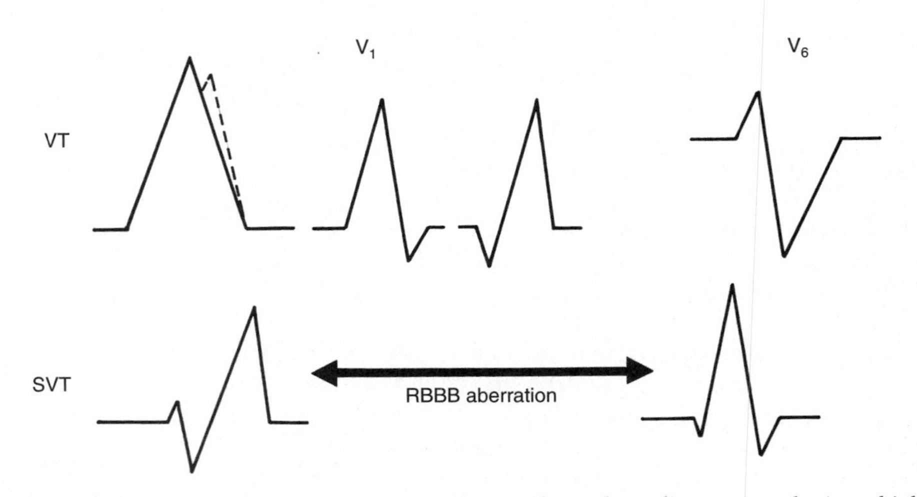

FIG. 14-8. Morphologic appearance in V_1-positive wide-complex tachycardia. A monophasic or biphasic complex indicates VT. A triphasic (rSR′) pattern indicates SVT. The "rabbit ear" clue (Rr′) in V_1 (initial peak taller) indicates VT. When the two peaks are reversed (rR′), a deep S (R/S ratio <1) indicates VT.

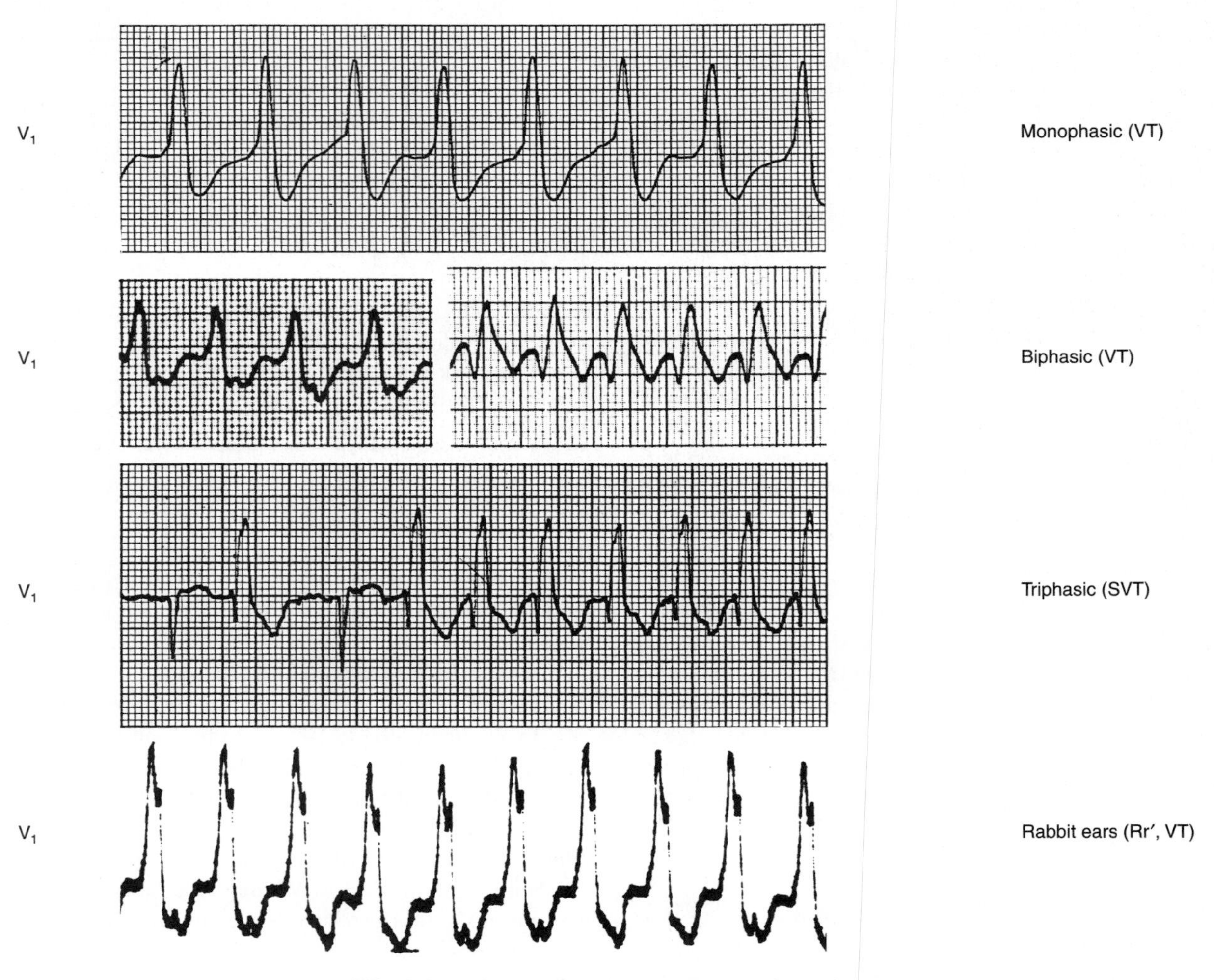

FIG. 14-9. Tachycardias with V_1-positive configuration.

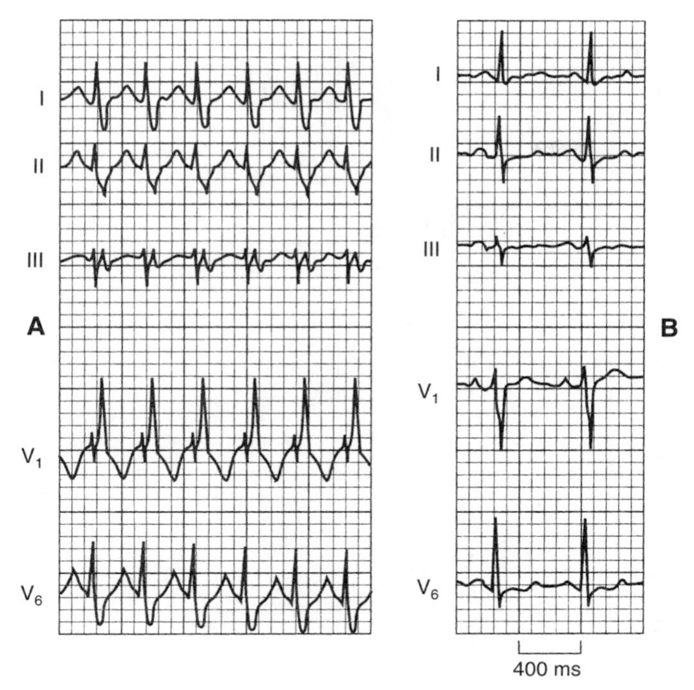

FIG. 14-10. **A,** SVT with RBBB aberration with, **B,** sinus rhythm from the same patient. (From Wellens HJJ. In Willerson JT, Cohn JN, editors: *Cardiovascular medicine,* New York, 1995, Churchill Livingstone.)

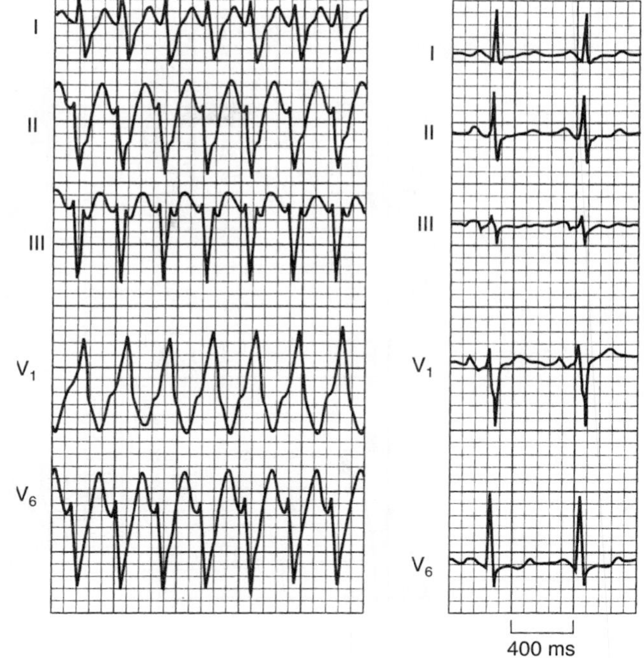

FIG. 14-11. VT in the same patient shown in Fig 14-10. The monophasic R wave in lead V_1, the superior axis, and the R/S ratio of less than 1 in lead V_6 are evident. (From Wellens HJJ. In Willerson JT, Cohn JN, editors: *Cardiovascular medicine,* New York, 1995, Churchill Livingstone.)

The monophasic or biphasic complex. An R, qR, or RS in lead V_1 is more common in VT. Fig. 14-11 illustrates sinus rhythm and VT with a monophasic R wave. It is possible for the monophasic or biphasic patterns to also occur in SVT, which emphasizes the systematic approach to the patient with all factors being evaluated.[13]

The rabbit ear sign. This pattern has two positive peaks in V_1; the initial peak is taller (Rr′; Figs. 14-8 and 14-9) and is generally considered diagnostic of VT. However, it is possible for this pattern to occur in supraventricular rhythms with RBBB and axis deviation. Fig. 14-12 illustrates this in a patient with anterior septal MI, RBBB (with two peaks in V_1, initial peak tallest), and hemiblock.

The opposite rabbit ear configuration with the initial peak shorter is shown in Figs. 14-13 and 14-14. This QRS configuration is not a helpful ECG sign because it is seen equally in both VT and SVT.

Value of V_6. When a positive QRS pattern in V_1 has a nondiagnostic rabbit ear configuration (rR′), lead V_6 may be of value. Because of the influence of the QRS axis on the shape of the QRS complex in V_6, the R/S ratio in that lead is helpful if the frontal plane axis is left; that is, in such a case an R/S ratio of less than 1 supports a diagnosis of VT. This finding is of no value if the axis is inferior (normal or right).[13]

V_1-Negative Broad QRS Tachycardia

Figs. 14-15 to 14-17 illustrate the patterns seen in V_1 and V_2 during broad QRS tachycardia when the QRS is negative in V_1[5,15]: broad R, slurred downstroke, delayed nadir, and any q in V_6. If the R wave is narrow in V_1 it is still necessary to check V_2 where the signs of VT may be present. Note in Fig. 14-18 that although the narrow little r wave in V_1 along with the swift, clean downstroke are signs of SVT, a glance at the slurred downstroke in V_2 confirms a diagnosis of VT.

Broad R. The wide R in V_1 or V_2 when the tachycardia is negative in V_1 is seen in more than 90% of VTs associated with inferior infarction and in only 25% of tachycardias associated with anterior infarction, in which case a QS complex is more common.[13] The broad R in V_1 or V_2 has 100% specificity, 36% sensitivity, and 100% predictive accuracy for VT.[5]

Slurred S downstroke. This clue usually occurs in ante-

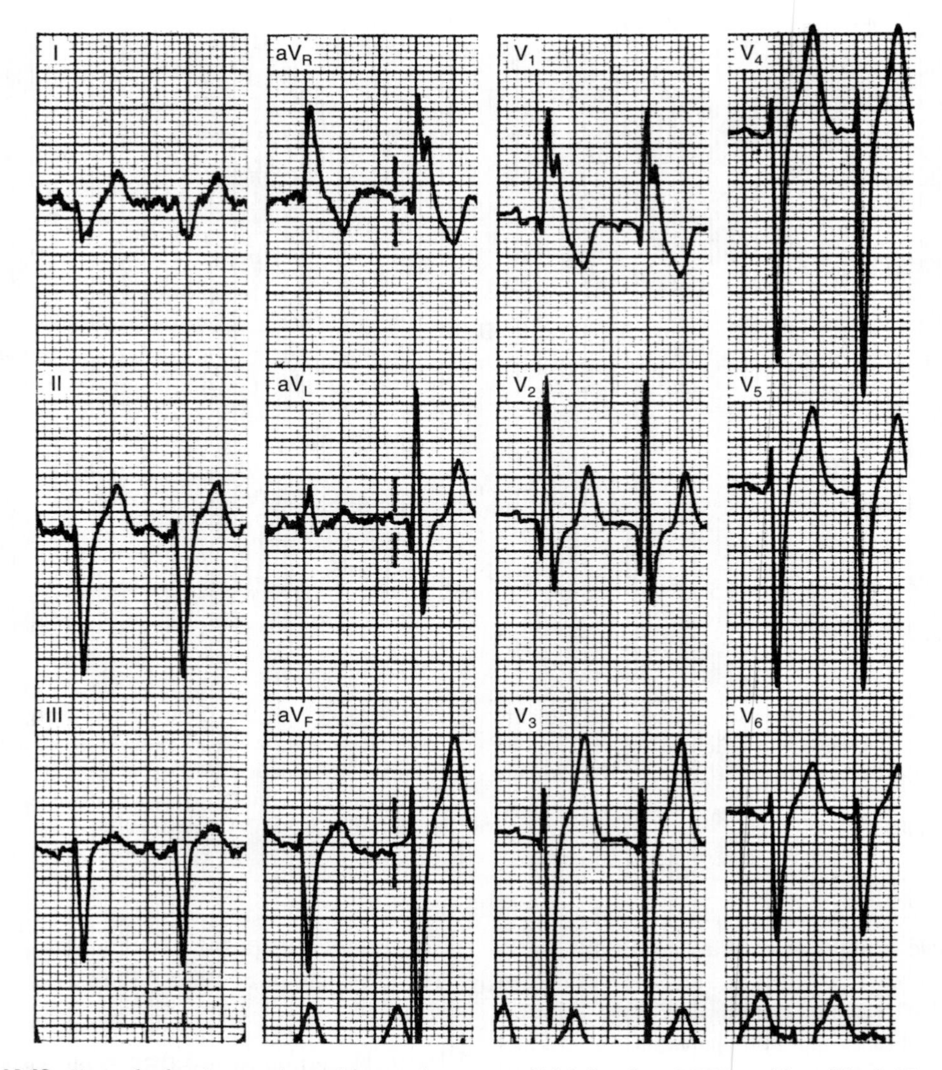

FIG. 14-12. Sinus rhythm in a patient with anterior myocardial infarction, RBBB, and hemiblock. Note the effect of the extreme axis deviation on the morphology of the V_1 QRS complex (Rr'). This "rabbit ear" sign usually indicates VT.

rior infarction and has 96% specificity, 36% sensitivity, and 97% predictive accuracy for VT.[5]

Delayed S nadir. The distance from the onset of the QRS to the lowest point of the S wave (its nadir) in V_1 or V_2 is more than 0.06 second. This finding is seen in two-thirds of patients who have V_1-negative VT. The delayed S nadir has 96% specificity, 63% sensitivity, and 98% predictive accuracy.[5]

Q in V_6. A Q wave in this lead *when V_1 is negative* suggests VT and is almost always present when the tachycardia originates from the anterior septum.[13] The Q wave can be deep, shallow, broad, narrow, or embryonic. Be careful not to apply this rule when V_1 is positive, in which case the tachycardia may be supraventricular. The presence of a Q in V_6 when V_1 is negative has 96% specificity, 55% sensitivity, and 98% predictive accuracy.

Combined criteria. When all four of these signs are present the specificity is 89%, sensitivity 100%, and predictive accuracy 96%.[5]

Limitations. The limitations associated with these ECG criteria for the differential diagnosis in V_1-negative broad QRS tachycardia include the following:

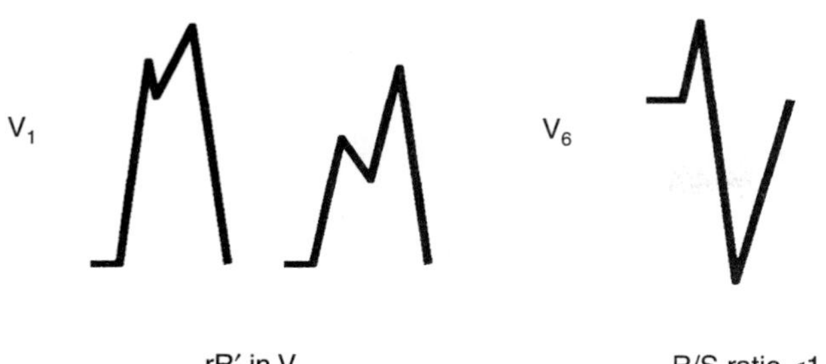

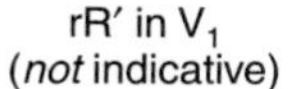

FIG. 14-13. In V_1 an rR' pattern of no help in the differential diagnosis of broad QRS tachycardia. However, if a deep S wave is seen in V_6 (R/S ratio <1), it is VT.

1. SVT with LBBB that looks like VT is found with preexistent LBBB and severe left ventricular fibrotic disease; a comparison with a tracing in sinus rhythm will permit the correct diagnosis.
2. Antidromic circus movement tachycardia with anterograde conduction over an accessory pathway inserting in the right ventricle produces a broad QRS tachycardia identical in morphology to V_1-negative VT.
3. Class IA (procainamide, quinidine, disopyramide) or class IC (encainide, flecainide, propafenone) drugs may broaden the R wave and produce a delayed S nadir in lead V_1 or V_2.

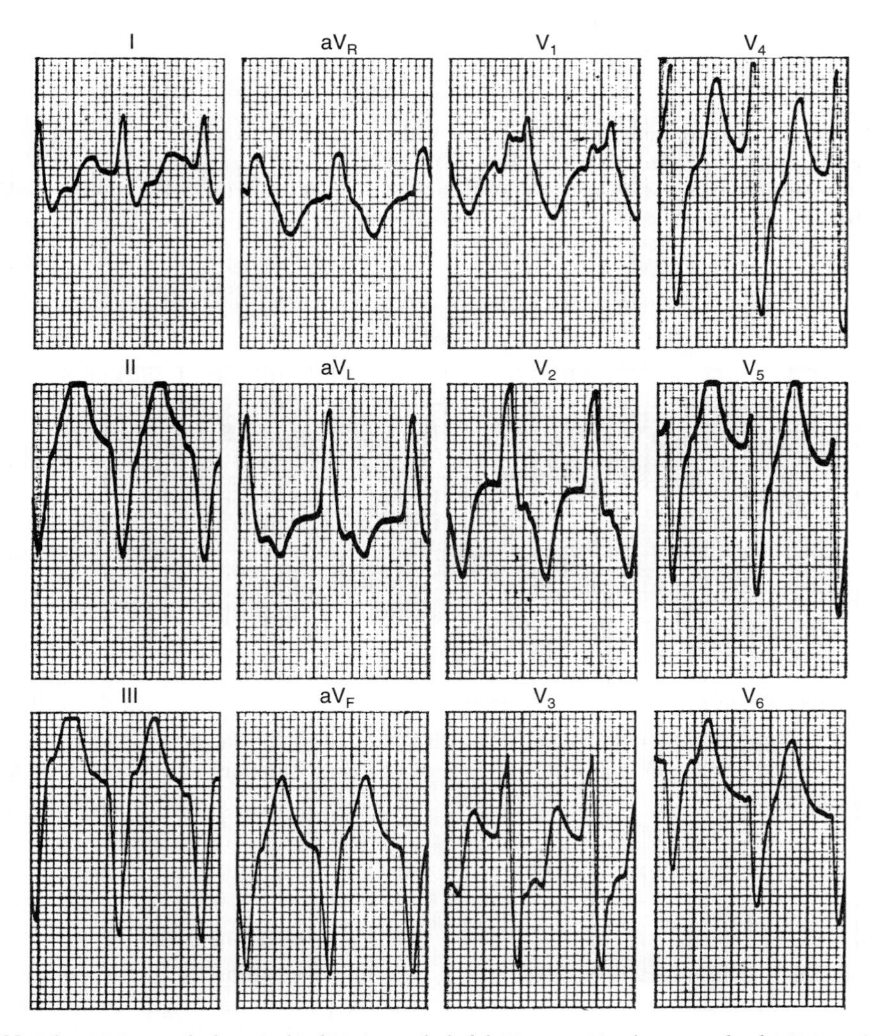

FIG. 14-14. The QRS morphology in lead V_1 is not helpful. However, in that same lead a P wave is seen in front of the first QRS but not in front of the next one. This is a sign of atrioventricular dissociation and diagnostic of VT. Another helpful clue is the R/S ratio in V_6. When the axis is left, as it is here, such a ratio supports a diagnosis of VT.

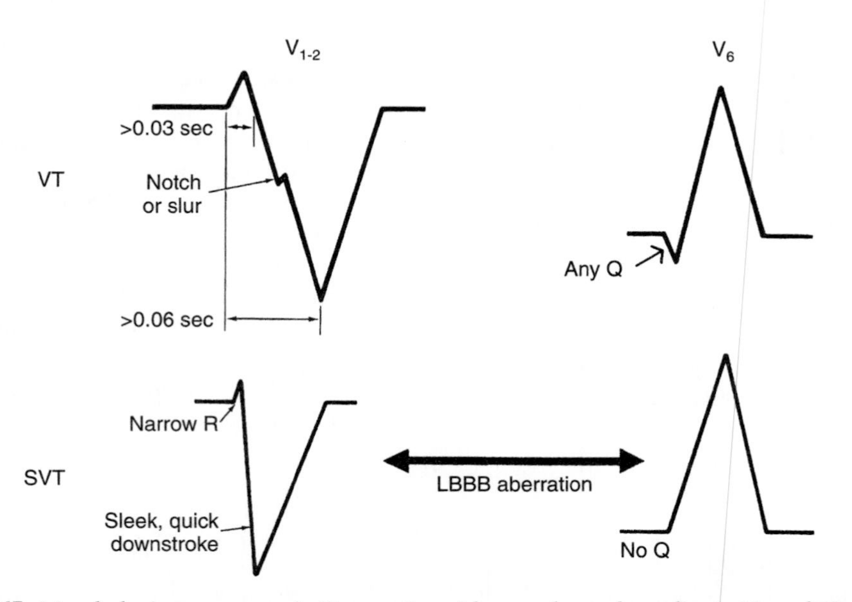

FIG. 14-15. Morphologic appearance in V_1-negative wide-complex tachycardia. In V_1 and V_2 a wide R, slurred S downstroke, or delayed S nadir indicates VT. In lead V_6 any Q (or q) wave indicates VT. In SVT there may be a small, narrow r wave in lead V_1 or V_2, and the S downstroke is quick and sleek. In SVT there is no Q or q in V_6 when V_1 is negative.

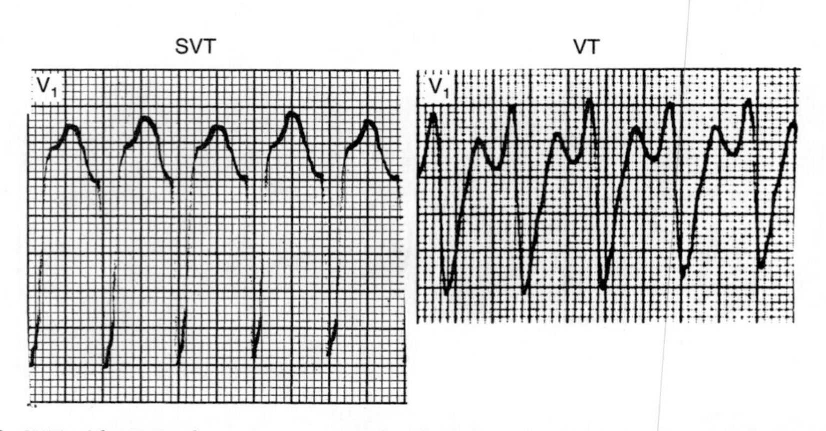

FIG. 14-16. SVT with LBBB aberration compared with V_1-negative VT. Note the typical physiologic LBBB pattern in the SVT (swift, clean S downstroke; QRS <0.14 second duration) as opposed to the fat R and delayed S nadir of the VT.

General Signs of VT

Although the broad QRS tachycardia is divided into V_1-positive and V_1-negative morphologies when making a differential diagnosis between aberration and ectopy, there are signs that are common to both V_1-positive and V_1-negative broad QRS tachycardia that indicate VT. They are listed in Box 14-3.

In Preexisting BBB

The two most difficult clinical settings in which to determine the origin of a broad QRS tachycardia are preexisting BBB and Wolff-Parkinson-White (WPW) syndrome. Figs. 14-19 and 14-20 illustrate the advantage to having a baseline 12-lead ECG, especially when there is preexisting BBB or ECG evidence of previous MI.

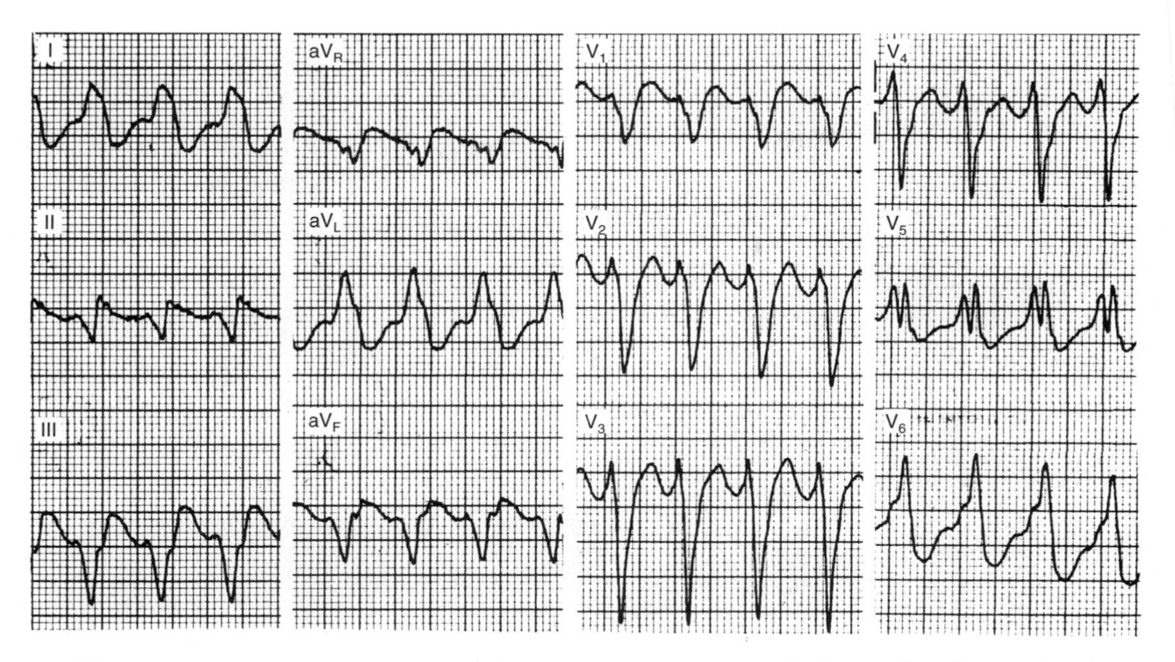

FIG. 14-17. In the V_1-negative pattern three features of VT can be seen. In leads V_1 and V_2 there is a broad R wave, a slurred S downstroke (V_1 only), and a delay from the beginning of the ventricular complex to the lowest point of the S wave (its nadir). The left axis deviation is not a helpful sign.

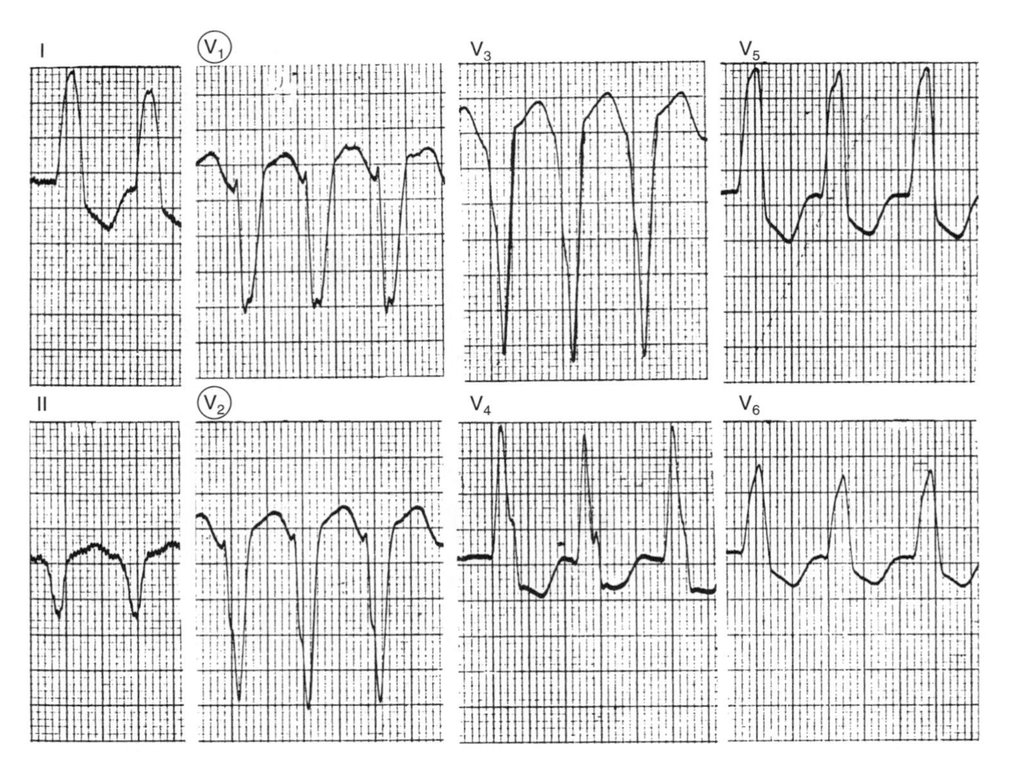

FIG. 14-18. VT. Although V_1 looks like SVT (narrow r and quick downstroke), lead V_2 shows a slurred downstroke, V_6 has a small q wave, V_4 shows signs of atrioventricular dissociation (the notch in the QRS of the second beat is a P wave), and the QRS is 0.16 second wide.

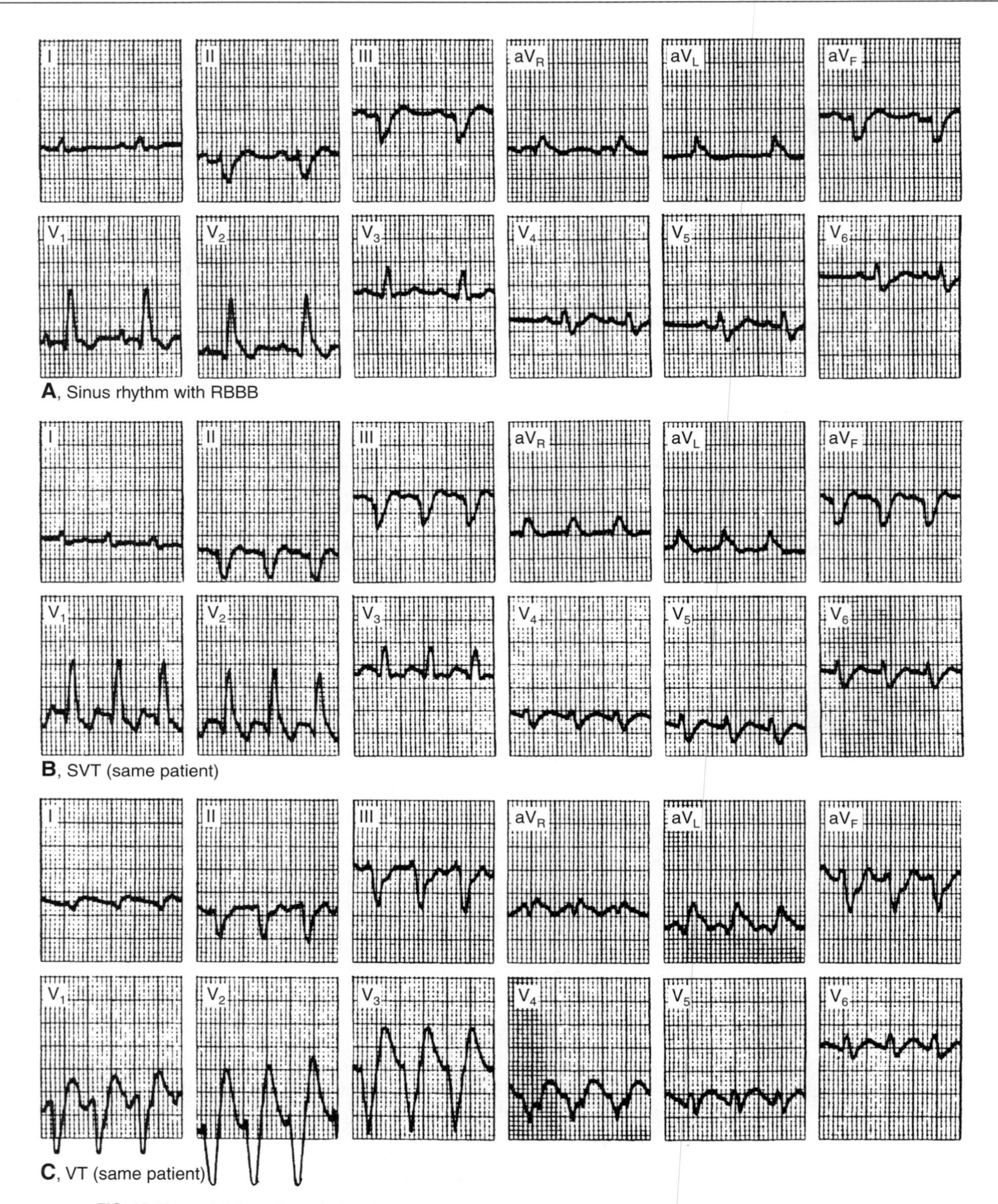

FIG. 14-19. **A-C,** The value of a baseline 12-lead ECG in the differential diagnosis of broad QRS tachycardia and preexisting BBB. Note that the patterns in SVT are virtually identical to those of sinus rhythm, whereas the patterns in VT are dramatically different. (Courtesy Hein J.J. Wellens, MD, Maastricht, The Netherlands.)

BOX 14-3. Common Indications of VT in V_1-Positive and V_1-Negative Broad QRS Tachycardia

- QRS morphology similar to previously seen PVCs
- Northwest axis
- Atrioventricular dissociation (physical and ECG signs)
- Retrograde conduction to the atria
- Ventricular fusion or capture beats
- Negative precordial concordance (diagnostic)
- Positive precordial concordance (strong indicator)
- Structural heart disease
- Prior myocardial infarction

The Value of a Vagal Maneuver

In Fig. 14-21, *A*, a broad QRS tachycardia seen in lead III responds to carotid sinus massage, revealing atrial flutter and pathologic LBBB, as confirmed by the sinus rhythm (Fig. 14-21, *B*).

QRS Axis

An abnormal axis is a strong indicator for VT and an axis in the northwest quadrant (−90 degrees to 180 degrees) is diagnostic, as is a right axis deviation in the presence of a V_1-negative configuration. The northwest axis is seen in Fig. 14-22 and is immediately recognized because leads I and aV_F are negative. Such an axis does not occur in SVT; it is an apical focus and therefore reliably distinguishes VT from SVT with aberration or accessory path-

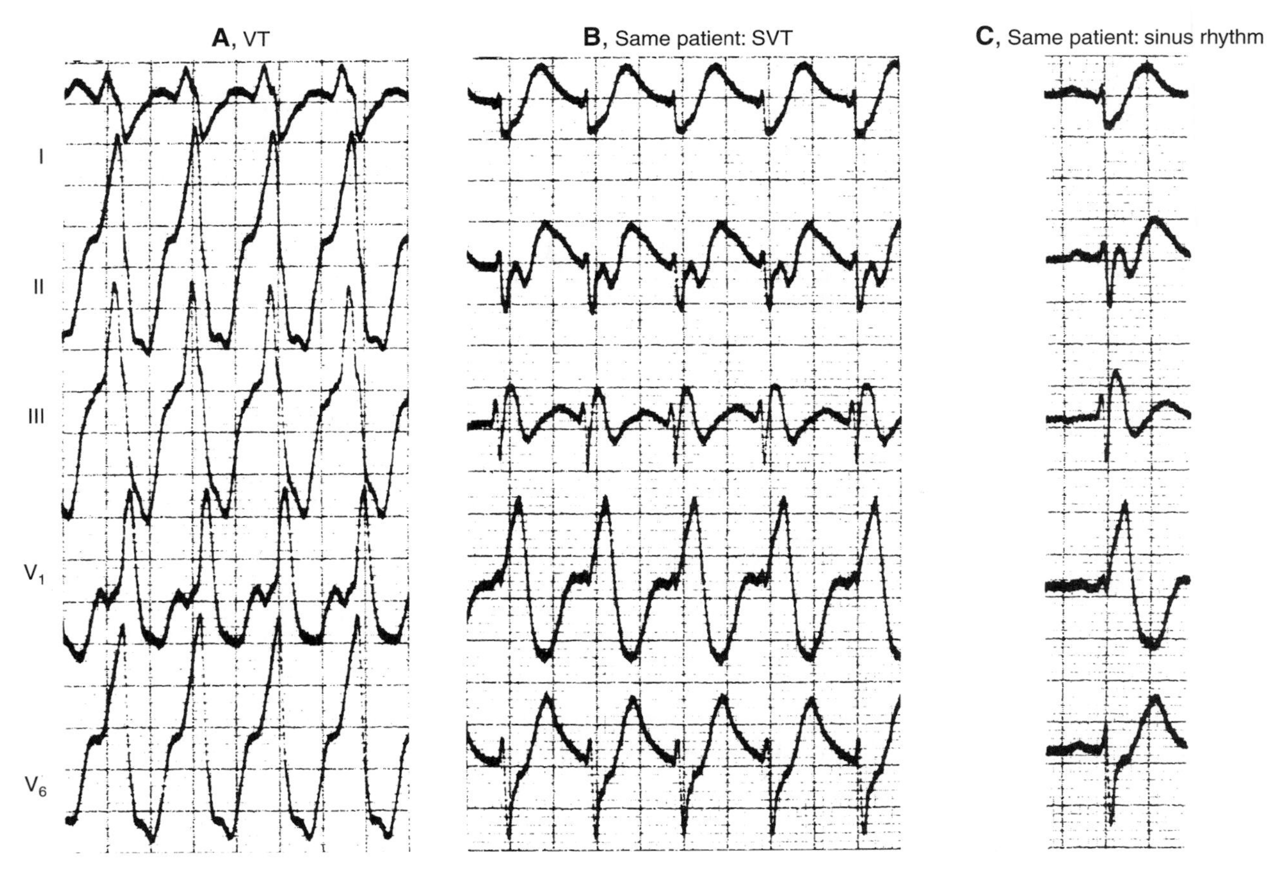

FIG. 14-20. ECGs from a 15-year-old boy who had complete correction of Fallot's tetralogy. The QRS patterns in V_1 of VT, SVT, and sinus rhythm are all positive. However, it is the patterns of SVT in **B** that are identical to those of the sinus rhythm seen in **C**. During programmed stimulation the tachycardia in **A** was found to be ventricular and the one in **B** originated in the AV node (SVT). These ECGs demonstrate the importance of careful comparison of wide QRS tachycardia with the ECG during sinus rhythm. (Courtesy Hein J.J. Wellens, MD, Maastricht, The Netherlands.)

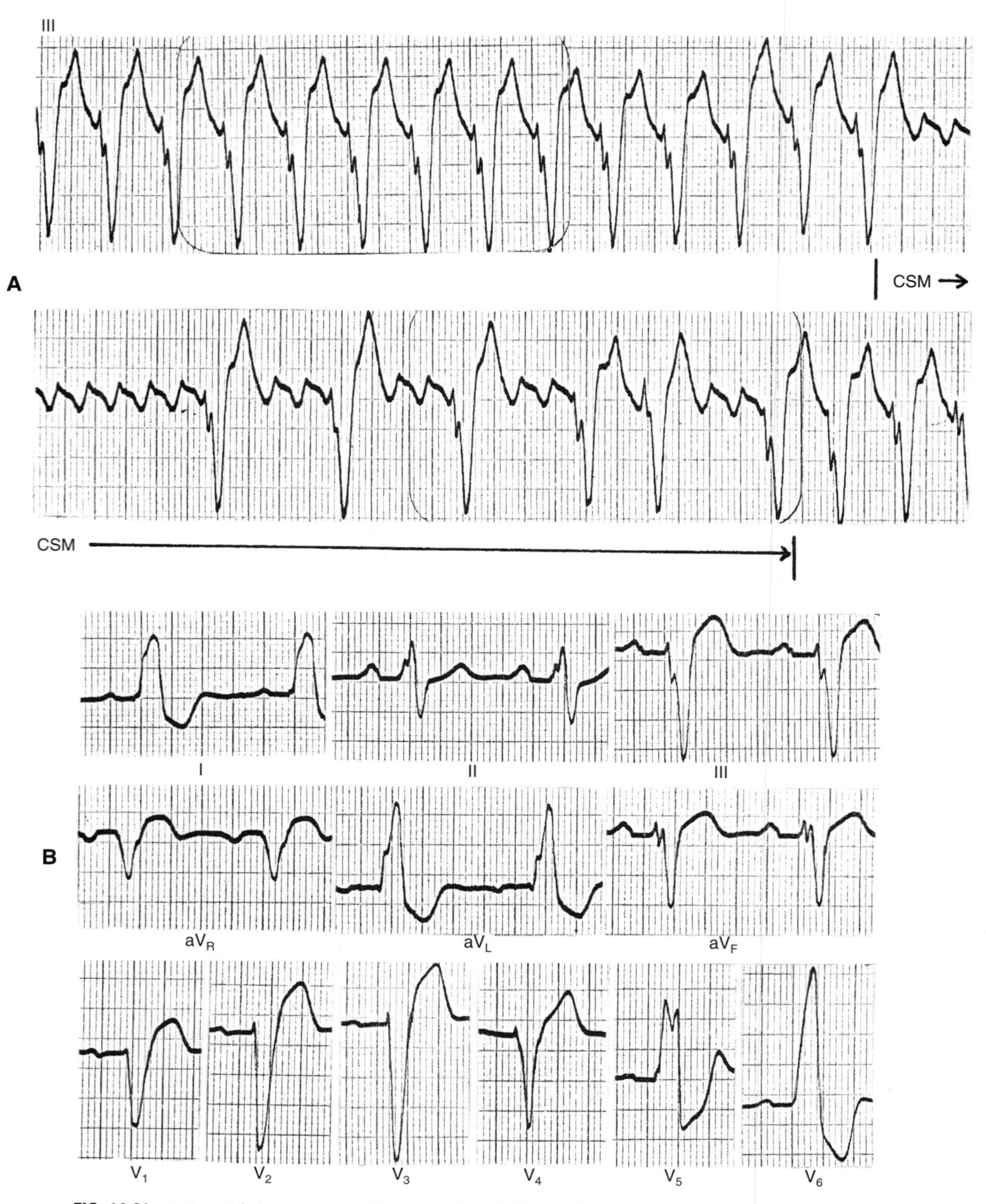

FIG. 14-21. **A**, Carotid sinus massage *(CSM)* in a broad QRS tachycardia clearly reveals atrial flutter and a pathologic BBB (still present after a long pause). **B**, The 12-lead ECG during sinus rhythm of the same patient confirms an underlying LBBB. (From Stein E: *The electrocardiogram. A self-study course in clinical electrocardiography,* Philadelphia, 1976, WB Saunders.)

way conduction. In this ECG AV dissociation is also very apparent in lead II with a P wave before the first QRS and after the second.

A study by Kindwall et al[5] found that when V_1 was negative, left axis deviation was not useful, being common to both VT and SVT with aberration. However, Akhtar et al[8] found that the combination of a negative complex in V_1 and right axis deviation was seen only in VT (nine patients), a fact also reported by Rosenbaum in 1969.[15] This pattern is shown in Fig. 14-23.

Clinical Correlations Regarding Axis[16]

Previous MI. When VT occurs in patients with a prior MI, the QRS axis in the frontal plane is usually abnormal. This is especially true when V_1 is positive. In such cases the axis is often superior (i.e., negative in aV_F).

Idiopathic VT. In the normal heart VT can have a normal axis, but most commonly there is a marked right axis deviation or the axis is directed superiorly.

Preexisting BBB. A markedly abnormal axis may occur in patients with preexisting BBB who have SVT.

Accessory pathways. Marked left axis deviation (left of –30 °) may be seen in SVT with conduction over a right-sided or posteroseptal accessory pathway, and marked right axis deviation may be seen in SVT with conduction over a left lateral accessory pathway.

Class IC drugs and QRS axis. Patients taking class IC drugs can have SVT with an axis to the left of –30 degrees.

ECG Signs of AV Dissociation

AV dissociation is often missed on the surface ECG. In one study[8] involving 150 patients with wide QRS tachycardia, AV dissociation was present in 67 patients (45%) but could be detected on the surface ECG in only 38 of those patients. The greatest danger is that the clinician may mistake T waves for P waves, a mistake that leads to an incorrect diagnosis and possibly lethal consequences. During the broad QRS tachycardia P waves can best be found by looking for a distortion in one cycle that cannot be found in another. For example, in Fig. 14-24 independent P waves can be seen throughout the tracing; four of them are marked. These P waves are found because they distort the ECG cycle differently each time; that is, after the first QRS there is a little nubbin that cannot be seen in the same place after the next QRS. Therefore this little nubbin cannot be part of the QRS or the T wave. It is undeniably a P wave. A long tracing is not always necessary to spot independent P waves. Look back at Fig. 14-14 and study the shapes seen in lead V_1. The QRS morphology itself is not helpful (two peaks with initial peak

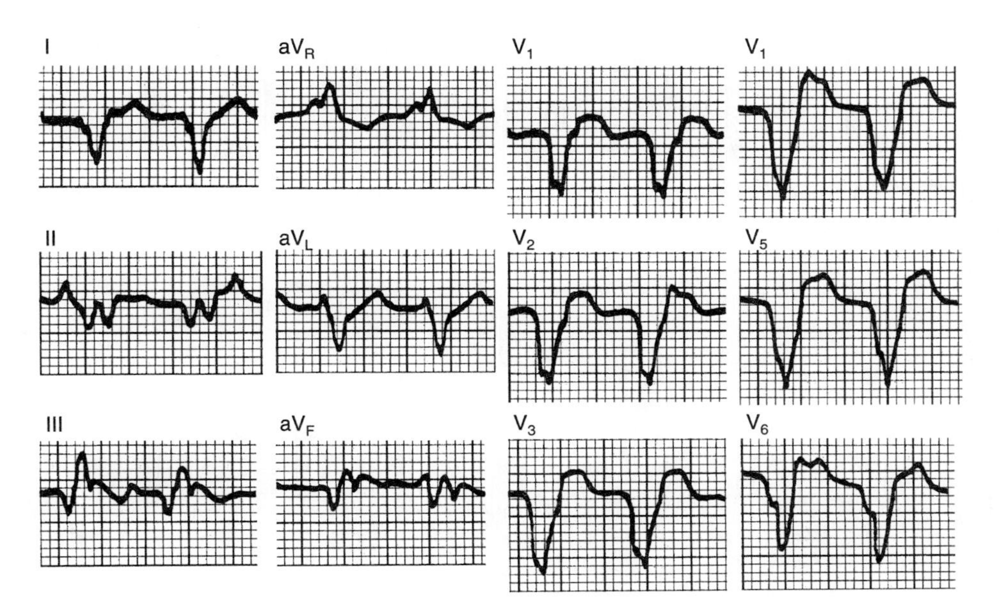

FIG. 14-22. Negative precordial concordance. The slurred downstroke in lead V_1 and the delayed S nadir in leads V_1 and V_2 (discussed on p. 180) are also evident. Note the two independent P waves easily seen in lead II (before the first complex and after the second); this is diagnostic of VT.

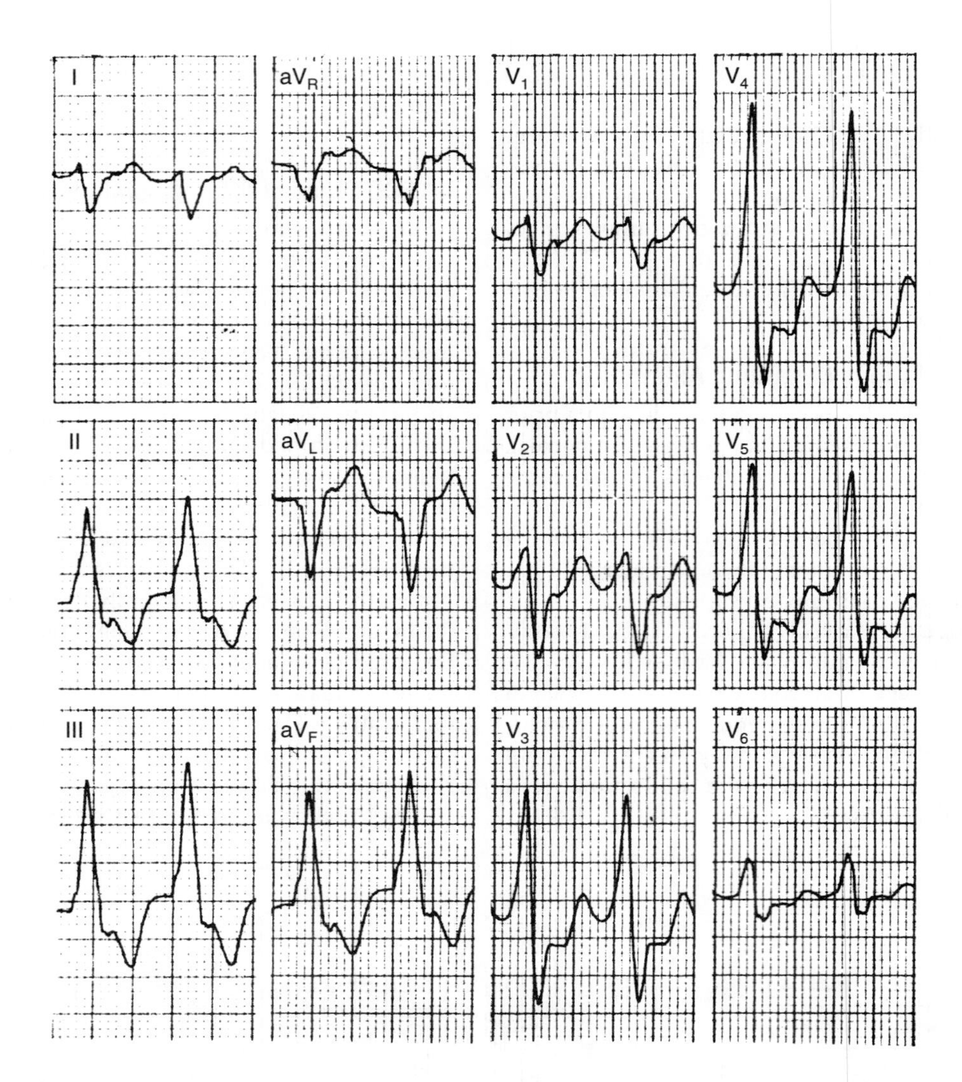

FIG. 14-23. VT. The slurred S downstroke in lead V_1, the broad R wave in V_2, and the delayed S nadir in both leads can be seen. When V_1 is negative, right axis deviation is diagnostic of VT.

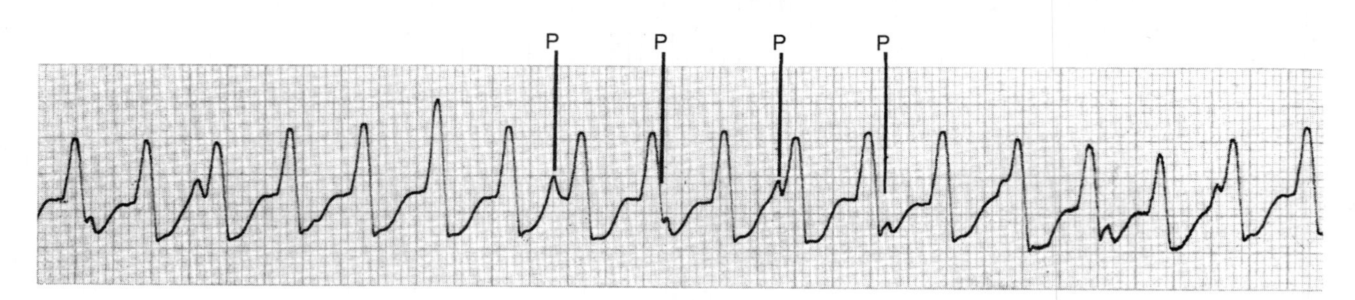

FIG. 14-24. AV dissociation. The regular, independent sinus P waves during the tachycardia can be seen. The P waves are easily found when a distortion is seen in the QRS, ST segment, or T wave of one cycle that is not seen in another.

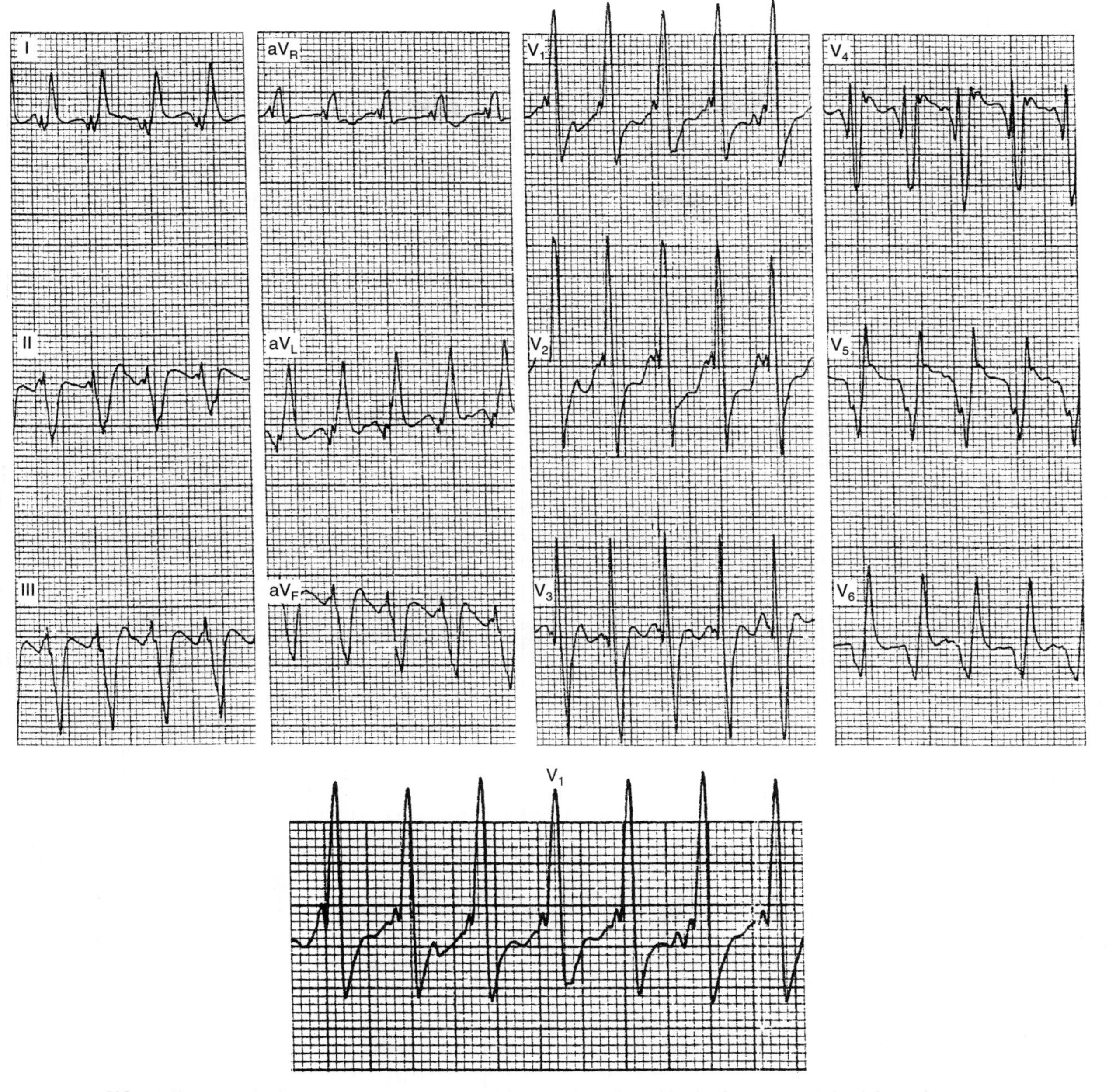

FIG. 14-25. Find the sinus P waves in this VT. They are best found by looking in each lead for a distortion in one cycle that is not found in another. This is nicely seen in leads V_1 and V_2, where there is a small positive deflection after the second QRS that is not seen in neighboring cycles. Another such distortion is in front of the sixth QRS.

shortest), but note the distortion in front of the first QRS that is not seen in the same place in front of the second QRS . . . sign of AV dissociation. This and the QS in V_6 secures the diagnosis of VT.

Exercise 1

The most common error when searching for P waves in a broad QRS tachycardia is to look for P waves as a consistent finding in every cycle; this leads to the costly error of mistaking T waves for P waves. For example, when examining the 12 leads seen in Fig. 14-25, the examiner looked in leads V_3 and V_4 among other leads and decided that there were P waves in front of every QRS and that this was SVT. Because of this uninformed and rash judgment, this patient received verapamil with devastating consequences.

Right approach. Look for P waves by searching for distortions in one cycle that are not seen in another. Such distortions are found in leads V_1, V_2, and V_3 at the end of the first QRS and at the beginning of the fifth QRS. These are independent P waves; there is AV dissociation and this is VT. You can also see a P wave distorting the second T wave in leads II and III. This distortion is identified as a P wave because the same distortion is not found in the neighboring T waves. The rR′ seen in V_1 is not a helpful clue.

Exercise 2

When evaluating Fig. 14-26, if the clinician is first looking for beat-to-beat deflections that look like P waves; little P-like nubbins in lead V_1 are easily found. If the decision to treat is made on this finding, the consequence to the patient may be loss of life.

Right approach. In assessing for AV dissociation, the informed examiner evaluates all leads in Fig. 14-26 looking

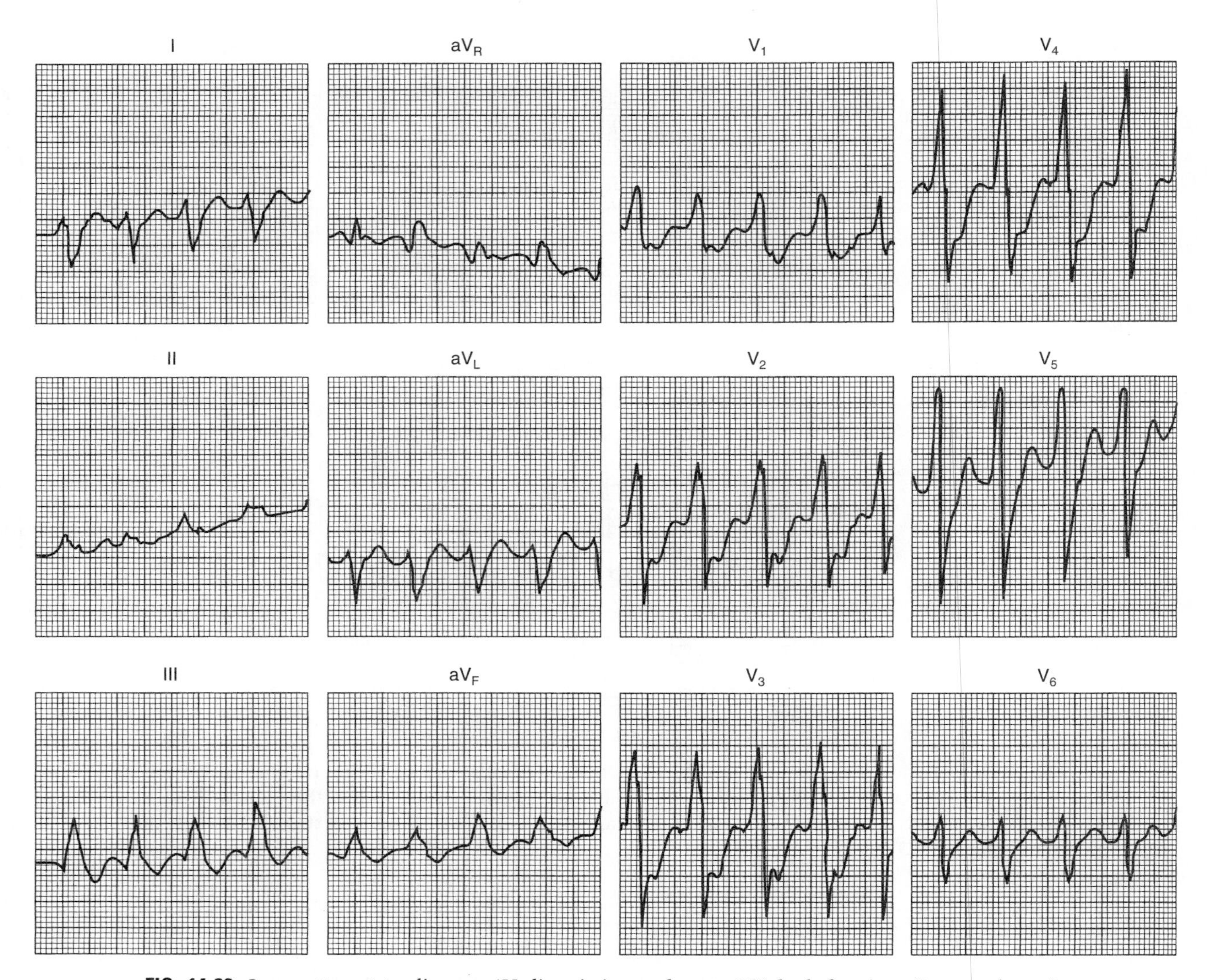

FIG. 14-26. In an attempt to discover AV dissociation and prove VT, look for sinus P waves (seen in lead II). There is a P wave between the first and second QRS complexes and one distorting the fourth QRS complex.

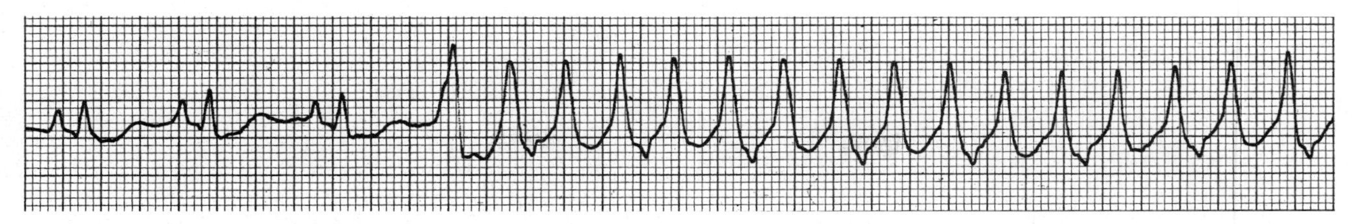

FIG. 14-27. VT with 2:1 retrograde conduction ratio. The retrograde P′ waves (negative in lead II) in every other T wave are diagnostic of VT. In approximately 50% of cases VT has some form of retrograde conduction to the atria.

for a distortion in one cycle that is not seen in another. This is found in leads I, II, and III, being most apparent in lead II. There is a sinus P wave before the second QRS and one distorting the last QRS. The P waves are independent; therefore, this is AV dissociation and the patient has VT. Of course, the R wave in V_1 also would have secured the diagnosis of VT. The right axis deviation suggests VT, but is not diagnostic.

Retrograde Conduction to the Atria During VT

Fifty percent of the time there is some form of retrograde conduction to the atria during VT. (The P′ waves are negative in leads II, III, and aV_F and positive in lead aV_R.) To visualize this on the ECG, however, ventriculoatrial (VA) conduction time must be sufficiently long so that the P′ waves occur outside the QRS complex. VA conduction with a 1:1 ratio is present in one fourth to one third of patients with VT at heart rates of less than 180 beats/min (without drugs). When the heart rate is more than 200 beats/min, 1:1 AV conduction is uncommon.[2]

Fig. 14-27 shows VT with 2:1 retrograde conduction. Note the negative P′ waves in every other T wave. Fig. 14-28 is VT with 4:3 retrograde Wenckebach conduction; look in leads II and III. Find the P′ wave between the third and fourth QRS; it is easy to spot because it is separate from the T wave. After identification of the P′ and the T in that cycle, it becomes evident that the preceding two T waves are dis-

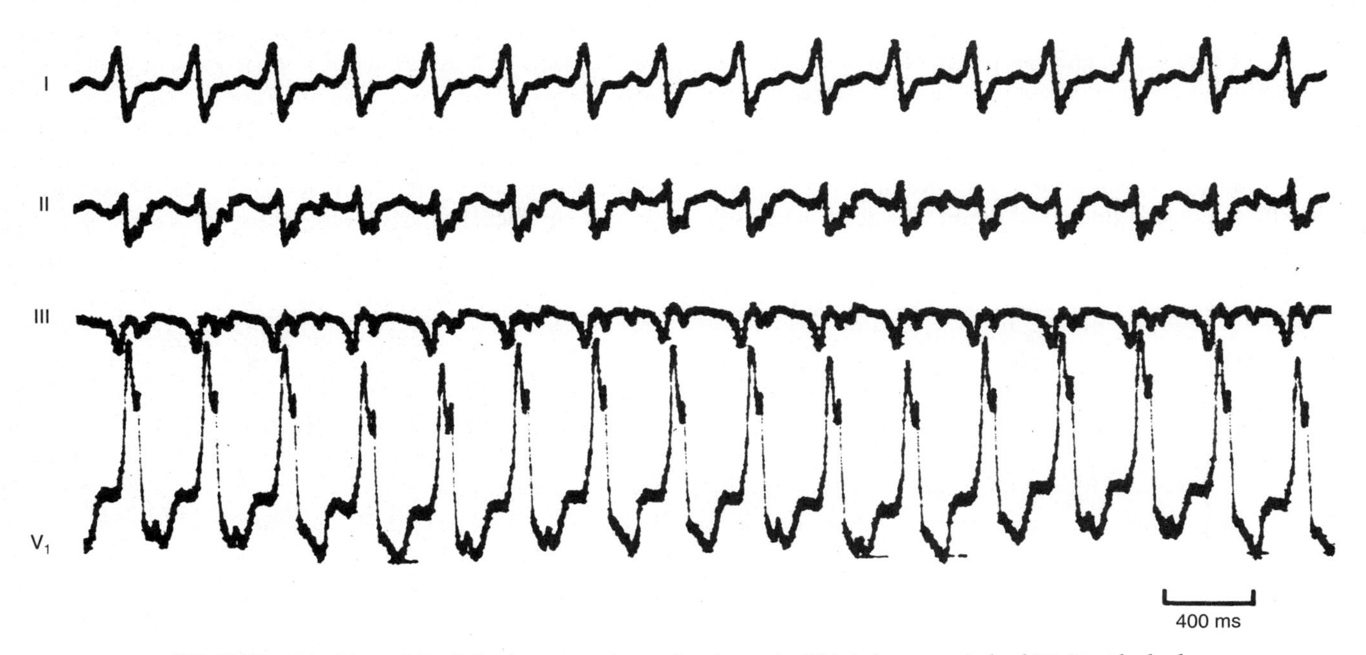

FIG. 14-28. VT with 4:3 Wenckebach retrograde conduction ratio. This is best seen in lead III. Start by looking between the third and fourth QRS complexes. The P wave seen there is not in the same place in the next cycle. You will now easily see the P waves distorting the first and second T waves and then note that there is no P wave at all in or near the fourth T wave. This sequence then repeats itself, with the RP becoming longer until ventriculoatrial conduction fails. (Courtesy Hein J.J. Wellens, MD, Maastricht, The Netherlands.)

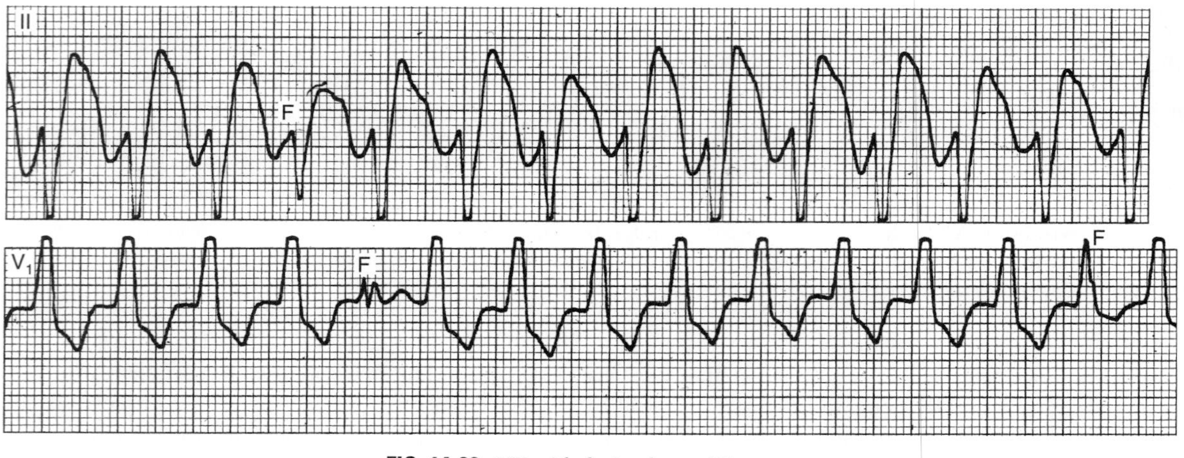

FIG. 14-29. VT with fusion beats *(F)*.

torted by P′ waves and that the cycle after the fourth QRS has no T wave at all. This Wenckebach sequence of lengthening RP′ intervals and then nonconduction is repeated. Other signs that support a diagnosis of VT in Fig. 14-28 are the left axis deviation, a very wide QRS, and the "rabbit ear" sign in lead V_1 (Rr′).

QRS Width

In the broad QRS tachycardia, a QRS duration of more than 0.14 second is highly suggestive of VT. Wellens[16] has shown in a study of 100 cases of SVT with aberration that a QRS width less than or equal to 0.14 second was present in all patients. He and his associates also studied 100 cases of VT and found that 59% had a QRS duration of more than 0.14 second. Akhtar et al[8] found "excellent" diagnostic accuracy for VT when they used a criterion for QRS duration of more than 0.14 second with a V_1-positive pattern and more than 0.16 second with a V_1-negative pattern.

Narrow Complexes During Broad QRS Tachycardia

When a narrow complex is seen during a broad QRS tachycardia, the possibilities include the following: capture or fusion, an echo beat, or conduction down the AV node-His-Purkinje axis during atrial fibrillation with an accessory pathway.

Capture and fusion beats. Capture beats occur when the position of a sinus impulse in the cardiac cycle of the VT is such that it is able to conduct to the ventricles, producing a narrow complex. It may capture the ventricles completely

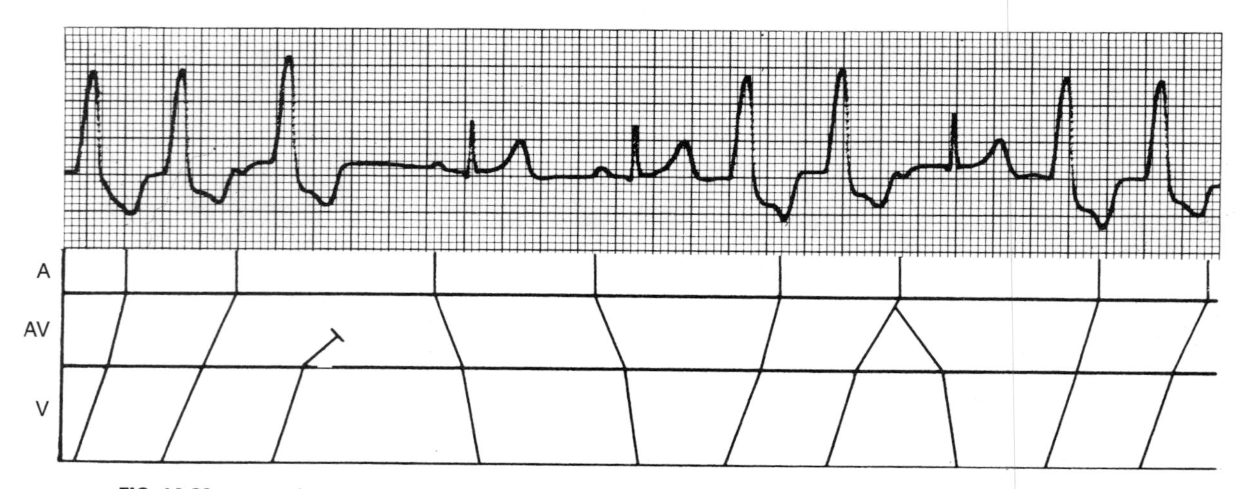

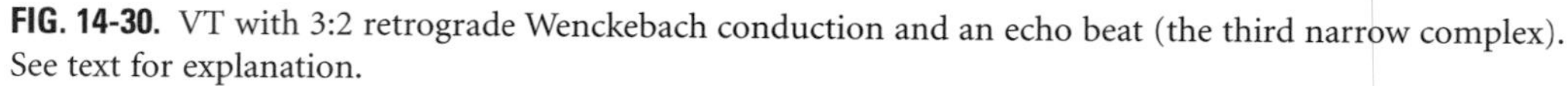

FIG. 14-30. VT with 3:2 retrograde Wenckebach conduction and an echo beat (the third narrow complex). See text for explanation.

or fuse with the ventricular impulse that is discharging at approximately the same time, creating a narrow beat. Fig. 14-29, *A* and *B*, show ventricular fusion *(F)* during VT. Another cause of ventricular fusion and a narrow complex is a second ventricular focus firing at the same time as the primary one. A fusion beat is a strong sign of VT. However, fusion beats are rarely seen and therefore have limited value.

Echo beats. During VT it is possible for the ventricular impulse to be conducted retrogradely into the atria. In fact, this happens approximately 50% of the time. Occasionally the retrograde atrial activity loops around and returns to the ventricles, producing a narrow complex. Fig. 14-30 is an example of VT with 3:2 retrograde Wenckebach conduction. After the first Wenckebach period (first three beats) there is a pause caused by absence of VA conduction of the third beat in the set. This allows the sinus node a couple of beats and then back again into VT with its retrograde Wenckebach. This time the second retrograde P′ wave returns to the ventricle to produce the echo beat, another narrow QRS complex. The laddergram helps one visualize the mechanism.

Concordant Pattern

The term *concordant pattern* refers to entirely positive or entirely negative QRS complexes in the precordial leads during the tachycardia.

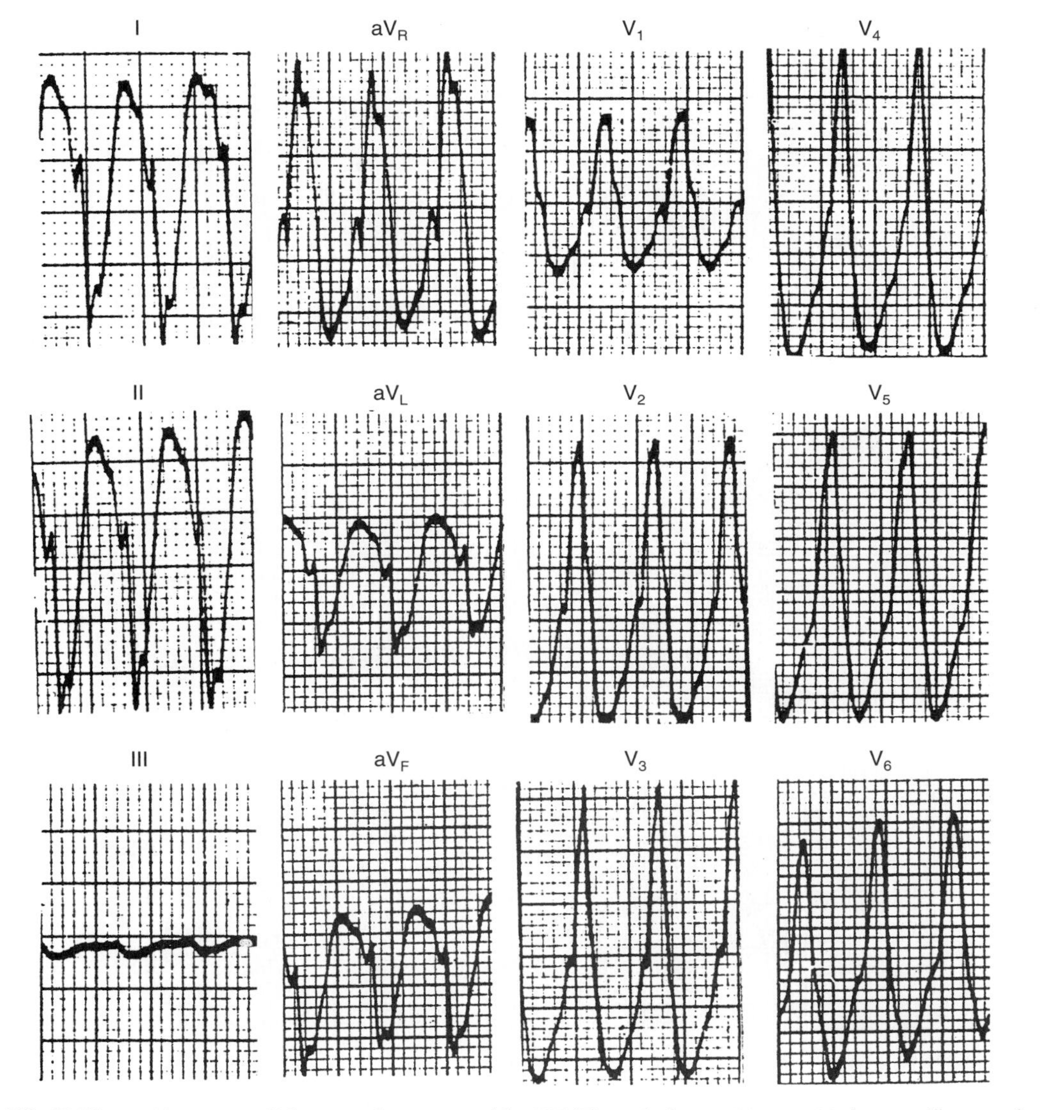

FIG. 14-31. Positive precordial concordance caused by VT. The axis from –90 to –180 degrees ("no man's land") can also be seen.

Negative precordial concordance, previously seen in Fig. 14-22, reflects a focus in the anteroapical left ventricle and is diagnostic of VT. This is because there is no accessory pathway location where conduction down the pathway would produce negative QRS complexes in all precordial leads.

Positive precordial concordance results when ventricular activation originates in the posterobasal left ventricle. Thus such a pattern can result both from VT with a focus in that region (Fig. 14-31) and from SVT with an accessory pathway located in that region (Fig. 14-32). However, because positive precordial concordance caused by SVT is rare, this finding should raise the level of suspicion for VT.

Other ECG Signs of VT

In 1991 Brugada et al[17] set forth four "new" rules for VT:

1. Absence of RS in all precordial leads
2. Delayed S nadir of more than 0.1 second in any RS lead
3. AV dissociation, fusion, or capture beats already mentioned

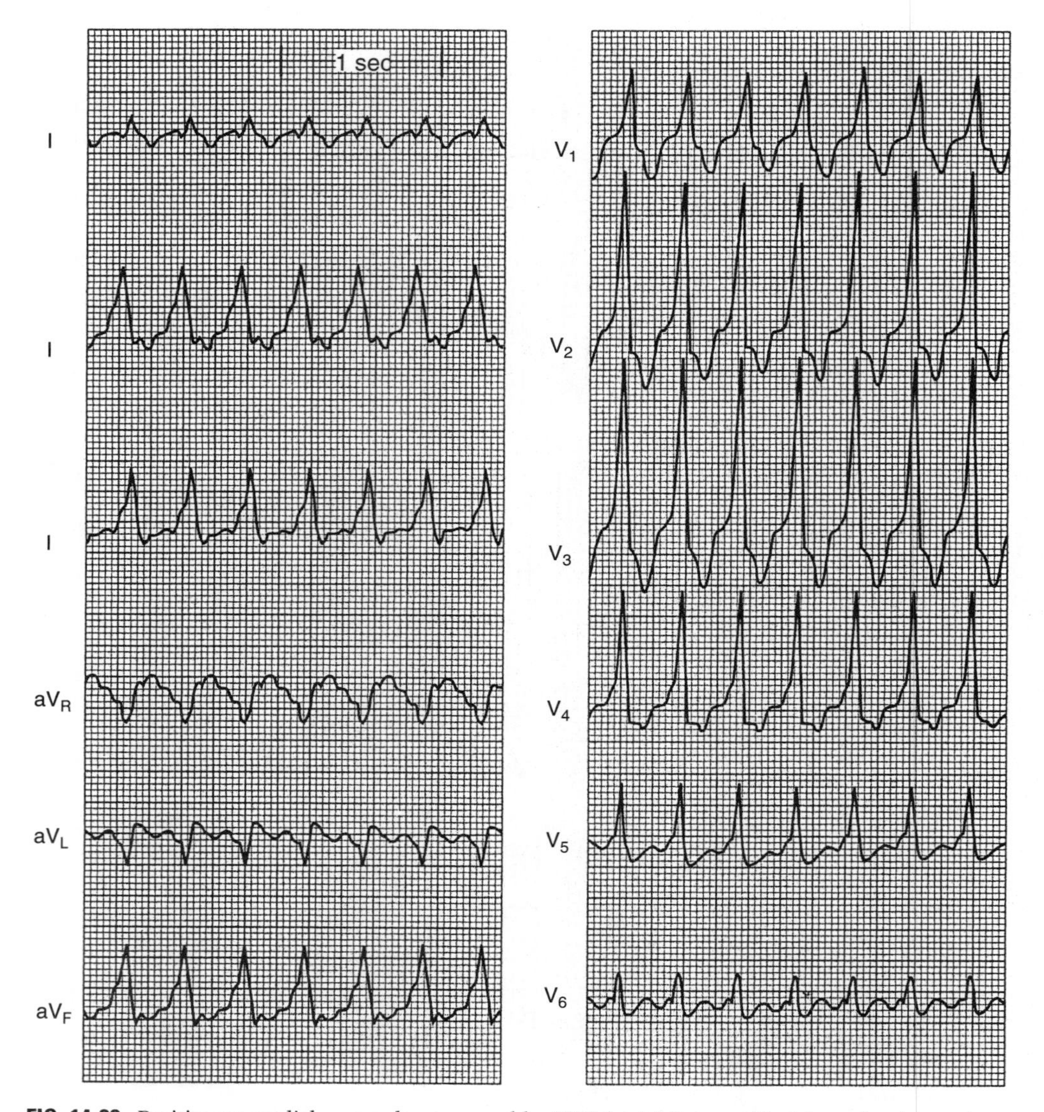

FIG. 14-32. Positive precordial concordance caused by SVT (atrial flutter with 2:1 conduction ratio over a left-sided accessory pathway). (From Wellens HJJ, Conover M: *The ECG in emergency decision making,* Philadelphia, 1992, WB Saunders.)

4. Morphologic clues in V_1 and V_6 already mentioned

The second point has limited usefulness because a delayed S nadir of more than 0.1 second may also occur in cases of SVT with conduction over an accessory pathway, administration of drugs that slow intraventricular conduction, and preexisting BBB—especially, LBBB.[16]

EMERGENCY RESPONSE TO BROAD QRS TACHYCARDIA[18]

If Hemodynamically Unstable

- Direct current cardioversion immediately
- Stabilize
- Evaluate systematically
- Diagnose

Examine the precardioversion and postcardioversion ECGs for mechanism, looking for signs of AV dissociation and a QRS morphologic clue to the origin of the tachycardia. It is important to remember that not all hemodynamically unstable patients with broad QRS tachycardia have VT. SVT with aberration is a definite possibility, in which case important decisions must be made about the differential diagnosis that still remains (i.e., the mechanism of the SVT).

If Hemodynamically Stable

- Evaluate systematically
- Diagnose
- Treat

Systematic Evaluation[18]

A good patient outcome for "now" and a long-term with the possibility of a cure is dependent on a systematic approach to a correct diagnosis.

1. Look for the physical signs of AV dissociation (cannon A waves in the jugular pulse, varying intensity of the first heart sound, and beat-to-beat changes in the systolic blood pressure).
2. Carefully and systematically evaluate the 12-lead ECG. If the baseline ECG is available, compare it with the QRS morphology during the tachycardia and determine if there is preexisting BBB, previous MI, or overt signs of WPW syndrome.
3. Perform a vagal maneuver; in some cases, this will terminate the tachycardia or reveal the mechanism (e.g., atrial flutter).
4. Obtain a history searching for evidence of previous MI, organic heart disease, known BBB, WPW syndrome, and drugs being taken. Class IA or IC drugs can cause VT.

If VT

1. Procainamide unless ischemia related (as in acute MI), then lidocaine; if unsuccessful:
2. Cardiovert
3. Examine and compare the ECG of VT with the postconversion ECG to discover mechanism

If SVT

1. Vagal stimulation; if unsuccessful:
2. Adenosine; if unsuccessful:
3. Procainamide; if unsuccessful:
4. Cardiovert
5. Examine and compare the ECG with broad QRS with the postconversion ECG to discover mechanism

If Irregular

Do not give digitalis or verapamil. Give intravenous procainamide unless torsades de pointes is present (see Chapter 26).

When the broad QRS tachycardia is irregular, special considerations are in order. There are three possibilities with three different and specific treatments:

- Torsades de pointes (see Chapter 26)
- Atrial fibrillation with BBB or atrial flutter with BBB and variable AV conduction (see Chapter 23)
- Atrial fibrillation with an accessory pathway or atrial flutter with an accessory pathway and variable AV conduction (see Chapter 21)

VT That Looks Like SVT

In some cases all rules regarding QRS morphology are defied. There are cases of VT that look like SVT with aberration; they are those that are idiopathic, or those caused by digitalis toxicity or bundle branch reentry. In these cases one is guided by the clinical picture (normal heart, digitalis toxicity, or cardiomyopathy). Table 14-1 summarizes the types of VT that look like VT, VT that looks like SVT, and SVT that looks like VT.

SVT That Looks Like VT

Likewise, some cases of SVT look exactly like VT; they are those that use an accessory pathway to enter the ventricles (atrial flutter, atrial fibrillation, or antidromic circus movement tachycardia).

When in Doubt[18]

When the diagnosis in wide-complex tachycardia remains uncertain after applying the rules described in this chapter, application of the following rules protects your patient from receiving the wrong drugs:

TABLE 14-1 Classification of Broad QRS Tachycardia

Type	ECG Morphology	Cure	Chapter
VT THAT LOOKS LIKE VT			
Torsades de pointes (drug-related)	Polymorphic	Discontinue culprit drug	26
Torsades de pointes (congenital)	Polymorphic		25
Polymorphous VT (ischemia-related)	Polymorphic		26
V_1 negative	V_1/V_2: broad R, slurred S downstroke, delayed S nadir; V_6: Q wave		13
V_1 positive	V_1: Rr′ (rabbit ear sign), monophasic or biphasic		13
VT THAT LOOKS LIKE SVT			
Idiopathic (normal heart)	LBBB, inferior axis (aV_F positive) RBBB, superior axis (aV_F negative)	RFA	13
Fascicular	RBBB, right or left axis deviation	Discontinue digitalis	15
Bundle branch reentry	Usually LBBB	RFA	13
SVT THAT LOOKS LIKE VT (MAY HAVE A HISTORY OF PALPITATIONS)			
Atrial fibrillation (preexcitation)	That of VT, irregular; rate >250 beats/min	RFA	21
Atrial flutter (preexcitation)	That of VT	RFA	21
Antidromic CMT	That of VT	RFA	21

ECG, Electrocardiogram; *VT,* ventricular tachycardia; *SVT,* supraventricular tachycardia; *LBBB,* left bundle branch block; *RFA,* radiofrequency ablation; *RBBB,* right bundle branch block; *CMT,* circus movement tachycardia (refers to AV reentry mechanism).

1. Do not give verapamil; give procainamide, unless there is a possibility that you are dealing with torsades de pointes.
2. When confronted with a wide QRS tachycardia that is greater than 200 beats/min and irregular, do not give digitalis or verapamil; give procainamide.[18]

Although both verapamil and procainamide have negative inotropic effects, procainamide causes the rate of the VT to slow, partially compensating for the fall in blood pressure.[19] Procainamide also blocks conduction in accessory pathways to interrupt AV reentry, blocks the retrograde fast pathway in the AV node to terminate PSVT caused by AV nodal reentry, and terminates nonischemic VT.[20]

SIGNS AND SYMPTOMS NOT USED IN THE DIFFERENTIAL DIAGNOSIS

In the differential diagnosis of broad QRS tachycardia there four conditions that cannot be used. They are hemodynamic age, status, ventricular rate, and rhythm (regularity or irregularity).

- **Age:** VT can occur at any age.
- **Hemodynamics:** Some patients are hemodynamically stable in spite of VT and hemodynamically compromised during SVT.
- **Heart rate:** Although SVT tends to be faster than VT, there is too much overlap for this to be a useful sign.
- **Regularity:** A regular, broad QRS tachycardia may be VT or SVT with BBB or conduction over an accessory pathway. Occasionally VT can be very irregular, especially when drug-induced (e.g., torsades de pointes; see Chapter 26).

SUMMARY

Monomorphic VT is usually regular and has a uniform beat-to-beat QRS morphologic appearance. It may be idiopathic, a reperfusion arrhythmia, or caused by ischemia, myocardial infarction, arrhythmogenic right ventricular dysplasia, or bundle branch reentry in patients with cardiomyopathy.

In SVT (sinus tachycardia, atrial tachycardia, atrial flutter, atrial, fibrillation, and AV nodal reentry) a broad QRS can occur because of functional BBB (aberrant ventricular conduction) or anterograde conduction over an accessory pathway. Therefore in regular broad QRS tachycardia it is important to differentiate between aberrant ventricular conduction and VT because of the different emergency treatments and clinical implications for the long term.

The emergency response to broad QRS tachycardia demands a calm, informed, and systematic approach. A hemodynamically unstable patient is cardioverted immediately. If stable, the 12-lead ECG is systematically evaluated, the physical signs of AV dissociation are searched for, and a history is taken questioning the presence of prior MI or structural heart disease.

Broad QRS tachycardia is classified according to its polarity in V_1 for the purposes of differentiating SVT with aberrancy from VT. After this division is made, the QRS morphology in V_1, and sometimes in V_2 and V_6 can accurately identify VT in 90% of cases. In V_1-negative patterns a broad R, slurred S downstroke, and delayed S nadir in V_1 or V_2, or both, or a Q wave in V_6 indicate VT. In V_1-positive patterns a monophasic R, biphasic pattern, or Rr′ in V_1 indicate VT.

Additional highly reliable ECG criteria for VT are AV dissociation, QRS duration greater than 0.14 second in V_1-positive patterns, QRS duration greater than 0.16 second in V_1-negative patterns, negative precordial concordance (diagnostic), positive precordial concordance (highly supportive), axis of –90 degrees to 180 degrees, V_1-negative patterns associated with right axis deviation, fusion or capture beats, and a QRS pattern that is different from sinus rhythm when there is preexisting BBB.

REFERENCES

1. Sandler JA, Marriott HJL: The differential morphology of anomalous ventricular complexes of RBBB type in lead V_1: ventricular ectopy versus aberration, *Circulation* 31:551, 1965.
2. Marriott HJL, Sandler JA: Criteria, old and new, for differentiation between ectopic ventricular beats and aberrant ventricular conduction in the presence of atrial fibrillation, *Prog Cardiovasc Dis* 9:18, 1966.
3. Marriott HJL: Differential diagnosis of supraventricular and ventricular tachycardia, *Geriatrics* 25:91, 1970.
4. Wellens HJJ, Bär FW, Vanagt EJ, Brugada P: Medical treatment of ventricular tachycardia: considerations in the selection of patients for surgical treatment, *Am J Cardiol* 49:186, 1982.
5. Kindwell KE, Brown J, Josephson ME: Electrocardiographic criteria for ventricular tachycardia in wide complex left bundle branch block morphology tachycardia, *Am J Cardiol* 61:1279, 1988.
6. Singer DH, Cohen HC: Aberrancy: electrophysiologic aspects and clinical correlations. In Mandel WJ, editor: *Cardiac arrhythmias,* Philadelphia, 1987, JB Lippincott.
7. Wellens HJJ, Ross DL, Farré J et al: Functional bundle branch block during supraventricular tachycardia in man: observations on mechanisms and their incidence. In Zipes D, Jalife J, editors: *Cardiac electrophysiology and arrhythmias,* New York, 1985, Grune and Stratton.
8. Akhtar M, Shenasa M, Jazayeri M et al: Wide QRS complex tachycardia: reappraisal of a common clinical problem, *Ann Intern Med* 109:905, 1988.
9. Wellens HJJ, Brugada P, Bär F: Diagnosis and treatment of the regular tachycardia with a narrow QRS complex. In Kulbertus HE, editors: *Medical management of cardiac arrhythmias,* Edinburgh, 1986, Churchill Livingstone.
10. Zipes DP: Specific arrhythmias: diagnosis and treatment. In Braunwald E, editor: *Heart disease,* ed 4, Philadelphia, 1992, WB Saunders.
11. Kojima S, Fujii T, Ohe T et al: Physiologic changes during supraventricular tachycardia and release of atrial naturetic peptide, *Am J Cardiol* 62:576, 1988.
12. Leitch JW, Klein GJ, Yee R et al: Syncope associated with supraventricular tachycardia; an expression of tachycardia rate or vasomotor response? *Circulation* 85:1064, 1992.
13. Josephson ME, Wellens HJJ: Differential diagnosis of supraventricular tachycardia, *Cardiol Clin* 8:411, 1990.
14. Tchou P, Young P, Mahmud R et al: Useful clinical criteria for the diagnosis of ventricular tachycardia, *Am J Med* 84:53, 1988.
15. Rosenbaum MB: Classification of ventricular extrasystoles according to form, *J Electrocardiol* 2:289, 1969.
16. Wellens HJJ: Wide QRS tachycardia. In Willerson JT, Cohn JN, editors: *Cardiovascular medicine,* New York, 1995, Churchill Livingstone.
17. Brugada P, Brugada J, Mont L et al: A new approach to the differential diagnosis of a regular tachycardia with a wide QRS complex, *Circulation* 83:1649, 1991.
18. Wellens HJJ, Conover M: *The ECG in emergency decision making,* Philadelphia, 1992, WB Saunders, p 37.
19. Marchlinski FE, Buxton AE, Vassallo JA et al: Comparative electrophysiologic effects of intravenous and oral procainamide in patients with sustained ventricular arrhythmias, *J Am Coll Cardiol* 4:1247, 1984.
20. Gorgels AP, van den Dool A, Hofs A et al: Procainamide is superior to lidocaine in terminating sustained ventricular tachycardia, *Circulation* 80:2590, 1989.

CHAPTER 15

Digitalis-Induced Arrhythmias

Digitalis toxicity remains a significant clinical problem, although the monitoring of serum digoxin levels, a better understanding of the pharmacokinetics, and introduction of alternate approaches for rate control have caused a decrease in its frequency.[1,2] Successful treatment depends on early recognition. However, the diagnosis of potentially life-threatening toxicity remains difficult because the clinical presentation is often subtle and nonspecific and the electrocardiographic (ECG) signs do not seem life-threatening until the final event. Because of the high mortality associated with digitalis toxicity it is imperative for those who care for patients taking digitalis to be familiar with ECG and physical signs of toxicity, mechanism, and treatment, and to establish a systematic diagnostic approach.

ECG RECOGNITION

When caring for a patient taking digitalis, be alert for these ECG features.[3]

Bradycardia when previously normal or fast
- Sinus bradycardia
- Sinoatrial block
- Atrioventricular (AV) block

Tachycardia when previously normal
- Atrial tachycardia with block
- Junctional tachycardia (rate, 70-140 beats/min)
- Fascicular ventricular tachycardia (VT)
- Double tachycardias (e.g., atrial and fascicular; atrial and junctional; atrial fibrillation and fascicular VT)

Unexpected regularity in atrial fibrillation
- Junctional tachycardia (rate, 70-140 beats/min)
- AV block with junctional escape (rate, less than 60 beats/min)

Group beating in atrial fibrillation
- Junctional tachycardia with Wenckebach exit block

Group beating in sinus rhythm
- Ventricular bigeminy
- Sinoatrial (SA) Wenckebach
- AV Wenckebach

Atrial flutter with
- AV dissociation
- High-degree AV block (bradycardia)

LIFE-THREATENING ARRHYTHMIAS

Life-threatening arrhythmias are as follows:

- Profound bradycardia
- Atrial tachycardia
- Junctional tachycardia
- Fascicular ventricular tachycardia

These arrhythmias of themselves are not difficult to diagnose. However, atrial tachycardia is often misdiagnosed as sinus tachycardia because the P′ wave looks like a sinus P wave. A digitalis-toxic junctional tachycardia is often ignored because its rate is only 70 to 140 beats/min and the QRS is narrow; unfortunately, the presence of AV dissociation often attracts more interest than the tachycardia that has caused it. Life-threatening fascicular VT is often misdiagnosed as junctional tachycardia with bundle branch block (BBB). Even the near-terminal bifascicular VT, although recognized as life-threatening, is mislabeled "bidirectional VT" and digitalis is not implicated. To complicate the ECG diagnosis even more, the arrhythmias of digitalis toxicity often appear in the company of another arrhythmia, as previously listed. If these arrhythmias are untreated, the mortality for any one of them is 100%.[4]

These very daunting clinical difficulties demand education and a systematic approach to the ECG, outlined in Box 15-1, and an evaluation of symptoms as reported by the patient and observed by the family.

SYSTEMATIC APPROACH

1. Talk to the patient and family regarding any noncardiac signs of digitalis intoxication (especially reduced visual acuity or red/green color distortions and personality changes), dosage, additional medication, and complaints.
2. Evaluate the atrial rhythm. Are there P waves? If so, what is the rate and the polarity of the P waves in leads II and aV_F? The P waves will be positive in those leads if atrial tachycardia is caused by digitalis.
3. Is there AV conduction? If so, what type (2:1 or AV Wenckebach)?
4. If there is no AV conduction, are the ventricular beats junctional or fascicular in origin? This is evaluated in lead V_1 or MCL_1.
5. If atrial fibrillation is present, is the rhythm appropriately irregular and not too slow? Or is there regularity or group beating? If the rhythm is regular, what is the morphologic appearance of the QRS in V_1? (right bundle branch block [RBBB] = fascicular VT; normal = junctional rhythm).

Note: Wenckebach conduction is lengthening conduction times until a beat is not conducted and the cycle begins again (p. 219). In sinus rhythm with AV Wenckebach the PR intervals can be seen and the signs of Wenckebach conduction are easily recognized (group beating, lengthening PRs, shortening RRs, and pauses less than twice the shortest cycle). During atrial fibrillation the PRs are of course absent, and the Wenckebach conduction takes place from a junctional or fascicular focus. Thus all of the ECG signs of Wenckebach are present except the PR intervals (group beating; or shortening RRs and pauses less than twice the shortest cycle).

SINUS BRADYCARDIA

Slowing of the sinus node rate by digitalis is mediated by the vagus nerve and by the direct effect of digitalis. Sinus bradycardia is often accompanied by a junctional escape rhythm, which is usually idiojunctional because of the blocking effect of digitalis on AV and ventriculoatrial conduction. Fig. 15-1 is sinus bradycardia with junctional escape. The junctional beats have a slightly different shape from the sinus conducted beats because of an offset focus in the AV junction.

BOX 15-1. Systematic Evaluation of the ECG for Digitalis Toxicity

P WAVE REGULARITY, RATE, AND POLARITY

If irregular, SA block?
If rate >120 beats/min, evaluate polarity in leads II and aV_F
Atrial tachycardia?

AV CONDUCTION

Signs of AV Wenckebach?
Signs of complete AV block?

AV JUNCTIONAL RHYTHM

Are all QRS complexes conducted?
If not, what is the rate of the AV junctional focus?
Is tachycardia paroxysmal or nonparoxysmal?
In nonparoxysmal and the rate is 70-130 beats/min—digitalis-toxic AV junctional tachycardia

FASCICULAR VENTRICULAR TACHYCARDIA

Are the ventricular complexes conducted from the atrium?
If not, what is the rate?
If 60-90 beats/min, suspect fascicular ventricular tachycardia
What is morphology in lead V_1?
If RBBB, what is the axis?
If abnormal—fascicular ventricular tachycardia

ATRIAL FIBRILLATION

Is the rhythm intermittently or completely regular?
What is the QRS morphology in lead V_1?
- If RBBB, suspect fascicular ventricular tachycardia resulting from digitalis toxicity
- If normal, suspect a junctional rhythm resulting from junctional tachycardia or AV block secondary to digitalis toxicity

ATRIAL FLUTTER

Does the flutter–R wave relationship have a pattern (fixed? alternative?)?
If not, is the ventricular rhythm regular?
If so—AV dissociation; assess ventricular rate and QRS morphology
- If ventricular rate <60 beats/min—atrial flutter with complete AV block
- If QRS is normal and rate 70-140 beats/min—atrial flutter with AV dissociation and AV junctional tachycardia resulting from digitalis toxicity
- If RBBB and rate 90-160 beats/min—atrial flutter, AV dissociation, and fascicular ventricular tachycardia resulting from digitalis toxicity

From Wellens HJJ, Conover M: *The ECG in emergency decision making*, Philadelphia, 1992, WB Saunders.

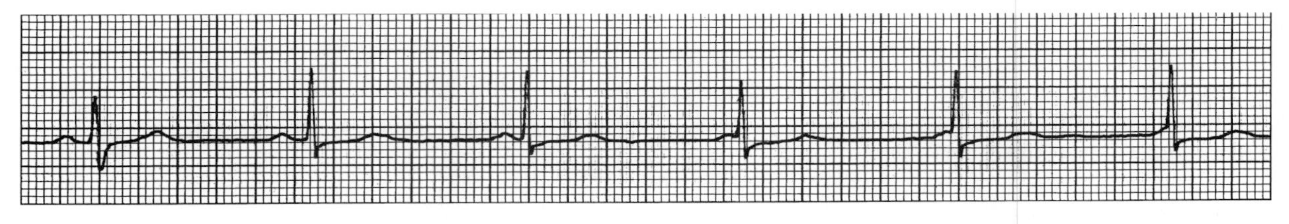

FIG. 15-1. Sinus bradycardia of 52 beats/min interrupted by a junctional escape rhythm of 54 beats/min. The junctional beats are easily spotted not only because the P wave begins to disappear as they overtake the sinus rhythm, but because they are shaped a little differently.

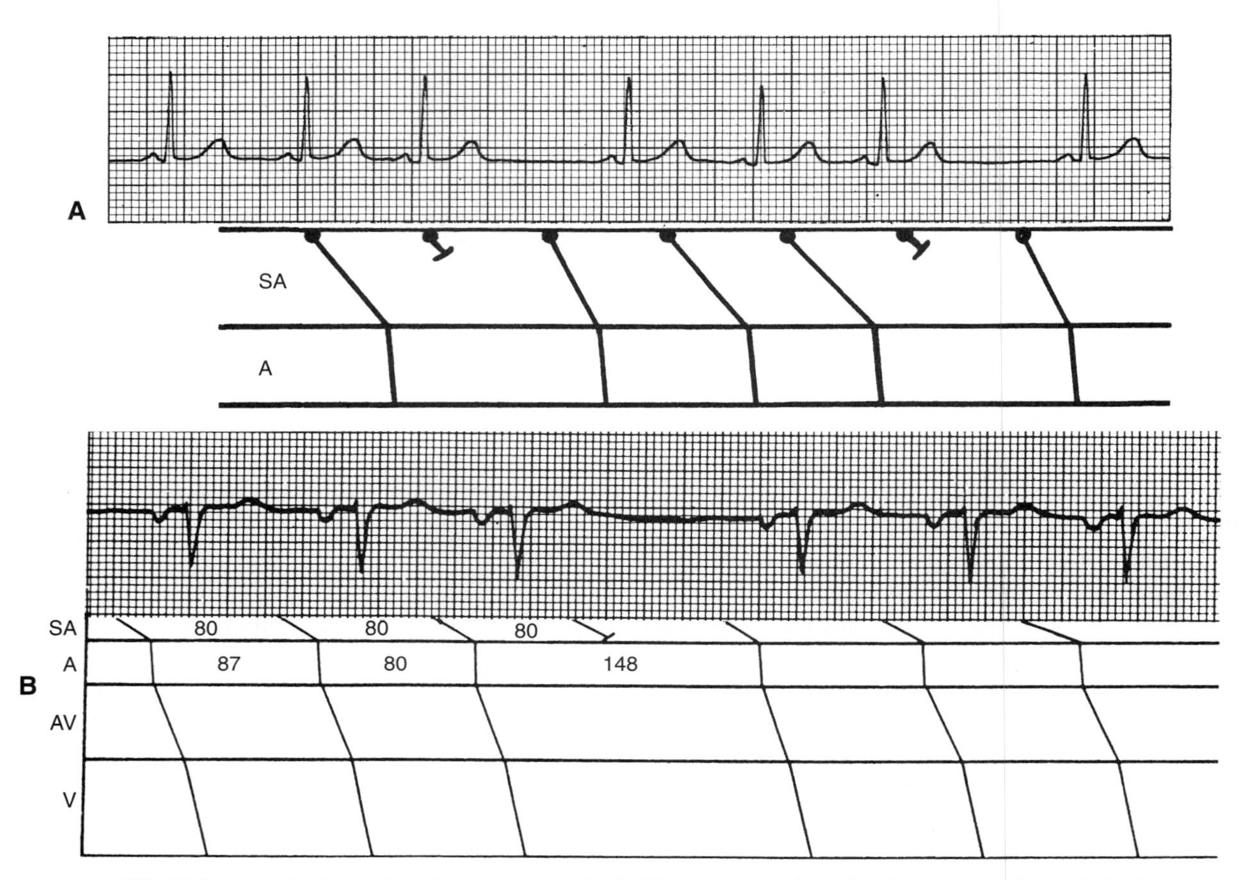

FIG. 15-2. **A** and **B**, Examples of 4:3 SA Wenckebach. These tracings show the classic signs of Wenckebach conduction: group beating, shortening RR intervals, and pauses less than twice the shortest cycle. However, because the PR intervals are short and all equal, the Wenckebach conduction must be higher in the conduction system between the sinus node and the atrial musculature. The laddergrams illustrate the regular sinus node discharge (SA tier) with SA conduction becoming longer and longer until it blocks, creating the tell-tale groups of P waves.

SA BLOCK

Digitalis, even in therapeutic doses, can impair the conduction of the sinus impulse to the atrial tissue. Such a block can be of the Wenckebach type, as demonstrated in Fig. 15-2, *A* and *B*. Sinoatrial Wenckebach is recognized by the same clues as AV Wenckebach except that the PR intervals are fixed (i.e., the same before and after the pause—unless of course AV Wenckebach is also present). Thus in SA Wenckebach, in addition to the fixed PR intervals, there is group beating, shortening RR intervals, and pauses less than twice the shortest cycle.

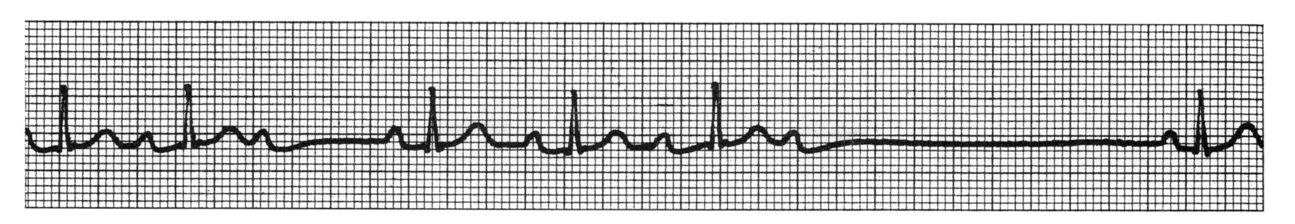

FIG. 15-3. SA block and AV Wenckebach. Absent P waves during the long pause indicates SA block. The group in the center of the tracing shows lengthening PR intervals with a 4:3 Wenckebach period. There are serious conduction problems at two levels—the sinus node and the AV node.

In Fig. 15-3 two levels of block are noted, SA and AV. In the center group, note the shortening PP intervals, an indication of SA Wenckebach, although the long pause is not typical. The PR intervals are not fixed as they would be in SA block; they lengthen with each cycle. The RR intervals shorten as they would in either SA or AV block. The first pause is less than twice the shortest cycle. Thus the signs of SA and AV Wenckebach are present.

ATRIOVENTRICULAR BLOCK

Fig. 15-4 shows sinus bradycardia and alarming prolongation of the PR interval during digitalis therapy—an early sign of toxicity. Fig. 15-5 is an example of life-threatening AV block during atrial fibrillation. There is also ventricular bigeminy.

ATRIAL TACHYCARDIA

Within 5 to 20 beats of the initiation of the tachycardias of digitalis intoxication a steady-state rate is usually established. This rate may vary slightly thereafter and increases along with the digoxin level, the arrhythmias of toxicity being dose-related.

In the atrial tachycardia of digitalis toxicity the focus is high in the right atrium, close to the sinus node. Therefore the P′ waves are identical in morphology or almost so to the sinus P waves, and are usually associated with AV block. The rhythm is exacerbated by hypokalemia.[5] As with other digitalis-related tachycardias, emergence is promoted by shortening of the cycle lengths of preceding beats and by catecholamines.

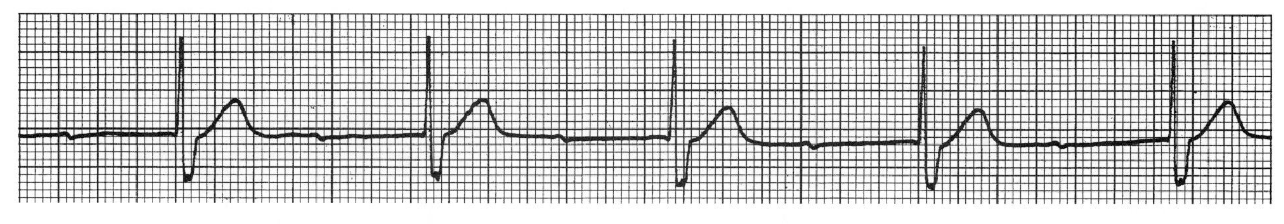

FIG. 15-4. Sinus bradycardia (47 beats/min) with a prolonged PR interval (0.48 second).

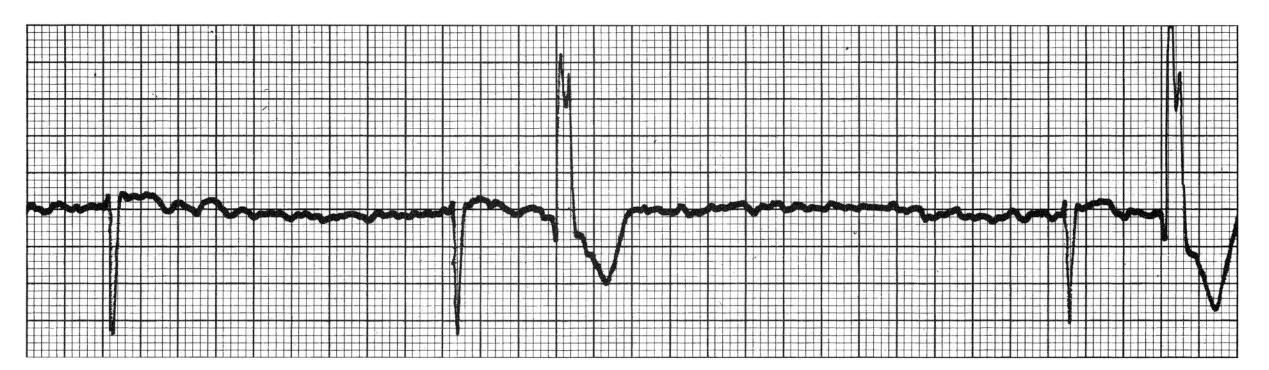

FIG. 15-5. Atrial fibrillation with AV block and ventricular bigeminy.

ECG Recognition

Atrial rate: 130 to 250 beats/min.

P waves: Similar in shape to sinus P waves (upright in leads II, III, and aV_F).

QRS complex: Narrow unless BBB is also present.

AV block: Usually present (2:1 or AV Wenckebach).

P′P′ intervals: Often ventriculophasic, that is, the P′P′ interval on either side of the R wave is shorter than the P′P′ interval without an R wave. This is a vagal effect. When the aortic pressure influences the baroreceptors of the carotid body, the next atrial cycle (without an R wave) is longer.[6]

Best lead: II (the P′ wave is upright and similar in shape to the sinus P wave).

Rhythm Variations: The Many Faces of Atrial Tachycardia

Atrial tachycardia is often combined with either AV block or another tachycardia (junctional or fascicular), causing a confusing ECG picture.

Atrial tachycardia with high-grade AV block. Fig. 15-6 shows a life-threatening bradycardia caused by high-grade AV block against a background of atrial tachycardia (130 beats/min) in an acute digitalis overdose (suicide attempt), recorded at admission to the emergency department. Fig. 15-6, *B*, shows conduction improvement after treatment with Fab fragments.

Conversion from atrial fibrillation with bradycardia to atrial tachycardia. Fig. 15-7 is an example of a life-threatening digitalis toxic tachycardia that was recognized late, but treated in time to avoid hemodynamic impairment. These tracings also demonstrate the dose dependence of the tachycardia and AV block.

In the first tracing, the patient who is taking digoxin and quinidine has atrial fibrillation and high-grade AV block. The toxicity is not noticed and medications are continued.

Six days later, in the second tracing, the patient converts to atrial tachycardia (167 beats/min) with 1:1 conduction. The conversion rhythm was misdiagnosed as sinus tachycardia and the digoxin continued.

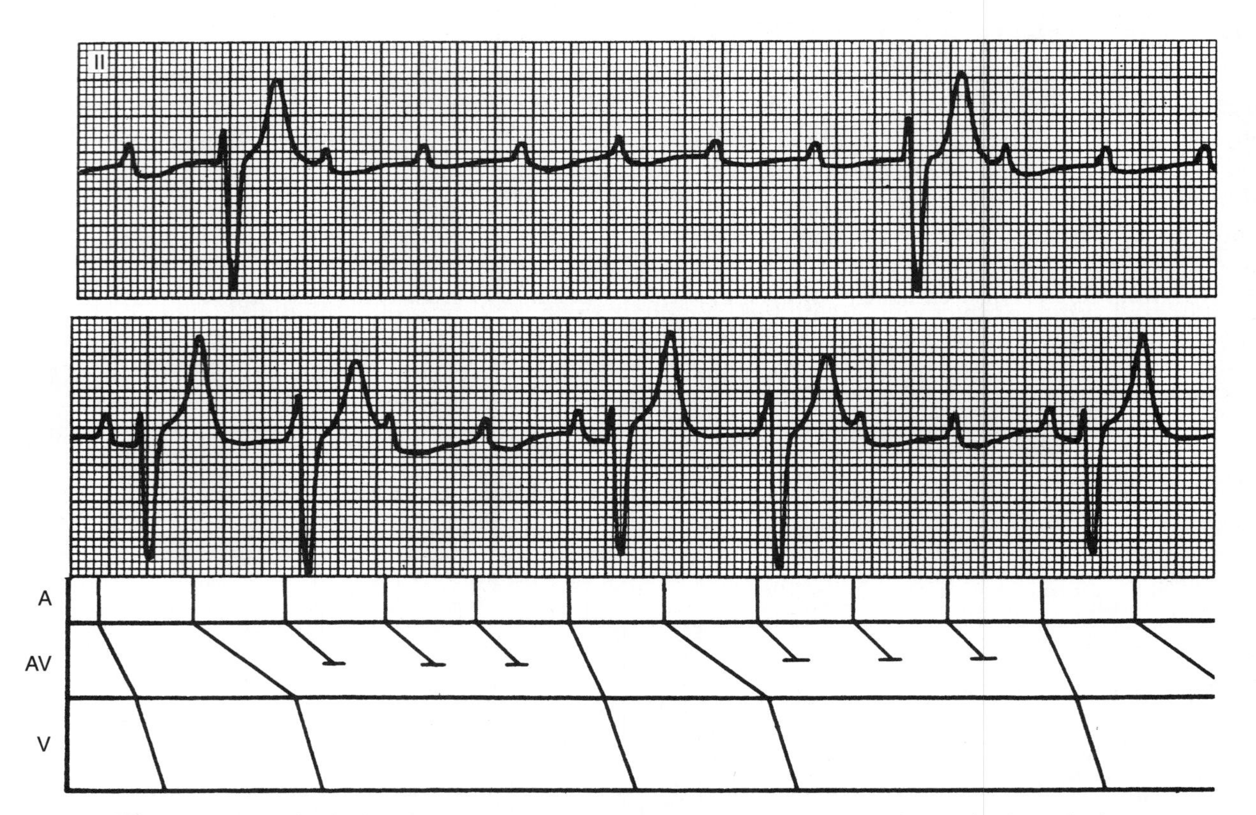

FIG. 15-6. The result of a digitalis overdose in a suicide attempt. *Top tracing,* Note the atrial tachycardia (130 beats/min); only two beats in the tracing are conducted because of the fixed prolonged PR intervals. *Bottom tracing,* After treatment with Digibind is under way the atrial tachycardia slows to a rate of 120 beats/min and conduction improves. The second and fourth complexes have what looks like an initial broad R wave, which is actually the P′ wave distorting the R. For every set of five P′ waves, only two are conducted with lengthening P′R intervals (a bigeminal rhythm).

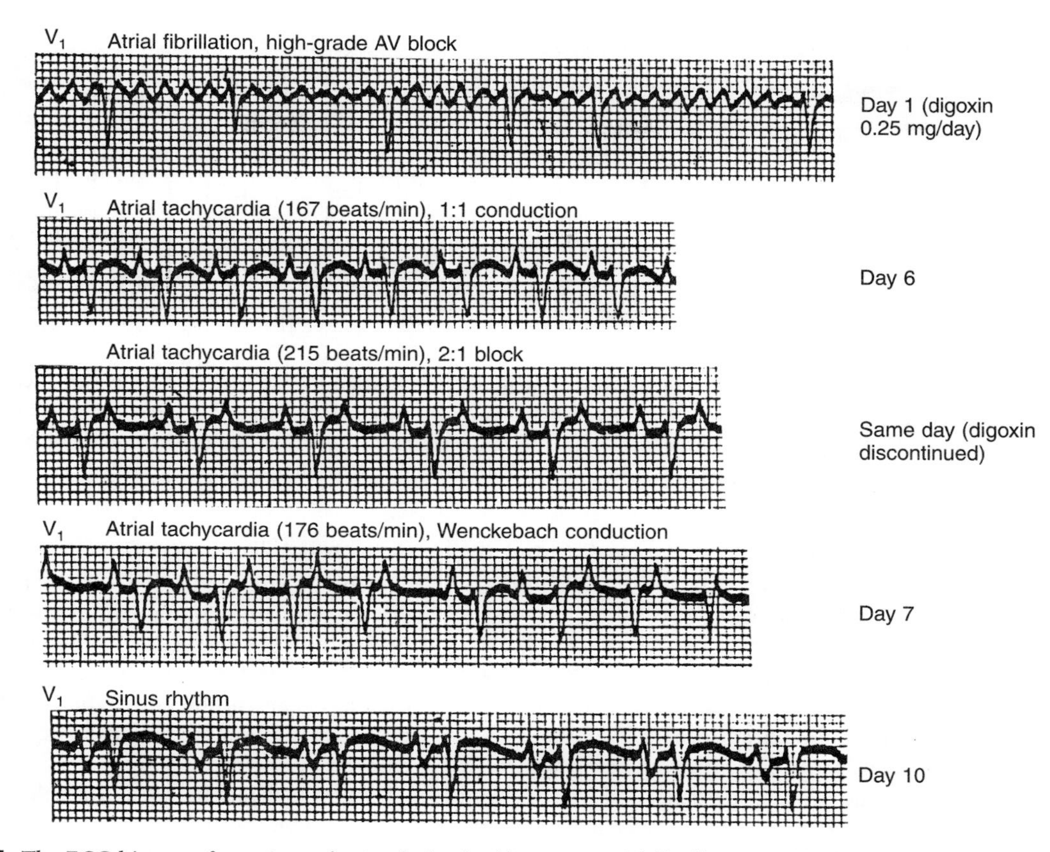

FIG. 15-7. The ECG history of a patient who is admitted with coarse atrial fibrillation and high-grade AV block caused by digitalis toxicity. See text for explanation.

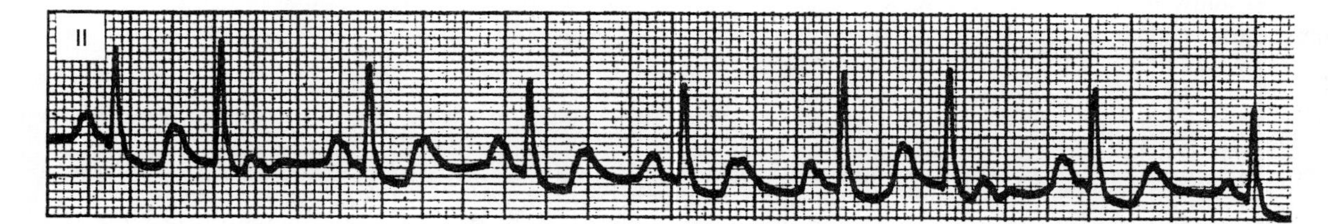

FIG. 15-8. Atrial tachycardia with 2:1 and Wenckebach conduction. See text for explanation. (Courtesy William P. Nelson, MD, Denver, Colo.)

Later the same day, as the digoxin blood level rises, the atrial rate increases from 167 to 215 beats/min, with *ventriculophasic PP intervals* and 2:1 block. This nicely illustrates the dose dependency of digoxin. At this point the problem is recognized and the digoxin discontinued.

The next day, with the drop in the digoxin level, the atrial rate slows to 176 beats/min and AV conduction improves in the form of a long and variable Wenckebach sequence (7:6 and 5:4). Of course, this means that the heart rate has jumped from 100 beats/min to approximately 150 beats/min; this is anticipated with the slower atrial rate and improved conduction.

Three days later, the rhythm has converted to sinus tachycardia and the patient is out of danger from intoxication with digoxin.

Atrial tachycardia with 2:1 and Wenckebach conduction. The tracing in Fig. 15-8 is another example of atrial tachycardia that was not immediately apparent. The patient was a 68-year-old man with chronic obstructive pulmonary disease and lung cancer. He was on digoxin 0.25 mg daily. A systematic approach will yield the diagnosis.

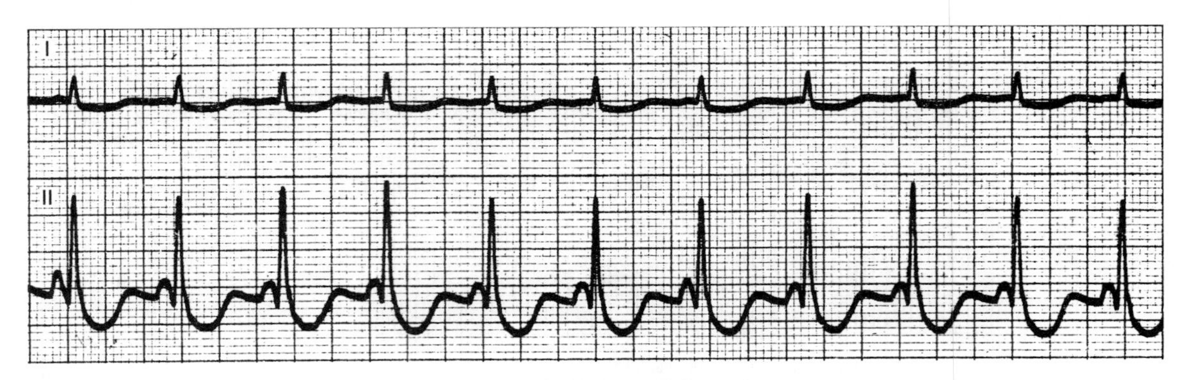

FIG. 15-9. Double tachycardia, atrial and junctional with isorhythmic AV dissociation. The P′ waves are very close to the QRS and are not seen in lead I because the mean atrial current is perpendicular to the axis of that lead. The atrial and junctional rates are 108 beats/min. Only when the two rates disagree will the AV dissociation become apparent. (Courtesy William P. Nelson, MD, Denver, Colo.)

1. What is the atrial rhythm? The P wave distorting the second ST segment gives a fix on the PP interval. The rest of the P waves can be found in T waves, in front of the R waves, and again in an ST segment. The atrial rate is 150 beats/min, and the P waves are upright in lead II, indicating atrial tachycardia as a result of digitalis intoxication.
2. Is there conduction? The irregular rhythm is your first clue to the presence of conduction. There is both 2:1 and Wenckebach 3:2 conduction.

Atrial tachycardia and junctional tachycardia. Fig. 15-9 shows a *double tachycardia.* The P′ waves in lead I are isoelectric and allow us to see the ventricular complexes as they are, narrow at a rate of 108 beats/min (junctional tachycardia). The P waves seem to pop out in lead II at exactly the same rate as that of the junctional tachycardia, clearly not conducting, and presenting the picture of isorhythmic AV dissociation. That is, the atria and ventricles are beating on their own, without interference from each other, and at the same rate. The main clinical concern is the recognition of digitalis toxicity and the appropriate emergency response.

Atrial tachycardia with 2:1 block deteriorating to 3:1. In Fig. 15-10, *A,* the atrial rate is 148 beats/min with 2:1 block in a patient with digitalis intoxication. In *B,* the atrial rate slows to 135 beats/min as the digoxin has been discontinued and the blood level is lowered; the conduction ratio, however, has deteriorated to 3:1 with a heart rate of 45 beats/min.

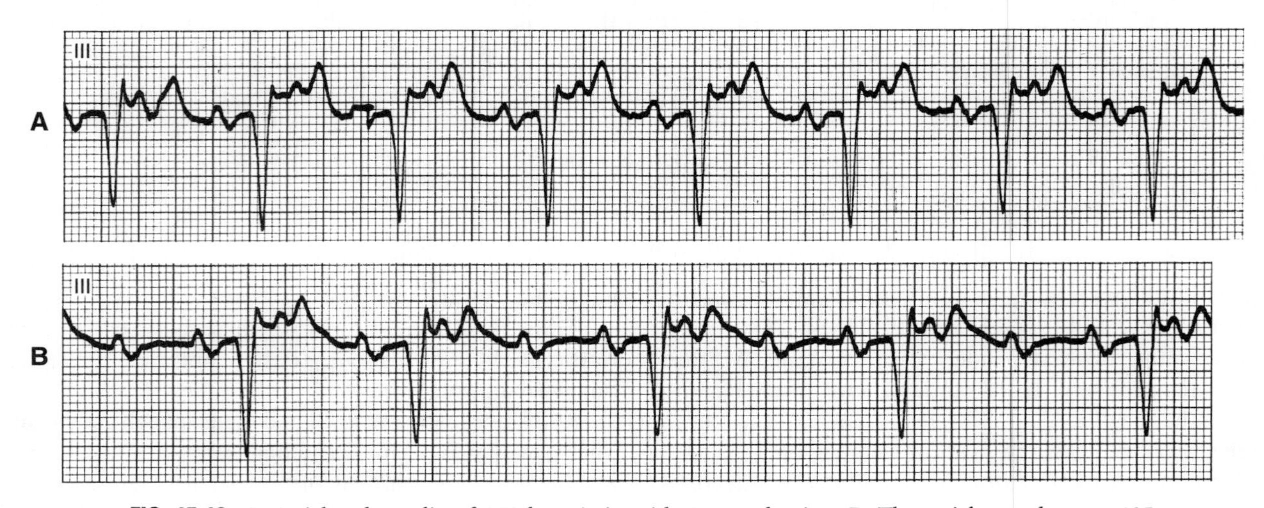

FIG. 15-10. **A,** Atrial tachycardia of 148 beats/min with 2:1 conduction. **B,** The atrial rate slows to 135 beats/min with 3:1 conduction.

JUNCTIONAL TACHYCARDIA

Digitalis overdose has long been considered the most common cause of junctional tachycardia. Other causes are myocardial infarction, cardiac surgery, rheumatic fever, and hypokalemia.

In digitalis-toxic junctional tachycardia the focus is in the nodal-His region. The activity of this focus will manifest itself when the sinus node allows it to, so that if the sinus rhythm is 70 beats/min, it will mask an accelerated junctional rate of 68 beats/min. Digitalis toxic junctional tachycardia rarely exceeds a rate of 140 beats/min. Because the mechanism is the same whether the rate is 70 or 140, the term "junctional tachycardia" is applied to point out that a junctional rate of 80 beats/min in a patient taking digitalis is just as alarming as a rate of 140 beat/min. The term "accelerated idiojunctional rhythm" (rate less than 100 beats/min) seems to mislead one to ignore a serious condition.

ECG Recognition

P waves: May or may not be present.

QRS complex: Narrow unless BBB is also present.

Junctional rate: 70 to 140 beats/min; increases with exercise but rarely exceeds 140 beats/min.

Carotid sinus massage: No effect or nodoventricular block.

Retrograde conduction: Absent because of the AV block created by the digitalis; therefore, AV dissociation is usually present and the term "idiojunctional" is applies.

Rhythm: Nonparoxysmal (gradual onset), then regular or in groups.

Best lead: V_1 (in this lead junctional tachycardia can be differentiated from fascicular VT).

Fig. 15-11 is a tracing of junctional tachycardia revealed at a rate of 74 beats/min when the sinus rhythm slows from 74 to 68 beats/min. AV dissociation is present after the third complex.

Rhythm Variations

During junctional tachycardia, Wenckebach conduction from the junctional pacemaker can occur. The result on the ECG is group beating, which may be missed if there is also atrial fibrillation. During atrial fibrillation the ECG recognition of digitalis toxicity is late because the compromised AV conduction cannot be seen and one must rely on the regularization of the rhythm or group beating for the first alarm. Therefore, in patients with atrial fibrillation it is especially important to pay attention to the physical signs of digitalis toxicity.

Atrial fibrillation with first signs of junctional tachycardia. Junctional tachycardia during atrial fibrillation is manifested by a regular rhythm. In atrial fibrillation the ventricular response should be irregular. Fig. 15-12 shows the development of junctional tachycardia in a patient with atrial fibrillation. The problem was not recognized until the junctional rate reached 92 beats/min (*C*). In *A*, the ventricular response to atrial fibrillation is irregular, as it should be. In *B*, it develops into a regular rhythm at 80 beats/min, a sign of digitalis toxicity that is often missed. When the rhythm is irregular and P waves absent, atrial fibrillation is easily recognized by most clinicians. However, when the rhythm is regular, mistakes are made because the regularity of the rhythm often causes the diagnosis of atrial fibrillation itself to be missed, let alone the problem of toxicity. This is a surprisingly consistent stumbling block. In *C*, the rate is

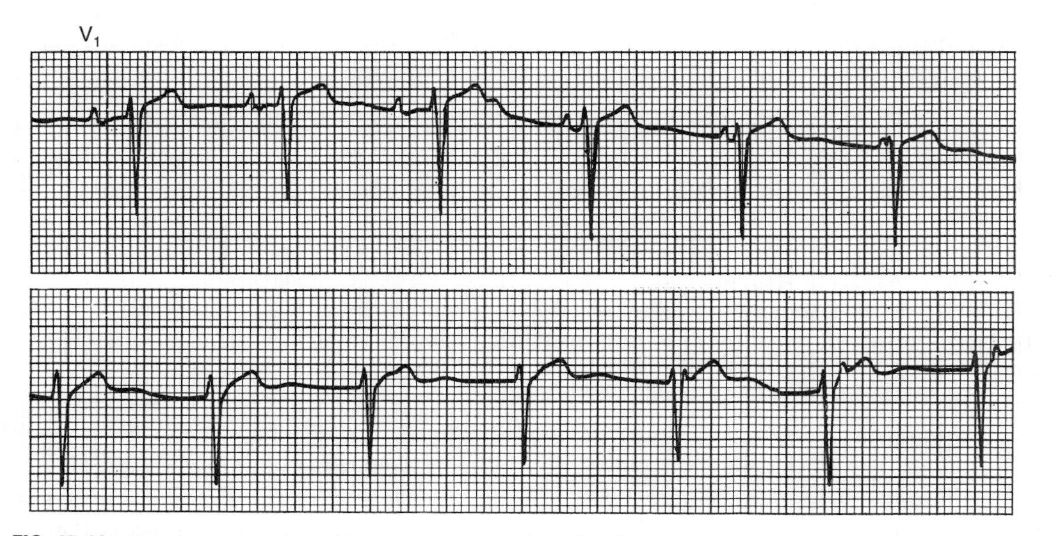

FIG. 15-11. Continuous tracings. Junctional tachycardia of 74 beats/min emerges when the sinus rhythm slows from 74 to 68 beats/min.

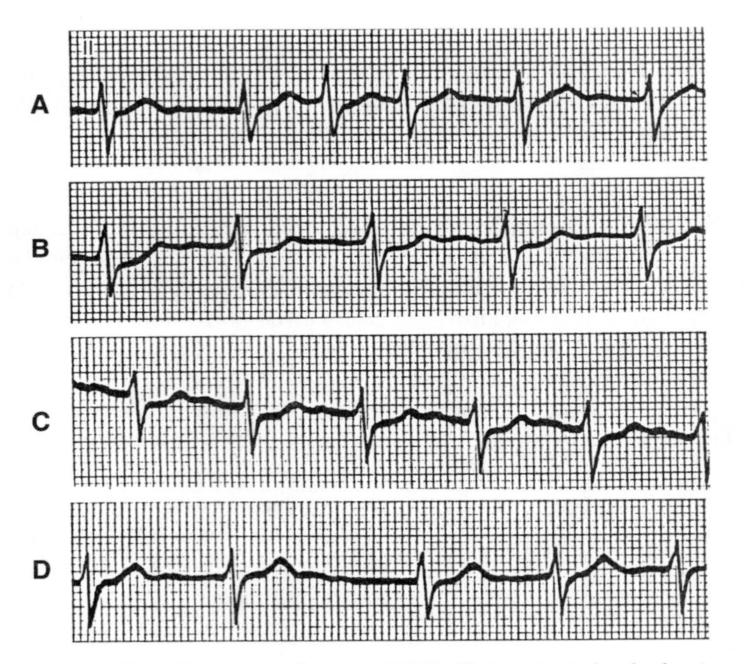

FIG. 15-12. The onset of digitalis toxicity during atrial fibrillation. In **A**, the rhythm is appropriately irregular. In **B**, 1 day later, the rhythm is regular at 80 beats/min and the problem is not recognized. In **C**, later the same day, the rhythm is still regular, but now the rate is 92 beats/min. The problem is recognized and the digitalis is discontinued. In **D**, the rhythm is again appropriately irregular and the patient is out of danger from digitalis toxicity.

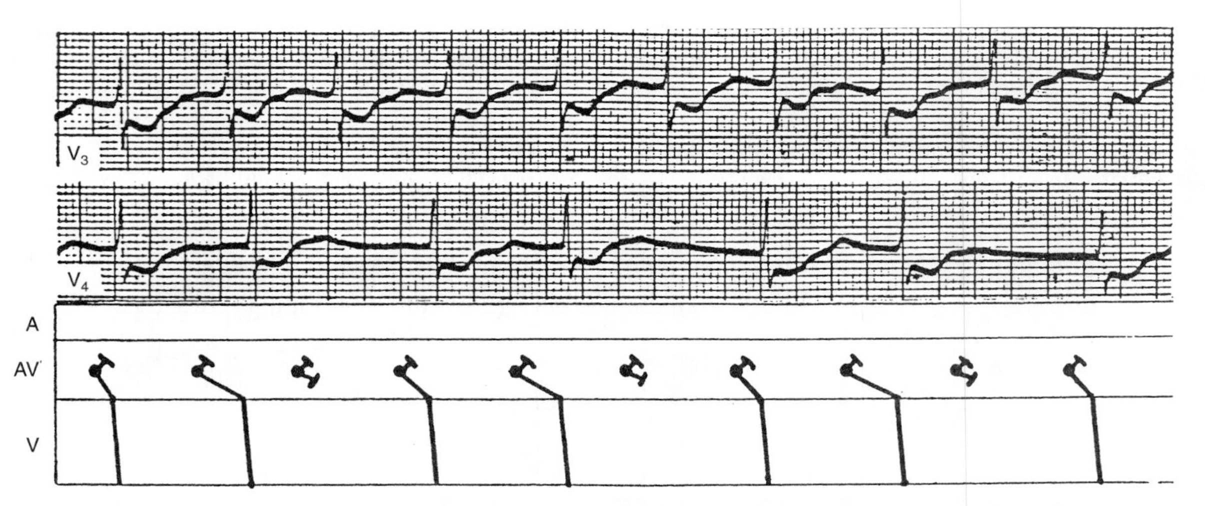

FIG. 15-13. Digitalis-toxic junctional tachycardia at 98 beats/min causes the rhythm to be regular in the top tracing. In the bottom tracing, in the same patient the junctional tachycardia develops a 3:2 Wenckebach conduction. (Courtesy Henry J.L. Marriott, MD, Riverview, Fla.)

approaching 100 beats/min, the problem is recognized, and the digitalis is discontinued. In *D,* the patient is no longer toxic, and the rhythm shows the appropriate irregularity of atrial fibrillation.

Atrial fibrillation with group beating. Even more of a stumbling block in atrial fibrillation is the recognition of junctional tachycardia when it is combined with Wenckebach exit block. In such a case the diagnostic ECG clue is *group beating,* usually in groups of two or three. In the top tracing of Fig. 15-13 the absence of P waves and the regular ventricular rhythm indicates atrial fibrillation with an independent junctional (narrow QRS) focus controlling the ventricles at a rate of 98 beats/min. In the bottom tracing P waves are still absent and there is group beating because of 3:2 Wenckebach exit block from the junctional focus; for every three junctional beats, two are conducted with lengthening conduction times from the junctional focus to the ventricles until the third concealed junctional beat is blocked.

In Figs. 15-14, *A, B,* and *C,* a similar situation is noted: absent P waves (atrial fibrillation) and groups of three (junctional tachycardia with 4:3 Wenckebach exit block). The additional signs of Wenckebach periods are the shortening RR intervals and pauses that are twice the shortest cycle. Note the digitalis effect ("dragging" down of the ST segment in *B* and *C*). It is important to be familiar with this fairly common mechanism reflecting digitalis toxicity in patients with atrial fibrillation because it is irregular (as atrial fibrillation should be) and the groups may not be noticed if not looked for. When an irregular rhythm occurs in groups it is sometimes called "regular irregularity" to distinguish it from the random irregularity of uncomplicated atrial fibrillation.

Atrial flutter with junctional tachycardia. When junctional tachycardia complicates atrial flutter there is of course AV dissociation. Its recognition is even more subtle

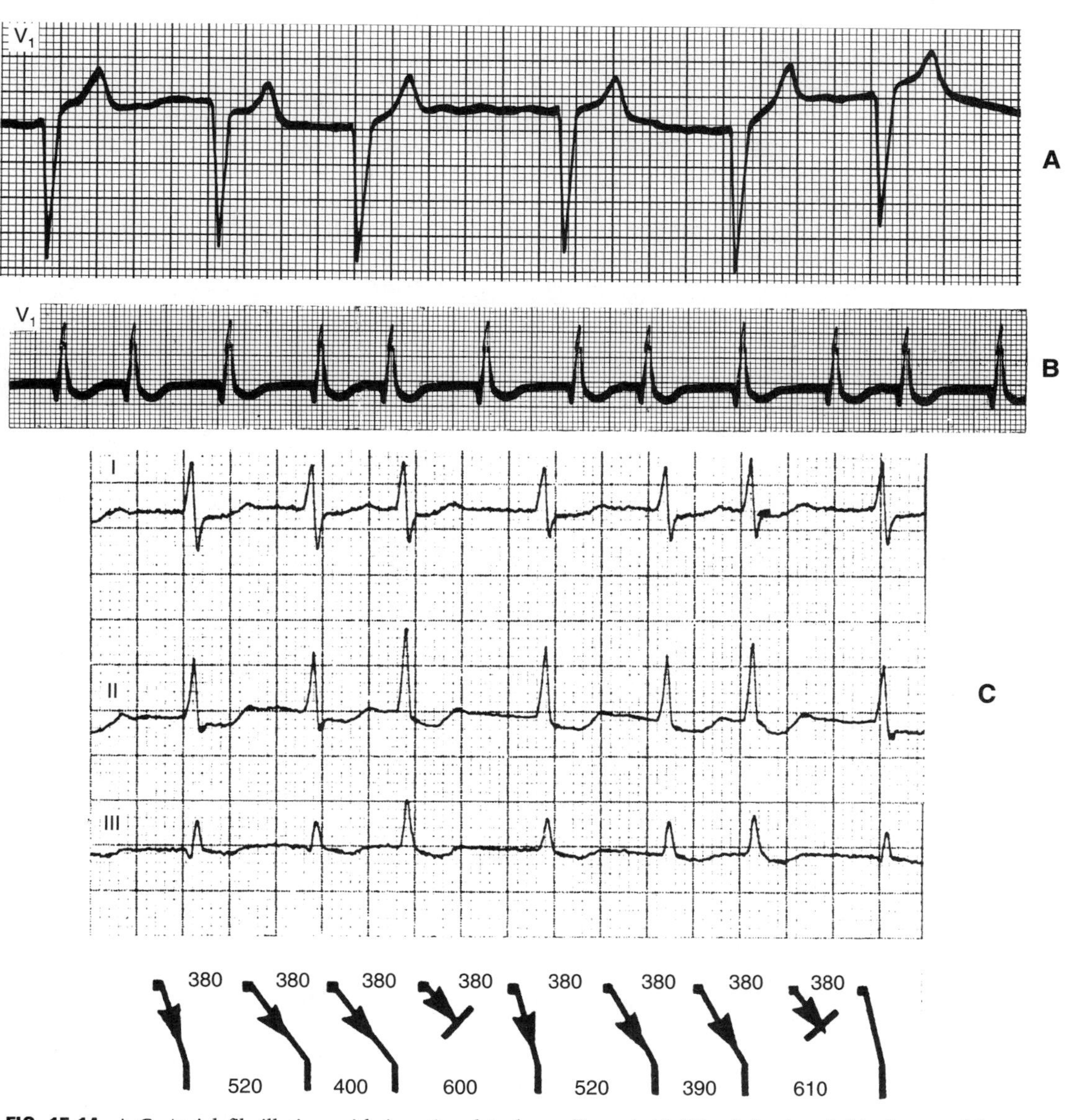

FIG. 15-14. **A-C.** Atrial fibrillation with junctional tachycardia and 4:3 Wenckebach exit block caused by excess digitalis. The group beating, shortening RR intervals, and pauses that are less than twice the shortest cycle are evident in both tracings. (**B** courtesy Henry J.L. Marriott, MD, Riverview, Fla; and **C** courtesy Hein J.J. Wellens, MD, Maastricht, The Netherlands.)

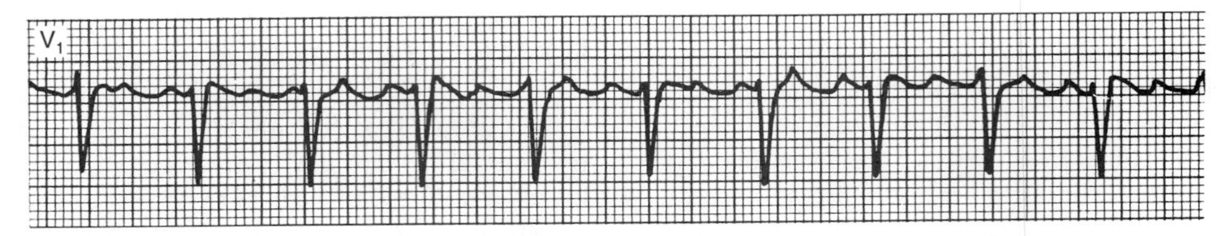

FIG. 15-15. Atrial flutter with junctional tachycardia. The regular ventricular rhythm (rate, 110 beats/min) is evident, yet the flutter waves have no fixed relationship to the QRS, a sign of AV dissociation. The narrow QRS indicates a junctional focus.

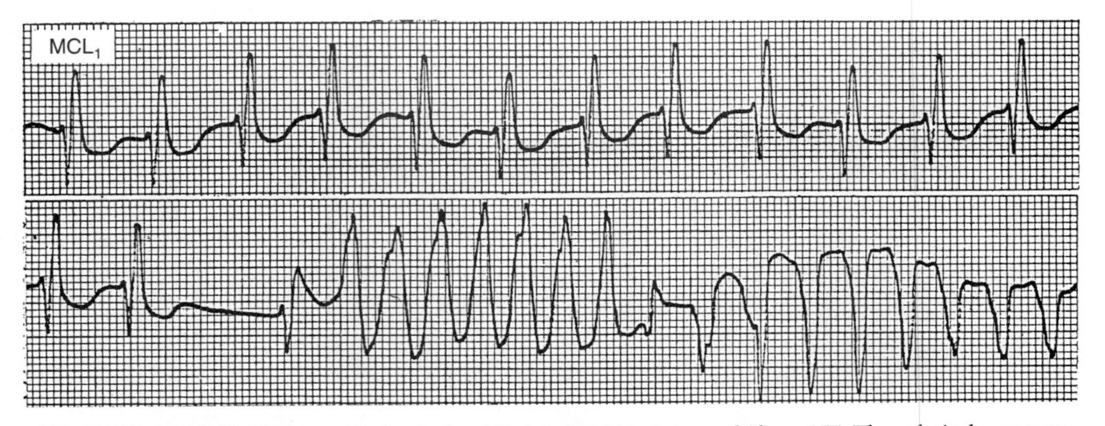

FIG. 15-16. Atrial fibrillation with fascicular VT deteriorating into multiform VT. The relatively narrow RBBB pattern (QRS, 0.12 second) is typical of this life-threatening arrhythmia. The sagging ST segment is an effect of digitalis. (Courtesy Henry J.L. Marriott, MD, Riverview, Fla.)

than when it occurs during atrial fibrillation. The toxicity may go on for days or even weeks without being recognized on the ECG. When AV dissociation occurs against a background of atrial flutter the ventricular rhythm is regular, but the flutter–R wave relationship is changing. In uncomplicated atrial flutter with 2:1 AV conduction there is a fixed flutter-R relationship. In Fig. 15-15 recorded in lead V_1 the P′ waves are positive peaks at regular intervals throughout the tracing. When the ventricular rhythm is regular, the flutter-QRS relationship should be fixed. In this case it varies—a sign of AV dissociation. The narrow QRS indicates junctional tachycardia.

FASCICULAR VT

Fascicular VT is one of the ventricular ectopic rhythms common to digitalis toxicity. Occasionally digitalis intoxication results in ventricular tachycardia, often originating in one of the fascicles of the left bundle branch and resulting in an RBBB pattern and axis deviation.

ECG Recognition

Rate: 90 to 160 beats/min.

QRS complex: 0.12 to 0.14 second. Configuration may change because of competition among Purkinje fibers for the pacing role or because of alternating fascicular foci (anterior and posterior).

QRS axis: Right or left; or alternating right and left, as in bifascicular VT.

Best leads: V_1, I, and II (V_1 for the RBBB pattern and I and II for the axis deviation).

Fig. 15-16 shows atrial fibrillation (no P waves) with fascicular VT that deteriorates into a multiform VT. The P waves are absent and an RBBB pattern with a QRS duration of 0.12 second is seen in MCL_1. This rhythm has commonly been mistaken for junctional tachycardia with RBBB aberration. The digitalis effect of a sagging ST segment is noticeable and is further illustrated in Fig. 15-17.

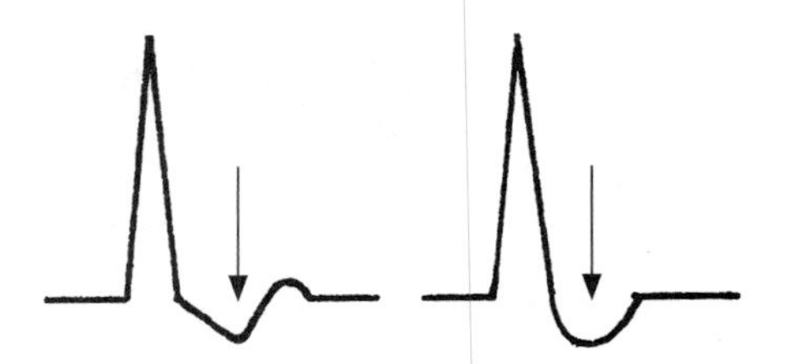

FIG. 15-17. The sagging ST segment known as the digitalis effect.

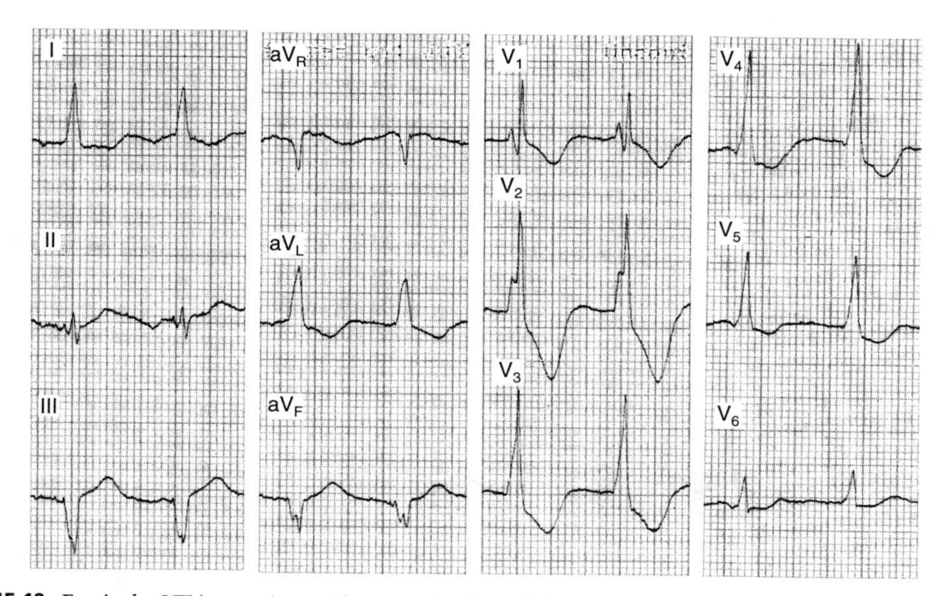

FIG. 15-18. Fascicular VT in a patient with congestive heart failure who was taking digitalis for chronic atrial fibrillation. Note the digitalis effect *(scooped-down ST segment),* the regular rhythm, the RBBB pattern in V_1, and left axis deviation, which indicate a posterior fascicular focus. (Courtesy Kathy Brown, RN, Okanogan, Wash.)

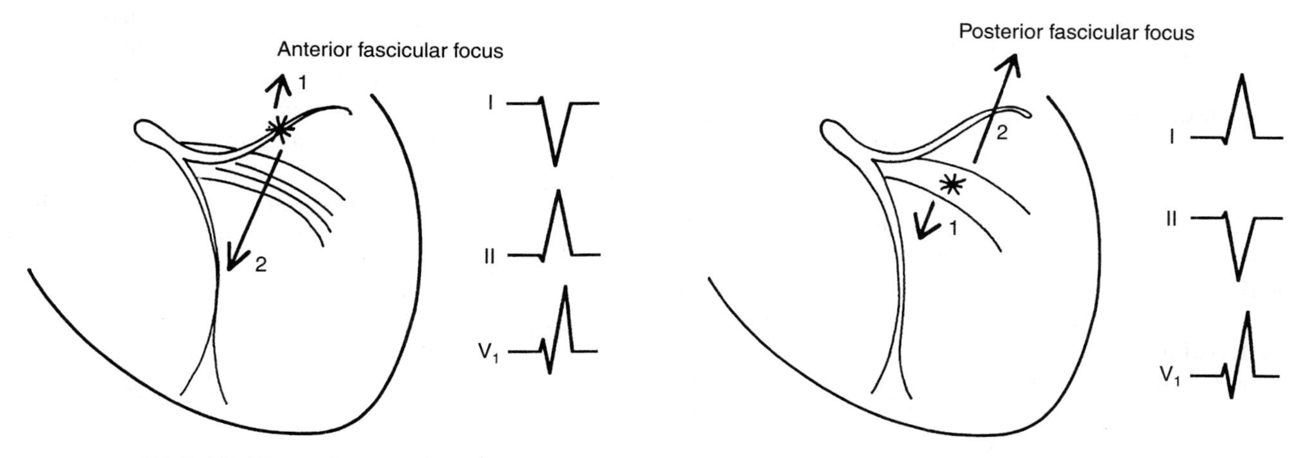

FIG. 15-19. The mechanism of the RBBB pattern and axis deviation in fascicular VT. In both cases the focus originates in the conduction system of the left ventricle, the right ventricle being the last to activate, producing an RBBB pattern. The axis deviation is caused by an impulse originating in one or the other fascicle.

Fig. 15-18 is a 12-lead ECG from a patient in congestive heart failure who was taking digitalis for chronic atrial fibrillation. Note the digitalis effect in the precordial leads (scooped-down ST segment) and the changing shape of the RBBB pattern in V_1, indicating competition among the Purkinje fibers for pacing function. The left axis deviation indicates a posterior fascicular focus.

Mechanism: The mechanisms of RBBB and axis deviation pattern in fascicular beats and rhythms are illustrated in Fig. 15-19. The RBBB pattern is not caused by a patho-

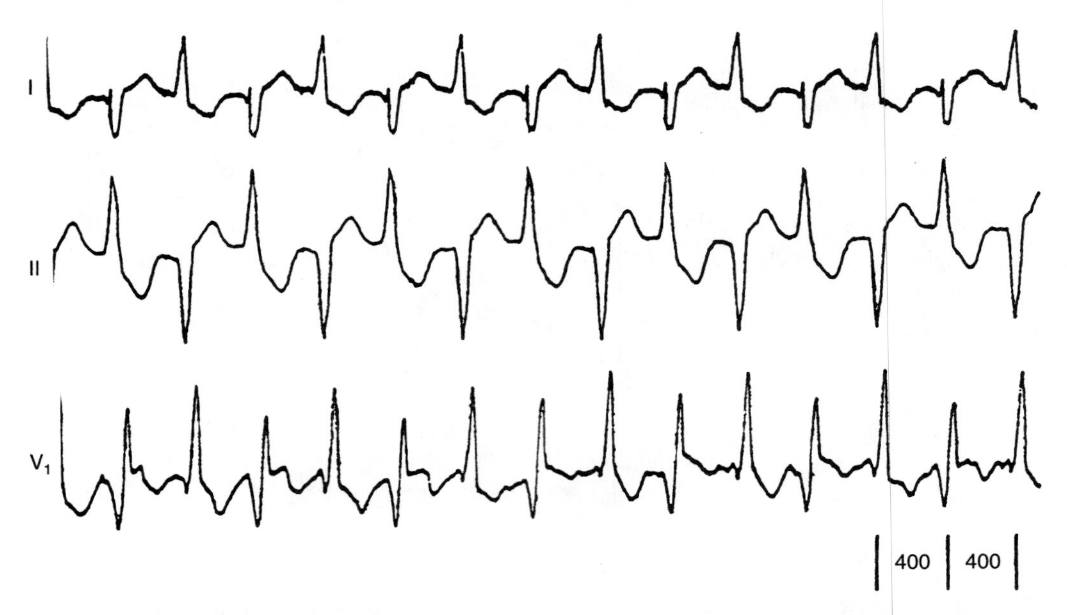

FIG. 15-20. Bifascicular VT in a patient with digitalis intoxication. Note the relatively narrow RBBB pattern (QRS, 0.12 second) and the alternating right and left axis deviation. The alternating heights of the QRS complex are caused by the switching axis. (Courtesy Hein J.J. Wellens, MD, Maastricht, The Netherlands.)

logic block in the right bundle branch, but by the origin of the rhythm in one of the fascicles of the left bundle branch, causing the right ventricle to be the last activated. However, because the impulse begins within the conduction system, the ventricular complex is not as wide as it is with other types of VT.

The axis deviation also occurs because of the location of the ectopic focus in the fascicles. A focus located in the anterior (superior) fascicle has a right axis deviation, and a focus located in the posterior (inferior) fascicle has a left axis deviation.

Fascicular VT reflects an advanced case of digitalis toxicity. When not associated with atrial fibrillation, there is often a double tachycardia (atrial and fascicular), or the focus alternates from the anterior to the posterior fascicle.

Rhythm Variations

Bifascicular VT. Fig. 15-20 is an example of bifascicular VT against a background of atrial fibrillation in a patient taking digoxin. First, note the absence of P waves (atrial fibrillation). Then evaluate the patterns in V_1; they are about 0.12 second in duration and, although there is alternans, each beat has an RBBB pattern. In a patient taking digoxin, this makes you think of fascicular VT. To confirm, check the QRS axis. The first beat has right axis deviation, an anterior fascicular focus; the second beat has left axis deviation, a posterior fascicular focus, and so on. This life-threatening form of VT has long been recognized as an arrhythmia that most often occurs in digitalis intoxication, especially in older patients and in those with severe myocardial disease.[6] Fig. 15-21 shows atrial fibrillation with bifascicular VT in a 90-year-old woman who was taking her daily dose of digoxin. When seen in the setting of digitalis excess, this arrhythmia is a sign of advanced toxic effects and has a poor prognosis.[7]

Fascicular VT and atrial tachycardia. Fig. 15-22 is another example of double tachycardia. The systematic approach outlined at the beginning of this chapter is most helpful in sorting this rhythm out.

1. What is the atrial rhythm? The P waves are upright in leads II and III at a rate of approximately 170 beats/min. This is atrial tachycardia.
2. Is there conduction? The regular ventricular rhythm without fixed PR intervals indicates that there is no conduction. Because of this, a third determination must be made.
3. Are the ventricular beats junctional or fascicular? Lead V_1 is the best lead to answer this question. The RBBB pattern (rSR′) in V_1 indicates that there is fascicular VT. This is a double tachycardia—atrial tachycardia and fascicular VT.

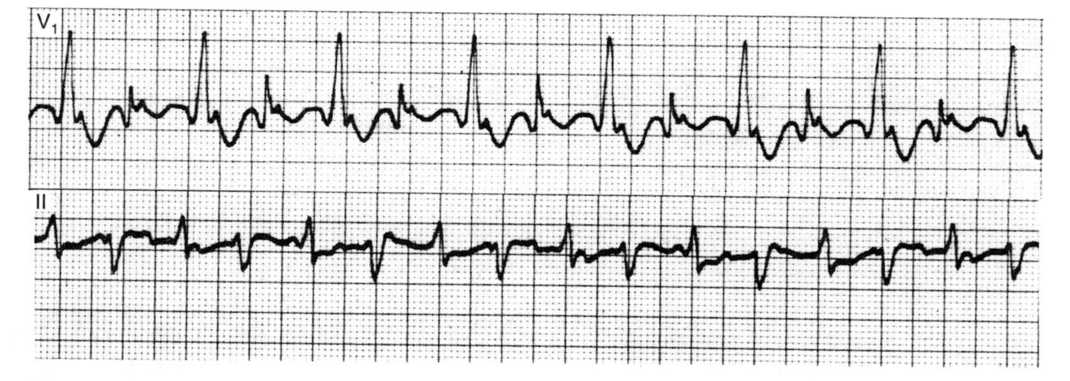

FIG. 15-21. Bifascicular VT. Note the RBBB pattern in V_1 with alternating heights caused by the QRS axis alternating from left to right.

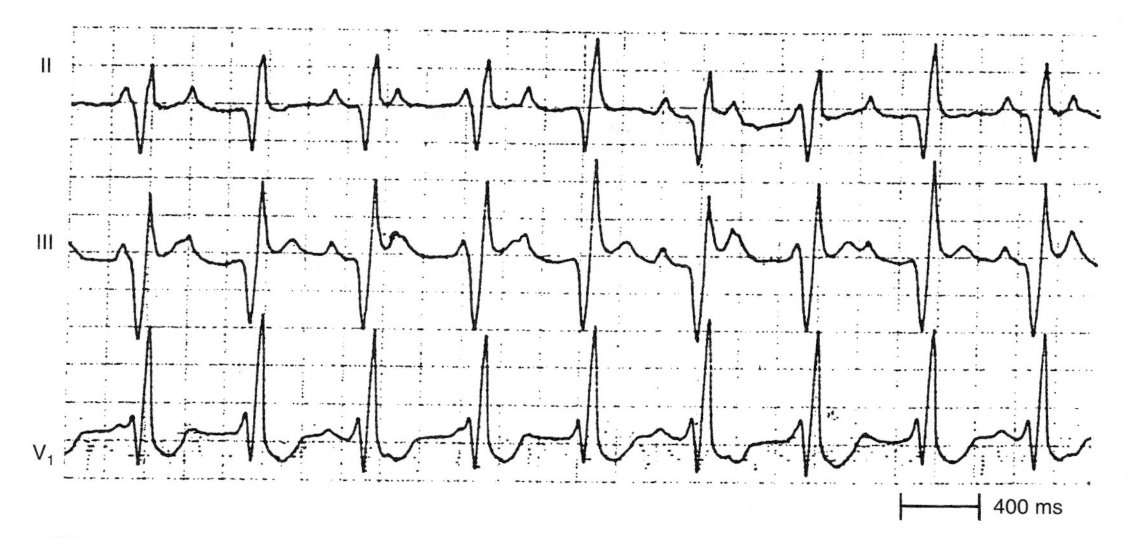

FIG. 15-22. Atrial tachycardia and fascicular ventricular tachycardia. See text for explanation. (Courtesy Hein J.J. Wellens, MD, Maastricht, The Netherlands.)

BIGEMINAL RHYTHMS

A bigeminal rhythm is the most characteristic form of the delayed afterdepolarization that is the mechanism of digitalis toxicity. The coupling interval remains fixed as long as the basic cycle length does not change. As the cycle length shortens, so do the coupling intervals. At a critical cycle length there may be sequences of tachycardia. Fig. 15-23 shows accelerated idioventricular rhythm with ventricular bigeminy, AV block, and AV dissociation in a child who was accidentally given a digitalis overdose.

MECHANISM

Digitalis is a cardiotonic steroid and a specific inhibitor of the sodium-potassium pump, which is responsible for establishing and maintaining the intracellular milieu that is vital to normal cardiac cellular function.[8] Thus it is easy to appreciate why there are often lethal consequences associated with chronic overdose and acute administration of high doses of digoxin. Although the effects of digoxin on the course of atrial fibrillation are controversial,[9,10] its potential proarrhythmic effects are specific and there are clinical indications that digoxin may cause a recurrence of atrial fibrillation,[11] in addition to its other proarrhythmic effects (see p. 85).

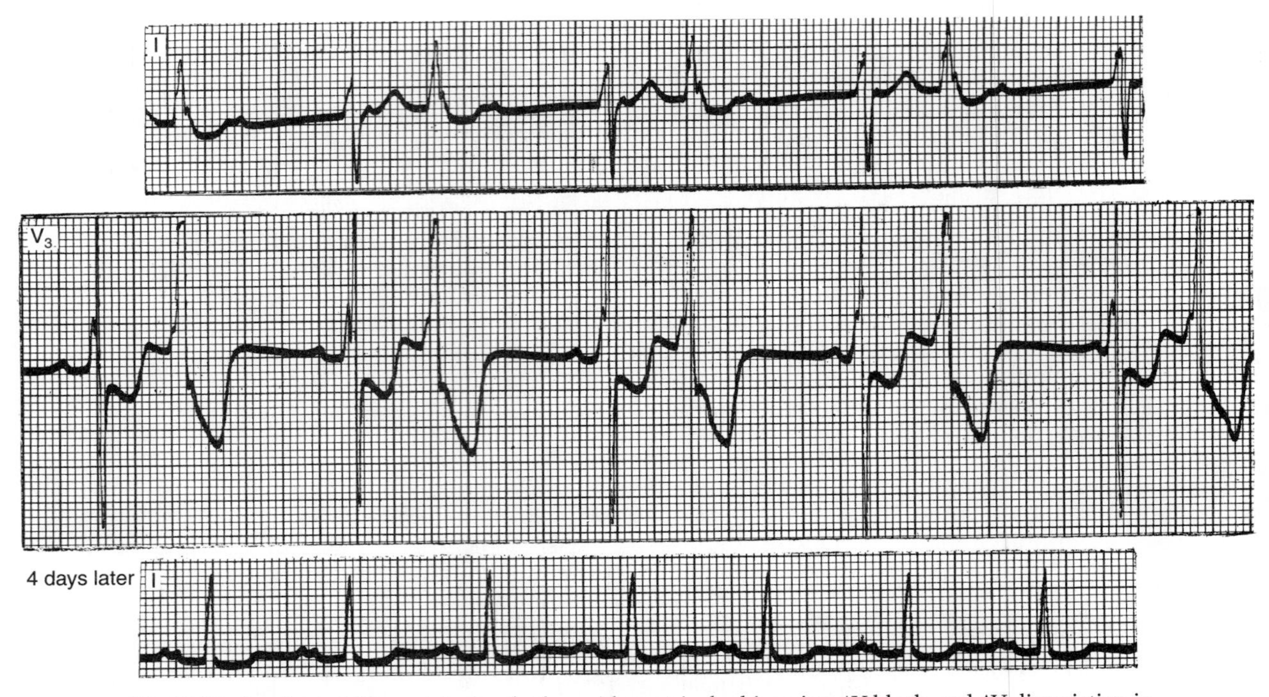

FIG. 15-23. Accelerated idioventricular rhythm with ventricular bigeminy, AV block, and AV dissociation in a 10-year-old who was mistakenly given a double dose of digitalis preparation after mitral valve surgery. The combined toxic effects of digitalis are evident. Digitalis was discontinued, and 4 days later the rhythm reverted to sinus with first-degree AV block. Note the P-mitrale in lead I. (From Marriott HJL, Conover M: *Advanced concepts in arrhythmias*, ed 3, St Louis, 1998, Mosby.)

Delayed Afterdepolarizations and Triggered Activity

Delayed afterdepolarizations and triggered activity are important in the genesis of digitalis-induced tachycardias. This mechanism may occur by itself or along with reentry or abnormal automaticity. An important feature of delayed afterdepolarizations is that they can be exacerbated by a shortening of the cycle length and by catecholamines. In fact, the tachycardias of digitalis intoxication occur more readily at faster intrinsic heart rates. As the heart rate increases, so does the amplitude of the delayed afterdepolarization. Finally it reaches threshold potential and induces ectopic action potentials. In addition, the rate of the tachycardia is faster if the prior heart rate was rapid.[12]

Other factors that influence the production of delayed afterdepolarizations are hypokalemia, hypercalcemia, hypomagnesemia, diuretics, ischemia, reperfusion, increased ventricular wall tension, and heart failure. All, of themselves, are capable of producing triggered activity caused by delayed afterdepolarizations. Catecholamines induce intracellular calcium overload, one of the factors in the production of delayed afterdepolarizations.[13]

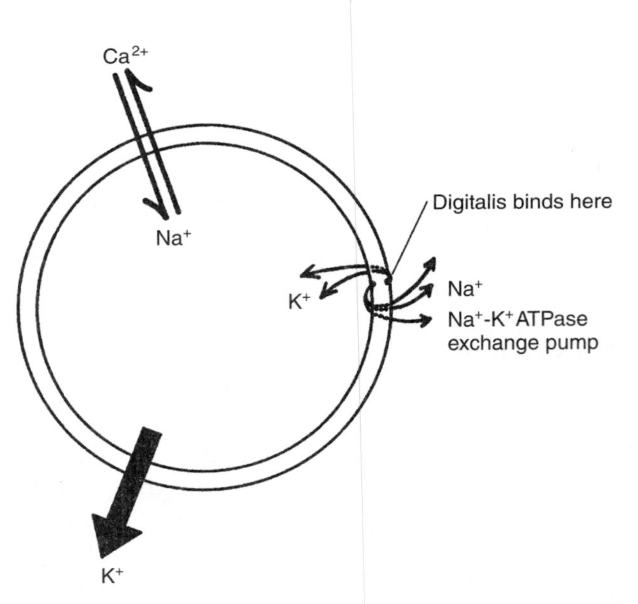

FIG. 15-24. The cellular action of digitalis. It competes with potassium (K^+) for a binding site on the membrane, poisoning the sodium-potassium (Na^+-K^+) pump and ultimately causing an increase in intracellular calcium (Ca^{2+}).

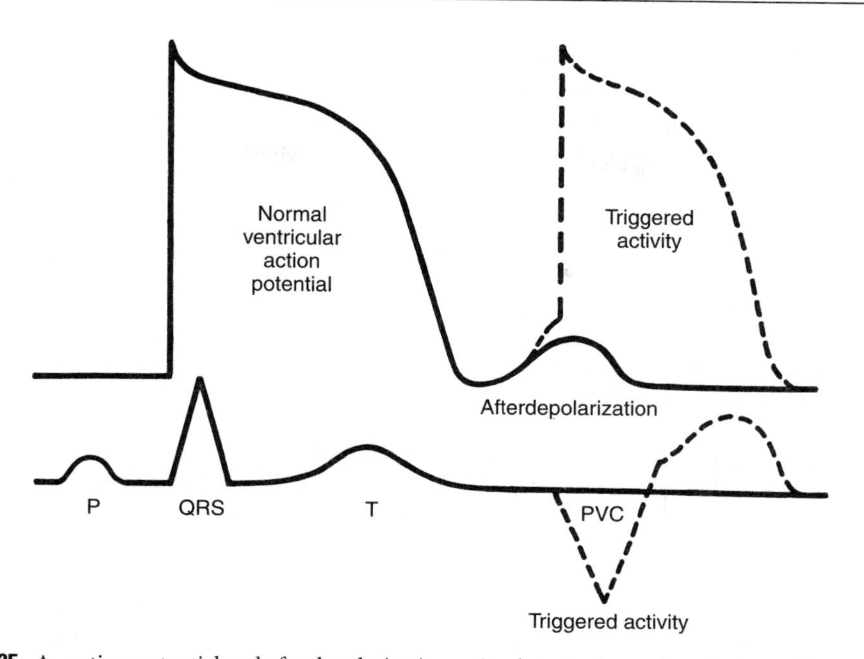

FIG. 15-25. An action potential and afterdepolarization as it relates to the surface electrocardiogram (ECG). The dotted lines represent the sequence of events that result when an afterdepolarization reaches threshold potential. The solid line represents cellular and ECG activity when the afterdepolarization does not reach threshold potential.

Delayed afterdepolarizations are oscillations in transmembrane potential that follow full repolarization of the membrane.[14] Such oscillations are the result of the poisoning of the sodium-potassium pump (Na^+-K^+ adenosine triphosphatase [ATPase]) by digitalis. The sequence of events that occur is as follows:

1. Digitalis competes with potassium for its binding site on the membrane (Fig. 15-24), disabling the Na^+-K^+ ATPase pump.
2. Sodium accumulates within the cell, and the exchange between sodium and calcium across the cell membrane is altered, as is the release of calcium from sarcoplasmic reticulum and other intracellular stores.
3. Calcium accumulates within the cell.
4. When the cell repolarizes, there is still free calcium within the cell.
5. This elicits a transient, inward sodium current. It is precisely this inward sodium current that causes the oscillation following the action potential.

Fig. 15-25 is a drawing of a normal action potential followed by a delayed afterdepolarization *(solid line)*. If this abnormal oscillation reaches threshold potential, an action potential results *(dotted line)*. This is a "triggered" beat because it is dependent on the preceding action potential.

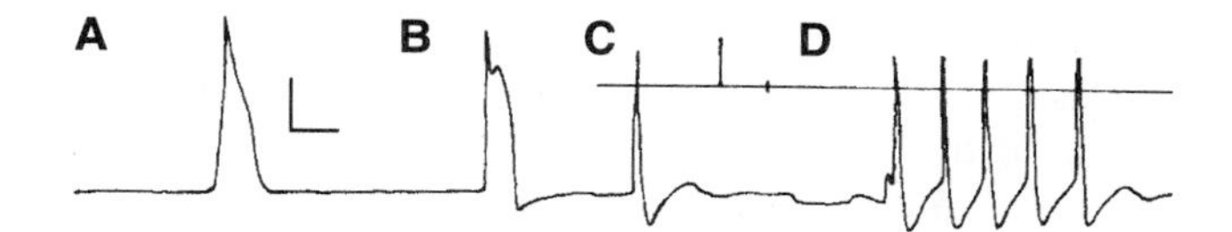

FIG. 15-26. **A**, Normal action potential compared with, **B** and **C**, an action potential followed by an afterdepolarization. **D**, Triggered activity. The first action potential is driven. Those that follow are triggered (i.e., they arise from delayed afterdepolarizations). (From Cranefield PF: *Circ Res* 41:415, 1977.)

The mechanism differs from the other arrhythmogenic mechanisms of automaticity or reentry (see Chapter 3). The normal action potential (Fig. 15-26, *A*) is compared with one followed by an afterdepolarization (Fig. 15-26, *B and C*) and a run of triggered activity (Fig. 15-26, *D*) that occurs when the afterdepolarization reaches threshold potential.

NONCARDIAC SIGNS OF DIGITALIS TOXICITY

The serum concentration of digitalis depends on many factors, including how much digitalis is bound to the membrane (where it cannot be measured). The ECG and the patient's symptoms are usually of more value in determining toxic effects.

Take a history that includes questions regarding neurologic symptoms such as headache, malaise, neuralgic pain, and pseudodementia (disorientation, memory lapses, hallucinations, nightmares, restlessness, insomnia, and listlessness).

Vision

The patient should be queried regarding reduced visual acuity and changes in the quality of color vision. Such symptoms are subtle and are not volunteered by the patient, often because they don't seem to relate to the cardiac problem. Questions from the examiner regarding the patient's assessment of the present quality of color television (especially the red and green colors), as compared with the past quality, may be revealing. One patient had recently purchased a new television set in a frustrated search for better picture quality. Other visual symptoms include scotomas and flickering halos.[15]

Gastrointestinal Symptoms

The gastrointestinal symptoms of digitalis intoxication (anorexia, nausea, and vomiting) are mediated by chemoreceptors in the medulla rather than by a direct irritant effect of digitalis on the gastrointestinal tract.[16]

EMERGENCY APPROACH

1. Discontinue the digitalis.[17]
2. Place the patient on bed rest. (Avoid sympathetic stimulation.)
3. Ensure continuous ECG monitoring.
4. Correct electrolyte abnormalities (maintain serum potassium levels of 4 mEq/L or more and pay attention to serum magnesium levels and the patient's acid-base status).
5. Provide active treatment of a rapid ventricular rhythm depending on the site of origin of the arrhythmia and its hemodynamic consequences.
6. Administer emergency intravenous Fab fragments of digoxin-specific antibodies if hemodynamic instability is present. If digoxin antibodies are not available, phenytoin may be used along with the placement of a ventricular pacing lead.
7. Provide ventricular pacing in cases of symptomatic bradycardia.
8. Reverse decompensated congestive heart failure or overt myocardial ischemia.

FACTORS THAT AFFECT DIGITALIS DOSAGE REQUIREMENTS

The frequently prescribed cardioactive drugs that interact with digitalis to cause a significant increase in serum digoxin concentration are quinidine,[18] amiodarone, verapamil, and diltiazem. Other factors that require a decrease in dosage of digoxin are renal disease, old age, hypothyroidism, small stature, chronic pulmonary disease, hypokalemia, hypomagnesemia, congestive heart failure, myocardial ischemia, and hypercalcemia.

Factors that require an increase in digoxin are malabsorption, antacids, neomycin, cholestyramine, colestipol, hyperthyroidism, hyperkalemia, reserpine, youth, and hypocalcemia.[3]

Drugs that do not appear to affect digoxin concentration are procainamide, disopyramide, mexiletine, flecainide, moricizine, and nifedipine.[6,17]

SUMMARY

Digitalis intoxication is diagnosed because of subjective and ECG symptoms; digoxin blood levels are used in conjunction with these findings. The ECG shows bradycardia (SA block or AV block); tachycardia (atrial, junctional, or fascicular); regularity in atrial fibrillation (junctional tachycardia or AV block with junctional escape); group beating in atrial fibrillation (junctional tachycardia with Wenckebach exit block); group beating in sinus rhythm (ventricular bigeminy, SA Wenckebach, or AV Wenckebach); or atrial flutter (with AV dissociation or high-degree AV block).

REFERENCES

1. Ma G, Brady WJ, Pollack M et al: Electrocardiographic manifestations: digitalis toxicity, *J Emerg Med* 20:145, 2001.
2. DiMarco JP: Adenosine and digoxin. In Zipes DP, Jalife J, editors: *Cardiac electrophysiology from cell to bedside,* Philadelphia, 2000, WB Saunders.
3. Vanagt EJ, Wellens HJJ: The electrocardiogram in digitalis intoxication. In Wellens HJJ, Kulbertus HE, editors: *What's new in electrocardiography?* The Hague, 1981, Martinus Nijhoff, pp 315-343.
4. Dreifus LS, McKnight EH, Katz M et al: Digitalis intolerance, *Geriatrics* 18:494, 1963.
5. Naccarelli GV, Shih HT, Jalal S: Clinical arrhythmias: mechanisms, clinical features, and management—supraventricular tachycardia. In Zipes DP, Jalife J, editors: *Cellular electrophysiology from cell to bedside,* ed 2, Philadelphia, 1995, WB Saunders.
6. Zipes DP: Specific arrhythmias: diagnosis and treatment. In Braunwald E, editor: *Heart disease,* ed 4, Philadelphia, 1992, WB Saunders.
7. Grimm W, Marchlinski FE: Accelerated idioventricular rhythm, bidirectional ventricular tachycardia. In Zipes DP, Jalife J, editors: *Cellular electrophysiology from cell to bedside,* ed 2, Philadelphia, 1995, WB Saunders.
8. Gadsby DC: The Na/K pump of cardiac myocytes. In Zipes DP, Jalife J, editors: *Cardiac electrophysiology from cell to bedside,* Philadelphia, 1990, WB Saunders.
9. Weiner P, Bassan MM, Jarchovsky J et al: Clinical course of acute atrial fibrillation treated with rapid digitalization, *Am Heart J* 105:223, 1983.
10. Rawles JM, Metcalfe MJ, Jennings K: Time of occurrence, duration and ventricular rate of paroxysmal atrial fibrillation: the effect of digoxin, *Br Heart J* 63:225, 1990.

11. Twileman RG, Van Gelder IC, Crijns HJ et al: Early recurrences of atrial fibrillation after electrical cardioversion: a result of fibrillation-induced electrical remodeling of the atria? *J Am Coll Cardiol* 31:167, 1998.
12. Rosen MR: Delayed afterdepolarizations induced by digitalis. In Rosen MR, Janse MJ, Wit AL, editors: *Cardiac electrophysiology,* Mount Kisco, NY, 1990, Futura.
13. Wit AL, Cranefield PF, Gadsby DC: Electrogenic sodium extrusion can stop triggered activity in the canine coronary sinus, *Circ Res* 49:1029, 1981.
14. Rosen MR: Cellular electrophysiology of digitalis toxicity, *J Am Coll Cardiol* 5:22A, 1985.
15. Nagai N, Ohde H, Betsuin Y et al: [Two cases of digitalis toxicity with reversible and severe decrease of visual acuity], *Nippon Ganka Gakkai Zasshi* 105:24, 2001.
16. Smith TW, Braunwald E, Kelly RA: The management of heart failure. In Braunwald E, editor: *Heart disease,* ed 4, Philadelphia, 1995, WB Saunders.
17. Wellens HJJ, Conover M: *The ECG in emergency decision making,* Philadelphia, 1992, WB Saunders.
18. Mordel A, Halkin H, Zulty L et al: Quinidine enhances digitalis toxicity at therapeutic serum digoxin levels, *Clin Pharmacol Ther* 53:457, 1993.

CHAPTER 16
Atrioventricular Block

Atrioventricular (AV) block is the term used to describe delayed conduction or nonconduction of an atrial impulse; it may be intermittent or persistent and is traditionally divided into three categories, first-, second-, and third-degree block. These designations are based purely on the electrocardiographic (ECG) characteristics rather than on lesion locations learned from the His bundle electrogram. In first-degree AV block the PR interval is prolonged. In second-degree AV block (type I, type II, and 2:1), some P waves are not conducted to the ventricles. In third-degree AV block there is no conduction between atria and ventricles.

Fig. 16-1 illustrates the possible anatomical locations of the different degrees of AV block. A more proximal block will have a narrow QRS and a better prognosis.

THE HIS BUNDLE ELECTROGRAM

The His bundle electrogram is an intracardiac recording of the electrical cardiac cycle. As such, its deflections reflect conduction time from sinus node depolarization to atrial activation; atrial activity; conduction time from atrial activity to activation of the bundle of His and from His activation to ventricular activation. These events are illustrated in Fig. 16-2.

With the introduction of the His bundle electrogram in 1969[1] the location of the pathology relative to the His

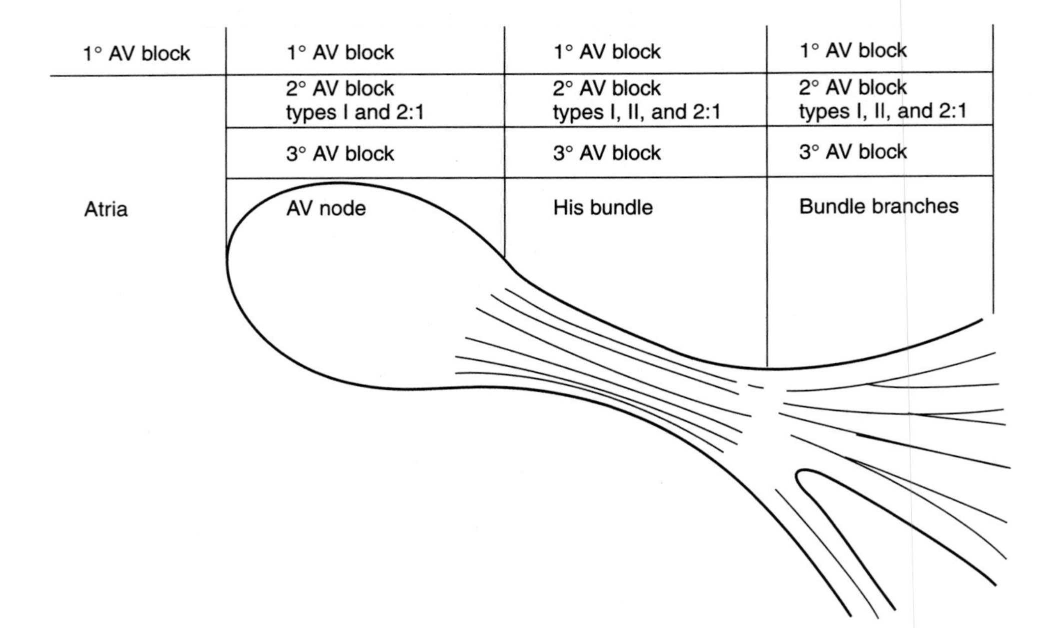

FIG. 16-1. The possible anatomic locations of the different degrees of AV block.

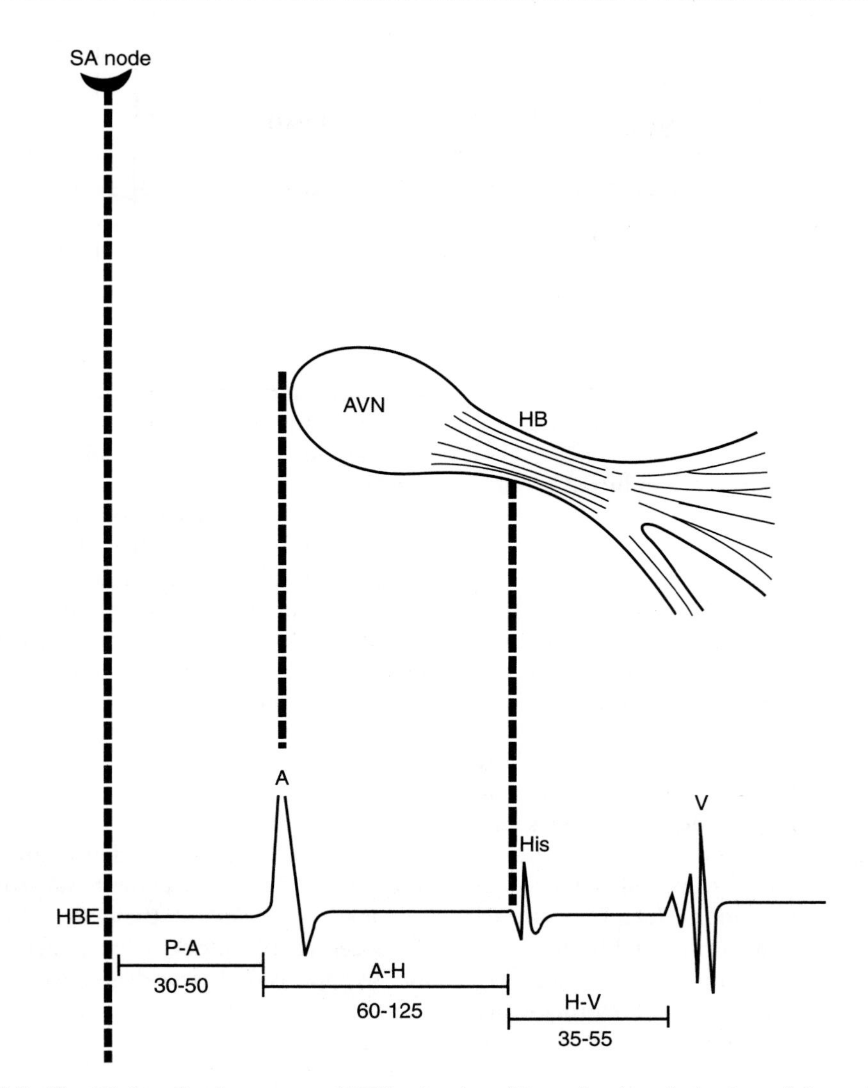

FIG. 16-2. The His bundle electrogram *(HBE)* related to AV conduction. Activation of the atria *(A)*, His bundle *(HB)*, and ventricles *(V)* can be clearly seen. The intervals between SA nodal and atrial activation (*P-A* interval), atrial and His bundle activation (*A-H* interval), and His bundle and ventricular activation (*H-V* interval) are deducted.

bundle became possible (proximal, within, or distal to the His bundle) and a more accurate prognosis could be made. Although the His bundle electrogram is not practical in clinical practice, it has allowed investigators to correlate its more precise localization of pathology with the findings on the surface ECG. Of course, although the level of block cannot be exactly determined by the surface ECG, much can be learned from the PR interval, QRS duration, and the response of the block to noninvasive interventions such as atropine, exercise, catecholamines, or vagal maneuvers (p. 132).

FIRST-DEGREE AV BLOCK

In the example of first-degree AV block in Fig. 16-3, the QRS is narrow, a hopeful prognostic sign.

ECG Recognition

PR interval: Longer than 0.20 second and may stretch to more than 0.60 second; does not change from beat to beat.

P waves: All P waves are conducted.

QRS complex: Normal in shape and duration unless there is another lesion lower in the conduction system. A

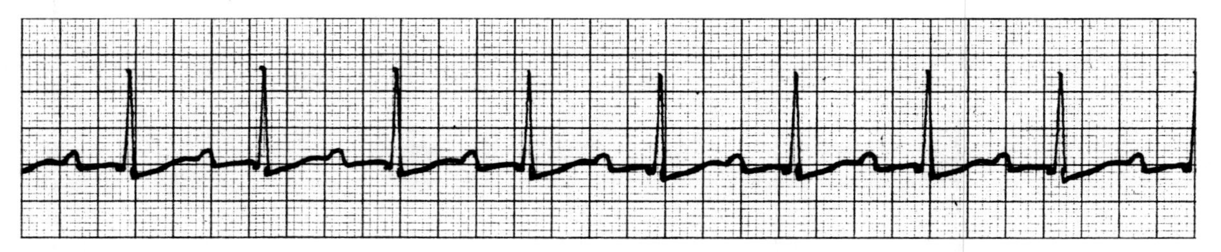

FIG. 16-3. First-degree AV block. The PR interval is 0.24 second.

narrow QRS associated with a prolonged PR interval indicates conduction delay within the AV node or bundle of His.

AV conduction: All sinus beats are conducted to the ventricles.

Mechanism

The term *first-degree AV block* is misleading in that there is a prolongation of conduction rather than an actual block in conduction. Fig. 16-4 illustrates the areas of the heart involved in forming the PR interval (the atria, the AV node, and the His-Purkinje system). The impulse invades the AV node early in the formation of the P wave. After this happens, the PR interval no longer depends on atrial conduction. As noted in Fig. 16-1 first-degree AV block can occur at any level of the atria or AV conduction system. However, the greatest part of the PR interval is due to the conduction time through the AV node, which is capable of lengthening that conduction time further and is most sensitive to provocation to do so in response to vagal stimulation, rapid ectopic atrial rates, or diseases. During sinus rhythm, AV nodal conduction works in tandem with the sinus rate, shortening with sinus tachycardia and lengthening with sinus bradycardia.

Mark Josephson, MD, has likened conduction through the AV node to the "stretch of a rubber band" as opposed to the all-or-none behavior of the His-Purkinje system. A prolongation of the PR interval to 0.28 second or more usually indicates AV nodal disease. However, the His bundle electrogram is the only definitive way to determine the level of block when the PR interval is prolonged. A His-ventricular (HV) interval of more than 55 ms indicates an AV nodal conduction delay, a subnodal conduction problem, or both.[2]

Causes

Prolonged PR intervals occur in up to 13% of patients with acute myocardial infarction (MI) (usually inferior); 75% of these patients subsequently have type I AV block, and half of these then have high-grade or third-degree AV block with a dependable junctional escape pacemaker.[3] First-degree AV block is also seen in individuals with no history of cardiac disease and in healthy children.[4]

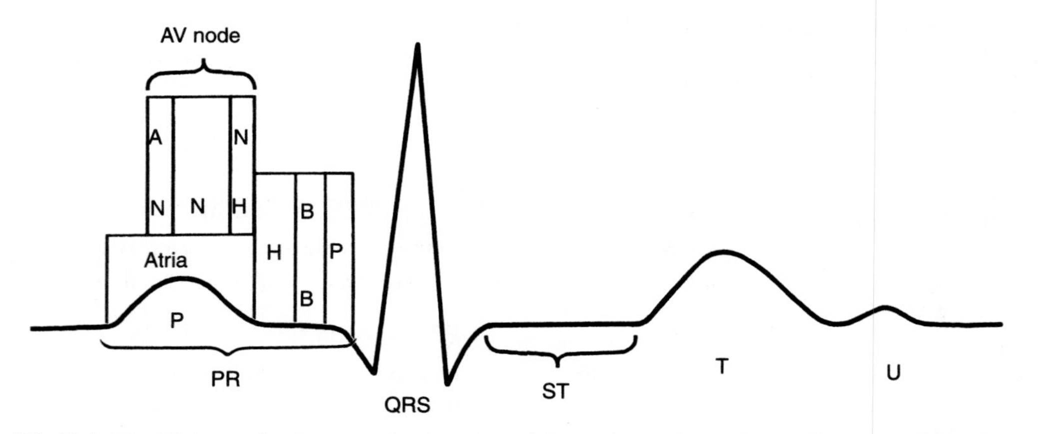

FIG. 16-4. The PR interval reflects conduction time of the cardiac impulse through the atria, AV node, His bundle *(H)*, bundle branches *(B)*, and Purkinje fibers *(P)*. When the PR interval is long, it is usually the result of conduction delay in the AV node. *AN,* Atrionodal; *N,* node; *NH,* nodal-His.

Clinical Implications

The clinical implications of a prolonged PR interval depend on the level of the lesion as determined by the HV interval of the His bundle electrogram (Fig. 16-2). When the QRS duration is normal, a PR of 0.28 second or more usually indicates AV nodal pathology.[2] However, as has been demonstrated by the His bundle electrogram, a PR that is not markedly prolonged may, in fact, be associated with disease in the His-Purkinje system, causing an alarmingly prolonged HV interval of greater than 100 ms.

Pediatrics

First-degree AV block in pediatrics is defined as a PR interval above the 98th percentile for age, a necessary accommodation because of the natural increase in the PR interval as the child grows.

In children taking digitalis the PR interval may become prolonged; unlike in adults, such a development may represent digitalis intoxication and the physician decreases the amount of the drug being taken.[5]

Bedside Diagnosis

At the bedside one may notice that in first-degree AV block the first heart sound diminishes in intensity with PR prolongation and that there is a long *A*- to *C*-wave interval in the jugular venous pulse.

Assessment of the jugular venous pulse. In examining the jugular pulse, the patient is positioned supine with the trunk at an angle of 15 to 45 degrees to the horizontal plane unless, of course, venous pressure is extremely high and the patient needs to sit upright. The right external jugular vein is the easiest to assess. Lighting should be oblique or tangential to the vein. Pulsation seen at the posterior border of the sternocleidomastoid muscle is a venous pulsation; the arterial pulsation is at the anterior border. Three separate pulsations can usually be identified in the venous pulse, as opposed to the artery, which has only one.

The *A* wave represents atrial contraction; when right atrial pressure rises, it is the most prominent. When the right atrium contracts against a closed tricuspid valve, "cannon *A* waves" can be seen.

The jugular *C* wave is thought to be caused by the onset of right ventricular contraction.

The jugular *V* wave reflects right atrial filling before the tricuspid valve has opened.[6]

Treatment

In adults the presence of first-degree AV block usually does not require therapy.

SECOND-DEGREE AV BLOCK

Second-degree AV block is divided into the following:

- Type I (AV Wenckebach or Mobitz type I)
- Type II (Mobitz type II)
- 2:1 AV block

Second-degree AV block is the nonconduction of some of the atrial impulses. The lesion may be in the AV node, within the bundle of His, or in the bundle branches as illustrated in Fig. 16-1. Each level of block has different clinical implications, treatment, and prognosis. The QRS duration helps localize the level of block to above (narrow QRS) or below (broad QRS) the branching portion of the bundle of His. A prolonged PR interval with a broad QRS would suggest a block in the bundle branches and either the AV node or the bundle of His.

Pediatrics. In children, second-degree AV block is similar to that seen in adults (i.e., type I with block in the AV node). When type II AV block is seen it is usually associated with bundle branch block (BBB) and possibly syncope.[7]

TYPE I AV BLOCK (AV WENCKEBACH)

In classic AV Wenckebach the PR lengthens until finally one P wave is not conducted, which produces a pause. This set is known as the "Wenckebach period." After the pause the sequence repeats itself, as shown in Figs. 16-5, *A* and *B*. In both tracings there are four P waves in each sequence; only three are conducted. This is called 4:3 Wenckebach.

ECG Recognition

Rhythm: Group beating.

PR intervals: Become progressively longer until one P wave is not conducted and the sequence begins again. The second PR in a sequence of 3 or more is often longest.

QRS complexes: Can be narrow or wide, although usually narrow. When broad, in addition to AV nodal pathology, there is pathology in the His-Purkinje system in 60% to 70% of cases.[8]

RR intervals: Typically shorten until there is a pause that is less than twice the shortest cycle. The shortening RR intervals result from the second PR interval having the largest increment of the set, causing the next R wave to be more delayed than the others in the group. The third PR interval of the group, although longer than the previous one, does not exhibit the same increment that the second in the series does. Nonetheless, it is not unusual for the pattern to be atypical.

Diagnostic maneuvers: When the conduction problem is

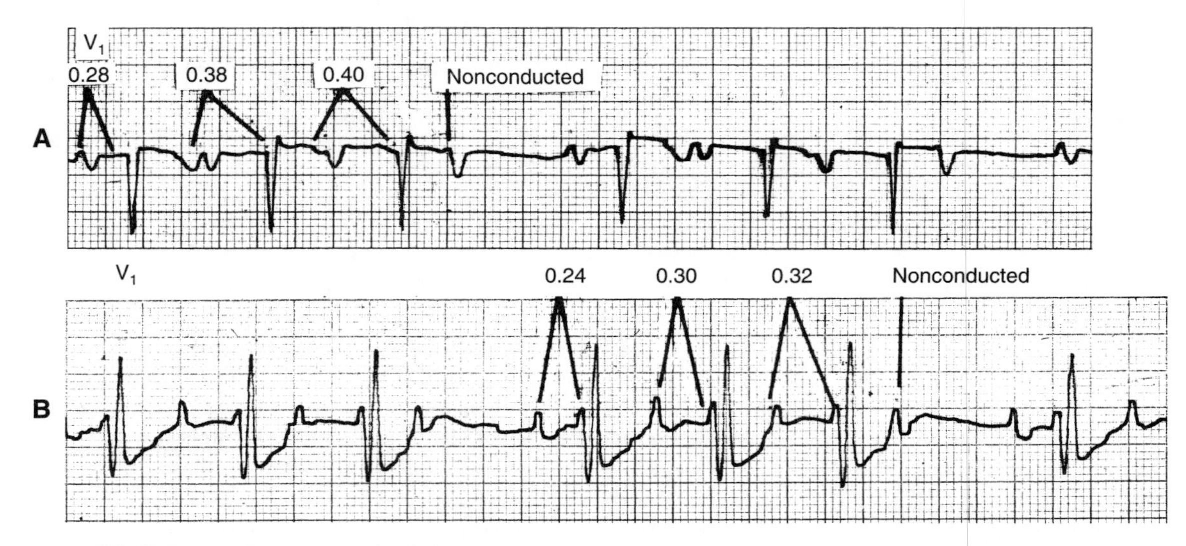

FIG. 16-5. **A** and **B,** Type I second-degree AV block (Wenckebach) is recognized because of the lengthening PR intervals, shortening RR intervals, dropped beats, and pauses less than twice the shortest cycle.

in the AV node, conduction will improve with atropine, exercise, or catecholamines (Table 16-1).

Distinguishing features:

- Group beating
- Lengthening PR intervals
- Pauses that are less than twice the shortest cycle
- Shortening RR intervals (when three or more P waves are consecutively conducted)

Rhythm Variations

Conduction ratio switch. Sometimes the conduction ratio switches between 2:1 and AV Wenckebach as seen in Fig. 16-6. When two beats in a row are conducted, the PR lengthens and a beat is dropped, a 3:2 Wenckebach.

Hidden Ps. When junctional escape beats or the conducted beat itself obscures a P wave the ECG picture can be confusing. In Fig. 16-7, *A,* the pause of the typical Wenckebach period is interrupted by a junctional escape beat (asterisk), which also obscures a sinus P wave. In Fig. 16-7, *B,* the dropped beat of a 5:4 Wenckebach period is obscured by the last conducted QRS of the sequence *(asterisk).*

Bigeminal patterns. AV Wenckebach with 3:2 conduction can sometimes resemble bigeminal premature atrial complexes (PACs) if the third P wave of the sequence (the nonconducted one) is not easily seen, as illustrated in Fig. 16-8, *A.* There is a common Wenckebach conduction ratio, 3:2, producing a bigeminal rhythm. The P waves are all sinus and right on time. The nonconducted P waves can be seen distorting the end of the T waves before the pauses. In Fig. 16-8, *B,* another bigeminal rhythm is illustrated. The PR intervals are lengthening as they would in AV Wenckebach. However, this bigeminal rhythm is caused by bigeminal PACs. The second P wave of the group is premature. Using the PP interval that is seen to measure off a sinus rhythm, you will find that the P wave after the pause is not on time. It is, in fact, late because of overdrive suppression.

AV Wenckebach with BBB. Fig. 16-9 is an example of 3:2 AV Wenckebach complicated by BBB.

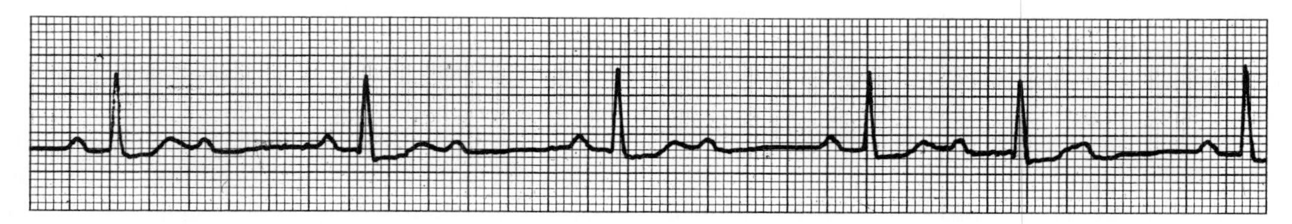

FIG. 16-6. Two-to-one AV block with a narrow QRS switches to 3:2 AV Wenckebach at the end of the tracing. The nonconducted P wave of the 3:2 Wenckebach sequence is in the last T wave.

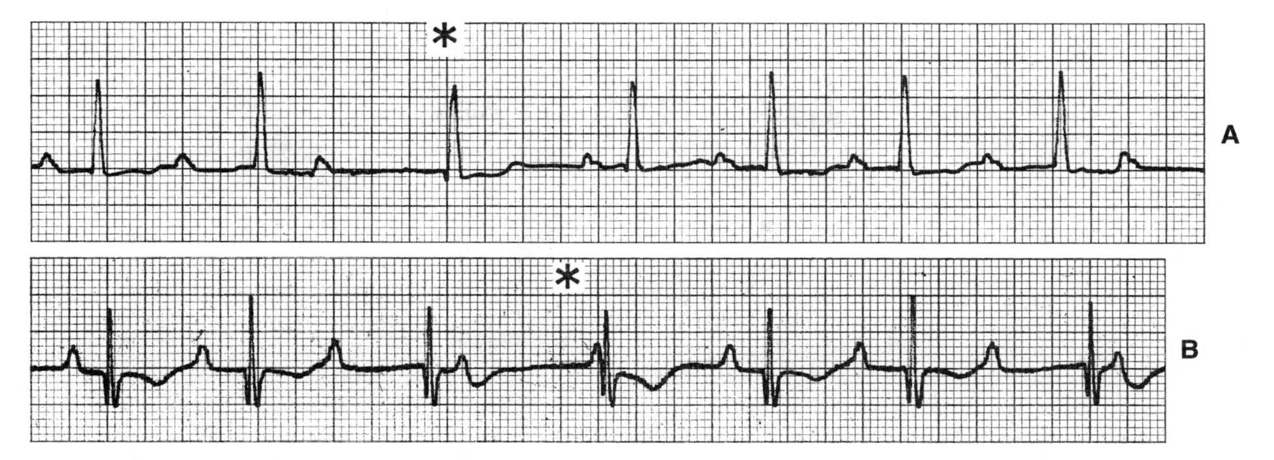

FIG. 16-7. **A,** The pause of the typical Wenckebach period is interrupted by a junctional escape beat (*), which also obscures a sinus P wave. **B,** The dropped beat of a 5:4 Wenckebach sequence is obscured by the last conducted QRS of the sequence (*).

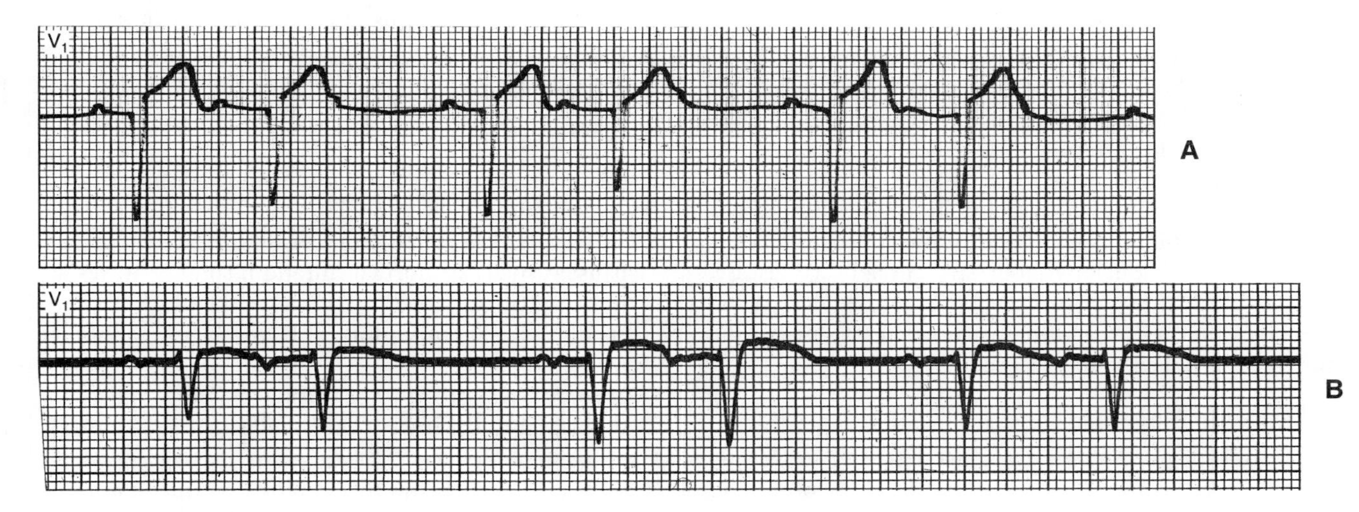

FIG. 16-8. Two bigeminal patterns with different causes. **A,** There is 3:2 AV Wenckebach. The P waves are on time, the PR lengthens, and there is a dropped beat. **B,** The second P of each group is a premature atrial complex, which, with its lengthened P′R interval, looks like a 3:2 Wenckebach period.

Mechanism

The disease in type I AV block is almost always in the AV node, rarely within the His bundle. The AV node normally has a slow-response action potential and slow conduction. Thus any depressive influence, such as digitalis or ischemia, easily compounds the normal situation, causing the PR to lengthen until one P wave is not conducted.

Causes

- Inferior MI
- Digitalis toxicity
- Acute myocarditis
- Drugs that prolong AV conduction
- Old age
- Following open heart surgery
- Ophthalmic beta blockers[9]

Clinical Implications

Organic heart disease. Chronic second-degree AV nodal block is usually benign unless associated with organic heart disease, in which case the prognosis is related to the underlying disease.

Inferior and right ventricular MI. Type I AV block with a narrow QRS complex is more benign than type II and

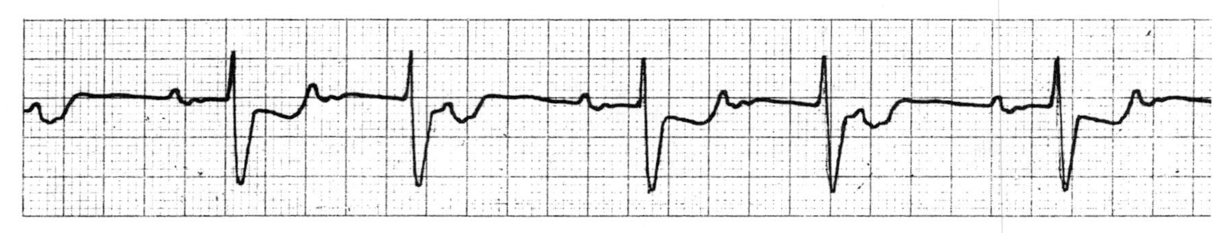

FIG. 16-9. An example of type I second-degree AV block. The 3:2 AV Wenckebach is complicated by BBB.

does not progress to a more advanced conduction problem. In the setting of acute inferior MI and right ventricular MI (elevated ST in lead V_4R) the development of type I AV block can be anticipated in that it occurs in approximately 45% of such patients. This combination places the patient at 2.5 times the risk of those who do not develop AV block.[2]

BBB. Type I AV block with BBB (Fig. 16-9) may be a manifestation of chronic conduction system disease and as such has a poor prognosis, requiring a permanent pacemaker even when the patient is asymptomatic.[8]

Trained athlete. AV Wenckebach also occurs as a normal condition in trained athletes and may be related to their enhanced vagal tone. It is possible for the block to become more profound, resulting in syncope or presyncope. At this point it is necessary for the athlete to "decondition." In individuals without structural heart disease, chronic block at the level of the AV node is benign. When the block is associated with structural heart disease, the prognosis is linked to the heart disease.[1]

Bedside Diagnosis

Second-degree AV block was first described in 1899 by Wenckebach[10] without benefit of the ECG, by observing the jugular venous pulse. The *A*- to *C*-wave interval widens until an *A* wave is not followed by a *V* wave. There is a pause, and the sequence begins again. As the PR interval lengthens, the first heart sound diminishes in intensity.

Treatment

When AV conduction problems occur in the setting of acute inferior MI they are usually transient and require observation only.[2]

TYPE II AV BLOCK

Type II AV block is identified when, in the face of a normal sinus rhythm and normal rate, there are nonconducted sinus P waves with all PR intervals identical (before and after a blocked impulse). The typical ECG of type II AV block is illustrated in Fig. 16-10.

ECG Recognition

Rhythm: irregular because of nonconducted sinus beats.

P waves: Sinus.

PR intervals: The same from beat to beat and after a pause; usually of normal duration; some P waves are not conducted. If the first PR after the block is shortened, the diagnosis of type II AV block cannot be made.[11]

QRS complexes: Broad (0.12 second or more) unless the problem is at the level of the bundle of His (Fig. 16-1).

Diagnostic maneuvers: Carotid sinus massage slows the sinus rate and may improve conduction when the lesion is His-Purkinje. Exercise, catecholamines, or administration of atropine in patients with His-Purkinje disease may increase the degree of AV block.

Distinguishing features:

- Normal sinus rhythm

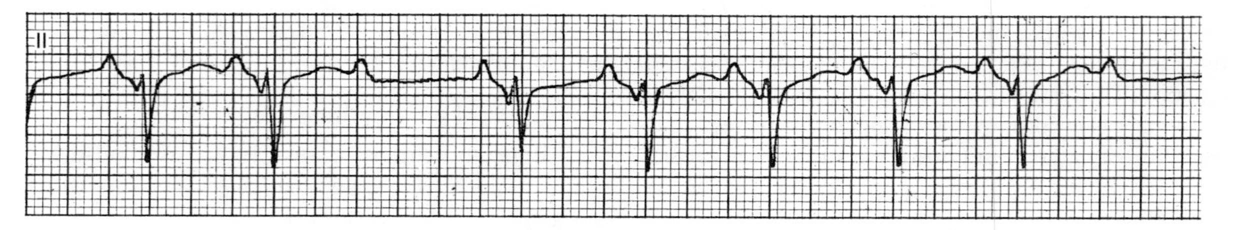

FIG. 16-10. Type II second-degree AV block with a broad QRS. Note that all PR intervals are the same. To make this diagnosis, it is important that the PR intervals on either side of the dropped beat be the same.

- Fixed PR intervals before and after a pause
- Broad QRS

Mechanism

Type II AV block reflects a lesion within or below the bundle of His. In Fig. 16-11, note the nonconducted sinus P waves, the fixed PR throughout the tracing, and the broad QRS, which are the hallmarks of type II second-degree AV block. The lesion may involve both bundle branches. Complete block of one bundle causes the ventricular complexes to be broad. Intermittent block of the other bundle causes dropped beats. Fig. 16-12 is an example of 2:1 AV block with a broad QRS revealing itself as type II with the onset of 1:1 conduction. Note that there is no change in the PR interval when 1:1 conduction commences. This tracing is from the same patient as in Fig. 16-10.

Causes

- Chronic fibrotic disease of the conduction system
- Anteroseptal MI

Clinical Implications

During acute MI in the thrombolytic era, the occurrence of type II second-degree AV block and complete AV block is associated with a high and independent risk of in-hospital death during acute MI.[12]

Type II AV block is not as common as type I and is a more serious condition; disease is lower in the conduction system (at the level of the bundle branches). It often is later associated with Adams-Stokes syncope and deteriorates into complete AV block. Its appearance in the setting of acute anteroseptal MI identifies a high-risk patient. Naccarelli et al[5] called this particular form of heart block "treacherous and unpredictable." If the AV conduction

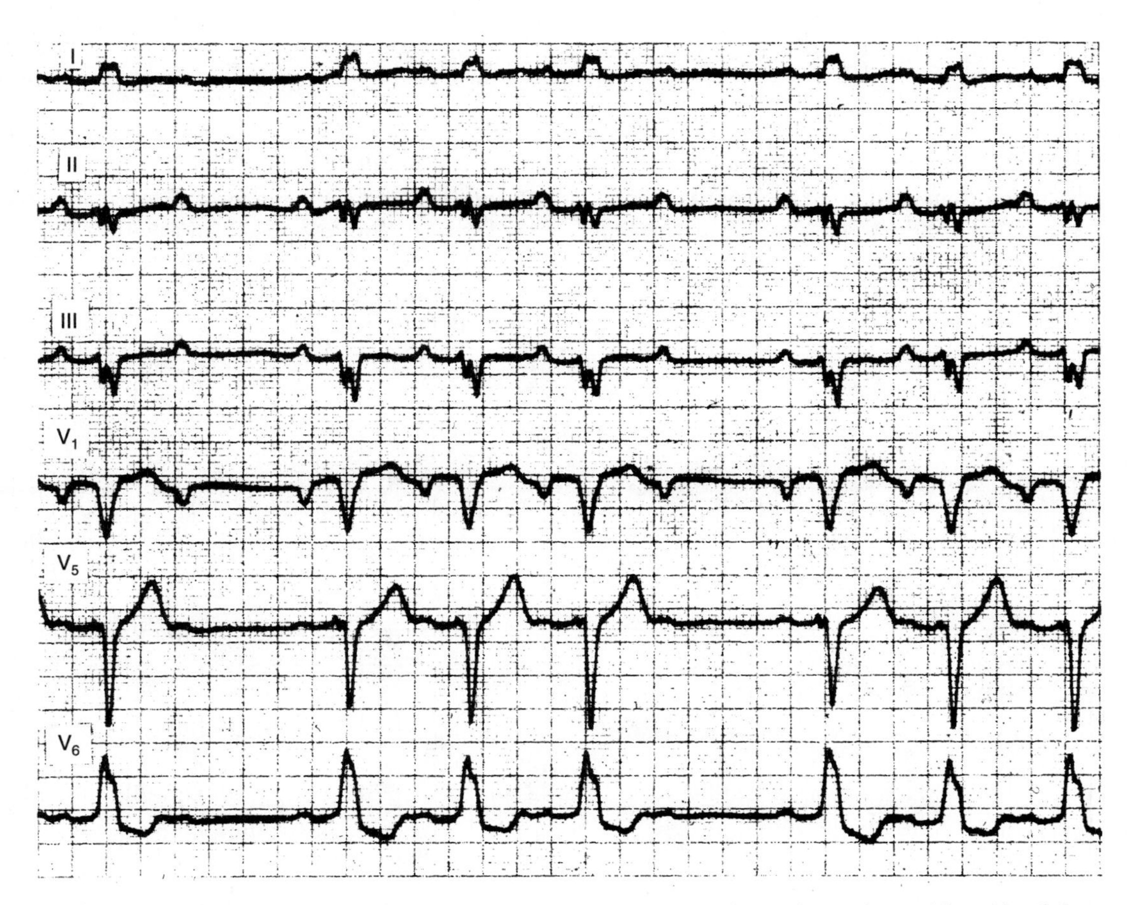

FIG. 16-11. Type II second-degree AV block with an LBBB pattern. The PR intervals on either side of the dropped beats are identical, although prolonged. The QRS is broad with an LBBB pattern indicating that the type II block is located in the right bundle branch. (Tracing courtesy Hein J.J. Wellens, MD.)

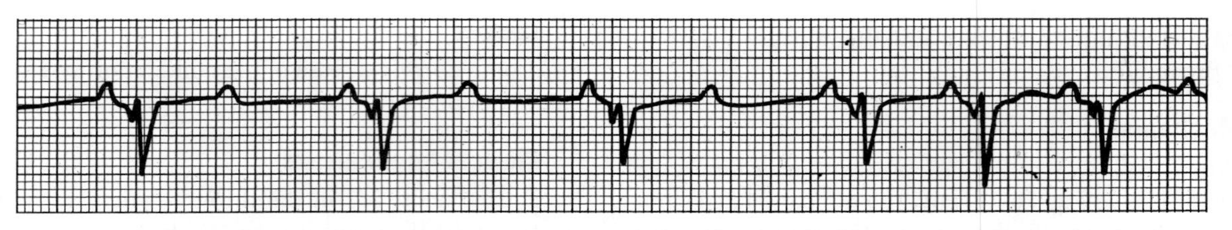

FIG. 16-12. Two-to-one AV block converting to 1:1 conduction. Note that all of the PR intervals are identical, indicating a type II AV block.

deteriorates further, the complete heart block that results has a slow ventricular escape rhythm, with its focus below the lesion in the bundle branches.

Bedside Diagnosis

In type II AV block the diagnosis can be made as in type I, by observing the neck veins. There are intermittent *A* waves not followed by *V* waves. Because the PR intervals are fixed, the first heart sound maintains a constant intensity. The patient may have a sense of the heart skipping a beat.

Treatment

When type II AV block is associated with syncope a temporary pacemaker is inserted. If the patient has chronic fibrotic disease of the conduction system, a permanent pacemaker is inserted. In anteroseptal MI with syncope, complete block is usually temporary, and implantation of a permanent pacemaker is rarely needed.[2]

TWO-TO-ONE AV BLOCK

Two-to-one second degree AV block can occur in either the AV node, the bundle of His, or the bundle branches. It is not described as type I or type II second-degree AV block because there are not two conducted P waves in a row to examine; thus, it is not known if the PR intervals are lengthening or fixed. It is of course possible that in 2:1 AV block one may eventually see two conducted beats in a row and thus reveal its "type."[13] The level of the lesion in 2:1 block can be determined by the width of the QRS (i.e., narrow if in the AV node or bundle of His; broad if in the bundle branches).

ECG Recognition

PR intervals: All the same; may be normal or prolonged. AV nodal disease is associated with a prolonged PR interval, whereas with subnodal disease the PR interval may be normal.

P waves: Sinus in origin.

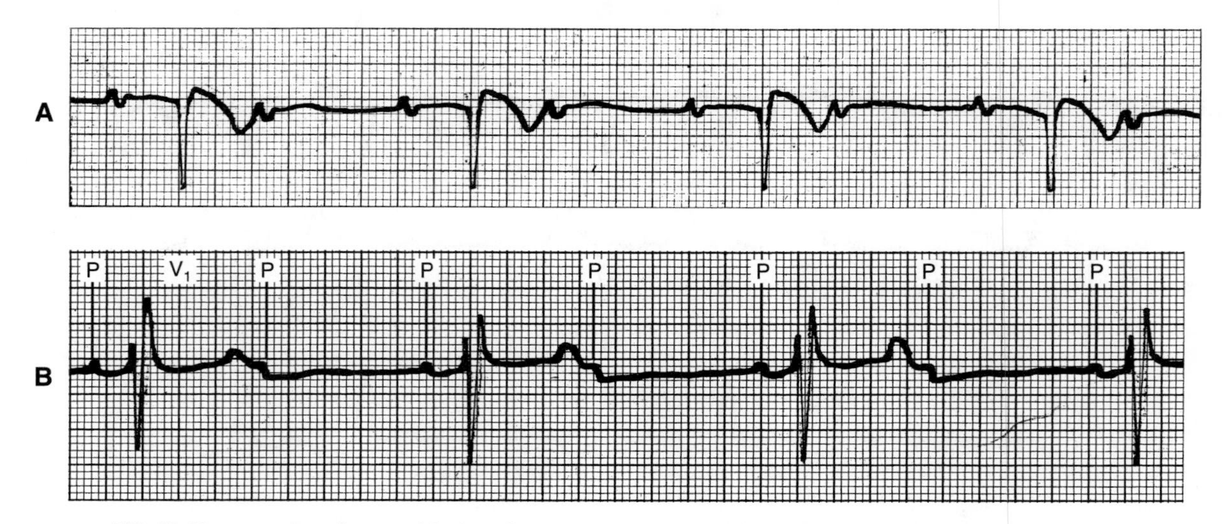

FIG. 16-13. Examples of 2:1 AV block with a narrow QRS and with a wide QRS. **A,** The PR interval of 0.40 second and the narrow QRS suggest an AV nodal problem. **B,** The relatively short PR interval (0.20 second) and the broad QRS suggest a subnodal problem. The sinus P waves are at regular intervals.

AV conduction: There are two sinus P waves for every QRS.

QRS complex: May be narrow or broad. A narrow QRS is associated with AV nodal disease, and a broad QRS with disease in the bundle branches. Fig. 16-13, *A* and *B*, are examples of 2:1 AV block with a narrow QRS and with a wide QRS. In *A*, the PR interval of 0.40 second and the narrow QRS suggest an AV nodal problem. In *B*, the relatively short PR interval (0.20 second) and the broad QRS suggest a subnodal problem.

Diagnostic maneuvers: When there is an *AV nodal lesion*, conduction improves with atropine, exercise, or catecholamines and worsens with carotid sinus massage. When there is a *subnodal lesion*, conduction worsens with atropine, exercise, or catecholamines and may improve when carotid sinus massage causes the sinus rate to slow.

Clinical Implications

The clinical implications depend on the level of block in the conduction system. AV nodal disease is associated with acute inferior wall MI and, although the block may be complete, a pacemaker is usually not necessary. Subnodal disease is associated with acute anterior MI, and the patient may have syncope or hemodynamic deterioration. A temporary pacemaker may be indicated in a symptomatic patient with a broad QRS.

The level of block may be determined by the diagnostic maneuvers described above or by a His bundle electrogram (see Fig. 16-2).

Symptoms

Two-to-one AV block may cause symptoms of bradycardia.

COMPLETE (THIRD-DEGREE) AV BLOCK

Third-degree AV block may be acquired or congenital, and is characterized by a complete failure of atrial impulses to be conducted to the ventricles. This is one form of AV dissociation, but keep in mind that not all AV dissociation is complete AV block (see Chapter 18).

ECG Recognition

Ventricular rate: Depends on the level of block. Block proximal to the His bundle has an escape ventricular rate of 40 to 50 beats/min; acquired complete AV block has a ventricular rate of less than 50 beats/min. The higher the focus is within the conduction system, the faster and more dependable the ventricular rhythm. In congenital AV block the escape rate may be greater than 50 beats/min.

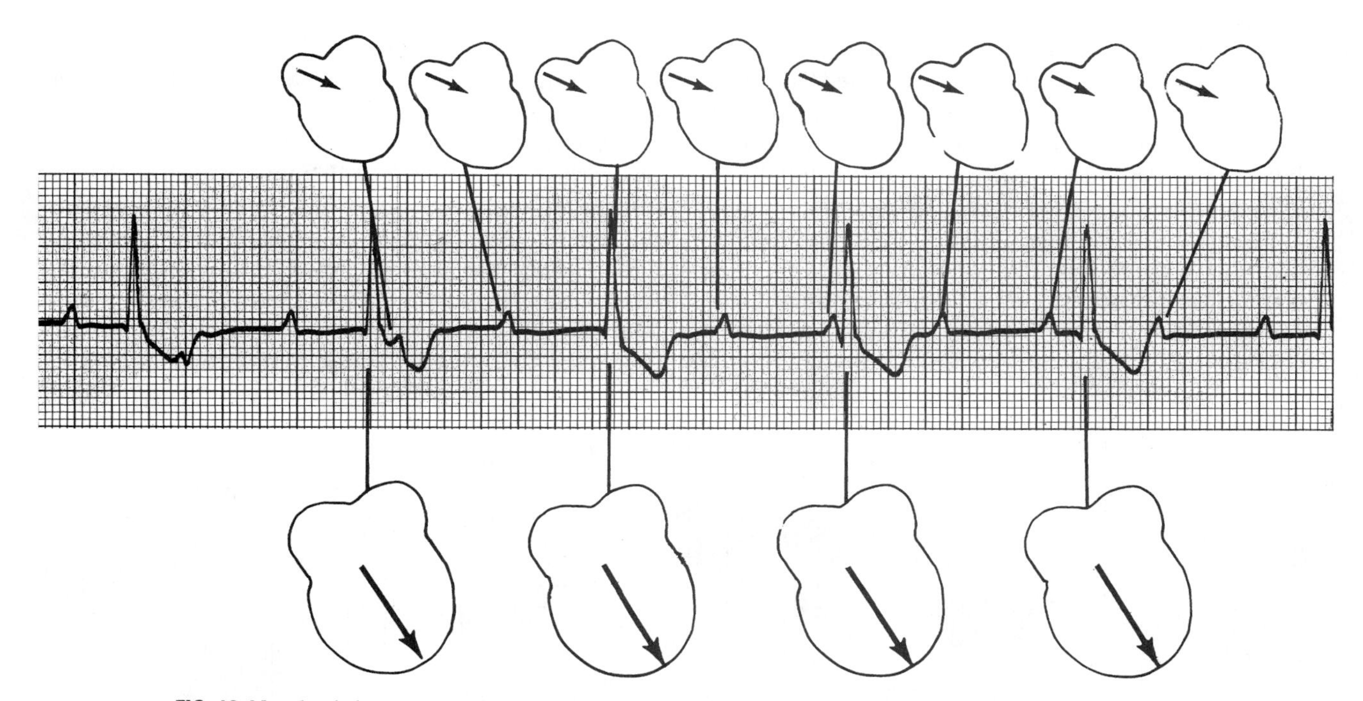

FIG. 16-14. Third-degree (complete) AV block with a junctional escape rhythm. The QRS is narrow, placing the conduction problem above the bundle branches. The sinus rate is 100 beats/min, and the junctional rate is 45 beats/min.

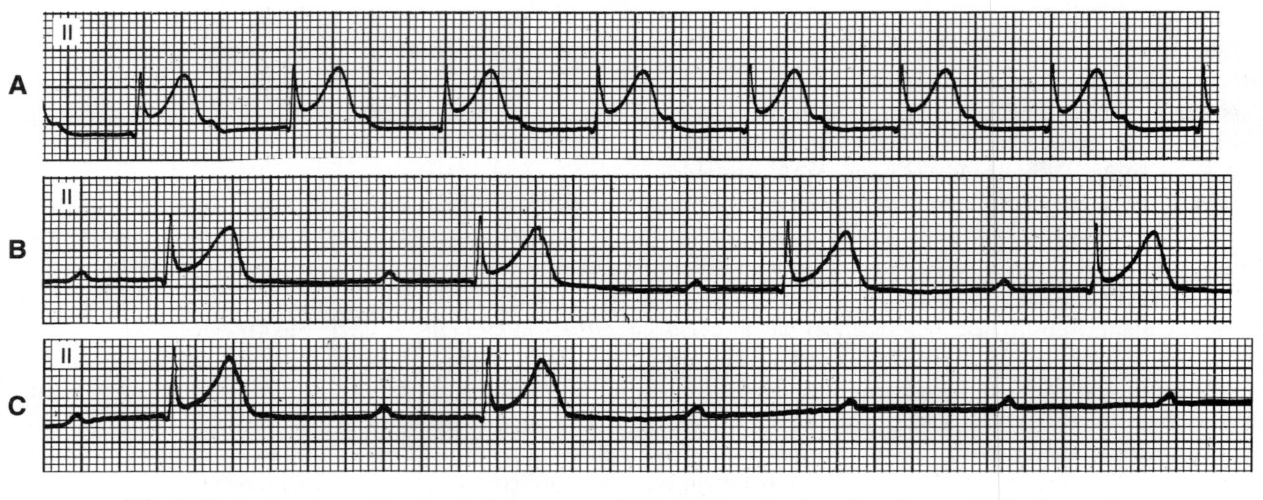

FIG. 16-15. **A,** A patient with acute inferior myocardial infarction develops first-degree AV block at a sinus rate of 74 beats/min. The PR interval is greater than 0.04 second. **B,** The AV block is 2:1, resulting in a heart rate of only 36 beats/min; the PR is 0.44 second. **C,** The 2:1 block abruptly converts to complete AV block without an escape pacemaker. (Courtesy Janet Bacon, RN, Eagle Creek, Ore.)

Rhythm: AV dissociation; regular ventricular rhythm; regular sinus rhythm unless there is atrial fibrillation or atrial flutter.

P waves: Sinus or ectopic (atrial fibrillation or atrial flutter).

QRS complex: Narrow or broad, depending on level of block. A focus above the bifurcation of the His bundle produces a narrow QRS (junctional escape rhythm); if associated with BBB, the QRS will of course be broad, but the rate dependable. A focus below the bundle of His produces a broad QRS (ventricular escape rhythm).

P/QRS relationship: None (AV dissociation).

Distinguishing features: AV dissociation when there is opportunity to conduct; a regular ventricular rhythm.

Rhythm Variations

Idiojunctional rhythm. Complete AV block with an idiojunctional rhythm is recognized because of narrow QRS complexes and AV dissociation. In Fig. 16-14 the P waves can be seen to occur regularly at a rate of 100 beats/min. They are totally independent of the ventricular rhythm (rate, 46 beats/min). The sinus node paces the atria, and the AV junction paces the ventricles.

Sudden, complete AV block. Fig. 16-15, *A-C*, is a sequence of tracings in lead II from a patient with acute inferior MI. In *A*, the PR interval of more than 0.24 second suggests an AV nodal lesion. In *B*, the AV block is now 2:1; in *C*, it deteriorates abruptly to complete AV block without an escape pacemaker. A precordial thump and isoproterenol (Isuprel) were followed by the emergency insertion of a pacemaker. The patient survived these frightening events.

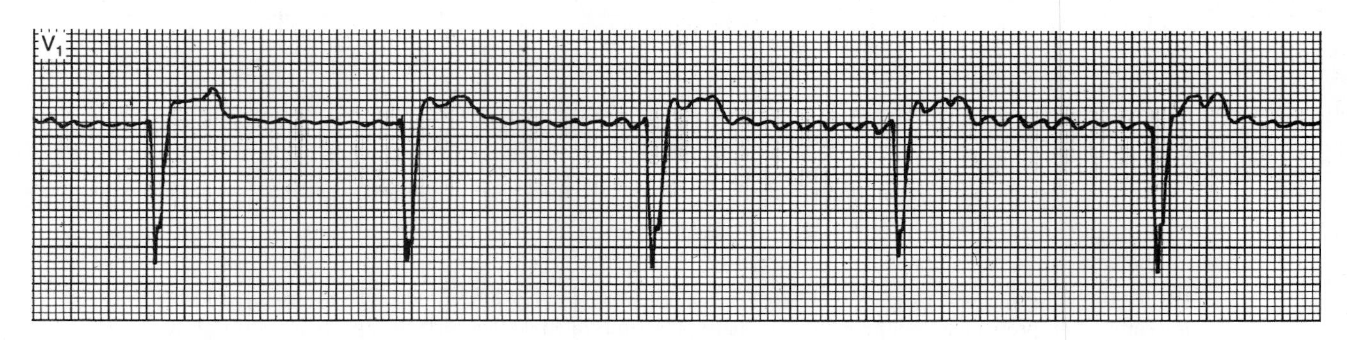

FIG. 16-16. Atrial fibrillation with complete AV block and an escape junctional rhythm of 45 beats/min.

Atrial fibrillation. Fig. 16-16 is an example of atrial fibrillation with complete AV block and a ventricular escape rhythm of 45 beats/min in a patient with acute anterior wall infarction. The diagnosis of complete AV block is made in atrial fibrillation when the ventricular response is absolutely regular and less than 50 beats/min. Other causes of regularity of the QRS complexes during atrial fibrillation are junctional tachycardia and fascicular ventricular tachycardia (see Chapter 15).

Clinical Implications

If complete AV block develops because of inferior wall MI, the escape pacemaker is usually junctional and a pacemaker is rarely required. However, the development of the block in this setting identifies a high-risk patient with more extensive infarction. Such a patient can be identified at admission by the observation of ST-segment elevation in lead V_4R (p. 351), which also indicates a proximal right coronary artery occlusion and right ventricular MI.

The incidence of third-degree AV block as a complication of acute MI is lower since the widespread use of thrombolytics. However, the prognosis for patients with acute MI and third-degree AV block, in spite of thrombolytic therapy, is significantly worse than it is for acute MI patients without complete AV block.[14]

Symptoms

Complete AV block may have all the symptoms of profound bradycardia, loss of atrial kick, and reduced cardiac output (presyncope, syncope, or angina).

Pediatrics

Complete AV block may be congenital and associated with maternal collagen vascular disease, or it may be secondary to surgery. In either case, there is usually a junctional escape rhythm.[7]

A common histologic finding is anatomic discontinuity between the atria and the AV node and between the AV node and the ventricles. Generally children are asymptomatic. Those in whom symptoms develop may require a pacemaker. The mortality rate is at its height in the neonatal period, is much lower during childhood and adolescence, and then increases slowly.[4]

Treatment

Complete AV block with a broad QRS usually requires a pacemaker. If the QRS is narrow, the cause of the block is ascertained before a decision is made to insert a pacemaker.

COMPLETE AV BLOCK WITH ALTERNATING BBB

The continuous tracing of lead II in Fig. 16-17 is an example of alternating BBB, a condition that carries with it the highest risk to develop third-degree AV block. In this patient, there is 2:1 block with a PR of 0.28 second, and presumably left bundle branch block (LBBB) alternating with 2:1 block, a PR of 0.32 second, and presumably right bundle branch block (RBBB). Unfortunately, leads V_1 and V_6 were not available in this patient. This ECG implies severe conduction abnormalities in both bundle branches and indicates the necessity for a permanent pacemaker.[2]

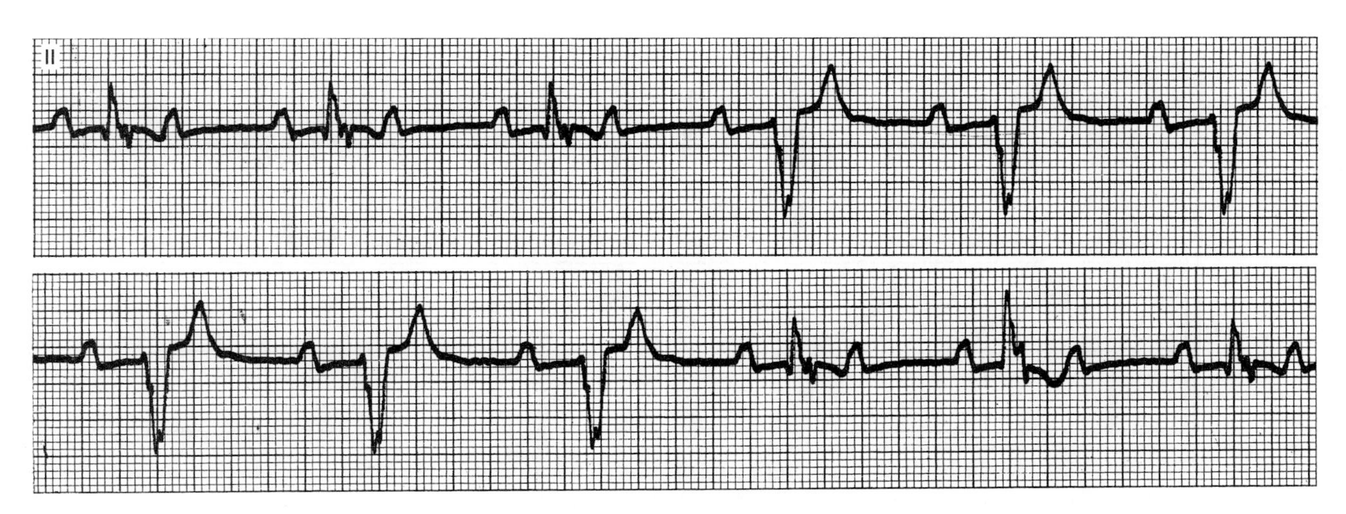

FIG. 16-17. Continuous tracings. In lead II it is difficult to tell which bundle branch is blocked. Presumably the tracing starts with 2:1 block and LBBB, then switches to 2:1 block with RBBB with hemiblock. The sinus rhythm is 100 beats/min. There are severe conduction problems in both bundle branches.

TABLE 16-1 Noninvasive Evaluation of Atrioventricular Block Level

Intervention		Type II (Subnodal)
Atropine	Improves	Worsens
Exercise	Improves	Worsens
Catecholamines	Improves	Worsens
Carotid sinus massage	Worsens	Improves

NONINVASIVE EVALUATION OF THE SITE OF BLOCK

Because AV nodal block has a better prognosis and different treatment than subnodal block, it is important to determine the location of the block. The ECG supplies much information: a prolonged PR interval implicates the AV node, and a prolonged QRS duration implicates the bundle branches. Interventions that slow or improve AV conduction are also helpful (Table 16-1). For example, if the sinus discharge and AV conduction are slowed with carotid sinus massage, the number of impulses reaching the bundle branches is fewer, so a block at that level should improve, whereas a block within the AV node would be compounded by such a maneuver. On the other hand, if the rate of the sinus node and the speed of AV conduction are increased with atropine, exercise, or catecholamines, impulses reach the bundle branches more frequently and would compound a block at that level, whereas a block at the AV node would be improved.[5] These three interventions tend to shorten the PR interval in both normal and diseased hearts.

CONCEALED JUNCTIONAL BEATS IMITATE SECOND-DEGREE AV BLOCK

Concealed junctional beats discharge the AV junction while both anterograde and retrograde conduction are blocked, and thus may imitate type I and type II second-degree AV block, as diagrammatically illustrated in Figs. 16-18 and 16-19.[15] Although concealed junctional beats are not seen on the surface ECG, its diagnosis may be extremely important in the management of the patient. Because the development of type II AV block is a widely accepted indication for a permanent implanted pacemaker, one has a serious responsibility to rule out concealed junctional extrasystoles. Additionally, the junctional beats themselves are thought to indicate significant junctional disease and should be recognized.

In Fig. 16-20, type II AV block is imitated when, at the end of the tracing, a single, concealed junctional beat suddenly prevents conduction of a sinus P wave. In the rhythm preceding this sudden, unexpected pause, the problem is suspected because of unexplained lengthening

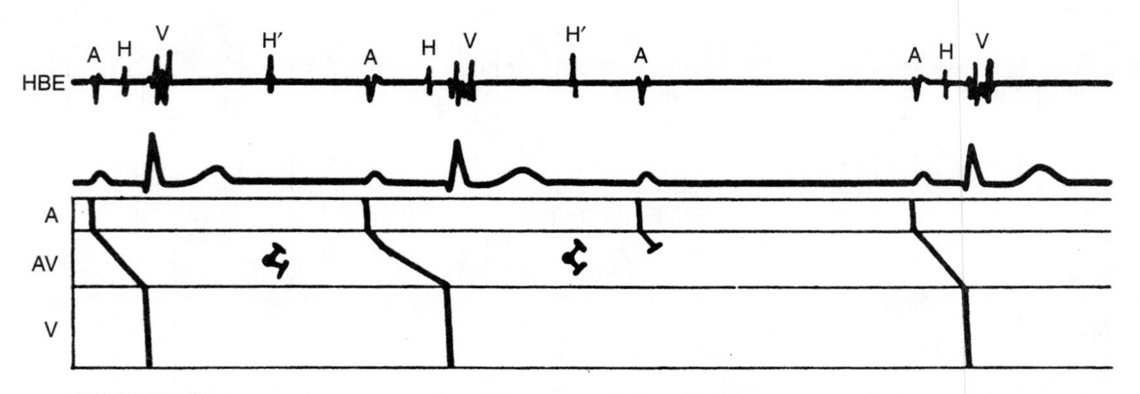

FIG. 16-18. Diagrammatic representation of how concealed junctional beats can imitate Wenckebach conduction. The first junctional beat (in the AV tier of the laddergram) lengthens the next PR interval and the AH interval on the His bundle electrogram *(HBE)*. The second junctional beat prevents conduction of the sinus impulse and simulates the dropped beat of a Wenckebach period. (From Marriott HJL, Conover M: *Advanced concepts in arrhythmias,* St Louis, 1998, Mosby, p 78.)

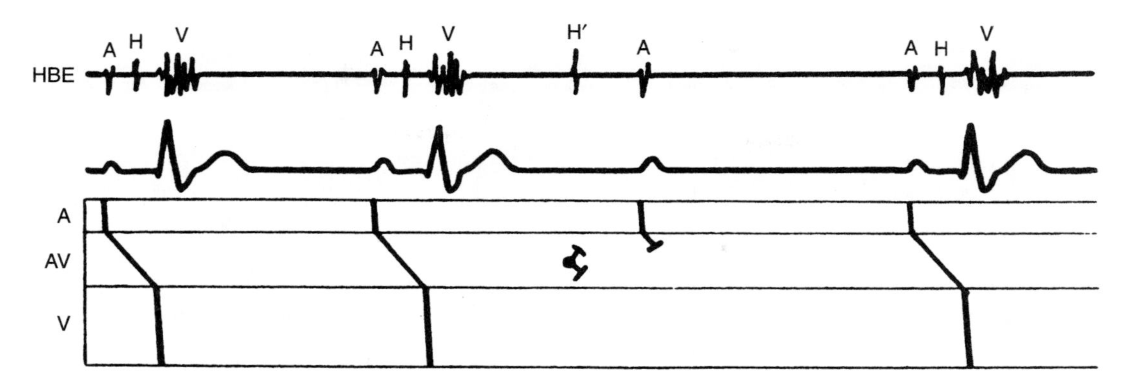

FIG. 16-19. Diagrammatic representation of how concealed junctional beats can mimic type II AV block. Without prior lengthening of the PR interval, the concealed junctional beat (AV tier of the laddergram) prevents conduction of the next sinus P wave. *HBE,* His bundle electrogram. (From Marriott HJL, Conover M: *Advanced concepts in arrhythmias,* St Louis, 1998, Mosby, p 78.)

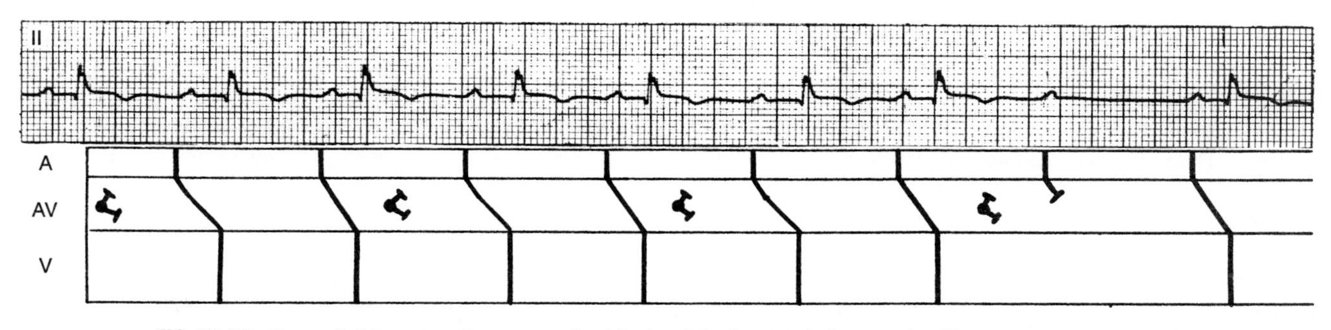

FIG. 16-20. Concealed junctional extrasystoles (depicted in the AV tier) every third beat cause unexplained PR prolongation followed by PR shortening. The last concealed junctional beat causes conduction from the sinus P wave to be blocked, simulating type II AV block. (From Marriott HJL, Conover M: *Advanced concepts in arrhythmias,* St Louis, 1998, Mosby, p 80.)

of PR intervals every third beat. Fig. 16-21 also demonstrates unexplained alternating PR lengthening and group beating.

ECG Clues to Concealed Junctional Extrasystoles

Although concealed junctional extrasystoles can be documented only with the aid of the His bundle electrogram, they can be strongly suspected from the following clues:

1. Abrupt, unexplained lengthening of the PR interval
2. The presence of apparent types I and II AV block in the same tracing (they rarely exist together)[8]
3. Apparent type II block in the presence of a normal QRS
4. The presence of manifest junctional extrasystoles elsewhere in the tracing

SUMMARY

AV block is conventionally divided into first-, second-, and third-degree block. The disease of first-degree AV block is commonly in the AV node, but may occur at any level, including the atria; it is recognized because the PR intervals are longer than 0.20 second. Second-degree AV block is divided into type I (Wenckebach), type II, and 2:1. Type I is recognized because of group beating, lengthening PR intervals, shortening RR intervals, and dropped beats with pauses less than twice the shortest cycle. Type II AV block is recognized because of dropped beats and normal and fixed PR intervals before and after the dropped beat. Two-to-one AV block is recognized because of a regular sinus or atrial rhythm, fixed PR intervals, and every other beat conducted. Prognosis and management is determined by the level of block in the conduction system. This can be determined noninvasively by observing AV conduction in

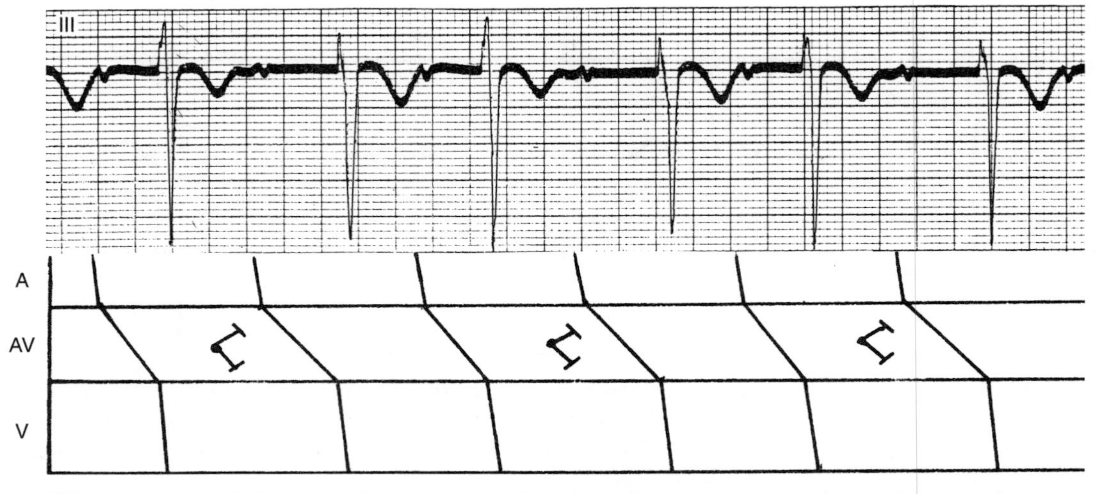

FIG. 16-21. Concealed junctional beats again explain alternating PR intervals and group beating. The junctional beats are depicted in the AV tier. (From Marriott HJL, Conover M: *Advanced concepts in arrhythmias,* St Louis, 1998, Mosby, p 80.)

response to atropine, exercise, catecholamines, and carotid sinus massage. Immediate pacemaker insertion is usually indicated only in complete AV block with a broad QRS complex.

REFERENCES

1. Scherlag BJ, Lau SH, Helfant RH et al: Catheter technique for recording bundle activity in man, *Circulation* 39:13, 1969.
2. Wellens HJJ, Conover M: *The ECG in emergency decision making,* Philadelphia, 1992, WB Saunders.
3. Lie KI, Durrer D: Acute and chronic aspects of conduction disturbances in acute myocardial infarction. In Befeler B, Lazzara R, Scherlag BJ, editors: *Selected topics in cardiac arrhythmias,* Mount Kisco, NY, 1980, Futura.
4. Zipes DP: Specific arrhythmias: diagnosis and treatment. In Braunwald E, editor: *Heart disease,* ed 4, Philadelphia, 1992, WB Saunders.
5. Naccarelli GV, Willerson JT, Blomquist CG: Recognition and physiologic treatment of cardiac arrhythmias and conduction disturbances. In Willerson JT, Cohn JN, editors: *Cardiovascular medicine,* New York, 1995, Churchill Livingstone.
6. Tilkian AG, Conover M: *Understanding heart sounds and murmurs with an introduction to lung sounds,* ed 4, Philadelphia, 2001, WB Saunders.
7. Chou TC, Knilans TK: *Electrocardiography in clinical practice adult and pediatrics,* ed 4, Philadelphia, 1996, WB Saunders.
8. Barold SS: Lingering misconceptions about type I second-degree atrioventricular block, *Am J Cardiol* 88:1018, 2001.
9. Rubin Lopez JM, Hevia Nava S, Veganzones Bayon A et al: [Atrioventricular block secondary to topical ophthalmic beta blockers], *Rev Esp Cardiol* 52:532, 1999.
10. Wenckebach KF: Zur Analyse des unregelmˇssigen Pulses. II. Ueber den regelmˇssig intermittirenden Puls, *Z Klin Med* 37:475, 1899.
11. Barold SS, Hayes DL: Second-degree atrioventricular block: a reappraisal, *Mayo Clin Proc* 76:44, 2001.
12. Escosteguy CC, Carvalho MD, Medronho RD: Bundle branch and atrioventricular block as complications of acute myocardial infarction in the thrombolytic era, *Arq Bras Cardiol* 76:291, 2001.
13. Barold SS: 2:1 Atrioventricular block: order from chaos, *Am J Emerg Med* 19:214, 2001.
14. Harpaz D, Behar S, Gottlieb S: Complete atrioventricular block complicating acute myocardial infarction in the thrombolytic era. SPRINT Study Group and the Israeli Thrombolytic Survey Group. Secondary Prevention Reinfarction Israeli Nifedipine Trial, *J Am Coll Cardiol* 34:1721, 1999.
15. Marriott HJL, Conover M: *Advanced concepts in arrhythmias,* St Louis, 1998, Mosby, pp 69-84.

CHAPTER 17

Potassium Derangements

Potassium is one of the body's major ions, with the kidney determining potassium homeostasis and excreting excess in the urine. Diuretics, vomiting, diaphoresis, and diarrhea can rapidly deplete the body of this vital ion (hypokalemia). Conversely, anuria can cause a potassium buildup (hyperkalemia). Both hypokalemia and hyperkalemia may produce serious arrhythmias and even death.

The reference range for serum potassium is 3.5 to 5 mEq/L; nearly 98% is intracellular.

MAJOR FUNCTIONS OF POTASSIUM

Potassium contributes to the following important antiarrhythmic functions:

- Prevents the action potential duration (and QT) from being too short or too long
- Accommodates rapid heart rates by shortening the QT interval
- Protects excitability in cases of hyperpolarization
- Slows the heart rate by increasing inward K^+ flux in response to parasympathetic stimulation

HYPOKALEMIA

Hypokalemia (less than 3.5 mEq/L) is the most frequent electrolytic disturbance in hospitalized patients and is sometimes familial.[1] It is estimated that 20% of patients are hypokalemic, although severe hypokalemia (less than 2.5 mEq/L) is relatively uncommon. Moderate hypokalemia is a serum level of 2.5 to 3 mEq/L.

ECG Recognition

- Progressive ST depression
- Progressive decrease in T wave amplitude
- Increased U wave amplitude

Advanced stage:

- U and T waves fuse
- Increased QRS amplitude
- Increased QRS duration
- Increased P wave amplitude
- Increased P wave duration
- PR interval usually slightly prolonged

Possible arrhythmias:

- Bradycardia or tachycardia
- Atrioventricular (AV) block
- Premature atrial or ventricular complexes
- Atrial flutter
- Exaggeration of toxic effects of digitalis
- Torsades de pointes
- Ventricular fibrillation
- Cardiac arrest

Fig. 17-1 is a schematic depiction of changes in the electrocardiogram (ECG) associated with progressive hypokalemia. Fig. 17-2 is an example of the ECG in a patient with a potassium level of 2.5 mEq/L. Note the ST depression and an exaggerated U wave that is beginning to fuse with the T wave. In Fig. 17-3 the potassium level is yet lower and the T and U waves have fused (best seen in V_2 to V_6), with the giant U wave larger than the T. There is ST segment depression and the amplitude of the QRS has increased.

Mechanism

Hypokalemia lengthens the QT interval, prolongs the action potential duration, and increases membrane automaticity.

Causes[2]

- Diuretics (thiazides, loop diuretics, and carbonic anhydrase inhibitors) produce kaliuresis and hypokalemia of variable severity
- Alcoholism (along with hyponatremia, hypophosphatemia, and hypomagnesemia)
- Pyloric stenosis and gastrointestinal suction and drainage
- Renal tubular acidosis (type I and type II)
- Primary or secondary hyperaldosteronism
- Magnesium depletion (loop diuretic, alcoholics, malabsorption syndrome, gentamicin, and cisplatin therapy)
- Ectopic adrenocorticotropic hormone production

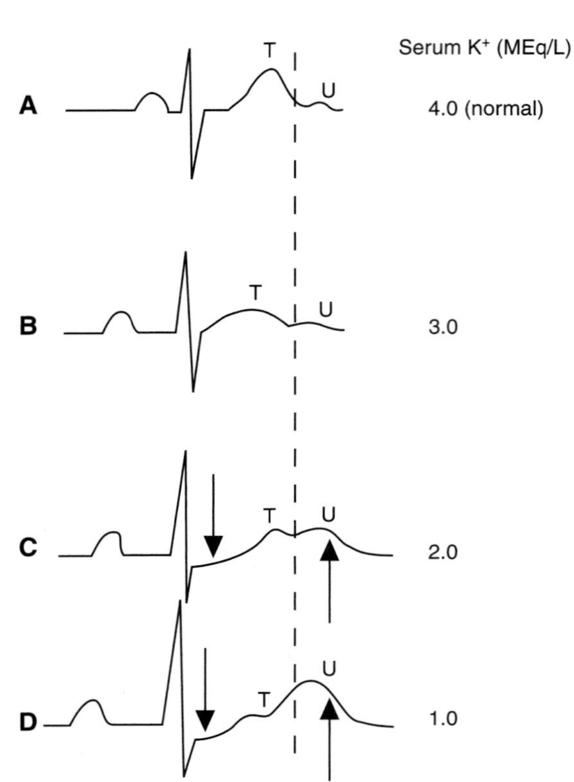

FIG. 17-1. T wave, U wave, and ST segment changes in progressive hypokalemia. **A,** At a normal serum concentration of 4 to 5.5 mEq/L the amplitude of the T wave is appreciably greater than that of the U wave. **B,** By the time the serum potassium level has dropped to 3 mEq/L, the T wave amplitude had decreased and the U wave increased, approaching the height of the T wave. **C** and **D,** With a further drop in the level of potassium the amplitude and duration of the QRS and the P wave increase, the PR may lengthen slightly, the ST segment becomes depressed (↓), and the U wave begins to tower over (↑) and fuse with the T wave.

- Antibiotics (penicillin, carbenicillin, gentamicin, and others)
- Genetic hypokalemia Liddle's syndrome, Bartter's syndrome, and Gitelmann's syndrome, tubular acidosis, hypokalemic periodic paralysis[1]
- Liquid protein diet
- Frequent ingestion of licorice
- Certain chewing tobaccos
- Trauma (decreases within 1 hour and returns to normal within 24 hours)
- Immune-related potassium losing nephropathy

Cellular shifts in potassium. In addition to the above mentioned causes, serum potassium level may be low because of a shift from the extracellular compartment into the intracellular compartment. This occurs because of the following:

1. Infusion of glucose
2. Infusion of alkali (potassium exchanges with hydrogen)
3. Infusion of large quantities of cortisol or glucocorticoids
4. Hypokalemic periodic paralysis
5. Adrenergic stimulation secondary to resuscitated ventricular fibrillation[3]

Clinical Implications

Hypokalemia causes arrhythmias by altered automaticity and reentry (because of slow conduction). If the level of extracellular K^+ is low, there is a tendency for the fibers of the specialized conduction system—and even fibers that do not normally possess the property of automaticity—to develop enhanced automaticity and automatic rhythms. The cell membrane becomes less and less negative until the cell is eventually nonexcitable.[4] Moreover, if digitalis is administered when the extracellular potassium is low, arrhythmogenicity is likely to be compounded. Digitalis and K^+ compete for membrane binding sites, and with less

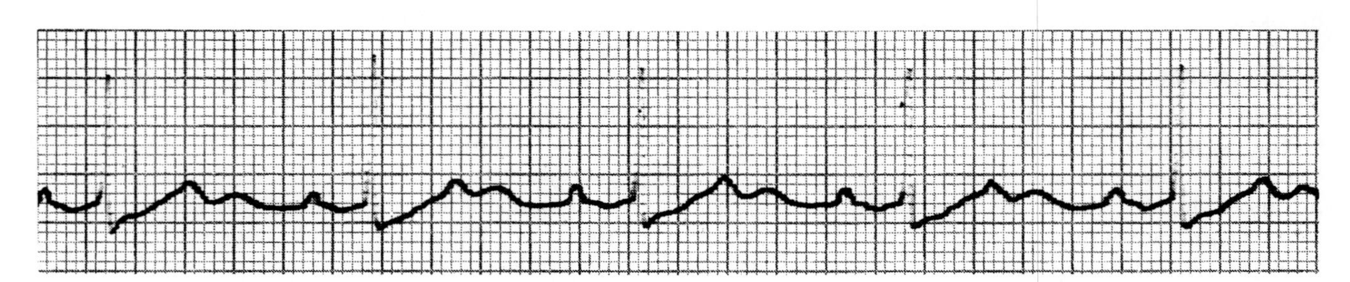

FIG. 17-2. Tracing from a patient with hypokalemia (serum K^+ level 2.5 mEq/L). The prominent U wave is beginning to fuse with the T wave, which is still the taller of the two.

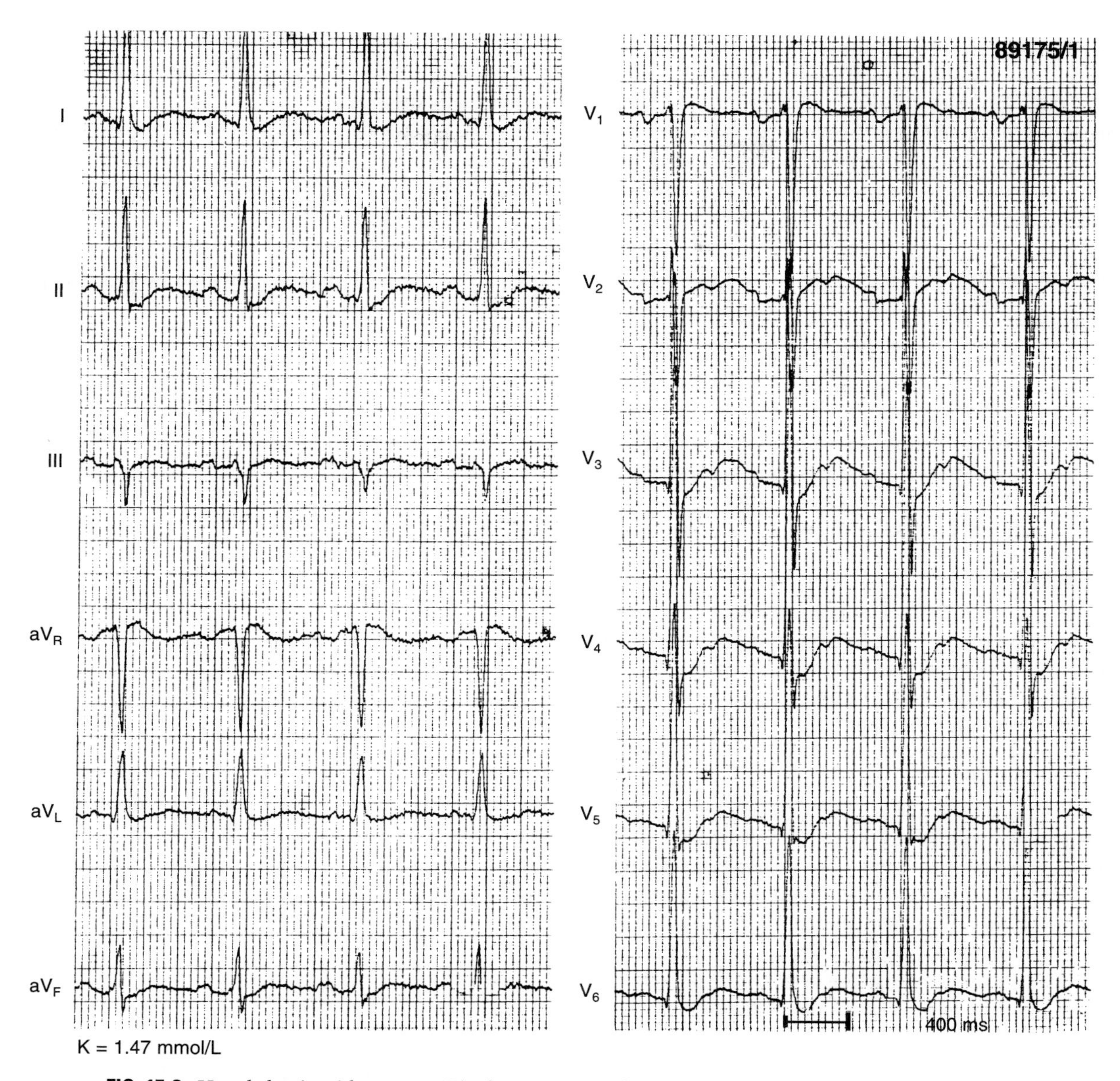

FIG. 17-3. Hypokalemia with a serum K^+ of 1.47 mEq/L. The giant U wave is best seen in V_2 to V_6. It towers over the T wave and has fused with it, although still definable. The QRS height and duration have increased and there is ST segment depression. (Courtesy Hein J.J. Wellens, MD, Maastricht, The Netherlands.)

K^+ in the extracellular fluid, more digitalis binds to the K^+ position on the membrane sodium-potassium pumps, augmenting digitalis intoxication.[5]

Signs and Symptoms

The following signs and symptoms of hypokalemia involve almost every system of the body:

Muscular: Weakness or cramping.
Neurologic: Tetany, decreased tendon reflexes.
Cerebral: Irritability, depression, lethargy, hallucinations, apathy, drowsiness, confusion, delirium, and coma (the electroencephalogram is usually normal).
Gastrointestinal: Nausea, vomiting, and ileus.
Carbohydrate metabolism: Impairment of glucose tolerance.

Renal: Symptoms result from the inability to concentrate urine (nocturia, polyuria, and polydipsia). Other renal manifestations of hypokalemia are related to the inability to maximally acidify urine because of stimulation of the production of massive amounts of renal ammonia by the hypokalemic kidney.
Pulmonary: Hypoventilation, respiratory distress, respiratory failure.
Cardiovascular: Hypotension, edema.

Treatment[6]

Moderate potassium deficiency. Treatment consists of an increased dietary intake of or supplementation with potassium salts when possible.

Severe potassium deficiency. Intravenous potassium chloride (40- to 60-mEq/L concentrations at 20 mEq/hr, approximately 200 to 250 mEq/day); continuous ECG monitoring. For treatment of torsades de pointes see Chapter 26.

HYPERKALEMIA

Hyperkalemia is one of the more common acute life-threatening metabolic emergencies seen in the emergency department. The patient's life is dependent in many cases on the emergency physician's or nurses' ability to recognize the ECG manifestations of hyperkalemia.[7]

ECG Recognition

Fig. 17-4 is a schematic depiction of typical ECG changes associated with progressive hyperkalemia. Note that as the condition worsens, the S wave ascends directly into the tall T wave (no ST segment). Slow conduction causes the ECG complexes and intervals to stretch out and flatten. The P wave flattens and the PR and QRS become prolonged. The ECG changes that occur as the degree of hyperkalemia progresses from mild to severe include the following.

Mild Hyperkalemia (Less Than 6.0 mEq/L)

P waves: Normal.
QRS: Normal.
T waves: Tall and tented at 5.7 mEq/L, often symmetric with a narrow base; usually best seen in leads II, III, V_2, and V_4. The corrected QT interval is not prolonged.[8]

Severe Hyperkalemia (Greater Than 6.0 mEq/L)

P wave: Amplitude decreases; duration increases until it eventually disappears.
QRS: Broadens; wide S waves in the left precordial leads.
QRS axis: Superior (left axis deviation).
ST segment: The terminal S wave becomes continuous with the tall tented T wave; a frequent early sign of severe hyperkalemia.

Fig. 17-5 is from a patient with a serum potassium level

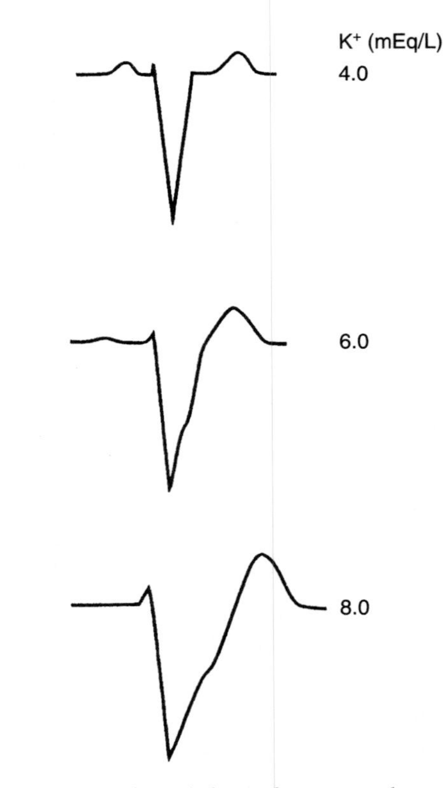

FIG. 17-4. Stages in hyperkalemia from normal potassium levels to mild and severe hyperkalemia. At 6 mEq/L the P wave flattens, PR lengthens, QRS broadens, and the ST segment disappears, with the S wave flowing into the tall tented T wave. At 8 mEq/L the P wave has disappeared and the QRS is even broader, with the S wave fusing with the T wave. (Courtesy Hein JJ Wellens, MD, Maastricht, The Netherlands.)

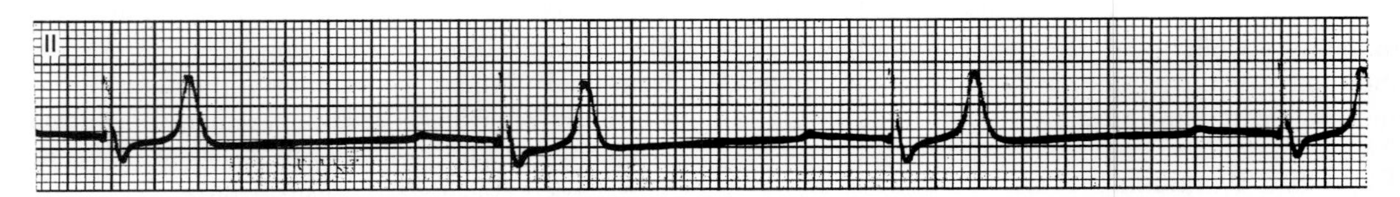

FIG. 17-5. Serum potassium level of 6.8 mEq/L (severe hyperkalemia). Note the tall tented T waves, wide P wave, broad QRS, and prolonged PR interval.

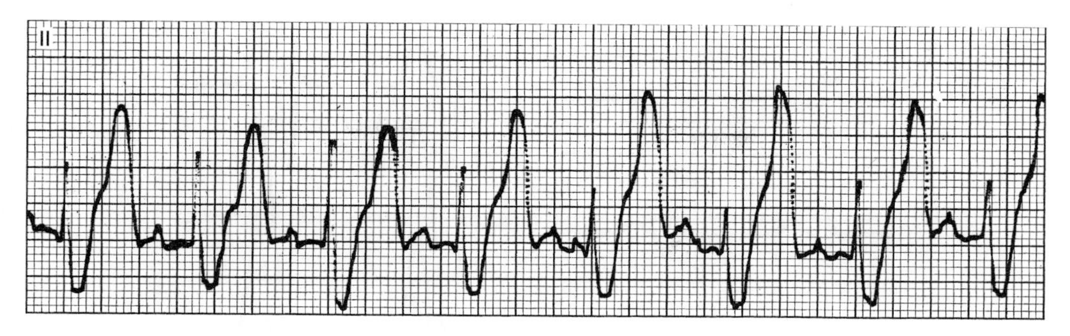

FIG. 17-6. Serum potassium level of 7.3 mEq/L. Note the distinctive ST segment as it loses itself in the tall tented T wave. The P wave is still intact. The QRS has widened to 0.20 second.

of 6.8 mEq/L, the beginning of severe hyperkalemia. The QRS is 0.15 second. Note the flattening of the P wave and long PR interval, and, of course, the tall tented T waves.

The patient whose ECG tracing you see in Fig. 17-6 had a potassium concentration of 7.3 mEq/L; the P wave has not yet flattened, but the distinctive merging of the ST segment with the tall tented T wave is apparent.

In Fig. 17-7, the potassium concentration is 8.3 mEq/L. Although the ST segment is still intact, the QRS has broadened, the P wave disappeared, and there is no mistaking the tall tented T wave and its clinical implications.

In Fig. 17-8, *A* and *B*, all 12 leads demonstrate before and after treatment of a case of severe hyperkalemia with a potassium plasma concentration of 8.4 mEq/L. In *A*, all of the signs of life-threatening hyperkalemia are present: broad QRS, absent ST segment, tall tented T waves, absent P waves, and left axis deviation. In *B*, the potassium levels are being restored to normal levels. Note the normal QRS axis and the reappearance of the P and ST segments.

It is interesting to note that there have been several reported cases of profound hyperkalemia without ECG manifestations.[9-11]

Causes[2]

- Renal failure, acute or chronic
- Angiotensin-converting enzyme (ACE) inhibitors; hyperkalemia is common in patients with chronic renal failure who are taking ACE inhibitors, the majority of whom have diabetes. A large number of patients with chronic renal failure require discontinuation of ACE inhibitors, depriving them of the renoprotective effects[12]
- Mineralocorticoid deficiency (Addison's disease, bilateral adrenalectomy, hypoaldosteronism)
- Congenital adrenal hyperplasia, primary defect in potassium excretion
- Cellular shift of potassium (tissue damage)
- Acidosis
- Digitalis overdose; hyperosmolality
- Succinylcholine, arginine infusion
- Oral or intravenous potassium intake
- Potassium containing drugs
- Transfusion
- Tourniquet (stasis) as opposed to free-flowing potassium levels[13]

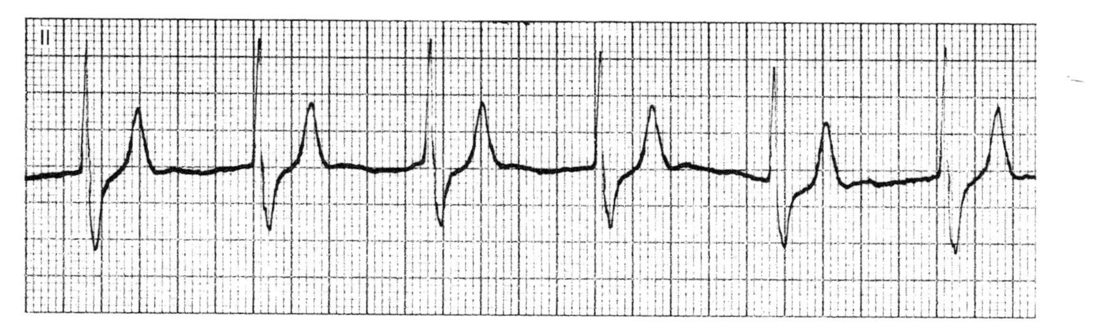

FIG. 17-7. Serum potassium level of 8.3 mEq/L. Although the ST segment is still distinct from the tall tented T wave, the QRS has broadened to 0.16 second and the P wave has disappeared.

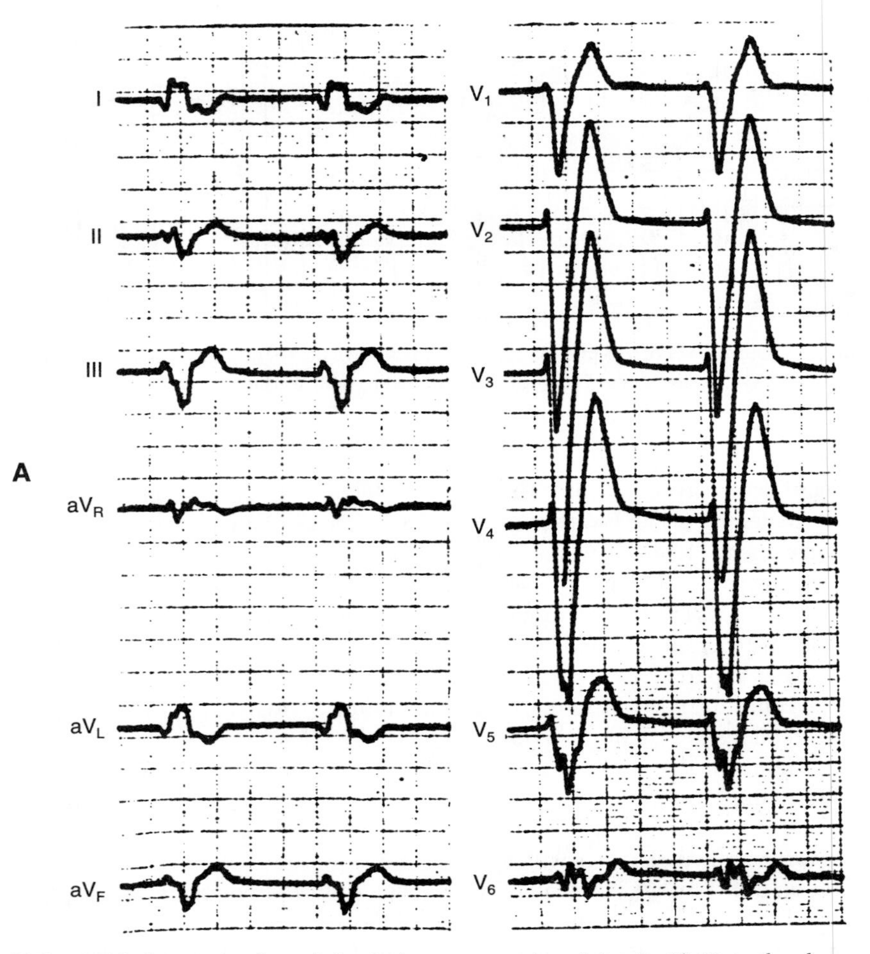

FIG. 17-8. **A,** Life-threatening hyperkalemia (serum potassium 8.3 mEq/L). Note the absence of P waves, broad QRS, left axis shift, lack of ST segment (in V_1 to V_5) and tall tented T waves. (Courtesy Hein J.J. Wellens, MD, Maastricht, The Netherlands.)

Continued

Clinical Implications

Hyperkalemia is associated with diabetes mellitus, diminished renal function, and the use of ACE inhibitors. An elevated serum potassium level in a hospitalized patient may be a marker for a significantly increased risk of death, which is due to underlying medical problems and is not a consequence of the hyperkalemia.[14]

Symptoms

Symptoms are fewer than those of hypokalemia, although the ECG is very helpful. Usually there is a history of diabetes, hypertension, or chronic renal failure.

Pediatrics

ECG findings are the same as in the adult. Plasma potassium levels are maintained between 3.5 and 4.5 mEq/L. Levels of 7.0 mEq/L can lead to significant hemodynamic and neurologic consequences. Levels exceeding 8.5 mEq/L cause respiratory paralysis and cardiac arrest.[15]

Treatment[6]

Mild hyperkalemia. Identify and eliminate the cause, if possible. The usual cause of hyperkalemia is renal disease.

Moderate or Severe Hyperkalemia

1. Intravenous infusion of 10 to 30 mL calcium gluconate (10%) over 1 to 5 minutes with constant ECG monitoring, which immediately and briefly alters the effects of the excess potassium on the cellular membranes without lowering the plasma potassium concentration.
2. Intravenous infusion of 200 to 500 mL of hypertonic glucose solution (10%) in 30 minutes, and 500 to

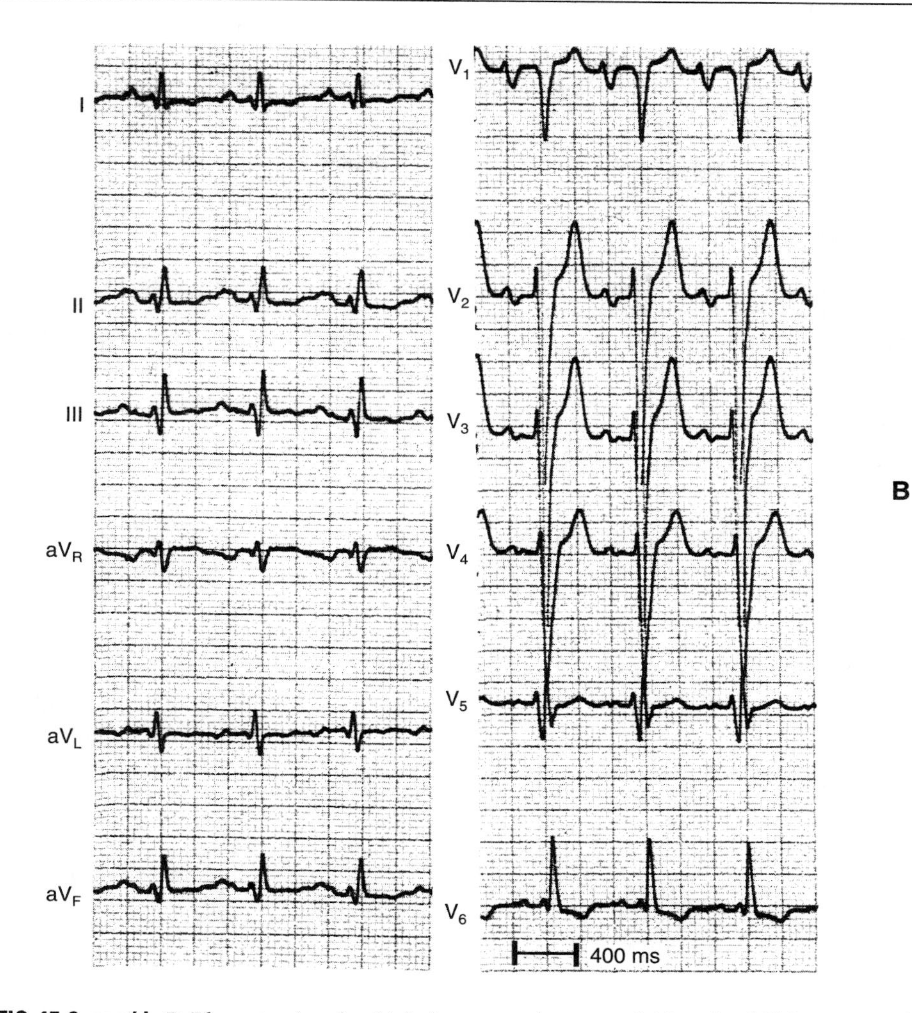

FIG. 17-8, cont'd. **B,** The potassium level is being restored to normal. Note the shift in QRS axis back to normal and the reemergence of the P wave and ST segment.

1000 mL over the next several hours. Glucose decreases the toxic effect of potassium by shifting potassium into the cells.

3. Sodium bicarbonate (2 to 3 ampules) may be added to 1 L of 5% dextrose in 0.9% saline, and will help to shift potassium into the cells even in patients who are not acidotic.
4. Administration of cation exchange resins (sodium polystyrene sulfonate) by retention enema; this may be repeated until potassium levels are within safe limits. Give oral doses of 20 g three or four times a day together with 20 mL of 70% sorbitol solution.
5. In cases of renal failure, initiate hemodialysis or peritoneal dialysis along with one of the treatments above.

SUMMARY

Potassium is one of the most important ions in the body, serving in many antiarrhythmic roles at the cellular level, including control of action potential duration at different heart rates, protection of the excitability of the cell in cases of hyperpolarization, and serving as an important link in parasympathetic stimulation.

REFERENCES

1. Goichot B: Genetic hypokalemia, *Rev Med Interne* 22:255, 2001.
2. Mandal AK: Hypokalemia and hyperkalemia, *Med Clinics N Am* 81:611, 1997.
3. Flaker GC: In cardiac arrest: is a low K or a high K "okay?" *J Cardiovasc Electrophysiol* 12:113, 2001.
4. Aronson RS: Delayed afterdepolarizations and pathological states. In

Rosen MR, Janse MJ, Wit AL, editors: *Cardiac electrophysiology,* Mount Kisco, NY, 1990, Futura.
5. Rosen MR: Cellular electrophysiology of digitalis toxicity, *J Am Coll Cardiol* 5:22A, 1985.
6. Wellens HJJ, Conover M: *The ECG in emergency decision making,* Philadelphia, 1992, WB Saunders.
7. Mattu A, Brady WJ, Robinson DA: Electrocardiographic manifestations of hyperkalemia, *Am J Emerg Med* 18:721, 2000.
8. Fisch C: Electrocardiography and vectorcardiography. In Braunwald E, editor: *Heart disease,* ed 4, Philadelphia, 1992, WB Saunders.
9. Martinez-Vea A, Bardaji A, Garcia C et al: Severe hyperkalemia with minimal electrocardiographic manifestations: a report of seven cases, *J Electrocardiol* 32:45, 1999.
10. Szerlip HM, Weiss J, Singer J: Profound hyperkalemia without ECG manifestations, *Am J Kidney Dis* 7:461, 1986.
11. Hylander B: Survival of extreme hyperkalemia, *Acta Med Scand* 221:121, 1987.
12. Ahuja TS, Freeman D Jr, Mahnken JD et al: Predictors of the development of hyperkalemia in patients using angiotensin-converting enzyme inhibitors, *Am J Nephrol* 20:268, 2000.
13. Wiederkehr MR, Moe OW: Factitious hyperkalemia, *Am J Kidney Dis* 36:1049, 2000.
14. Stevens MS, Dunlay RW: Hyperkalemia in hospitalized patients, *Int Urol Nephrol* 32:177, 2000.
15. Lieh-Lai M: Hyperkalemia, *eMedicine J* 2(9), Sept 13, 2001.

CHAPTER 18

Atrioventricular Dissociation

Atrioventricular (AV) dissociation is the independent beating of atria and ventricles. Table 18-1 summarizes the atrial and ventricular rhythms and the combinations that are possible in AV dissociation.

ECG RECOGNITION

Heart rate: That of the ventricular pacemaker.

Rhythm: Usually regular, but may be irregular if there is occasional conduction (capture).

P waves: May or may not be present depending on atrial activation (sinus rhythm, atrial tachycardia, atrial flutter, atrial fibrillation).

PR interval: No conduction between atria and ventricles.

PP intervals: Regular.

QRS complex: Narrow or broad depending (junctional or ventricular pacemaker).

Distinguishing features: Independently beating atria and ventricles; in some cases, the P waves may appear to "walk into" R waves as the PR interval becomes shorter and shorter.

RHYTHM VARIATIONS

Sinus Bradycardia and Junctional Escape

The tracings in Fig. 18-1 are of AV dissociation caused by sinus bradycardia; the strips are continuous. The sinus rate is 57 beats/min and the junctional escape rate is 58 beats/min. After the first complex, which is conducted (capture; *C*), the slightly faster junctional escape focus take over to pace the ventricles. Notice how the P waves seem to be "walking" into the QRS and appearing on the other side. At the end of the second tracing the sinus node accelerates to 68 beats/min; the last beat is a capture beat (*C*). Because of the two conducted beats, this rhythm is known as *AV dissociation with capture.*

Mechanism. When the sinus node slows to a rate below that of the AV junction, a junctional escape rhythm normally takes over as pacemaker of the ventricles. With the combination of sinus bradycardia and AV dissociation there is a drop in cardiac output because of the loss of atrial kick before the QRS; this is the stimulus for a faster sinus rhythm. Sinus bradycardia with junctional escape is often seen in trained athletes because of their marked sinus bradycardia.

If the junctional focus does not have retrograde conduction to the atria, the rhythm qualifies as AV dissociation and the term *idiojunctional rhythm* is sometimes used. When there is retrograde conduction, the junctional rhythm is not "idio" (independent) and the atria and the ventricles are not dissociated; they are associated retrogradely. A junctional escape rhythm with a rate of 56 beats/min and retrograde conduction to the atria is shown in Fig. 18-2. These retrograde beats are depolarizing the

TABLE 18-1 Atrial and Ventricular Rhythms of AV Dissociation

Atria	Ventricles
Sinus rhythm	Complete atrioventricular block and junctional escape
Atrial tachycardia	Junctional tachycardia (65-140 beats/min)
Atrial fibrillation	Junctional tachycardia with Wenckebach
Atrial flutter	Ventricular escape rhythm
	Accelerated idioventricular rhythm
	Fascicular VT

Any combination between the two columns is possible.

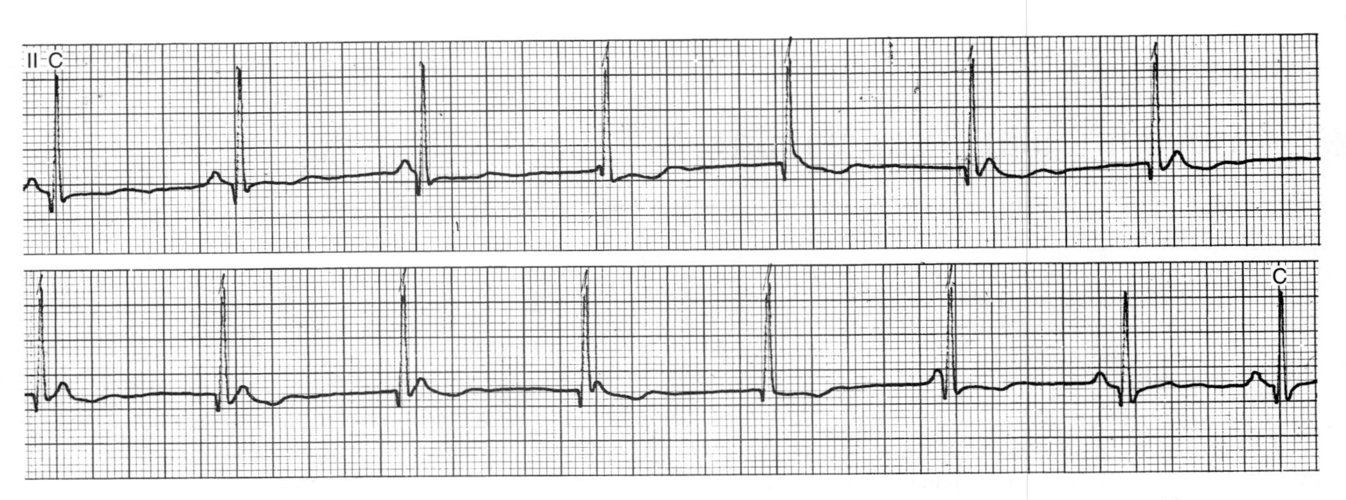

FIG. 18-1. Continuous tracings. Sinus bradycardia with junctional escape. This is AV dissociation with capture; only the first and the last beats are conducted (capture; *C*). The sinus rate is 57 beats/min, slightly slower than the junctional escape rhythm of 58 beats/min.

sinus node and exerting overdrive suppression. Thus, in spite of the bradycardia and the drop in cardiac output (atria and ventricles are beating simultaneously), the sinus node does not regain control. This may be overcome by exercise.

Clinical implications. The clinical implications of AV dissociation resulting from bradycardia are those of the bradycardia and the loss of the atrial contribution to ventricular filling (the atrial kick). If the patient is tolerating this arrhythmia (has no symptoms related to hemodynamic impairment), no intervention is indicated.

Junctional Tachycardia During Sinus Rhythm

In Fig. 18-3 the sinus rate is 74 beats/min. In spite of this adequate sinus rate, the AV junctional focus takes over at the same rate, which is too fast for a junctional focus, and therefore is a "tachycardia," often called an *accelerated idiojunctional rhythm*. The first beat is conducted with a PR of 0.17 second. The second beat is not conducted (PR 0.16 second) so that the junctional focus is beginning to manifest itself. The third beat is again conducted with a PR of 0.17 second. Thereafter the junctional focus takes over at a rate of 73 beats/min with the sinus node at a rate of 72 beats/min, placing the P waves in and out the other side of the QRS.

Mechanism. When the AV junction accelerates its firing rate, it may assume the pacing of the ventricles, especially during sinus bradycardia, but even in the face of an adequate sinus rhythm. If there is no retrograde conduction to the atria, AV dissociation results. The sinus node or an atrial rhythm paces the atria, and the junctional focus paces the ventricles. A common cause of junctional tachycardia (rate approximately 65-140 beats/min) with AV dissociation is digitalis intoxication.

Clinical implications. The clinical implications of AV dissociation caused by junctional tachycardia are those of the accelerated focus and the hemodynamic consequences of the arrhythmia. If digitalis intoxication is a factor, digitalis should be discontinued and the patient should be confined to bed (no sympathetic stimulation). Potassium

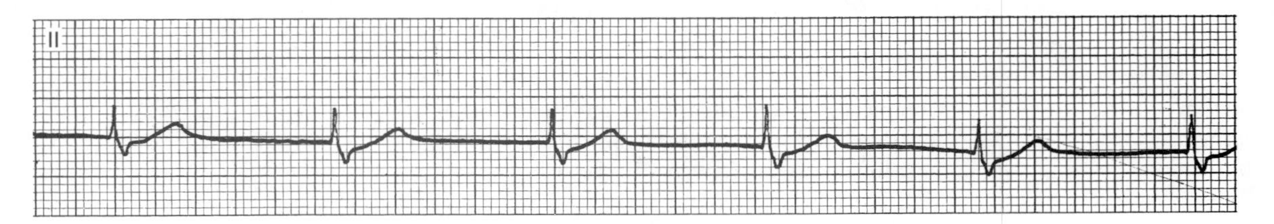

FIG. 18-2. Junctional escape with retrograde conduction. The junctional rate is 56 beats/min. The retrograde P′ wave is the negative deflection immediately after the QRS (at first glance it may look like an S wave). The sinus node is not pacing because it is slow and is being retrogradely activated by the junctional focus.

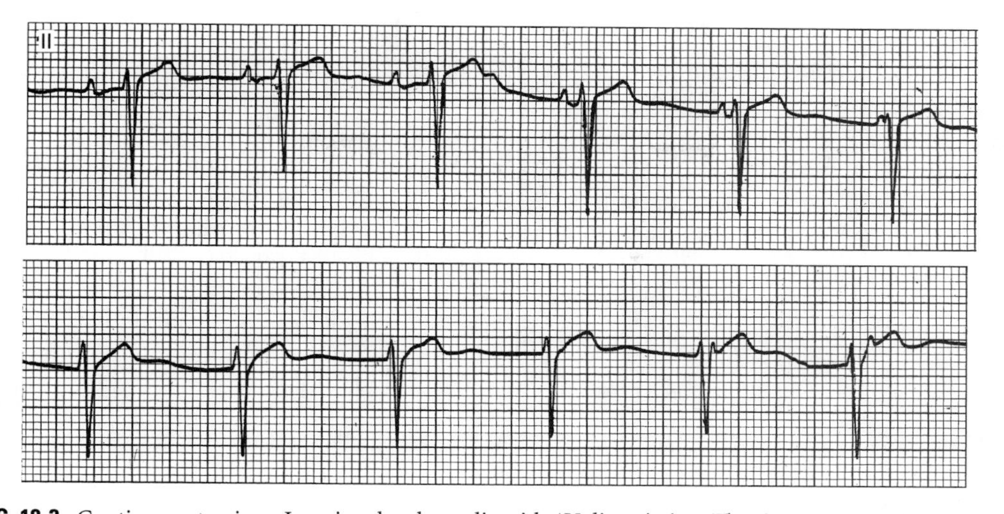

FIG. 18-3. Continuous tracings. Junctional tachycardia with AV dissociation. The sinus rate is 74 beats/min. The junctional rate is accelerated (73 beats/min). Slight slowing of the sinus rhythm allows the accelerated junctional focus to take over. Note that the second PR interval is shorter than the first; this is a junctional beat. The third beat is conducted with a PR of 0.17 second. The remaining beats are junctional with the P wave hiding in the QRS and T. In the last two beats the P looks like an r′.

levels should be checked and corrected. Another precipitating factor may be excessive catecholamines.

Junctional Tachycardia During Atrial Flutter

When AV dissociation occurs during atrial flutter it is because of junctional tachycardia, complete heart block, or an accelerated idioventricular rhythm. Fig. 18-4 is an example of atrial flutter with AV dissociation caused by junctional tachycardia. The patient was a 58-year-old woman who was given a supplemental dose of digoxin before surgery. AV dissociation during atrial flutter is an arrhythmia that is not easily spotted because the rhythm in atrial flutter is often normally regular, although it can be irregular. When the ventricular rhythm is regular in the setting of atrial flutter, it means a fixed conduction ratio (2:1; 4:1) and as such the flutter–R wave relationship should be fixed. In Fig. 18-4 you will note that with a regular ventricular rhythm of 115 beats/min, the flutter wave in front of the QRS is changing each time. The diagnosis is atrial flutter with junctional tachycardia secondary to digitalis toxicity.

Accelerated Idioventricular Rhythm

Fig. 18-5 shows AV dissociation caused by an accelerated idioventricular rhythm at a rate of 75 beats/min. The fourth (and perhaps the third) and fifth beats are ventricular fusion beats, as is the last beat in this continuous tracing. The rhythm begins with a long coupling interval, a typical beginning for this reperfusion arrhythmia. An accelerated idioventricular rhythm that reflects reperfusion typically shows the following:

1. Three or more successive ventricular ectopic beats
2. A rate of 50 to 120 beats/min
3. A long coupling interval to begin with
4. AV dissociation

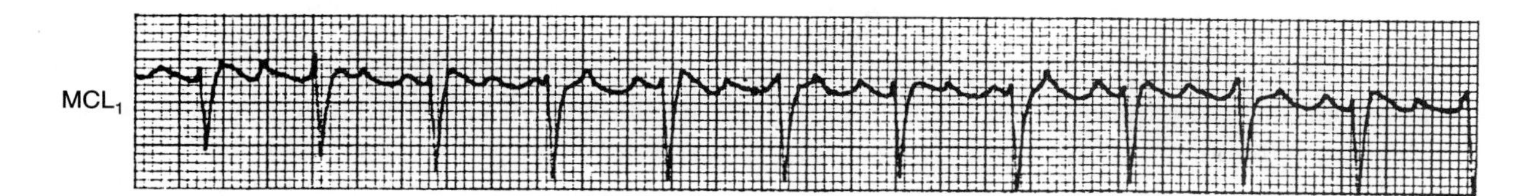

FIG. 18-4. Atrial flutter and junctional tachycardia caused by digoxin excess. Note the regular junctional rhythm with no fixed relationship between the flutter waves and the QRS, indicating AV dissociation. (Courtesy William P. Nelson, MD.)

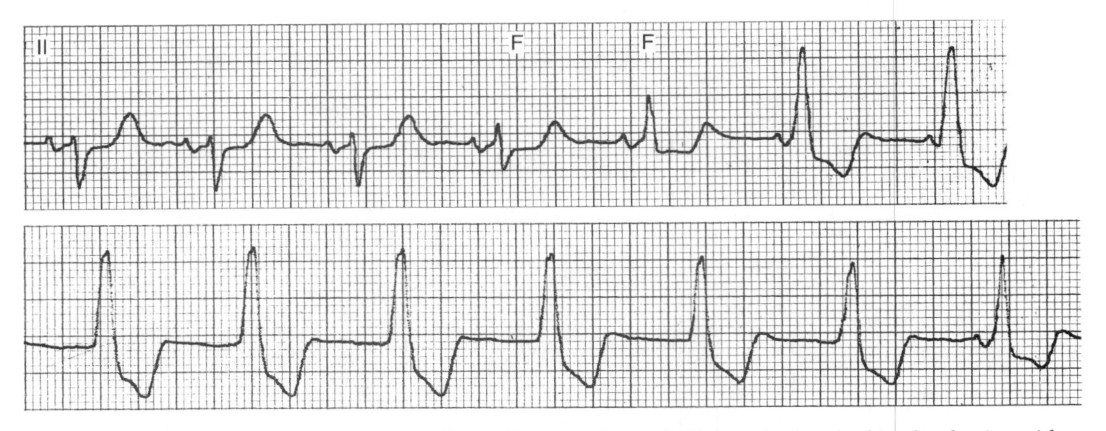

FIG. 18-5. Continuous tracings. Sinus rhythm with an accelerated idioventricular rhythm that begins with two fusion beats (*F*).

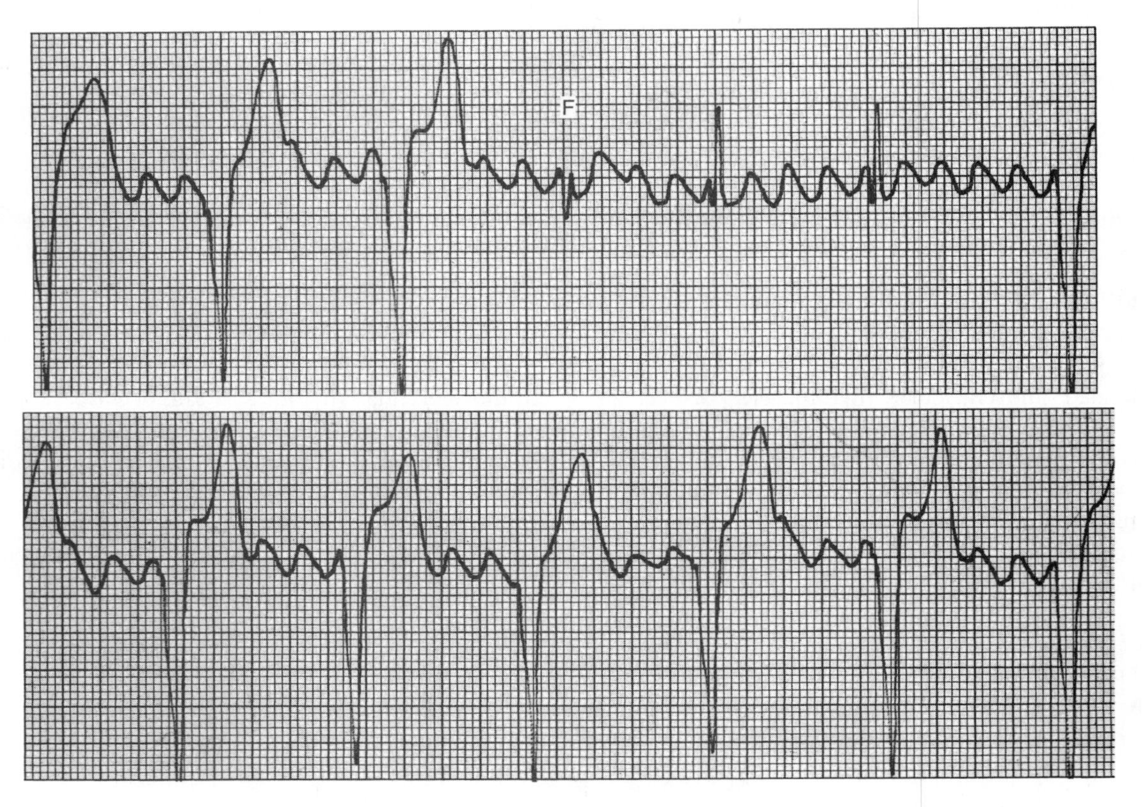

FIG. 18-6. Atrial flutter with an accelerated idioventricular rhythm and one fusion beat (*F*).

Fig. 18-6 is an interesting tracing of atrial flutter with an accelerated idioventricular rhythm. In the top tracing there are three capture beats, the first of which is a fusion beat (*F*). In the bottom tracing the signs of AV dissociation during atrial flutter can be seen. The flutter–R wave relationship is changing with every ventricular beat.

Mechanism. When a ventricular pacemaker accelerates to a rate greater than that of the sinus node, AV dissociation may result or there may be 1:1 retrograde conduction to the atria and therefore no AV dissociation. When the rate of a ventricular focus is greater than 40 beats/min, it is accelerated but does not become evident until its rate

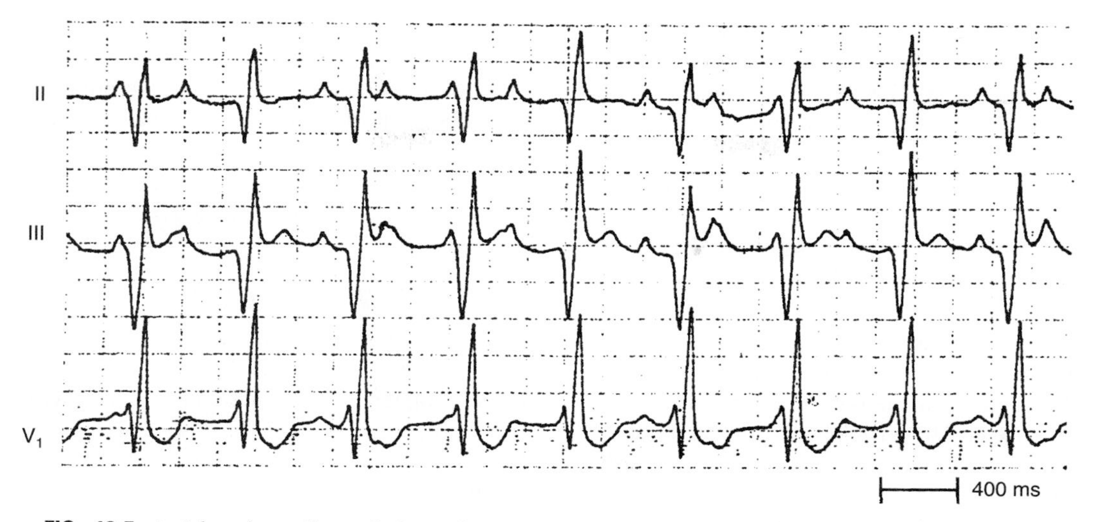

FIG. 18-7. Atrial tachycardia and fascicular VT. (Courtesy Hein J.J. Wellens, MD, Maastricht, The Netherlands.)

exceeds that of the sinus node. For this reason fusion beats are usually at the beginning and end of the run of ventricular beats.

Clinical implications. Accelerated idioventricular rhythm with atrioventricular dissociation is often seen in the setting of acute myocardial infarction during reperfusion. No treatment is necessary unless associated with hemodynamic impairment.

Physical signs. When the ventricular rate is faster than the atrial rate, the intensity of the first heart sound increases as the PR interval shortens until finally there is a very loud sound ("bruit de canon") followed by a sudden softening in intensity. As the P waves "march through" the QRS, atrial and ventricular contractions coincide, causing a giant A wave in the jugular pulse.

Atrial Tachycardia and Fascicular VT

Fig. 18-7 is a double tachycardia of digitalis toxicity. The P waves are upright in leads II and III at a rate of approximately 170 beats/min. The upright Ps in lead II are typical of the atrial tachycardia of digitalis toxicity (see Chapter 15). The ventricular rhythm is regular but the PR intervals are not fixed; therefore, there is AV dissociation. A look at V1 identifies the ventricular rhythm as fascicular ventricular tachycardia (VT) (right bundle branch block pattern and axis deviation).

AV Block

Complete AV block is recognized on the electrocardiogram (ECG) because of total absence of conduction in the face of opportunities to conduct; that is, the rates of both pacemakers are not too fast. Fig. 18-8 is a tracing from a patient with complete AV block. The sinus rate is 100 beats/min, and the idioventricular rhythm is discharging at 46 beats/min.

Mechanism. Total AV block is included here for completeness. It is discussed more fully in Chapter 16. The term *complete AV block or third-degree AV block* implies the

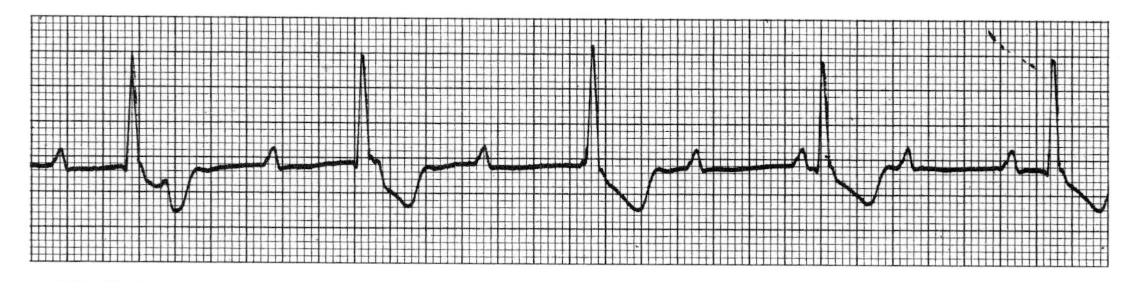

FIG. 18-8. Complete AV block always results in AV dissociation. The sinus rate is 100 beats/min; the ventricular escape rhythm is 46 beats/min.

existence of a pathologic obstruction to conduction; the term *AV dissociation* does not necessarily indicate inability to conduct. The dissociation between the atria and the ventricles could be due to any number of reasons—physiologic or pathologic. Thus although complete AV block causes AV dissociation, AV dissociation is not necessarily complete AV block.

Clinical implications. The clinical implications of complete AV block depend on where the block is located. If it occurs early in the setting of inferior wall myocardial infarction, it is transient and thought to be the result of increased parasympathetic tone or sudden ischemia that is relieved by the opening of the collateral circulation. This type of block responds to atropine or isoproterenol. AV block that occurs late in the course of the myocardial infarction appears to be the result of metabolic alteration within the AV node caused by ischemia. A pacemaker may be indicated if there is hemodynamic impairment. In the setting of acute anterior wall myocardial infarction the clinical implications of complete AV block are ominous because the block is usually at the level of the bundle branches and requires a pacemaker.

Digitalis-Induced AV Dissociation

The AV dissociation caused by digitalis excess has been covered in Chapter 15 and is reviewed here. The development of AV dissociation is compounded by the fact that digitalis prolongs and may block AV nodal conduction. The arrhythmias that result in AV dissociation that one can expect to see in patients taking an excess of digitalis are as follows:

- Sinus bradycardia and junctional tachycardia
- Sinus bradycardia and fascicular VT
- Normal sinus rhythm and junctional tachycardia (see Fig. 18-3)
- Atrial tachycardia and junctional tachycardia
- Atrial tachycardia and fascicular VT (see Fig. 18-7)
- Atrial fibrillation and junctional tachycardia (regular rhythm)
- Atrial fibrillation and junctional tachycardia with Wenckebach exit block (irregular rhythm [i.e., group beating])
- Atrial fibrillation and complete AV block with junctional escape
- Atrial flutter and junctional tachycardia (see Fig. 18-4)
- Atrial flutter and junctional tachycardia with Wenckebach exit block
- Atrial flutter and fascicular VT
- Atrial flutter and complete AV block with junctional escape

CAUSES OF AV DISSOCIATION

1. Sinus bradycardia (Chapter 6)
2. Junctional or ventricular focus accelerated (Chapter 10)
3. Pathology in the AV junction preventing AV conduction (Chapter 16)
4. Digitalis toxicity (Chapter 15)
5. Ventricular tachycardia (Chapter 13)

PHYSICAL FINDINGS

1. Irregular cannon A waves in the jugular pulse
2. Varying intensity of the first heart sound
3. Beat-to-beat changes in systolic blood pressure

Any of the preceding clues indicates AV dissociation, although the absence of these clues does not rule out AV dissociation. For example, in atrial fibrillation with VT there is AV dissociation without its usual physical or ECG signs. The physiologic aspects of the physical signs of AV dissociation have already been discussed on pp. 176-177.

TREATMENT

AV dissociation itself is not treated because it is merely a symptom. The physician treats the underlying cause of the AV dissociation. For example, the treatment of VT with AV dissociation differs vastly from that of AV dissociation caused by complete AV block or sinus bradycardia and junctional tachycardia caused by digitalis intoxication.

SUMMARY

AV dissociation is always the result of another condition such as sinus bradycardia, an accelerated lower pacemaker, VT, or AV block. The clinical implications are evaluated according to the primary condition.

CHAPTER 19

Fusion Beats and Parasystole

VENTRICULAR FUSION

In electrocardiography the term *fusion* is used to indicate that currents from two different sources have collided within the muscle mass of either the ventricular chambers (ventricular fusion) or the atrial chambers (atrial fusion). Ventricular fusion beats are often seen at the beginning and end of an accelerated idioventricular rhythm, and are, in fact, a requirement for the diagnosis of ventricular parasystole. When seen during a broad QRS tachycardia, a fusion beat is virtually diagnostic of ventricular tachycardia (VT). Rarely, a ventricular fusion beat may occur during sinus rhythm with bundle branch block and thus masquerade as VT.

ECG Recognition

QRS complex: The principal electrocardiographic (ECG) sign of ventricular fusion is that a QRS complex differs from the dominant rhythm. This difference varies according to how much tissue each current source has captured. Some of the clues are that a QRS complex during sinus rhythm or during VT takes on a different shape; the difference can be slight or marked. The QRS is in some degree narrower, broader, shorter, or taller than the dominant rhythm. When the sinus-conducted beat and the ventricular ectopic beat capture equal amounts of ventricular myocardium the QRS may, as you will see, be isoelectric.

PR interval: The PR interval may be shorter or of the same duration as that of the underlying sinus rhythm because ventricular fusion can take place as long as the sinus impulse is still traveling when the ectopic impulse discharges (same PR as the sinus rhythm), or as long as the sinus impulse can enter the ventricles before the ectopic one is finished (shorter PR).

Rhythm Variations

Accelerated idioventricular rhythm. In the continuous tracing of Fig. 19-1 the beginning of an accelerated idioventricular rhythm can be seen. The sinus rate at the

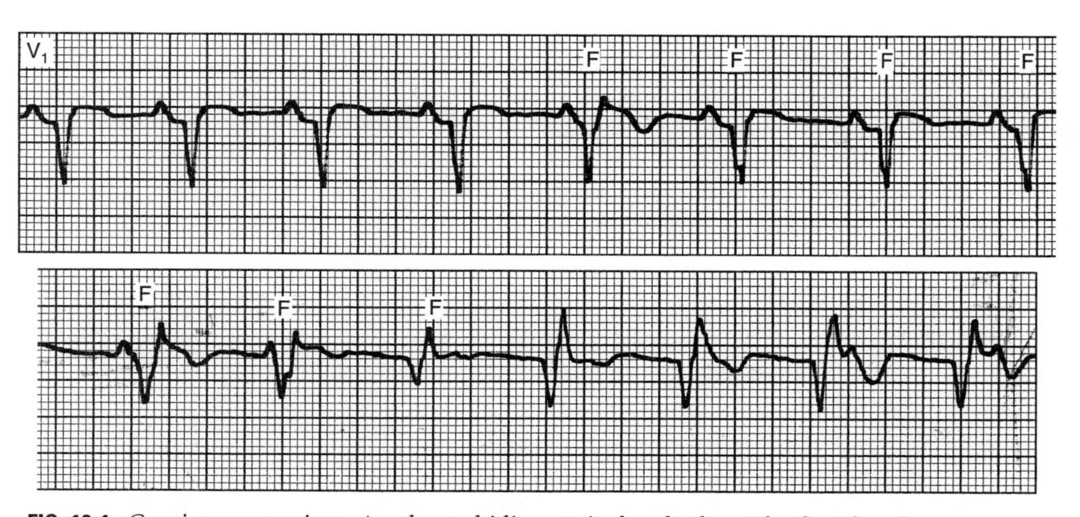

FIG. 19-1. Continuous tracings. Accelerated idioventricular rhythm. The first four beats are pure sinus-conducted beats. Thereafter seven fusion *(F)* beats introduce an accelerated idioventricular rhythm, which manifests itself because the sinus rhythm slows from 88 to 77 beats/min (sinus arrhythmia). The rate of the ventricular rhythm is 82 beats/min.

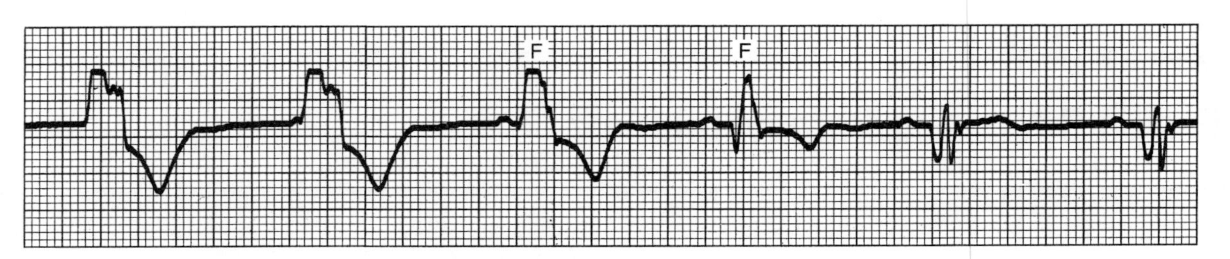

FIG. 19-2. Accelerated idioventricular rhythm. The sinus P wave distorts the beginning of the second beat and emerges from the third beat to partially capture the ventricles (fusion; *F*). Note the slightly different shape of this beat. The fourth beat is also a fusion beat.

beginning of the tracing is 88 beats/min, which is fast enough to dominate the rate of 82 in the ventricular ectopic focus. However, when the sinus rate drops to 77 beats/min (sinus arrhythmia), the ventricular focus discharges, finds part of the ventricles nonrefractory, and fuses with the descending sinus conducted impulse. There are seven fusion beats, after which the P wave is within the QRS, distorting the ventricular ectopic complex. The first four beats of the tracing are purely sinus-conducted, the last four are purely ventricular ectopic, and in between there are different degrees of fusion as the ventricular ectopic focus captures more and more of the ventricular myocardium.

Fig. 19-2 shows an accelerated idioventricular rhythm; the P wave can be seen emerging from the second broad beat and changing the shape of the QRS slightly. The next two beats are fusion beats, and then the sinus rhythm takes over.

Ventricular tachycardia. The broad QRS tachycardia in Fig. 19-3 has two fusion beats, which is virtually diagnostic of VT. This clue has limited usefulness because it usually occurs during relatively slow rhythms. The rate of this VT is 110 beats/min. The fusion occurs when there is atrioventricular (AV) dissociation and a well-placed P wave is able to conduct at least partially to the ventricles. It is possible, however, to also have a narrow beat during the broad QRS tachycardia of atrial fibrillation with conduction over an accessory pathway (Wolff-Parkinson-White syndrome) and the AV node at the same time. The rhythm in this case would be irregular.

Isoelectric fusion beat. There probably is no other tracing as confusing to look at as that of a bigeminal end-diastolic premature ventricular complex (PVC) because such beats are usually fusion beats. Such a tracing is shown in Fig. 19-4. Some complexes are so isoelectric that only the T wave can be seen. If you "walk out" the P waves, you will find them to be right on time.

Bigeminal end diastolic PVCs. In Fig. 19-5 it is the tall broad beats that are pure sinus-conducted beats and small, narrow, alternate beats that represent bigeminal end diastolic PVCs and fusion beats. There are two clues: (1) the first two beats in the top tracing are clearly sinus-conducted with a broad QRS; (2) the PR is fixed in all of the tall broad beats, whereas it varies in the small alternate beats, as is common with end diastolic fusion beats.

ATRIAL FUSION

Atrial fusion beats occur when an ectopic atrial focus and the sinus node or two atrial foci discharge simultaneously or almost simultaneously.

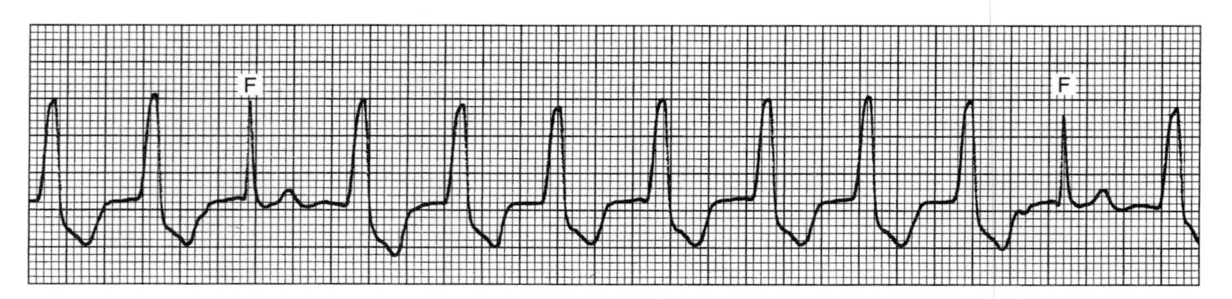

FIG. 19-3. Ventricular tachycardia with two fusion beats *(F)*.

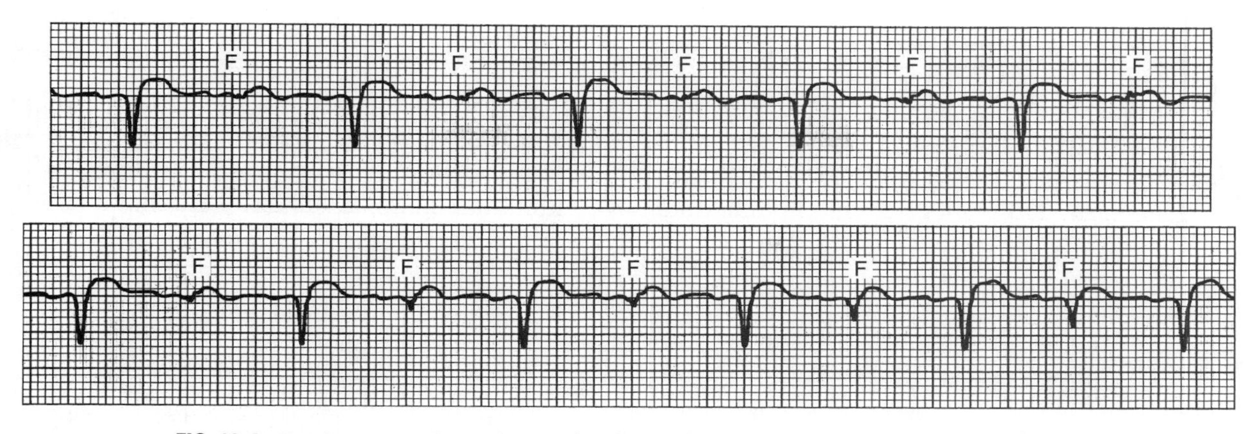

FIG. 19-4. Continuous tracings. Bigeminal end diastolic PVCs, all of which are fusion beats *(F)*.

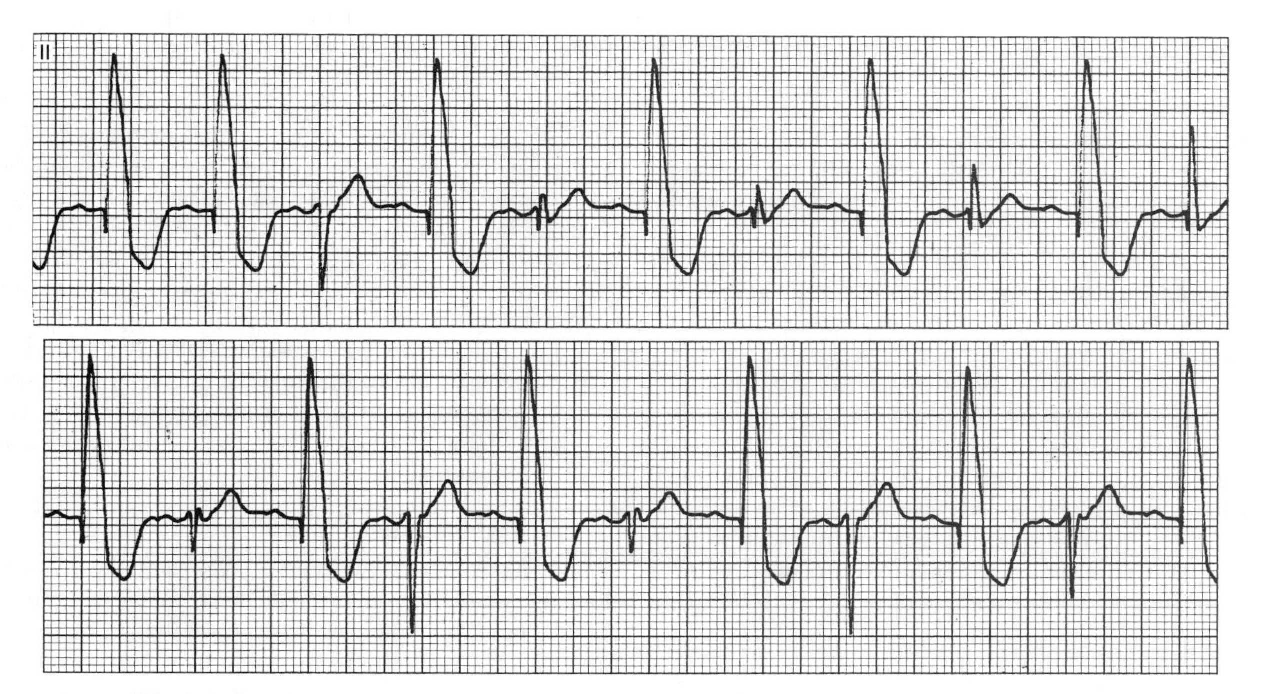

FIG. 19-5. Bigeminal end diastolic PVCs. Here again, all of the PVCs cause fusion with the sinus-conducted impulse, causing them to be varied in shape, polarity, and width. Note that it is the tall broad beats that have a fixed PR interval and represent the basic sinus rhythm with bundle branch block.

ECG Recognition

Atrial fusion occurs when there is a pacemaker shift and is recognized because it has a different shape from the P waves before and after the shift.

Fig. 19-6, *A,* is an example of a pacemaker shift from a sinus rhythm to a junctional rhythm with atrial fusion in between. Fig 19-6, *B,* shows the opposite shift (i.e., junctional rhythm to sinus rhythm with atrial fusion in between).

PARASYSTOLE

A parasystolic rhythm results from an ectopic focus surrounded by an area that protects it from discharge by the depolarizations of the surrounding tissue. Such a focus

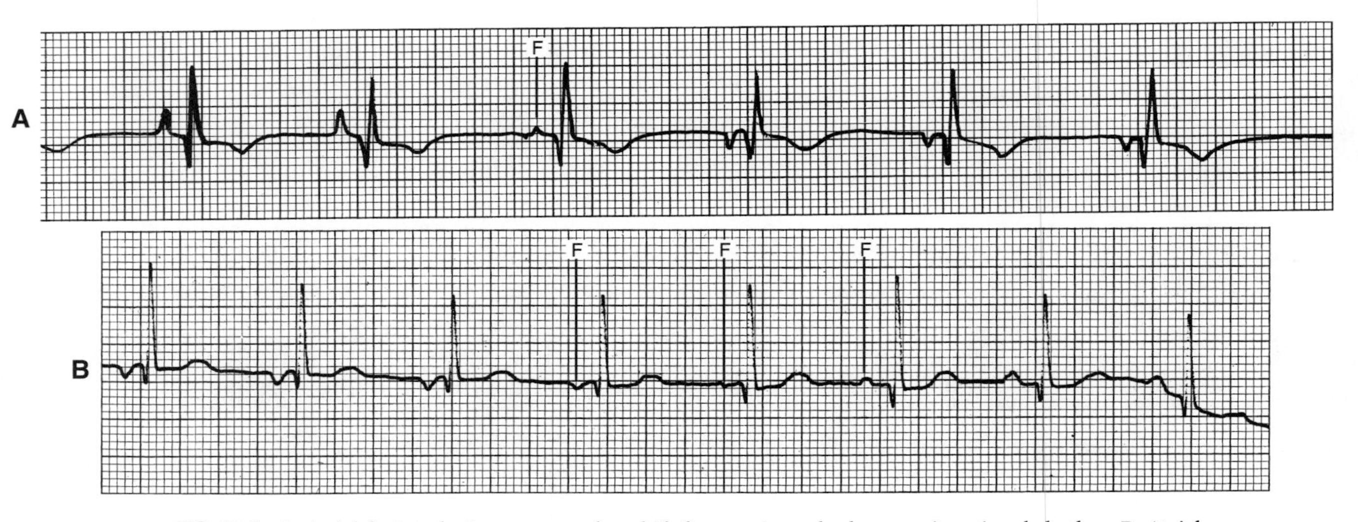

FIG. 19-6. **A**, Atrial fusion during a pacemaker shift from a sinus rhythm to a junctional rhythm. **B**, Atrial fusion during a pacemaker shift from a junctional rhythm to sinus rhythm with atrial fusion in between.

can originate anywhere in the heart (sinoatrial [SA] node, atria, AV junction, ventricles), the most common location being ventricular. Two forms of parasystole have been described: "pure" and modulated.

Pure parasystole is sometimes called "traditional" or "classic" and is usually described as (1) continuous (with or without exit block) or (2) intermittent. In the past, such a parasystolic focus was believed to be completely protected by an area of depressed excitability (entrance block) and uninfluenced by surrounding depolarizations. However, since the initial microelectrode studies of Jalife and Moe,[1] many investigators have shown that such an assumption cannot be made. If impulses can exit across such a depressed zone, it is likely that the parasystolic focus is subject to some degree of modulation by electrotonic depolarizations arising in the surrounding tissue.[1-3]

ECG Recognition

No fixed coupling: Ventricular ectopic beats are often exactly coupled to the preceding complex. The parasystolic beat is usually not linked to a preceding beat; it is independent. An exception is when the nonparasystolic rhythm modifies the parasystolic rate so that there is exact coupling (entrainment)—that is, the parasystolic rate is changed so that it equals the nonparasystolic rate.[2]

Fusion beats: An occasional fusion beat is also a feature of parasystole, given a long enough tracing. If the parasystole is ventricular, the fusion beats result because the ectopic focus discharges just before or just as the sinus-conducted beat enters the ventricles. If the parasystole is atrial, fusion beats result because the ectopic focus discharges at the same time as or just before the sinus node. The fusion beats, obviously happenstance, are not necessary for making the diagnosis of parasystole.

Interectopic intervals: Some of the time the parasystolic focus may beat without being influenced electronically by the sinus (or dominant) rhythm, causing the interectopic intervals to be mathematically related (pure parasystole). Most of the time the interectopic interval is irregular, especially when examined in a tracing that covers a long period, as with Holter recordings (modulated parasystole).[2]

Pure Parasystole

When the interectopic interval is constant, the minimal time interval between interectopic beats is an exact multiple of longer time intervals. After what appears to be the minimal interval in a suspected tracing has been identified, the parasystolic rhythm can be "walked out." When the ventricles (or the atria in the case of atrial parasystole) are nonrefractory, an ectopic complex appears. Failure of the parasystolic impulse to appear when expected is called "exit block."

Fig. 19-7 is an example of pure ventricular parasystole. The ventricular ectopic beats have variable coupling intervals, there is a fusion complex *(F)*, and the interectopic intervals are multiples of a common denominator. However, given a longer tracing, modulation of the rhythm would probably be demonstrated. This perfect symmetry of the ectopic beats is found only when the atrial and ventricular rates are constant (i.e., paced).[2]

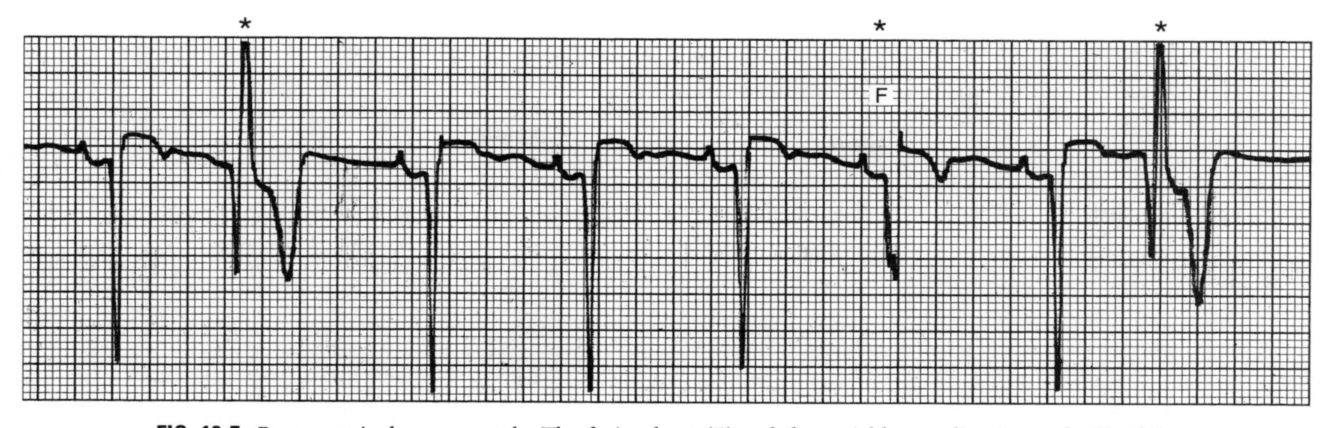

FIG. 19-7. Pure ventricular parasystole. The fusion beat *(F)* and the variable coupling intervals (*) of the ectopic beats are evident. The interectopic intervals have a common denominator.

Figs. 19-8 and 19-9 are examples of pure atrial parasystole and are less common and more difficult to diagnose than the ventricular variety. In Fig. 19-9, a diagnosis is even more difficult because the parasystolic P waves are almost identical in shape to the sinus P waves. Parasystole originating in the SA node has been described.[1] The tracing in Fig. 19-8 is of atrial parasystole and may well be such a case. It fulfills the criteria given: (1) premature P waves having contour identical to sinus P waves, (2) variable coupling intervals, and (3) PP intervals of the parasystolic-sinus pair not longer than the PP intervals of the sinus rhythm.

Modulated Parasystole

A parasystolic focus is said to be modulated when its protection is partial and its regular rhythm is disrupted by impulses arising in the surrounding tissues. In such a case, subthreshold electrotonic depolarizations are transmitted across the depressed barrier, prolonging or shortening the parasystolic cycle, depending on the amplitude of the electrotonic event and the relationship of the parasystolic and sinus beats to each other. If the sinus beat occurs early in phase 4 of the parasystolic rhythm, the next parasystolic beat is delayed. If the sinus beat occurs late in phase 4 of the parasystolic rhythm, the next parasystolic beat is early

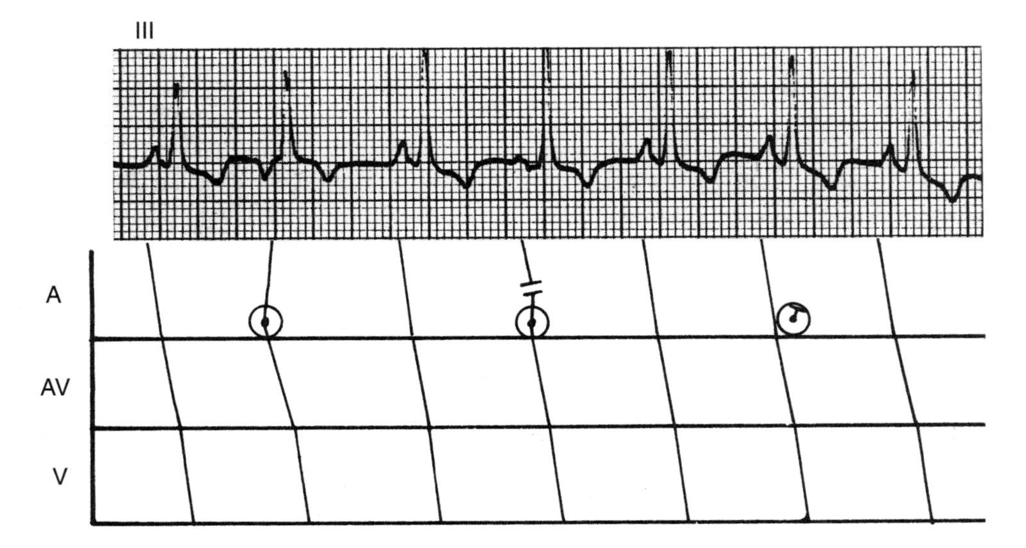

FIG. 19-8. Atrial parasystole. Note the two visible atrial ectopic beats with no fixed coupling, the second of which is a fusion beat. The third atrial ectopic beat may be hidden by the second QRS from the end. (From the Alan Lindsay Collection, Salt Lake City, Utah.)

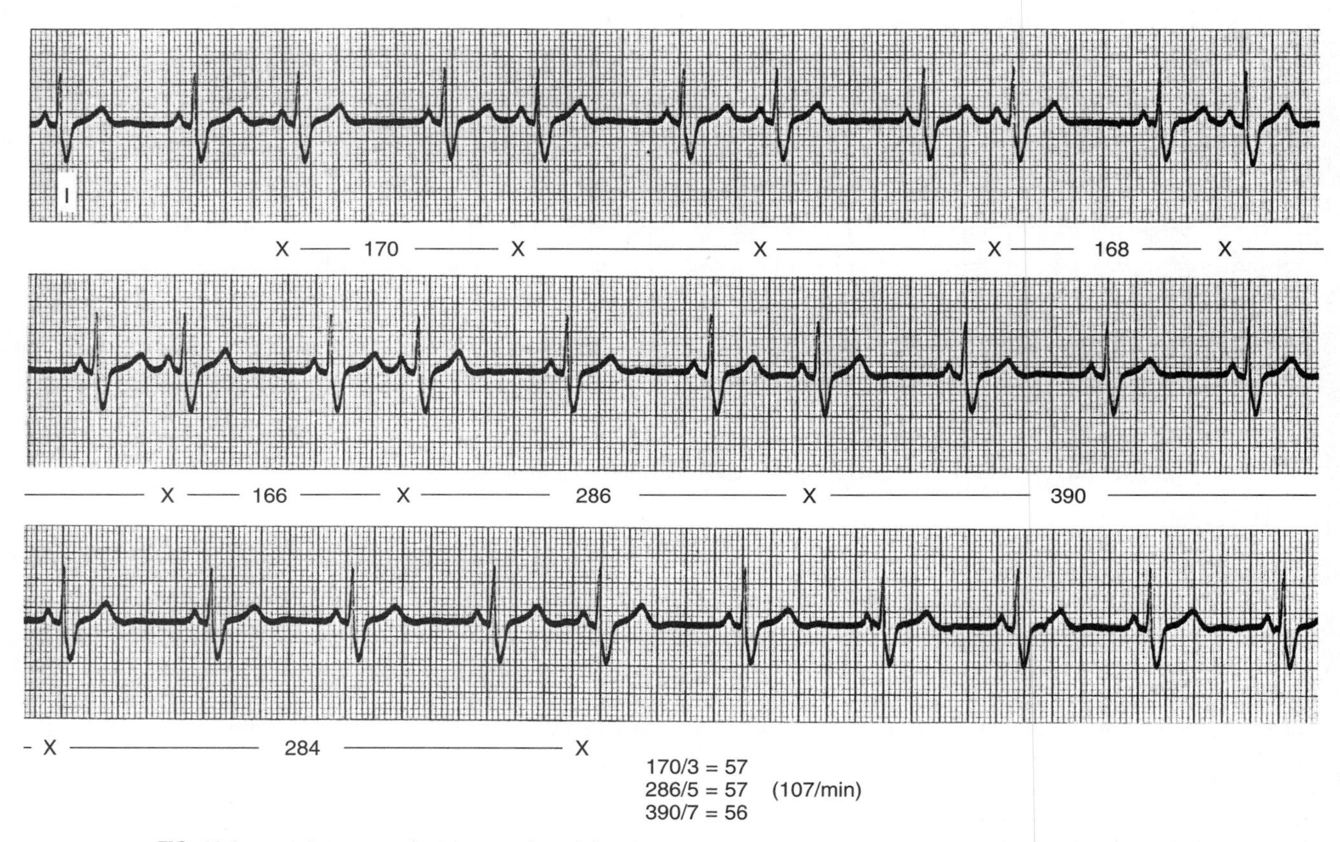

FIG. 19-9. Atrial parasystole (sinoatrial nodal). The parasystolic P waves *(X)* are identical in shape to the sinus P waves, there is no exact coupling, the interectopic intervals have a common denominator, and the parasystolic P wave resets the sinus node. (From the Alan Lindsay Collection, Salt Lake City, Utah.)

because it is captured by the invading impulse. The latter occurs because late in phase 4 the parasystolic focus is closer to threshold potential and a partial depolarization at this time across the zone of protection causes the parasystolic focus to fire prematurely.[2,4-7] In fact, a parasystolic focus can actually be entrained by the dominant pacemaker, causing fixed coupling of the parasystolic beat to the sinus beat.[4-6]

An example of modulated parasystole is shown in Fig. 19-10. The intrinsic cycle length of the ectopic parasystolic pacemaker is assumed to be 1300 ms. Modulation of the pacemaker was assessed only in bigeminal and trigeminal groupings. There are few examples of modulated parasystole and even of pure parasystole, not because it is rare, but most likely because of the difficulty making the diagnosis given its complexities and probably because of its benign nature. I have only one very faded tracing (see Fig. 19-10) of modulated ventricular parasystole that was analyzed for me by Charles Antzelevitch, PhD, Derge Sicouri, MD, and William Gans.

Mechanism

Parasystole may be caused by a focus of normal or altered automaticity or triggered activity (early or delayed afterdepolarizations). This focus is surrounded by an area of protection, an abnormality that should not be confused with normal refractoriness. A variety of mechanisms has been postulated to explain the protected zone surrounding the ectopic focus. Although the ectopic focus is protected, it is not totally immune to the electrical activity going on around it and may change its rhythm because of what is called *electrotonic modulation.* When an impulse meets with the area of protection around the parasystolic focus, electrotonic potentials may be transmitted across the depressed tissue and may cause the ectopic focus to be delayed or accelerated. A beat that arrives early in diastole may cause the parasystolic discharge to be delayed. If the beat arrives late, the parasystolic discharge may be early.[1-3,8-10]

In addition to the preceding findings, experimental studies by Jalife and Moe[10] and others[1,2,7-13] showed that coupled beats can result from parasystolic rhythms and

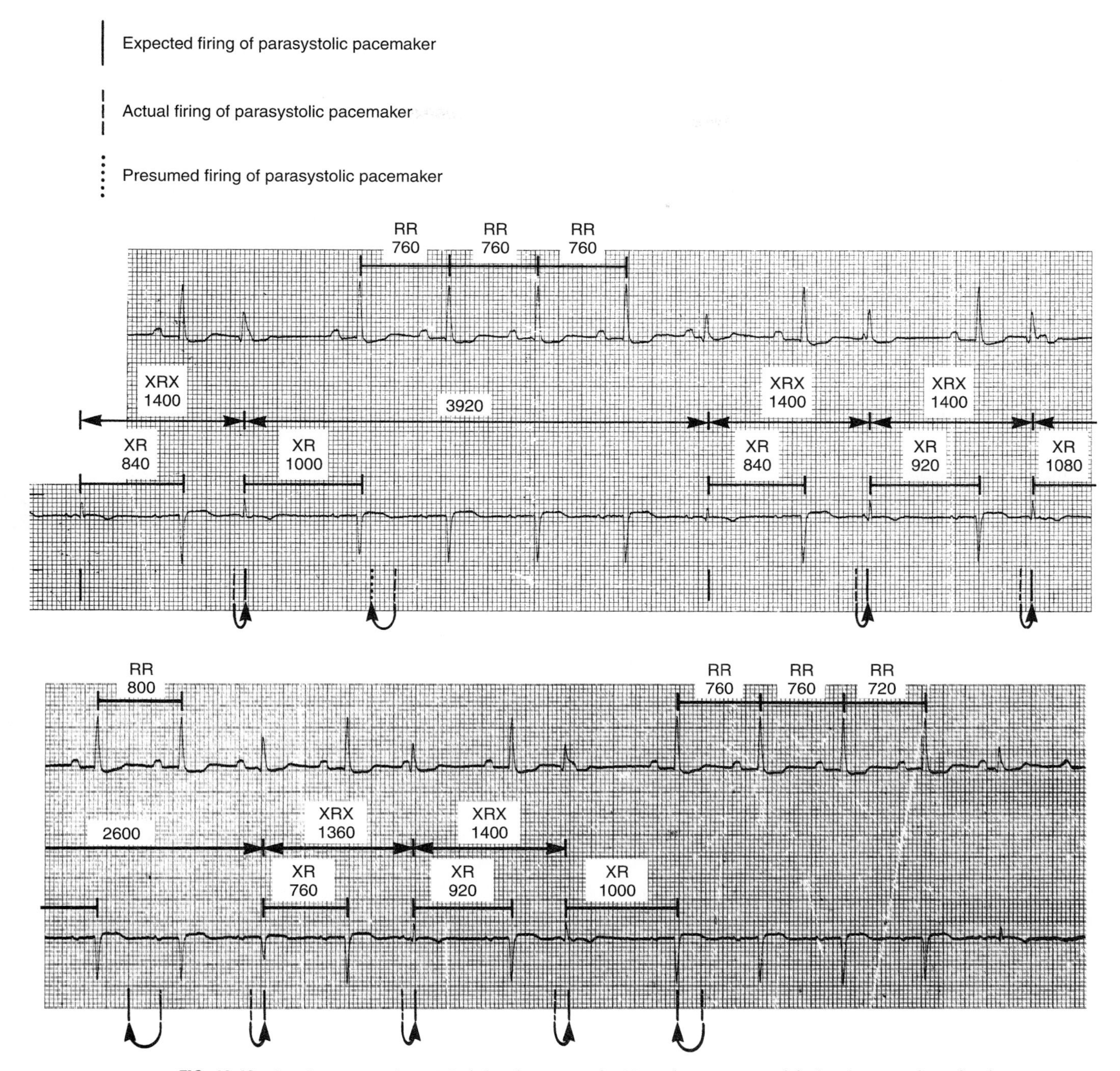

FIG. 19-10. Continuous tracings. Modulated parasystole. Note the presence of fusion beats and no fixed coupling of the ventricular ectopic beats, which are features typical of ventricular parasystole. The interectopic intervals, however, are not multiples because the rhythm of the parasystolic focus is influenced by subthreshold current being transmitted across the area of protection. Expected firing, actual firing, and presumed firing times of the parasystolic focus are identified. *RR*, R wave to R wave (i.e., the interval between the two sinus conducted beats); *XRX*, interectopic intervals, with *X* indicating the ectopic beats and *R* indicating the underlying rhythm; *XR*, the distance between a parasystolic beat and the next sinus conducted beat. I am grateful to Charles Antzelevitch, PhD, Derge Sicouri, MD; and William Gans for their expert analysis of this figure. (Tracing courtesy Carol Fuller, RN, Portland, Ore.)

that the parasystolic focus could be modulated by a slight change in heart rate, ectopic pacemaker rate, level of block, and position of the parasystolic pacemaker relative to the block border.

Clinical Implications

Empirically the parasystolic rhythm is benign and is generally not treated. Although it would appear that the ventricular ectopic beats that are not precisely coupled to normal beats may easily fall on the T wave, in clinical practice this has not been the case. One report described ventricular fibrillation in a modulated parasystole with supernormal excitability.[14]

SUMMARY

Fusion beats, which can occur within the atria or the ventricles, are the result of the presence of two opposing currents within the same chamber. Usually one is normal and the other ectopic. The collision of forces results in an ECG complex that looks neither normal nor ectopic but is something in between, often narrower and of lesser amplitude than either the normal or the ectopic beat.

A parasystolic rhythm is usually benign and results from an ectopic focus surrounded by an area of protection that may be "pure" or modulated by the electrical activity around it. Parasystole may occur in any area of the heart.

REFERENCES

1. Jalife J, Moe GK: Effects of electrotonic potentials on pacemaker activity of canine Purkinje fibers in relation to parasystole, *Circ Res* 39:801, 1976.
2. Castellanos A, Saoudi N, Moleiro F, Myerburg RJ: Parasystole. In Zipes DP, Jalife J, editors: *Cardiac electrophysiology from cell to bedside,* ed 3, Philadelphia, 2000, WB Saunders, pp 690-695.
3. Saoudi N, Letac B, Castellanos A: An electronic model for evaluating the dynamics of perfect pure parasystole in the human heart, *Am J Cardiol* 75:739, 1995.
4. Antzelevitch C, Jalife J, Moe GK: Electrotonic modulation of pacemaker activity: further biological and mathematical observations on the behavior of modulated parasystole, *Circulation* 66:1225, 1982.
5. Jalife J, Antzelevitch C, Moe GK: The case for modulated parasystole, *PACE Pacing Clin Electrophysiol* 5:811, 1982.
6. Moe GK, Antzelevitch C, Jalife J: Premature contractions: reentrant or parasystolic? In Harrison DC, editor: *Cardiac arrhythmias,* Boston, 1981, GK Hall.
7. Moe GK, Jalife J, Mueller WJ, Moe B: A mathematical model of parasystole and its application to clinical arrhythmias, *Circulation* 56:968, 1977.
8. Wit AL: Cellular electrophysiologic mechanisms of cardiac arrhythmias, *Ann NY Acad Sci* 432:1, 1986.
9. Ferrier GR, Rosenthal JE: Automaticity and entrance block induced by focal depolarization of mammalian ventricular tissues, *Circ Res* 47:238, 1980.
10. Jalife J, Moe GK: A biologic model of parasystole, *Am J Cardiol* 43:761, 1979.
11. Moe GK, Jalife J: An appraisal of "efficacy" in the treatment of ventricular premature beats, *Life Sci* 22:1189, 1978.
12. Rosenthal JE, Ferrier GR: Contribution of variable entrance and exit block in protected foci to arrhythmogenesis in isolated ventricular tissues, *Circulation* 67:1, 1983.
13. Antzelevitch C, Bernstein MJ, Feldman HN, Moe GK: Parasystole, reentry and tachycardia: a canine preparation of cardiac arrhythmias occurring across inexcitable segments of tissue, *Circulation* 68:1101, 1983.
14. Robles de Medina EO, Delmar M, Sicouri S, Jalife J: Modulated parasystole as a mechanism of ventricular ectopic activity leading to ventricular fibrillation, *Am J Cardiol* 63:1326, 1989.

CHAPTER 20
The Athlete's ECG

Intense physical training is associated with a variety of electrocardiographic (ECG) patterns that are considered a consequence of physiologic adaptations of the heart to hemodynamic load induced by chronic exercise conditioning. It is important for the clinician to be aware of the benign nature of such ECG patterns, but also to recognize possible pathologic ECG changes that require further investigation, such as hypertrophic cardiomyopathy or arrhythmogenic right ventricular cardiomyopathy, which represent the most common causes of sudden death in young competitive athletes.[1]

Although abnormal ECG patterns representing physiologic adaptation to intense training can be found in many trained athletes, they are not consistently present in all athletes, even in those undergoing intensive exercise, training, and participating in premier competitive events. In fact, such abnormal ECG patterns are more likely to be found in male athletes with a history of years of endurance training. Such a history aids the physician in the differential diagnosis between physiologic and pathologic ECG changes.[2] ECG variants usually seen in trained athletes are summarized in Boxes 20-1 and 20-2 and described in the following section.

SINUS BRADYCARDIA AND SINUS ARRHYTHMIA

In the athlete's ECG, sinus bradycardia and sinus arrhythmia are the most common findings. Junctional escape rhythms may be seen during the slow phase of the sinus arrhythmia. In athletes engaged in endurance sports (such as rowing, swimming, bicycling, and long-distance running) sinus bradycardia is usually more pronounced in those with a superior level of training. In some highly conditioned athletes sinus bradycardia and sinus arrhythmia are present even during normal daily activity as a result of predominance of vagal tone with relative reduction in sympathetic tone induced by aerobic physical training.

Fig. 20-1 is an ECG from a very fit 20-year-old male endurance athlete. His cross-training consists of the fol-

BOX 20-1. ECG Changes Due to Heightened Resting Vagal Tone

- Sinus bradycardia (<60 beats/min, and often <50 beats/min)
- Sinus arrhythmia
- Prolonged PR interval (>0.20 second)
- Wenckebach (second degree, type I) AV block in athletes who usually also have first-degree AV block
- Junctional escape rhythms
- Tall T waves
- Prominent U waves

BOX 20-2. ECG Changes Associated with Physiologic Cardiac Remodeling

- Coronary sinus
- Increased P wave amplitude
- Notched P waves
- Increased QRS voltage (R and/or S wave amplitude in precordial leads larger than 30 mm)
- Early repolarization pattern
- T wave inversion
- Incomplete RBBB pattern
- QRS axis between 0 and 90 degrees

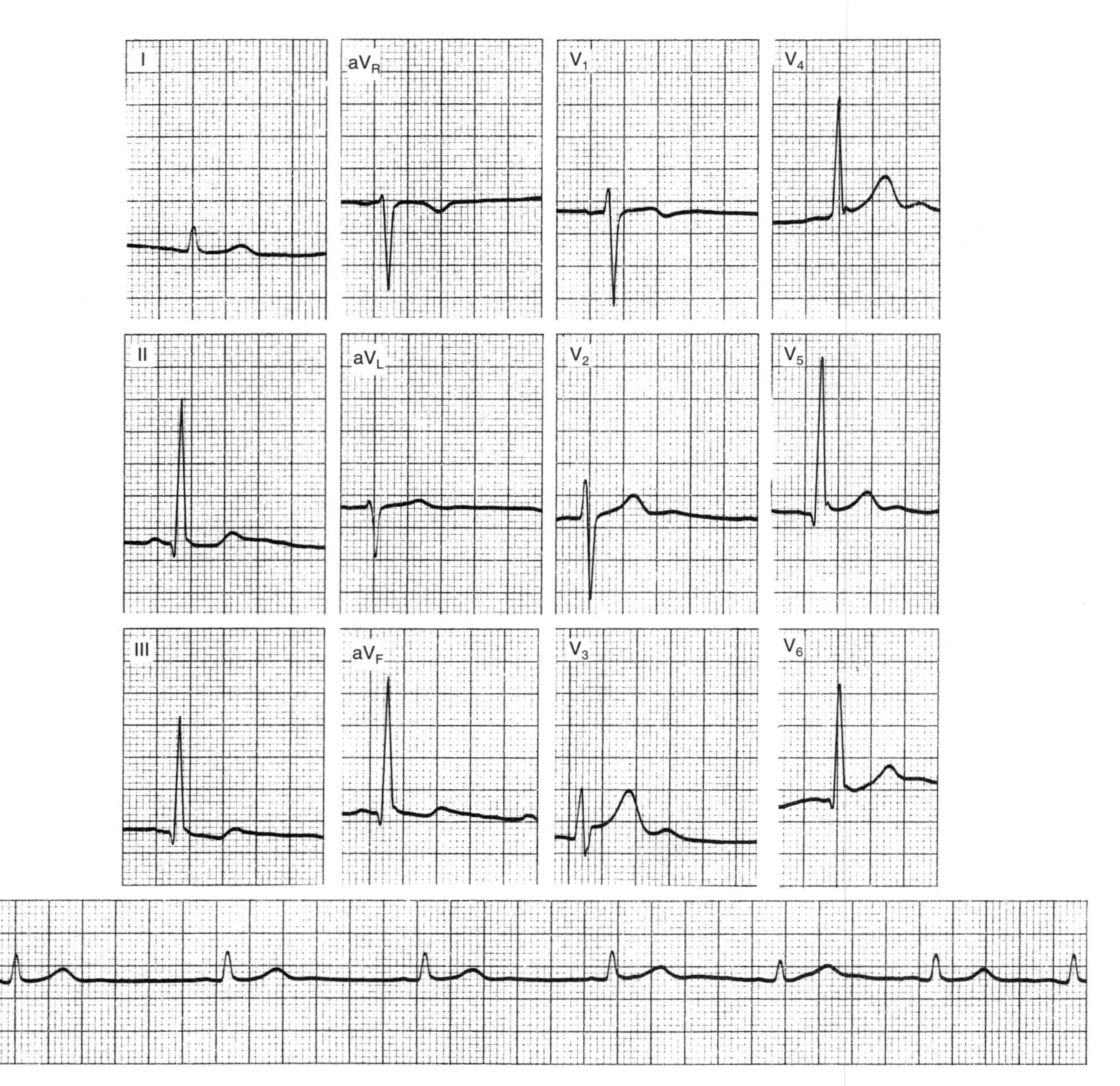

FIG. 20-1. A 12-lead ECG from a 20-year-old endurance athlete. Note the sinus bradycardia of less than 50 beats/min in the slowest part of his sinus arrhythmia and the vertical QRS axis. The early repolarization pattern is seen in the left precordial leads with ST segment elevation in leads V_3 and V_4 and J point elevation in V_4 to V_6.

lowing routine two to three times a week: 3-mile run, 15- to 20-mile bike ride, 60 to 90 minutes of jumping rope, and 4,000 meters of rowing.

Figs. 20-2 and 20-3 are preexercise and postexercise ECGs in a 27-year-old Olympic male triathlete and a 53-year-old male swimmer, respectively, undergoing regular training since childhood. The postexercise ECGs of both athletes were taken after a 3,500-meter swim competing with each other. Preexercise and postexercise ECGs demonstrate a dramatic difference in heart rate, as would be expected, and diffuse changes in ECG patterns. The athlete whose ECG is noted in Fig. 20-3 was an All-American in the 1,650-yard freestyle at the University of California, Berkeley, and a consistent top five finisher at National

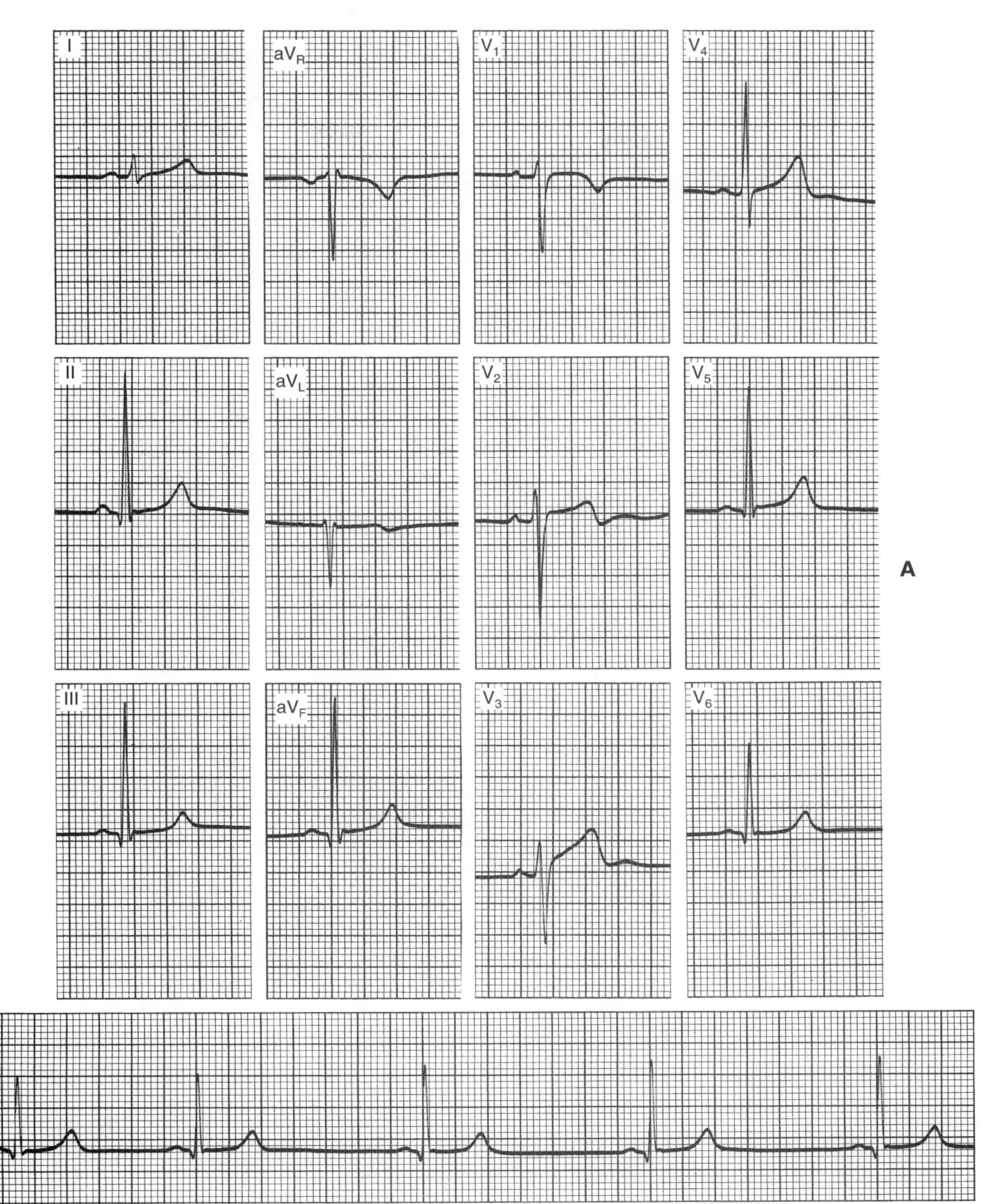

FIG. 20-2. A, Preexercise ECGs from a 27-year-old male Olympic triathlete. The PR, QRS, QTc, and QRS axes all are normal. Other findings typical of a highly trained athlete are sinus bradycardia and sinus arrhythmia, widely notched P waves in the limb leads, and early repolarization pattern (ST elevation in V_3 and V_4). The T wave is normally inverted in V_1, and the peaked, tall T waves seen in V_4 and V_5 are normal for an athlete. There are q waves in standard leads II, III, and aV_F.

Continued

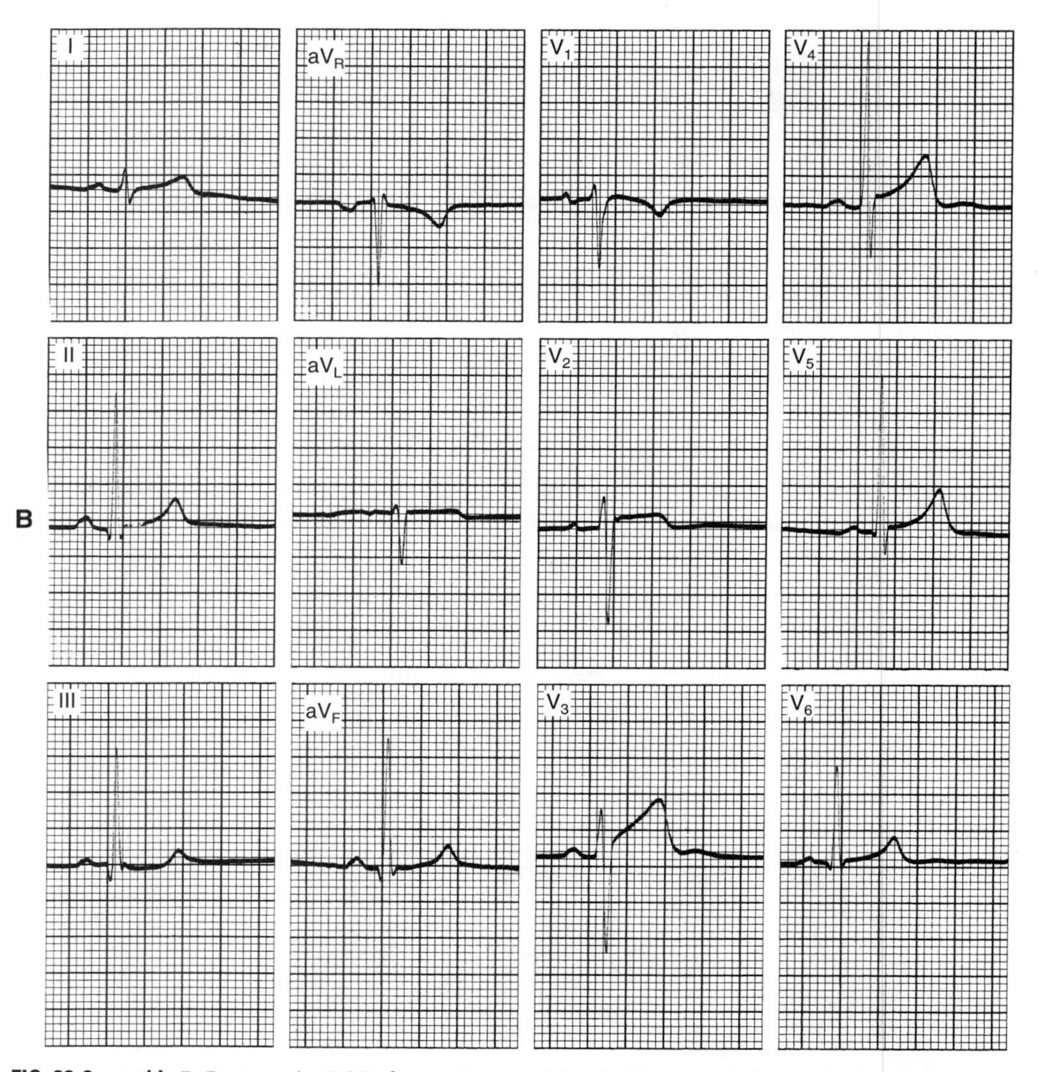

FIG. 20-2, cont'd. **B**, Postexercise ECGs from a 27-year-old male Olympic triathlete. The PR, QRS, QTc, and QRS axes all are normal. Other findings typical of a highly trained athlete are sinus bradycardia and sinus arrhythmia, widely notched P waves in the limb leads, and early repolarization pattern (ST elevation in V_3 and V_4). The T wave is normally inverted in V_1, and the peaked, tall T waves seen in V_4 and V_5 are normal for an athlete. There are q waves in standard leads II, III, and aV_F.

Masters Championship pool and open water swims for the last 30 years. Among his most notable open water swims are 26 Alcatraz crossings plus two round trips and 25 Golden Gate crossings.

Fig. 20-4 is a resting ECG from a 30-year-old male champion of Brazilian jiu jitsu (two-time World Champion; two-time Pan-American Champion; and four-time U.S. Open Champion). This ECG demonstrates the dramatic difference between the ECG patterns of the endurance disciplines (cycling, cross-country skiing, swimming, rowing) and the technical disciplines (equestrian, alpine skiing, jiu jitsu) in which distinctly abnormal ECGs are not seen.[3]

P WAVES

Another ECG sign of an athletic heart is the notched P wave, as already seen in Fig. 20-3, *B*. P waves may also be tall. Nakamoto found notched P waves in 18 of 25 marathon runners both before and after exercise.

Although the two atria activate sequentially, this activa-

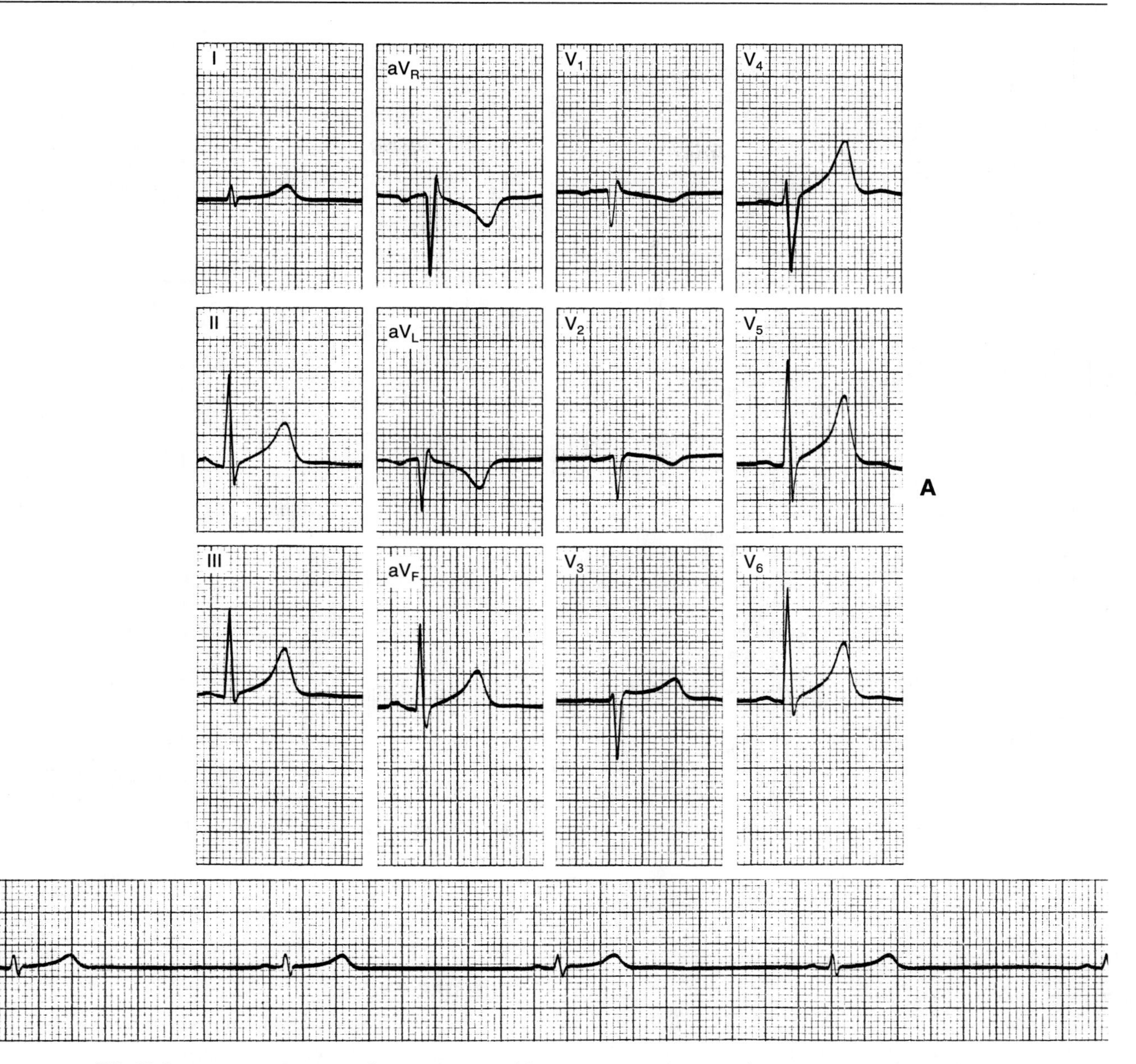

FIG. 20-3. A, Preexercise ECGs from a 53-year-old competitive swimmer. The resting ECG shows sinus bradycardia (36 beats/min), a vertical QRS axis (+80 degrees), early repolarization pattern in the precordial leads V_3 to V_6, and poor R wave progression in precordial leads V_1 to V_4. The postexercise ECG shows an increased heart rate (60 beats/min) and a widely notched P wave.

Continued

tion is reflected in a smooth P wave in the normal heart. When activation in the atria is delayed (such as in the case of atrial enlargement), the two separate events, right and left atrial activation, can be distinguished and slight notching of the P wave is evident.

ATRIOVENTRICULAR BLOCK

First-degree atrioventricular (AV) block with a PR interval of 0.20 second or more and AV Wenckebach (second degree, type I) has, along with sinus bradycardia, been attributed to enhanced vagal tone in trained athletes and

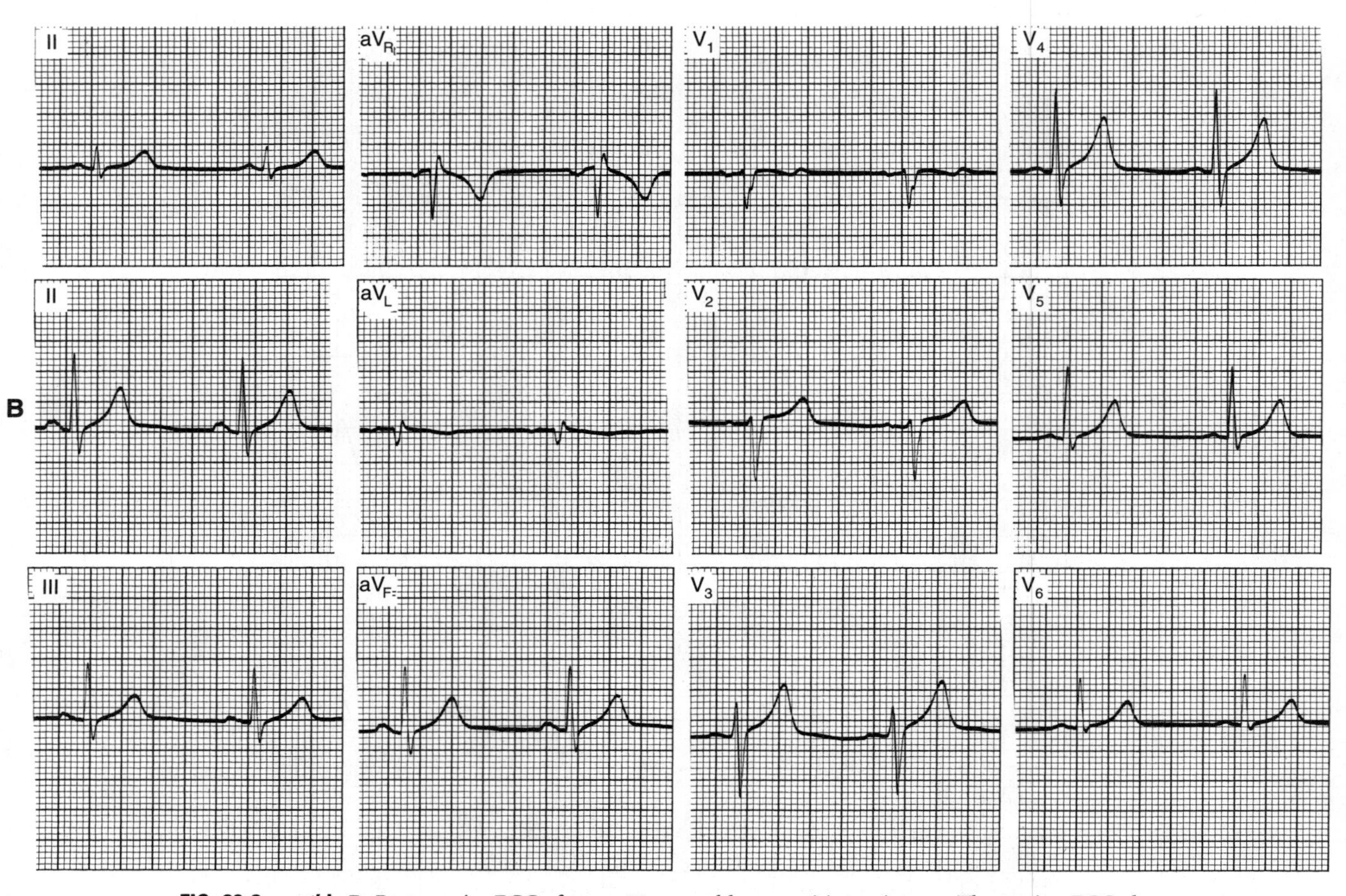

FIG. 20-3, cont'd. B, Postexercise ECGs from a 53-year-old competitive swimmer. The resting ECG shows sinus bradycardia (36 beats/min), a vertical QRS axis (+80 degrees), early repolarization pattern in the precordial leads V_3 to V_6, and poor R wave progression in precordial leads V_1 to V_4. The postexercise ECG shows an increased heart rate (60 beats/min) and a widely notched P wave.

typically normalizes during exercise or after complete deconditioning. Although prolonged AV conduction is common, advanced second- and third-degree atrioventricular blocks are not, and when present, the possibility of underlying heart disease must be excluded.

Q WAVES

Small q waves in an athlete's ECG are compatible with, but not necessarily indicative of, cardiovascular disease. Normal q waves reflect normal septal activation. They are seen in leads I, aV_L, and V_6 and are less than 0.04 second in duration and less than 25% of the amplitude of the R wave. In the electrically horizontal heart, normal septal q waves may also appear in leads V_4 and V_5; in the electrically vertical heart, they may appear in leads II, III, and aV_F, as seen in Fig. 20-4.

HIGH QRS VOLTAGE

High QRS voltage is common among athletes engaged in dynamic training, and when seen on the ECG does not imply, per se, the diagnosis of pathologic left ventricular hypertrophy. The ECG in Fig. 20-5, *A*, shows a pattern consistent with physiologic left ventricular hypertrophy in a 41-year-old female athlete with a history, since the age of 6 years, of swimming, running, and other strenuous physical exercise, and who presently is a serious competitive amateur triathlete. For comparison, the ECG seen in Fig. 20-5, *B*, shows instead, a pattern of pathologic left ventricular hypertrophy.

INCOMPLETE RIGHT BUNDLE BRANCH BLOCK

Incomplete right bundle branch block (RBBB) is a common finding in trained athletes; its significance is not

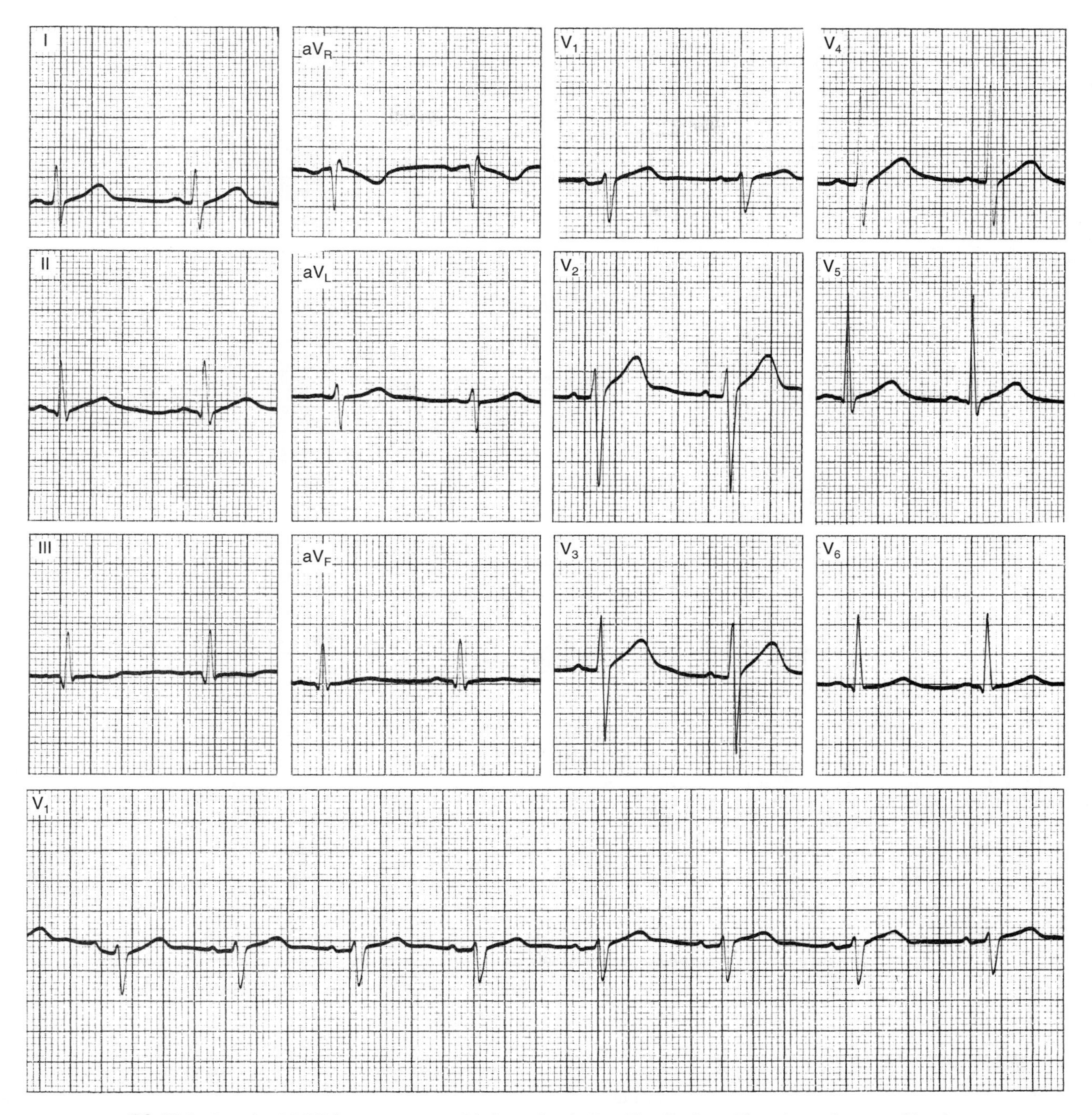

FIG. 20-4. A 12-lead ECG from a 30-year-old champion in Brazilian jiu jitsu. There is an absence of bradycardia, no signs of left ventricular hypertrophy, and only a mild ST segment elevation in V_2 to V_3.

completely defined, but is likely related to the delayed activation of the basal segments of the right ventricle. On the other hand, the findings of complete RBBB (QRS longer than 0.12 second), left bundle branch block, and fascicular block are rare in athletes and would prompt cardiac evaluation for underlying structural heart disease.

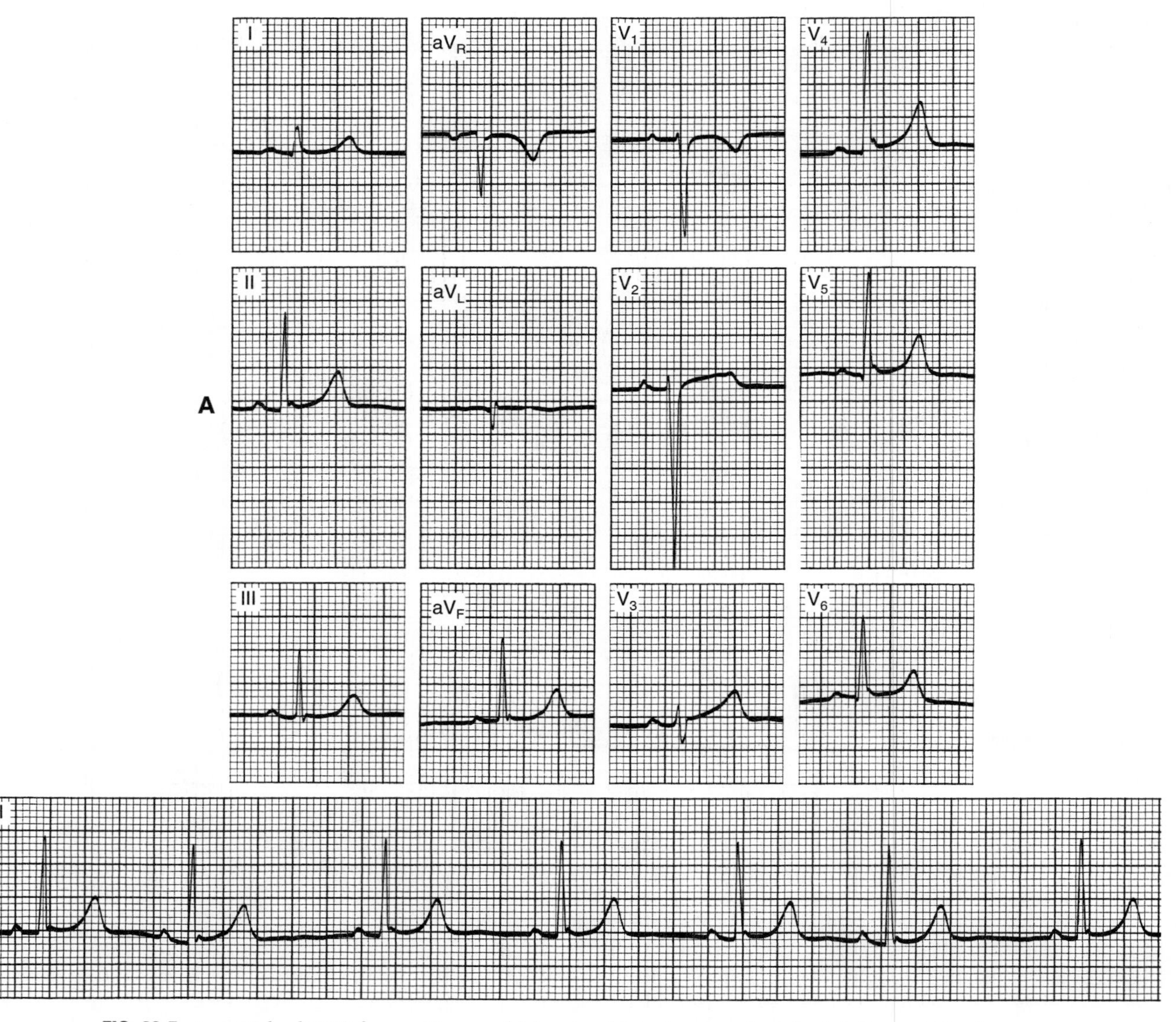

FIG. 20-5. **A,** A 12-lead ECG from a 41-year-old female athlete showing physiologic left ventricular hypertrophy. Note the increased S wave voltage in precordial lead V_2 with a sharp transition in precordial lead V_3. There is only a mild elevation of the J point in precordial lead V_2. No other ECG abnormalities are evident.

Continued

EARLY REPOLARIZATION SYNDROME

The early repolarization syndrome, manifesting with elevation of the J point and ST segment, is almost always the rule in the athlete's ECG, as shown in Fig. 20-6.

Mechanism

The elevated J point is the result of a distinct difference in the shapes of the epicardial and endocardial action potentials, causing a small voltage gradient at the end of the depolarization process (end of the QRS). Thus a current flows between the two myocardial layers, reflected on the ECG as a slight J point elevation and ST segment elevation. In athletes, the maximal ST elevation may occasionally be as high as in patients with the Brugada syndrome.[4,5]

Differential Diagnosis

The elevated ST segment of the early repolarization syndrome may mimic those observed in patients with myocardial ischemia and Brugada syndrome.

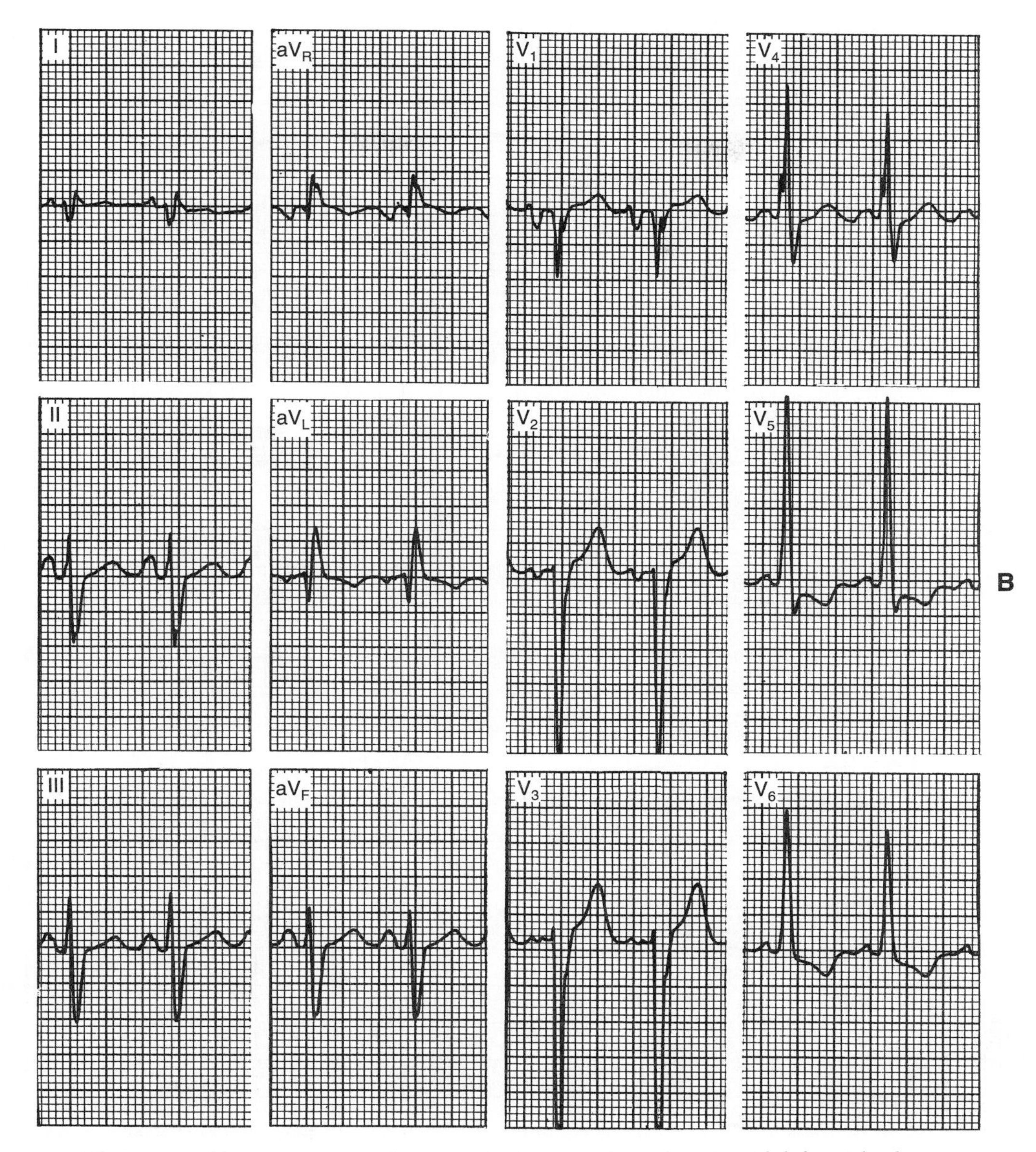

FIG. 20-5, cont'd. **B,** Pathologic left ventricular hypertrophy and strain with left atrial enlargement.

Brugada syndrome. Both the early repolarization syndrome seen in most athletes and Brugada syndrome seen in young, often asymptomatic, individuals manifest with elevated J points in right precordial leads and elevated ST segments. Electrocardiographically, the two conditions differ significantly from each other; however, Brugada syndrome can be missed if the individual's condition is not clearly manifested on the ECG and a family history is not taken, or if the observer is uninformed regarding this condition and fails to recognize an overt ECG pattern.

Brugada syndrome is an inherited arrhythmogenic syndrome caused by mutation of the cardiac voltage-dependent Na^+ channel gene SCN5A, which upsets the repolarization process and causes the J point to be elevated to such an extent that in V_1 it looks like a terminal R′ (i.e., RBBB) and in extreme cases the elevated J point and ST segment plunges into an inverted terminal T wave. As in the early repolarization syndrome, there is a difference in the shapes of the right ventricular epicardial and endocardial action potentials, in this case the result of mutation of

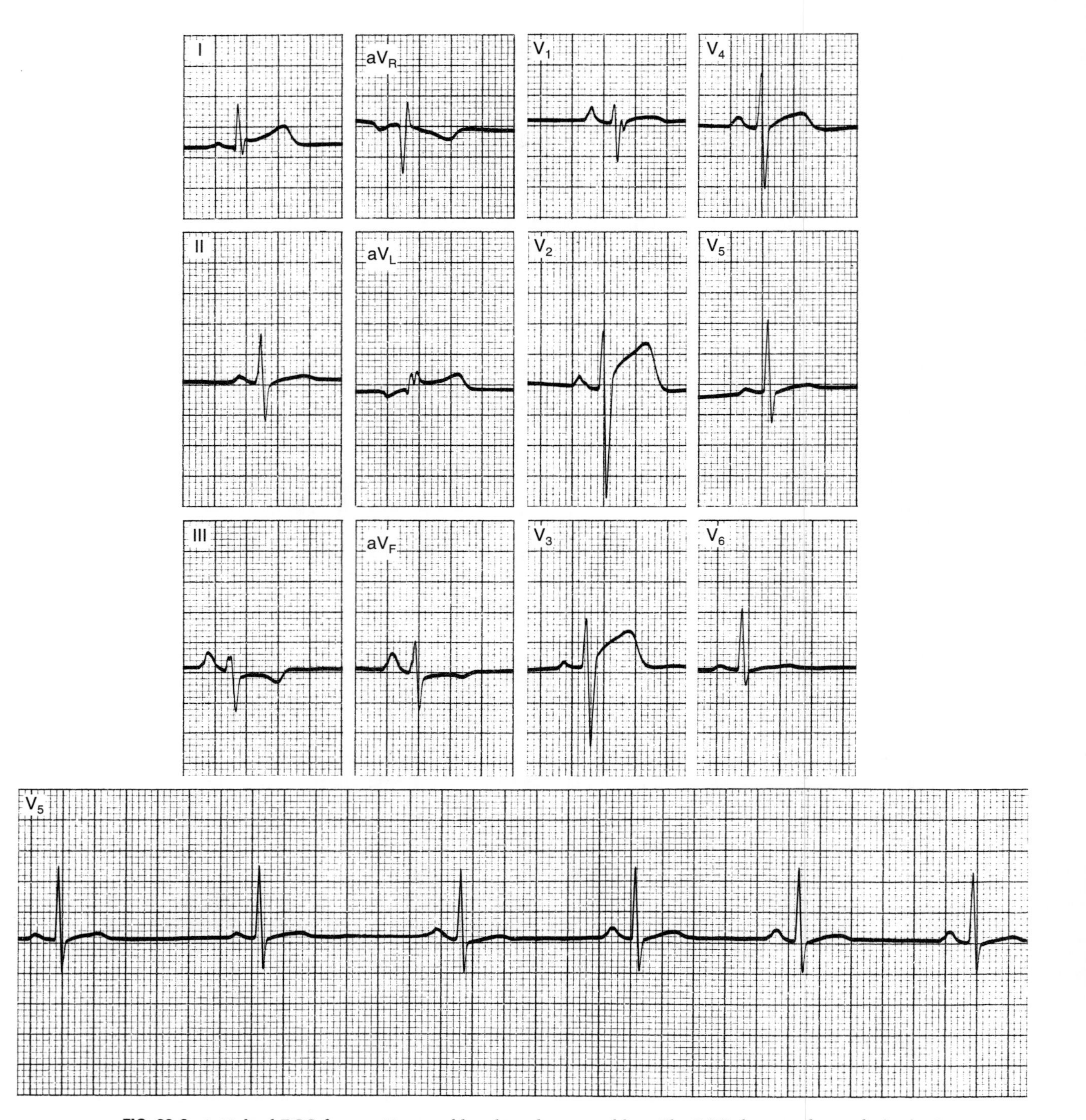

FIG. 20-6. A 12-lead ECG from a 45-year-old male endurance athlete. The ECG shows early repolarization (ST elevation) in leads I, aV_L, and V_2 to V_4. Other findings are sinus bradycardia (52 beats/min); biatrial enlargement (P wave duration: 0.12 second; P wave height: 3 mm in III and aV_F); and biventricular hypertrophy reflected by a QRS of 0.12 second, frontal plane axis of –30 degrees, and late activation of both right (late R in aV_R) and left ventricles (late R in aV_L). The initial QRS slurring in II and aV_F is not unusual in the hypertrophied ventricle and does not indicate preexcitation. (With thanks to Hein J.J. Wellens, MD, Maastricht, The Netherlands, for his expert evaluation.)

a gene that controls Na^+ channels. This causes a large voltage gradient at the end of the QRS resulting in a larger current flow than that usually seen in the early repolarization syndrome. A very tall J wave and ST segment elevation thus appears in right precordial leads V_1 and V_2.

In Fig. 20-7 the elevated J point of *(A)* Brugada syndrome and *(B)* the early repolarization syndrome are compared; they are clearly different. In the more vulnerable cases of Brugada syndrome the J point is markedly elevated and then seems to dive into a negative T wave. The overt cases may be picked up with ECG screening; the concealed or intermittent forms may be suspected because of the symptoms of nonfatal ventricular tachycardia or a family history of sudden death. The ECG manifestation of concealed or intermittent Brugada syndrome can be unmasked by administration of a Na^+ channel blocker, such as intravenous ajmaline, flecainide, or procainamide. This syndrome is discussed at length in Chapter 27.

PREMATURE BEATS

Premature atrial and ventricular complexes are commonly seen in athletes, although they rarely cause symptoms and usually are not clinically important, unless associated with structural heart disease.

ECG FINDINGS IN 1,005 OLYMPIC ATHLETES

Pelliccia et al at the Institute of Sports Science in Rome[6] were in a unique position to directly compare ECG patterns with cardiac morphology as assessed by echocardiography in a large group of consecutive athletes, aged 24 ± 6 years, who were participating in 38 sporting disciplines as members of the Italian national teams. Men were more likely than women to have an abnormal ECG, especially with regard to the R and S wave voltages and the presence of abnormal Q waves. Normal ECGs were found in 78% of the women and 55% of the men. There were also more abnormal ECGs in cyclists (35%), cross-country skiers (30%), and rowers (20%) than in other disciplines. The notable ECG patterns were assigned to one of three subgroups depending on the presence of one or more of the ECG criteria listed in Box 20-3.

Although abnormal ECGs were found in 40% of the athletes, only 5% were associated with presence of structural cardiac diseases. When cardiac disease was not a

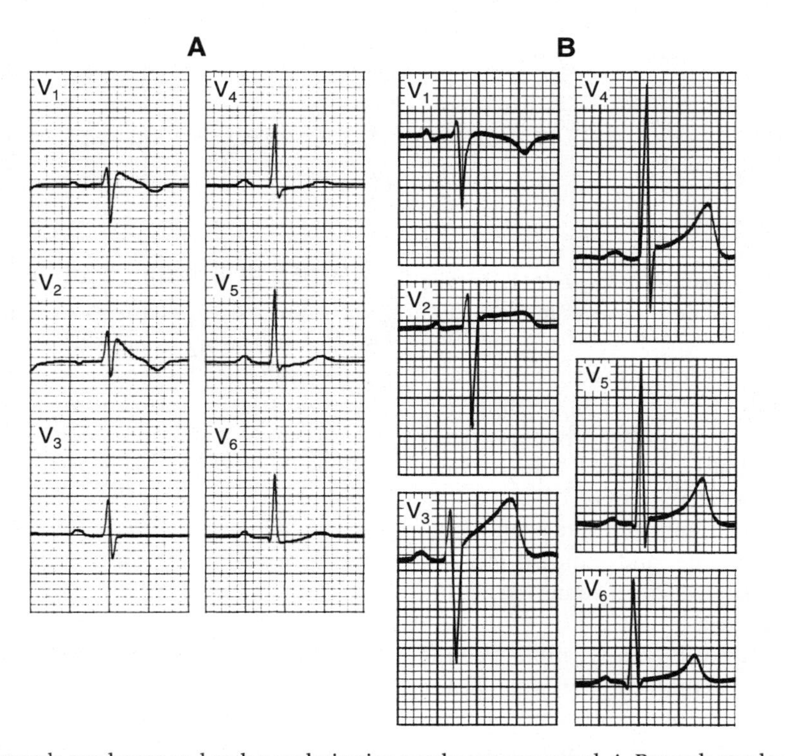

FIG. 20-7. Brugada syndrome and early repolarization syndrome compared. **A,** Brugada syndrome. Note the elevated J point, typically seen in the right precordial leads V_1 and V_2. From the peak of the J point, the ST segment swoops into a negative T wave. The higher the J point and the deeper the T, the more vulnerable the patient is. **B,** Early repolarization syndrome. Note the elevated J point in precordial leads V_3 and V_4 and the positive T wave.

BOX 20-3. Notable ECG Patterns in 1,005 Olympic Athletes

DISTINCTLY ABNORMAL ECG (14%); STRONGLY SUGGESTIVE OF CARDIOVASCULAR DISEASE

- R or S wave >35 mm in any lead
- Q >4 mm deep in more than one lead
- Early repolarization pattern with deeply inverted T wave >2 mm in more than one lead (with exclusion of standard lead III)
- Left bundle branch block pattern
- Marked axis deviation (i.e., to the left of –30 degrees or to the right of +110 degrees)
- Short PR (<0.12 second) and delta wave with QRS >0.10 second (overt WPW syndrome)

MILDLY ABNORMAL ECG (26%); COMPATIBLE WITH THE PRESENCE OF CARDIOVASCULAR DISEASE

- R or S wave 30 to 34 mm in any lead
- Q wave 2-3 mm deep in more than one lead
- Early repolarization pattern with flat, minimally inverted, or tall (>15 mm) T waves in more than one lead
- Poor R wave progression in V_1 to V_3
- RBBB (>0.12 second in V_1 and V_2)
- Right atrial enlargement (peaked P of >2.5 mm in II, III, V_1)
- Left atrial enlargement (prolonged positive P in II and/or deep, prolonged negative P in V_1)
- Short PR interval (<0.12 second)

NORMAL ECG OR MINOR ALTERATIONS (60%); PART OF ATHLETE'S HEART SYNDROME

- PR interval >0.20 second
- Mildly increased R or S wave (25-29 mm)
- Early repolarization pattern (ST elevation >2 mm in >2 leads)
- Incomplete RBBB in V_1 and V_2 (QRS <0.12 second)
- Sinus bradycardia (<60 beats/min)

Adapted from Pelliccia A, Maron BJ, Culasso F et al: Clinical significance of abnormal electrocardiographic patterns in trained athletes, *Circulation* 102(3):278-284, 2000.

factor, male gender and participation in an endurance type of sport were deemed responsible for the abnormal ECG patterns.

It should be noted that the low prevalence of cardiac disease was anticipated in this large group of Olympic athletes because almost all of them had been prescreened before admittance to the Italian national teams. Those found to have structural heart disease were, of course, not accepted. Therefore in trained amateur and professional athletes competing at local, state, and national levels, a larger number of abnormal ECGs reflecting structural heart disease would be expected.

Of the 1,005 athletes in the Italian Olympic training program approximately 5% had markedly abnormal ECGs, instinctively suggesting the presence of structural cardiovascular disease but without evidence of cardiac disease or morphologic changes. The cause of these false-positive ECGs is not known, although Pellicia et al could not exclude that they represent the result of long-term, intense athletic training.

CAUSES OF SUDDEN CARDIAC DEATH IN ATHLETES

Although the acute risk of sudden cardiac death is enhanced during intense sports training or competition, regular physical training results in an overall cardioprotective effect. In fact, physical inactivity and sedentary lifestyle are recognized as major risk factors for the development of coronary heart disease, adverse cardiovascular events, and mortality.[7]

Sudden death is a rare event in the young athlete, with the most common causes in subjects younger than 35 years of age being *hypertrophic cardiomyopathy* and *arrhythmogenic right ventricular cardiomyopathy*. In individuals older than 35 years of age, *atherosclerotic coronary artery disease* accounts for the vast majority of deaths, usually related to activities such as distance running, racquet sports, and isometric exertion such as weight-lifting. Other rare causes of sudden death in athletes are congenital anomalies of the coronary vessels, Wolff-Parkinson-White (WPW) syndrome, congenital long QT syndrome, myocarditis, dilated cardiomyopathy, and Marfan syndrome.

HYPERTROPHIC CARDIOMYOPATHY

Hypertrophic cardiomyopathy is a familial autosomal dominant disorder involving almost 200 mutations in genes encoding proteins for the cardiac sarcomere.[8] The ventricular hypertrophy in this disease occurs in the absence of left ventricular cavity dilatation, unlike the physiologic changes in the athlete's heart. This condition is difficult to identify by history and physical examination. In one study[9] only 21% had symptoms of cardiovascular disease before their death.

ECG Suspicion

The ECG in both the athlete and the patient with hypertrophic cardiomyopathy is significantly altered, rendering the ECG not always useful, especially when evaluated without careful clinical and echocardiographic examinations. The ECG signs that favor a diagnosis of hypertrophic cardiomyopathy are as follows:

- Prominent Q waves
- S in V_1 + R in V_5 >35 mm
- ST depression of more than 1.5 mm in the left precordial leads
- Deep negative T wave in the left precordial leads
- Left axis deviation
- Left atrial enlargement
- Ventricular or atrial arrhythmias at rest or during a maximal exercise test

The ECG in Fig. 20-8 shows a borderline ECG that may be compatible with either a physiologic or a pathologic cardiac condition. Note the tall R wave in left precordial leads, ST segment depression, and a negative T wave. Also evident are ST segment elevation in right precordial leads associated with an incomplete RBBB pattern.

Differential Diagnosis

The increase in left ventricular mass observed in competitive athletes known as the "athlete's heart" is the result of an increase in left ventricular diastolic cavity dimension rather than increased wall thickness. In a small percentage of athletes, mainly those training in rowing sports, the increased cavity dimension is associated with increased ventricular wall thickness significant enough to require a differentiation from hypertrophic cardiomyopathy.[10]

Left ventricular wall thickness. In echocardiographic studies of 947 athletes, Pelliccia et al[11] found that only 16 had wall thicknesses of 13 mm or more; none more than 16 mm. Of these 16 athletes, 15 were rowers or canoeists and 1 was a cyclist. All 16 athletes had achieved a distinguished level, 8 being among the top three in the world in their sport.

The enhanced wall thickness seen in these athletes was associated with an enlarged left ventricular cavity. Because of these findings, it was concluded that intense training, mainly in rowing, increases left ventricular wall thickness, in some as much as 15 to 16 mm, beyond which, when associated with a nondilated left ventricular cavity, the athlete is likely to have primary forms of pathologic hypertrophy, such as hypertrophic cardiomyopathy.

In the population studied, it is believed that the

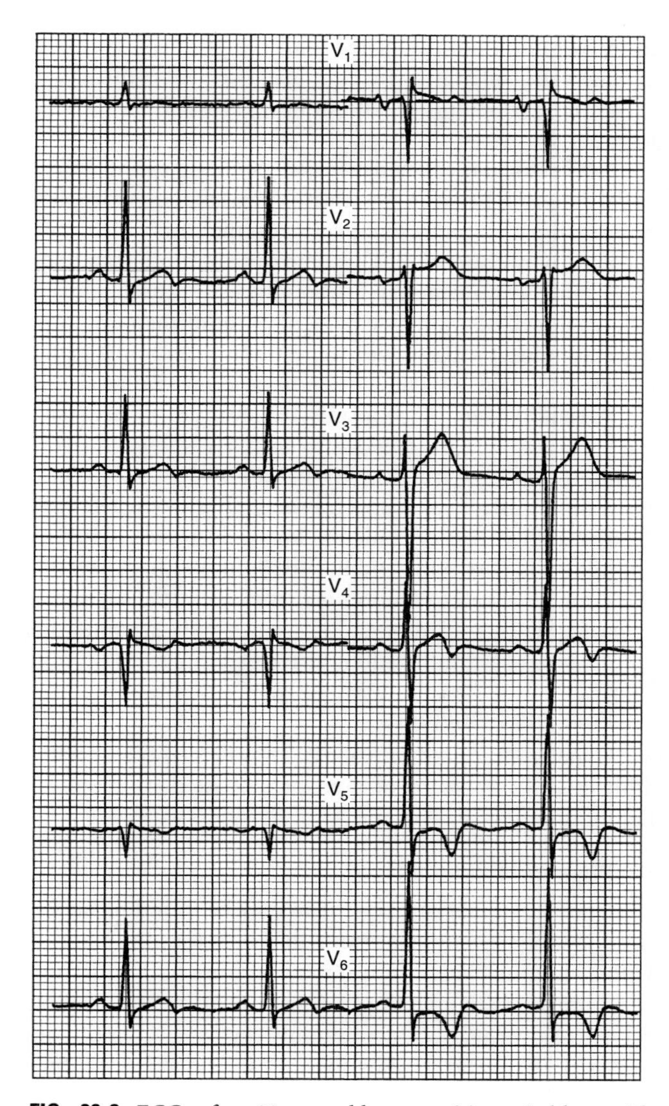

FIG. 20-8. ECG of a 29-year-old competitive triathlete with incomplete RBBB, moderate ST elevation in right precordial leads and marked ST depression in left precordial leads with deep negative T waves, and a positive Sokolow index (S in V_1 + R in V_5 > 35 mm). (From Claessens P, Claessens C, Claessens M et al: Physiological or pseudophysiologic ECG changes in endurance-trained athletes, *Heart Vessels* 15:181-190, 2000.)

increased wall thickness was found almost exclusively in rowers at the elite level because of their increased cardiac output in response to demanding isometric and isotonic exercise performed against resistance. Generally, the total fitness of elite rowers is exemplary, even when compared to canoeists, because of the full lower extremity and hip involvement required of their sport.[12]

Although in the majority of patients with hypertrophic cardiomyopathy, left ventricular wall thickness is marked, in a minority of such patients it is mild (in the range of 13 to 15 mm) and not associated with symptoms, presenting a diagnostic dilemma. In this instance, left ventricular cavity dimension and deconditioning are useful in the differential diagnosis.

Left ventricular cavity dimension. Sometimes the differential diagnosis between the athlete's heart and hypertrophic cardiomyopathy can be made solely on the basis of left ventricular cavity dimension. This is because in more than one-third of highly trained male athletes the left ventricular diastolic cavity dimension is enlarged to more than 55 mm, whereas in most patients with hypertrophic cardiomyopathy (unless end-stage) this dimension is less than 45 mm.

Deconditioning. The most useful means of differentiating hypertrophic cardiomyopathy from an athlete's heart is an interruption of training for at least 3 months.[13] When the trained athlete interrupts training, physiologic left ventricular cavity size or wall thickness decreases, whereas pathologic hypertrophy and hypertrophic cardiomyopathy does not. This determination is made by careful examination of serial echocardiographic studies and presumes the compliance of the athlete to interrupt training.

Possible Symptoms

Hypertrophic cardiomyopathy may be suspected in any athlete with symptoms of exertional chest pain, dyspnea, lightheadedness, or syncope.

Physical Examination

Upon examination the athlete may be found to have a harsh systolic ejection murmur that increases in intensity with a sustained Valsalva or it may decrease with squatting and increase with standing; a fourth heart sound may be present. However, not uncommonly the physical examination is negative and the diagnosis is confirmed by echocardiography.

ARRHYTHMOGENIC RIGHT VENTRICULAR CARDIOMYOPATHY

Arrhythmogenic right ventricular cardiomyopathy[14] is a myocardial disease that is familial in about 50% of cases and is characterized by fibro-fatty replacement of the right ventricular myocardium. A large proportion of young individuals with arrhythmogenic right ventricular disease has an abnormal ECG and late potentials in the signal-averaged ECG.

ECG Recognition

The ECG is an initial diagnostic test that is useful, but not highly sensitive; a normal ECG does not exclude the possibility of arrhythmogenic right ventricular cardiomyopathy. The most frequent ECG abnormalities include the following:

T waves: Inverted in V_1 through V_3.

QRS morphology during sinus rhythm:

- Incomplete or complete RBBB pattern reflecting conduction delays through the right ventricle
- Epsilon wave (a notch in the terminal portion of the QRS in V_1 reflecting delayed right ventricular activation; Fig. 20-9)

QRS duration: Prolonged to more than 0.11 second in leads V_1 and V_2 as compared to the shorter QRS duration in V_6, as illustrated in Fig. 20-10.

QT interval: Prolonged to more than 0.44 second in right precordial leads.

QRS morphology of premature ventricular complexes or during ventricular tachycardia (VT): V_1-negative pattern with a ventricular ectopic morphology (see Chapter 14) and superior axis (left or northwest).

Pathophysiology

The degenerative process begins with a genetic predisposition to fatty infiltration of the right ventricular myocardium from which it eventually degenerates into a fibrofatty form that, over time, involves both ventricles. In

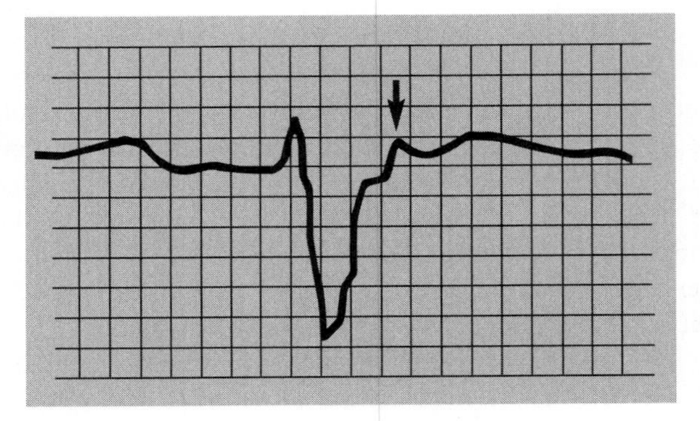

FIG. 20-9. The epsilon wave in lead V_1 *(arrow)* is highly specific for arrhythmogenic right ventricular cardiomyopathy. It is followed by a saddleback pattern of ST segment, another ECG sign seen in arrhythmogenic right ventricular cardiomyopathy. (Courtesy Andrea Naiall, MD, Cleveland Clinic Foundation.)

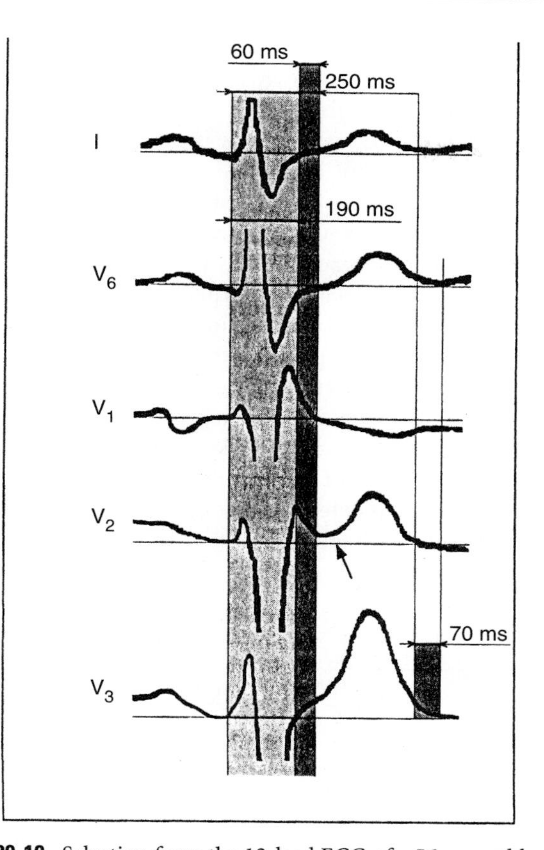

FIG. 20-10. Selection from the 12-lead ECG of a 56-year-old man who had the histologic diagnosis of arrhythmogenic right ventricular dysplasia that could be suspected by the analysis of the ECG. The ECG showed an RSR′ pattern in right ventricular precordial leads with a QRS complex of 250 ms in V_1 or V_2 as compared with 190 ms in lead V_6, suggesting the pattern of parietal block superimposed on a complete RBBB. Note the saddleback pattern of ST segment in lead V_2 *(arrow)* frequently seen in patients with arrhythmogenic right ventricular dysplasia. (From Fontaine G, Tonet J, Frank R: Ventricular tachycardia in arrhythmogenic right ventricular dysplasia. In Zipes DP, Jalife J, editors: *Cardiac electrophysiology from cell to bedside,* Philadelphia, 2000, WB Saunders, p 549.)

its terminal stage it is clinically indistinguishable from dilated cardiomyopathy.

Symptoms

There is a variety of symptoms (usually related to episodes of VT), such as palpitations, dizzy spells, blurred vision, syncope, malaise, or abrupt extreme weakness in an individual who is apparently in good health. However, not uncommonly, sudden death may be the first clinical manifestation of this disease in association with exercise.

Treatment

Treatment is controversial with options that include antiarrhythmic drugs, radiofrequency ablation, or an implantable cardioverter-defibrillator.[15] Cardiac transplantation may ultimately be an option in cases of progressive biventricular failure.

CONGENITAL CORONARY ARTERY ANOMALIES

In young athletes, congenital coronary artery anomalies are not uncommonly associated with sudden death, probably precipitated by myocardial ischemia. Such coronary anomalies are rarely identified during life, often because of insufficient clinical suspicion. However, because anomalous coronary artery origin *can be treated surgically,* timely clinical identification is crucial.

In retrospective postmortem evaluation of the medical records of young competitive athletes who died suddenly, Basso et al[16] identified 27 with congenital coronary artery anomalies, 23 with left main coronary artery originating from the right aortic sinus, and 4 with right coronary artery originating from the left sinus. Fifteen of these athletes (55%) had no premonitory symptoms or cardiovascular testing during life. In the remaining 12 athletes (45%) aged 16 ± 7, all cardiovascular tests were normal, including 12-lead ECG in 9 of the athletes, stress ECG with maximal exercise in 6 of the athletes, and cardiac morphology and function by two-dimensional echocardiography in 2 of the athletes.

With no help from the usual cardiovascular tests, one is left with the premonitory symptoms of a possibly life-ending congenital abnormality to be recognized by alert physical trainers. Those symptoms were reported in only 10 of the 27 athletes. Thus 17 deaths could not have been anticipated, but in the remaining 10, an alertness to athlete's symptoms results in further testing. Those symptoms include syncope in four (exertional in three) 3 to 24 months before death and chest pain in five (exertional in three)—all single episodes within the 2 years of their death. The results of this study have important implications for screening of competitive athletes and suggest that a history of exertional syncope or chest pain requires exclusion of congenital coronary artery anomalies of wrong aortic sinus origin in young competitive athletes.[16]

WPW SYNDROME

WPW syndrome is a congenital and curable cause of sudden unexpected death in which an accessory pathway connects an atrium with a ventricle. The accessory pathway may conduct anterogradely and retrogradely and under the right conditions provides one arm of a reentry circuit to produce paroxysmal supraventricular tachycardia (PSVT).

Atrial fibrillation may be a fatal arrhythmia depending on the refractory period of the accessory pathway, which varies considerably relative to location.[17]

There are three functional types of accessory pathways: overt, latent, and concealed. In *overt* WPW, there is an initial slurring of the beginning of the QRS called a *delta wave*. This early beginning of the QRS produces a *short PR interval* and a *prolonged QRS*.

A *latent* accessory pathway is capable on anterograde conduction, but the impulse does not arrive in the ventricle before it traverses the AV node and His bundle, thus the 12-lead ECG is normal. This is the most dangerous type for the athlete because although prescreening may have been done, the accessory pathway cannot be detected. Hopefully, the first arrhythmia that such an athlete experiences will be PSVT, prompting further investigation. However, in some patients, the first arrhythmia experienced is atrial fibrillation. If the refractory period of the accessory pathway is short, the ventricular rate may exceed 300 beats/min. This is a life-threatening arrhythmia.

A *concealed* accessory pathway is capable only of retrograde conduction. This individual is not in danger of sudden death in the event of atrial fibrillation. However, retrograde conduction can support a reentry mechanism using the AV node anterogradely. Thus the person with a concealed accessory pathway may experience bouts of PSVT. In the case of symptomatic individuals with either a latent or concealed accessory pathway there is need for a differential diagnosis between the circus movement tachycardia of WPW and AV nodal reentry tachycardia.

The risk of sudden death makes it prudent to perform a cardiac evaluation of each athlete with a diagnosis of WPW syndrome to determine the refractory period of the accessory pathway in the event that the individual's first

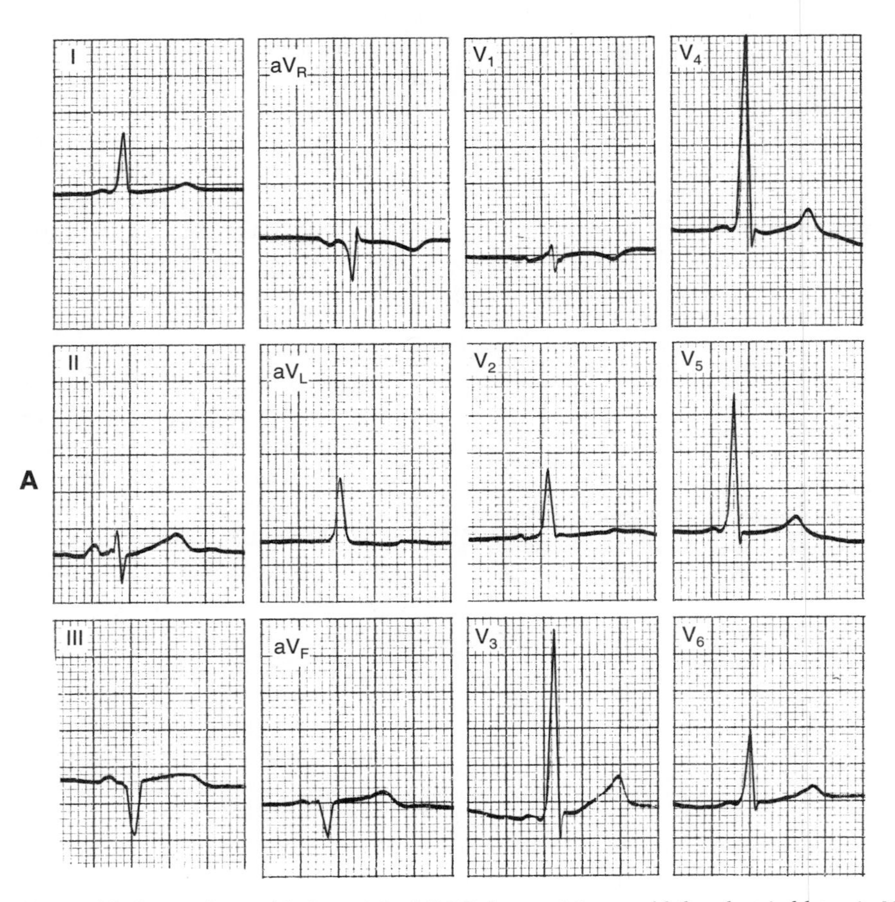

FIG. 20-11. Preablation and postablation 12-lead ECG from a 26-year-old female triathlete. **A,** Note the short PR of 0.08 second and the delta waves seen best in precordial leads V_3 to V_6 and in leads I and II. The delta wave is the initial slow beginning (slurring) of the QRS that accounts for the short PR interval and the QRS duration of 0.10 second.

Continued

arrhythmia would be atrial fibrillation. Such an evaluation can be done with electrophysiologic studies that would also allow radiofrequency ablation of the accessory pathway.

Symptomatic individuals with overt ECG signs of WPW should not participate in athletics until the accessory pathway has been ablated. Symptomatic individuals with a normal ECG should not participate in athletics until a complete cardiac evaluation has been performed to determine the mechanism responsible for the symptoms (i.e., AV nodal reentry or circus movement tachycardia using a latent or concealed accessory pathway). Such individuals should also be instructed in several vagal maneuvers and demonstrate that the instructions have been understood and they know how to do them.

Although the PSVT of AV nodal reentry or that associated with WPW syndrome are not life-threatening they are not without their price and may precipitate atrial fibrillation. WPW syndrome, its mechanism, types, ECG recognition, emergency response, and cure are discussed in detail and illustrated in Chapter 21.

Figs. 20-11, *A* and *B*, are from a 26-year-old female triathlete before and after radiofrequency ablation of her right posteroseptal accessory pathway. Although symptomatic, she did not present herself to me because of her symptoms, but simply as an athlete responding to my request for ECGs for this chapter. She had never had an ECG before the one seen in Fig. 20-11, *A*. Her palpitations were frequent, even at rest. When she was running, her heart rate would accelerate inappropriately and she would feel like her "lungs were being crushed." On one occasion after competing, her heart racing, she presented herself to the first aid tent and was told to "go sit under a tree," that she was probably "having a heat stroke." After ablation, her professional athletic career "took off." This case supports prescreening and exposes the fact that some physical trainers are not informed regarding alarming symptoms.

CONGENITAL LONG QT SYNDROME

Congenital long QT (LQT) syndrome is a group of inherited disorders affecting cardiac repolarization and resulting in a prolonged QT interval and T wave abnormalities. As with the acquired (drug-related) form of LQT syndrome, the congenital form may cause torsades de pointes, ventricular fibrillation, and sudden death. Unlike the acquired form, the congenital form may be precipitated by a variety of circumstances such as exercise, emotion, rest, or sudden arousal, depending on the affected gene. (Congenital LQT syndrome is briefly reviewed here; please see Chapter 25 for a full description of genetics, T wave patterns, and mechanisms.)

ECG Recognition

QTc interval: Range: 0.41 second to more than 0.60 second. The congenital form of LQT syndrome may have a normal QTc.[18] Thus this measurement may not be diagnostic in nonsymptomatic members of an affect-

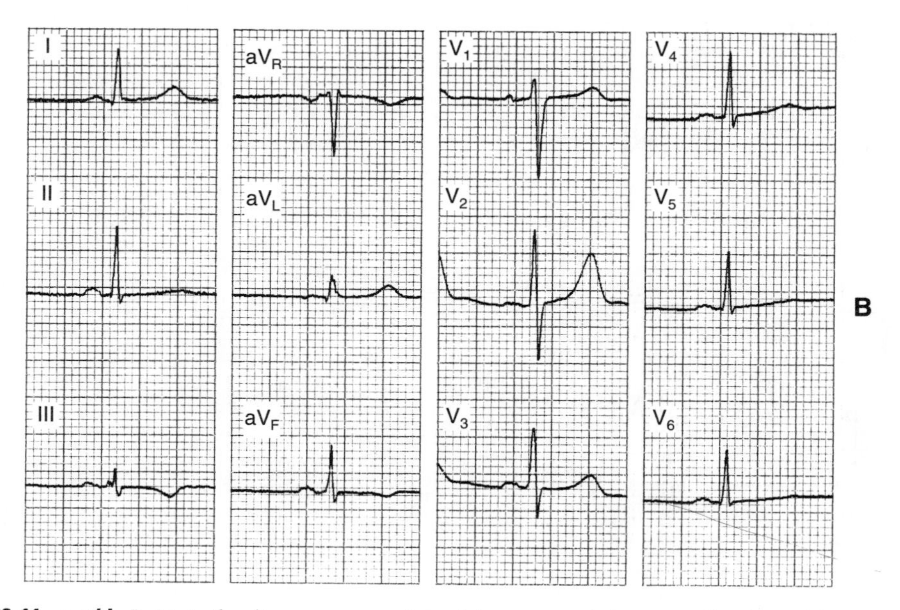

FIG. 20-11, cont'd. B, Note the disappearance of the delta wave and the normalization of the QRS interval and pattern. The inverted T wave seen in lead III is a common immediate postablation finding, especially with right-sided accessory pathways. It resolved in 3 weeks.

ed family. Fig. 20-12, *A*, is an example of congenital LQT syndrome in a 20-year-old woman with a history of recurrent syncope. The rhythm strip shows torsades de pointes, the terminal event of her life.

U waves: Often prominent.

T wave morphology: Varies, may be normal or bizarre, broad-based, late onset, bifid or alternating in polarity (T wave alternans).

Torsades de pointes: The life-threatening VT known as torsades de pointes (Chapter 25) is seen in the rhythm strip of Fig. 20-12, *B*. In most adults with congenital LQT syndrome, torsades de pointes is preceded by a pause. In children, who often have a more severe form of the disease, the onset of torsades de pointes is typically not pause-dependent.

Mechanism

The congenital LQT syndrome is the result of gene mutations that cause a disruption of the flow of ions across the cardiac cell membranes during repolarization.

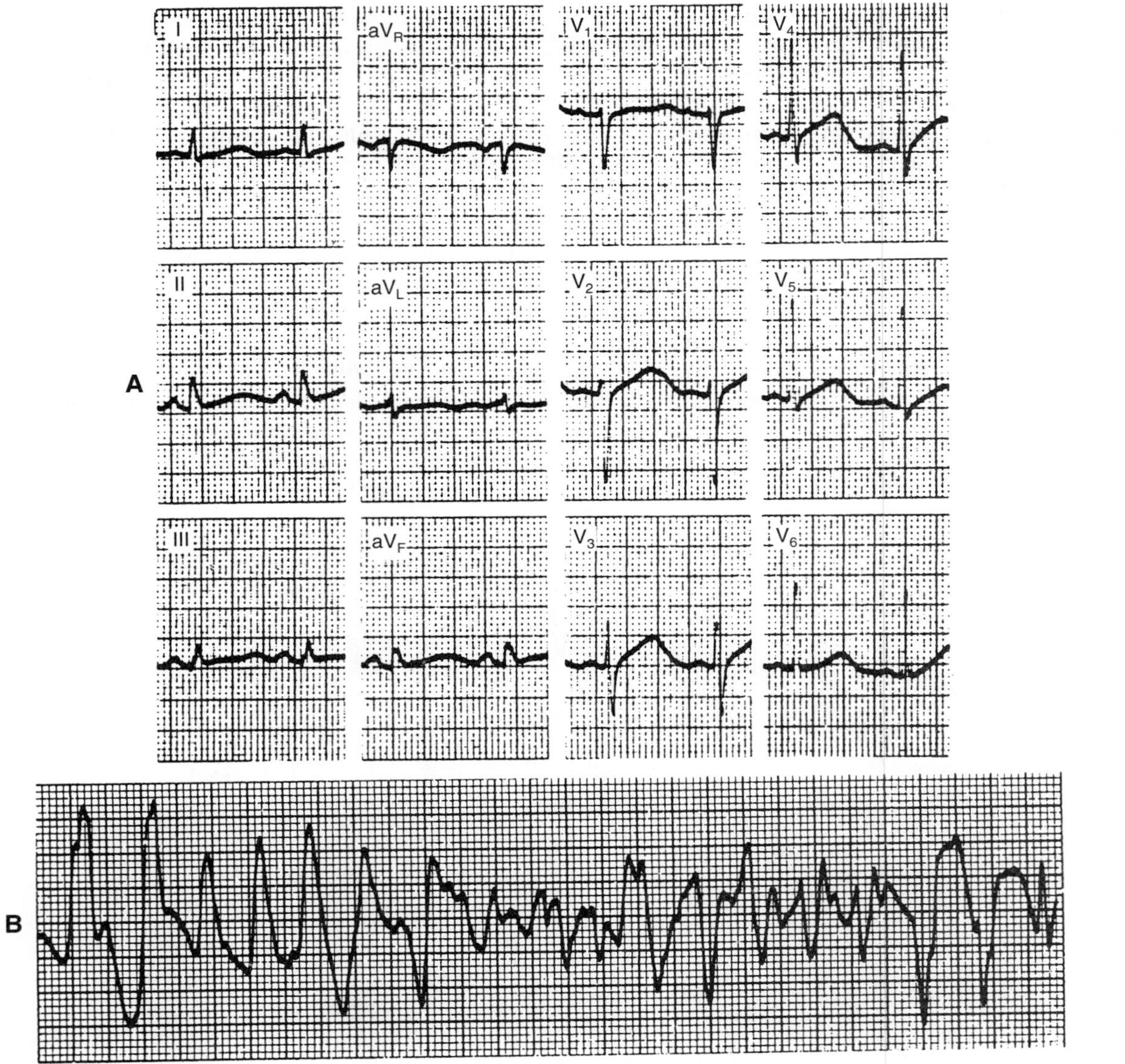

FIG. 20-12. **A,** The 12-lead ECG of congenital long QT syndrome in a 20-year-old woman with a history of recurrent syncope. Her QTc was 0.61 second. **B,** Torsades de pointes in the same patient. The patient died on the same day the 12-lead ECG was obtained. (From Chou TC: *Electrocardiography in clinical practice; adult and pediatric*, Philadelphia, 1996, WB Saunders, p 56.)

Signs and Symptoms

- Unexpected sudden death or cardiac arrest in an apparently healthy child or young adult during sleep, and especially during exercise or emotional stress
- Syncope of sudden onset without warning, during exercise, upon being startled by an alarm clock, when very excited (e.g., during an argument), causing a precipitous, hard, injury-producing fall to the ground.[19]

SUMMARY

There are many ECG variations seen in athletes that reflect the adaptation of their hearts to intense physical training rather than to a pathologic process. It is important to recognize these ECG variations in the athlete and to be able to differentiate them from the pathologic ones. In trained athletes P wave amplitude and morphology, PR intervals, QRS voltage amplitude and shape, ST segments, and T wave changes may mimic pathologic conditions. It is important to be aware of an individual's physical conditioning and recognize these common changes when evaluating his or her ECG. Failure to do so may label a healthy athlete with a cardiac problem and have a tremendous emotional and life-changing impact, whereas failure to recognize a true pathologic condition could prove life-threatening.

REFERENCES

1. Maron BJ, Epstein SE, Roberts WC: Causes of sudden death in the competitive athlete, *J Am Coll Cardiol* 7:204-214, 1986.
2. Urhausen A, Kindermann W: Sports-specific adaptations and differentiation of the athlete's heart, *Sports Med* 28:237-244, 1999.
3. Pelliccia A, Maron BJ, Culasso F et al: Clinical significance of abnormal electrocardiographic patterns in trained athletes, *Circulation* 102(3):278-284, 2000.
4. Antzelevitch C: The Brugada syndrome: ionic basis and arrhythmia mechanisms, *J Cardiovasc Electrophysiol* 12:268-272, 2001.
5. Bianco M, Bria S, Gianfelici A et al: Does early repolarization in the athlete have analogies with the Brugada syndrome? *Eur Heart J* 22:504-510, 2001.
6. Pelliccia A, Maron BJ: Athlete's heart electrocardiogram mimicking hypertrophic cardiomyopathy, *Curr Cardiol Rep* 3:147-151, 2001.
7. Maron BJ, Araujo CG, Thompson PD et al: Recommendations for pre-participation screening and the assessment of cardiovascular disease in masters athletes: an advisory for healthcare professionals from the Working Groups of the World Heart Federation, the International Federation of Sports Medicine, and the American Heart Association Committee on Exercise, Cardiac Rehabilitation, and Prevention, *Circulation* 103:327-334, 2001.
8. Maron BJ: Cardiovascular risks to young persons on the athletic field, *Ann Intern Med* 129:379-386, 1998.
9. Maron BJ, Shirani J, Poliac LC et al: Sudden death in young competitive athletes: clinical, demographic, and pathological profiles, *JAMA* 276:199-204, 1996.
10. Maron BJ, Pelliccia A, Spirito P: Cardiac disease in young trained athletes. Insights into methods for distinguishing athlete's heart from structural heart disease, with particular emphasis on hypertrophic cardiomyopathy, *Circulation* 91:1596-1601, 1995.
11. Pelliccia A, Maron BJ, Spataro A et al: The upper limit of physiologic cardiac hypertrophy in highly trained elite athletes, *N Engl J Med* 324:295-301, 1991.
12. Glassman G: Personal communication, January 2002.
13. Maron BJ, Pelliccia A, Spataro A et al: Reduction in left ventricular wall thickness after deconditioning in highly trained Olympic athletes, *Br Heart J* 69:125-128, 1993.
14. Mcrae AT III, Chung MK, Asher CR: Arrhythmogenic right ventricular cardiomyopathy: a cause of sudden death in young people, *Cleveland Clinic J Med* 69:459-466, 2001.
15. Pinski SL: The right ventricular tachycardias, *J Electrocardiol* 33(Suppl):103-114, 2000.
16. Basso C, Maron BJ, Corrado D, Thiene G: Clinical profile of congenital coronary artery anomalies with origin from the wrong aortic sinus leading to sudden death in young competitive athletes, *J Am Coll Cardiol* 35:1493-1501, 2000.
17. Duckeck W, Kuck KH: Syncope in supraventricular tachycardia. Incidence, pathomechanism and consequences, *Herz* 18:175-181, 1993.
18. Roden DM: Torsades de pointes, *Clin Cardiol* 16:683, 1993.
19. Vincent GM: The long QT syndrome. In Parmley WW, Chatterjee K, editors: *Cardiology physiology, pharmacology, diagnosis,* Philadelphia, 2000, Lippincott-Raven.

PART III

ABNORMAL 12-LEAD ELECTROCARDIOGRAMS

CHAPTER 21

Wolff-Parkinson-White Syndrome

Wolff-Parkinson-White (WPW) syndrome is a group of electrocardiographic (ECG) findings reflecting preexcitation (short PR, delta wave, and broad QRS) and associated with the occurrence of supraventricular tachycardia, most commonly in the form of paroxysmal supraventricular tachycardia (PSVT) or atrial fibrillation. The anatomical substrate for these ECG findings and symptoms is an accessory pathway connecting atria and ventricle. As you will see, the accessory pathway and its associated tachycardias can also be present without the ECG findings of the syndrome (latent or concealed accessory pathways).

HISTORICAL BACKGROUND

In 1930 Wolff et al[1] described bundle branch block with a short PR interval in healthy young people prone to PSVT. At the time the ECG findings were not linked to an extra atrioventricular (AV) connection. However, as early as 1876, Paladino had described AV connections. In 1893 Kent[2] described AV connections in normal hearts that were located anteriorly, adjacent to the fibrous ring of the tricuspid valve. We now know that AV connections can exist all around the fibrous rings. In 1932 and 1933 Holzman and Scherf[3] in Germany and Wolferth and Wood[4] in the United States hypothesized that the AV connection described by Kent transmitted impulses from atria to ventricles and was responsible for the short PR interval and broad QRS complex of the WPW syndrome. By 1943 and 1944 Wood, Wolferth, and Geckeler[5] and Ohnell[6] linked the ECG findings of short PR and broad QRS with postmortem histologic confirmation of the presence of accessory AV connections on the both sides of the heart.

ECG RECOGNITION

A 12-lead ECG showing the ECG features of WPW syndrome is shown in Fig. 21-1.

PR interval: Less than 0.12 second.

QRS complex: A delta wave is present, which causes the QRS to be broader than 0.10 second. A negative delta wave looks like a pathologic Q wave, as shown in leads II, III, and aV_F of Fig. 21-1.

T wave: Secondary repolarization changes may be present. Because ventricular depolarization does not follow a normal sequence and is delayed, the repolarization process may also be out of sequence, causing secondary T wave changes. The extent of these changes depends on the degree and the area of preexcitation.

Associated arrhythmias: PSVT and atrial fibrillation.

Distinguishing features: Short PRs, delta waves, and a history of PSVT.

MECHANISMS

The short PR interval in WPW syndrome is the result of accelerated AV conduction across an accessory pathway (Fig. 21-2). The sinus impulse enters the ventricle via a strand of cardiac muscle that does not involve the AV node or the His-Purkinje system. Because this strand of cardiac muscle has faster conduction than the AV node, the PR interval is short. The shortest normal PR intervals according to age are shown in Table 21-1.

Delta Wave

The delta wave is the initial slurring of the QRS complex (a slow beginning) caused by the early arrival of the supraventricular impulse into the ventricle via the accesso-

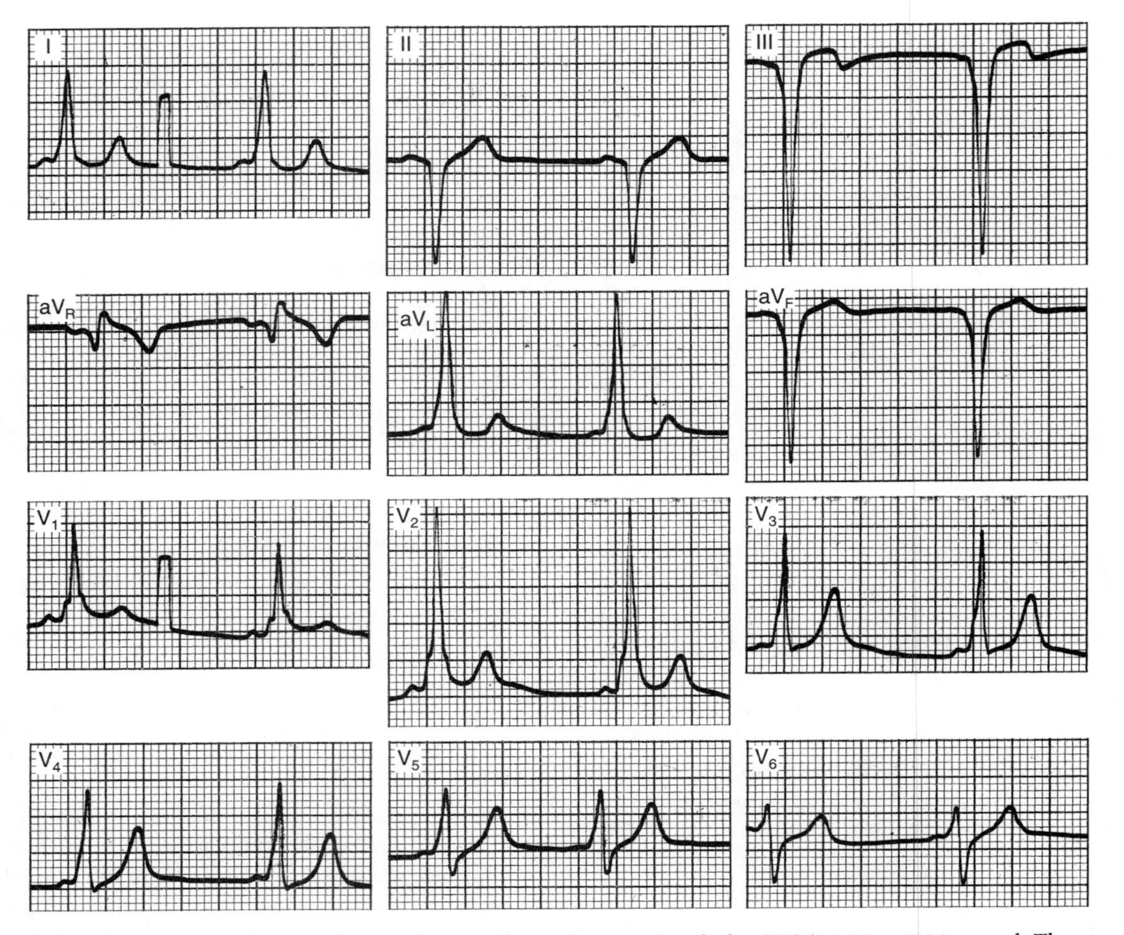

FIG. 21-1. Wolff-Parkinson-White syndrome. The PR is 0.08 second; the QRS is 0.13 to 0.14 second. The delta wave is well-defined in leads V_1 and V_2 but is visible in all leads except II, in which it is isoelectric (PR 0.12 second; QRS 0.08 second). The QS complexes in the inferior leads mimic inferior myocardial infarction. The tall R waves in V_1 and R wave regression across the precordial leads mimic right ventricular hypertrophy. However, there is no mistaking the short PRs and delta waves. (Tracing courtesy Ara Tilkian, MD, Mission Hills, Calif.)

ry pathway (preexcitation). When the sinus impulse arrives in the ventricle in this manner, it is outside the conduction system when it begins its journey (an "ectopic beginning").

Polarity. The mechanism of delta wave polarity is illustrated in Fig. 21-3. Its polarity depends on the orientation of the preexcitation forces to the axis of the lead in question. An isoelectric delta wave is the result of the delta forces being perpendicular to the axis of a lead, as seen in lead II of Fig. 21-1. If delta forces are flowing away from the positive electrode, the delta wave will be negative in that lead, producing an abnormal Q wave, simulating myocardial infarction (MI).

Size. The size of the delta wave depends on many factors but is ultimately the result of the time difference between the arrival of the sinus impulse in the ventricles via the accessory pathway and its arrival via the AV node and His bundle.

Ventricular Fusion

If the normal impulse should happen to be traveling within the ventricles at the same time as the delta force (Fig. 21-3), the QRS complex would be a fusion beat. This occurs in all cases except maximal preexcitation.

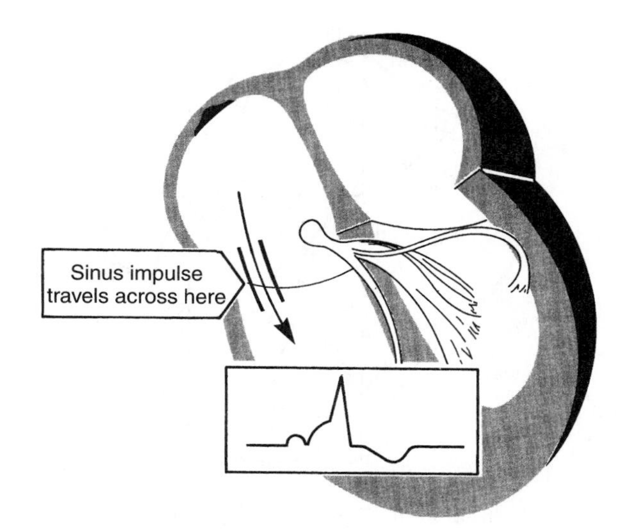

FIG. 21-2. In Wolff-Parkinson-White syndrome the impulse arrives early in the ventricles through an accessory pathway, causing a short PR interval. The initial ventricular forces begin at the ventricular insertion of the accessory pathway, traveling in myocardial tissue, as opposed to a rapid route in the conduction system. This causes the delta wave (initial slurring of the QRS). There may also be secondary ST-T segment changes. The accessory pathway is a small fiber; it is diagrammatically illustrated.

T Wave Changes after Ablation ("Cardiac Memory")

With termination of preexcitation, secondary repolarization changes immediately disappear and the T wave axis after ablation of the accessory pathway approximates that of the QRS before ablation (not observed with concealed accessory pathways). The negative T waves that result are sometimes called "cardiac memory." The T wave axis correlates in magnitude directly with the change in QRS axis and inversely with the anterograde effective refractory period in the accessory pathway.[7] The inverted T waves that result may last 3 to 6 weeks postablation and are seen more frequently with right-sided accessory pathways than with left.[8]

ACCESSORY PATHWAYS

An accessory pathway (bypass tract) is an extra muscle bundle composed of working myocardial tissue[9] that forms a connection between atria and ventricles outside the conduction[10] system, often resulting in the ECG manifestation of WPW syndrome. Other AV connections are rare, not easily recognized on the surface ECG, and are only demonstrated with sophisticated intracardiac studies.[11]

Location

The general locations of accessory pathways are assigned to the right and left ventricles (free walls and posteroseptal) and the septum (right anterior and intermediate or midseptal). In the era of catheter ablation this classification is expanded to include arbitrary designations such as right and left anterolateral and posterolateral; right and left posterior; and para-Hisian. The most common location is left lateral, followed by the right lateral and posterior septum.

Intermediate septal bypass tracts are located along the tricuspid annulus between the coronary sinus os and the region of the His bundle; the AV node is also located in this region so that radiofrequency ablation of intermediate septal pathways carries with it an increased risk for development of complete heart block.[12] Almost 50% of intermediate septal bypass tracts studied[13] exhibit unusual properties that distinguish them from those in other locations, in that they have a conduction delay during atrial pacing as opposed to the constant anterograde conduction of pathways in other locations. The pathways may be single or multiple, active or inactive, and may possess the capability of conducting in both anterograde and retrograde directions (WPW syndrome); only retrograde (concealed accessory pathway); or only anterograde.

Locating the Accessory Pathway During Sinus Rhythm

In approximately 60% to 70% of patients with an accessory pathway the diagnosis can be made by a knowledgeable examiner from the surface ECG when the patient

TABLE 21-1 Shortest Normal PR Intervals and Longest Normal QRS Complexes According to Age

Age	PR (sec)	QRS (sec)
0-6 mo	0.08	0.06
6 mo–3 yr	0.08	0.08
3-5 yr	0.10	0.08
5-16 yr	0.10	0.09
>16 yr	0.12	0.10

Modified from Ferrer MI: *Electrocardiographic notebook,* ed 4, Mount Kisco, NY, 1973, Futura.

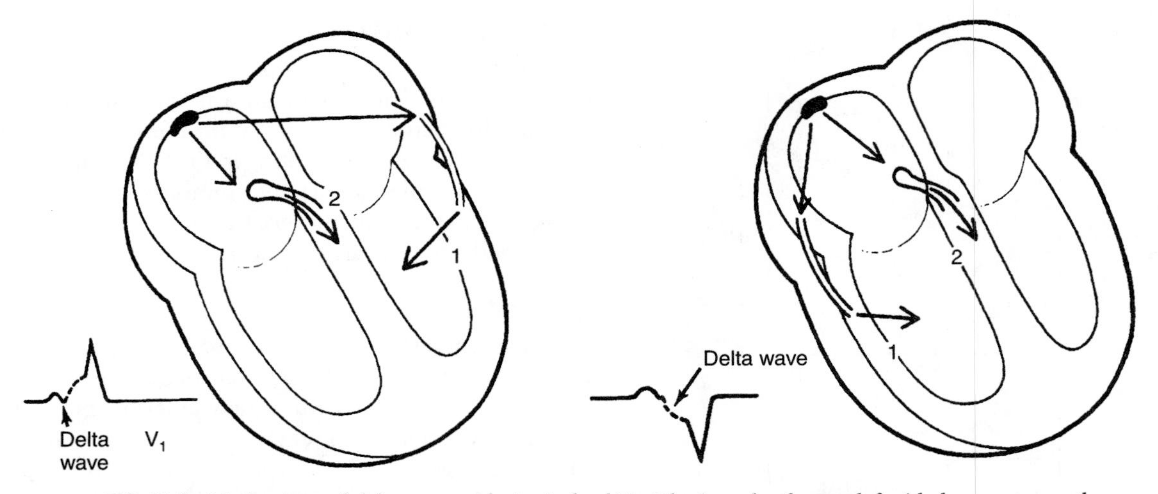

FIG. 21-3. Mechanism of delta wave polarity in lead V_1. The impulse from a left-sided accessory pathway travels toward V_1, producing a positive delta wave, whereas the impulse from a right sided accessory pathway travels away from V_1, producing a negative delta wave.

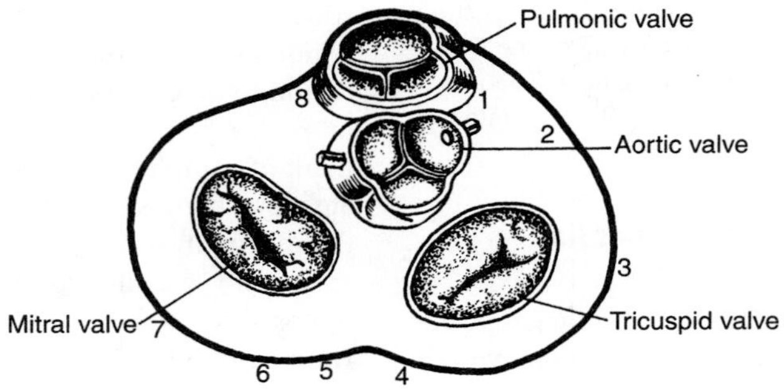

Pulmonic valve
Aortic valve
Tricuspid valve
Mitral valve
1 2 3 4 5 6 7 8

Delta wave polarity

	I	II	III	aV_R	aV_L	aV_F	V_1	V_2	V_3	V_4	V_5	V_6
1	+	+	+	−		+			+	+	+	+
2	+	+	−	−	+	−		+	+	+	+	+
3	+		−	−	+			+	+	+	+	+
4	+	−	−	−	+	−		+	+	+	+	+
5	+	−	−	−	+	−	+	+	+	+	+	+
6	+	+		−		+	+	+	+	+	+	+
7	−		+		−	+	+	+	+	+	−	−
8	−	+	+	−	−	+	+	+	+	+	+	+

FIG. 21-4. Locating the accessory pathway from the delta wave polarity. (Courtesy H.J.J. Wellens, MD, Maastricht, The Netherlands.)

is in sinus rhythm and some degree of preexcitation is present. The remainder of cases is concealed or latent. In such cases the presence and even the location of the accessory pathway can be determined by an informed examiner from the P′ wave axis during circus movement tachycardia (CMT). In antidromic CMT and in atrial flutter, the diagnosis may require intracardiac recordings. Fig. 21-4 offers a method for localizing the accessory pathway during sinus rhythm by evaluating the polarity of the delta wave in the 12-lead ECG.

Fig. 21-5 offers another approach in which the polarity of the QRS in V_1 is determined, placing the accessory pathway in the right or left ventricles or in anteroseptal or midseptal locations. Then the polarity of the delta wave in certain leads further pinpoints the location as right or left posteroseptal or right or left lateral.[14]

Conduction Properties

In one study the conduction properties of accessory pathways were demonstrated by electrophysiologic studies of 931 symptomatic patients with 1,016 accessory pathways.[15] Accessory pathways were capable of anterograde or retrograde conduction in the following distribution:

- Anterograde and retrograde conduction, 44.1% (447)
- Only retrograde conduction (concealed accessory pathways), 51.6% (525)
- Only anterograde conduction, 4.3% (44)

Both anterograde and retrograde conduction. Individuals with accessory pathways possessing the capability of both anterograde and retrograde conduction may have either a normal ECG (latent accessory pathway) or a typical WPW syndrome ECG (short PR, delta wave) and are candidates for PSVT in the forms of orthodromic or antidromic CMT and for the life-threatening ventricular rates that result when atrial fibrillation or atrial flutter is conducted over an accessory pathway.

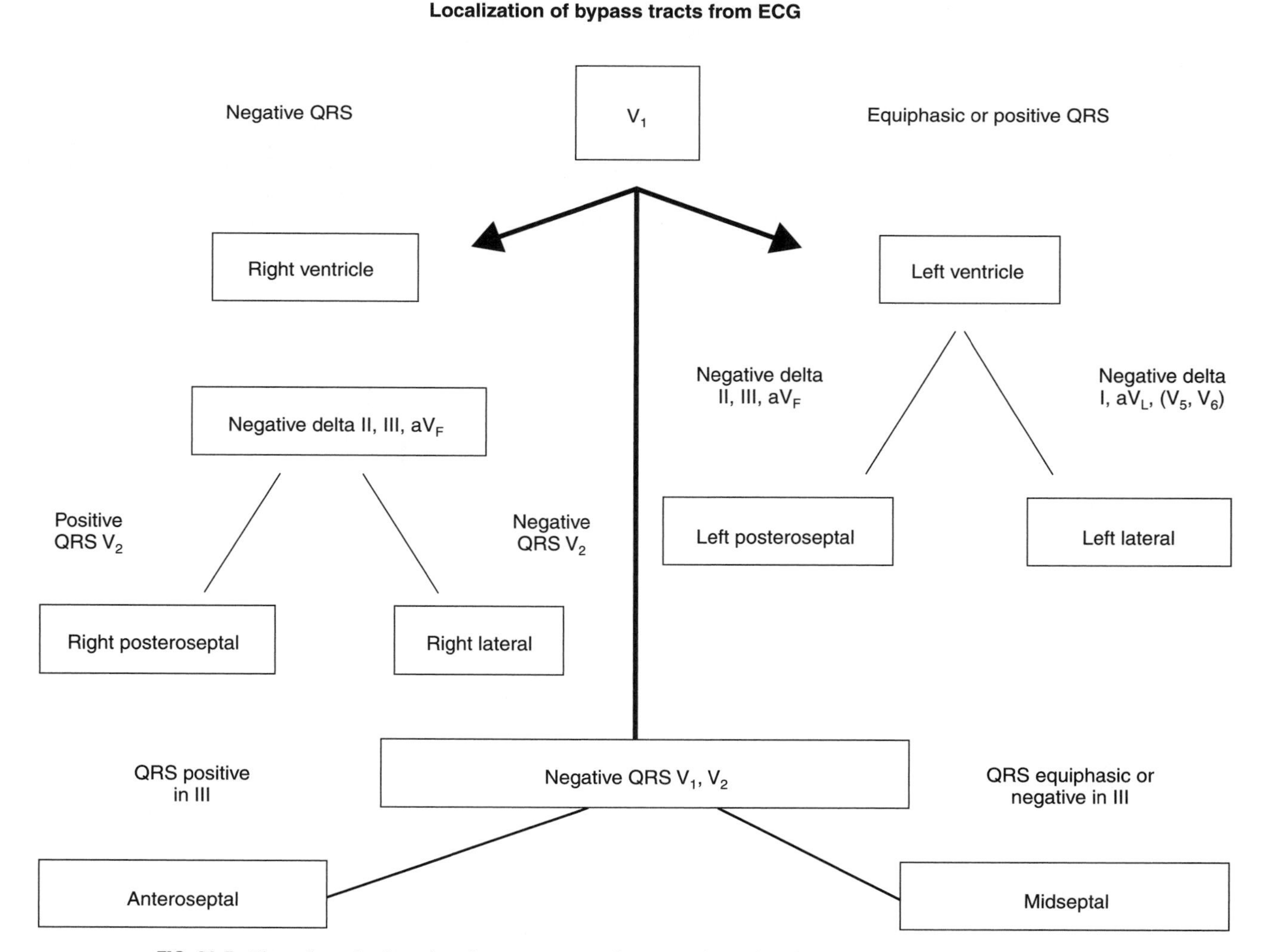

FIG. 21-5. Flow chart for locating the accessory pathway. Midseptal pathway is also known as intermediate pathway. (Courtesy G.V. Reddy, MD, FAAC, Wilmington, Del.)

Only retrograde conduction (no preexcitation; concealed). When only retrograde conduction is possible in the accessory pathway, the PR intervals and QRS complexes are of normal duration and the pathway is called *concealed*. These individuals may be symptomatic with orthodromic CMT, in which case the current travels down the AV node and up the accessory pathway. They are, however, protected from the life-threatening ventricular rates associated with atrial fibrillation with anterograde conduction over the accessory pathway.

The diagnosis can be made from the ECG taken during PSVT, usually recorded in the emergency department. The ECG signs of the AV reentry mechanism using a concealed accessory pathway are the same as those seen in overt WPW syndrome (p. 125). The concealed accessory pathway (no anterograde conduction) should not be confused with the latent accessory pathway, which is capable of anterograde conduction.

Only anterograde conduction. When only anterograde conduction is possible in the accessory pathway, the ECG signs of WPW may be present. However, orthodromic CMT is not possible without retrograde conduction in the accessory pathway. This situation may deprive the person of the usual warning sign (PSVT) that a problem exists. Their first arrhythmia may be atrial fibrillation with heart rates approaching 300 beats/min. In one study of 1,016 accessory pathways,[15] 4.3% (44) of the accessory pathways had only anterograde conduction.

Latent accessory pathways. Not mentioned in this study are the accessory pathways that are capable of both anterograde and retrograde conduction, although the ECG is normal. This mechanism is demonstrated later in Fig. 21-12 on p. 284.

Estimating the Refractory Period

Any degree of preexcitation is possible. However, it is not the size of the delta wave but the duration of the refractory period of the accessory pathway in the anterograde direction that identifies high-risk patients. This duration varies considerably among patients and is influenced by sympathetic tone.[16]

Wellens[17] has described three noninvasive ways of estimating the adequacy of the refractory period of the accessory pathway in the anterograde direction. When any one of the following three conditions is present, the refractory period in the accessory pathway is considered long enough to protect the patient from excessive ventricular rates should atrial fibrillation develop.

1. Preexcitation is intermittent.
2. Preexcitation disappears (not just lessens) with exercise (as a result of the catecholamines), Wellens[11] exhorts care in this interpretation because sympathetic stimulation during exercise speeds up AV nodal conduction and may diminish the area of preexcitation. Concurrent multiple ECG leads should be recorded with attention to the ECG after exercise. In cases of exercise-induced block in the accessory pathway, upon resumption of conduction through this pathway a sudden marked change in the ECG takes place.
3. The PR and QRS normalize following intravenous administration of procainamide (10 mg/kg body weight over 5 minutes).

Note: Before using procainamide for this purpose, hypertrophic cardiomyopathy is ruled out by echocardiogram. Because procainamide prolongs the refractory period of both the accessory pathway and the His-Purkinje system, it is given in a setting where complete heart block can be managed.[11]

VARIATIONS IN PREEXCITATION

During sinus rhythm WPW syndrome may manifest with different degrees of preexcitation (i.e., different delta wave durations) depending on intra-atrial conduction time, accessory pathway time, and AV nodal conduction time.

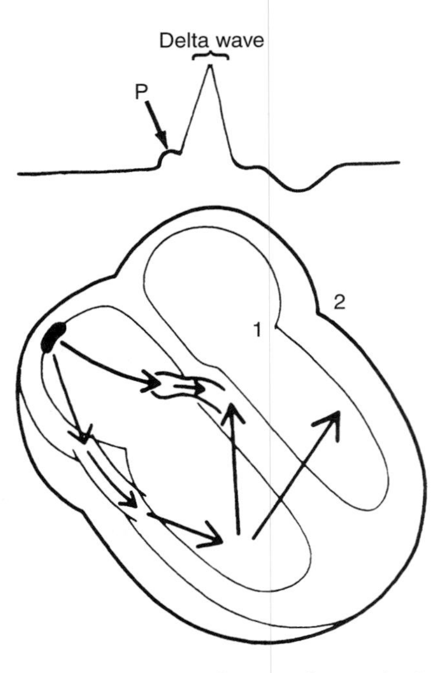

FIG. 21-6. The mechanism of maximal preexcitation. The ventricles are activated only by the delta force.

Maximal Preexcitation

The mechanism of maximal preexcitation is illustrated in Fig. 21-6. The 12-lead ECG in Fig. 21-7 is from Eric, a 36-year-old male who is an elite athlete (cyclist) and has been competitive for 22 years. His ECG shows nearly maximal preexcitation (i.e., virtually the entire QRS is created by the delta force with no or little contribution from nodal-His activation). The PR is only 0.06 second, and the QRS 0.16 second. He had an underlying sinus arrhythmia and sinus bradycardia of 46 to 52 beats/min because of his athleticism. The T wave in many leads is inverted, a normal result of abnormal ventricular depolarization. The ECG signs of ventricular hypertrophy are not diagnosed in WPW syndrome because the altered sequence of activation may mimic the ECG signs of ventricular hypertrophy.[18] Eric's symptoms of PSVT began when he was a teenager, but have become less frequent in recent years. However, when he does go into PSVT it is very difficult for him to

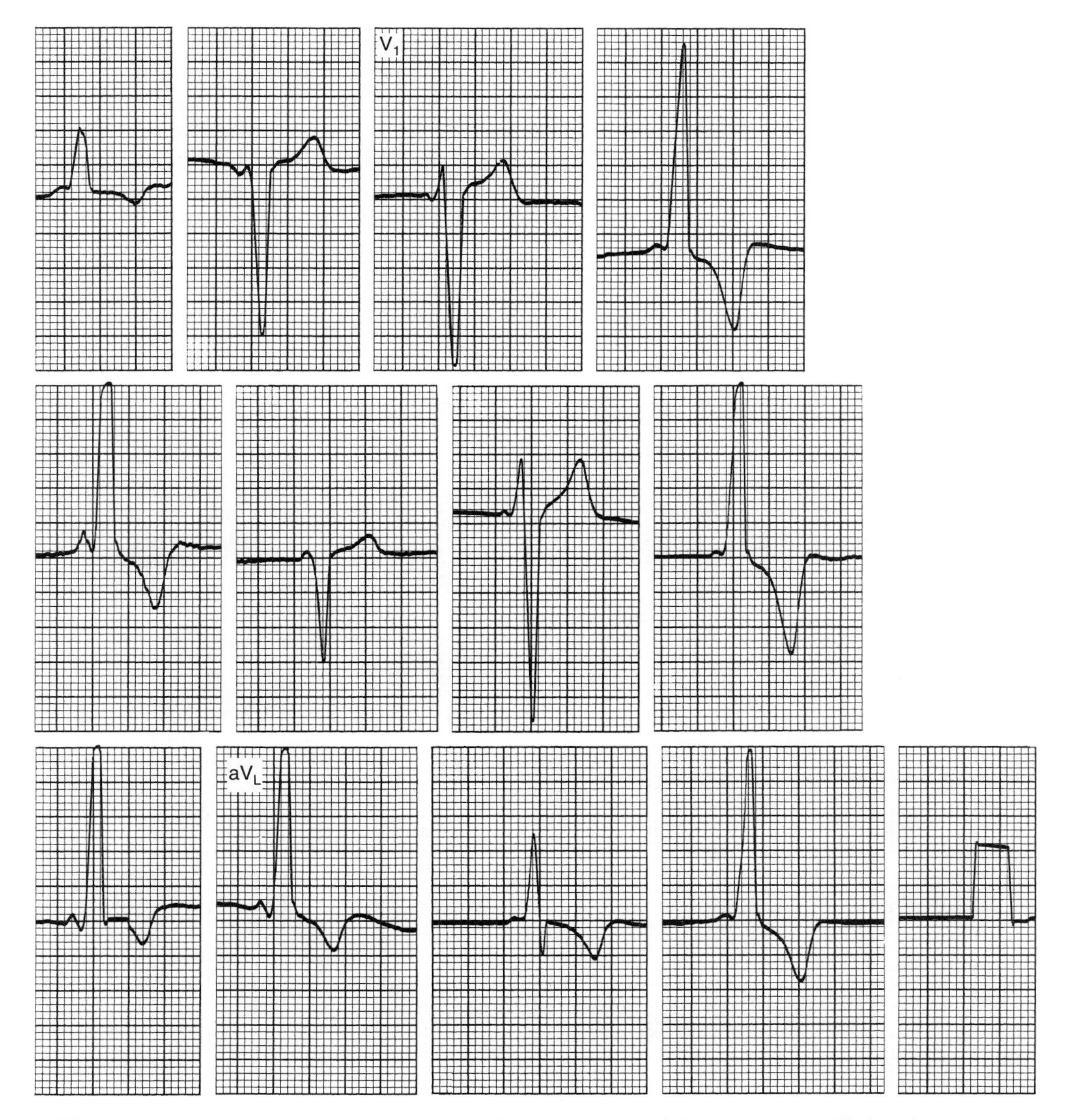

FIG. 21-7. Maximal preexcitation. PR, 0.06 second; QRS, 0.16 second. (Courtesy Eric Wilhelm, elite category I amateur cyclist, Santa Cruz, Calif.)

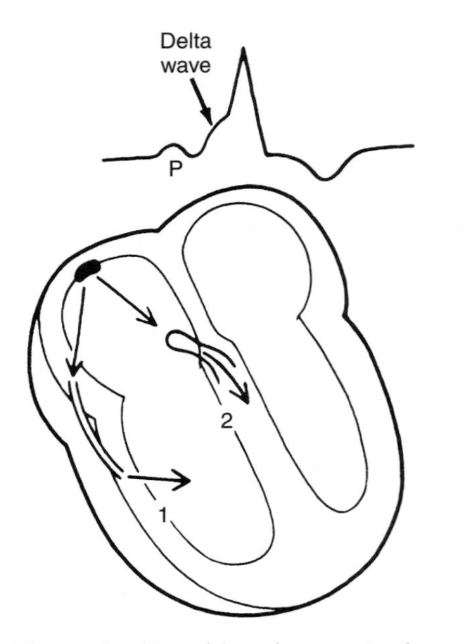

FIG. 21-8. The mechanism of less than maximal preexcitation resulting in a fusion beat.

terminate the arrhythmia even using a variety of vagal maneuvers; at this writing he is awaiting a cure with radiofrequency ablation.

Less Than Maximal Preexcitation

The mechanism of less than maximal preexcitation is illustrated in Fig. 21-8. Examples are noted in Fig. 21-9, *A* and *B*. Because the delta force does not capture the entire ventricle before nodal-His activation, all QRS complexes are fusion beats (i.e., the normal impulses traveling down the His bundle fuse with the early impulse coming from the accessory pathway). Fig. 21-9, *A*, is from Sarah, a 26-year-old professional triathlete; *B* is from Melanie, a 31-year-old professional cyclist. Both women were symptomatic with debilitating PSVT, but Sarah had not seen a cardiologist or even dreamed that her problems lay in her heart. Both women have had their right-sided accessory pathway ablated and are back participating actively and "better than ever" in their sport without fear of abnormally rapid heart rates.

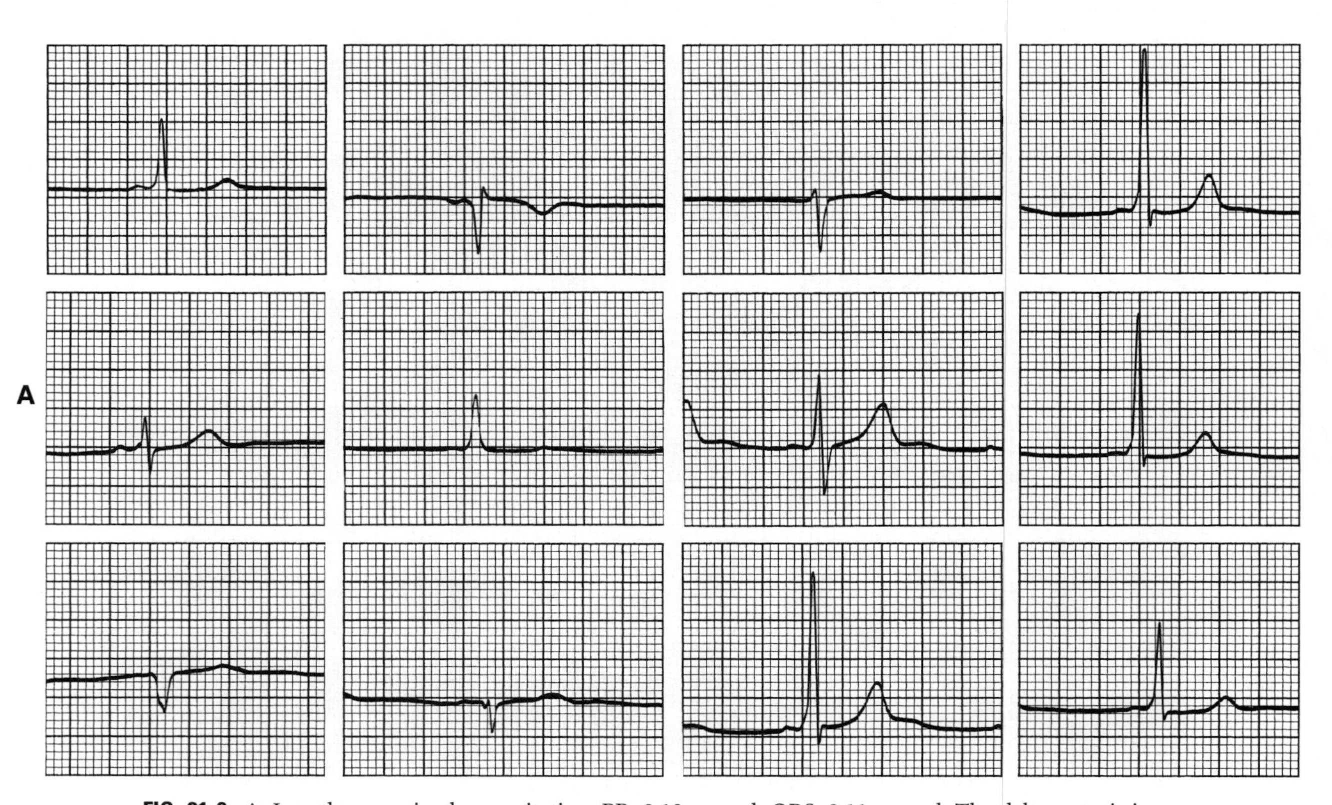

FIG. 21-9. A, Less than maximal preexcitation. PR, 0.10 second; QRS, 0.11 second. The delta wave is isoelectric in V_1 and aV_F but is visible in the other leads. (Courtesy Sarah Kerlin, Santa Cruz, Calif.)

Continued

Minimal Preexcitation

The mechanism of minimal preexcitation is illustrated in Fig. 21-10. Michele's ECG, seen in Fig. 21-11, is an example of minimal preexcitation. The delta waves, a slightly slow beginning to the QRS, are best seen in leads I, and V_3 to V_5. Michele is a 32-year-old recent mother of one, who knew she had WPW, but at the time of the diagnosis declined surgery (first-line treatment at the time). She has recently had radiofrequency ablation of her left-sided accessory pathway and is free of arrhythmias.

In Fig. 21-11 one has to search all the leads for the short PR interval and the delta wave. Note that in leads II, III, aV_F, and V_1 the PR is 0.12 to 0.14 second (normal), although the presence of abnormal Q waves (actually delta waves) in the inferior leads in this young patient makes one suspicious. However, in leads V_2 to V_6 the delta wave becomes a little more apparent.

No Preexcitation

The mechanism of no preexcitation in a patient with an accessory pathway that is capable of anterograde conduction is shown in Fig. 21-12. During sinus rhythm

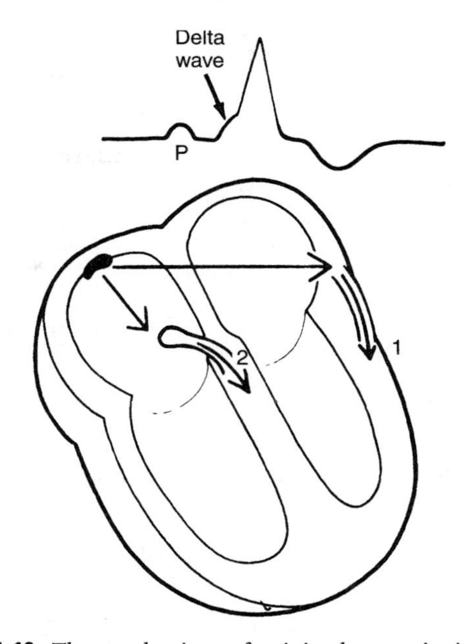

FIG. 21-10. The mechanism of minimal preexcitation; as the degree of preexcitation becomes less, the delta wave becomes smaller.

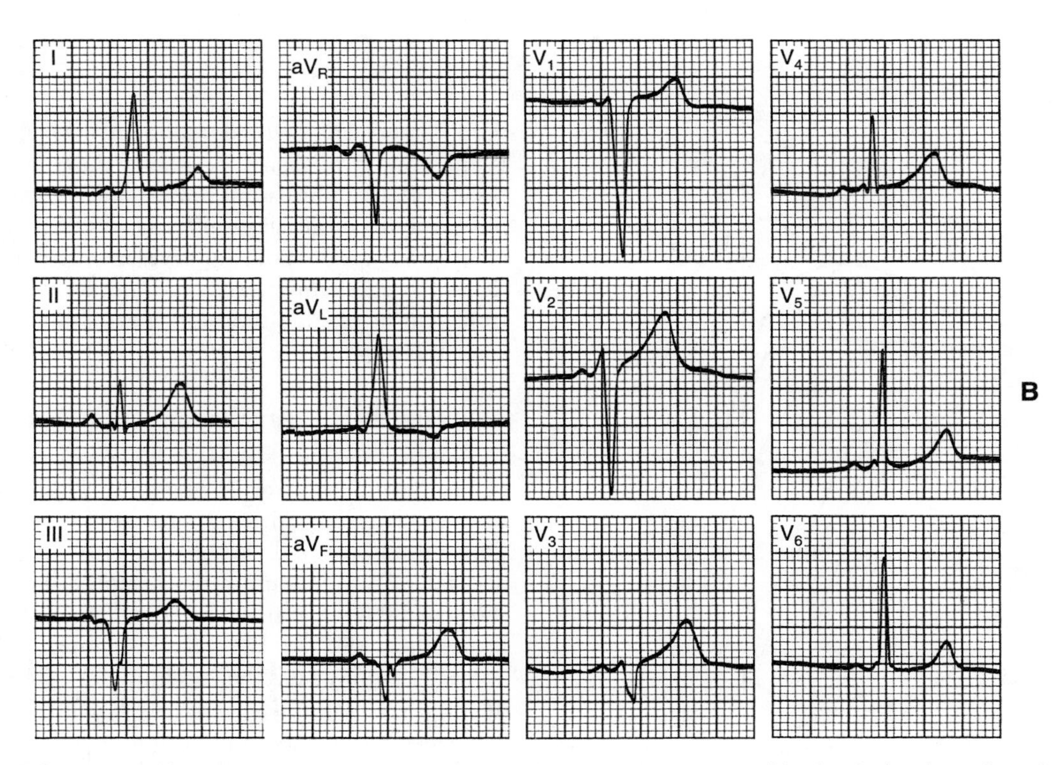

FIG. 21-9, cont'd. **B**, The PR is 0.12 second, but the delta wave is apparent in all leads. The heightened vagal tone in this professional cyclist would account for the normal PR interval in the face of preexcitation. (Courtesy Melanie Dominguez, Santa Cruz, Calif.)

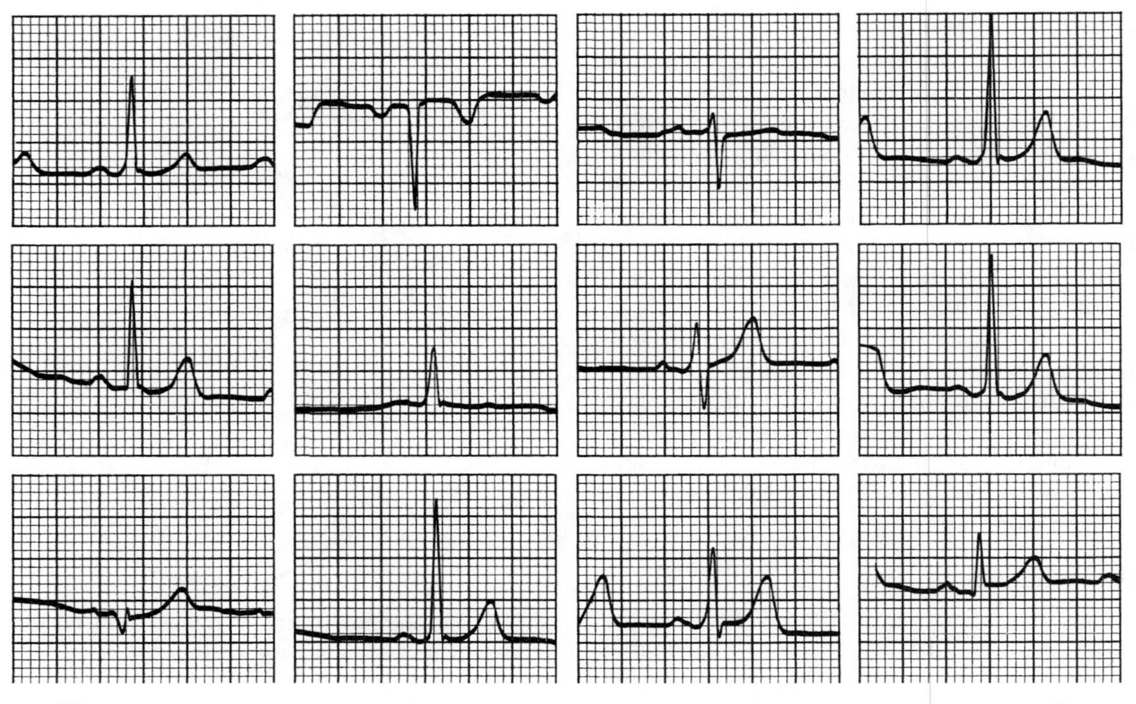

FIG. 21-11. Minimal preexcitation. PR, 0.13 second; in V_4, QRS: 0.11 second. (Courtesy Michele Ignoffo, Santa Cruz, Calif.)

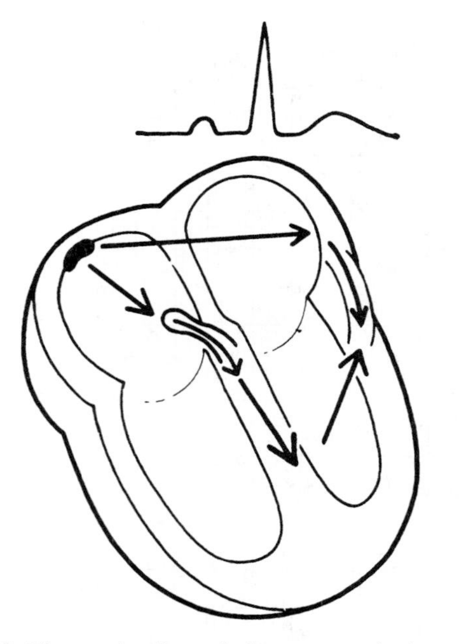

FIG. 21-12. The mechanism of absent preexcitation associated with an accessory pathway. The journey of the sinus impulse through the atria and down the accessory pathway is longer than through the normal route.

the PR interval and QRS duration are normal. The tracing at the bottom of Fig. 21-13 shows the potentially lethal results of atrial fibrillation in this same patient because of the existence of an accessory pathway that is capable of anterograde conduction, but never manifested itself on the ECG. The mechanism, ECG recognition, and emergency treatment of this life-threatening arrhythmia will be discussed shortly.

Intermittent Preexcitation

Intermittent preexcitation demonstrates the concept of the "latent" accessory pathway. In Fig. 21-14 there is sinus bradycardia with a PR interval of 0.16 second and a QRS of 0.08 second. When the cycle length shortens because of a premature atrial complex (PAC), note the shortened P′R interval and the appearance of a delta wave in the third and the last beats. Obviously this patient's accessory pathway has the capability for anterograde conduction, yet has no delta wave until conditions are optimal. Generally, this is an indication of a longer refractory period in the accessory pathway. Intermittent conduction may be the reason for previously dormant accessory pathways manifesting themselves clinically following radiofre-

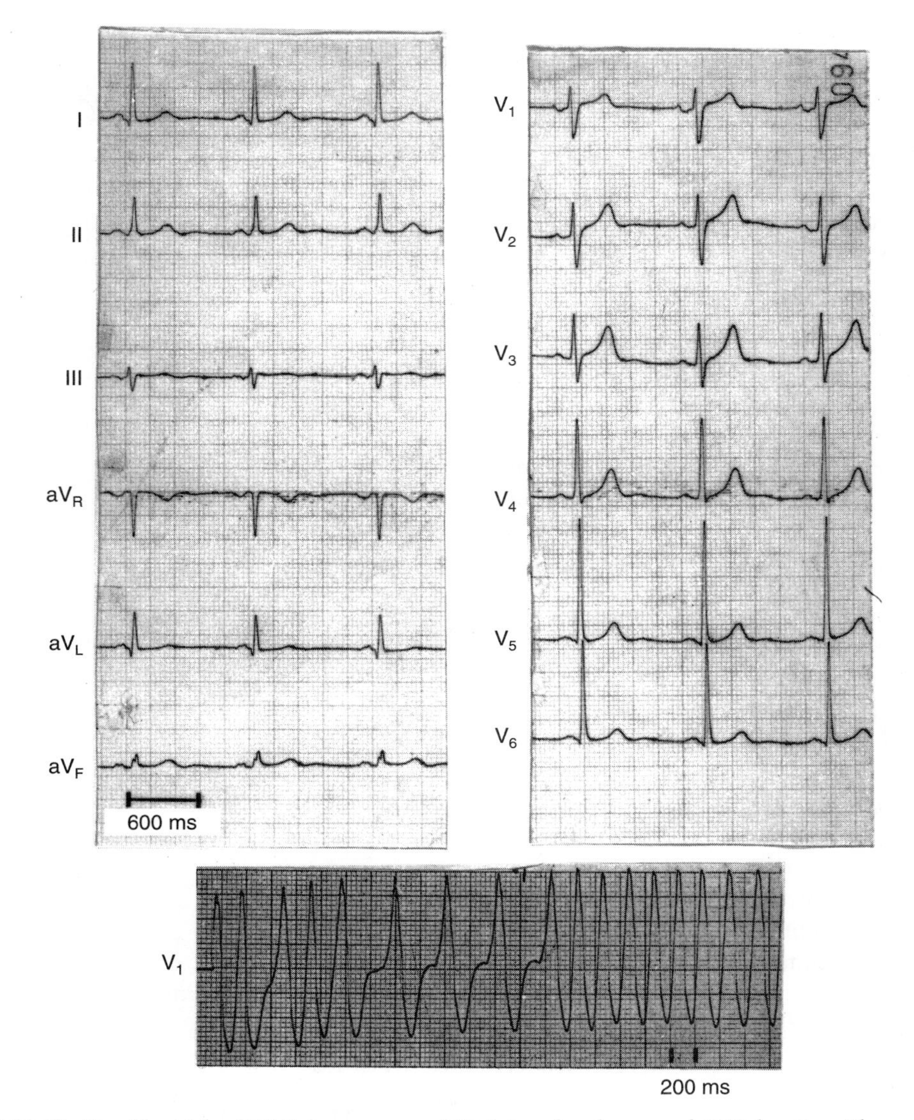

FIG. 21-13. *Top,* The 12-lead ECG shows a normal PR interval and a normal QRS duration. The patient was admitted for an attack of atrial fibrillation *(bottom tracing)* with a very high ventricular heart rate because of conduction from the atrium to the ventricles over an accessory pathway. (Courtesy Hein J.J. Wellens, MD, Maastricht, The Netherlands.)

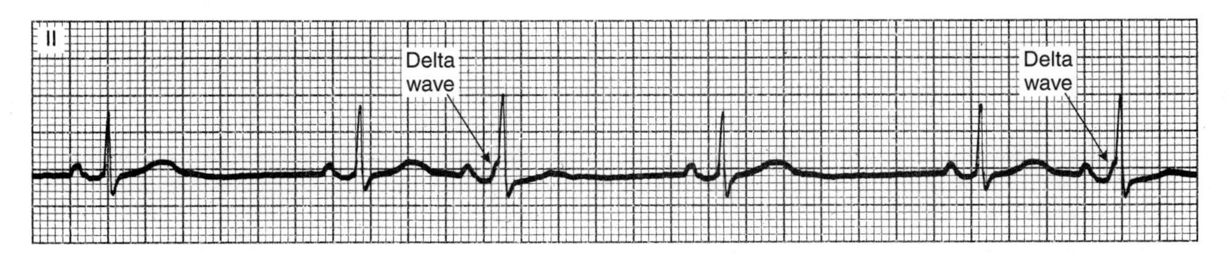

FIG. 21-14. Intermittent preexcitation. In this tracing of sinus bradycardia there are two PACs with a short P′R interval followed by a delta wave in a broad QRS.

quency ablation of an electrocardiographically overt pathway (incidence 4.2%).[19]

CAUSES

During early fetal development the heart is a single chamber; the atrial myocardium is continuous with the ventricular myocardium. The four chambers are formed with the invagination of the atrial and ventricular septa and the regression of muscle bands around the heart concomitantly with the formation of the annulus fibrosus (AV ring), which is normally a continuous sheet of fibrous tissue separating the atria from the ventricles. Accessory pathways are the result of faulty development of the AV ring, which may occur at almost any point around the annulus fibrosus as strands of normal myocardium bridge this insulating fibrous division between atria and ventricles. Fig. 21-15 is a diagrammatic representation of a left-sided accessory pathway.

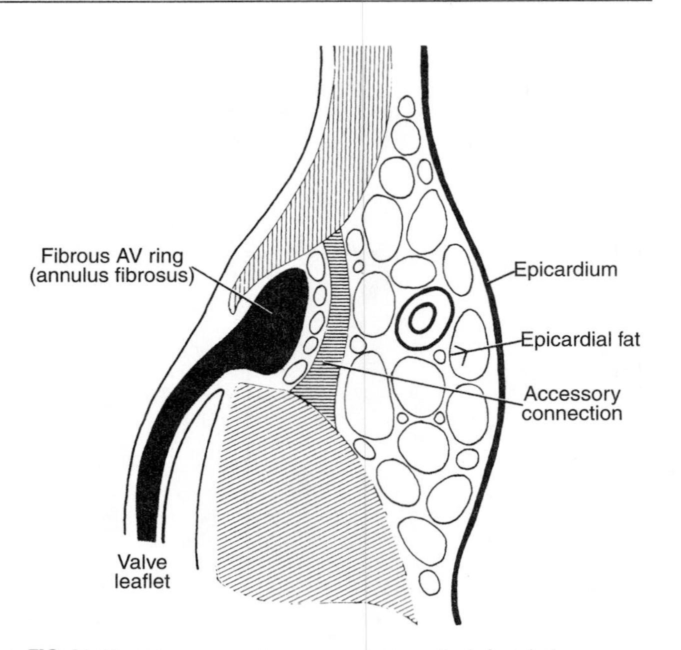

FIG. 21-15. Diagrammatic representation of a left-sided accessory AV connection. The connection skirts through the epicardial fat, being outside the fibrous AV ring. (From Becker AE et al: *Circulation* 57:870, 1978.)

Genetics

In 1990 Wellens et al[20] suggested that the WPW syndrome is inherited as an autosomal dominant trait. The observation was made that family members of patients with WPW syndrome have a four times greater chance of having an accessory pathway than do people without a family history.[21] It is now known that a familial form of WPW syndrome occurs in association with hypertrophic cardiomyopathy and intraventricular conduction abnormalities. Because of this, identification of WPW in more than one family member prompts clinical evaluation of relatives for additional findings of ventricular hypertrophy or conduction abnormalities.[22,23]

CLINICAL IMPLICATIONS

The clinical implications of WPW syndrome are the associated arrhythmias that significantly compromise quality of life and may even cause death. A cure is available in the form of radiofrequency ablation.

The estimated incidence of WPW syndrome is reported to be 0.1% to 0.3% of the general population, with an annual incidence of new cases 4 per 100,000 population. It is reportedly twice as common in men as in women. However, it may be that the condition is underreported. Many individuals with WPW syndrome who have experienced PSVT do not seek medical attention unless the PSVT cannot be terminated or they are in atrial fibrillation. Additionally, even when symptomatic individuals do seek attention in emergency departments, their condition may not be noted for the following reasons:

1. The 12-lead ECG during the tachycardia is not examined closely by an informed clinician for its diagnostic clues.
2. The 12-lead ECG after termination of the tachycardia is normal (concealed or latent accessory pathway), misleading the clinician.
3. The delta wave is so small that it is not noticed during sinus rhythm.

DIFFERENTIAL DIAGNOSIS

In WPW syndrome, because of the multiple possible location sites for the accessory pathway and the different degrees of preexcitation (minimal to maximal), the ECG pattern may resemble that of ventricular hypertrophy or MI.[15]

Ventricular Hypertrophy

A *right-sided accessory pathway* may direct the delta force toward the left, amplifying the R waves in left chest leads and simulating left ventricular hypertrophy.

A *left-sided accessory pathway* may direct the delta force toward the right, amplifying the R waves in right chest leads and simulating right ventricular hypertrophy.

Myocardial Infarction

A *left lateral accessory pathway* directing the delta force toward the right may cause Q waves in lateral limb-leads, simulating high lateral MI.

A *posteroseptal accessory pathway* directing the delta force superiorly may cause prominent Q waves in inferior limb leads simulating inferior MI.[18]

ARRHYTHMIAS IN WPW SYNDROME

The most frequently occurring arrhythmias in patients with WPW syndrome are (1) orthodromic circus movement tachycardia (CMT) using the AV node anterogradely and an accessory pathway retrogradely, and (2) atrial fibrillation. In a series of 407 patients with WPW syndrome and cardiac arrhythmias, 265 had CMT, 76 had atrial fibrillation, and 66 had both.[25] Other arrhythmias are, of course, possible; antidromic CMT, atrial flutter, and atrial tachycardia also result in rapid ventricular rates with a broad QRS because of AV conduction via the accessory pathway.

PAROXYSMAL SUPRAVENTRICULAR TACHYCARDIA

In all patients presenting with PSVT an accurate diagnosis depends on the following:

1. Recording an adequate number of leads (at least I, II, III, V_1, and V_6) during PSVT and the same leads for comparison during sinus rhythm; the comparison helps locate the P′ waves during the tachycardia and determine their position relative to the QRS
2. Taking a good history
3. Performing electrophysiologic studies

Symptoms

Symptoms include feelings of palpitations, nervousness, polyuria, anxiety, angina, heart failure, syncope, or shock, depending on the duration and rate of the tachycardia and whether there is structural heart disease. These and other subjective symptoms during CMT are listed in Table 21-2.

Syncope in patients with WPW syndrome may help to identify those at risk for ventricular fibrillation due to rapid conduction over an accessory pathway during atrial fibrillation. When this symptom occurred in young patients (<25 years) with WPW syndrome, it was found to be associated with a short anterograde refractory period (<220 ms) of the pathway.[26]

Differential Diagnosis

The location of the P′ wave is the key to the differential diagnosis in PSVT (AV nodal reentry tachycardia [AVNRT] vs CMT). Compare the location of the P′ waves in Figs. 21-16, *A-D*. PSVT has been covered in detail in Chapter 11; its differential diagnosis on the ECG is briefly reviewed here.

AVNRT. When the impulse passes down the slow atrial-nodal pathway to enter the AV node, it returns to the atria by the fast atrial nodal pathway at the same time that it passes down to activate the ventricles, placing the P′ waves within the QRS (Fig. 21-16, *A*). In many cases the P′ will distort the end of the QRS, looking like S waves in the inferior leads and r′ waves in V_1 (Fig. 21-16, *B*).

There is an uncommon form of AVNRT in which the impulse uses the fast atrial-nodal pathway anterogradely and return to the atrial by the slow pathway.

Orthodromic CMT using a rapidly conducting accessory pathway. This is the most common arrhythmia in symptomatic patients with WPW syndrome. It is the mechanism in approximately 40% of all cases of symptomatic PSVT and is itself 15 times more common than antidromic CMT.[11]

When the impulse passes down the AV node (orthodromic) and up a rapidly conducting accessory pathway, the retrograde P′ wave immediately follows the narrow

TABLE 21-2 Subjective Symptoms During Paroxysmal Circus Movement Tachycardia (69 Patients)

Symptom	No. of Patients (%)
Palpitations	67 (97)
Dyspnea	40 (57)
Anginal pain	39 (56)
Perspiration	38 (55)
Fatigue	28 (41)
Anxiety	20 (30)
Dizziness	20 (30)
Polyuria	18 (26)

From Wellens HJJ et al: In Mandel WJ, editor *Cardiac arrhythmias: their mechanisms, diagnosis and management,* Philadelphia, 1980, JB Lippincott.

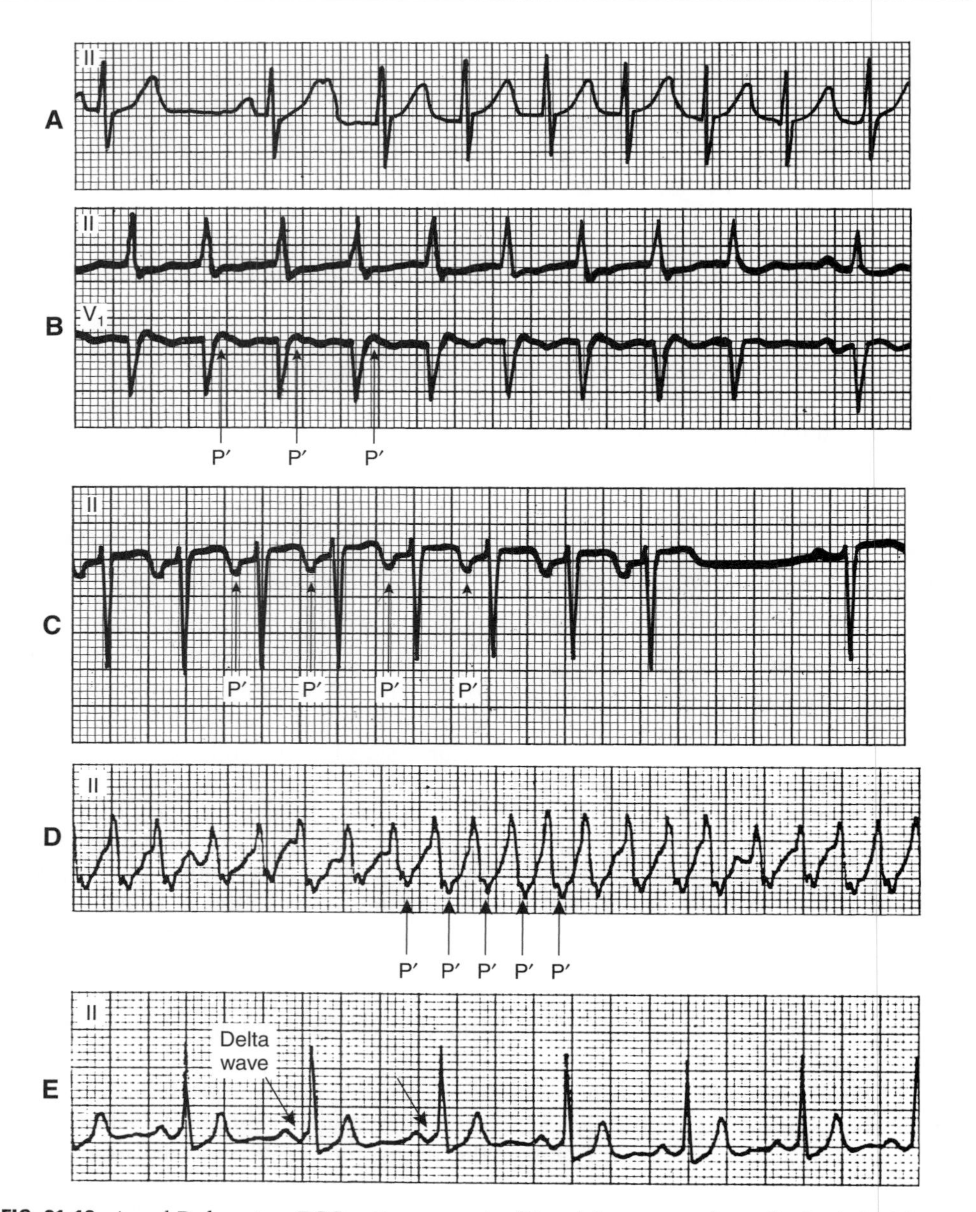

FIG. 21-16. **A** and **B** show two ECG patterns seen in AV nodal reentry tachycardia. In **A** the P′ wave is not seen because it is hidden within the QRS. In **B** the end of the P′ wave peeks out at the end of the QRS, looking like an S wave in lead II and an r′ wave in V_1. **C** is an example of a circus movement tachycardia that uses a slowly conducting accessory pathway; the impulse passes down the AV node to produce a narrow QRS and up the slowly conducing accessory pathway to produce a negative P′ wave in lead II with the RP′ greater than the P′R. **D** and **E** are tachycardia and sinus rhythm tracings from a patient with Wolff-Parkinson-White syndrome and a rapidly conducting accessory pathway. The P′ wave always immediately follows the QRS. Note the delta wave during sinus rhythm.

QRS and can be found in the ST segment (Fig. 21-16, *D*). The polarity of the P′ wave depends on the location of the accessory pathway. For example, a left lateral accessory pathway would result in a negative P′ wave in lead I; often there is QRS alternans.

Other ECG signs of CMT are QRS alternans, aberrant ventricular conduction, and heart rate during aberrancy slower than without aberrancy.

Orthodromic CMT using a slowly conducting accessory pathway. When the impulse passes down the AV node and up a slowly conducting accessory pathway, the retrograde P′ wave is at a distance from its QRS and appears immediately in front of the next QRS. This type of CMT is persistent (constantly reoccurring). Because the impulse travels from the area of the AV node where the pathway is inserted, the P′ waves in II, III, and aV_F are negative (Fig. 21-16, *C*), and in lead I they are isoelectric. In some publications this persistent CMT is called "incessant junctional tachycardia," although it is not always unceasing; there are occasional interruptions by the sinus rhythm.

CMT with two accessory pathways. CMT using two accessory pathways is another rare form of PSVT in which the QRS complexes are broad. Anterograde conduction is down one accessory pathway, and retrograde conduction is up another, producing a rhythm that is identical to VT. The mechanism is illustrated in Fig. 21-17.

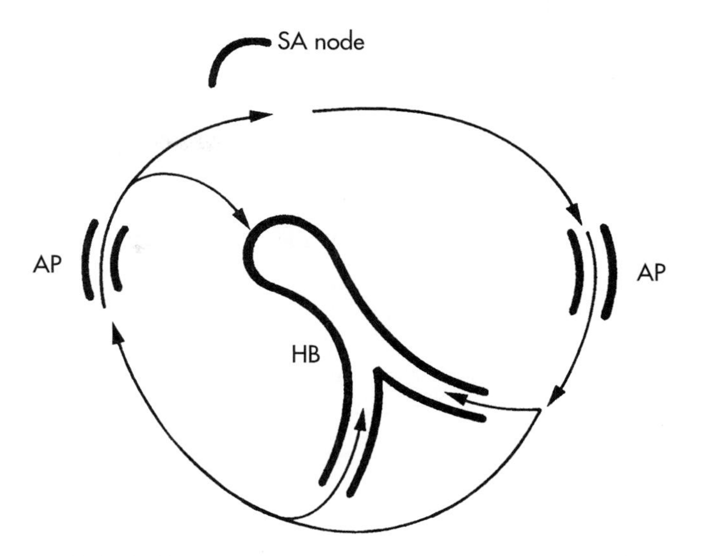

FIG. 21-17. A schematic representation of the mechanism of circus movement tachycardia using two accessory pathways. The resulting rhythm is identical to that of VT. *AP*, Accessory pathway; *HB*, His bundle.

Emergency Response to PSVT

The clinical approach to each of the more common types of PSVT differs, but the emergency treatment is the same. Therefore, when faced with PSVT, do the following:

1. Immediately secure an ECG in at least four leads (I, II, III, and V_1); these are the most helpful leads in making the differential diagnosis.
2. Terminate the arrhythmia and record another ECG.
3. Stabilize your patient and make him or her comfortable.
4. Systematically evaluate the ECG during and after the PSVT.

ANTIDROMIC CMT (BROAD QRS)

In patients with WPW syndrome, there are two mechanisms that use the accessory pathway during PSVT: (1) down the AV node (orthodromic) and up the accessory pathway, resulting in a narrow QRS tachycardia; and (2) up the AV node (antidromic) and down the accessory pathway, resulting in a broad QRS tachycardia identical in morphology to ventricular tachycardia (VT). The presence of antidromic CMT is associated with multiple accessory pathways.[15,27] Electrophysiologic studies are necessary to rule out VT. The ECGs from a patient with antidromic CMT caused by anterograde conduction down a left free wall accessory pathway are seen in Fig. 21-18.

ECG Recognition

Rate: 150 to 250 beats/min.

QRS complex: Broad. As one would expect, the shape of the ventricular complexes exactly mimics those of VT because the ventricles are being activated solely from the ventricular insertion of the accessory pathway.

Rhythm: Usually regular; however, it may be slightly irregular because retrograde conduction times vary through the fascicles of the left bundle branch to the atria. This fact may help to distinguish this type of broad QRS tachycardia from VT, which is regular 75% of the time, but may serve to confuse it with atrial fibrillation with conduction over an accessory pathway, which looks like VT but is irregular.

P waves: Although P′ waves usually are present after every QRS complex, they are not seen during this tachycardia because of the width of the QRS.

Main diagnostic feature: A broad QRS tachycardia with slow initial forces caused by excitation outside of the conduction system is the main diagnostic feature.

Mechanism

The mechanism of antidromic CMT is schematically illustrated in Fig. 21-19. Note that anterograde conduction proceeds down the accessory pathway and that initial forces are in the ventricular myocardium, where conduction is slower than it is in the conduction system. Initial penetration of the ventricle via an accessory pathway causes a relatively slow beginning to the broad QRS. Antidromic CMT begins as does orthodromic CMT, with a critically timed PAC, premature ventricular complex, a critical sinus rate, or because of a drug.

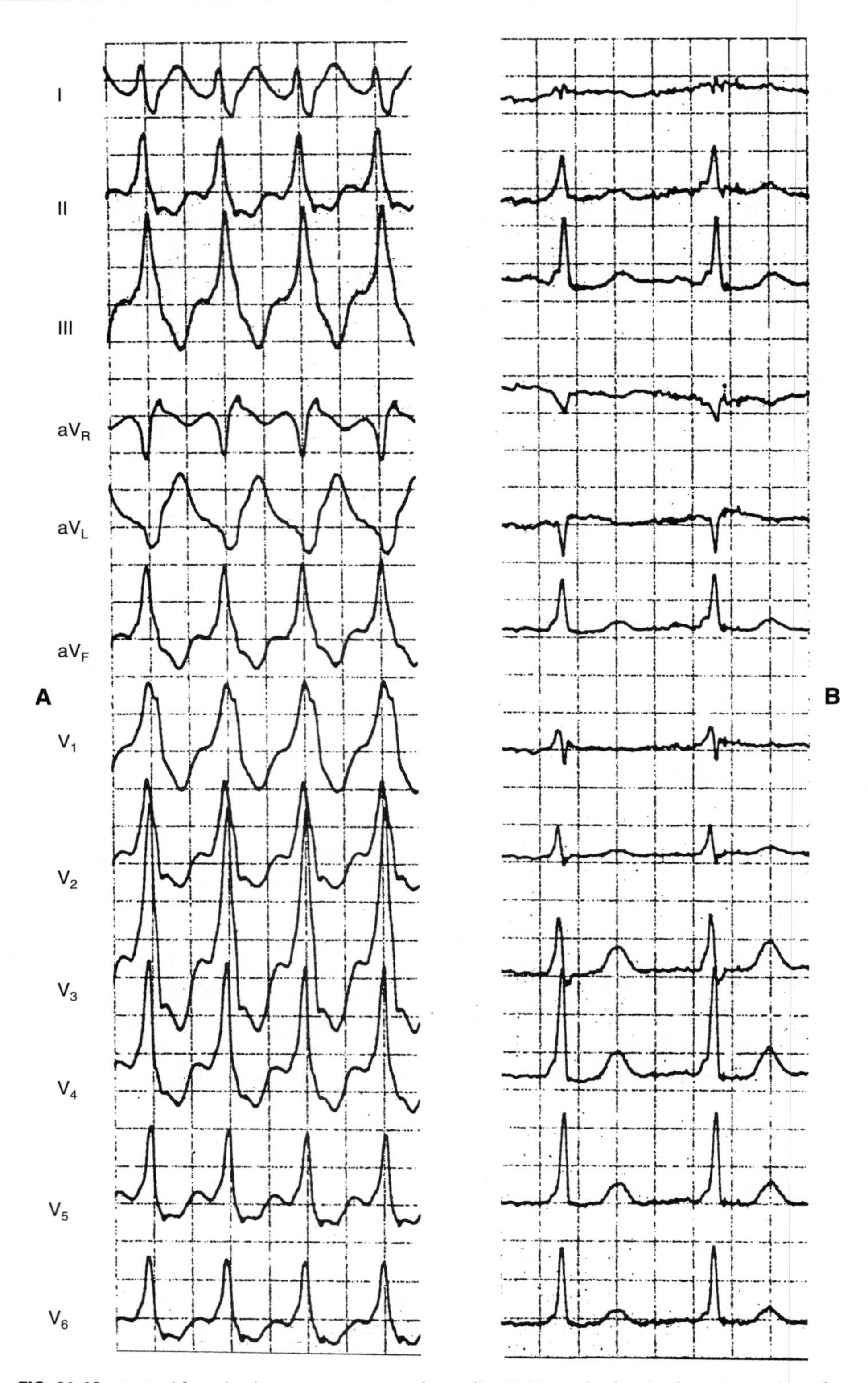

FIG. 21-18. **A**, Antidromic circus movement tachycardia. **B**, Sinus rhythm in the same patient shows a short PR interval and a delta wave caused by a left free wall accessory pathway. (Courtesy Hein J.J. Wellens, MD, Maastricht, The Netherlands.)

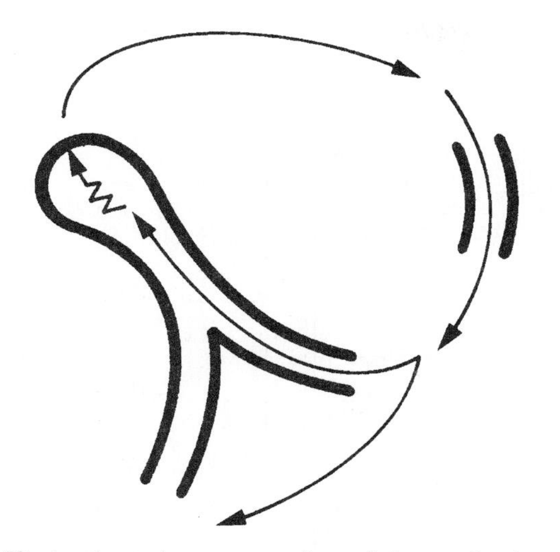

FIG. 21-19. A schematic representation of the mechanism of antidromic circus movement tachycardia. Anterograde conduction is down the accessory pathway, and initial ventricular forces are outside the conduction system, which explains the wide QRS with the relatively slow beginning.

Emergency Treatment

The treatment for antidromic CMT is the same as for that of orthodromic CMT (p. 130). The diagnostic challenge is that antidromic CMT is identical in morphologic appearance to VT.

ATRIAL FIBRILLATION

Atrial fibrillation occurs in 10% to 32% of patients with WPW syndrome and may precipitate ventricular fibrillation, especially when the accessory pathway has a short anterograde refractory period (<250 ms). In patients with concealed accessory pathways (no anterograde conduction) atrial fibrillation is rare (3%).[28]

ECG Recognition

Rate: Fast—usually more than 200 beats/min—and often more than 300 beats/min.
QRS complex: Broad; pattern is that of VT.
Rhythm: Irregular.
Main diagnostic features: A fast, broad, irregular (FBI) rhythm is a red flag for this life-threatening arrhythmia. If it were not for its irregularity, this broad QRS tachycardia would be identical to VT.

Fig. 21-20 is a 12-lead ECG tracing from a patient with atrial fibrillation and AV conduction over an accessory pathway. A sinus rhythm strip in lead II is shown. Note the FBI features recorded after cardioversion. Note the typical ECG features of WPW syndrome—short PR, broad QRS, and delta wave.

The tracings from an 18-year-old man in this potentially lethal case (Fig. 21-21) dramatically illustrate the potentially lethal arrhythmia that can occur in a patient with a latent accessory pathway. This patient did not respond to procainamide, which would indicate a long refractory period in the accessory pathway. In the 12-lead ECG during sinus rhythm recorded after cardioversion (Fig. 21-22) the delta waves are subtle. In II, III, and aV_F they look like q waves. In V_3, V_4, and V_5 there is a slightly slow beginning to the QRS, and the PR interval is only 0.09 second. The young man was referred for radiofrequency ablation of his accessory pathway.

Mechanism

The mechanism of atrial fibrillation with conduction over an accessory pathway is diagrammatically illustrated in Fig. 21-23 with the typical ECG tracing. Procainamide blocks the accessory pathway and is the first response for a hemodynamically stable with this arrhythmia.

When an accessory pathway is present, a very rapid ventricular response is possible. The mechanisms of the FBI features of atrial fibrillation in WPW syndrome follow.

Fast. The ventricular rate exceeds 200 beats/min. The following factors determine the ventricular rate during atrial fibrillation[11]:

1. Refractory period duration of the accessory pathway in the anterograde direction.
2. Refractory period of the AV node.
3. Refractory period of the ventricle.
4. Concealed anterograde and retrograde penetration into the accessory pathway and the AV node.[25]
5. Sympathetic stimulation shortens the refractory period of the accessory pathway and accelerates the ventricular rate.[29] It is important to terminate this tachycardia promptly and in the meantime to reassure the patient. There is a reflex sympathetic response to the fall in blood pressure that is associated with atrial fibrillation and the very rapid ventricular rate. Anxiety adds to this response.

If the refractory period of the accessory pathway is

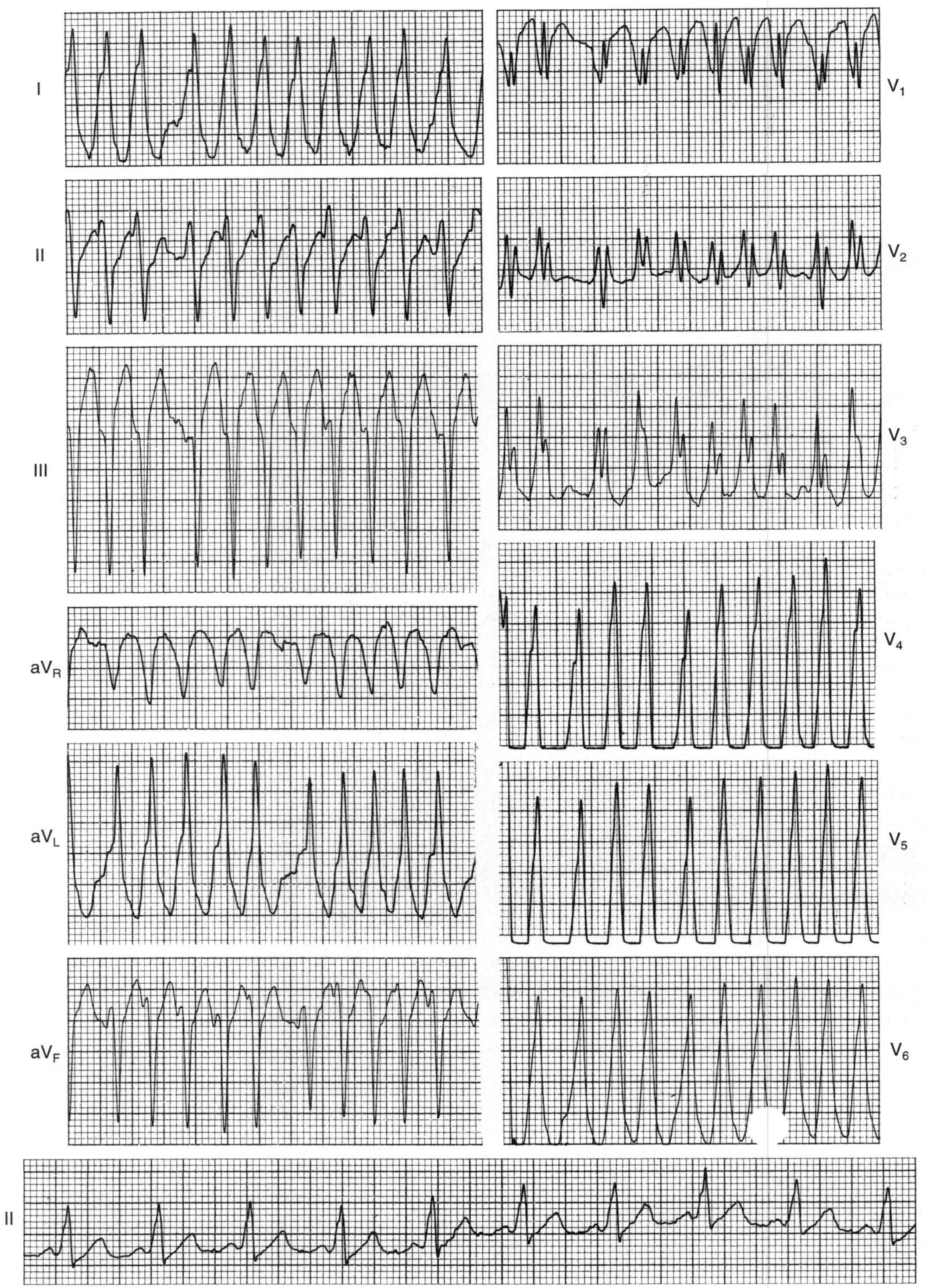

FIG. 21-20. A 12-lead ECG showing atrial fibrillation with conduction over an accessory pathway. Although the QRS has the shape of VT, the rhythm is irregular, typical of this mechanism. The lead II rhythm strip was taken after conversion to sinus rhythm. Note the short PR interval, delta wave, and broad QRS complex typical of overt Wolff-Parkinson-White syndrome. (Courtesy Ara Tilkian, MD, Van Nuys, Calif.)

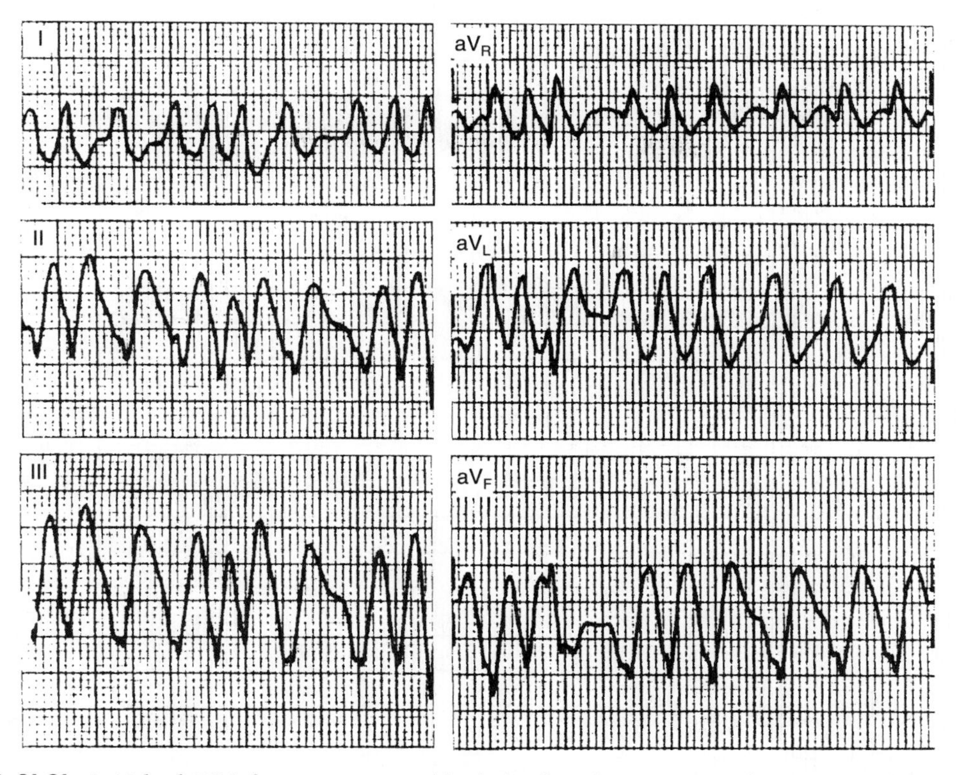

FIG. 21-21. A 12-lead ECG from an 18-year-old admitted to the emergency department. The signs of atrial fibrillation with conduction over an accessory pathway are the fast rate, broad QRS, and irregular rhythm.

short, the heart rate exceeds 300 beats/min. This is a life-threatening arrhythmia that may deteriorate into ventricular fibrillation.

Broad. The QRS complex is broad (it looks just like VT) because ventricular activation is initiated outside the normal conduction system. (Remember that this is not a reentry circuit and that it is the accessory pathway that must be blocked, not the AV node.)

Irregular. The rhythm is irregular because of rapid stimulation from the fibrillating atria, concealed conduction into the accessory pathway, and perhaps also because of changing refractoriness of the accessory pathway. This irregularity, which is typical, distinguishes atrial fibrillation with conduction over an accessory pathway from VT, which is usually regular.

Cause

Spontaneous degeneration of CMT has been reported to represent the most frequent mode of initiation of atrial fibrillation during electrophysiologic study (up to 64% of episodes). Hemodynamic changes during tachycardia may lead to increased sympathetic tone, hypoxemia, or increased tension of the atrial wall, thus triggering atrial fibrillation.

Emergency Treatment

Cardiovert if hemodynamically unstable.

When a fast, broad, irregular rhythm is encountered in the emergency setting, do the following:

1. Obtain a 12-lead ECG during the tachycardia and one during sinus rhythm after conversion.
2. Administer procainamide 10 mg/kg body weight over 5 minutes. If procainamide does not slow down the rhythm and block the accessory pathway (complexes will become narrow as they pass down the AV node), the next step is as follows.
3. Cardiovert if procainamide does not slow the ventricular response or if the patient at any time becomes hemodynamically unstable. After conversion to a sinus rhythm the patient is referred to a center skilled in the treatment of patients with

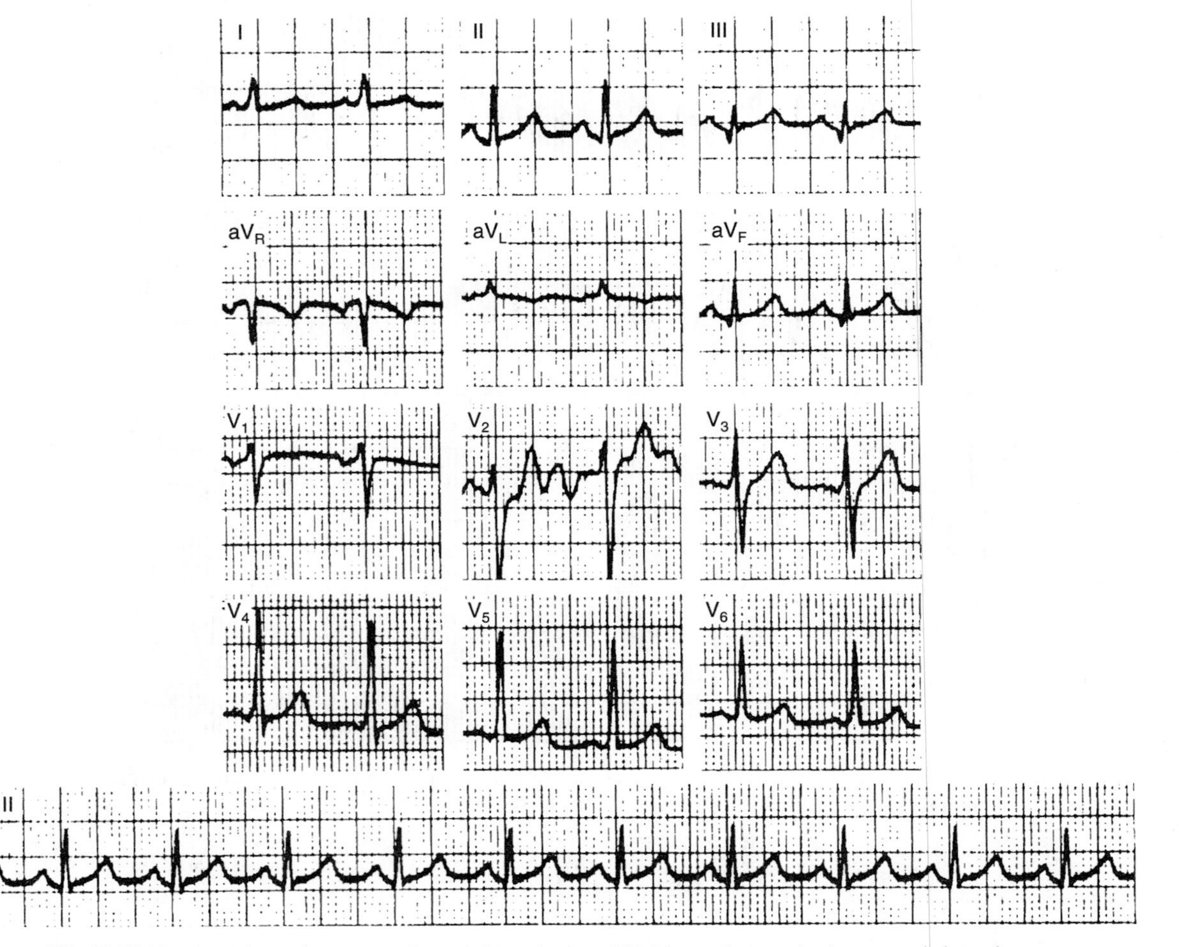

FIG. 21-22. Same patient after conversion to sinus rhythm. The signs of preexcitation are subtle and easy to miss. This young man had been symptomatic since the age of 8 years. (Courtesy Kathleen Hester, RN, and Cathy Stark, RN, Concord, Calif.)

WPW syndrome. If procainamide did not work, this referral is in an emergency basis because the patient cannot be protected from recurrence.

Atrial Fibrillation with Two Accessory Pathways

As illustrated in Fig. 21-24, when atrial fibrillation occurs in a patient with two accessory pathways, conduction into the ventricles has three pathways, the AV node and the two accessory pathways. This results in an irregular rhythm and broad QRS complexes of different shapes, depending on which pathway activates the ventricles first. There would also be fusion beats. Fig. 21-25 illustrates the ECG during atrial fibrillation in a patient with both right-sided and left-sided accessory pathways.

CURATIVE RADIOFREQUENCY CATHETER ABLATION

The most important steps in the management of a patient with WPW syndrome are its *recognition and referral* to an experienced electrophysiologist for curative catheter ablation,[30] after which 90% to 95% of patients are free of the associated arrhythmias.[28] In patients with WPW syndrome, atrial fibrillation can be lethal and has a lifetime risk of sudden death of about 4%. Although the risk is relatively low, when combined with the morbidity associated with recurrent tachycardias, the widespread use of catheter ablation therapy to eliminate accessory pathway conduction is justified. Pharmacologic therapy is reserved for those rare patients who do not respond to catheter ablation or do not wish to undergo the procedure.[30]

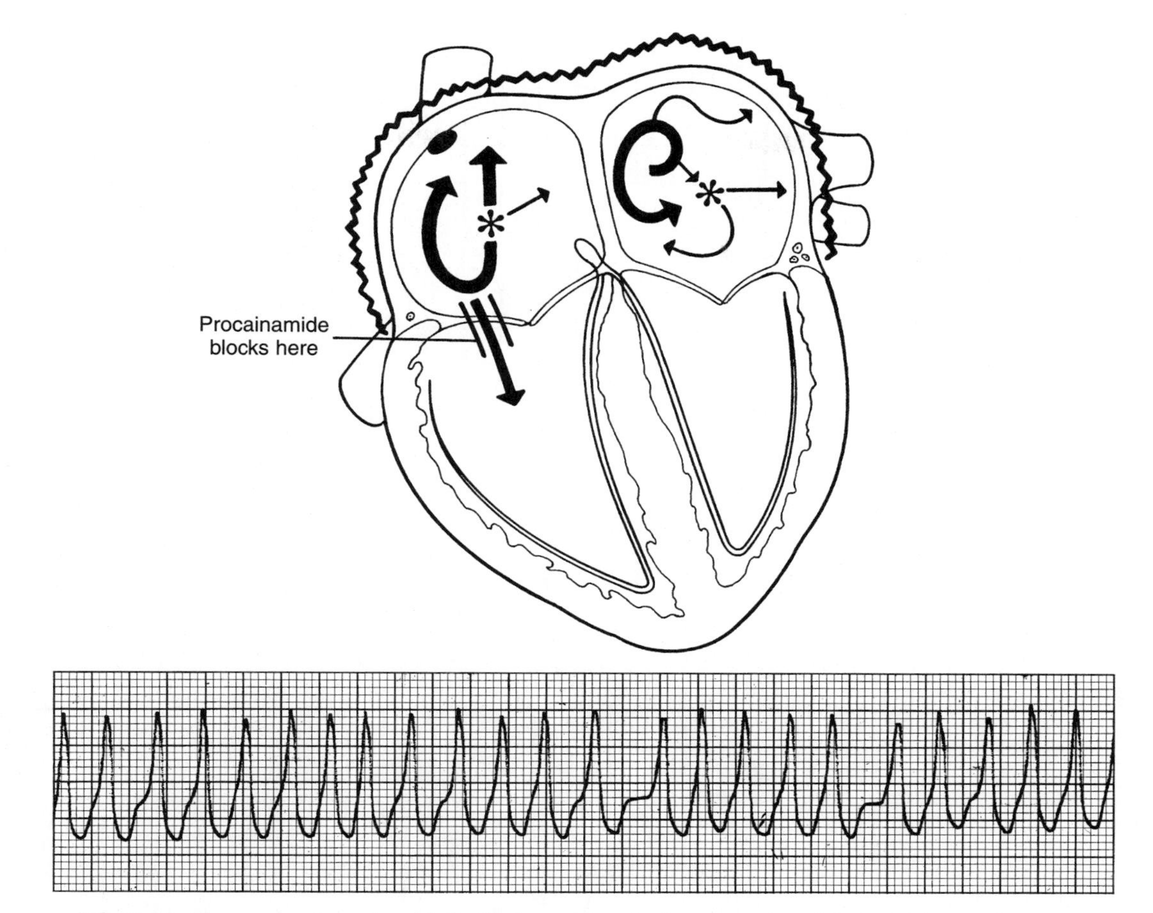

FIG. 21-23. The mechanism of atrial fibrillation with a single accessory pathway and the resultant ECG. Emergency response for a hemodynamically stable patient is procainamide to block the accessory pathway.

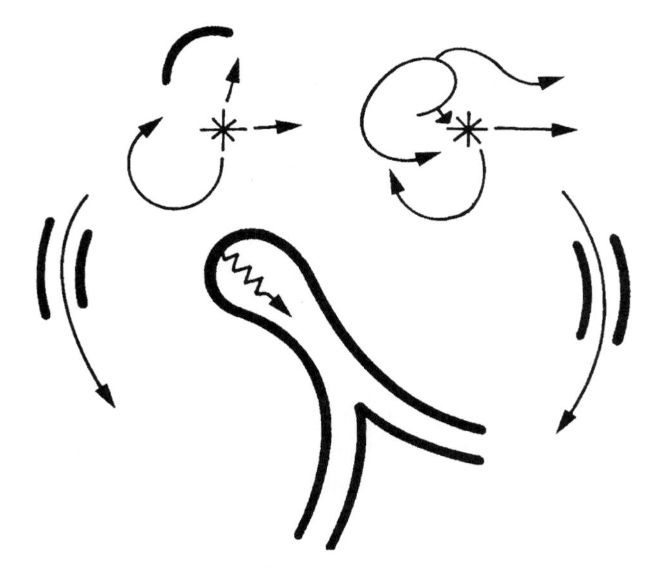

FIG. 21-24. A representation of the mechanism of atrial fibrillation with conduction down a right-sided and left-sided accessory pathway.

Pediatrics

Children have a different natural history and age-related risks for radiofrequency ablation of accessory pathways than adults, leaving physicians with less certainty about the recommendations for radiofrequency ablation as a therapeutic option for WPW syndrome in children as opposed to adults. Vignati et al[24] suggest that ablation should be avoided before the age of 5 or 6 years and that the procedure should become first-line treatment for symptomatic patients older than 12 years of age. These investigators found that when the peak incidence of the onset of PSVT occurred during infancy

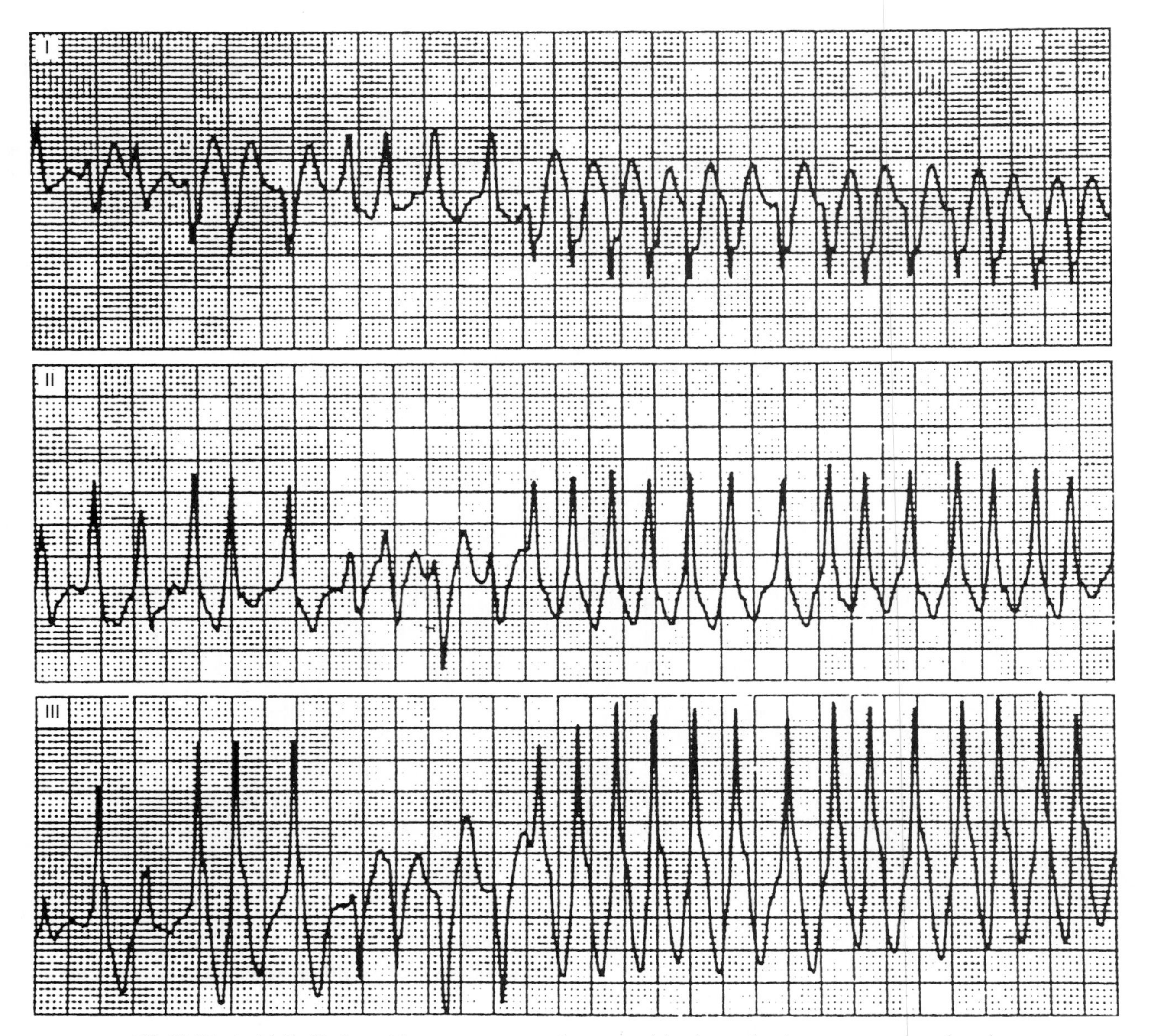

FIG. 21-25. Atrial fibrillation with two accessory pathways resulting in conduction over one, then the other, and fusion beats when the two pathways conduct simultaneously.

that it often disappeared spontaneously (53%). This only occurred in 12% of cases when the PSVT first appeared after 12 years of age. The same correlation existed with the induction of atrial fibrillation. In children younger than 6 years of age the risk was low as opposed to those older than 12 years of age, in whom the risk was highest.

Beginnings

The excitement over the early use of radiofrequency ablation was well-justified. Radiofrequency energy was being applied successfully in neurosurgery as early as 1970[31] and 1975,[32] and in dermatologic oncology in 1980.[33] The first experimental use of transvenous radiofrequency energy in the heart was between 1985 and 1988, when Huang and colleagues[34-36] introduced the use of radiofrequency current to successfully ablate the AV junction in a canine model.

In 1987 Jackman et al[37,38] demonstrated in dogs that radiofrequency current could be used to selectively destroy myocardial tissue in the anatomic location where some accessory pathways lie (underneath the tricuspid and mitral valve annulus at the AV junction between the atrium and ventricle). Soon after, this technique was to replace the open chest surgical ablation as a cure for patients with WPW syndrome.[39-41] Over the years investigators the catheter electrodes and energy delivery system has been improved.

Radiofrequency ablation involves the use of unmodulated, high-frequency alternating current through tissue to cause heat, cell desiccation, and coagulation necrosis for the purpose of destroying troublesome areas and pathways in the heart. The closed electrical circuit required for cardiac ablation is achieved by a radiofrequency generator, connecting leads, and unipolar or bipolar electrodes.

Repeat Sessions

Nearly 25% percent of repeat radiofrequency ablation sessions in patients initially thought to have a single accessory pathway are caused by the late manifestation of an additional accessory pathway; intermittent concealed conduction appears to be a likely explanation for this phenomenon.[42] Recurrence of conduction in an accessory pathway already ablated is less than 5%.[42]

The recurrence rate of paroxysmal atrial fibrillation after successful radiofrequency ablation of accessory pathways shows an age-related increase, being low in patients younger than 50 years of age (12%) and high in the older patients.[43]

MAHAIM PATHWAYS[44]

In 1941 Mahaim and Winston[45] described anomalous tracts between the lower AV node or bundle of His and the ventricles. However, the majority of these pathways has been found to be long right atriofascicular pathways capable of only anterograde conduction. They are involved in antidromic AV reciprocating (Mahaim) tachycardia with a left bundle branch block morphology.

Mechanism of Associated PSVT

Fig. 21-26 is an ECG during sinus rhythm *(A)* and during tachycardia *(B)* in a patient with a nodoventricular fiber running from the AV node to the posteroinferior part of the right ventricle. The mechanism is diagramed in Fig. 21-27.

Clinical Implications

Mahaim fibers that exhibit decremental AV node-like conduction properties are unusual—comprising less than 3% of accessory pathways—and are frequently associated with Ebstein's anomaly, additional AV accessory pathways, and dual AV nodal pathway conduction. True nodoventricular or nodofascicular Mahaim pathways usually also capable of only anterograde conduction appear to be rare and are associated with tachycardia of left bundle branch block morphology not distinguishable from the preexcitation pattern of right atriofascicular pathways. Fasciculoventricular Mahaim pathways have never been reported to be involved in a tachycardia circuit.

Treatment

Radiofrequency ablation of right atriofascicular pathways is reported to be safe and highly effective in patients with Mahaim pathways. Hluchy et al[44] report successful radiofrequency ablation of unusual Mahaim pathways (concealed nodoventricular, nodofascicular, and left anterograde atriofascicular) was performed without impairing the normal AV conduction system.

SHORT PR NORMAL QRS SYNDROME

In 1938 by Clerc et al[46] reported a syndrome of short PR intervals, normal QRS durations, and a tendency to PSVT, thus this clinical picture is sometimes called Clerc-Levy-Cristeco syndrome. However, it is best known because of the emphasis given it by the work of Lown et al,[47] who in 1952 reported that 11 patients with a short PR interval and a normal QRS complex had a much greater incidence of PSVT than did individuals with a normal PR interval. Thus the short PR syndrome is sometimes called the *Lown-Ganong-Levine syndrome* or short PR-normal qRS syndrome.

Note that (1) the syndrome is not said to exist simply because the PR is short. Supraventricular tachycardia (AV reciprocating tachycardia, atrial fibrillation, or atrial flutter) must also be documented and (2) a short PR interval may reflect error in measurement, a lower limit of normal, a child or an adolescent, increased heart rate, enhanced sympathetic activity, or ectopic atrial or junctional rhythms.

Fig. 21-28 is a 12-lead ECG tracing from an individual

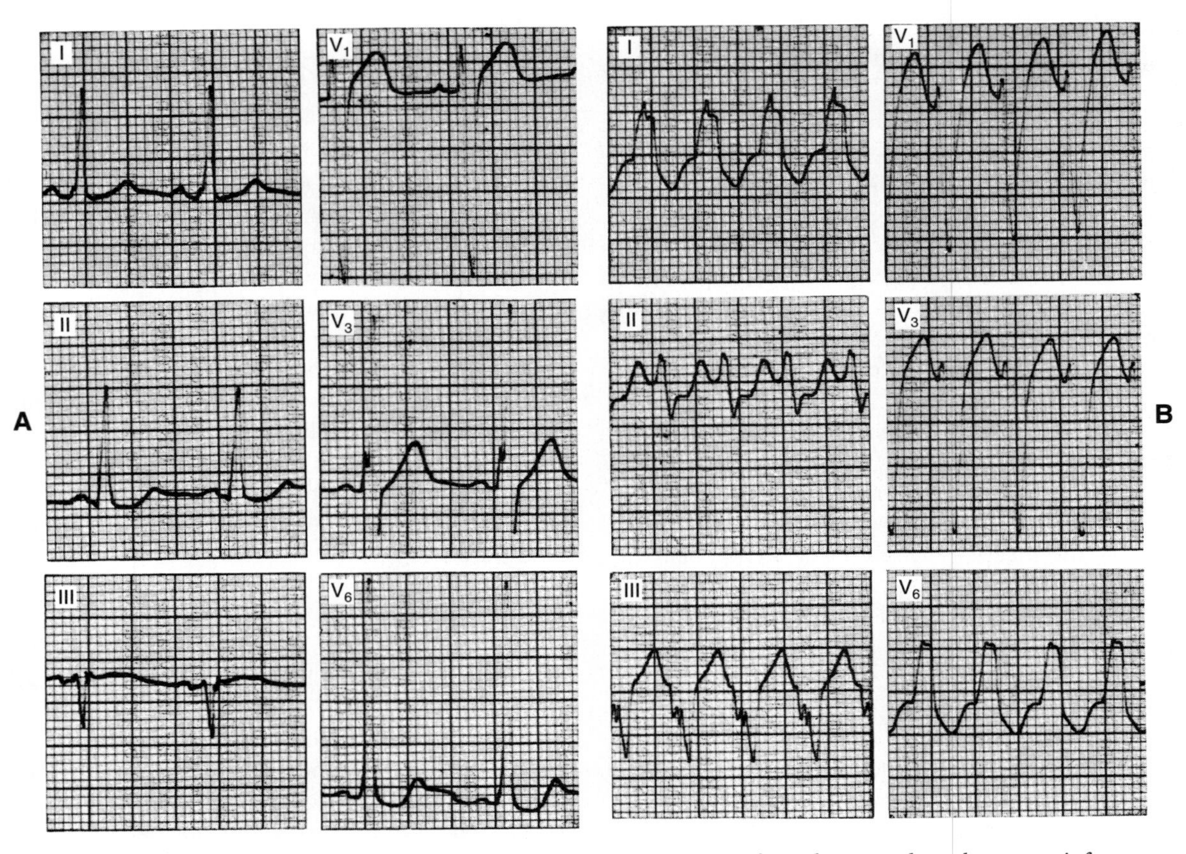

FIG. 21-26. A patient with a nodoventricular (Mahaim) fiber running from the AV node to the posteroinferior part of the right ventricle. **A** is the ECG during sinus rhythm; **B** is the ECG during the reentry tachycardia. The ventricle is activated exclusively by way of the nodoventricular fiber. (From Wellens HJJ et al: The differentiation between ventricular tachycardia and supraventricular tachycardia with aberrant conduction: the value of the 12-lead electrocardiogram. In Wellens HJJ, Kulbertus HE, editors: *What's new in electrocardiography*, The Hague, 1981, Martinus Nijhoff, p 197.)

with Lown-Ganong-Levine syndrome. Note that the PR interval in this case is so short that there is no PR segment and that the QRS duration is normal.

SUMMARY

WPW syndrome is a group of ECG findings (short PR, delta wave, and broad QRS) associated with the occurrence

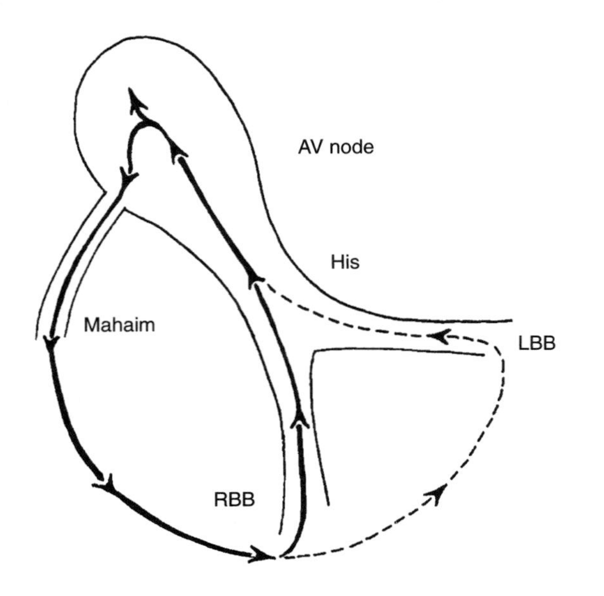

FIG. 21-27. Schematic representation of the reentry circuit underlying a reciprocating tachycardia. This reentry circuit uses a nodoventricular fiber. The nodoventricular fiber may insert into either the right ventricle or the right bundle branch *(RBB)*. The retrograde return circuit can conceivably be completed by either the right bundle branch or the left bundle branch *(LBB)*. A portion of the reentry loop is confined to the AV node, and the atrium does not form a necessary link in the loop. (From Gallagher JJ et al: *Circulation* 64:176, 1981.)

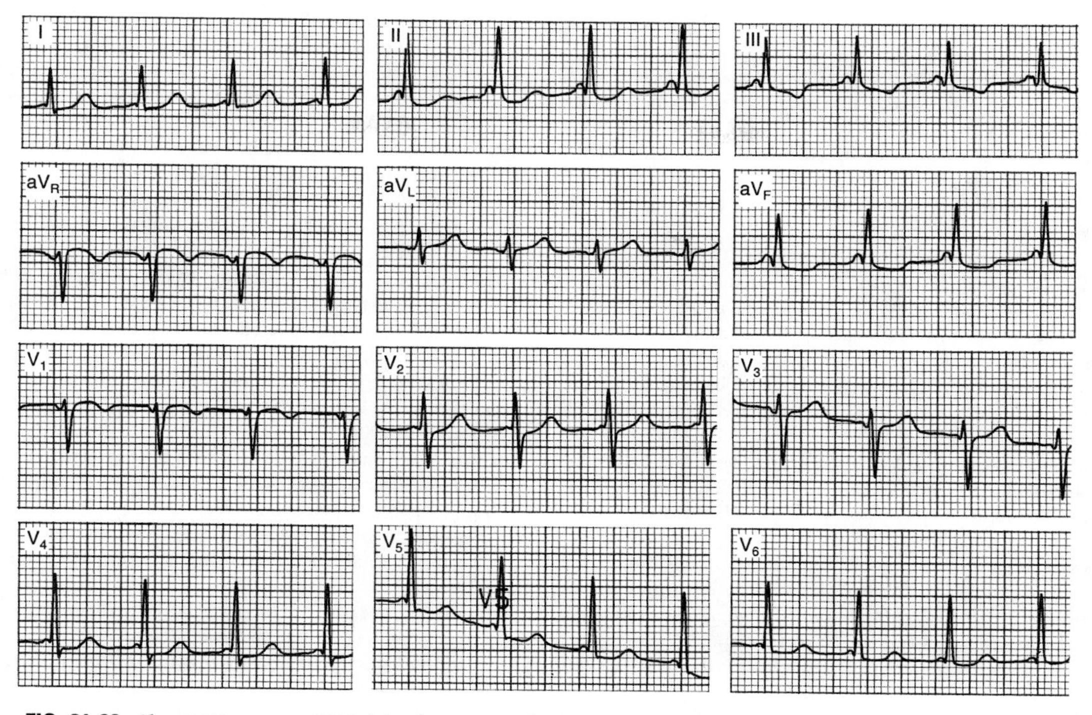

FIG. 21-28. Short PR narrow QRS (also known as the Lown-Ganong-Levine or Clerc-Levy-Critesco syndrome). Note the short PR (0.04 second) and narrow QRS (0.08 second). (Courtesy Dixie Lee Hacker-Summers, Anchorage, Alaska.)

of tachycardias. The most important steps in the management of a patient with WPW syndrome are its *recognition and referral* to an experienced electrophysiologist for curative catheter ablation, after which 90% to 95% of patients are free of the associated arrhythmias.

The two most common arrhythmias of WPW syndrome are PSVT and atrial fibrillation. In PSVT there is a differential diagnosis between circus movement tachycardia using an accessory pathway and AV nodal reentry tachycardia (Chapter 11). Atrial fibrillation in the presence of an anterogradely conducting accessory pathway can be lethal. Although the risk is relatively low (4%), when combined with the morbidity associated with recurrent tachycardias, the widespread use of radiofrequency catheter ablation to eliminate accessory pathway conduction is justified.

Accessory pathways capable of anterograde conduction may exist in patients who do not manifest the ECG signs of preexcitation but who have the same tendencies to develop CMT and life-threatening atrial fibrillation (latent accessory pathways). Accessory pathways capable of only retrograde conduction are called "concealed." Patients with concealed accessory pathways, although prone to orthodromic CMT, would not have excessively rapid heart rates should atrial fibrillation develop because retrograde accessory pathway conduction is not possible.

REFERENCES

1. Wolff L, Parkinson J, White P et al: Bundle-branch block with short P-R interval in healthy young people prone to paroxysmal tachycardia, *Am Heart J* 5:685, 1930.
2. Kent AFS: Researches on structure and function of mammalian heart, *J Physiol* 14:233, 1893.
3. Holzman M, Scherf D: Uber Elektrokardiogramme mit vorkurzten vorhol Kammer-Distanz und positiven P-Zacken, *Z Klin Med* 121:404, 1932.
4. Wolferth CC, Wood FC: The mechanism of production of short P-R intervals and prolonged QRS complexes in patients with presumably undamaged hearts. Hypothesis of an accessory pathway of auriculoventricular conduction (bundle of Kent), *Am Heart J* 8:297, 1933.
5. Wood FC, Wolferth CC, Geckeler GD: Histological demonstration of accessory muscular connections between auricle and ventricle in a case of short P-R interval and prolonged QRS complex, *Am Heart J* 25:454, 1943.
6. Ohnell RF: Preexcitation: a cardiac abnormality, *Acta Med Scand (Suppl)* 152:74, 1944.
7. Herweg B, Fisher JD, Ilercil A et al: Cardiac memory after radiofrequency ablation of accessory pathways: the post-ablation T wave does

not forget the pre-excited QRS, *J Interv Card Electrophysiol* 3:263-372, 1999.
8. Coelho L, Elvas L, Ventura M et al: Repolarization abnormalities after catheter ablation of differently located overt accessory pathways, *Rev Port Cardiol* 19:553-565, 2000.
9. Hiss RG, Lamb LE: Electrocardiographic findings in 122,043 individuals, *Circulation* 25:947, 1962.
10. Smith RF: The Wolff-Parkinson-White syndrome as an aviation risk, *Circulation* 29:672, 1964.
11. Wellens HJJ: Pre-excitation. In Willerson JT, Cohn JN, editors: *Cardiovascular medicine,* New York, 1995, Churchill Livingstone.
12. Kuck KH, Schluter M, Gursoy S: Preservation of atrioventricular nodal conduction during radiofrequency current catheter ablation of midseptal accessory pathways, *Circulation* 86:1743-1752, 1992.
13. Coppess MA, Altemose GT, Jayachandran JV et al: Unusual features of intermediate septal bypass tracts, *J Cardiovasc Electrophysiol* 11:730-735, 2000.
14. Personal communication: G. Veerender Reddy, December 2001.
15. Yi-Jen Chen, Shih-Ann Chen, Ching-Tai Tai et al: Long term results of radiofrequency catheter ablation in patients with Wolff-Parkinson-White syndrome. *Chin Med J* 59:78-87, 1997.
16. Wellens HJJ, Bruguda P: Value of programmed stimulation of the heart in patients with Wolff-Parkinson-White syndrome. In Josephson ME, Wellens HJJ, editors: *Tachycardias: mechanisms, diagnosis, treatment,* Philadelphia, 1984, Lea & Febiger.
17. Wellens HJJ: Wolff-Parkinson-White syndrome. Part I, *Mod Concepts Cardiovasc Dis* 52:53, 1983.
18. Khan IA; Shaw IS: Pseudo ventricular hypertrophy and pseudo myocardial infarction in Wolff-Parkinson-White syndrome, *Am J Emerg Med* 18:807-809, 2000.
19. Schluter M, Cappato R, Ouyang F et al: Clinical recurrences after successful accessory pathway ablation: the role of "dormant" accessory pathways, *J Cardiovasc Electrophysiol* 8:1366-1372, 1997.
20. Wellens HJJ, Brugada P, Penn OC et al: Pre-excitation syndromes. In Zipes DP, Jalife J, editors: *Cardiac electrophysiology,* Philadelphia, 1990, WB Saunders.
21. Vidaillet HJ, Pressley JC, Henke E et al: Familial occurrence of accessory atrioventricular pathways (pre-excitation syndrome), *N Engl J Med* 34:65, 1987.
22. Mehdirad AA, Fatkin D, DiMarco JP et al: Electrophysiologic characteristics of accessory atrioventricular connections in an inherited form of Wolff-Parkinson-White syndrome, *J Cardiovasc Electrophysiol* 10:629-635, 1999.
23. Gollob MH, Green MS, Tang AS et al: Identification of a gene responsible for familial Wolff-Parkinson-White syndrome, *N Engl J Med* 344:1823-1831, 2001.
24. Vignati G, Balla E, Mauri L et al: Clinical and electrophysiologic evolution of the Wolff-Parkinson-White syndrome in children: impact on approaches to management, *Cardiol Young* 10:367-375, 2000.
25. Josephson ME, Wellens HJJ: Differential diagnosis of supraventricular tachycardia, *Cardiol Clin* 8:411, 1990.
26. Duckeck W, Kuck KH: [Syncope in supraventricular tachycardia. Incidence, pathomechanism and consequences], *Herz* 18:175-181, 1993.
27. Wellens HJJ, Josephson ME: *Diagnosis of difficult arrhythmias,* Miami, 1987, Medtronic.
28. Duckeck W, Kuck KH: [Atrial fibrillation in Wolff-Parkinson-White syndrome. Development and therapy], *Herz* 18:60-66, 1993.
29. Wellens HJJ, Brugada P, Roy D et al: Effect of isoproterenol on the antegrade refractory period of the accessory pathway in patients with Wolff-Parkinson-White syndrome, *Am J Cardiol* 50:180, 1982.
30. Sharma AD, O'Neill PG: Wolff-Parkinson-White syndrome, *Curr Treat Options Cardiovasc Med* 1:117-126, 1999.
31. Fox JL: Experimental relationship of radiofrequency electrical current and lesion size for application to percutaneous cordotomy, *J Neurosurg* 33:415-421, 1970.
32. Pawl RP: Percutaneous radiofrequency electrocoagulation in the control of chronic pain, *Surg Clin North Am* 55:167-179, 1975.
33. Dickson JA, Calderwood SK: Temperature range and selective sensitivity of tumors to hyperthermia: a critical review, *Ann NY Acad Sci* 335:180-205, 1980.
34. Huang SK, Jordan N, Graham A et al: Closed-chest catheter desiccation of atrioventricular junction using radiofrequency energy—a new method of catheter ablation [abstract]. *Circulation* 72:III-389, 1985.
35. Huang SK, Bharati S, Lev M, Marcus FI: Electrophysiologic and histologic observations of chronic atrioventricular block induced by closed-chest catheter desiccation with radiofrequency energy, *PACE* 10:805-816, 1987.
36. Huang SK, Graham AR, Bharati S et al: Short-and long-term effects of transcatheter ablation of the coronary sinus by radiofrequency energy, *Circulation* 78:416-427, 1988.
37. Jackman WM, Kick K-H, Naccarelli GV, et al: Catheter ablation at the tricuspid annulus using radiofrequency current in canines [abstract], *J Am Coll Cardiol* 9:99A, 1987.
38. Jackman WM, Kuck KH, Naccarelli GV et al: Radiofrequency current directed across the mitral valve annulus with a bipolar epicardial-endocardial catheter electrode configuration in dogs, *Circulation* 78:1288, 1988.
39. Jackman WM, Wang W, Friday KJ et al: Catheter ablation of accessory atrioventricular pathways (Wolff-Parkinson-White syndrome) by radiofrequency current, *N Engl J Med* 324:1605, 1991.
40. Calkins H, Souza J, El-Atassi R et al: Diagnosis and cure of the Wolff-Parkinson-White syndrome of paroxysmal supraventricular tachycardias during a single electrophysiologic test, *N Engl J Med* 324:1612, 1991.
41. Schluter M, Geiger M, Siebels J et al: Catheter ablation using radiofrequency current to cure symptomatic patients with tachyarrhythmias related to an accessory atrioventricular pathway, *Circulation* 84:1644, 1991.
42. Schluter M, Schluter CA, Cappato R et al: [Anatomic distribution, conduction properties and recurrences after ablation of multiple in comparison with single accessory conduction pathways], *Z Kardiol* 86:221-230, 1997.
43. Dagres N, Clague JR, Lottkamp H et al: Impact of radiofrequency catheter ablation of accessory pathways on the frequency of atrial fibrillation during long-term follow-up; High recurrence rate of atrial fibrillation in patients older than 50 years of age, *Eur Heart J* 22:423-427, 2001.
44. Hluchy J: Mahaim fibers: electrophysiologic characteristics and radiofrequency ablation, *Z Kardiol* 89 (Suppl):136-143, 2000.
45. Mahaim I, Winston RM: Recherches d'anatomie comparee et de pathologie experimentale sur les connexions hautes du faisceau de His-Tawara, *Cardiologia* 5:189, 1941.
46. Clerc A, Levy R, Critesco C: A propos du raccourcissement permanent de l'espace P-R de l'≥ctrocardiogramme sans d≥formation du complexe ventriculaire, *Arch Mal Coeur* 31:569, 1938.
47. Lown B, Ganong WF, Levine SA: The syndrome of short P-R interval, normal QRS complex and paroxysmal rapid heart activation, *Circulation* 5:693, 1952.

CHAPTER 22

Wellens Syndrome

Wellens syndrome consists of specific ST-T wave changes in V_2 and V_3 during the *pain-free period* in a patient with unstable angina, indicating critical stenosis high in the left anterior descending (LAD) coronary artery. Recognition of such a pattern and confirmation by subsequent cardiac catheterization identify the need for bypass grafting or percutaneous transluminal coronary angioplasty. Such intervention would prevent the development of extensive anterior wall myocardial infarction (MI). In view of the large area of the ventricle at risk, the recognition of this electrocardiogram (ECG) pattern takes on critical importance.

- Prior angina
- Progressive, deep, symmetric T wave inversion
- Little or no enzyme elevation
- Little or no ST elevation
- No loss of R wave progression

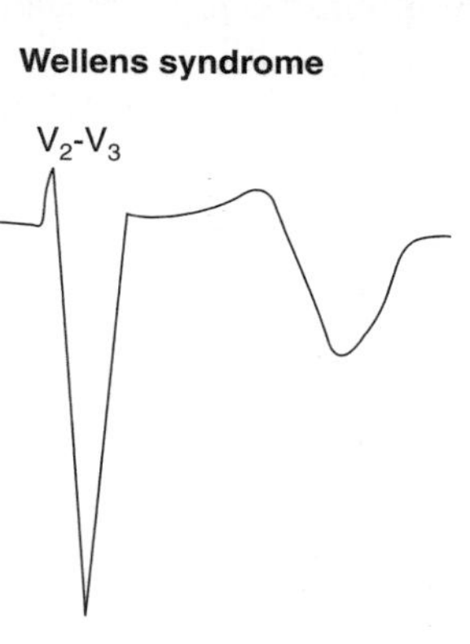

HISTORICAL BACKGROUND

In 1981 and 1982 and again in 1985, 1986, and 1989 the Wellens group in Maastricht, The Netherlands, described in lectures[1,2] and publications[2-4] criteria by which critical stenosis high in the left anterior descending coronary artery could be diagnosed from specific ST-T segment changes on or shortly after admission to the hospital. The initial published study[3] involved 145 consecutive patients who were admitted because of unstable angina, of whom 26 had what is now recognized as Wellens syndrome, the classic pattern for critical proximal LAD coronary artery stenosis and imminent (mean period, 8.5 days) extensive anterior wall MI. Another study reported on 180 consecutive patients with unstable angina who had this distinctive, easily recognized ECG pattern.[4] The term *Wellens syndrome* has become an expedient way of communicating the need for urgency. Many patients with unstable angina have benefited from these important studies by the Wellens group.

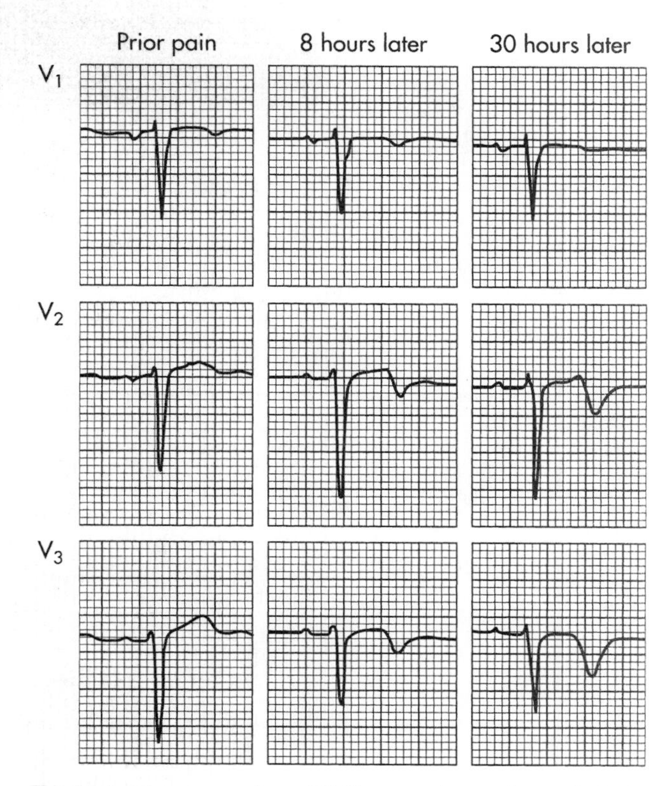

FIG. 22-1. The progression of Wellens syndrome from admission in the emergency department to 30 hours later, before angiography. Note the dramatic changes in the T waves of V_2 and V_3 compared to the insignificant changes in V_2.

ECG RECOGNITION (PAIN-FREE)

- Progressive, deep T wave inversion in V_2 and V_3 during pain-free periods
- Little or no ST segment elevation (<1 mm); the ST segments in leads V_2 and V_3 turn down into negative T waves at an ST-T angle of 60 to 90 degrees. If the T wave is also inverted in V_1, this angle is wider
- No loss of precordial R wave progression

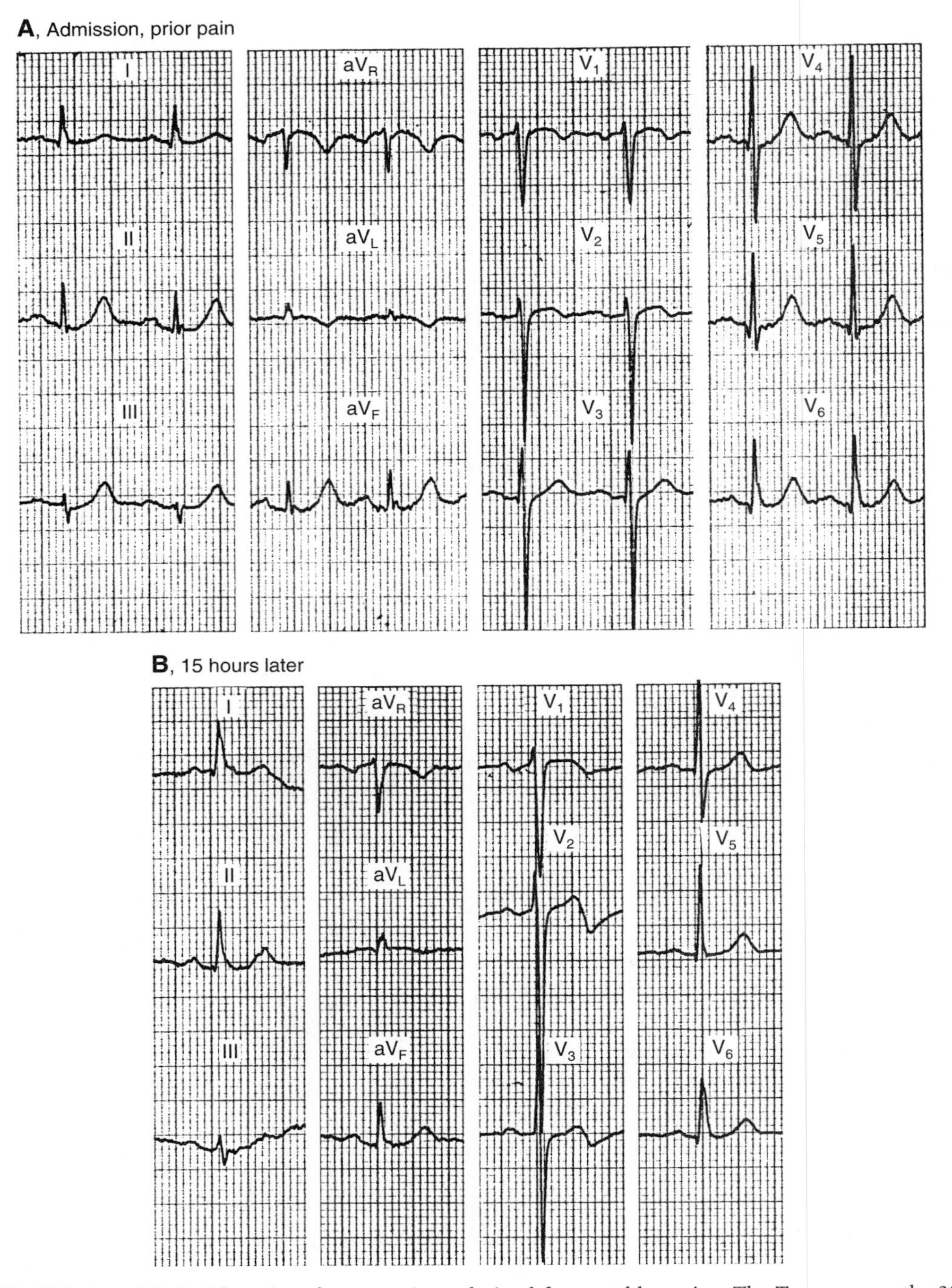

FIG. 22-2. **A** and **B**, Serial tracings from a patient admitted for unstable angina. The T waves over the 30 hours before angiography demonstrate the progressive, deep, symmetric inversion of the T wave typical of Wellens syndrome.

Continued

Fig. 22-1 is a series of ECGs showing V_1, V_2, and V_3 from a patient admitted for unstable angina. His angiogram showed 98% occlusion of the LAD. Note that the T wave in V_1 changed very little and was not diagnostic, whereas the T waves in V_2 and V_3 were changing dramatically and diagnostically. Enzymes were not elevated.

Although leads V_2 and V_3 are the diagnostic leads for Wellens syndrome, the T wave inversion is not necessarily limited to those leads. In a study involving 180 patients, the ST-T segment abnormalities seen in V_2 and V_3 were also found in lead V_1 in 121 patients, in lead V_4 in 136 patients, and sometimes in leads V_5 and V_6.[4]

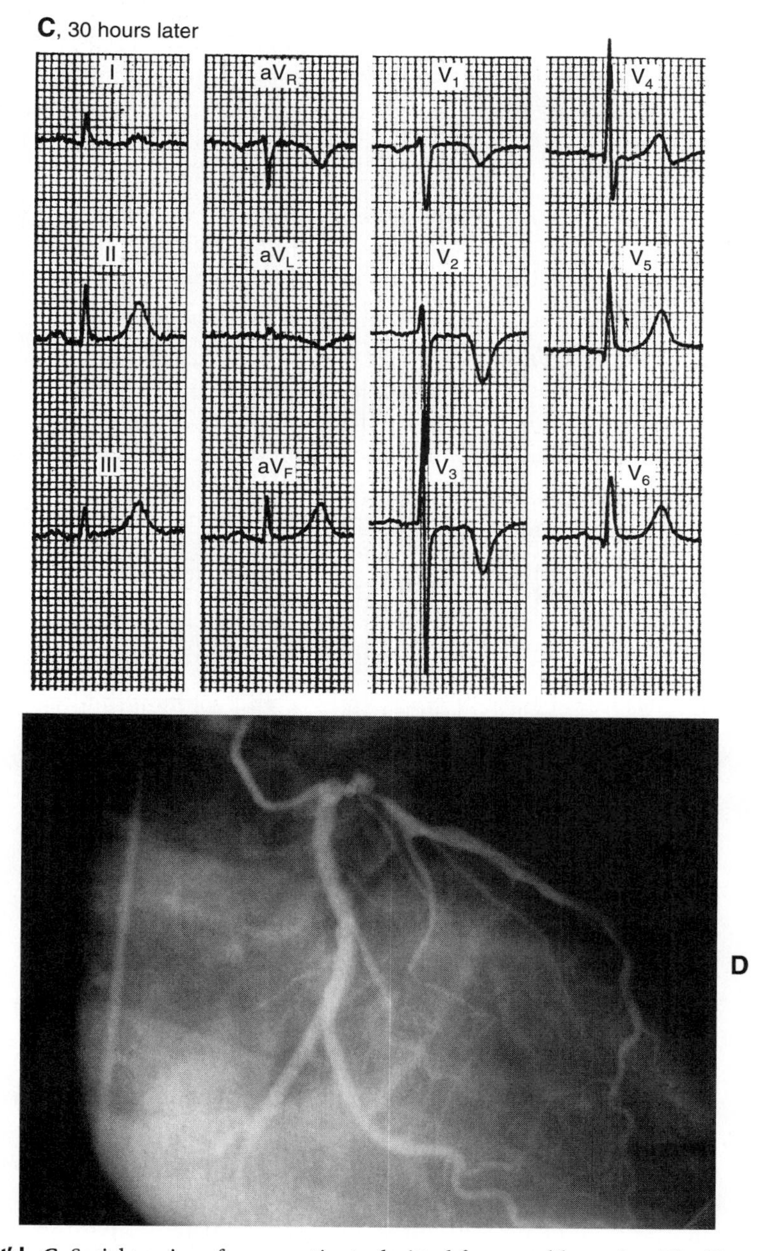

FIG. 22-2, cont'd. C, Serial tracings from a patient admitted for unstable angina. The T wave over the 30 hours before angiography demonstrate the progressive, deep, symmetric inversion of the T wave typical of Wellens syndrome. **D**, Angiogram from the same patient. (Courtesy Morgan Carroll, BSN, Kingman, Ariz.)

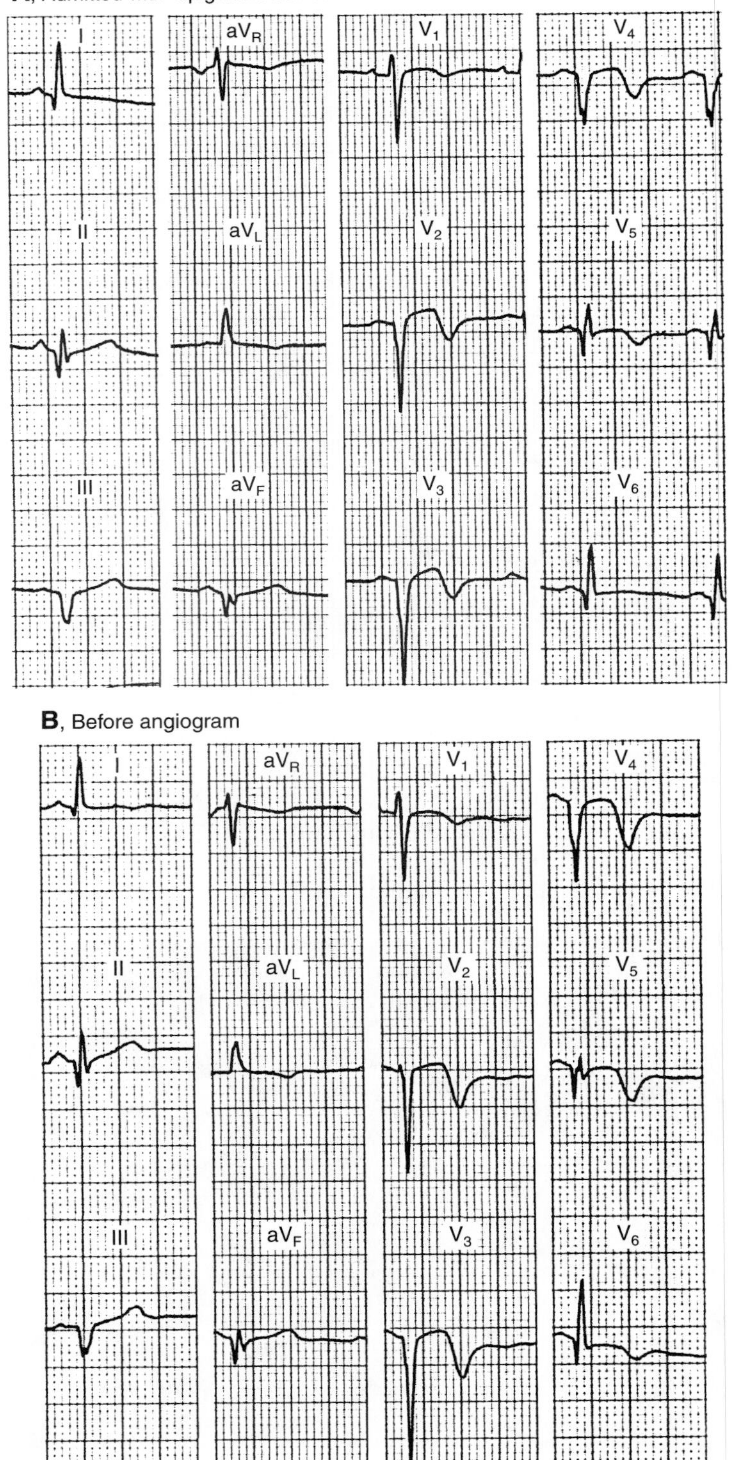

FIG. 22-3. A and B, Wellens syndrome in a patient with an old inferior and anterior myocardial infarction and apical aneurysm. The tracings were taken over 3 days. (Courtesy Sue Prather, RN, Kirksville, Mo.)

The series of 12-lead ECGs in Fig. 22-2 is from a patient admitted for unstable angina. In the admission 12-lead ECG the depression at the end of the T wave in leads V_1 and V_2 is not yet diagnostic. However, in a patient with prior chest pain you are alerted to the possibility of Wellens syndrome and carefully watch V_2 and V_3. The ECG in Fig. 22-2, *B*, from the same patient taken 15 hours after admission, is typical for Wellens syndrome. At this point an emergency angiogram should be done to confirm the diagnosis and determine management. Thirty hours after admission the patient is in the cardiac catheterization laboratory, his T waves in leads V_2 and V_3 are deeply and symmetrically inverted. The angiogram is shown in Fig. 22-2, *D*. There is critical occlusion of the proximal LAD.

The 68-year-old man whose ECG is seen in Fig. 22-3, *A* and *B*, was admitted with "epigastric distress." He had an old inferior and anterior wall MI and an apical aneurysm. Monitoring the patient on lead V_2, the nurse was alerted to the signs of Wellens syndrome. An arteriogram revealed 98% occlusion of the LAD. He was discharged after bypass and removal of the aneurysm.

Fig. 22-4 is an example of a less common pattern in Wellens syndrome in which a positive T wave plunges into a symmetrically negative terminal portion. This pattern was found in 44 of the 204 patients in the study by the Wellens group.[4]

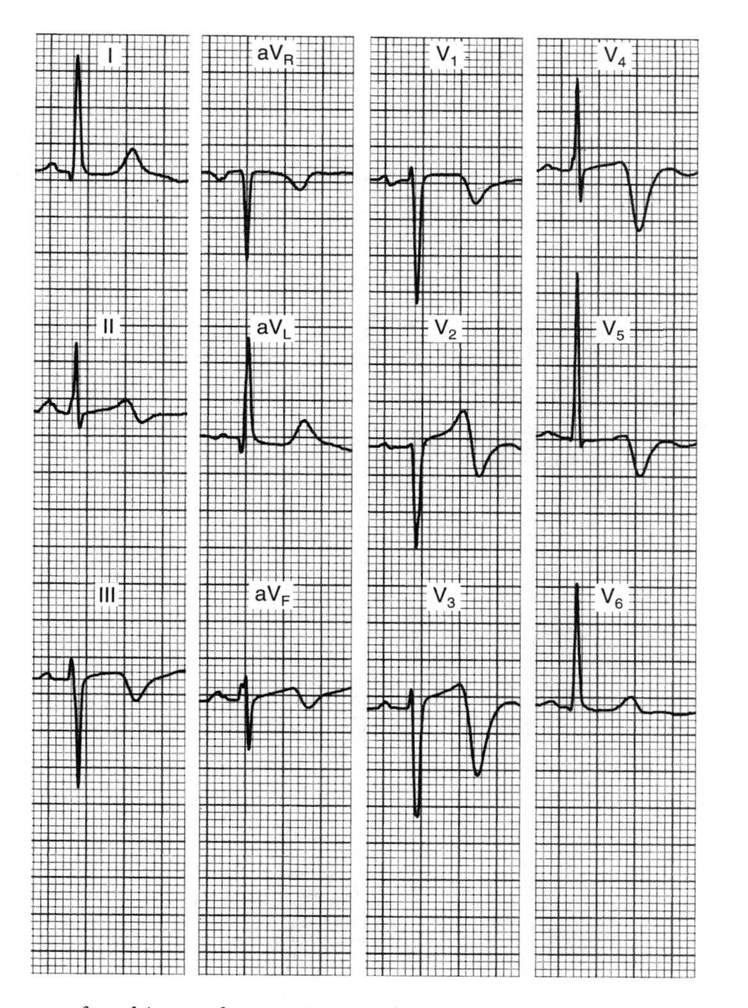

FIG. 22-4. ECG pattern found in 44 of 204 patients in the study by the Wellens group. (Courtesy Jerilyn Briten, RN, Nampa, Idaho.)

Time Frame

The typical ECG findings in Wellens syndrome were present:

- At admission or developed shortly thereafter in 60% of the 180 patients
- Within 24 hours in the majority of the remainder of patients
- Within 2 to 5 days in a few patients

In the study by the Wellens group,[4] patients who had ECG signs at the time of admission had a longer duration of unstable angina and had a higher incidence of collateral vessels than did patients whose ECG signs developed later.

The 12-lead ECG in Fig. 22-5 was recorded on admission to the emergency department. The patient was a 51-year-old woman who complained of chest pain. The ECG changes of Wellens syndrome were present on admission; cardiac catheterization revealed 99% occlusion of the proximal LAD. This patient required an airlift because of the time factor concern. There was 99% occlusion of the proximal LAD.

Fig. 22-6 shows a series of 12-lead ECGs taken from a 90-year-old woman for whom the cardiac catheterization would have itself carried too great a risk. The time span from admission to massive anterior wall MI was 12 hours. Her admission tracing already shows dramatic signs of reperfusion. These tracings represent the 12-hour span without pain (Fig. 22-6, *A*), with pain (Fig. 22-6, *B*), and after having sustained anterior wall MI, right bundle branch block, and anterior hemiblock (Fig. 22-6, *C*). It was difficult for all who were caring for her during this time, knowing that at any time the proximal LAD would finally occlude irreversibly. It was also a wake-up call for those who may ignore this syndrome.

ECG DURING PAIN

Below is a series of ECGs from a 35-year-old woman who was complaining of "epigastric pain." Upon admission signs of critical proximal LAD stenosis were noted. During pain the ST segment is elevated in V_1 to V_3. Following pain the signs of reperfusion are present (Wellens syndrome). As you can see in the tracings, inverted T wave in V_2 and V_3 is a sign of reperfusion after a transient narrowing of the proximal LAD coronary artery. During chest pain these T wave changes are replaced by positive T waves with either ST-segment

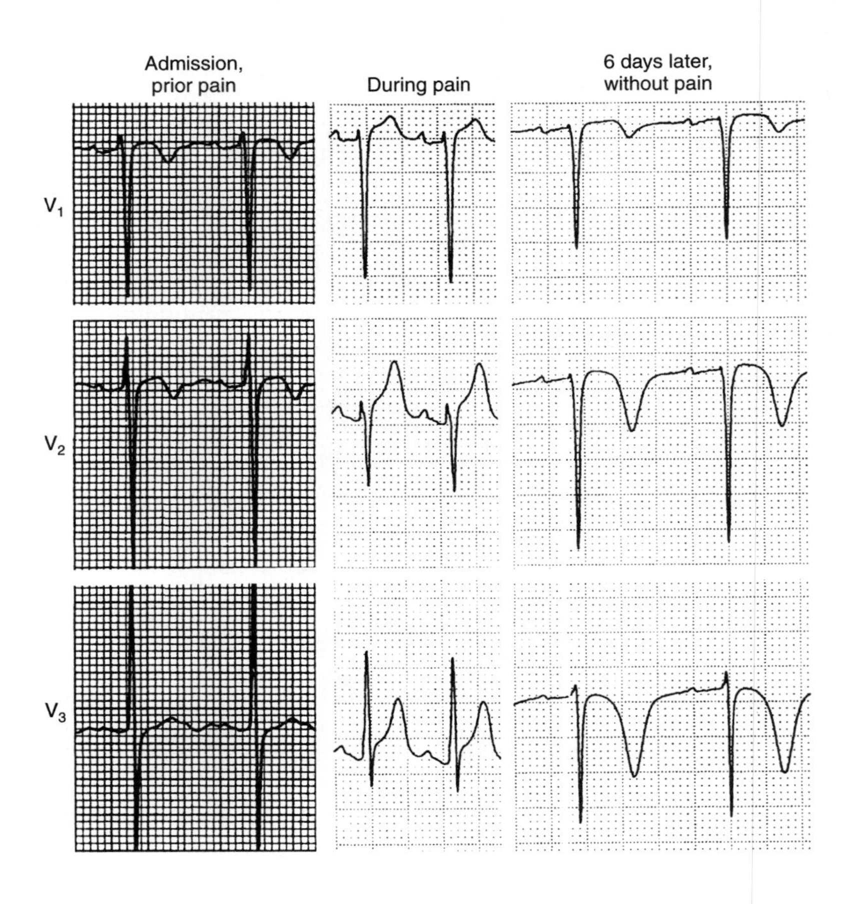

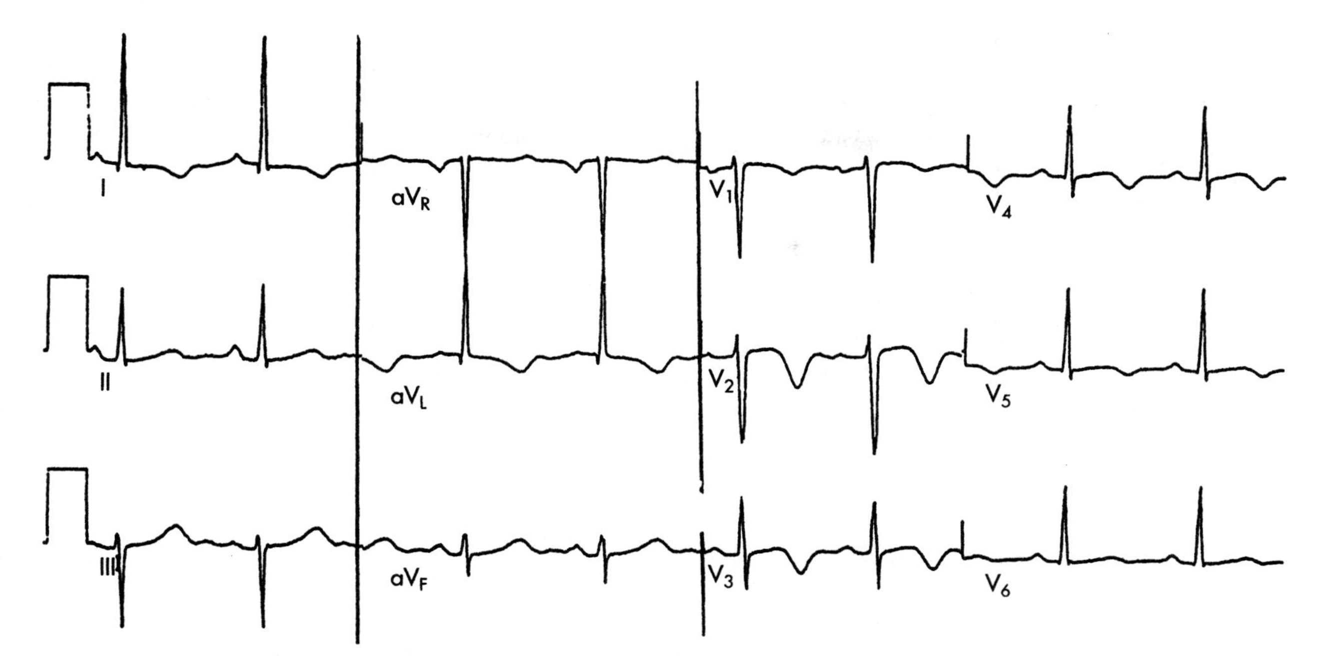

FIG. 22-5. Wellens syndrome. The 12-lead ECG was obtained in the emergency department, and the diagnosis made by Rebecca Fuller, RN, of Monterey, Calif. The patient was flown to San Jose, Calif, for cardiac catheterization. There was 99% occlusion of the proximal left anterior descending.

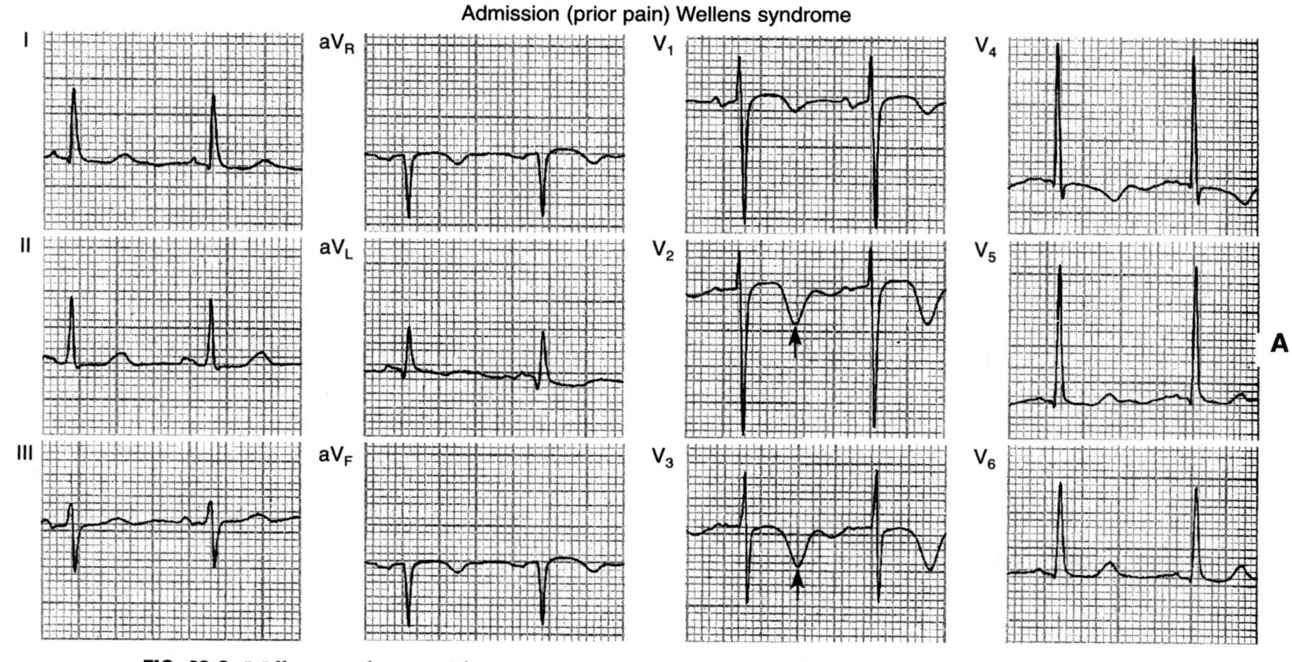

FIG. 22-6. Wellens syndrome with progression to anterior myocardial infarction *(MI)* within a 12-hour period. **A,** Admission ECG (prior pain).

Continued

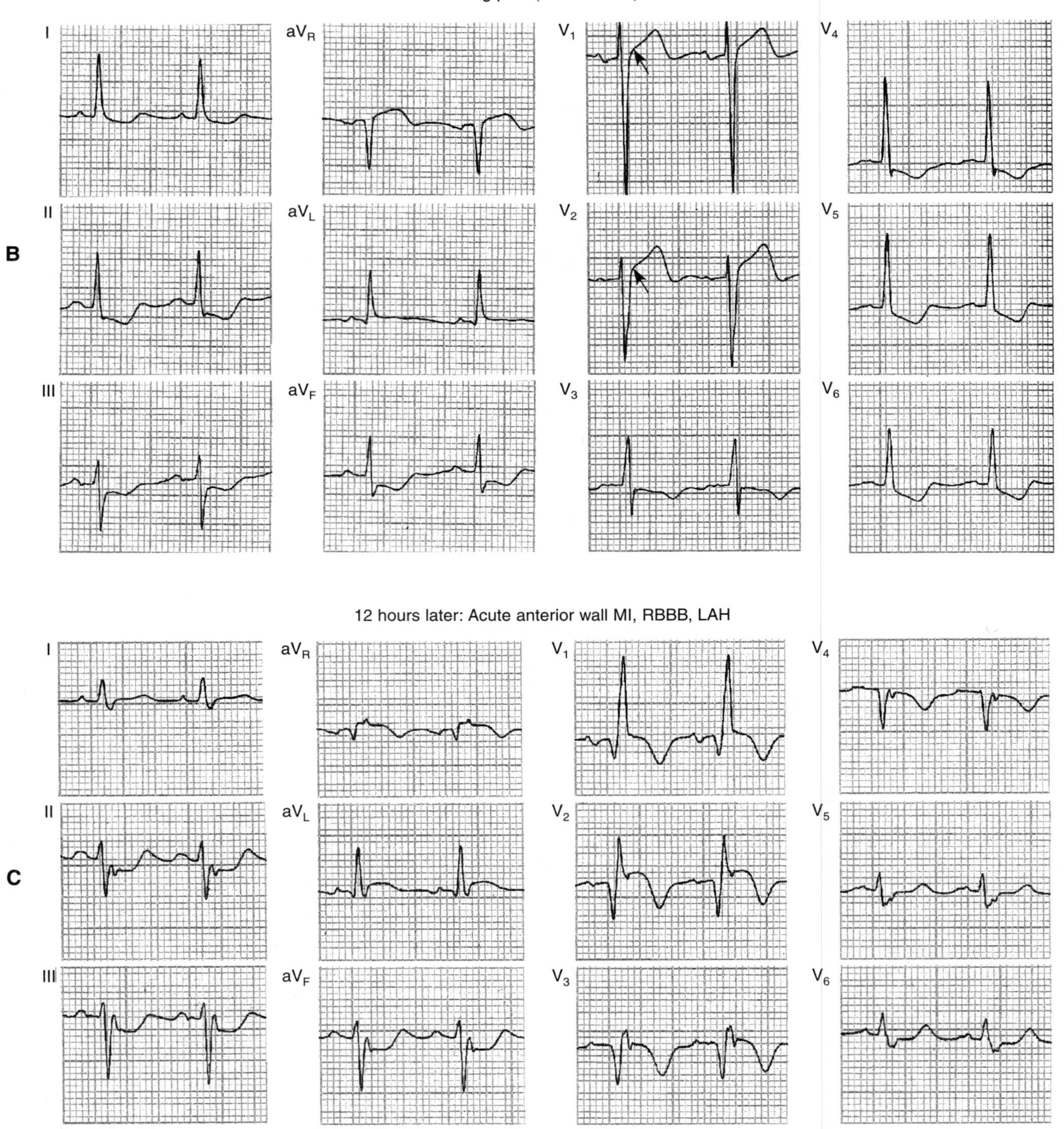

FIG. 22-6, cont'd. **B**, During pain. **C**, Anterior MI, right bundle branch block *(RBBB)* and anterior hemiblock *(LAH)*. The diagnosis of Wellens syndrome was made by Mary E. Thomas, RN, of South Whitley, Ind, but because of the patient's advanced age there was no cardiac catheterization.

elevation or depression. During this time the coronary vessel is critically narrowed or occluding; the T wave inversion of Wellens syndrome represents reperfusion.

The ECG series shown in Fig. 22-7 is from a 69-year-old man with unstable angina who was admitted to the coronary care unit. His admission tracing showed Wellens syndrome. Note that 8 hours later, during pain, there is ST-segment elevation as the coronary vessel critically narrows or occludes. Ten hours later he was without pain prior to coronary artery bypass surgery. Note that the T waves in V_2 and V_3 have deepened, showing signs of reperfusion. His cardiac catheterization revealed 95% occlusion of the proximal LAD and 90% occlusion of the right coronary and circumflex arteries. He was discharged on his sixth hospital day without complications. During the evolution of the dramatic changes taking place in leads V_2 and V_3, lead II remained the same and V_1 was not diagnostic, again emphasizing that patients with unstable angina must be monitored on lead V_2 or V_3.

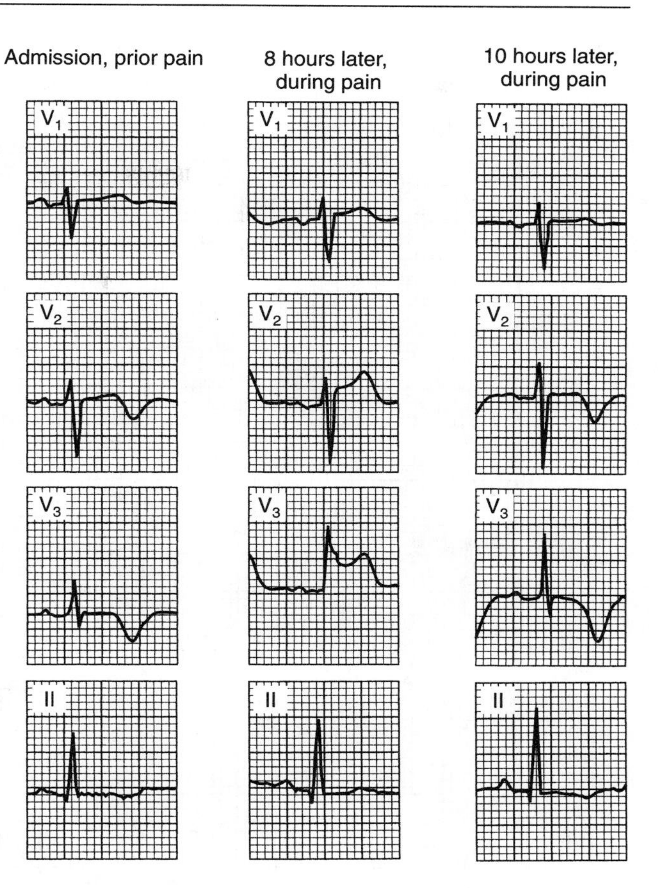

FIG. 22-7. Wellens syndrome on admission. The creatine kinase was 97, and the patient is without pain at the time. Eight hours later the patient is in pain; note the elevated ST segments in V_2 and V_3. Ten hours later, before bypass surgery, he is without pain and his ECG shows signs of reperfusion. These dramatic events are not seen on the usual monitoring leads of V_1 and II. (Courtesy Darlene Boomhower, RN, La Mirada, Calif.)

DIAGNOSTIC MONITORING LEADS

Often patients with unstable angina are admitted to telemetry units where nurses may not have the capability of monitoring on multiple leads. In such cases or in the intensive care unit or coronary care unit where this is also the situation, the choice of monitoring leads is very important. It is not sufficient to admit the patient, monitor on lead V_1 or II, and await the next day's routine 12-lead ECG. Fig. 22-8 illustrates the obvious development of Wellens syndrome in leads V_2 and V_3 whereas leads V_1 and II remain virtually unchanged.

If a unipolar V_2 or V_3 lead is not available for monitoring, the bipolar modified chest lead (MCL) MCL_2 or MCL_3 should be used. Fig. 22-9 demonstrates the use of MCL_3 to monitor a patient who was admitted with unstable angina. The 12-lead ECG obtained on admission showed no signs of an occluding coronary artery or reperfusion. The patient was monitored on MCL_3. When the T wave inverted, an emergency 12-lead ECG was ordered, the physician was called, and the patient was flown from Le Grande, Ore, to Portland. Cardiac catheterization revealed 95% occlusion of the proximal LAD.

EMERGENCY ANGIOGRAPHY

Because patients with Wellens syndrome without intervention may be imminently destined for massive anterior wall MI, emergency angiography to identify candidates for early revascularization is justified. The morbidity and mortality resulting from cardiac catheterization and revascularization surgery are less than those resulting from extensive anterior wall MI. In the past, in patients with the ECG findings that are now recognized as Wellens syndrome the condition had been diagnosed as either nontransmural or subendocardial ischemia (in the absence of enzyme changes) or subendocardial infarction of the anterior wall in the presence of slight enzyme elevation. However, patients with Wellens syndrome have not yet had the acute episode of MI.

LEFT MAIN AND THREE-VESSEL CORONARY ARTERY DISEASE

Left main and three-vessel coronary artery disease can be diagnosed in patients with unstable angina from specific ST-T segment changes in the 12-lead ECG

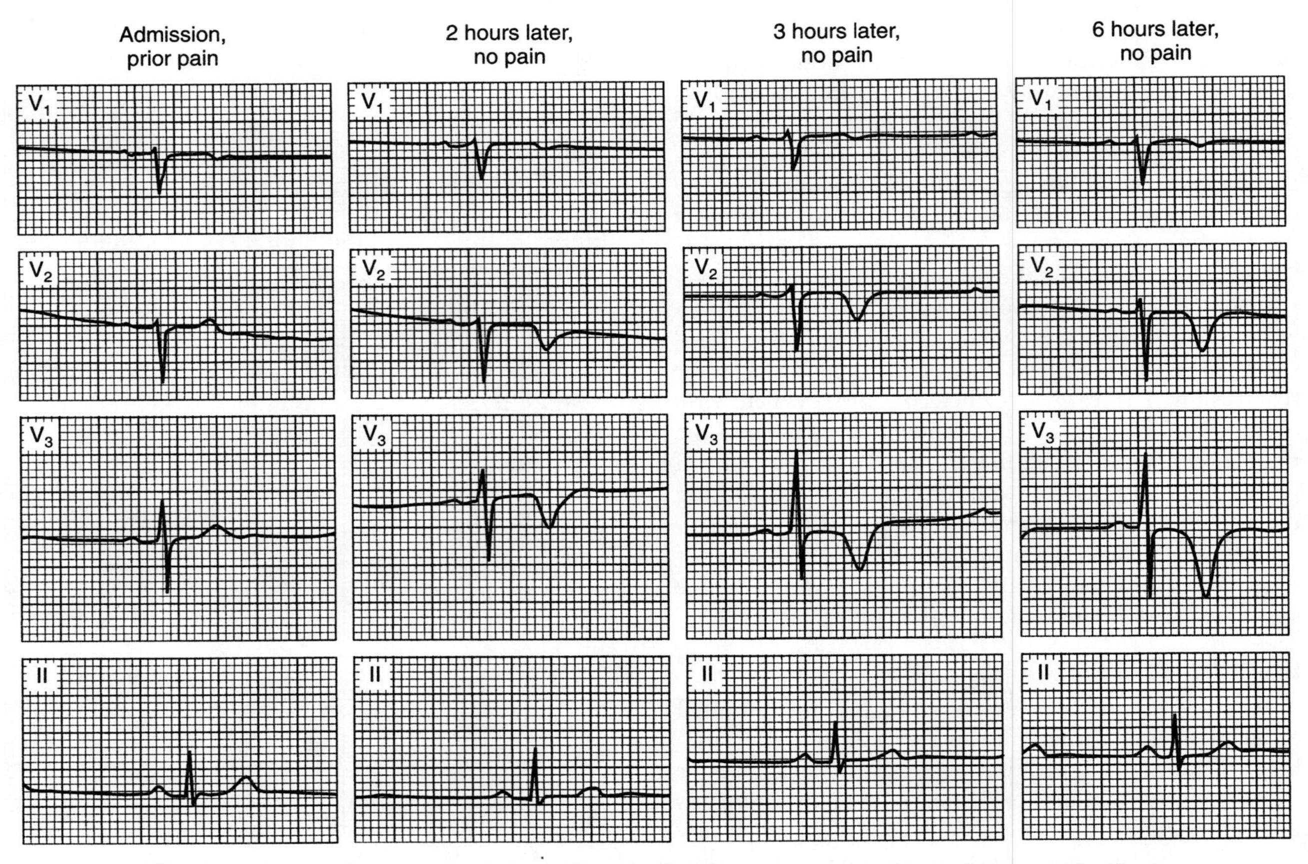

FIG. 22-8. The two diagnostic leads for Wellens syndrome are unquestionably leads V_2 and V_3. Classic picture of progressive, symmetric, deep inversion of the T wave in leads V_2 and V_3 in a patient with 97% occlusion of the proximal left anterior descending. The T waves in leads V_1 and II do not change significantly.

(Fig. 22-10). It is important to recognize this ECG pattern so that emergency cardiac catheterization can be performed and the myocardium revascularized before infarction occurs.

ECG Recognition

- ST elevation in aV_R and V_1
- ST depression in eight or more leads

Record a 12-lead ECG during chest pain because the tracing may be normal during a pain-free period. It is important to record the 12-lead ECG when the patient has pain. In a study involving 125 patients with left main coronary artery disease it was found that 25% have a normal ECG when they are without pain, even with as much as 91% to 99% occlusion of the left main coronary artery. In the same study the most frequently seen ECG pattern was ST depression in leads V_3 to V_5 and ST elevation in leads V_1 and aV_R. Lead V_4 showed ST depression in 67% of patients.[5,6]

UNSTABLE ANGINA

Unstable angina is cardiac pain caused by severe transient myocardial ischemia resulting from severe coronary narrowing or coronary occlusion.

Incidence

Unstable angina has become the most frequent indication for admission to most coronary care units, being responsible for more than 570,000 hospitalizations annu-

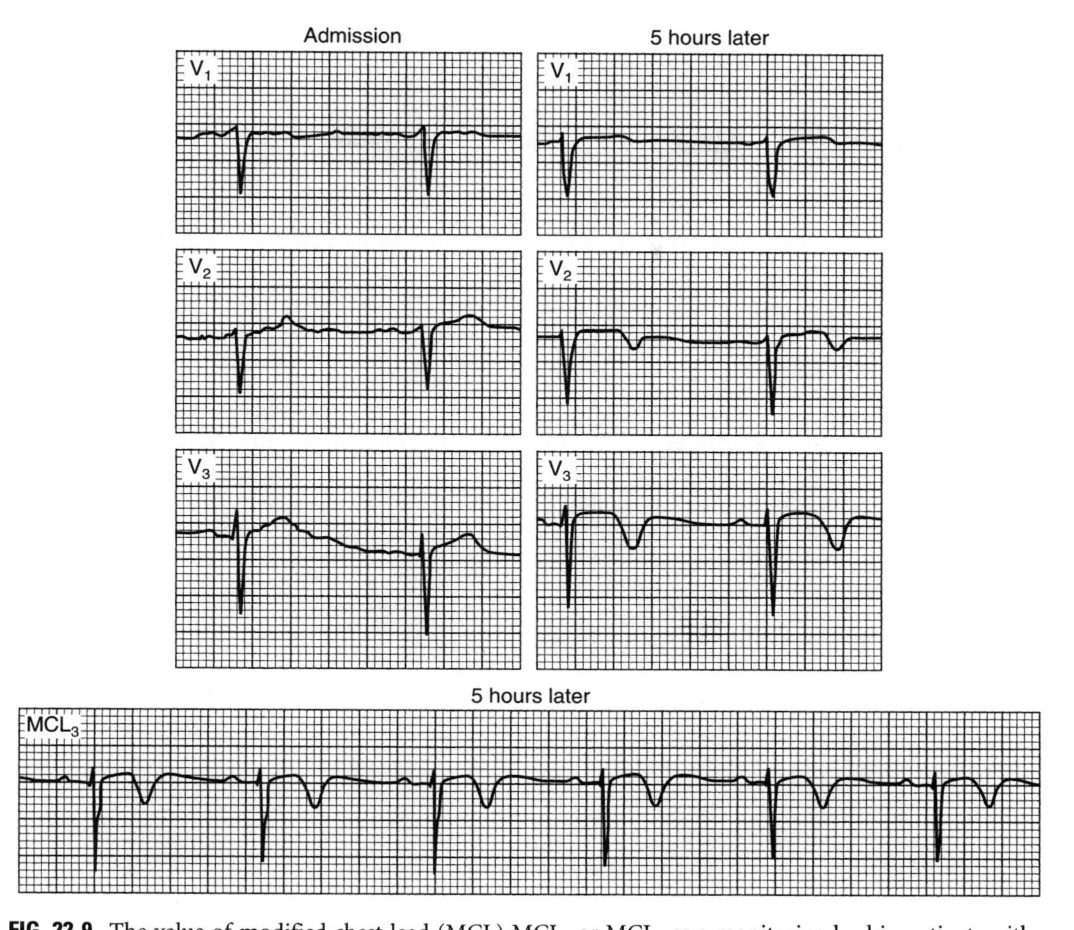

FIG. 22-9. The value of modified chest lead (MCL) MCL_2 or MCL_3 as a monitoring lead in patients with unstable angina. The patient was admitted with unstable angina. Five hours later the monitoring lead, MCL_3, showed Wellens syndrome and an emergency 12-lead ECG was obtained, confirming the diagnosis. Cardiac catheterization revealed 95% occlusion of the proximal left anterior descending, total right coronary artery occlusion, and 50% occlusion in both the left main and the circumflex coronary artery. The diagnosis was made from the monitoring lead MCL_3 and the serial 12-lead ECGs by B.J. Brown, RN, and Norma Follett, RN, of Le Grande, Ore.

ally in the United States. In more than 70,000 of those hospitalized with unstable angina, MI develops, and some people die suddenly. Of the patients admitted with acute MI, 30% to 60% have unstable angina before they reach the hospital.[7]

Type of Pain

- Recent onset
- Sudden worsening of preexisting angina
- Occurs after a pain-free period
- Stuttering recurrence over days and weeks

Identifying Characteristics

- Not "momentary" in duration
- Occurs at rest or is brought on by minimal exertion, commonly by walking or use of the arms
- Patient may describe "walking through" or "walking off" the pain
- During pain, blood pressure and heart rate are usually elevated, S_3 gallop is heard, and the patient resists lying down
- Relieved by sublingual nitroglycerin within a few (less than 5) minutes

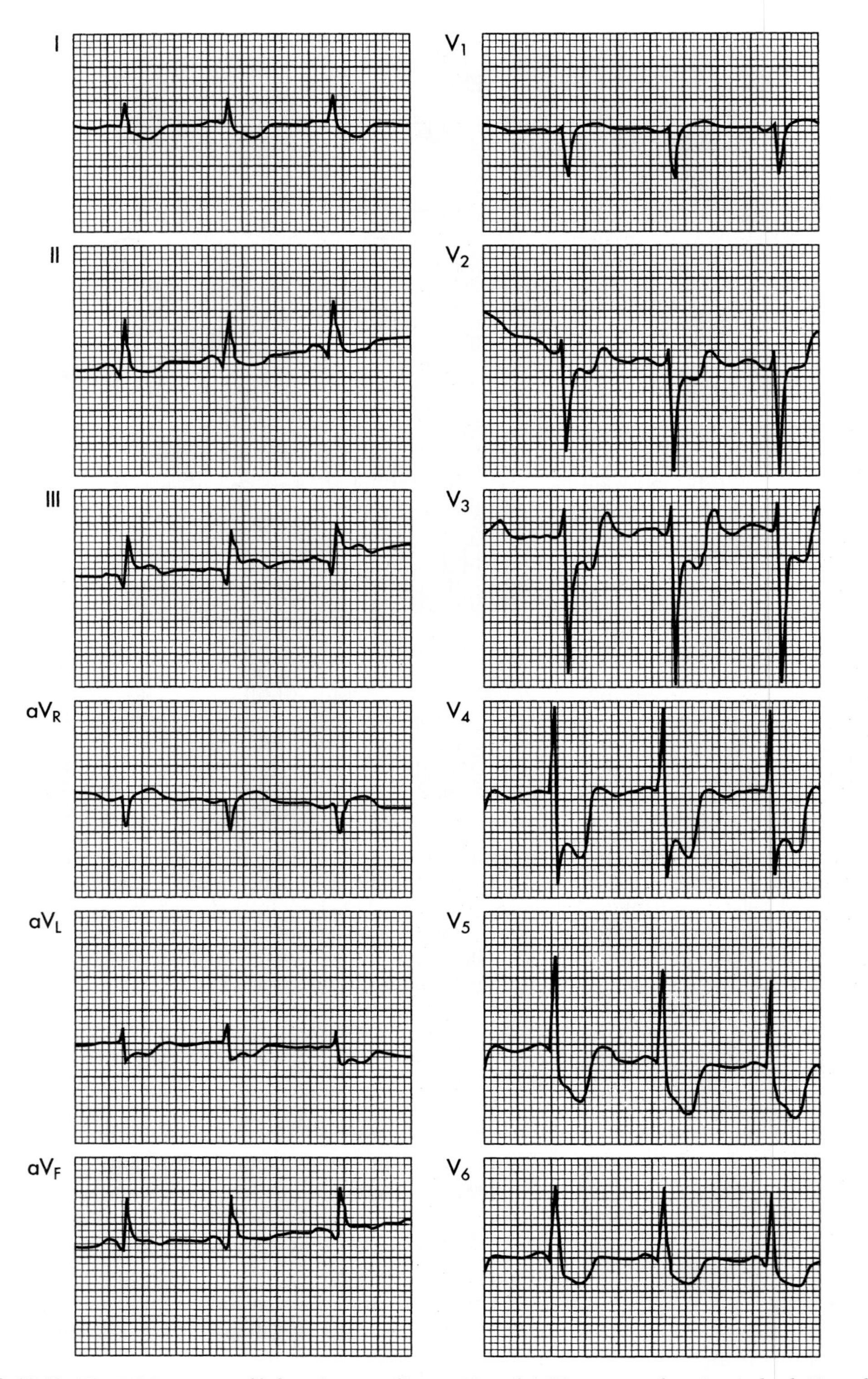

FIG. 22-10. The ECG pattern of left main stem disease. Note the ST segment elevation in leads V_1 and aV_R and the ST segment depression in the remainder of the precordial leads and in leads I, II, and aV_L. The patient had an old inferior myocardial infarction. (From Wellens HJJ, Conover M: *The ECG in emergency decision making*, Philadelphia, 1992, WB Saunders.)

Anginal Pain

Anginal pain may radiate to the following:

- Any region above the waist
- Epigastric location (may confuse the diagnosis)
- Medial aspect of arms and the mandible (most characteristic location)
- Retrosternal area (highly specific)

Note: Localization of the pain to small areas is unusual.

Patients' Common Descriptions of Anginal Pain

- Tightness, heaviness, squeezing, choking, aching, burning, a weight, or numbness
- Duration: "Lasts about 2 minutes" (patients tend to overestimate)
- Builds up gradually, plateaus, and subsides gradually

Words and phrases patients use to describe angina pectoris[8] include the following (with thanks to J. Willis Hurst, MD):

- "A red hot poker"
- "A shoe box in my chest"
- "A toothache"
- "Hot flame in the upper part of my mouth"
- "An elephant on my chest"
- "Jaw pain"
- "Arthritis" (shoulder, elbow, or wrists)
- "A bad feeling in the upper portion of my back"
- "Tracheitis"
- "A good feeling in my chest—like I used to have in my side when I ran as a child"
- "Sternal whisper"
- "Dryness in my throat produced by effort or emotional stress"
- "Smoke in my chest"
- "Someone choking me from behind"

One patient in Hurst's study described severe, moderate, and mild discomfort as follows:

Severe discomfort: "A large fish hook stuck under my jaw" (hung up and suspended from a scaffold)
Moderate discomfort: "A small fish hook caught in my lower jaw"
Mild discomfort: "A needle and thread being pulled between two lower teeth"

Pain That Is Not Anginal

- Occurs after, rather than during, exertion
- Caused by talking
- Caused by "lying on the left side"
- Occurs after, rather than during, coitus
- Precipitated exclusively by emotion
- Associated with palpitations, precordial tenderness, lightheadedness, or dysphagia
- "Sharp" (anginal pain is not sticking or needlelike)

Pathogenesis

Plaque fissure. During the pain of unstable angina there is increased thrombin generation. The most widely proposed mechanism for the increased thrombin formation that heralds the onset of the acute event is plaque fissure. The complicated events after plaque fissure are the

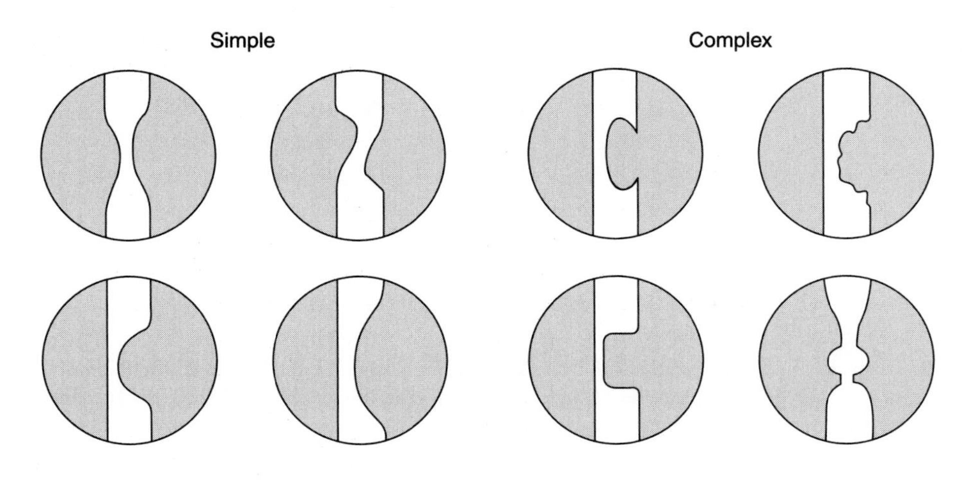

FIG. 22-11. Schema of the most common coronary lesion geometries found at angiography (discrete simple versus discrete complex lesions). (From Ambrose JA, Israel DH: *Am J Cardiol* 68:78B, 1991.)

following: exposure of endothelial collagen and its prothrombotic substrates to flowing blood, platelet aggregation, release of a vasospastic substance, coagulation, and thrombus formation.

A fibrous cap covers the atherosclerotic plaque. Thinning of this cap causes its delicate latticework of collagen to tear, usually at the junction of its attachment to normal intima, producing a fissure into the plaque. This tear constitutes an injury to the artery, which responds with the formation of a platelet-rich thrombus. The deeper the injury, the more layers of platelet deposition. For example, a mild injury such as endothelial denudation would result in a single layer of platelet deposition as long as the event was not accompanied by severe stenosis, which itself is a stimulus for enhanced platelet deposition. A deep injury, such as a tear into the internal elastic lamina of the artery or into the plaque fissure, results in platelet deposition within milliseconds; total occlusion may occur within minutes. The occluding lesion is typically complex with irregular, ragged borders (Fig. 22-11).[9]

After the tearing event several things can happen to the thrombus, as illustrated in Fig. 22-12.

In Fig. 22-12, *A,* the tear gets bigger until the lumen of the vessel occludes, resulting in acute MI and perhaps sudden death. In Fig. 22-12, *B,* it partially and perhaps critically obstructs the lumen, resulting in unstable angina with or without non–Q-wave MI and perhaps sudden death. In Fig. 22-12, *C,* it may be incorporated into the lesion and the fissure may heal over, resulting in no symptoms. In Fig. 22-12, *D,* it may become organized and may produce more symptoms. In Fig. 22-12, *E,* the thrombus may embolize.[10]

Transient intermittent lymphocyte activation. Doubts have arisen about the concept of plaque fissure being responsible for the events leading to unstable angina. The hypothesis is that the events precipitating unstable angina represent an acute, transient inflammatory state caused by lymphocyte activation that is intermittently triggered by unknown factors. Thus the string of events leading to the unstable pain is proposed to be exposure of

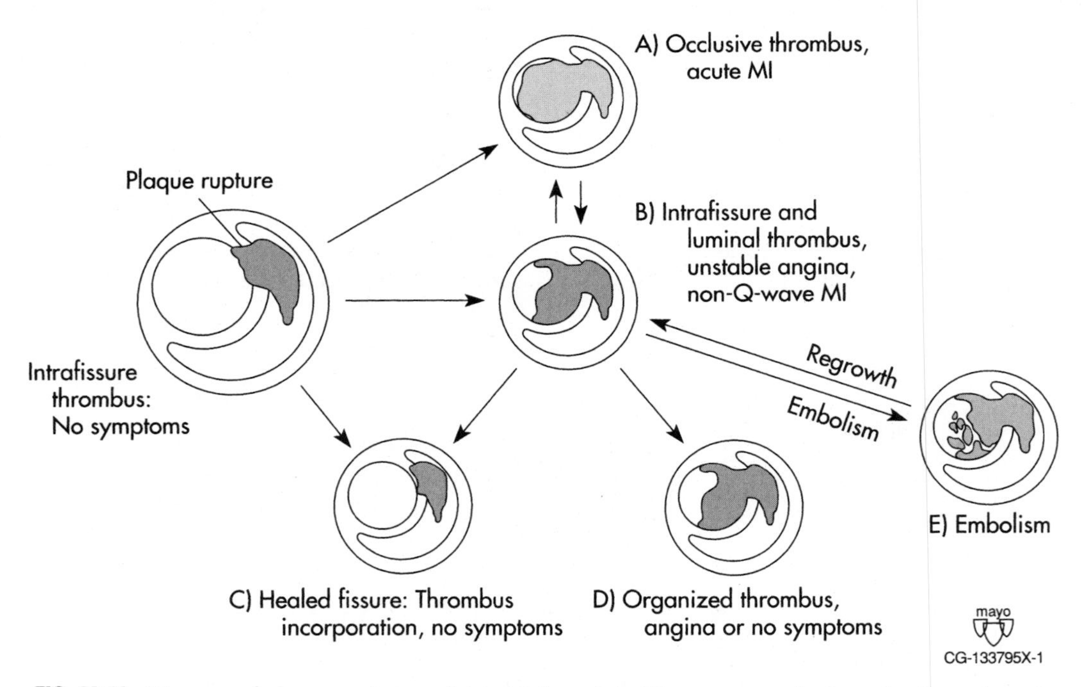

FIG. 22-12. Diagram of plaque rupture and arterial thrombus. Plaque rupture leads to the formation of a fissure. Flowing blood contacts intraarterial structures and forms an intrafissure thrombus. The thrombus may progress to a luminal thrombus causing, *A,* total occlusion, often associated with transmural or Q wave myocardial infarction *(MI)*. *B,* Incomplete occlusion resulting in unstable angina or non–Q-wave MI. *B* and *C,* The intraluminal thrombus may undergo endogenous lysis with healing of the fissure and no progression of disease or symptoms. *D,* The intraluminal thrombus may organize, leading to progression of disease with or without subsequent symptoms. *E,* A piece of thrombus may embolize distally. (From Chesebro JH, Zoldhelyi P, Fuster V: *Am J Cardiol* 68:2B, 1991.)

lymphocytes to an inducer that triggers monocyte activation, increased thrombin generation, and thrombin formation.[11]

SUMMARY

Wellens syndrome reflects reperfusion during unstable angina in the pain-free period and includes the ECG findings of progressive, symmetric T wave inversion in leads V_2 and V_3 with no loss of precordial R wave and little or no enzyme elevation. Severe left main and three-vessel coronary artery disease is recognized because of ST elevation in two leads (V_1 and aV_R) and ST depression in eight other leads.

Although the ECG changes that are diagnostic of critical proximal LAD coronary artery stenosis are best recognized *outside* the episode of anginal pain, the abnormalities suggestive of severe left main or three-vessel coronary artery disease are most marked on the ECG recorded *during* an attack of chest pain.

This chapter has also discussed unstable angina and ECG patterns that are typical either of critical proximal LAD coronary artery stenosis (Wellens syndrome) or of left main or three-vessel coronary artery disease. Because revascularization procedures are now readily available, it is important to know how to recognize these ECG patterns so that emergency coronary arteriography can be performed to identify patients who are candidates for bypass graft or coronary angioplasty.

REFERENCES

1. Wellens HJJ: Characteristic electrocardiographic pattern indicating a critical stenosis high in left anterior descending coronary artery in patients admitted because of impending myocardial infarction. Paper presented at the Symposium on New Strategies in the Management of Ischemic Heart Disease, Scottsdale, Ariz, January 24-26, 1981.
2. Wellens HJJ: The electrocardiogram 80 years after Einthoven: the Bishop Lecture. Presented at the annual meeting of the American College of Cardiology, Anaheim, Calif, March 1985.
3. de Zwaan C, B˚r RWHM, Wellens HJJ: Characteristic electrocardiographic pattern indicating a critical stenosis high in left anterior descending coronary artery in patients admitted because of impending myocardial infarction, *Am Heart J* 103:730, 1982.
4. de Zwaan C, B˚r FW, Janssen JHA et al: Angiographic and clinical characteristics of patients with unstable angina showing an ECG pattern indicating critical narrowing of the proximal LAD coronary artery, *Am Heart J* 117:657, 1989.
5. Gorgels AP, Vos MA, B˚r FW et al: An electrocardiographic pattern, characteristic for extensive myocardial ischemia, *Circulation* (Suppl 2)78:1682, 1988.
6. Atie J, Brugada P, Smeets JLRM et al: Electrocardiographic findings during and outside an episode of chest pain in patients with left main coronary artery disease, *Circulation* 80:154, 1989.
7. Wilcox I: Risk of adverse outcome in patients admitted to the coronary care unit with suspected unstable angina pectoris, *Am J Cardiol* 64:845, 1989.
8. Hurst JW, Logue RB: Angina pectoris: words patients use and overlooked precipitating events, *Heart Dis Stroke* 2:89, 1993.
9. Ambrose JA, Israel DH: Angiography in unstable angina, *Am J Cardiol* 68:78B, 1991.
10. Chesebro JH, Zoldhelyi P, Fuster V: Pathogenesis of thrombosis in unstable angina, *Am J Cardiol* 68:2B, 1991.
11. Neri Serneri GG, Abbate R, Gori AM et al: Transient intermittent lymphocyte activation is responsible for the instability of angina, *Circulation* 86:790, 1992.

CHAPTER 23

Bundle Branch Block and Hemiblock

One of the most distinctive examples of intraventricular conduction defect is the delay or obstruction of impulse conduction in one of the bundle branches. This chapter describes the anatomy, clinical implications, prognosis, mechanisms, and electrocardiographic (ECG) patterns in bundle branch block (BBB) and hemiblock in acute myocardial infarction (MI) and in MI in its chronic form.

THE TRIFASCICULAR SPECIALIZED CONDUCTION SYSTEM

Fig. 23-1 illustrates the specialized conduction system: right bundle branch and left bundle branch with its two main fascicles (anterior and posterior). A third division (septal) sends out connecting branches between the anterior and posterior fascicles. Note the broad, ribbonlike posterior fascicle and the long, thin anterior one that is similar in shape and position to the right bundle branch. Three divisions of the left bundle branch were described and illustrated by Tawara in 1906[1] and then cast aside. Until the late 1960s, only two divisions, the right and left bundle branches, were described. From 1968 to 1973 Rosenbaum et al[2-5] described the intraventricular conduction system as trifascicular (right bundle branch and the two distinct divisions of the left bundle branch) and coined the term *hemiblock* for the condition when conduction to half of the left ventricle is impaired. Rosenbaum's work gave clinicians a new insight into previously unexplained ECG phenomena and stimulated research into the electrical activation of the intraventricular conduction system. From this work evolved the terms *left anterior hemiblock, left posterior hemiblock, bifascicular block,* and *trifascicular block,* which have been widely used.

In 1972 Demoulin and Kulbertus[6] reminded us of the validity of Tawara's original 1906 model of the left bundle branch as having three divisions instead of the two described by Rosenbaum. A left bundle branch lesion is hardly ever confined solely to a distinct anterior or posterior division. Most of the time there is a network of septal fibers between the two main left branches that may be

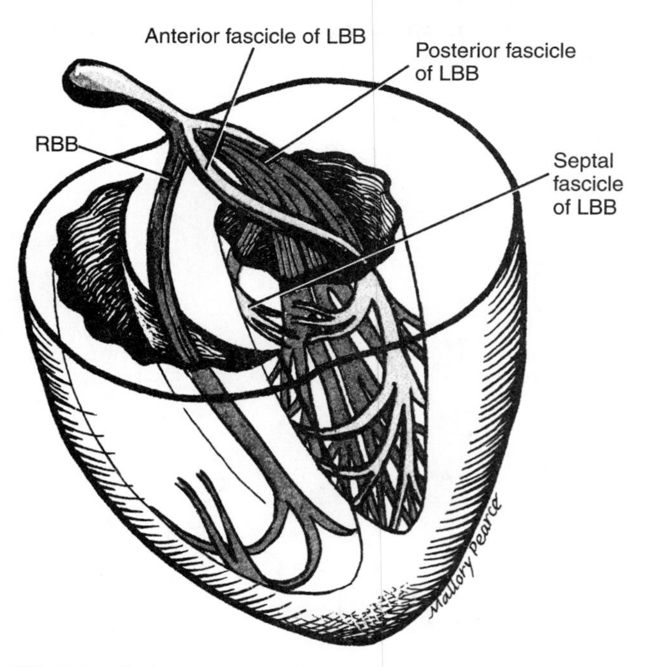

FIG. 23-1. The intraventricular conductive system shown through transparent walls. Note the anterior positions and similar constructions of the right bundle branch *(RBB)* and the anterior fascicle of the left bundle branch *(LBB).*

involved as well. However, the concept of two distinct divisions is useful in electrocardiography and clinical practice and continues to be employed to explain the axis shifts seen in acute MI.

BLOOD SUPPLY TO THE CONDUCTION SYSTEM

There are two main arterial systems supplying the conduction system. The left anterior descending (LAD) coronary artery supplies the anterior wall of the heart and the anterior two thirds of the septum. Its septal branch is the main blood supply to the proximal right bundle branch and anterior division of the left bundle branch and is vulnerable in anteroseptal MI. The posterior division of the left bundle branch has two blood supplies, the LAD and the right coronary artery (RCA). The posterior descending coronary artery is the RCA in 90% of individuals. It supplies the posterior third of the septum, and its atrioventricular (AV) nodal branch is the main blood supply to the AV node and bundle of His. Thus, acquired right bundle branch block (RBBB) is more common in anterior wall MI and left bundle branch block (LBBB) in inferior wall MI.[7]

CHRONIC BBB

Chronic BBB is rare in the young, but is a common finding in the elderly, becoming more common with age. Prognosis is related to the cardiac status. In patients with chronic BBB, widespread fibrosis is often present, especially if left fascicular block is also present. Diseases associated with BBB are coronary artery disease, hypertension, aortic valve disease, idiopathic degenerative diseases of the conduction system, and cardiomyopathy.

PEDIATRICS

When found in conjunction with congenital cardiac abnormalities, BBB is usually not accompanied by heart disease and has an excellent prognosis. During surgery for congenital heart abnormalities the bundle branches (especially the right) are frequently damaged. Surgical repairs in which this finding is common are for ventricular septal defects, atrial septal defect, tetralogy of Fallot (50% to 100%), and complex intraventricular procedures such as the combination of ventricular septal defect, transposition of the great arteries, and pulmonary stenosis. Left axis deviation (left anterior hemiblock) is also present in up to 25% of postsurgical patients.[8]

PHYSICAL FINDINGS

In patients with complete RBBB, because of a delay in the pulmonic component of the second heart sound, persistent splitting is noted; that is, the two components (aortic second sound [A_2] and pulmonic second sound [P_2]) are split on both inspiration and expiration but continue to exhibit normal respiratory changes. (The split is more marked during inspiration.) In patients with complete LBBB (or a right ventricular pacemaker), the right side of the ventricular septum is activated before the left, causing paradoxical (reversed) splitting of the second heart sound.[9-10] That is, the two components of the second heart sound separate during expiration and become single during inspiration.

COMPARISON OF RBBB AND LBBB IN LEAD V_1

BBB causes the heart to be activated in a very lopsided manner—one ventricle after the other instead of both together. This characteristic is clearly reflected in lead V_1. Note in Fig. 23-2 that normally the deflection resulting from activation of the right ventricle is buried in that from the left ventricle, resulting in a narrow rS complex in V_1. However, in RBBB the deflection representing right ventricular activation is delayed and becomes prominent, resulting in a broad terminal R′ wave and the typical rSR′ complex (Fig. 23-2, *A*). In LBBB, activation of both ventricles is also in sequence, but from right to left, resulting in a broad negaive complex in V_1 (Fig. 23-2, *B*).

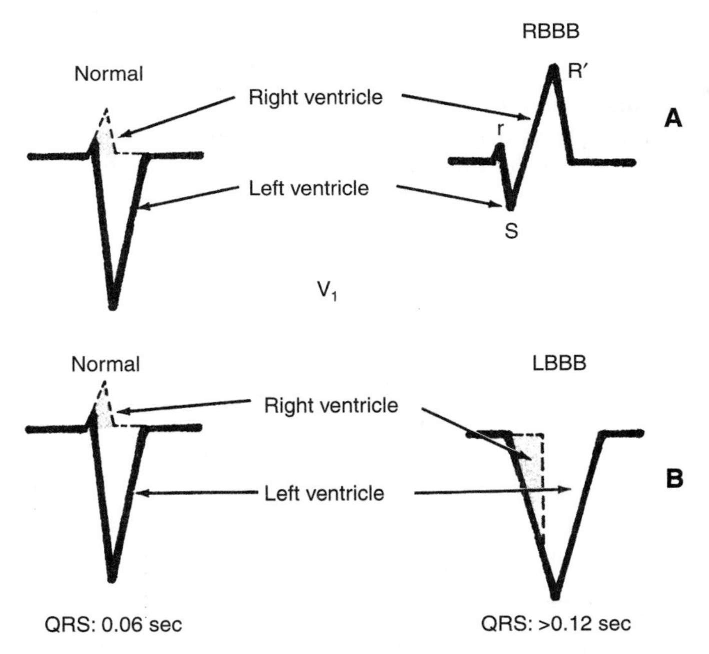

FIG. 23-2. The ventricular complexes of **A**, RBBB and, **B**, LBBB are compared with the normal complex in lead V_1. The *dotted lines* indicate hidden events on the ECG. For example, right ventricular activation is normally effaced by left ventricular activation.

INTRINSICOID DEFLECTION

The intrinsicoid deflection is analogous to the intrinsic deflection, which is impractical because it requires direct epicardial lead placement. The time from the beginning of ventricular activation (onset of the QRS complex) to that point at which the impulse arrives under a particular electrode is called the *ventricular activation time,* and the downward deflection that follows is the *intrinsicoid deflection* (the peak of the R wave). Because V_1 is over the right ventricle and V_6 is over the left, we look to those two leads for the ventricular activation time for the right and the left ventricles, respectively.

Normally the impulse arrives over the thin-walled right ventricle early (0.02 second); at that point, the graph in V_1 begins its downstroke. Because the left ventricular wall is thicker than the right wall, it takes longer for the impulse to arrive under the V_6 electrode, and the graph peaks later (within 0.04 second). The onset of normal intrinsicoid deflections for the right and left ventricles is shown in Fig. 23-3. The ventricular activation times and the intrinsicoid deflections for some of the possible patterns of RBBB are shown in Fig. 23-4.

T WAVE CHANGES IN BBB

Because depolarization is abnormal in BBB, so is repolarization. Thus the T wave is expected to be opposite in polarity to the terminal component of the QRS complex. This is known as a secondary change because it is a normal consequence of the BBB. If the direction of the T wave is the same as that of the terminal component of the QRS complex, myocardial disease is suspected.

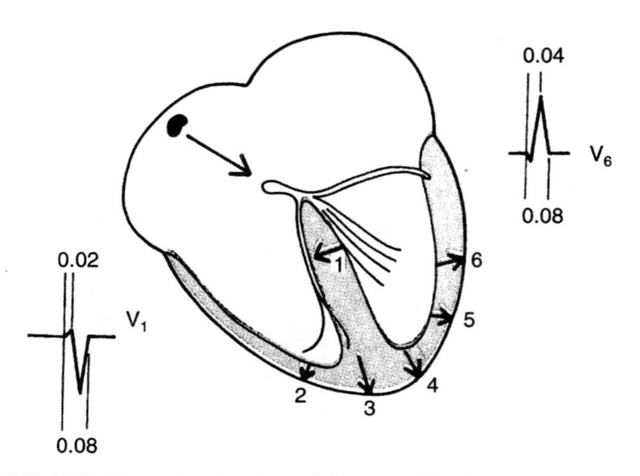

FIG. 23-3. Normal activation of the ventricles *(arrows 1 to 6)* as reflected in leads V_1 and V_6.

RIGHT BUNDLE BRANCH BLOCK

ECG Recognition Without MI

QRS duration: 0.11 second or more.

Intrinsicoid deflection: Late in V_1 (0.07 second or more), the hallmark of RBBB (Fig. 23-4).

T wave polarity: Opposite in polarity to the terminal portion of the QRS.

Leads I, aV_L, and V_6: Terminal S wave.

Lead V_1: Triphasic complex (rSR′).

Lead V_6: Triphasic complex (qRS).

ECG Recognition with MI

Lead V_1: Biphasic complex (QR) along with the clinical picture of MI.

Mechanism Without MI

1. Septal activation proceeds normally and on time, producing an initial r wave in lead V_1 and a little q wave in lead V_6.
2. Septal activation is followed by normal activation of the left ventricle, producing an S wave in V_1 and an R wave in V_6; these two events comprise the first 40 ms of activation and closely resemble the normal.
3. The right ventricle is activated last and abnormally, with the impulse gaining access from the edges of the septal border and slowly sweeping across the right ventricle from left to right. This diagnostic portion of ventricular activation is nonuniform, late, and synchronous.[11] This produces the hallmark of RBBB—a late R wave in V_1 and an S wave in V_6. Thus the triphasic pattern in these two leads is formed.

Fig. 23-5 shows RBBB without MI. Note the triphasic patterns in V_1 and V_6 and the broad terminal S wave in leads I, aV_L, and V_6. Often the amplitude of the initial r wave is increased in RBBB in lead V_1 because normal septal

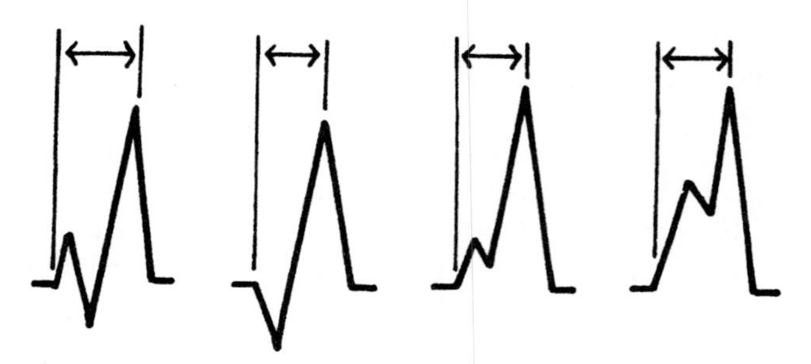

FIG. 23-4. Ventricular activation times *(arrows)* and intrinsicoid deflections in different patterns of RBBB. The QRS is broad, and although the patterns differ slightly, they have in common a ventricular activation time of 0.07 second or more.

activation involves a contribution from both sides of the septum with left-to-right activation dominating and a modest initial r wave is produced. When the right bundle branch is blocked, activation of the septum is exclusively from left to right, producing a larger initial R wave. For the same reason the S wave is markedly reduced in lead V_1 in RBBB, even though this is the component reflecting the large left ventricular mean vector. The S wave reduction in lead V_1 occurs because the now stronger septal current opposes left ventricular activation. Thus some of the left ventricular forces are canceled out, producing a smaller S wave.

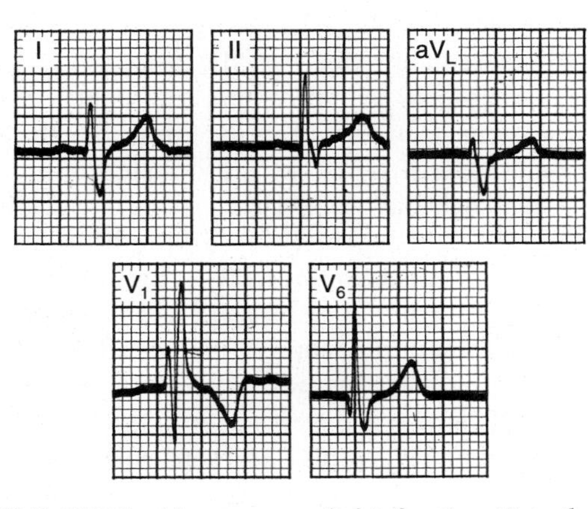

FIG. 23-5. RBBB without myocardial infarction. Note the classic rSR′ pattern in V_1 and the normal septal q waves and abnormal S waves in leads I, aV_L, and V_6.

Mechanism with MI

ECG patterns in V_1 without and with MI are compared in Fig. 23-6. In both cases the two ventricles are activated one after the other instead of together, as they normally are.

1. Septal activation does not take place because of necrotic and injured tissue. Initial forces are left ventricular, producing a Q wave in lead V_1.
2. Initial left ventricular forces are followed by late activation of the right ventricle, producing an R wave in V_1. Fig. 23-7 demonstrates in V_1 the onset of RBBB in a patient with anteroseptal MI.

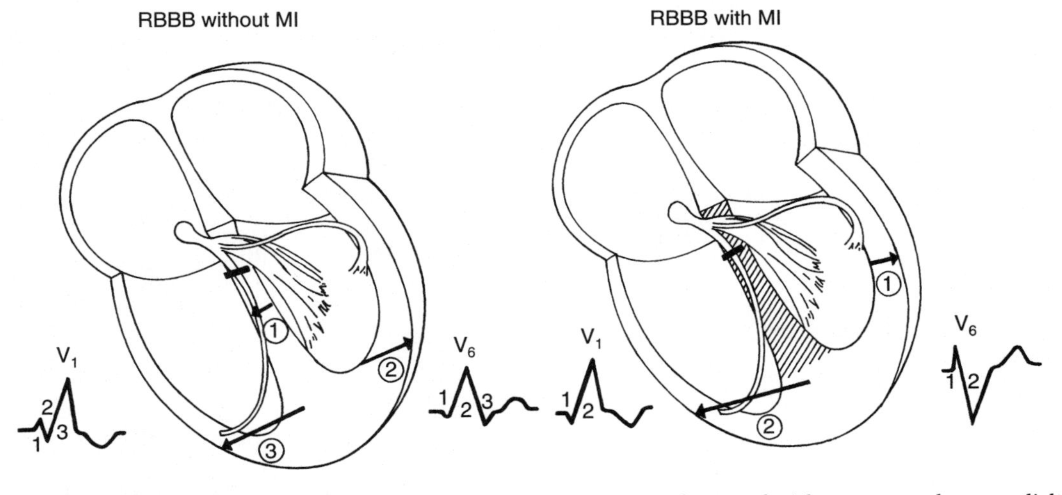

FIG. 23-6. Sequences in the activation of the ventricles in RBBB without and with anteroseptal myocardial infarction *(MI)*. In one, septal activation is intact; in the other, it is not.

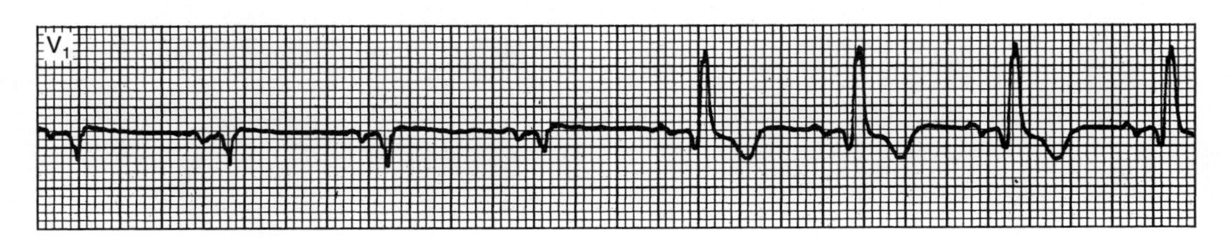

FIG. 23-7. The onset of RBBB in a patient with anteroseptal myocardial infarction.

Fig. 23-8 is a 12-lead ECG of RBBB with acute anteroseptal MI. Note the absence of the initial r wave in lead V_1; there is a Q wave instead. The patient also has left anterior hemiblock. Mortality is very high with such a pattern, which indicates a proximal LAD occlusion. Fig. 23-9 is from a 70-year-old woman with a history of paroxysmal atrial fibrillation who is healthy and active and has never had MI. With an RBBB pattern in V_1, there is no initial r wave. There is a prolonged PR interval and left axis deviation, all of which would indicate high risk had this occurred in the setting of acute anterior MI, emphasizing the importance of correlating the ECG with the clinical picture and the patient's history.

Causes

RBBB may result from advancing coronary artery disease, pulmonary hypertension, inflammatory or infiltrative diseases of the myocardium, or congenital lesions involving the septum. It may also be found in about 0.2% to 0.6% of individuals without evidence of heart disease.

Clinical Implications

Without underlying heart disease. In the U.S. Air Force, 394 air crewmen with RBBB were studied using cardiac catheterization, electrophysiologic study of the conduction system, and noninvasive workups; 94% had no evidence of underlying heart disease. When a noninvasive cardiac workup of aviation personnel with RBBB is negative they are considered physically qualified for duty.[12]

In acute anterior MI. When RBBB or hemiblock is acquired because of anterior wall MI, it signifies an occlusion in the proximal LAD coronary artery and extensive myocardial damage. In such cases there is a high chance of developing complete AV block, and despite the transient nature of the block and prophylactic pacing, the death rate is significantly higher than it would have been had this complication not occurred. Mortality is high even if complete AV block does not develop. Death results not from the AV block, but from pump failure. If pump failure does not cause death within the first few days, there is a 30% chance that death will come 1 to 3 weeks later in the form of sustained ventricular tachycardia or ventricular fibrillation.

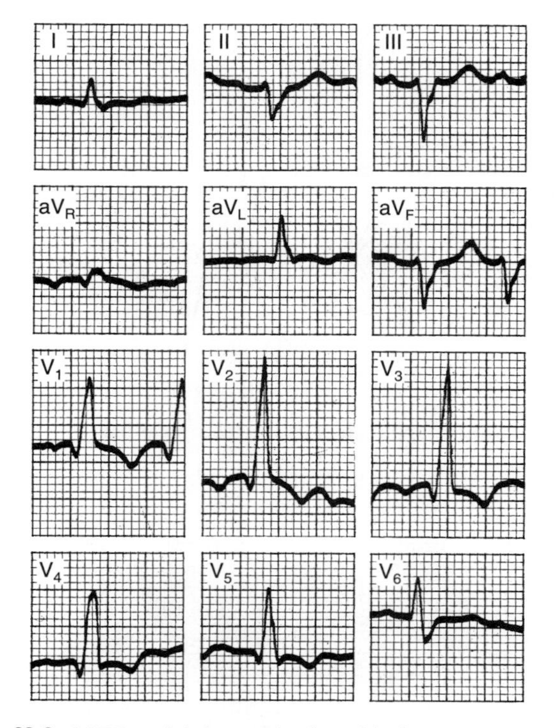

FIG. 23-8. RBBB and left anterior hemiblock in a patient with acute anteroseptal myocardial infarction.

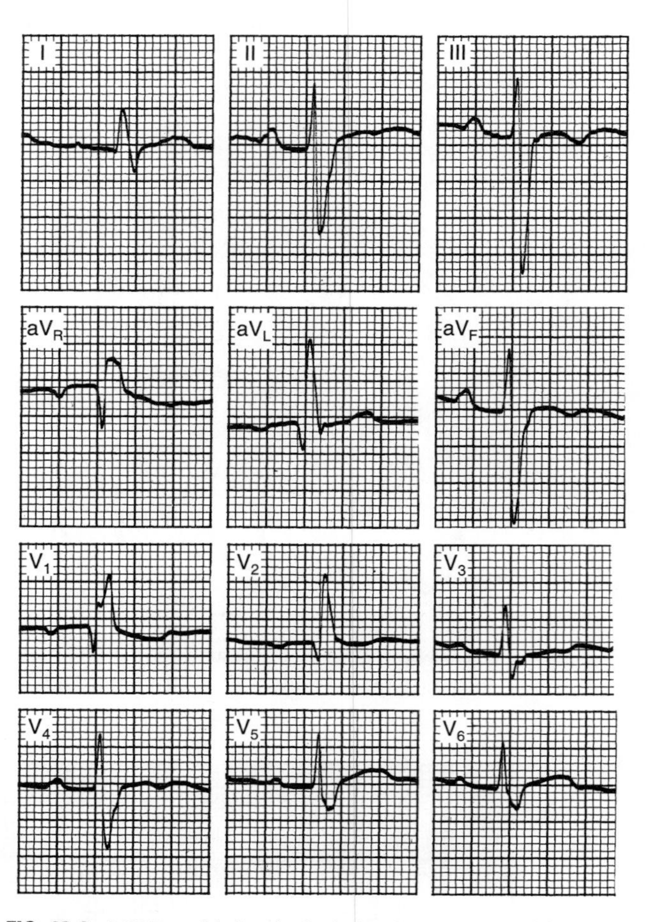

FIG. 23-9. RBBB and left axis deviation in a 70-year-old woman who has never had a myocardial infarction. Note the q wave in V_1 and V_2 and the left axis deviation.

However, if the BBB existed before the infarction, the in-hospital mortality is lower. These dire predictions emphasize the importance of early recognition and intervention in patients admitted with chest pain in order to prevent extensive myocardial damage.

Determining on admission whether a BBB is new or preexisting is a challenge. One group[13] found that BBB present on admission in a patient with acute anterior wall MI at an age older than 70 years and with the classic triphasic rSR′ pattern in lead V_1 (rather than a QR pattern) favors preexistent RBBB. When inferior wall MI is associated with preexistent RBBB, hospital mortality is not affected.[7]

After elective coronary artery bypass graft. The occurrence of new RBBB after elective coronary artery bypass graft is indicative of perioperative myocardial necrosis and thus serves as a valuable tool for the diagnosis of new, perioperative ischemic events.[14]

Hypertrophic cardiomyopathy. RBBB with negative T waves in left precordial leads strongly indicates hypertrophic cardiomyopathy.[15]

Incomplete RBBB

In incomplete RBBB the QRS morphologic appearance is that of RBBB (rSR′) and the QRS duration of less than 0.12 second.

Fig. 23-10, *A*, is an example of incomplete RBBB; the QRS is 0.11 second. In Fig. 23-10, *B*, the QRS durations differ in complete and incomplete RBBB. The narrower QRS complexes follow pauses. There are two premature atrial contractions (one conducted [hidden in second T wave] and the other not conducted), producing pauses; after the pauses the QRS duration is only 0.10 second, but the morphologic appearance is that of RBBB. After shorter cycles the duration of the QRS increases to 0.12 second as the R′ wave broadens.

Fig. 23-11, *A* and *B*, are examples of normal conduction after the compensatory pause afforded by a premature ventricular complex. In these three patients normal conduction is possible if the bundle in question has a long enough rest.

Incomplete BBB in athletes. The incidence of incomplete RBBB in all athletes is about 14% and is related to an increase in muscle mass of the right ventricular tip. After athletic activity is discontinued, the RBBB pattern disappears. Other bundle branch and fascicular blocks are extremely rare.[16]

LEFT BUNDLE BRANCH BLOCK

ECG Recognition Without MI

QRS duration: 0.12 second or more, depending on the presence of associated ischemic heart disease or prior MI.

QRS in I, aV_L, and V_6: A wide R wave with a plateau or notched summit (no q wave and no S wave).

QRS in V_1: QS or an rS pattern, and the downstroke of the S wave is swift and clean.

Intrinsicoid deflection: Delayed in left precordial leads (0.08 to 0.12 second after the onset of QRS).

T wave: Secondary abnormalities (opposite in polarity to the QRS complex).

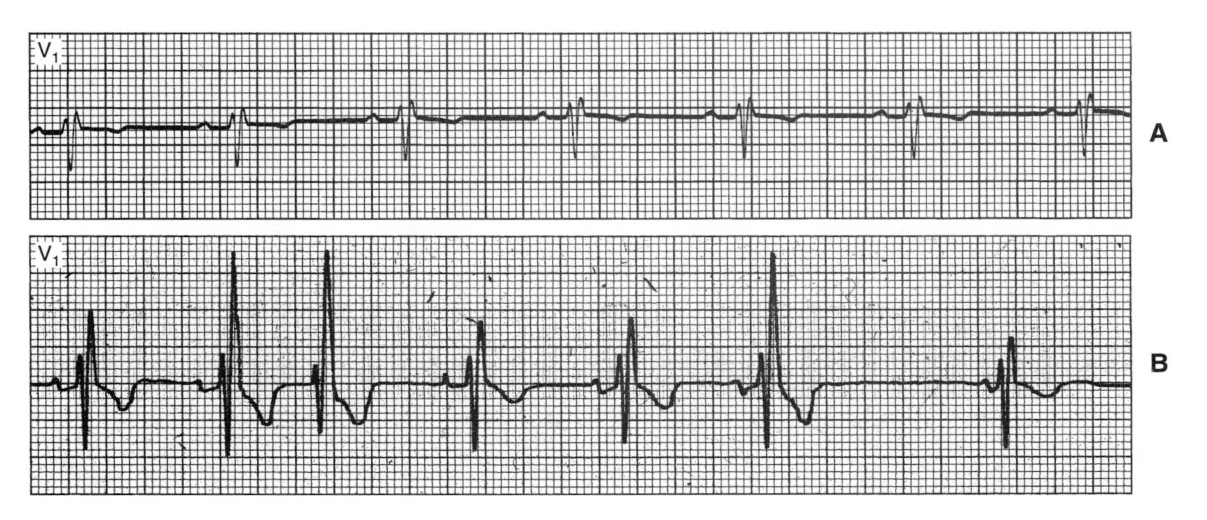

FIG. 23-10. **A**, Incomplete RBBB; the QRS is 0.11 second. **B**, Complete and incomplete RBBB patterns in lead V_1. There is a premature atrial complex in the second and sixth T waves. Because of the pause that follows these premature atrial complexes, the degree of RBBB is less.

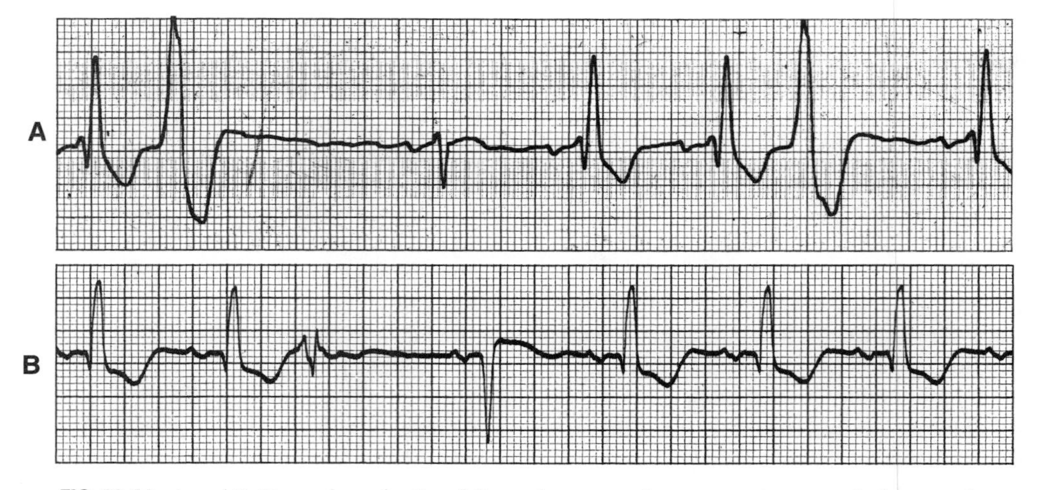

FIG. 23-11. **A** and **B**, Normal conduction follows the pause after a premature ventricular complex.

The classic 12-lead pattern of LBBB without anteroseptal MI is shown in Fig. 23-12. The right ventricle and the septum are activated simultaneously, followed immediately by left ventricular activation. Right ventricular activation is not seen. Thus the dominant current flow is away from lead V_1 (a negative deflection) and toward lead V_6 (a positive deflection). The ST segment is slightly elevated, and the T wave is opposite in polarity to that of the ventricular complex. Lead V_6 has no q wave and no S wave; it is totally positive.

ECG Recognition with MI

V_1 often has a tall, narrow r wave; V_5 or V_6 has a q wave.

Wackers et al[17] found the five most valuable ECG criteria for a diagnosis of acute MI associated with LBBB to be as follows:

1. Serial ECG changes (sensitivity 67%); a single ECG is of restricted value
2. ST segment elevation (sensitivity 54%)
3. Abnormal Q waves (sensitivity 31%)
4. Cabrera's sign (i.e., notching of 0.05 second in the ascending limb of the S wave in leads V_3 and V_4 [sensitivity 27%])
5. An R wave in V_1 and a Q wave in V_6. A 12-lead ECG showing LBBB with anteroseptal MI is seen in Fig. 23-13. In the absence of septal activation, right ventricular activation can be seen and is reflected by the tall, skinny R wave in V_1 and the abnormal Q wave in V_5 and V_6

Additionally, it is helpful to note that patients with new LBBB and suspected ischemia are five times more likely to have acute MI than patients with LBBB of chronic or unknown duration.[18]

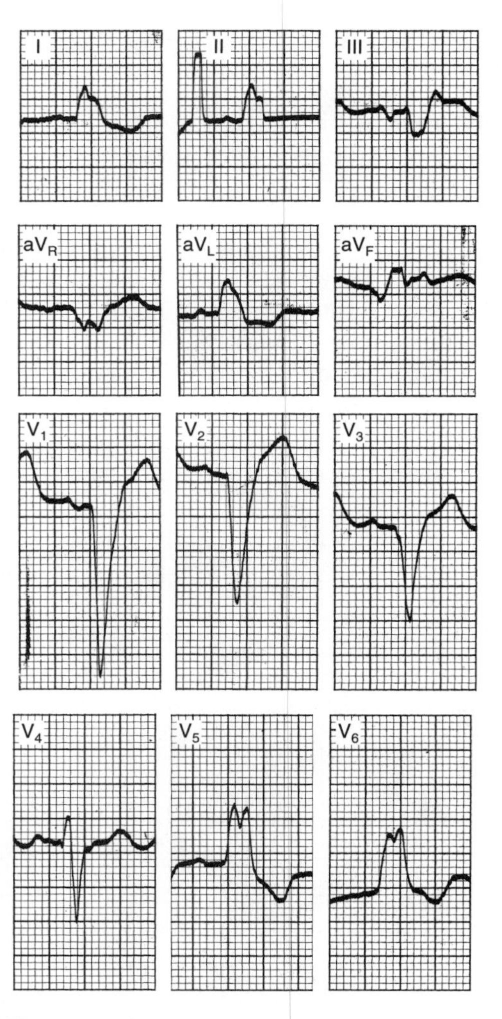

FIG. 23-12. LBBB without anteroseptal myocardial infarction. Note the absence of a tall R wave in V_1 and the absence of a q wave in V_6.

Three strategies that may help in the correct ECG interpretation of LBBB with MI are as follows:

1. Serial ECGs demonstrating ischemic changes
2. Comparison to previous ECGs
3. Knowledge of the expected ST segment and T wave morphologies in uncomplicated LBBB and thus the ability to recognize ischemic changes[19]

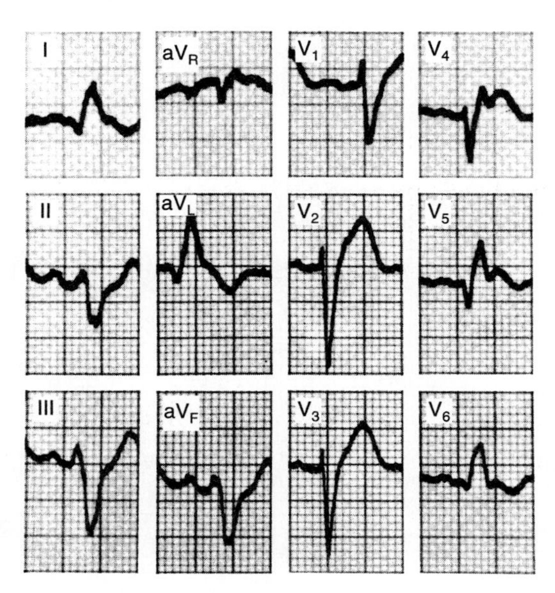

FIG. 23-13. LBBB and anteroseptal MI. The Q wave in lead V_5 and V_6 and the R wave in lead V_1 are evident. (From Lyon LJ: *Basic electrocardiography handbook*, New York, 1977, Van Nostrand Reinhold.)

Mechanism

Without MI. Ventricular activation begins when the impulse enters the right ventricle via the right bundle branch, moving to the right ventricular wall and from right to left across the septum simultaneously. The impulse then travels from the septum into its connections with the anterior and posterior walls of the left ventricle. Anterior and posterior wave fronts move around the left ventricular wall to meet and depolarize the posterior or lateral areas last.[20]

With left axis deviation. In patients with marked left axis deviation and LBBB the current moves toward the left shoulder and upper back probably because the left anterior fascicle is more impaired distally than is the posterior fascicle and therefore fails to complete terminal activation of the anterobasal left ventricle as is would in LBBB without left axis deviation.[21]

With MI. In LBBB with MI, septal activation does not take place because of necrotic and injured tissue. Initial forces are right ventricular, producing a tall, thin R wave in lead V_1 and a Q wave in V_6. The left ventricle is activated next, producing a deep S wave in lead V_1 and an R wave in V_6.

Fig. 23-14 compares the mechanisms of ventricular activation in LBBB without and with acute anteroseptal MI. In both cases the ventricles are activated from right to left.

It is difficult to recognize MI when it is associated with LBBB because initial forces and left ventricular activation are not normal. Not only are the two ventricles activated sequentially (the right and then the left) instead of simultaneously, activation of the left ventricle does not take the normal pathway, being activated from the right bundle

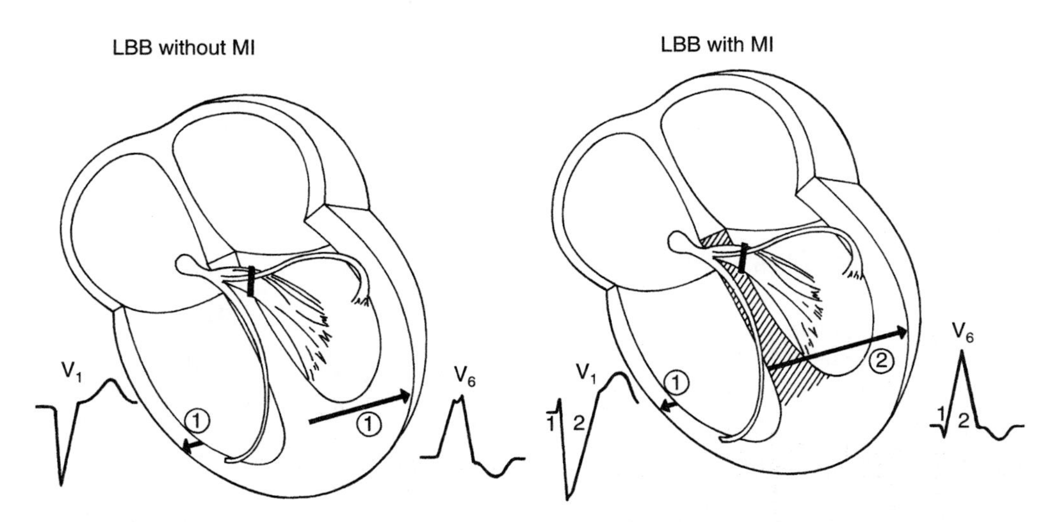

FIG. 23-14. Sequences in the activation of the ventricles in LBBB without and with anteroseptal myocardial infarction *(MI).*

branch. Thus areas in the left ventricle that usually produce initial QRS forces are now activated at the end of the QRS, rendering the traditional ECG signs of ischemia and MI inappropriate.[19]

Causes

The most common causes of LBBB are coronary artery disease, hypertensive heart disease (or both), idiopathic dilated and secondary cardiomyopathy, advanced cases of rheumatic heart disease, calcific aortic stenosis, and Lev disease (sclerosis and calcification of the left side of the cardiac skeleton). In the absence of detectable heart disease, LBBB may be caused by primary degenerative disease of the conduction system or it may be benign.[20]

Clinical Implications

The left bundle branch receives its blood supply from both the left and the right coronary arteries. Thus the appearance of LBBB usually indicates a severe lesion with involvement of both coronary arteries.

Left axis deviation. In individuals with LBBB (Fig. 23-15), left axis deviation reportedly has a 41.9% sensitivity and a 91.6% specificity for the presence of organic heart disease, a statistically significant difference from patients with a normal axis. Aortic valve disease in patients with LBBB seems to be frequently accompanied by left axis deviation.[21]

Underlying cardiac disease. Grady et al[22] found that exercise-induced LBBB independently predicts a higher risk of death and major cardiac events.

In the Framingham study[23] the associated ECG findings correlated with the prevalence of systemic hypertension, cardiomegaly, coronary heart disease, and congestive heart failure. The findings were as follows:

1. A QRS axis of 0 degrees or to the left of 0 degrees (heart enlargement, coronary disease, and congestive heart failure)
2. P wave pattern of left atrial enlargement (hypertension and possible cardiac enlargement)
3. Inverted T wave in lead V_6 in the first tracing after the development of LBBB; when the T wave was upright or biphasic in this lead in the Framingham study, the patients remained free of associated cardiovascular abnormalities
4. Abnormal ECG before onset of LBBB

In this study patients (1) without the axis shift, (2) without abnormal P morphologic appearance, and (3) without abnormal ECG before development of LBBB were six times more likely to remain free of all cardiovascular disease than were the 47 other patients who had one or more of these three ECG findings.

Myocardial infarction. Prognosis worsens when LBBB and MI coexist, whether or not the LBBB was preexisting or was a consequence of the infarction.[13] Over the last decade, this fact has spurred on the search for a reliable ECG clue to the presence of acute MI in patients presenting with LBBB.

Wide QRS. The QRS duration has a significant inverse relationship with ejection fraction and prolongation of QRS duration to 0.17 second or more in the presence of LBBB is a marker of significant left ventricular systolic dysfunction.[24]

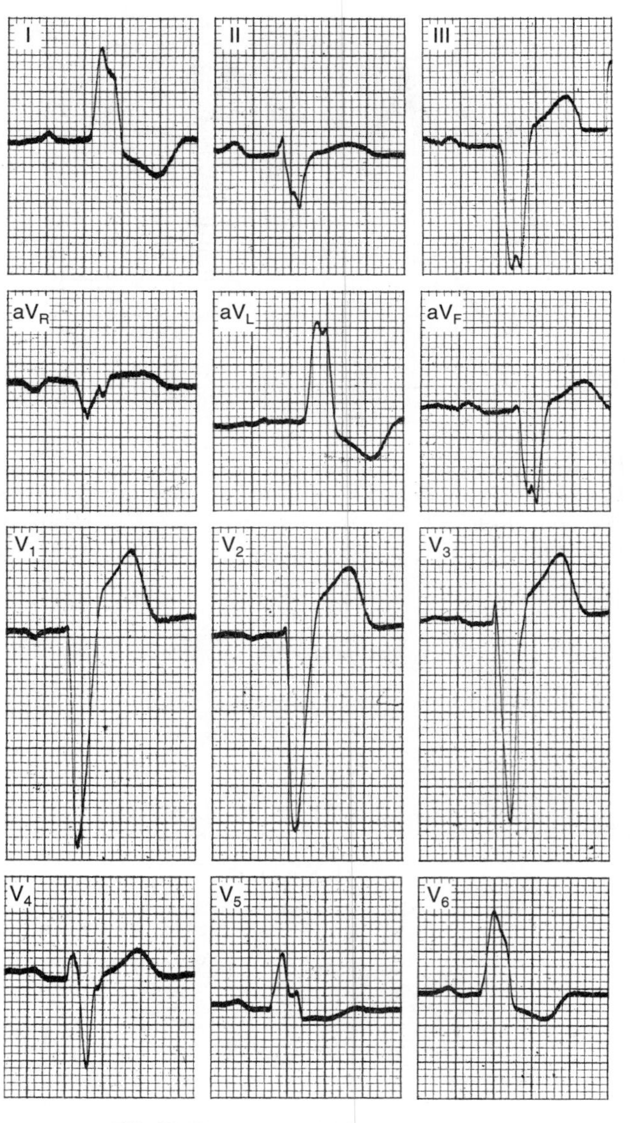

FIG. 23-15. LBBB and left axis deviation.

Chronic LBBB. When LBBB is found on a routine ECG, it is usually associated with hypertensive ischemic, primary, or degenerative myocardial disease, which may be manifested on clinical examination, or it may not be associated with serious cardiac disease at all. The Framingham study has concluded that when LBBB is newly acquired, the presence of underlying disease can be established by evaluating associated ECG findings such as QRS axis, P wave morphologic appearance, polarity of the T wave in lead V_6, and tracings made before the LBBB.

Hemodynamic effects. LBBB is associated with asynchronous myocardial activation with profound hemodynamic effects.

Dilated cardiomyopathy. When LBBB is associated with dilated cardiomyopathy, there is progressive left ventricular dilatation and mitral regurgitation. Patients with dilated cardiomyopathy and LBBB are more likely to have a nonischemic etiology, profound left ventricular dilatation, lower ejection fraction, increased symptomatology, and shorter survival than are individuals with normal intraventricular conduction.[25]

Treatment

The recommendations of the American College of Cardiology/American Heart Association are that, in the absence of contraindications, acute reperfusion therapy should be used in all patients with LBBB who have the clinical presentations indicative of acute MI.[26]

This approach protects patients with chest pain. However, Shlipak et al[27] studied the clinical features, treatment, and in-hospital survival of 29,585 acute MI patients with LBBB. Nearly half of them do not present with chest pain and are therefore less likely to receive optimal therapy, placing them at increased risk of death.

ALTERNATING RBBB AND LBBB

Alternating RBBB and LBBB indicates disease in both bundles. Sometimes, only a one-sided BBB (which may be incomplete) is evident, and the block on the other side will not be seen until it is unmasked by an increase in the sinus rate. Such is the case in Fig. 23-16. At the onset of the tracing there is RBBB. When the cycle length shortens a little, the left bundle blocks (rate-related LBBB). However, because the block in the right bundle was incomplete, the impulse now can proceed slowly down the right bundle (long PR interval with LBBB). The next sinus beat is blocked (the P wave is hidden in the LBBB complexes), then conduction resumes down the left bundle branch, and this cycle continues to produce a bigeminal pattern of LBBB with a long PR interval and RBBB with a short PR interval.

ANTERIOR HEMIBLOCK

There is no right-sided hemiblock. Therefore the shorter term *anterior hemiblock* is often used instead of *left anterior hemiblock*. Another term in common usage is *anterior fascicular block*.

Because the anterior fascicle of the conduction system is relatively thin and lies in the turbulent outflow tract, and because the anterior fascicle has only one blood supply, it is vulnerable to injury and block.

ECG Recognition

ECG findings associated with anterior hemiblock include the following:

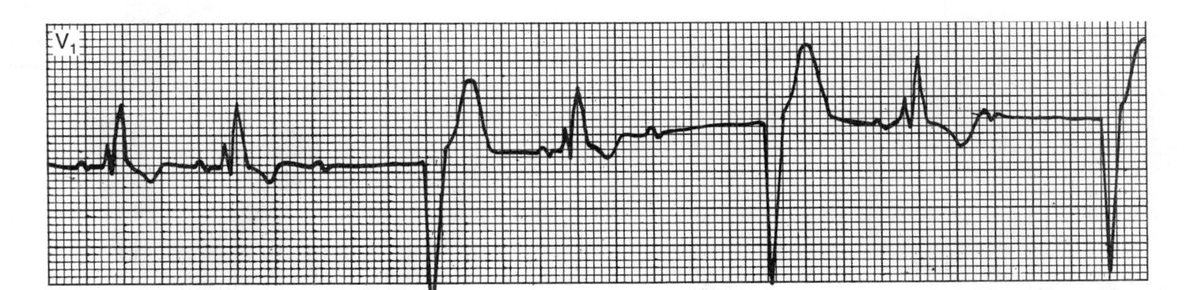

FIG. 23-16. Alternating LBBB and RBBB. In the first two beats there is RBBB. The left bundle is able to conduct as long as the rate is slow enough. When the rate speeds up, the left bundle blocks, unmasking the slow conduction through the right bundle branch (note the long PR interval with the LBBB beats). The next P wave (hidden) blocks in both bundles, and the sequence begins again: (1) a short PR interval and conduction over the left bundle (RBBB), (2) block in the left bundle and slow conduction over the right bundle (LBBB with a long PR interval), and (3) block in both bundles (hidden P wave). (Courtesy Hein J.J. Wellens, MD, Maastricht, The Netherlands.)

QRS axis: Left; –40 degrees or greater.

QRS duration: Normal (lengthens an average of 25 ms).

QRS morphologic appearance: Small q waves in leads I and aV_L (may be seen but are not necessary for the diagnosis and are caused by the shift of initial forces [first 0.02 second] inferiorly and to the right). There are small initial r waves in leads II and III.

Fig. 23-17 is from a patient with acute anterior MI and anterior hemiblock. Note the marked left axis deviation, the normal QRS duration, the small q wave in leads I and aV_L, and the small r wave in the inferior leads.

Mechanism

A block in the anterior fascicle is illustrated in Fig. 23-18; the block causes marked left axis deviation because the impulse activates the left ventricle through the posterior fascicle, spreading upward and to the left.

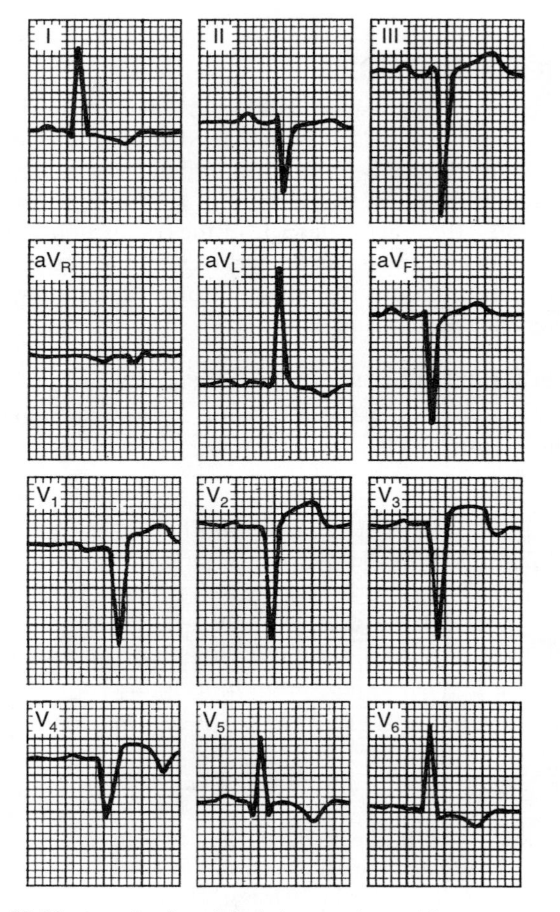

FIG. 23-17. Anterior hemiblock in a patient with acute anterior myocardial infarction. The abnormal left axis deviation (greater than –30 degrees), the normal QRS duration, and the q waves in leads I and aV_L can be seen.

Clinical Implications

The anterior fascicle can receive its blood supply solely from the septal branch of the LAD coronary artery or may also be supplied by the AV nodal artery, a branch of the right coronary artery in 90% of individuals, which explains why, although left anterior hemiblock is considerably more common in acute anterior MI, it is also seen in the setting of inferior MI. Of all the conduction defects associated with acute MI, isolated left anterior hemiblock carries the lowest hospital mortality.

Differential Diagnosis

Inferior wall myocardial infarction. Inferior wall MI and anterior hemiblock may occur together, especially if some portion of the anterior wall is also involved or if the AV nodal artery supplies the proximal bundle branches. In some cases anterior hemiblock may obscure the signs of inferior wall infarction by abolishing the diagnostic Q waves in the inferior leads (II, III, and aV_F). The diagnosis of the combination of inferior MI and anterior hemiblock is also difficult because both abnormalities can result in left axis deviation. The degree of axis shift is helpful in the differential diagnosis because a large inferior infarction without anterior hemiblock can only produce a left axis shift of less than –30 degrees caused by loss of electrical forces

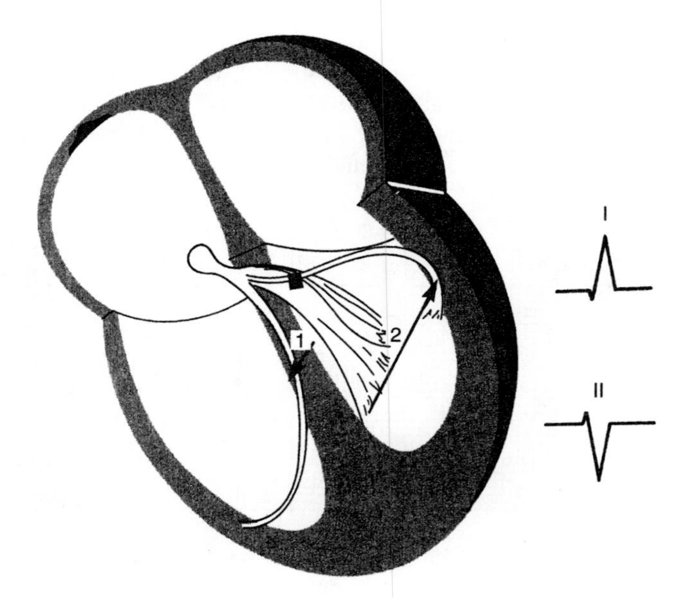

FIG. 23-18. The mechanism of the left axis deviation in anterior hemiblock. When the anterior fascicle is blocked, initial forces are septal (q wave in leads I and aV_L and r wave in lead II). The left ventricle is then activated through the posteroinferior fascicle, causing left axis deviation.

from the inferior wall; however, if the axis is as far left as –60 degrees, hemiblock is almost certainly complicating the inferior wall MI.[4]

A helpful clue to the presence of anterior hemiblock is the following: with or without inferior wall infarction, anterior hemiblock will produce a deep S wave in lead II, but never a terminal r wave.[28] In lead aV_R there is commonly a terminal r or R wave with anterior hemiblock. Warner et al[29] have proposed the following criteria for the diagnosis of inferior MI and anterior hemiblock based on the relations between portions of the vectorcardiographic QRS loop in the frontal plane and the corresponding portions of the QRS complexes recorded by the limb leads: a terminal R wave in aV_R and aV_L with the peak of the R wave later in aV_R than in aV_L and a Q wave present in lead II (can be of any magnitude). In leads aV_R and aV_L measure the distance from the beginning of the QRS complex to the peak of the R wave. These leads must be simultaneous because the onset of the QRS may differ slightly from lead to lead as a result of isoelectric initial forces in one lead and not in the other.

Anterior wall MI. Anterior wall MI may also be masked by anterior hemiblock because of a small r wave in leads V_1 and V_2, which obscures the diagnostic QS wave. It may be that a low-lying V_1 electrode is recording an r wave because initial forces in anterior hemiblock are inferior and to the right. Moving the electrode up reveals the QS wave of anterior wall MI in the right chest leads.

POSTERIOR HEMIBLOCK

The shorter term *posterior hemiblock* is often used instead of *left posterior hemiblock.* Another term in common usage is *posterior fascicular block.*

The posterior division of the left bundle block, first division to branch from the bundle of His, is the conduction system for the posteroinferior wall of the left ventricle and the septum. It receives its blood supply from both the anterior descending left and the posterior descending coronary artery.

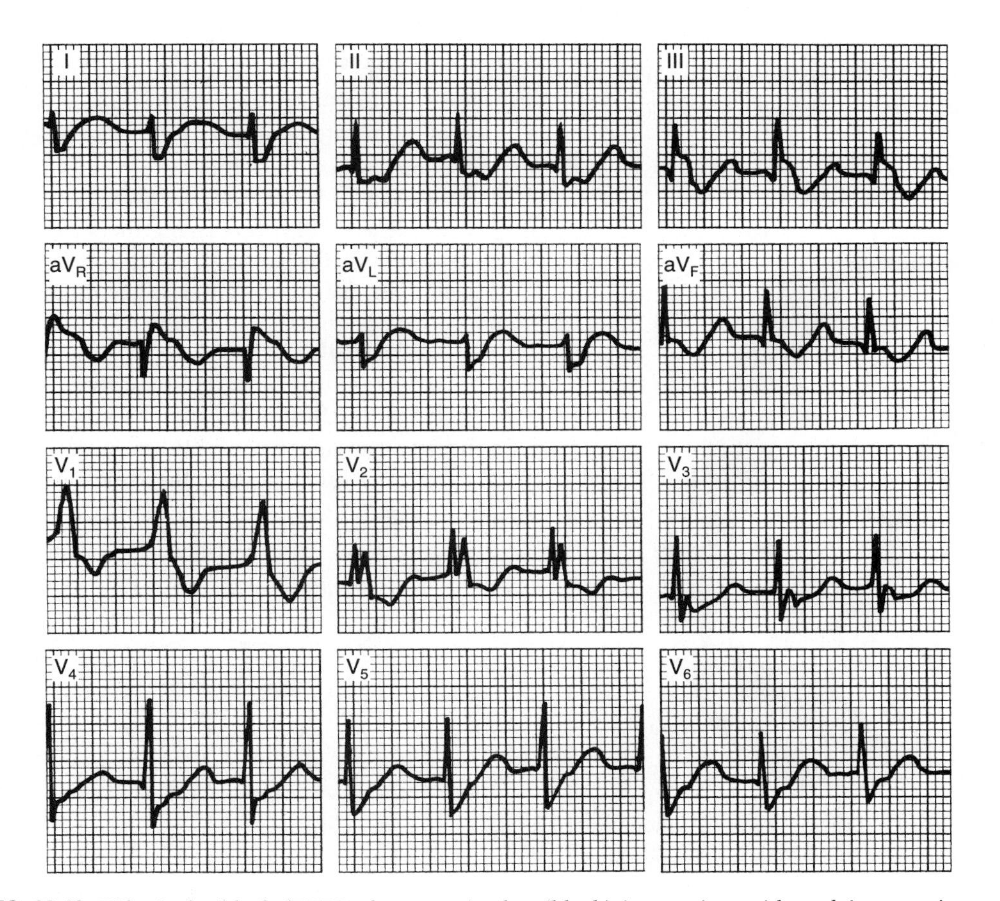

FIG. 23-19. Bifascicular block (RBBB plus posterior hemiblock) in a patient with evolving anterior wall myocardial infarction. The abnormal right axis deviation and the small r wave in leads I and aV_L, as well as small q waves in the inferior leads, are evident.

ECG Recognition

ECG findings associated with posterior hemiblock include the following:

- Right axis deviation of approximately +120 degrees
- q wave in leads II, III, and aV_F
- r wave in leads I and aV_L

When RBBB and right axis deviation are encountered, the diagnosis is always one of exclusion, distinguishing the acute from the chronic state and ruling out right ventricular hypertrophy. Fig. 23-19 is from a patient with both posterior hemiblock and RBBB (bifascicular block). Note the right axis deviation, the q wave in the inferior leads, and the r wave in leads I and aV_L.

Mechanism

A block in the posterior fascicle is illustrated in Fig. 23-20. It causes marked right axis deviation because the impulse activates the left ventricle through the anterior fascicle, spreading downward and to the right and causing lead I to be mainly negative and leads II, III, and aV_F to be mainly positive. The initial forces (the first 0.02 second) travel upward and leftward from the anterior papillary muscle. This is why there is a small initial r wave in leads I and aV_L and a q wave in leads II, III, and aV_F.

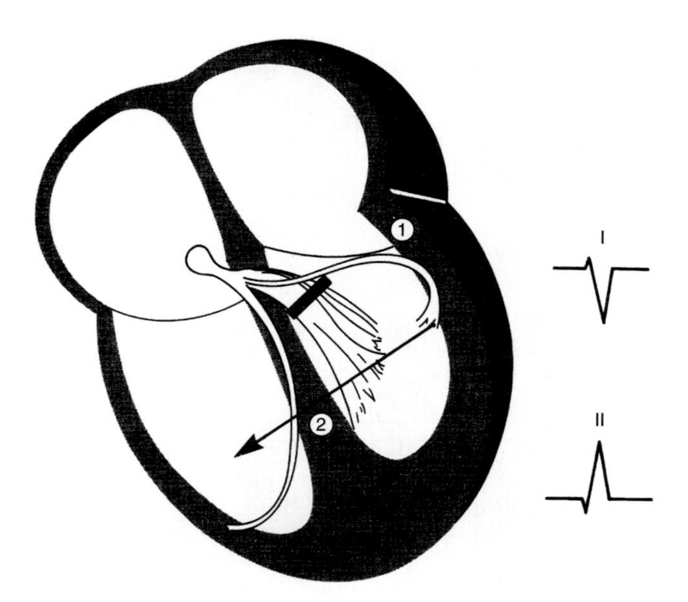

FIG. 23-20. The mechanism of the right axis deviation in posterior hemiblock. When the posterior fascicle is blocked, initial forces are toward the high, lateral left ventricle (r wave in leads I and aV_L and q wave in lead II). The remainder of the left ventricle is then activated through the anterior fascicle, causing right axis deviation.

Clinical Implications

Because of the width and the dual blood supply of the posterior fascicle, it is rarely completely compromised. If left posterior hemiblock does occur in the setting of acute MI (incidence, 1.1%), it is almost always associated with RBBB and carries a poor prognosis (hospital mortality, 71.3%).

HEMIBLOCK WITH RBBB (BIFASCICULAR BLOCK)

ECG Recognition

ECG findings associated with bifascicular block include the following:

- Pattern of RBBB with left axis deviation (RBBB plus anterior hemiblock)
- Pattern of RBBB with right axis deviation (RBBB plus posterior hemiblock) in the setting of acute MI and after having ruled out right ventricular hypertrophy

It is possible for anterior hemiblock to obscure the ECG signs of RBBB, especially if the chest electrodes are placed too low. In such cases the R′ wave in lead V_1 and the telltale S waves in leads I and aV_L are abolished. You may be able to unmask the RBBB by placing the V_1 electrode one interspace above the conventional position or slightly to the right. This may reveal the classic terminal R′ wave of RBBB.

Mechanism

In the setting of acute MI, anterior hemiblock is associated with RBBB more often than is posterior hemiblock because the right bundle and the anterior fascicle are similar in structure and share the same blood supply.

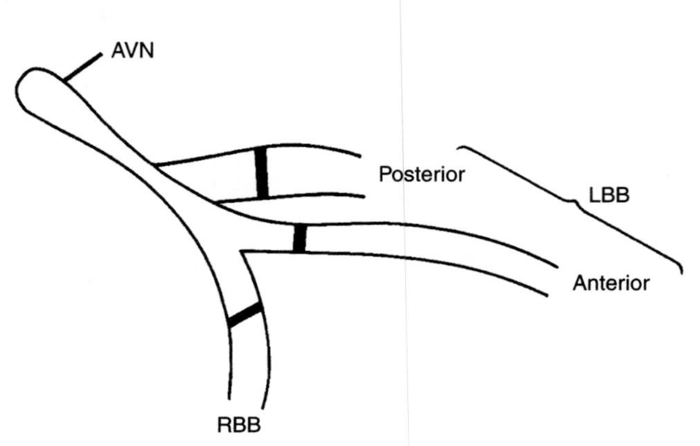

FIG. 23-21. Trifascicular block. *AVN,* Atrioventricular node; *LBB,* left bundle branch; *RBB,* right bundle branch.

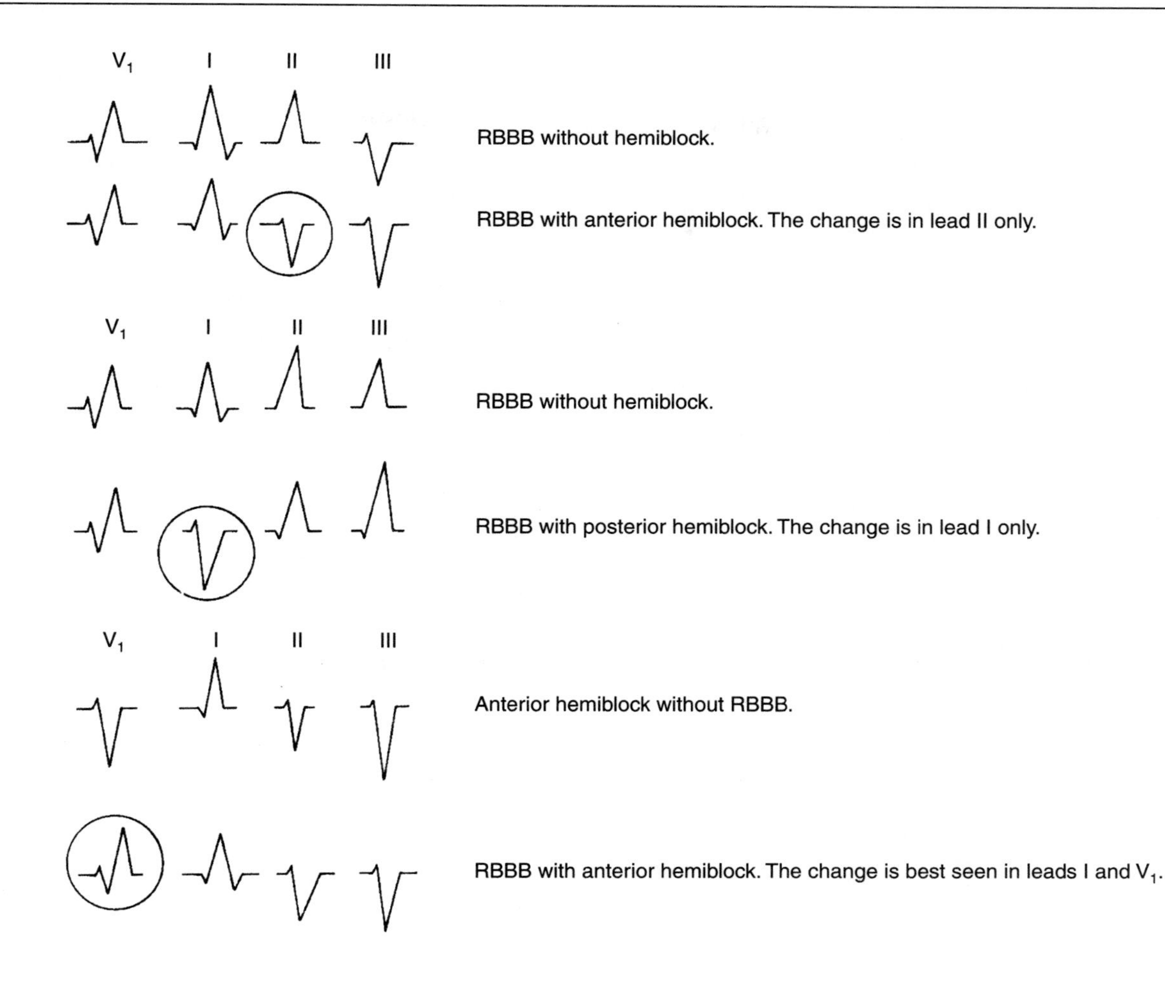

BEST LEADS FOR AXIS SHIFTS AND FOR RBBB

The decision on which leads to use for monitoring may be different from patient to patient, depending on the clinical setting (see Chapter 30). In anterior MI, among other things, we look for the development of RBBB and hemiblock. Leads I and II are best for detecting hemiblock; there will be an axis shift. Left axis shift can be detected in lead II. Right axis shift is seen best in lead I. RBBB is best detected in lead V_1. In the presence of anterior hemiblock, when the QRS complex may broaden only slightly more, V_1 is the best lead for seeing RBBB because of the development of a broad terminal R′.

TRIFASCICULAR BLOCK

Fig. 23-21 illustrates that the trifascicular block is located simultaneously in the three main fascicles of the intraventricular conduction system: the right bundle branch and the anterior and posterior divisions of the left bundle branch. If the block in all three of the fascicles is complete, the escape pacemaker is in the ventricles below the lesions. Thus the ventricular rate is that of a ventricular escape focus. If there is complete block in two fascicles and incomplete block in the third fascicle, AV conduction takes place, but usually with a prolonged PR interval. For example, RBBB, anterior hemiblock, and first-degree block may qualify as trifascicular if the first-degree block is in the posterior fascicle. AV nodal disease is also a possibility.

Fig. 23-22, *A*, was obtained in lead II from a patient with acute anterior wall MI. Lead II is the best lead for observing a shift of the axis to the left; there is abnormal left axis beyond –30 degrees every third beat; the QRS complex is broad, probably indicative of BBB; and the PR interval is long. Fig. 23-22, *B*, is from the same patient and shows trifascicular block as follows: (1) complete block of the right bundle (RBBB), (2) complete block of the anterior fascicle of the left bundle (left anterior hemiblock), and (3) a long PR interval, presumably the result of partial block of the posterior fascicle.

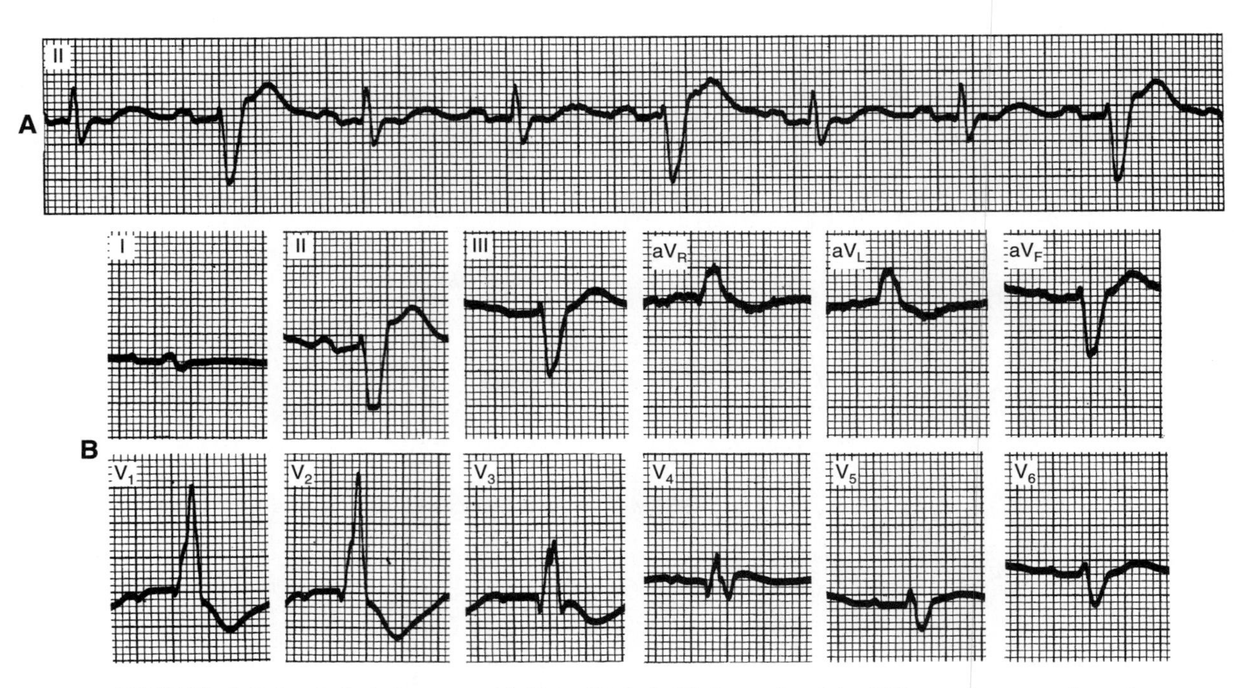

FIG. 23-22. **A**, Left axis deviation every third beat. Both the PR interval and the QRS complex are prolonged. **B**, Same patient, later. There is anterior wall myocardial infarction, and the intermittent left anterior hemiblock is now continuous. RBBB and a long PR interval (trifascicular block) are present.

TABLE 23-1 Electrocardiographic Recognition of Bundle Branch Block

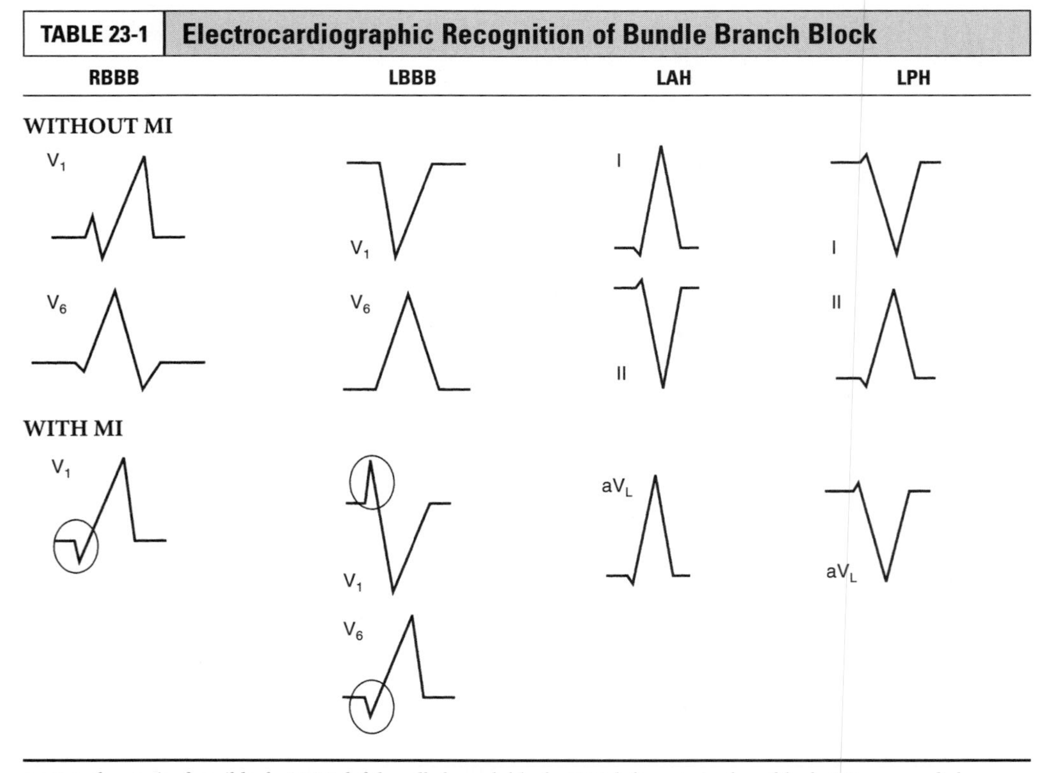

LAH, Left anterior hemiblock; *LBBB*, left bundle branch block; *LPH*, left posterior hemiblock; *MI*, myocardial infarction; *RBBB*, right bundle branch block.

SUMMARY

The importance of recognizing BBB and hemiblock lies in the rapid identification of high-risk patients with acute MI. An appreciation for the mechanism of pathologic BBB adds to depth in the understanding of the 12-lead ECG and leads to a facility in recognizing functional BBB (RBBB or LBBB pattern) in the broad QRS tachycardia and in other critical clinical situations. Table 23-1 summarizes the ECG recognition of BBB and hemiblock and compares the patterns of RBBB and LBBB with and without anteroseptal MI and of anterior and posterior hemiblock.

REFERENCES

1. Tawara S: Das Reitzleitungssystem des Sˇugtierherzensm, Jena, 1906, Gustav Fischer.
2. Rosenbaum MB: Types of right bundle branch block and their clinical significance, *J Electrocardiol* 2:197, 1969.
3. Rosenbaum MB, Elizari MV, Lazzari JO: Intraventricular trifascicular blocks: review of the literature and classification, *Am Heart J* 78:450, 1969.
4. Rosenbaum MB, Yesuron J, Lazzari JO, Elizari MV: Left anterior hemiblock obscuring the diagnosis of right bundle branch block, *Circulation* 48:298, 1973.
5. Rosenbaum MB, Elizari MV, Lazzari JO: *The hemiblocks,* Oldsmar, Fla, 1970, Tampa Tracings.
6. Demoulin JC, Kulbertus HE: Histopathological examination of the concept of left hemiblock, *Br Heart J* 34:807, 1972.
7. Wellens HJJ: Atrioventricular nodal and subnodal conduction disturbances. In Willerson JT, Cohn JN, editors: *Cardiovascular medicine,* New York, 1995, Churchill Livingstone.
8. Perry JC, Garson A Jr: Arrhythmias following surgery for congenital heart disease. In Zipes DP, Jalife J, editors: *Cardiac electrophysiology from cell to bedside,* ed 2, Philadelphia, 1995, WB Saunders.
9. Perloff JK: Heart sounds and murmurs: physiological mechanisms. In Braunwald E, editor: *Heart disease,* ed 4, Philadelphia, 1992, WB Saunders.
10. Tilkian A, Conover M: *Understanding heart sounds and murmurs,* ed 4, Philadelphia, 2001, WB Saunders.
11. Flowers NC, Horan LG: Body surface potential mapping. In Zipes DP, Jalife J, editors: *Cardiac electrophysiology from cell to bedside,* ed 3, Philadelphia, 2000, WB Saunders.
12. *United States Naval Flight Surgeon's Manual,* ed 3, Iowa City, 1991, University of Iowa.
13. Lie KI, Wellens HJJ, Schuilenburg RM: Bundle branch block and acute myocardial infarction. In Wellens HJJ, Lie KI, Janse MJ, editors: *The conduction system of the heart: structure, function and clinical implications,* The Hague, 1976. Martinus Nijhoff.
14. Seitelberger R, Wild T, Serbecic N et al: Significance of right bundle branch block in the diagnosis of myocardial ischemia in patients undergoing coronary artery bypass grafting, *Eur J Cardiothorac Surg* 18:187-193, 2000.
15. Suzuki J, Shin WS, Shimamoto R et al: Clinical implication of left precordial T wave inversions in the presence of complete right bundle branch block, *Jpn Heart J* 40:745-753, 1999.
16. Langdeau JB, Blier L, Turcotte H et al: Electrocardiographic findings in athletes: the prevalence of left ventricular hypertrophy and conduction defects, *Can J Cardiol* 17:655-659, 2001.
17. Wackers FJT, Lie KI, David G et al: Assessment of the value of electrocardiographic signs for myocardial infarction in left bundle branch block. In Wellens HJJ, Kulbertus HE, editors: *What's new in electrocardiography,* The Hague, The Netherlands, 1981, Martinus Nijhoff.
18. Li SF, Walden PL, Marcilla O, Gallagher EJ: Electrocardiographic diagnosis of myocardial infarction in patients with left bundle branch block. *Ann Emerg Med* 36:561-565, 2000.
19. Wellens HJJ: Acute myocardial infarction and left bundle-branch block—can we lift the veil? *N Engl J Med* 334:528-529, 1996.
20. Chou TC, Knilans TK: *Electrocardiography in clinical practice, adult and pediatric,* ed 4, Philadelphia, 1996, WB Saunders.
21. Parharidis G, Nouskas J, Efthimiadis G et al: Complete left bundle branch block with left QRS axis deviation: defining its clinical importance, *Acta Cardiol* 52:295-303, 1997.
22. Grady TA, Chiu AC, Snader CE et al: Prognostic significance of exercise-induced left bundle-branch block, *JAMA* 279:153-156, 1998.
23. Schneider JF, Thomas HE Jr, McNamara PM, Kannel WB: Clinical-electrocardiographic correlates of newly acquired left bundle branch block: the Framingham study, *Am J Cardiol* 55:1332, 1985.
24. Das MK, Cheriparambil K, Bedi A et al: Prolonged QRS duration (QRS Δ170 ms) and left axis deviation in the presence of left bundle branch block: a marker of poor left ventricular systolic function? *Am Heart J* 142:756-759, 2001.
25. Littmann L, Symanski JD: Hemodynamic implications of left bundle branch block, *J Electrocardiol* 33(Suppl):115-121, 2000.
26. Ryan TJ, Anderson JL, Antman EM et al: ACC/AHA guidelines for the management of patients with acute myocardial infarction: executive summary. *Circulation* 94:2341-2350, 1996.
27. Shlipak MG, Go AS, Frederick PD et al: Treatment and outcomes of left bundle-branch block patients with myocardial infarction who present without chest pain. National Registry of Myocardial Infarction 2 Investigators. *J Am Coll Cardiol* 36:706-712, 2000.
28. Marriott HJL: *Practical electrocardiography,* Baltimore, 1983, Williams & Wilkins.
29. Warner RA, Reger M, Hill NE et al: Electrocardiographic criteria for the diagnosis of combined inferior myocardial infarction and left anterior hemiblock, *Am J Cardiol* 51:718, 1983.

CHAPTER 24

Acute Myocardial Infarction

The 12-lead electrocardiogram (ECG) remains the most important diagnostic tool in the evaluation of patients with acute phase of cardiac ischemia. The ECG also plays an important role in risk stratification of acute myocardial infarct patients and in the early recognition of reperfusion. Precise bedside ECG interpretation is important because in response to ECG findings, in the appropriate clinical context, immediate management strategies are initiated, and the physician is guided in the choice of reperfusion therapy (thrombolysis, primary angioplasty, or combination therapy). To this end, the physician's emergency response to an acute episode of cardiac ischemia involves evaluation of the QRS complex, ST segment, and T wave, seeking answers to three questions[1]:

1. Does the patient have acute ST segment elevation myocardial infarction (MI), non–Q wave MI, acute coronary syndrome or unstable angina?
2. How much myocardium is at risk?
3. Which artery is the culprit?

All emergency, prehospital, and critical care unit health care professionals should know how to use the ECG to identify patients with acute MI and the subgroups at high risk for MI, institute urgent and appropriate treatment, and recognize the ECG signs of successful and unsuccessful reperfusion.

MI REDEFINED

In July 1999 the European Society of Cardiology and the American College of Cardiology[2] convened a group of experts whose purpose it was to redefine myocardial infarction.

BOX 24-1. Aspects of Myocardial Infarction by Different Techniques

PATHOLOGY
- Myocardial cell death

BIOCHEMISTRY
- Markers of myocardial cell death (blood samples)

ELECTROCARDIOGRAM
- Evidence of myocardial ischemia (ST-T segment changes)
- Evidence of loss of electrically functioning cardiac tissue (Q waves)

IMAGING
- Reduction or loss of tissue perfusion
- Cardiac wall motion abnormalities

From The Joint European Society of Cardiology/American College of Cardiology Committee: Myocardial infarction redefined—a consensus document of the joint European Society of Cardiology/American College of Cardiology Committee for the redefinition of myocardial infarction, *J Am Coll Cardiol* 36:959-969, 2000.

BOX 24-2. Electrocardiogram Changes Indicative of Myocarcial Ischemia That May Progress to Myocardial Infarction

PRESENCE OF ST SEGMENT ELEVATION

- New or presumed new ST segment elevation at the J point in two or more contiguous* leads with the cutoff points 0.2 mV or more in leads V_1, V_2, or V_3 and 0.1 mV or more in other leads

ABSENCE OF ST SEGMENT ELEVATION

- ST segment depression
- T wave abnormalities only

From The Joint European Society of Cardiology/American College of Cardiology Committee: Myocardial infarction redefined—a consensus document of the joint European Society of Cardiology/American College of Cardiology Committee for the redefinition of myocardial infarction, *J Am Coll Cardiol* 36:959-969, 2000.

*Contiguous leads in the frontal plane are defined by the lead sequence: aV_L—I—inverted aV_R—II—aV_F—III.

The four techniques used to evaluate myocardial ischemia and cell death are listed in Box 24-1. The sensitivity and specificity of each differs markedly. The ECG changes listed in Box 24-2 determine the diagnosis of myocardial ischemia, but do not of themselves define MI.

Acute, Evolving, or Recent MI

The diagnosis for an acute, evolving, or recent MI is satisfied if there is a typical rise and fall of the *markers of myocardial necrosis* (i.e., the rise and gradual fall of troponin) or the more rapid rise and fall of creatinine kinase isoenzyme (CK-MB), along with at least one of the following:

1. Ischemic symptoms
2. Development of pathologic Q waves (necrosis)
3. ST segment elevation or depression (ischemia)
4. Pathologic findings of acute MI

Note: During the very early phases of acute MI, *hyperacute T waves* (tall, peaked T waves) have been noted.

Microinfarction

A normal ECG does not rule out the diagnosis of MI. The European Society of Cardiology and the American College of Cardiology's group of experts[2] accepted the concept of a small MI that may not show the ECG signs of myocardial necrosis and formerly may have been labeled stable or unstable angina. This concept was accepted because current technology using sensitive markers such as troponin is able to identify myocardial necrosis of less than 1 g. Further clarification of the clinical significance of this is needed.

ECG Changes in Established MI

The following are the ECG changes seen in the standard 12-lead ECG in the absence of other conditions that would produce an abnormal QRS, such as bundle branch block (BBB), left ventricular hypertrophy, Wolff-Parkinson-White syndrome, or immediately after coronary artery bypass graft surgery. They are as follows:

- Any Q wave in leads V_1 through V_3
- Q waves of 30 ms (0.03 second) or more in any two of the following contiguous leads: I, II, aV_L, aV_F, V_4, or V_6

Detection of Reinfarction or Extension of an Infarct

The timing of reinfarction may be difficult to determine using troponin levels as a guide because the elevated levels of troponin can persist for 7 to 10 days. In such cases, sequential samples of CK-MB may help to determine the timing of the new infarct or infarct extension.

The wisdom and clinical value of redefining MI using these very sensitive myocardial markers have been questioned. Opposing comments have also been published by a cochairman of the epidemiology group that participated in the consensus process. Further debate on this topic is expected.[3,4]

PATHOPHYSIOLOGY OF THE EVOLVING MI

The unstable atherosclerotic plaque with plaque rupture and thrombus formation is the underlying pathophysiology of acute MI. Inflammation may be a key component, lasting up to 6 months after unstable angina or non–Q wave MI.[5]

The stable plaque may cause coronary arterial stenosis and may not be large enough to cause obstruction to blood flow. Most atherosclerotic plaques are stable, progressing slowly by buildup of lipid and macrophage complexes and do not become the site of thrombus formation and total occlusion. The unstable plaque on the other hand, builds rapidly, frequently because of hemorrhage within the plaque itself. These events generally do not cause acute MI but may present as unstable angina.

If the plaque is injured, ulcerates, or ruptures, it becomes a site for platelet aggregation, fibrin deposition, spasm, and thrombus formation. This active thrombus is the substrate and the anatomic and pathophysiologic basis of acute coronary syndromes and acute MI. If the active thrombus is only partially or intermittently occluding the coronary artery, the patient may present with unstable angina, acute coronary insufficiency, or non–Q wave MI. If the active thrombus totally occludes the vessel and stays occlusive, it usually causes the onset of acute MI with acute ST segment elevation and evolution into a Q wave MI.

After coronary occlusion, cellular changes in the myocardium begin immediately. Within 10 seconds aerobic metabolism ceases and systolic contraction stops. If the ischemic condition is severe or prolonged, the area of ischemic tissue becomes more and more severely injured, cell functions cease, and necrosis begins within about 45 minutes, becoming complete by about 6 hours after injury. The resultant cellular pathophysiologic condition may produce life-threatening ventricular arrhythmias, especially in the first 15 to 30 minutes after coronary occlusion.

Injured (ischemic) tissue is unable to contract (accounting for the systolic stretch during the acute stage of MI) but the left ventricle may be able to remain in a depressed but salvageable condition (myocardial stunning) for some time and may return to normal function if flow is reestablished or collateral circulation develops and blood flow improves. If the blood flow to the myocardium is greatly compromised because of a severely stenotic coronary artery, contractile function is reduced as a compensatory mechanism (myocardial hibernation). Stunned myocardium is viable; however, if ischemia is severe and prolonged, cell death is inevitable. Fig. 24-1 demonstrates the pathologic process after a coronary occlusion and compares subendocardial and transmural infarctions. The surface ECG does not consistently distinguish between the two types of infarcts.

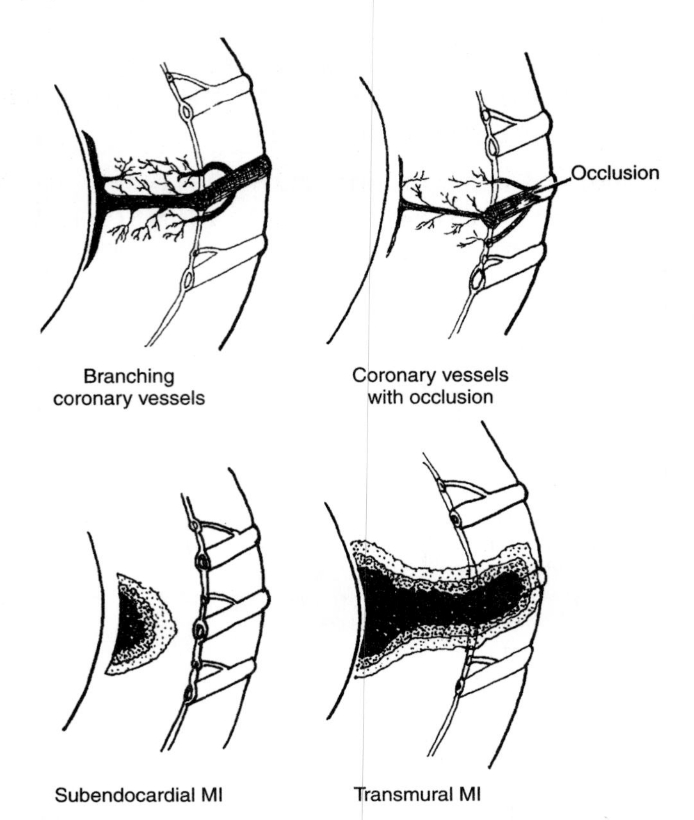

FIG. 24-1. A branching coronary vessel shown without and with occlusion and the resulting pathologic conditions.

BLOOD SUPPLY TO THE MYOCARDIUM AND CONDUCTION SYSTEM

The coronary arteries and their major divisions are illustrated in Fig. 24-2. When the right coronary artery (RCA) provides the posterior descending branch, the term *dominant RCA* is used. When it is the left coronary artery (LCA) that provides the posterior descending branch, the term *dominant LCA* is used. Occlusion of the dominant RCA results in inferior MI. High-risk patients with inferior MI have proximal RCA occlusion in a dominant RCA, right ventricular MI, and atrioventricular (AV) block. Occlusion of the left anterior descending (LAD) coronary artery results in anterior MI. High-risk patients with LAD coronary artery occlusion have a proximal occlusion, right bundle branch block (RBBB), or hemiblock. Table 24-1 summarizes the features of AV conduction disturbances complicating acute MI.

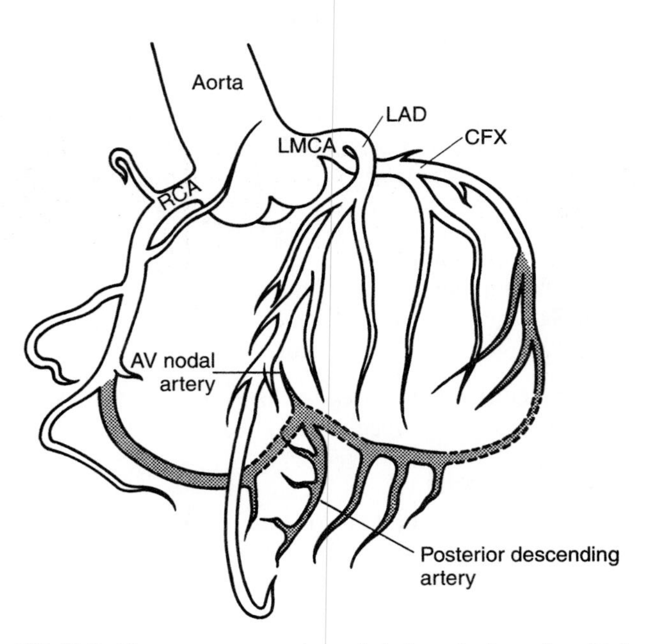

FIG. 24-2. The coronary arteries and their major branches. Right coronary artery *(RCA)*, left main coronary artery *(LMCA)*, left anterior descending *(LAD)* coronary artery, and circumflex *(CFX)* artery.

TABLE 24-1 Features of Atrioventricular Conduction Disturbances Complicating Acute Myocardial Infarction

Feature	Acute Inferior MI	Acute Anterior MI
Site of block	AV node	Bundle branches
Artery involved	RCA	LAD
Escape rhythm	Narrow QRS; HR: 40-60 beats/min; dependable	Wide QRS; HR: <40 beats/min; undependable
Duration of block	Transient	Transient
Increase in hospital mortality (compared with same infarct location without block)	2.5 times	4 times

From Wellens HJJ, Conover M: *The ECG in emergency decision making,* Philadelphia, 1991, WB Saunders.
MI, Myocardial infarction; *AV,* atrioventricular; *RCA,* right coronary artery; *LAD,* left anterior descending (coronary artery); *HR,* heart rate.

Right Coronary Artery

In 90% of individuals the posterior descending branch of the RCA supplies the posterior third of the interventricular septum and the posterior division of the left bundle branch (posterior fascicle). The RCA's AV nodal branch supplies the AV node and the proximal part of the bundle of His. Hence 20% of patients with acute inferior MI have high-degree AV nodal block. Rarely the AV nodal artery may also supply the proximal bundle branches and, again rarely, the distal His bundle and the proximal bundle branches. The RCA also supplies the right and left ventricles and, in some individuals, the posterolateral wall of the left ventricle.[6]

Left Coronary Artery

The LCA divides into the LAD branch and the circumflex artery. It is the LAD coronary artery that supplies the anterior and anterolateral walls of the heart and two thirds of the interventricular septum. In most hearts, the first septal perforator from the LAD coronary artery provides the blood supply for the distal bundle of His and the proximal bundle branches. In individuals with a dominant LCA the posterior descending branch of the left bundle and the AV node are supplied by the distal branch of the circumflex coronary artery. The circumflex artery and its obtuse marginal branches supply the posterolateral wall of the left ventricle and, in some patients, the inferior wall of the left ventricle.

ECG SIGNS OF ACUTE MI

The ECG signs of acute MI are as follows:

- T wave changes (ischemia)
- ST segment displacement (injury)
- Abnormal Q waves (cellular death)

Although oversimplified, this classification, first described in humans in 1920,[7] is useful in clinical practice. Almost immediately after coronary artery occlusion, there are T wave changes (initially peaked T waves followed by T wave inversion) in the leads reflecting the involved surface; there is also a loss of R wave amplitude. These events are accompanied by a maximal elevation of the ST segment. As the pathologic condition progresses, the typically coved, elevated ST segment gradually evolves into inverted, symmetrical T waves. Abnormal Q waves appear as early as 2 hours after the onset of chest pain in some patients and are usually fully developed within 12 to 24 hours. This evolution of the ECG in patients with acute MI is dramatically altered with successful reperfusion (angioplasty or thrombolytic therapy). Early signs include rapid reduction in ST segment elevation and resolution of conduction abnormalities.

T WAVES

T waves, along with the ST segment, reflect repolarization of the myocardium.

Normal T Waves

Normal T waves are asymmetric, rounded, and have the same polarity as the terminal QRS. Although the process of depolarization proceeds from endocardium to epicardium, the process of repolarization proceeds in the opposite direction (epicardium to endocardium). Thus T waves normally are inverted in lead aV_R and may be inverted or upright in V_1. They vary in leads V_2 and III, and they are normally positive in leads aV_L and aV_F but may be inverted if the QRS is less than 6 mm tall in those leads.

Ischemic T Wave

In contrast to the asymmetric, rounded normal T wave, the progressively deepening T wave inversion of ischemia is symmetric and pointed. As the infarction evolves, the inverted T waves are preceded by upwardly coved ST segments in the leads reflecting the injured myocardium. Inverted T waves in the leads adjacent to the injury reflect acute ischemia. For example, a patient with acute anterior MI may have ST elevation in leads V_1 to V_4 and T wave inversion in leads V_5 and V_6.

During subendocardial ischemia the sequence just described for the normal T wave remains unchanged; that is, repolarization proceeds from epicardium to endocardium (positive T wave). In subepicardial ischemia conduction is slowed in the epicardium, preventing it from initiating the repolarization process first. Instead, the process begins in the endocardium, resulting in an inverted T wave. T wave inversion of itself is by no means specific, since it may occur for many reasons.

Ischemia of Unstable Angina

In patients with unstable angina or acute coronary syndrome there can be deep, symmetric inversion of the T waves without loss of R waves in the precordial leads and with little or no cardiac enzyme or troponin elevation. These patients frequently have not yet had their infarction. Wall motion abnormalities may be observed on echocardiography in the absence of definite infarction—myocardial stunning. Such ECG signs may indicate critical proximal LAD coronary artery stenosis with possible brief periods of total occlusion and then spontaneous reperfusion (Wellens syndrome; see Chapter 22) and generally call for aggressive intervention, which may include emergency angiography and possible revascularization. Similar pathology in a dominant right coronary artery may produce these ECG changes in the inferior leads.

Hyperacute T Waves

Marked T wave peaking may be present in the very early stages of acute MI, usually in association with ST elevation. The ECGs in Fig. 24-3, *A* and *B*, were taken 3 days apart. Note the tall, peaked T waves in leads V_1 to V_4 preceding the development of Q waves and elevated ST segments 3 days later.

In some patients with unstable angina, marked T wave

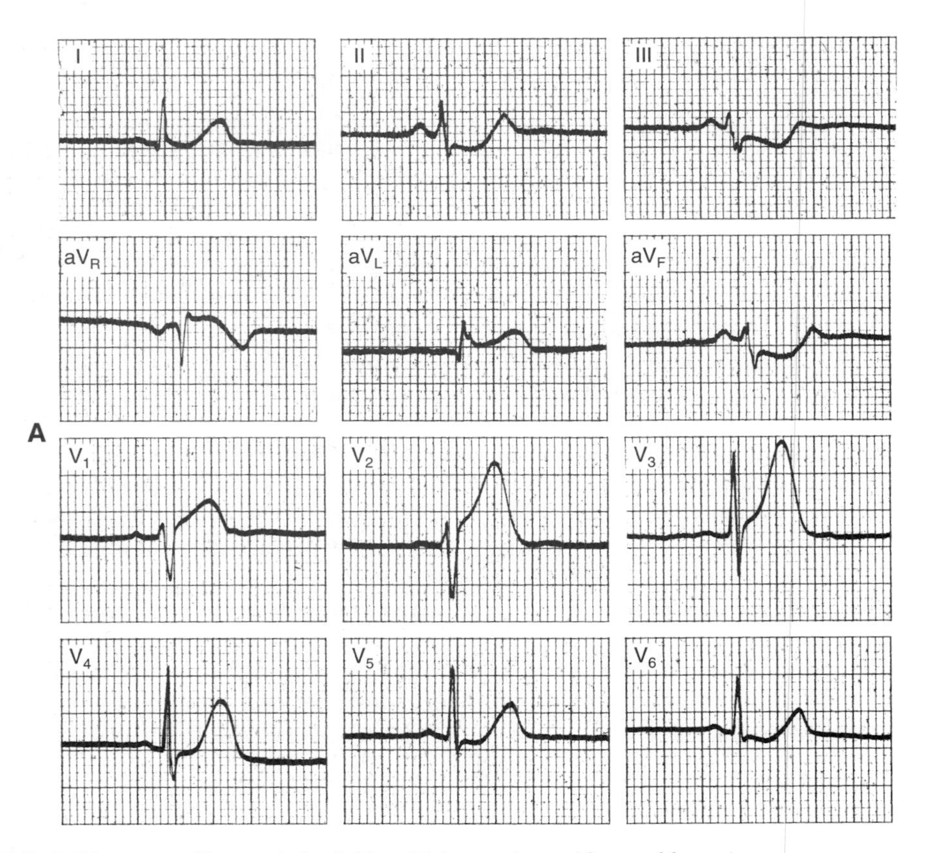

FIG. 24-3. A, Hyperacute T waves in leads V_1 to V_4 in a patient with unstable angina.

Continued

peaking may be noted (hyperacute T waves) before the development of deeply inverted symmetric T waves in V_2 and V_3 (Wellens syndrome, Chapter 22). Peaked T waves, as with ST elevation, are indicative of acute occlusion. This occlusion could be the result of plaque rupture that is causing spasm, thrombus, platelet aggregation, or a combination of these. If the occlusion is total and unrelieved, it evolves into MI. If it is total but transient, there are varying degrees of ST segment and T wave abnormalities and deep T wave inversion. The approximate time frame for the occlusion and appearance of ECG changes is as follows:

Less than 1 to 2 minutes: No ECG change
5 to 30 minutes: ST segment elevation, peaked T waves, followed by T wave inversion
More than 1 hour: Frequent infarction (persistent ST elevation and perhaps Q waves)

T Wave Inversions from Causes Other Than Myocardial Ischemia/Infarct

Juvenile T waves. T wave inversion may occur as a normal variant in the right-side to midchest leads of children (the juvenile T wave pattern) and may persist to adulthood.

The athlete's T waves. In the athlete's heart the T waves may be peaked, tall, biphasic, isoelectric, or even frankly inverted. T wave inversion in the precordial or limb leads have been seen in up to 30% of endurance athletes. These T wave changes may normalize with exercise or with isoproterenol infusion. The clinical setting is the basis for distinguishing T wave changes in the athlete's heart from metabolic or ischemic causes.[8]

After periods of abnormal depolarization. When the ventricles are depolarized abnormally, as they are in ventricular tachycardia, Wolff-Parkinson-White syndrome

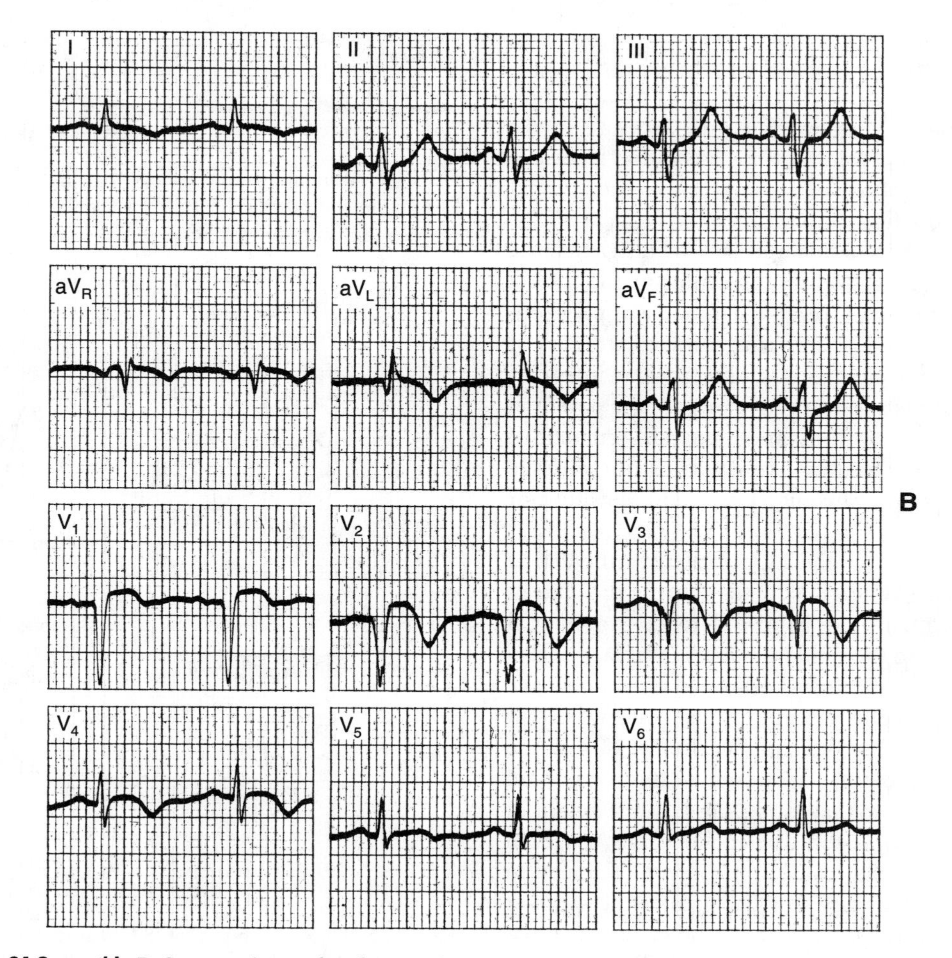

FIG. 24-3, cont'd. **B**, Same patient 3 days later with acute anteroseptal acute myocardial infarction.

with supraventricular tachycardia, paced ventricular rhythm, and BBB, the T wave is opposite in polarity to the terminal QRS. Thus the T wave is inverted when the ventricular complex ends in an R wave, but is upright when it ends in an S wave. These T wave inversions may persist for many hours after the resolution of abnormal depolarization.

Other causes. Deeply inverted, wide, blunted T waves may be seen in some cases of acute pulmonary embolism, acute cerebrovascular accident such as subarachnoid bleeding, major stroke, or central nervous system trauma.

ST SEGMENT

During the ST segment all layers of the myocardium are at the same electrical potential; this is phase 2 (the plateau) of the action potential (p. 9). Thus in the normal heart during this time there is no current flow between areas of the heart, leaving the ST segment isoelectric. This is not the case when the myocardium is acutely injured.

Acute Injury

New ST segment elevation of 1 mm or more in the limb leads and 2 mm or more in the precordial leads is a powerful diagnostic feature of acute MI, as is the appearance of a new conduction defect.[9]

Because of severe ischemia and lack of nutrients, the tissue immediately surrounding the center of the infarct is nonfunctional but may receive a blood supply from collateral circulation. This supply is sufficient to keep it alive but insufficient to maintain membrane integrity. The injured tissue has a less negative membrane potential from the healthy myocardium, and a current (current of injury) flows from the healthy tissue to the injured tissue during the ST segment, causing ST segment elevation or depression.

Fig. 24-4, *A,* illustrates the ECG related to the action potential in the normal heart. Note that during the plateau of the action potential there is no difference in potential (where the dashed and the solid lines fuse). This lack of difference produces a normal isoelectric ST segment, and the normal sequence of repolarization results in a T wave that is the same polarity as the QRS complex. In Fig. 24-4, *B,* the ischemic tissue has a membrane potential that is reduced to –60 mV and less. Note that in Fig. 24-4, *B,* the height of the action potential with the dashed line does not even reach the normal plateau, causing a current of injury to displace the ST segment upward. The greater the number of ischemic and injured cells present, the greater the displacement of the ST segment. Fig. 24-5 illustrates the different types of ST elevation in acute MI—concave, convex, oblique, and plateau shaped. The "tombstoning" ECG is illustrated in Fig. 24-14 and Fig. 24-15.

Prognostic Significance of ST Depression in Lateral Leads

Among 432 patients with a first acute MI without Q waves or ST segment elevation of 1 mm or more, Barrabés et al[10] found that ST segment depression in the lateral leads (I, aV_L, V_5, and V_6) on hospital admission predicts a poor in-hospital outcome. These patients had higher rates of death, severe heart failure, and angina with ECG changes

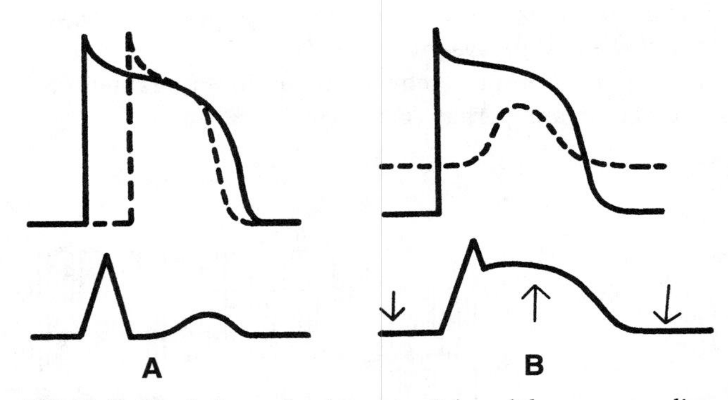

FIG. 24-4. Simulations of action potentials and the corresponding ECG from the normal heart (**A**) are compared with those from the ischemic and injured heart (**B**).

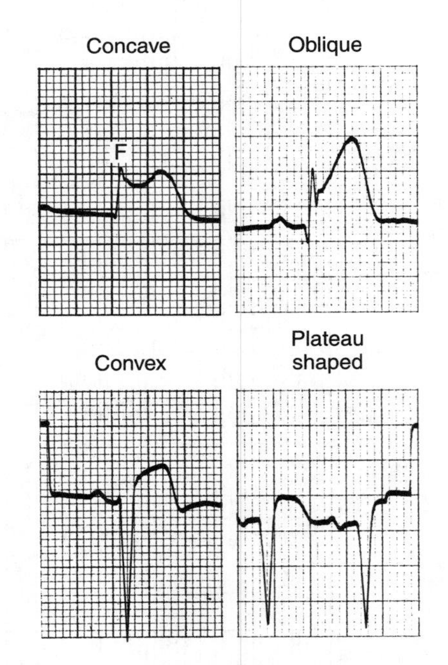

FIG. 24-5. Different types of ST segment elevations in acute myocardial infarction.

than did patients without this finding, even though they had similar peak creatine kinase and MB fraction levels.

ST-T Changes Not Caused by MI

Not all ST-T changes are caused by MI. They may be the result of unstable angina, acute pulmonary embolism, ventricular aneurysm, pericarditis, artifact, or the physiologic early repolarization syndrome of a trained athlete.

Prinzmetal's angina. Prinzmetal's angina is caused by reversible severe coronary artery spasm and is characterized by an episode of chest pain associated with ST elevation that reverts to normal within a matter of minutes. In such cases, ST elevation indicates total occlusion and cessation of blood flow through the epicardial coronary artery. If the duration of the occlusion is short (usually minutes), the ST elevation resolves. This is the cause of the ECG pattern seen in Prinzmetal's angina. However, such a sequence is not necessarily associated with pain; it can be painless. There are two possibilities for the mechanism of the occlusion: (1) Severe spasm leading to total occlusion in an artery that shows no luminal narrowing on angiography or (2) spasm superimposed on a fixed atherosclerotic obstruction, leading to 100% occlusion. If, on the other hand, the total occlusion is prolonged (20 to 40 minutes), the ST elevation does not resolve, enzyme levels rise, infarction develops, T waves become abnormal, and Q waves may develop.

Thus Prinzmetal's angina differs from an acute infarction: Prinzmetal's angina is a temporary, reversible condition caused primarily by spasm and does not involve an acute thrombus, whereas in MI acute thrombus is primary, spasm may be contributing, and the occlusion is not self-limited.

Critical proximal coronary artery stenosis. The ST segment may elevate during pain in some patients with unstable angina and critical proximal coronary artery stenosis. The ST segment may be only slightly elevated or not at all elevated and there may be deep, symmetric T wave inversion (see Chapter 22). ST segment elevation usually accompanies transient total occlusion of the vessel. The changes may occur in the absence of chest pain (silent ischemia).

Left main and three-vessel coronary artery disease. The more common type of unstable angina than Prinzmetal's angina is associated with diffuse depression of the ST segment, especially in leads V_3 and V_4, and ST elevation in leads aV_R and V_1. These ECG findings have frequently been shown to represent extensive myocardial ischemia and are commonly associated with left main or three-vessel coronary artery disease (see Chapter 22). Aggressive medical therapy followed by urgent coronary arteriography and, frequently, revascularization are required.[11]

Acute pulmonary embolism. ST segment elevation may be seen in acute pulmonary embolism in the leads reflecting the dilated right ventricle, V_1 and aV_R. When the ST elevation in V_1 is associated with an RBBB pattern and a positive T wave, it should raise the suspicion of acute pulmonary embolism. In acute pulmonary embolism, troponin may be elevated, presumably secondary to right ventricular insult or pressure overload (see p. 404).

Ventricular aneurysm. Ventricular aneurysm causes ST segment elevation to persist after acute infarction. The ST elevation is caused by a current of injury generated from the myocardial cells bordering the aneurysm.

Acute pericarditis. ST elevation in pericarditis is often associated with pleuritic-type chest pain and is not accompanied by reciprocal ST changes. Frequently the ST segment elevation is diffuse, involving multiple leads, and is accompanied by an increased sinus rate. The pericardium is electrically silent and does not contribute to ECG changes. Thus these ECG changes usually reflect inflammatory involvement of the epicardium.

Early repolarization syndrome. Along with the T wave changes already mentioned, J point elevation (see Chapter 20) and ST segment elevation are frequently found in the athlete and, as with the T wave changes, may normalize with exercise. Early repolarization has elevated, upward, concave ST segments, located commonly in precordial leads, with reciprocal depression in a right chest lead; tall, peaked, and slightly asymmetrical notched T waves; and a slur on the R wave. Other ECG features are vertical axis, shorter and depressed PR interval, counterclockwise rotation of the heart (p. 18), and U waves. The J wave may be confused with the ECG changes of acute pericarditis and with acute MI because of the associated ST segment elevation. However, as with T wave changes in an athlete's ECG, the clinical setting helps in the differential diagnosis. Additionally the J point changes in the athlete's ECG are localized as opposed to the global changes in pericarditis. The athlete's heart at rest is in sinus bradycardia and sometimes sinus arrhythmia, whereas in pericarditis there usually is sinus tachycardia.[8]

Artifact. ST segment elevation may be caused by the low-frequency filter on the cardiac monitor or by poor electrode contact. Overdamping of the ECG stylus is another cause of ST elevation. It is recognized in the standardization artifact, which is slurred on its upstroke.

Nonspecific ST-T changes. *Nonspecific* describes ST-T changes that are outside the range of normal, including minor deviations of the ST segment, flattening of the T wave, and slight T wave inversions. Such changes should be

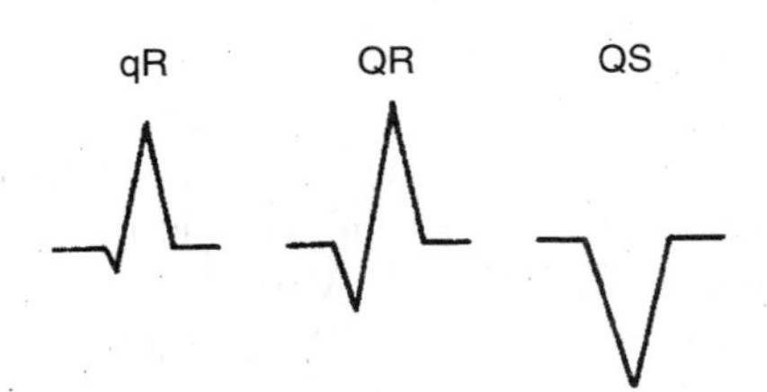

FIG. 24-6. Designation of the components of the QRS according to size and sequence. Lowercase type is used when the component is small.

monitored continuously in patients with unstable angina. Critical proximal LAD coronary artery stenosis is often initially manifested in these patients with a very slight negativity at the end of the T wave in leads V_1 to V_3.

Q WAVES

A Q wave is a negative deflection that, when present, is the first component of the ventricular complex. An uppercase or a lowercase letter is used to indicate the size of the Q wave. Fig. 24-6 illustrates the differences between q and Q waves.

Normal Q Waves

Normal q waves reflect normal septal activation. They are narrow and small and are usually seen in leads I, aV_L, and V_6. The dominant current in the interventricular septum is from left to right. Thus the leads that record these initial forces have left-to-right lead axes with the positive electrode on the left side of the body, that is, leads I, aV_L, and V_6.

The axis of lead I is straight across the shoulders. Lead aV_L has an axis from the left shoulder to the center of the electrical field of the heart. Lead V_6 has an axis from a midaxillary position to the center of the electrical field of the heart. Fig. 24-7 illustrates the relationship of these three lead axes to normal septal forces. In leads I, aV_L, and V_6, septal forces move away from the positive electrode, producing a small q wave. In the electrically horizontal heart, normal septal q waves may also appear in leads V_4 and V_5, and in the electrically vertical heart, in leads II, III, and aV_F.

Pathologic Q Waves

Lead V_4: 0.02 second or more
Leads I, II, aVL, V_5, or V_6: 0.03 second or more
Leads V_1 to V_3: Present at any width (i.e., loss of R wave)[12,13]

Abnormal Q waves, the classic diagnostic feature of myocardial necrosis, are identified when there is an

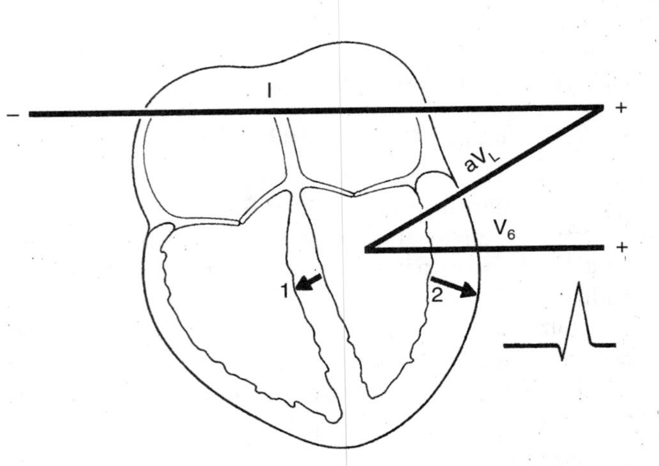

FIG. 24-7. Orientation of the initial QRS forces (septal) to the axes of leads I, aV_L, and V_6.

increase in duration and depth of normal Q waves or the appearance of "new" Q waves (not present in previous tracings). Thus changes in pattern may be just as significant as the size of the Q wave. Possible processes for the appearance of pathologic Q waves are the following:

1. When electrically inactive tissue is present under the electrode, it records from the opposite wall of the heart (as if looking through a window).
2. When there is inactive tissue under the electrode, the wavefront must travel long distances around the inactive tissue. Abnormal Q waves reflect this delay. The larger and deeper the lesion, the larger the Q wave.[17]
3. When there is conduction delay in the zone under the electrode, as in the early stages of acute MI, pathologic Q waves may appear. Thus, even with new pathologic Q waves, thrombolysis can still accomplish significant myocardial salvage, even after several hours of delay from the onset of pain.

Q Waves from Causes Other Than Myocardial Infarction

Q waves are not always a sign of necrotic myocardial tissue. They may be the result of other conditions such as acute pulmonary embolism, infiltrative myocardial disease, interventricular conduction problems, ventricular hypertrophy, or they may be a normal variant.

Acute pulmonary embolism. Following acute pulmonary embolism (see Chapter 28) a q wave often appears in leads V_1, III, and aV_F accompanied by T wave changes that are sometimes seen in the precordial leads. Given the clinical presentation of chest pain and dyspnea, such patients may be misdiagnosed as having acute MI. The occasionally elevated troponin in acute pulmonary embolism may further complicate the differential diagnosis (see p. 405).

Infiltrative myocardial disease. In conditions such as amyloidosis, muscular dystrophy, and any other type of myocardial disease that causes a loss of electrical potentials and an inability to depolarize, abnormal Q waves may be seen.

Intraventricular conduction problems. Abnormal Q waves may be seen when intraventricular conduction is abnormal, such as in BBB and Wolff-Parkinson-White syndrome.

Ventricular hypertrophy. In the leads facing the ventricle opposite the hypertrophy, reciprocal Q waves may be seen. These may be prominent in hypertrophic cardiomyopathy.

Normal variant. A QS complex may be normal in lead V_1 but rarely occurs in leads V_1 and V_2, simulating anteroseptal MI. A QS complex may also be a normal finding in leads III and aV_F. In the electrically vertical heart there may be a QS or Qr pattern in aV_L, simulating lateral wall infarction; the difference is that there are no other signs of MI, including ST segment abnormalities, abnormal Q waves, or loss of R waves in the other lateral leads, I, V_5, and V_6.

ACUTE ECG REFLECTING RISK

When faced with a patient with acute chest pain, clinicians must distinguish acute MI from all other causes of acute chest pain. If acute MI is suspected, decisions regarding treatment, including reperfusion strategy, are then made based on ECG changes, including ST segment elevation or left bundle branch block (LBBB). If the ECG does not indicate acute MI the physician must decide whether or not to admit the patient to the cardiac care unit on the basis of suspected unstable high-risk ischemia or acute MI without ECG changes. The history and physical examination, in combination with the ECG and cardiac markers (troponin) or enzymes (CK-MB), remain the key tool for the diagnosis of acute MI.[1]

Chest Pain and the Probability of Acute MI

Three features noted on admission that increase the probability of acute MI are as follows:

- New ST segment elevation
- New Q wave
- Chest pain radiating to both arms simultaneously

Of lesser likelihood to increase that probability are the presence of a third heart sound and hypotension.

Features that decrease the probability of acute MI are as follows:

- A normal ECG (the incidence of acute MI with a normal ECG is 3.7%)[14]
- Sharp, stabbing, or positional chest pain that is pleuritic[9]

Terminal QRS and Myocardial Damage

Distortion of the terminal part of the QRS on the admission ECG in patients with acute MI may indicate severe myocardial damage[18,19] (i.e., lower left ventricular [LV] ejection fraction, more reduced regional wall motion, and less improvement in regional wall motion in the infarct region at both 1 and 6 months) after acute MI than patients without this pattern.

Distortion of the terminal QRS is defined as follows:

- Elevation of the J point at 50% or more of the R wave amplitude in leads with a qR configuration
- Absence of s waves in leads that should have an Rs configuration

BBB and Hemiblock

The development of BBB and hemiblock help to identify high-risk patients with acute anterior MI. These conduction problems are recognized on ECG in leads V_1, I, and II. Such findings are an independent marker of poor prognosis in patients with acute anterior MI and generally reflect an extension of myocardial injury.

TIMI RISK SCORE ON ADMISSION

The Thrombolysis in Myocardial Infarction (TIMI) group have presented risk assessment scoring system derived from the multivariable analysis of nearly 15,000 patients with ST segment elevation. This can be done at the bedside at the time of admission of a patient with acute MI.[15,16]

The score may vary from 0 to 14 possible points, with a graded increase in mortality from 0.8% (risk score 0) to 35.9% (risk score >8 points). In patients who survived 30 days the mortality at 1 year increases from 1% (risk score 0) to 17.2% (risk score >8 points).

Age 65 to 74 years = 2 points
Age >7 = 3 points
Systolic blood pressure <100 mm Hg = 3 points
Heart rate >100 beats/min = 2 points
Killip (see the following section) class 2 to 4 = 2 points
Anterior ST elevation or left bundle branch block = 1 point

Diabetes, history of hypertension, or history of angina = 1 point
Weight <67 kg = 1 point
Time to treatment >4 hours = 1 point

KILLIP SCORING SYSTEM[17]

Class I: Absence of rales over the lung fields and absence of a third heart sound
Class II: Presence of rales over 50% of the lung fields or the presence of a third heart sound
Class III: Rales over more than 50% of the lung fields, with the patient often presenting in pulmonary edema
Class IV: Cardiogenic shock

Mortality rises dramatically through the classes from I to IV.

LOCATING THE INFARCT

The location of acute ischemic or infarcted areas is not difficult to determine by ECG when it involves initial QRS forces (Q waves appear in leads reflecting the infarct). Diagnostic difficulties may arise when terminal instead of initial forces are affected, as in the posterobasal acute MI or when LBBB and MI coexist.[1]

The key to locating the infarct is an understanding of the surfaces of the heart and their reflecting leads. Although it is almost always possible to identify the location of an anterior, lateral, or inferior infarction on the ECG, apical locations are difficult, if not impossible, to determine. The sensitivity of the ECG in localizing apical acute MI is very low. At times there are Q waves in precordial leads V_1 to V_4, and at other times, in the inferior leads. One source defines *apical MI* as Q waves present in leads II, III, and aV_L and one or more of the leads V_1 to V_4.[20]

Echocardiography has proved invaluable in both the diagnosis and the localization of acute MI, especially when the clinical and ECG findings are not diagnostic or if complications of acute MI are suspected.

In Fig. 24-8 the cylinder of the left ventricle is portioned into anterior, septal, lateral, and inferior surfaces. The base of the heart is part of all of these surfaces. The anterior base of the left ventricle is the anterior septum. The inferior base is called *posterior*. The leads reflecting these surfaces are discussed under their headings.

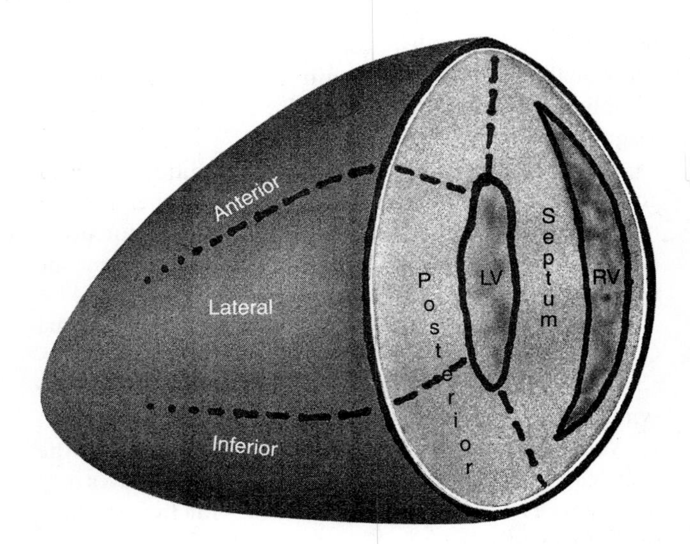

FIG. 24-8. The surfaces of the heart. Note that involvement of the anterior segment may extend to the septum (anteroseptal myocardial infarction) and the lateral wall (anterolateral). The inferior segment may extend to the posterior wall (inferoposterior), the lateral wall (inferolateral), or both (inferoposterolateral), and the right ventricle *(RV)*. *LV,* Left ventricle.

ANTERIOR MI

The anterior wall includes its lateral borders and the interventricular septum. Anterior MI results from an occlusion of the proximal LAD coronary artery and may involve a combined blockage of the LAD coronary artery and RCA or left circumflex artery. The infarction may extend from the anterior wall into the septum (anteroseptal infarction) and to the left base, free wall, or apex; such infarctions are grouped under the term *anterolateral* or *extensive anterior MI.*

Reflecting Leads

Anterior: V_3 and V_4
Anteroseptal: V_1 to V_4
Lateral: I, aV_L, and V_6
Anterolateral: I, aV_L, and V_3 to V_6
Extensive anterior: I, aV_L, and V_1 to V_6
High lateral: I and aV_L

Fig. 24-9 illustrates the proximity of the precordial leads to the anterior heart as follows:

- V_1 is over the anterior right ventricular surface
- V_2 and V_3 span the septum
- V_3 and V_4 are over the anterior wall of the left ventricle
- V_5 and V_6 reflect the anterior and lateral walls of the heart, with leads I and aV_L reflecting the high lateral wall

Right-sided chest leads V_{3R} to V_{6R} are also illustrated (Fig. 24-9). As you will see, V_{4R} is useful in acute inferior

MI in identifying high-risk patients and right ventricular MI.

Fig. 24-10 is a diagram of muscle involved in an extensive anterolateral wall infarction and the relationship of the reflecting leads. Note that leads I and aV_L are close to the base of the heart. Fig. 24-11 shows a more circumspect anteroseptal infarction.

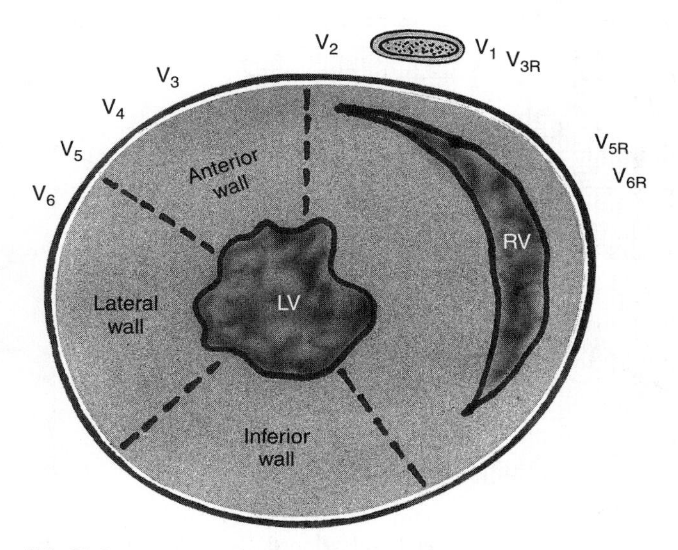

FIG. 24-9. Location of left and right precordial leads. Note the proximity of these leads to the surface of the ventricles. Leads V_2 and V_3 span the septum; leads V_2 to V_4 are over the anterior wall; and V_5 to V_6 are over the lateral wall. Lead V_{4R} is the best right-side precordial lead for detecting right ventricular acute myocardial infarction. *LV,* Left ventricle; *RV,* right ventricle.

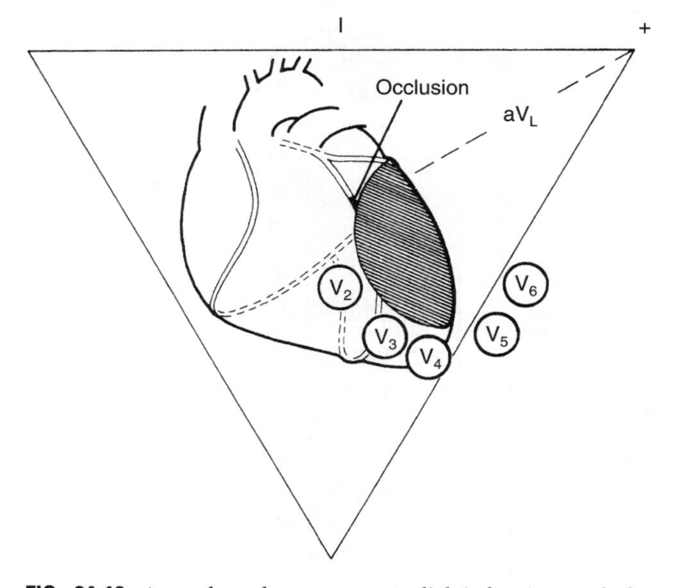

FIG. 24-10. Anterolateral acute myocardial infarction and the reflecting leads.

ECG Recognition

1. ST segment elevation in the precordial leads; leads I and aV_L may also be involved. In general, the more leads involved and the higher the ST segment, the bigger the infarction.
2. Loss of R wave progression (loss of anterior forces).
3. Symmetric T wave inversion from an ST segment that is coved upward.

In Fig. 24-12 there are Q (QS) waves in leads V_1 to V_4 and ST elevation in leads V_1 to V_6 (anteroseptal and anterolateral).

The Q waves in leads III and aV_F reveal an old inferior MI. The left-axis deviation indicates left anterior hemiblock in this clinical setting. In Fig. 24-13 the ECG signs of acute MI are seen in all of the superior leads (V_1 to V_6, I, and aV_L).

Predicting the Site of Occlusion in Acute Anterior MI

In acute anterior MI the more proximal the occlusion in the left anterior descending coronary artery, the less favorable the prognosis. The Wellens group,[21] in a study involving 100 patients with first acute anterior MI demonstrated that the ECG is of value not only in predicting the LAD occlusion site, but also in predicting the culprit lesion in its major side branches (first septal perforator or first diagonal branch). Strong predictors of occlusion were described as follows.

Proximal LAD to the first septal perforator

- ST elevation in lead aV_R
- Complete right bundle branch block

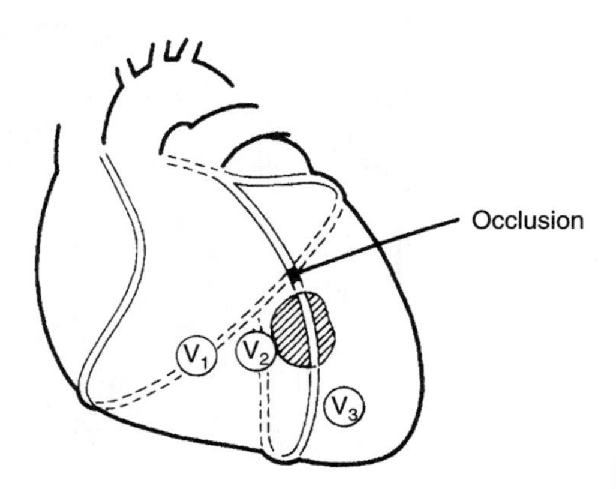

FIG. 24-11. Anteroseptal acute myocardial infarction and the reflecting leads.

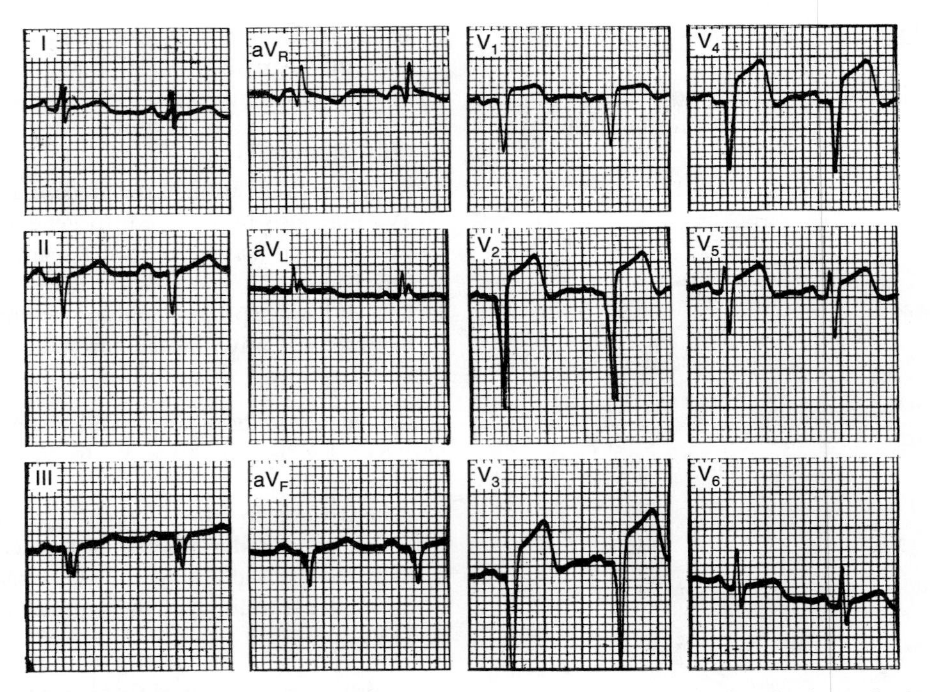

FIG. 24-12. Anterior acute myocardial infarction. The loss of R wave progression from lead V_1 to lead V_4 and the ST segment elevation are evident. Limb leads show that anterior hemiblock has developed. (Note the negative complex in lead II.) Hemiblock and development of right bundle branch block identify high-risk patients.

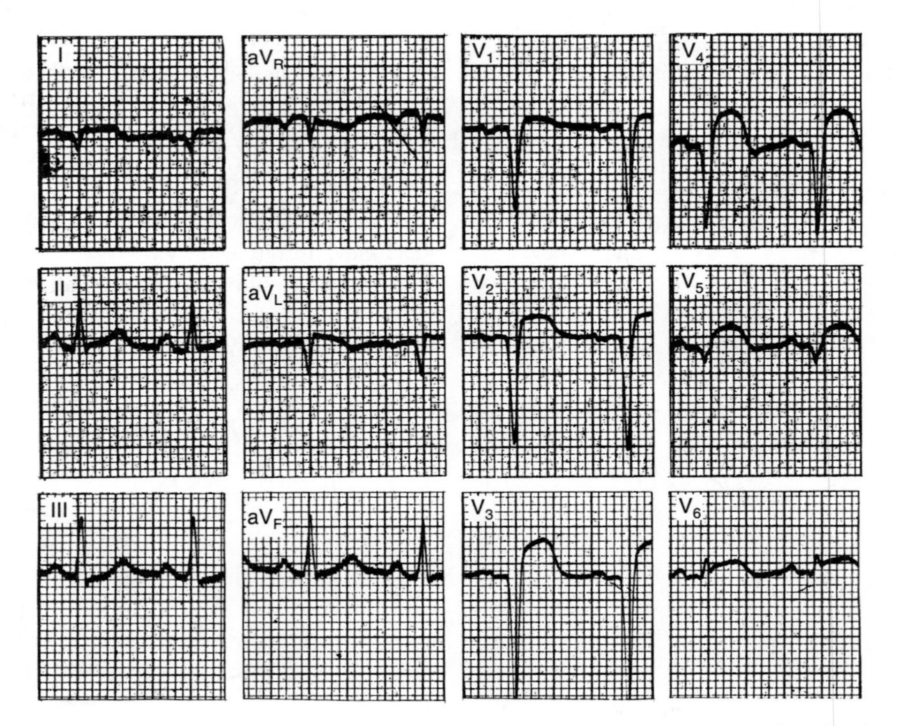

FIG. 24-13. Anterolateral acute myocardial infarction. The loss of R wave progression from lead V_1 to lead V_6 and the ST segment elevation in those leads are evident.

- ST depression in lead V_5
- ST elevation in V_1 greater than 2.5 mm
- Inferior ST depression
- ST depression in III greater than the ST elevation in aV_L[22]

Distal to the first septal perforator

- Abnormal Q waves in V_4 through V_6
- Absence of inferior ST depression

Proximal to the first diagonal branch

- Abnormal Q wave in lead aV_L
- ST elevation in aV_L[23]
- Inferior ST depression (leads II, III, and aV_F)

Distal to the first diagonal branch

- ST depression in aV_L
- Absence of inferior ST depression

Small conal branch of the RCA that does not reach the interventricular septum[24]

- ST elevation in V_1

"Tombstoning." The tombstone pattern seen on admission is associated with severe coronary artery disease involving the proximal LAD. Figs. 24-14, *B* and *D*, show the ECG pattern of the tombstoning ECG in acute anterior MI compared to the nontombstoning ECG. The features of the tombstoning ECG are examined more closely in Fig. 24-15:

1. The R wave is either absent or, if present, its duration is less than 0.04 second with a minimal amplitude; there is no trough following the R wave
2. The ST segment is convex upward and merges with the descending limb of the R wave or the ascending limb of the QS/QR wave
3. The peak of the convex ST segment is higher than whatever remains of the R wave
4. The convex ST segment merges with the ascending limb of the following T wave

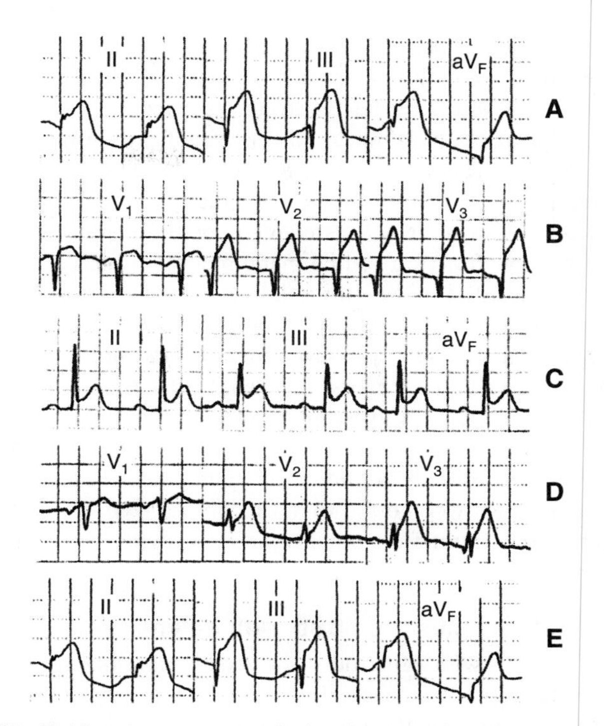

FIG. 24-14. ECG patterns and classification of tombstoning. **A,** Tombstoning ECG of an inferior acute MI. **B,** Tombstoning ECG of an anterior acute myocardial infarction (MI). **C,** Nontombstoning ECG of an inferior acute MI. **D,** Nontombstoning ECG of an anterior acute MI. **E,** Borderline ECG of an inferior acute MI. (From Guo XH, Yap YG, Chen LJ et al: Correlation of coronary angiography with "tombstoning" electrocardiographic pattern in patients after acute myocardial infarction, *Clin Cardiol* 23:347-352, 2000.)

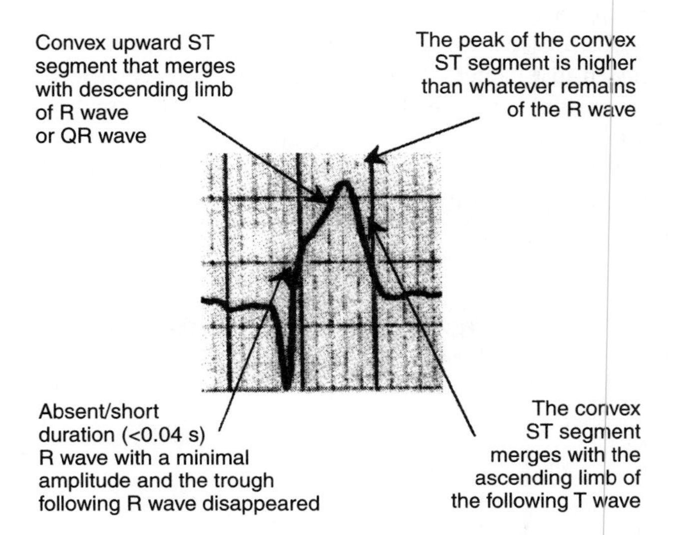

FIG. 24-15. The features of the tombstoning ECG. (From Guo XH, Yap YG, Chen LJ et al: Correlation of coronary angiography with "tombstoning" electrocardiographic pattern in patients after acute myocardial infarction, *Clin Cardiol* 23:347-352, 2000.)

Q Waves in Acute Anterior Versus Inferior MI

Among patients with acute anterior MI, abnormal Q waves on the admission ECG are associated with higher peak CK-MB, higher prevalence of heart failure, and increased mortality. The same is however, not true for patients with inferior MI.[25]

Left Ventricular Function after Q Wave Anterior MI

Patients with reduced left ventricular function and ventricular enlargement after Q wave anterior MI are at significantly greater risk for congestive heart failure and cardiac death than are those without these conditions.[26] Nevertheless, with current aggressive medical treatment, combined with reperfusion strategies, partial recovery of ventricular function may occur in a significant proportion of patients. The recovery may take several weeks and is best evaluated by follow-up echocardiography.

At 1 year after MI, assessment of the degree of left ventricular function can be made by evaluating the time required for T wave normalization in the leads with abnormal Q waves. Patients whose T waves invert after admission and are still inverted after 12 months have been shown to have worse left ventricular function than patients whose T waves are inverted on admission but normalize early. Remarkably, patients whose T waves remain positive throughout the acute and the recovery phases of MI were found to have a poorer recovery of left ventricular function than patients with persistent negative T waves.[27]

ECG Diagnosis of RBBB with Anterior Septal MI

Patients with BBB and suspected MI have been shown to receive suboptimal treatment because the infarction is often obscured by the BBB.[28] However, you will see that it is MI with LBBB rather than MI with RBBB that is difficult to recognize.

RBBB without MI is recognized because of a broad QRS with an rSR′ pattern in lead V_1. Initial forces (septal and left ventricular) are normal, thus there is an rS complex in V_1; it is the terminal forces that are late (activation of the right ventricle), thus the terminal R wave in V_1 results in an rSR′ pattern.

RBBB with MI has already been illustrated and discussed in Chapter 23. It is recognized when septal forces are missing (no initial r wave in V_1); the terminal late R wave will of course still be apparent in V_1. Thus, instead of the usual rSR′ pattern, the initial little septal r wave will be missing, resulting in a broad QR pattern in lead V_1, as shown in Fig. 24-16. Of course, one must correlate the ECG with the clinical picture since the initial little r wave in V_1 may normally be absent. Fig. 24-17 shows the serial tracings of a patient with acute anterolateral MI in whom left anterior hemiblock (Fig. 24-17, *B*) and RBBB (Fig. 24-17, *C*) subsequently develop. In Fig. 24-17, *C*, the typical rSR′ pattern of uncomplicated RBBB is replaced by a QR pattern.

Fig. 24-18 shows anterior MI with RBBB, there is no hemiblock. (Note the normal axis.) In Fig. 24-19 there are anterior MI (Q waves in leads V_1 and V_2), RBBB (late

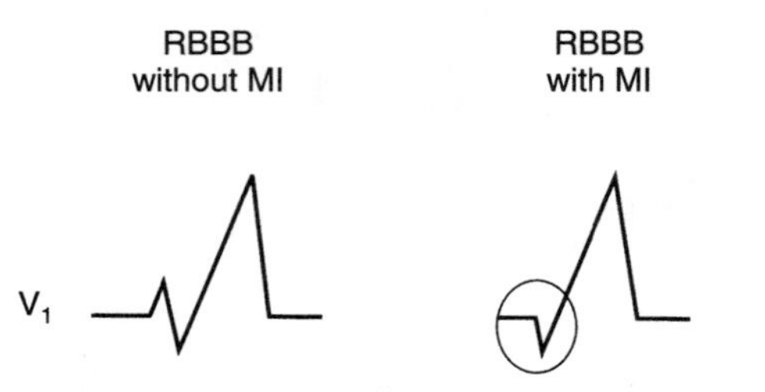

FIG. 24-16. Patterns of right bundle branch block *(RBBB)* without and with anteroseptal myocardial infarction *(MI)* compared in lead V_1.

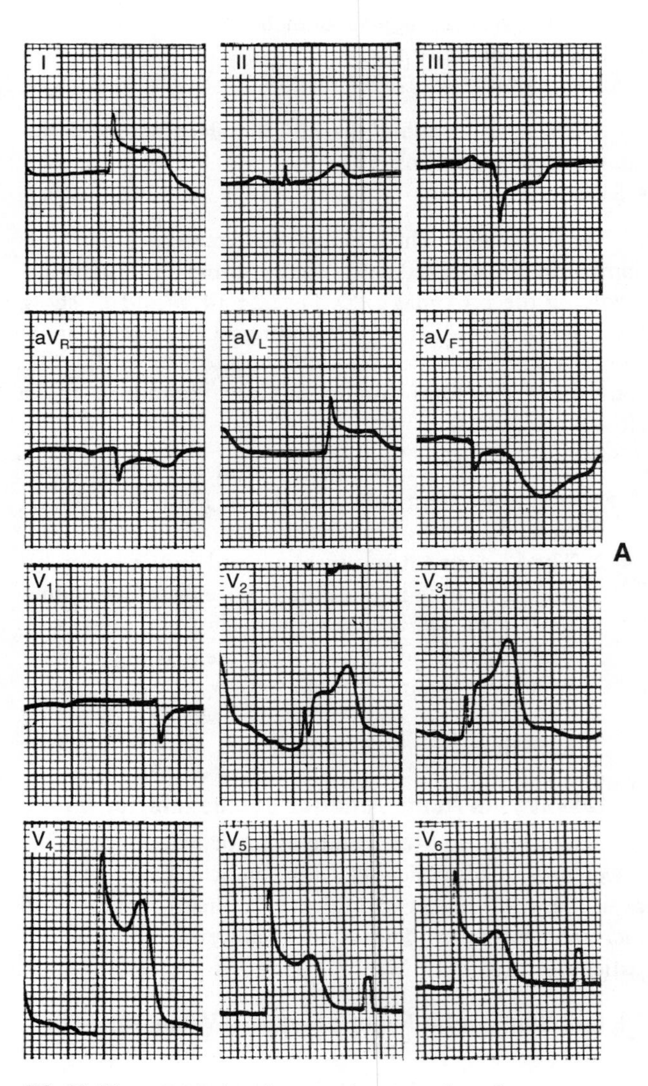

FIG. 24-17. **A**, ECG showing massive anterolateral acute myocardial infarction. The ST elevation is evident in all the superior leads.

Continued

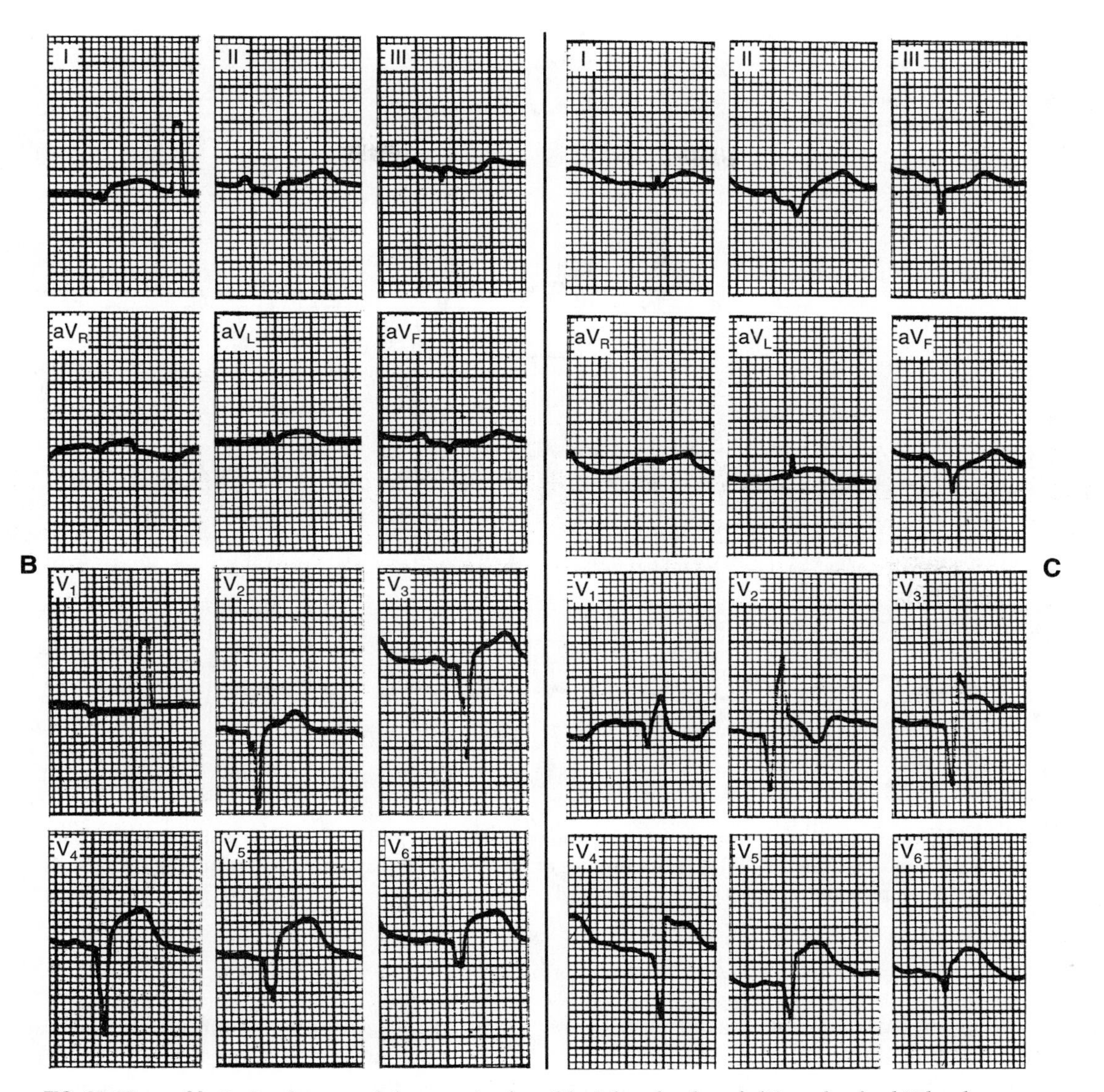

FIG. 24-17, cont'd. **B**, On the second day anterior hemiblock has developed. (Note that lead II has become negative.) **C**, By the third day RBBB has developed. (Courtesy Peggy McKnight, RN, Las Vegas.)

R wave in V_1), and left anterior hemiblock (extreme left-axis deviation).

Immediately recognizing and reporting the development of BBB or hemiblock in patients with acute anterior MI is extremely important. Such a finding identifies a high-risk patient and is an indication for aggressive therapy.

ECG Diagnosis of LBBB with Anterior Septal MI

Prognosis worsens when LBBB and MI coexist, whether or not the LBBB was preexisting or is a consequence of the infarction.[29] Over the last decade, this fact has spurred the search for a reliable ECG clue to the presence of acute MI in patients presenting with LBBB. It is helpful, however, to note that patients with new LBBB and suspected ischemia are five times more likely to have acute MI than patients with LBBB of chronic or unknown duration.[30]

It is not a diagnostic challenge to recognize MI when associated with RBBB because initial forces are septal and left ventricular, and the criteria for normal activation still applies (p. 318). It is, however, difficult and sometimes

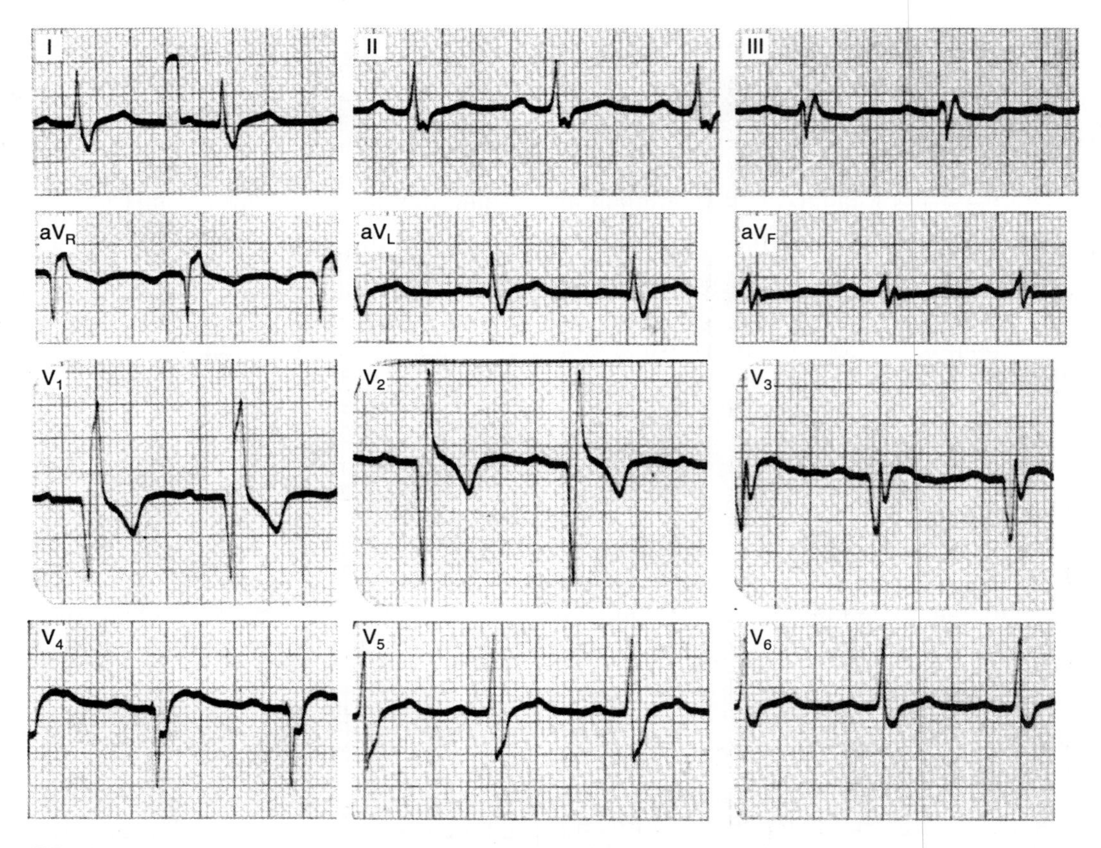

FIG. 24-18. Anteroseptal acute myocardial infarction with RBBB. In lead V_1 the absence of the initial r wave is typical of uncomplicated RBBB. The appearance of RBBB identifies a high-risk patient. The QRS axis is normal; therefore, hemiblock has not yet developed.

impossible to recognize MI when it is associated with LBBB because initial forces and left ventricular activation are not normal. Not only are the two ventricles activated sequentially (the right and then the left) instead of simultaneously, activation of the left ventricle does not take the normal pathway, being activated from the right bundle branch. Thus areas in the left ventricle that usually produce initial QRS forces are now activated at the end of the QRS, rendering the traditional ECG signs of ischemia and MI inappropriate. Strategies that may help in the correct ECG interpretation of LBBB with MI are listed on p. 323.[1]

It is useful to remember the pragmatic words of Wellens: "The evidence favors an aggressive approach to the treatment of the patient admitted with chest pain suggestive of acute cardiac ischemia and left bundle branch block."[1] The recommendations of the American College of Cardiology/American Heart Association are that, in the absence of contraindications, acute reperfusion therapy should be used in all patients with LBBB who have the clinical presentations indicative of acute MI.[31]

This approach protects patients with chest pain. However, Shlipak et al[32] studied the clinical features, treatment and in-hospital survival of 29,585 acute MI patients with LBBB. Nearly half of them do not present with chest pain and are therefore less likely to receive optimal therapy, placing them at increased risk of death.

ECG criteria

1. Serial ECG changes (sensitivity 67%); a single ECG is of restricted value
2. ST segment elevation (sensitivity 54%)
3. Abnormal Q waves (sensitivity 31%)
4. Cabrera's sign (i.e., notching of 0.05 second in the ascending limb of the S wave in leads V_3 and V_4 [sensitivity 27%])

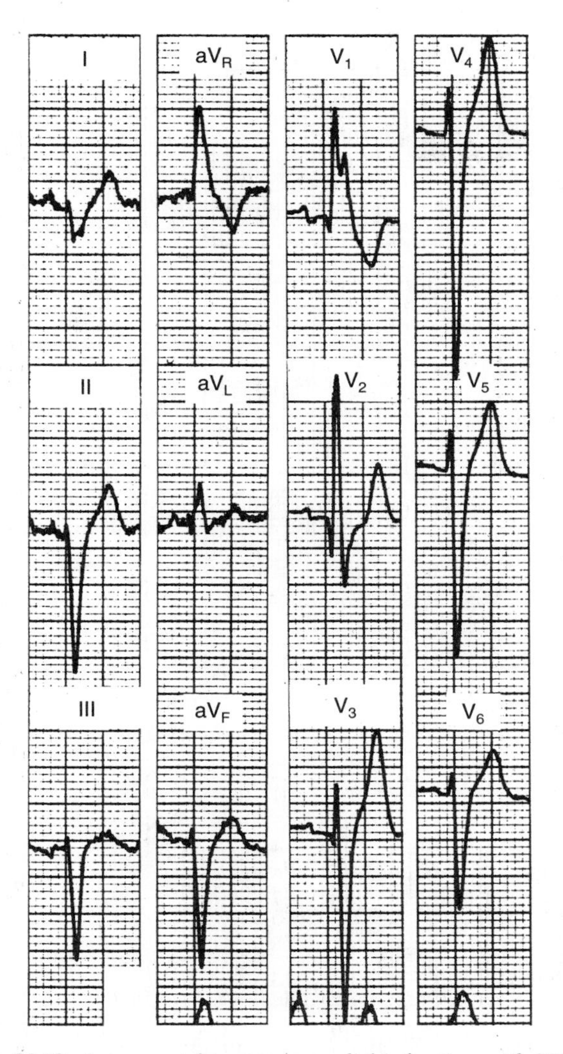

FIG. 24-19. Anteroseptal acute myocardial infarction with RBBB and hemiblock. There is a Q wave in leads V_1 to V_3, along with a broad R wave. There is also left anterior hemiblock, as evidenced by the extreme left axis deviation. These ECG signs identify a high-risk patient.

5. An R wave in V_1 and a Q wave in V_6, as shown in Fig. 24-20 and Fig. 24-21 (sensitivity 20%; but with a specificity of 100% for anteroseptal MI); the mechanism has already been illustrated and discussed in Chapter 23

Additional ECG Signs of Acute MI in Patients with LBBB

Three recently described ECG criteria for recognizing acute MI in patients with LBBB have been published by Sgarbossa et al.[34] They are (1) ST segment elevation of 1

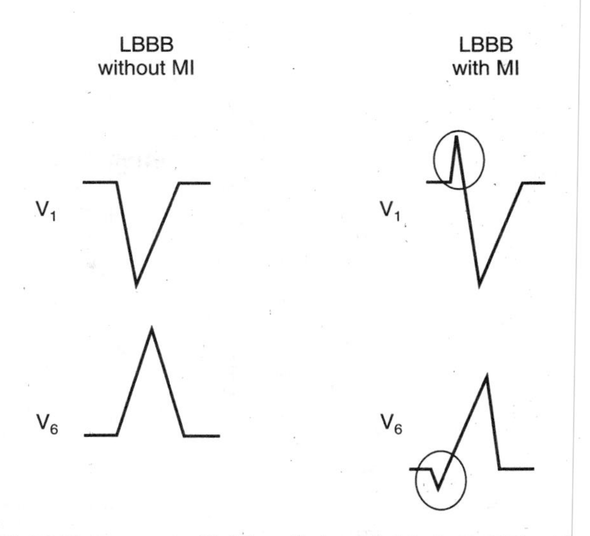

FIG. 24-20. Patterns of left bundle branch block *(LBBB)* without and with anteroseptal myocardial infarction *(MI)* compared in lead V_1.

mm or more in the presence of a positive QRS complex; (2) ST segment depression of 1 mm or more in lead V_1, V_2, or V_3; and (3) ST segment elevation of 5 mm or more in the presence of a negative QRS complex.

Li et al[30] found that only the first criterion (ST elevation of 1 mm or more when the QRS is positive) demonstrated a clinically useful likelihood ratio. Additionally, Wellens[1] has pointed out that these three criteria, although useful, may not represent the acute stage of severe cardiac ischemia because confirmation for the presence of acute MI was made by enzyme measurements in patients from the GUSTO-1 study (Global Utilization of Streptokinase and Tissue Plasminogen Activator for Occluded Coronary Arteries).

NON–Q WAVE ACUTE MI

A non–Q wave acute MI results when an active thrombus partially or transiently occludes a coronary artery. When critical reductions in myocardial blood flow persist for more than 2 hours, the infarct is usually transmural. Large non–Q wave acute MI is associated with greater prolongation of the QTc and QT dispersion compared with Q wave acute MI,[35] both of which provide the milieu for arrhythmias.

ECG Recognition

Fig. 24-22 shows non–Q wave anterior MI; there is ST segment depression in leads V_1 to V_6 and T wave inversion in leads I, aV_L, and V_2 to V_6. Helpful indicators in differen-

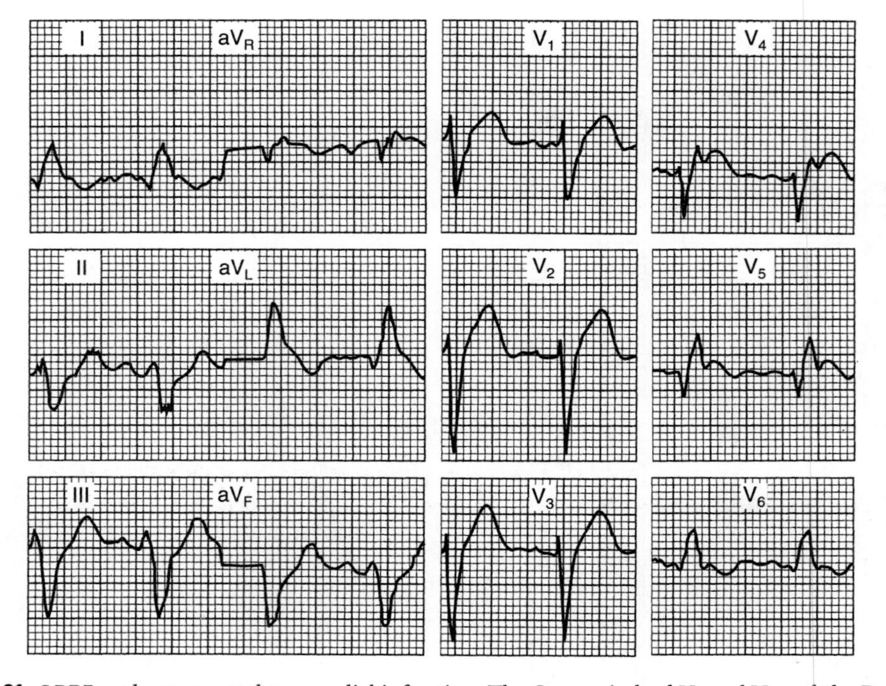

FIG. 24-21. LBBB and anteroseptal myocardial infarction. The Q wave in lead V_5 and V_6 and the R wave in lead V_1 are signs of MI complicated by LBBB. (From Lyon LJ: *Basic electrocardiography handbook,* New York, 1977, Van Nosstrand Reinhold.)

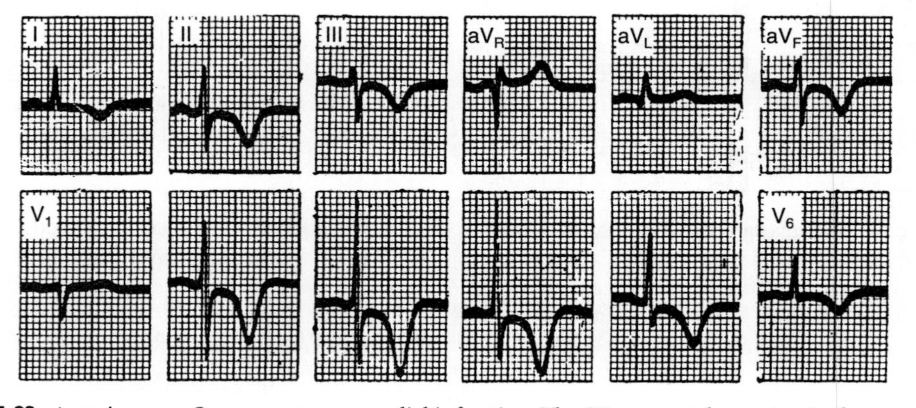

FIG. 24-22. Anterior non–Q wave acute myocardial infarction. The ST segment depression in the precordial leads and the T wave inversions in leads I, aV_L, and V_2 to V_6 are evident. (From Boden WE, Kleiger RE, Gibson RS et al: *Am J Cardiol* 59:782, 1987.)

tiating this type of acute MI from posterior MI are (1) the degree of enzyme elevation (larger in acute posterior MI) and (2) the degree of ST segment depression (more marked in acute posterior MI).

In contrast to Q wave MI, in which there is a classic, evolving ECG pattern of ST elevation followed by development of Q waves in leads overlying the necrosis, there is not a specific ECG pattern in non–Q wave MI; the diagnosis is based on the ECG and characteristic elevations of myocardial markers (troponin) or cardiac enzymes (CK-MB).

Clinical Implications

A study reflecting the years 1975-1997 of patients with non–Q wave acute MI does not show the impressive declines in the incidence, in-hospital, and long-term mortality associated with Q wave acute MI. On the contrary, non–Q wave acute MI is increasing in frequency and has the same in-hospital mortality now as it did 22 years ago.[36]

Differential Diagnosis

In the chronic stage of MI the polarity of the T waves in the leads with Q waves differentiates between transmural and nontransmural MI.

Persistent negative T waves in leads with Q waves. Transmural infarction consisting of a thin fibrotic layer.

Positive T waves in leads with Q waves. Nontransmural infarction containing viable myocardium within the layer of the ventricular wall under the electrodes.[37]

Prognosis

Patients with acute non–Q wave MI have a smaller infarct size, better residual left ventricular function, and lower in-hospital mortality than do patients with Q wave infarction. Nonetheless, long-term survival is the same or less than that of patients with Q wave infarction. The factors related to mortality in the 1 year follow-up data for 515 patients surviving acute non–Q wave MI were persistent ST segment depression, a history of congestive heart failure, older age, and ST segment elevation at discharge.[38] Patients without ST segment depression had approximately half the mortality of those with ST segment depression.

Haim et al[39] evaluated early and long-term prognosis of patients with a first non–Q wave acute MI in relation to infarct location. Among patients with anterior MI (compared to inferior/lateral acute MI) in-hospital complications were more common and there was a higher rate of in-hospital and 5-year postdischarge mortality. Cardiac death or the recurrence within a year of acute MI was significantly higher among the anterior MI group than the inferior/lateral acute MI group.

INFERIOR MI

The inferior wall of the heart rests on the diaphragm and is opposite to the anterior wall, which is superior. It is contiguous with the right ventricle, the posterior base of the heart, the lateral wall, and the apex. Inferior MI results from an occlusion of the posterior descending coronary artery, which is usually a terminal branch of the RCA, but in a small number of patients (10%) may arise from the circumflex artery. An occlusion of the proximal RCA results in a large infarction involving not only the inferior wall, but the right ventricle and the AV node.

Reflecting Leads

Inferior MI: II, III, and aV_F (the inferior leads)
Inferolateral MI: II, III, aV_F, I, aV_L, and V_5
Inferior and right ventricular MI: II, III, aV_F, and V_{4R}

ECG Recognition

Indicators include ST segment elevation, development of Q waves, and symmetric T wave inversion in the inferior leads. Tombstoning in acute inferior MI is seen in Fig. 24-14, *A*, and is compared with nontombstoning in acute inferior MI in Fig. 24-14, *C*.

Coexisting ECG Findings Identifying High-Risk Patients

Identification of high-risk patients is important because of the critical need to initiate immediate reperfusion therapy—intravenous thrombolytics or coronary angioplasty. There are five ECG findings indicating high-risk in inferior MI:

1. ST segment elevation in lead V_{4R} of 1 mm or more has a high sensitivity and specificity for detecting right ventricular MI and identifying the site of occlusion in the proximal RCA. The ST segment elevation in V_{4R} usually disappears within 10 to 12 hours after the onset of pain; thus it is important to record this lead on admission
2. Complete AV block
3. Anterior precordial ST depression
4. ST elevation in lead V_6 with Q wave acute inferior MI indicates a larger infarct and greater incidence of major arrhythmias and pericardial involvement[40]
5. ST depression in V_4 through V_6 indicates high prevalence of multivessel coronary artery disease with frequent need for revascularization. The absence of this finding suggests absence of multivessel coronary artery disease

Using V_{4R} to Identify the Culprit Lesion

Recording lead V_{4R} in patients with acute inferior MI makes it possible to identify the occlusion sites. Fig. 24-23 illustrates the V_{4R} morphology, pinpointing the following occlusion sites:

Proximal right coronary artery: ST segment is elevated 1 mm or more.
Distal right coronary artery: ST segment is not elevated but coves into a positive T wave.
Circumflex coronary artery: T wave is inverted.

Evaluate the 12-lead ECG in Fig. 24-24 and identify the

coronary artery involved. Further identify a proximal or distal occlusion.

Using Leads II and III to Identify the Culprit Lesion

Comparison of the ST segment elevation in leads II and III can also help differentiate between RCA occlusion and circumflex occlusion as follows.

RCA occlusion. ST segment elevation in lead III is greater than in lead II. Fig. 24-25, *A*, illustrates the location of the infarcted and injured myocardium when the RCA is occluded. Note that the ST segment injury current *(arrow)* is more closely aligned with the axis of lead III than it is with lead II, causing the ST segment to be highest in lead III (Fig. 24-25, *B*). Additionally, the ST segment injury current is between the axes of these two leads, causing ST elevation to be dramatic.

Circumflex artery occlusion. ST segment elevation in lead II is greater than in lead III. Fig. 24-26, *A*, illustrates the location of the infarcted and injured myocardium when the circumflex artery is occluded. Note that the ST vector *(arrow)* is more closely aligned with the axis of lead II and actually remote from that of lead III, causing the ST segment to be highest in lead II (Fig. 24-26, *B*). Additionally, the total ST elevation in the inferior leads is smaller than that seen in RCA occlusion (given the same amount of infarcted tissue) because the injury current is between the axes of leads I and II (more remote from lead

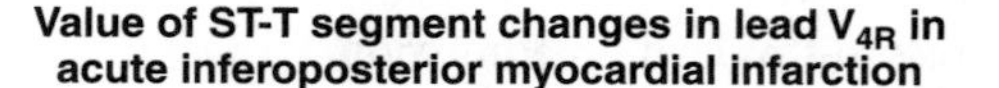

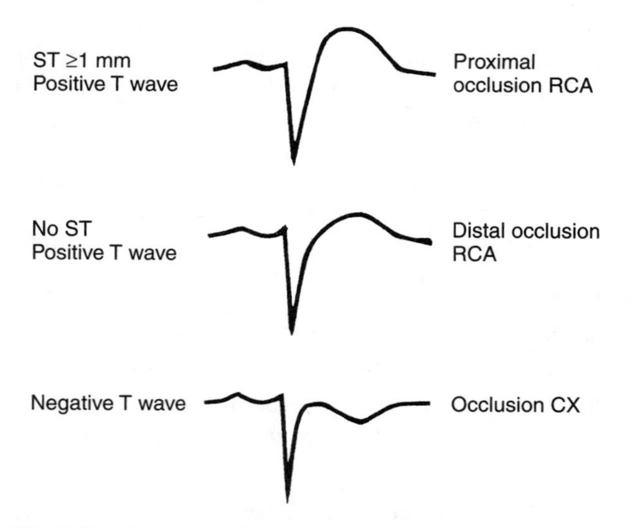

FIG. 24-23. Three possible patterns in lead V_{4R} in patients during the early hours of acute inferior myocardial infarction. These patterns identify the location of the occlusion. *RCA*, Right coronary artery; *CX*, circumflex coronary artery. (From Wellens HJJ, Conover M: *The ECG in emergency decision making,* Philadelphia, 1991, WB Saunders.)

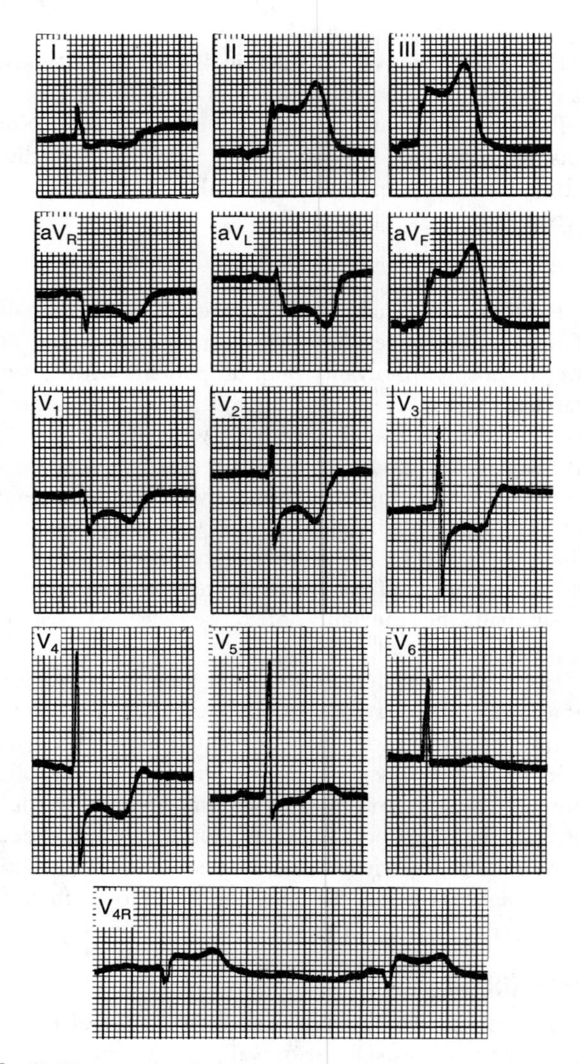

FIG. 24-24. Acute inferior and right ventricular myocardial infarction. The ST segment elevation is evident in leads II, III, aV_F, and V_{4R}. The ST segment elevation in V_{4R} identifies a patient with a proximal right coronary artery occlusion and right ventricular acute myocardial infarction who is at high risk for AV block. The right coronary artery is also identified as the culprit lesion by comparing the ST segment elevation in leads II and III; higher elevation in lead III than in lead II denotes right coronary artery occlusion. (Courtesy William P. Nelson, MD.)

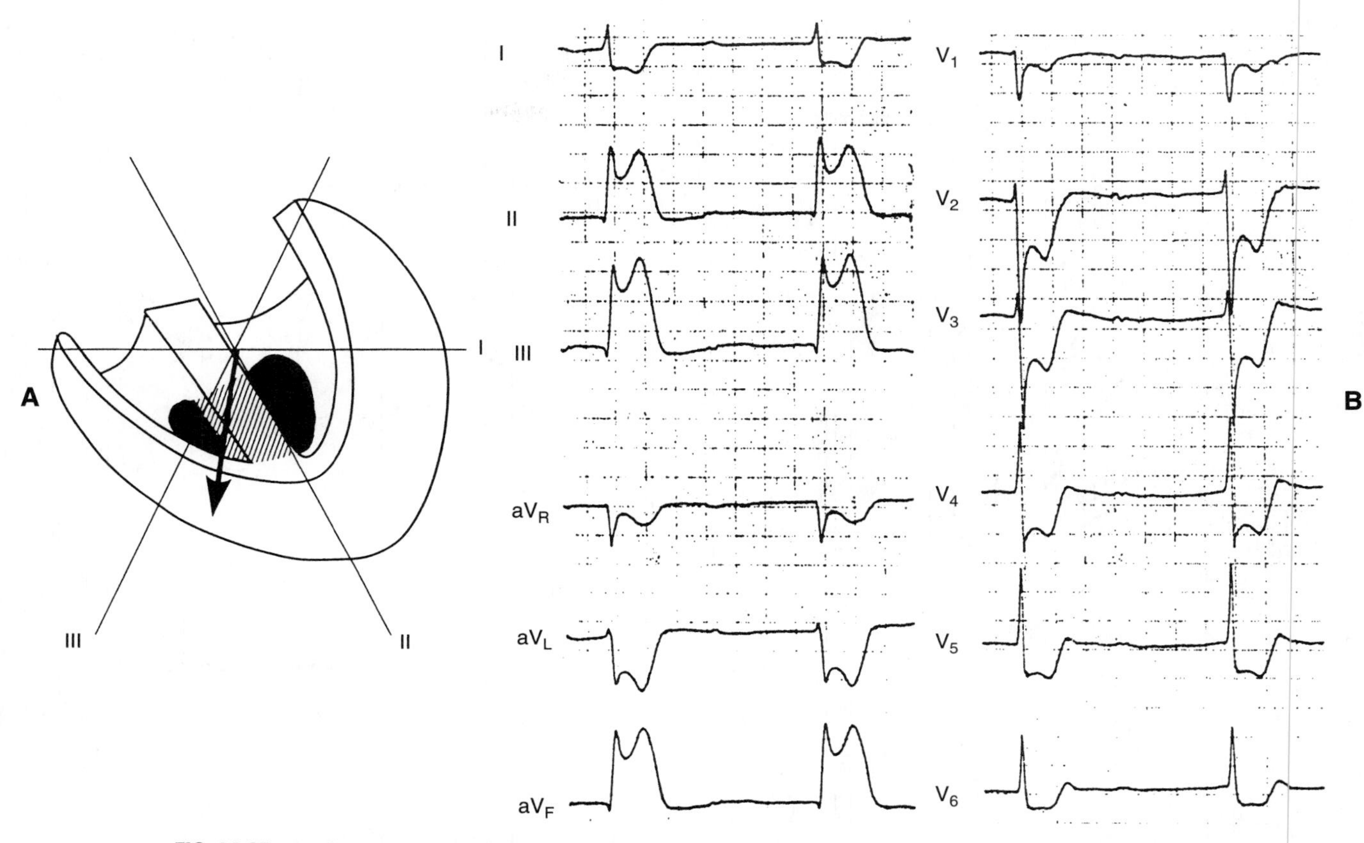

FIG. 24-25. **A**, The approximate locations of the infarcted and injured myocardium when an occlusion of the right coronary artery causes acute inferior myocardial infarction. The *arrow* represents the current of injury; note its approximation to the lead axis of III compared to lead II. **B**, This causes the ST segment to be elevated more in lead II than in lead III. (Courtesy Hein J.J. Wellens, MD, Maastricht, The Netherlands.)

III). These changes contribute to the difficulty of recognizing acute circumflex occlusion, which may resolve with less aggressive treatment.

Associated Conduction Abnormalities

AV block occurs frequently in the setting of acute inferior MI and seems to indicate a larger infarct and increased mortality. Although with thrombolytic therapy the mortality rate of patients with AV block is somewhat lower than that of patients in the prethrombolytic era, the rate still remains relatively high. Mortality 1 year after discharge is increased in patients in whom AV block developed within 24 hours after thrombolytic therapy but not in those who had AV block before treatment.[41]

Second-degree AV block. Conduction abnormalities at the AV nodal level can be expected in the form of second-degree AV block (usually type I) and complete AV block with a junctional escape pacemaker. Such conduction abnormalities occur in 20% of patients with acute inferior MI, are the result of proximal RCA occlusion, and identify a patient with right ventricular infarction who is at higher risk had AV block not been present. In such cases the in-hospital mortality rate is 23%, or 2.5 times that of inferior wall infarction without AV block.

Third-degree AV block. When third-degree heart block is present, the average mortality rate is 29%. This high mortality reflects a more proximal occlusion and more muscle damage.

Other causes of AV block in acute inferior MI may be high vagal tone, release of potassium and adenosine from inside the cells (both of which can cause heart block), and the presence of concomitant stenosis of the proximal LAD coronary artery, which would compromise the septal per-

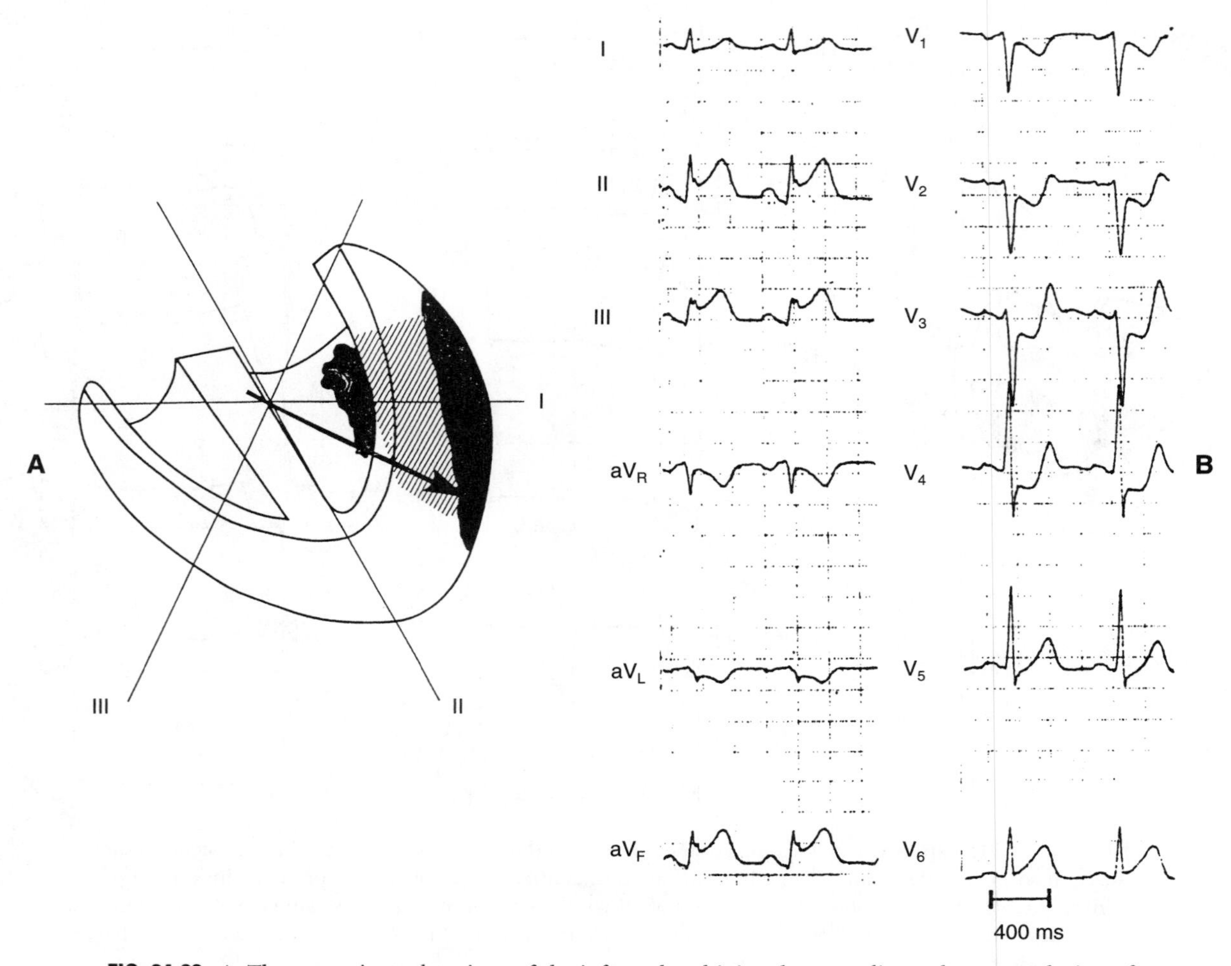

FIG. 24-26. **A**, The approximate locations of the infarcted and injured myocardium when an occlusion of the circumflex coronary artery causes inferior acute myocardial infarction. The *arrow* represents the current of injury; note its approximation to the lead axis of II compared to lead III. **B**, This causes the ST segment to be elevated more in lead III than in lead II. (Courtesy Hein J.J. Wellens, MD, Maastricht, The Netherlands.)

forators and their rich network of collateral vessels that reach toward the AV nodal artery.

ECG Diagnosis of Healed Inferior MI with LBBB

The ECG diagnosis of healed inferior MI in patients with LBBB can be made with the presence in lead aV_F of either diagnostic Q waves (30 ms or more) or diagnostic T wave inversion (i.e., complete T inversion or biphasic waves with initial, predominantly negative deflection [sensitivity of 86%; specificity 91%]).[42]

RIGHT VENTRICULAR INFARCTION

Right ventricular infarction should be suspected in any patient with acute inferior MI, being associated with it in as many as 50% of cases. Although the damage to the right ventricle may not be large enough to produce significant hemodynamic changes (i.e., hypotension, elevated jugular venous pulse, and occasionally shock), the potential of right ventricular MI should be recognized to avoid inappropriate therapy, such as diuretics, that will further lower right heart preload, reduce cardiac output, and aggravate hypotension.

ECG Recognition

The ST segment elevation of 1 mm or more in lead V_{4R} as a sign of acute right ventricular MI has already been illustrated and discussed.

Recording Lead V_{4R} in the Coronary Care Unit

The value of V_{4R} in the detection of right ventricular MI was described by Erhardt et al in 1976[43] and has been repeatedly validated over the years.[44-48] If lead V_{4R} is not routinely recorded on the 12-lead ECG at admission, it can be easily recorded on admission to the coronary care unit (CCU). Assuming that leads I, II, and III are in place (Einthoven's triangle), you now have the option to record any of the right- or left-side chest leads. Place the V_1 electrode on the right side of the chest at the midclavicular line in the fifth intercostal space. Select V_1 to be recorded and label the tracing V_{4R}. Any of the V electrodes can be used to record V_{4R} as long as the recording is made of that particular V-lead and relabeled V_{4R}. Lead V_{4R} may also be simulated using bipolar chest leads (negative electrode on the left shoulder; positive electrode in V_{4R} position).

Development of AV Block

One common complication of right ventricular infarction with inferior MI is the development of AV block. If the block is complete (third-degree AV block), the blood pressure falls precipitously and mortality is quite high. In such cases it is important to maintain AV synchrony because of the preload problem for the ventricles. If atrial fibrillation develops, it is generally poorly tolerated and direct current cardioversion is attempted early in its course.

Pathophysiology

Right ventricular infarction occurs exclusively in patients with transmural infarction of the inferior-posterior wall with extension into the right ventricular free wall. Although the culprit lesion is usually the proximal RCA, a mid-RCA occlusion (before any large right ventricular branches) may also cause right ventricular infarction; rarely is a dominant circumflex artery involved. Isolated right ventricular infarction is seen in 3% to 5% of cases of MI (autopsy-proven), usually associated with chronic lung disease and right ventricular hypertrophy.[49]

Cardiogenic shock. Only 5% to 10% of patients with right ventricular infarction have hemodynamic symptoms. If the patient develops cardiogenic shock, the mortality rate may exceed 35%. Hypotension and cardiogenic shock occur when ischemia is enough to decrease right ventricular compliance and cause volume (pressure) overload in the right ventricle. Within a closed pericardial space this changes the curvature of the septum, which shifts to the left, increasing left ventricular end-diastolic pressure and decreasing left ventricular compliance and cardiac output. Right ventricular dilatation also produces an increased intrapericardial pressure, further aggravating the decrease in LV compliance.[48] The dramatic decrease in LV preload results in a hemodynamic situation consistent with LV tamponade. Because of this, patients with hemodynamic compromise caused by right ventricular infarction may have elevated jugular venous pressure of 10 mm or more, a positive Kussmaul's venous sign (inspiratory increase in jugular venous distention), and clear lung fields. Data from hemodynamic monitoring can be characteristic and can aid in the treatment of these patients.

Differential Diagnosis

Anteroseptal MI. Right ventricular infarction may be erroneously interpreted as an anteroseptal MI because of ST elevation in leads V_1 through V_4. The differential diagnosis can be made because of the differences in the ST axis.[50,51] In inferior right ventricular MI the ST axis is inferior, to the right, and anterior. In anteroseptal MI the ST axis is superior, to the left, and anterior.

Summary of Acute Inferior and Right Ventricular MI

Right ventricular infarction is common in inferior MI and carries with it a poor prognosis because of serious hemodynamic consequences and increased incidence of life-threatening arrhythmias and AV block. In most patients this high-risk indicator is not recognized by physical signs. However, a recording of lead V_{4R} is a simple, promptly available means of establishing the presence of right ventricular infarction. Such an ECG assessment should be routinely performed in all patients with acute inferior MI.

Following are observations made regarding right ventricular infarction in the last two decades. Some of these were already mentioned and are summarized here:

1. Right ventricular infarction is present in 19% to 51% of patients with acute inferior MI (postmortem studies).[52,53]
2. In most patients with right ventricular infarction the condition does not manifest itself with its hemodynamic picture.
3. The presence of right ventricular infarction is a strong, independent prognostic predictor of life-threatening postinfarction tachyarrhythmias, AV

block (45%), and poor short- and long-term outcome after inferior MI.[54,55]

4. Early diagnosis of right ventricular infarction helps prevent mismanagement; use of diuretics, nitroglycerin, and morphine is avoided because they decrease right heart preload. Even in patients who do not present with hypotension, therapy that further lowers right ventricular preload is avoided.
5. Effective reperfusion with angioplasty or thrombolysis improves the ischemic and hemodynamic condition and right ventricular function improves

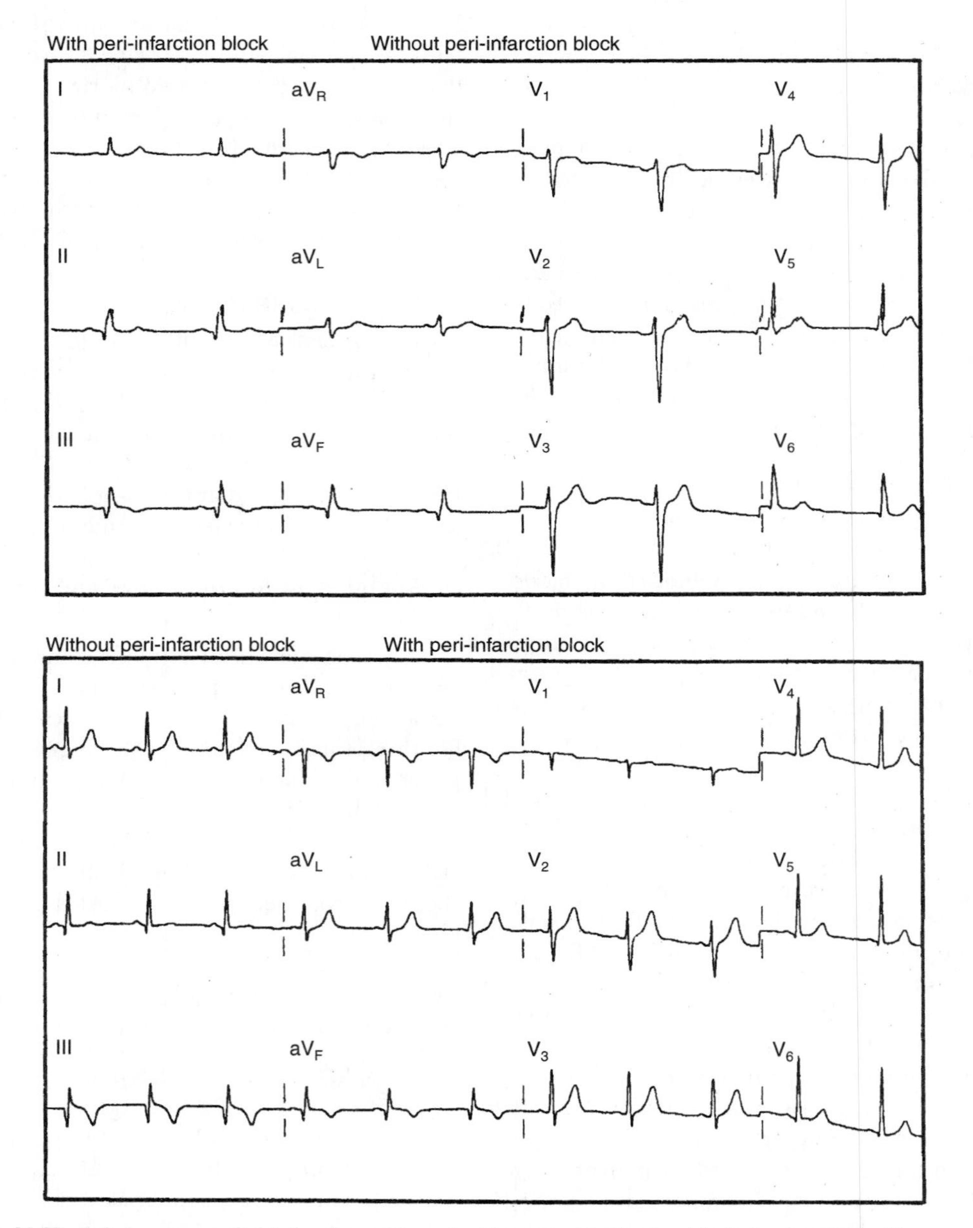

FIG. 24-27. Inferior myocardial infarction with and without peri-infarction block. In the ECG without peri-infarction block, note the narrow QRS (duration, 0.09 second) and the sharp descending limb of the R wave in leads II, III, and aV_F. In the ECG with peri-infarction block, note the broadened QRS (duration, 0.11 to 0.12 second) and the distortion of the descending limb of the R wave in leads II, III, and aV_F. Also, in lead I the QRS complex is narrow. (From Flowers NC, Horan LG, Wylds AC: *Am J Cardiol* 66:568, 1990.)

rapidly. If cared for carefully, these patients improve in a few days as collateral flow increases and ischemia resolves.

6. In the 5% of patients who have serious hemodynamic compromise, knowledgeable medical treatment guided by hemodynamic monitoring help to avoid acute tamponade caused by the right ventricular volume overload.
7. Early diagnosis allows anticipation of conduction problems and arrhythmias, which are aggressively treated.
8. Lead V_{4R} has high sensitivity, specificity, and predictive accuracy in diagnosing right ventricular infarction.

PERI-INFARCTION BLOCK IN INFERIOR MI

Peri-infarction block is the ECG manifestation of slowed conduction and delayed activation of fibers in association with or near the acute MI zone. It is possible that the ECG recognition of this condition may identify patients after acute MI who are at greater risk for sustained VT.[56,57]

History

It is necessary to explain the historical evolution of the term *peri-infarction block* because the meaning taken is that of the original application in 1950, not that of later authors who equated it with hemiblock.

Peri-infarction block was described in 1950,[58] when it was recognized that although the electrodes close to and adjacent to the infarction could have a QRS duration of 0.11 second or more, the electrodes in remote zones could have a normal QRS duration. The anatomic basis was demonstrated in the early studies by direct recordings from infarcted myocardium. When the electrode was over the center of the infarction, there was a QS pattern; when it was moved to the peri-infarction zone, there was a QR complex. Soon after these initial studies, peri-infarction block was wrongly equated with left anterior fascicular block. Rosenbaum et al[59] later correctly refuted this usage, but by this time the concept of peri-infarction block became one with hemiblock and slipped into oblivion. In 1985 an editorial by Scherlag et al[60] suggested a link between the original concept of peri-infarction block and ventricular late potentials. The study by Flowers et al[56] in 1990 demonstrated such a link.

ECG Recognition

Fig. 24-27 compares the 12-lead ECG from patients with and without peri-infarction block. Both patients have inferior MI with Q waves in leads II, III, and aV_F. However, the ECG without peri-infarction block has a narrow QRS complex in all leads, whereas the patient with peri-infarction block has a narrow QRS complex in all leads except II, III, and aV_F, which is caused by a distortion of the terminal forces.

Fig. 24-28 is a magnification of lead II in both patients. Note the broadening of the QRS complex in the peri-infarction block caused by a slurring of the downstroke of the R wave as compared to the swift downstroke of the R wave in the patient without peri-infarction block.

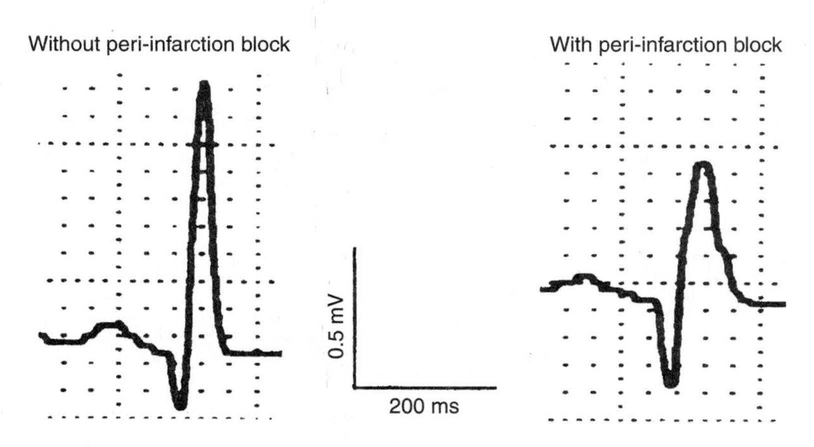

FIG. 24-28. A magnified lead II complex from each ECG shown in Fig. 24-27. The contrast is evident between the sharpness of the descending limb of the R wave in the patient without peri-infarction block *(left)* and the slurred descent of the R wave in the patient with peri-infarction block *(right)*. (From Flowers NC et al: *Am J Cardiol* 66:568, 1990.)

Clinical Significance

The data from the study by Flowers et al[56] showed that patients who have had acute MI with the ECG pattern described for peri-infarction block may be at greater risk for sustained ventricular tachycardia. There is apparently a link between the presence of the ECG pattern of peri-infarction block in inferior MI and ventricular late potentials, which are in turn linked to an increased risk for sustained ventricular tachycardia and ventricular fibrillation.

INFEROLATERAL MI

Reflecting leads: Leads III, aV_F, V_5, V_6, I, and aV_L

ECG Recognition

- Leads II, III, and aV_F reflect the inferior wall
- Leads I, aV_L, V_5, and V_6 reflect the lateral wall
- ST segment elevation
- Q waves
- Inverted T waves

Fig. 24-29 shows an acute inferolateral acute MI.

ECG Identification of High-Risk Patients

1. ST segment elevation in lead V_{4R} (proximal RCA occlusion and right ventricular infarction)
2. Complete AV block

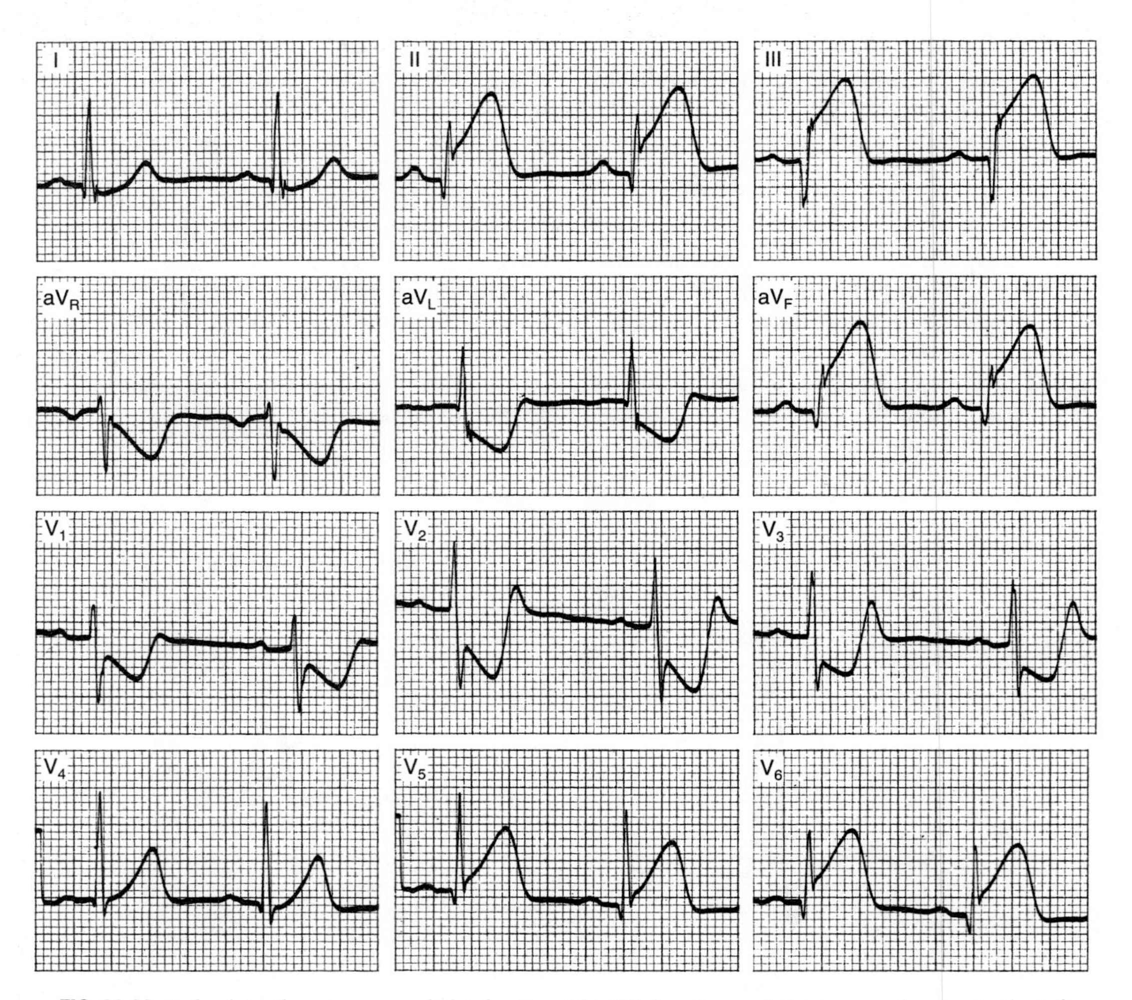

FIG. 24-29. Inferolateral acute myocardial infarction. The ST elevation and Q waves can be seen in the inferior leads and in leads V_5 and V_6. The ST segment is higher in lead III than in II; this is a right coronary artery occlusion.

3. Anterior precordial ST segment depression (posteroseptal involvement)

ACUTE POSTERIOR WALL MI

Reflecting Leads

Acute stage: Leads V_3 and V_4
Evolving stage: Lead V_1

ECG Recognition

Acute stage: Horizontally depressed ST segments are seen in leads V_3 and V_4.
Evolving stage: ST segment depression resolves, and a tall R wave appears in leads V_1 or V_2. Q waves and ST segment elevation in leads V_7 to V_9.[61,62]

Because it is the endocardial surface of the posterior wall of the heart that faces the precordial leads (as opposed to the epicardial surface of the anterior wall), the ECG signs of acute posterior wall infarction are reversed (reciprocal changes). Therefore when evaluating for acute posterior wall acute MI, one looks especially in precordial leads for a depressed ST segment. In the acute stage the ST segment is typically horizontally depressed, especially in leads V_3 to V_4. As the infarction evolves, the ST segment depression gives way to an R wave in lead V_1. The R wave is, of course, a Q wave infarction seen in reverse. Sometimes the ST segment depression is downsloping.

Recording Leads V_7, V_8, and V_9

After the 12-lead ECG is recorded, the three left chest electrodes can be moved to the following:

1. The posterior axillary line (V_7)
2. The level of the tip of the left scapula (V_8)
3. Just to the left of the vertebrae (V_9)

Differential Diagnosis

The possibility of recovery from MI by reperfusion techniques has made the diagnosis of acute transmural posterior wall MI important. It has been shown that leads V_7 to V_9 are simple and accurate means of making this diagnosis and in differentiating posterior wall MI from other causes of tall R waves in V_1 to V_2.

Q waves and ST segment elevation in these three leads are diagnostic of acute posterior wall MI.[61] Table 24-2 lists the causes and diagnostic clues of tall R waves in V_1.

ATRIAL INFARCTION

Reflecting leads: Leads I, II, and III and leads V_1, V_2, V_5, and V_6

ECG Recognition

One of the following is present:

- PR-segment elevation is greater than 0.5 mm in leads V_5 and V_6 with PR segment depression in leads V_1 and V_2
- PR segment elevation is greater than 0.5 mm in lead I with PR-segment depression in leads II and III
- PR segment depression is greater than 1.5 mm in precordial leads and greater than 1.2 mm in leads I, II, and III, combined with atrial arrhythmias
- P waves may also be abnormal in shape (W-shaped, M-shaped, notched, or irregular in configuration)

TABLE 24-2 Causes and Diagnosis of Tall R Waves in V_1

Diagnosis	Confirmatory Clues
True posterior infarct	ST depression, tall T V_1-V_2 **V_7-V_9:** Q waves and ST elevation
Right ventricular hypertrophy	RAD, RAE; secondary ST-Ts **V_7-V_9:** Normal
Ventricular septal hypertrophy	Associated Q waves, LVH **V_7-V_9:** Normal or deep
RBBB	Wide QRS, Broad S in V_6, R peaks late in V_1 **V_7-V_9:** Normal or broad S
Wolff-Parkinson-White syndrome	Short PR, delta wave **V_7-V_9:** Normal or short PR and delta wave
Normal variant	No other abnormalities

Adapted from Casas RE, Marriott HJL, Glancy DL: Value of leads V_7-V_9 in diagnosing posterior wall acute myocardial infarction and other causes of tall R waves in V_1-V_2, *Am J Cardiol* 80:508-509, 1997.

RAD, Right axis deviation; *RAE,* right atrial enlargement; LVH, left ventricular hypertrophy; *RBBB,* right bundle branch block.

Clinical Implications

Atrial infarction occurs in 17% of cases of acute MI (necropsy findings). Because supraventricular arrhythmias often complicate atrial infarctions, its ECG recognition may influence the choice of therapy during the early stages of infarction.

Differential Diagnosis

Pericarditis, sympathetic stimulation, and atrial overloading that is due to left ventricular failure are also causes of PR segment depression.

EMERGENCY APPROACH TO ACUTE MI

The focus of prehospital and emergency management of patients with acute MI is on rapid identification and treatment. It is well-known that early effective reperfusion via intravenous (IV) thrombolysis or angioplasty improves LV function and survival rates in patients with acute MI.[63,64] More important than the specific method of reperfusion used is its early application. Time delays to treatment may occur with patient behavior as well as inefficiencies in prehospital and hospital emergency medical system, although patient-related delays are more significant.[65]

THROMBOLYTIC THERAPY

Thrombolytic therapy can successfully be delivered in freestanding emergency departments, ambulatory health care centers, physicians' offices, ambulances, and even at patients' homes, whereas angioplasty approach requires a cardiac catheterization facility and a trained coronary intervention team.

Given the importance of early treatment, Braunwald[66] suggested that to obtain maximal benefit, paramedics, nurses, emergency medical technicians, and physicians' assistants should be trained in the recognition of candidates for thrombolysis and in the delivery of therapy.

After thrombolytic treatment has begun, the patient's care is best managed in a facility equipped with cardiac catheterization laboratory and a cardiac intervention team to deal with patients who do not respond to thrombolysis or reocclude after initial reperfusion.

The recent development of bolus thrombolytic agents is a notable advance in thrombolytic therapy because of ease of administration and the potential it holds for prehospital treatment. The first available bolus thrombolytic agent has been reteplase (rPA). Others are lanoteplase (nPA) and tenecteplase (TNK-tPA). The long half-life of these agents permits rapid infusion with a duration of action similar to the first- and second-generation thrombolytic agents, which require IV infusion and careful monitoring.[67,68]

Prompt IV Thrombolysis

The value of thrombolytic therapy is highly time-dependent, being most beneficial when administered within 1 to 4 hours of the onset of pain; the earlier the better. These benefits are proportionally reduced the later the treatment. These facts place the focus of both prehospital and emergency department management of patients with acute MI on rapid identification and treatment.[65,69] The requirements for such an optimal program are as follows:

1. Well-trained emergency medical staff and paramedics with a physician-directed plan for quick effective response. When thrombolytic therapy is to be initiated in the field, evaluation of the patient is carried out quickly. Patients with chest pain or tightness, acute epigastric distress, or other symptoms of acute MI are placed on established protocol; any contraindications to thrombolysis are noted. The patient's status and ECG are transmitted via cellular telephone to the emergency department for physician guidance. Even if thrombolytics are not administered in the field, transmitting the ECG from the field to the emergency department of itself is a benefit to the patient whose ECG is diagnostic of acute MI because it markedly reduces the time delay between the arrival at the hospital and the starting of thrombolysis.[70]
2. The base hospital should have facilities for emergency cardiac catheterization, angioplasty, and cardiac surgery. If such facilities are not available and if the patient's condition requires emergency intervention, the patient should be promptly transferred.
3. At the hospital the emergency team is ready to respond, having been alerted by the mobile unit. One hospital using prehospital evaluation for acute MI and administration of thrombolysis found a threefold increase in the termination of the ischemic process, compared with the in-hospital program of a nearby hospital.[71]
4. A "stat" 12-lead ECG with lead V_{4R} is obtained. Cardiac monitoring is continuous, vital signs are recorded frequently, and a physician sees the patient within the first few minutes of arrival. Delays of any kind should not be permitted in the admission and evaluation of these patients.
5. From the 13-lead ECG (12 standard leads plus lead

V_{4R}) and the clinical assessment, high-risk patients are promptly identified. Stat echocardiography may be used selectively but should not cause any delay in the initiation of treatment.

6. For patients with acute MI without contraindication to thrombolytic therapy, IV thrombolytic therapy is initiated by a trained emergency department physician and the staff if this has not already been done by paramedics en route to the hospital. If the facilities and experienced team are available, the first choice of reperfusion therapy may be primary angioplasty, bypassing the use of thrombolytic therapy. If systemic IV thrombolytic therapy is contraindicated or considered too hazardous, or when early large acute MI is suspected or the patient is in cardiogenic shock, emergency angioplasty is the best alternative.
7. In rural areas where hospitals do not have special cardiac facilities or physicians trained in emergency cardiac care, a protocol should be established for telephone communication with nearby medical centers. Protocol for initiating thrombolytic therapy in patients from rural hospitals before transferring them to metropolitan centers has been shown to be safe and effective.

Current emphasis is on reducing delays by administering thrombolytic therapy in the field with the implementation of one of the following possible basic protocols:

1. A physician-operated mobile intensive care unit (ICU)
2. Prehospital physician evaluation followed by activation of the mobile ICU
3. Paramedic evaluation with cellular ECG transmission

The special task force[72] of the American College of Cardiology and the American Heart Association, from which most of these guidelines have been taken, advises that in the critical setting of acute MI there should be no unnecessary delays in initiating treatment, such as those consumed by "administrative procedures, for example, establishing insurance coverage" and "prolonged efforts to consult with the patient's private physician." Such delays "must not be allowed to occur" and are "inappropriate." Other causes for delay also occur. For example, patients with chest pain sometimes wait their turn in busy emergency departments. Once admitted, there may be additional delay while a cardiologist is found to evaluate the need for thrombolysis. Sometimes therapy is not initiated until the patient is transferred to the CCU. The sum of these delays reduces the potential benefit of thrombolysis. Evaluation of these delays by emergency department directors and hospital administrators is the first step in eliminating them. The goal is to start the IV thrombolytic treatment in the proper candidate within 30 minutes of arrival to the emergency care setting or proceed to primary angioplasty within 60 minutes of arrival in the emergency department.

ST Segment Scoring to Identify Patients Who Would Benefit Most from Thrombolytic Therapy

In 1987[73] and 1990[74] the Wellens group in Maastricht published their studies regarding the outcome of thrombolytic therapy and presented a simple system of ST segment scoring to identify patients most likely to benefit. The greatest reduction in infarct by thrombolytic therapy is accomplished in patients with the largest infarctions. On the ECG the size of the infarction is reflected in the amount of ST segment elevation and depression, and the number of leads involved. These conclusions prompted the Wellens group to develop an ST scoring system to help identify patients most likely to benefit from thrombolytic therapy.

ST score; anterior MI. Add the total amount of ST elevation in millimeters in V_1 to V_6. High score is 12 mm or more (extensive anterior MI). Low score is less than 12 mm.[73]

ST score; inferior MI. Add the total amount of ST elevation in millimeters in II, III, and aV_F. High score is 7 mm or more (extensive anterior MI). Low score is less than 7 mm.

Candidates most likely to profit from thrombolytic therapy can be identified when this scoring system is coupled with the time from the onset of pain and the presence or absence of Q waves. Thus the following patients profit from thrombolysis:[73]

- High ST score at less than 2 hours: all patients with acute MI
- High ST score at 2 to 4 hours: all patients with anterior MI
- High ST score at 2 to 4 hours: inferior MI without Q waves
- Low ST score up to 4 hours: anterior MI with Q waves

CONTRAINDICATIONS TO THROMBOLYTIC THERAPY

Contraindications to thrombolytic therapy may be absolute, relatively major, or relatively minor.

Absolute Contraindications

In such cases as those listed here, other reperfusion strategies are considered, such as percutaneous transluminal coronary angioplasty (PTCA) or coronary artery bypass surgery:

- Altered consciousness
- Active internal bleeding
- Suspected aortic dissection or pericarditis
- Recent head trauma
- Known spinal cord or cerebral arteriovenous malformation or tumor
- Known previous *hemorrhagic* cerebrovascular accident
- Intracranial or intraspinal surgery within 2 months
- Trauma or surgery within 2 weeks that could result in bleeding into a closed space
- Persistent blood pressure greater than 200/120 mm Hg
- Pregnancy
- Previous allergy to streptokinase product (other thrombolytic agents may be used)

Relatively Major Contraindications (Individual Evaluation of Risk Versus Benefit)

- Active peptic ulcer disease (recent)
- Gastrointestinal or genitourinary hemorrhage
- History of ischemic or embolic cerebrovascular accident
- Current use of oral anticoagulants with therapeutic INR (international normalized ratio)
- Known bleeding disorder
- Major trauma or surgery within 2 weeks
- History of chronic uncontrolled hypertension (diastolic blood pressure greater than 100 mm Hg, treated or untreated)
- Subclavian or internal jugular venous cannulation or puncture of central noncompressible vessel
- Prolonged, traumatic cardiopulmonary resuscitation (CPR)
- Unwitnessed syncope or fall with potential central nervous system trauma

In instances when these contraindications have paramount importance, such as very recent trauma, surgery, or active peptic ulcer disease with recent bleeding, they become absolute contraindications when weighed against a less than life-threatening and evolving acute MI.

Relatively Minor Contraindications

- Brief nontraumatic CPR
- Diabetic retinopathy
- Endocarditis

PRIMARY PTCA

In settings of acute high-risk MI, primary PTCA (angioplasty without thrombolysis) is being used with increasing frequency because it can achieve prompt reperfusion and avoid the hemorrhagic risks of thrombolysis. Primary PTCA provides a small-to-moderate, short-term clinical advantage over thrombolytic therapy with tissue plasminogen activator.[75] This approach assumes the availability of a well-staffed, well-equipped cardiac catheterization laboratory and the ability to mobilize the team within 1 hour and achieve reperfusion within 2 hours.

Rescue angioplasty is the use of angioplasty after an unsuccessful attempt with thrombolytic therapy. Such would be the case when thrombolysis was the chosen reperfusion strategy. If successful reperfusion is not promptly achieved, angioplasty remains an alternative.

Combination Therapy

Recent research in acute MI has focused on combination therapy: combining reduced-dose thrombolytic treatment with IIb/IIIa inhibitors, with study results showing equivalency of this combination treatment but no superiority to using thrombolytic therapy alone.[76] Studies are in progress exploring the potential benefits of combining thrombolytic therapy along with IIb/IIIa inhibitors with immediate infarct angioplasty.

FOLLOW-UP CARE

The follow-up care of the MI patient must be individualized, factoring in the degree of LV damage, differentiation of MI versus myocardial stunning, presence or absence of multivessel disease, and degree of reperfusion and flow established in the infarct vessel.

ECG Monitoring and Medical Treatment

If the patient survives the first few hours of acute MI, continuous ECG monitoring and ongoing medical treatment is required because of the risk of late-appearing arrhythmias.

Swan-Ganz Catheter with Pacing Electrodes

For patients with hemodynamic instability or conduction abnormalities, a Swan-Ganz catheter with pacing electrodes may be inserted to gather information about pump function and permit emergency treatment.

After Reperfusion Therapy

After reperfusion therapy, heparin is continued for a few days in the absence of contraindications. Other proven effective interventions include continuation of aspirin and the use of beta blockers, angiotensin-converting enzyme inhibitors, statins for cholesterol lowering, and possibly intravenous magnesium in the acute phase of treatment. Clopidogrel (Plavix) in addition to aspirin may give added protection.[77] Detailed discussion of these treatments is beyond the scope of this book.

ECG PREDICTION OF SUCCESSFUL REPERFUSION THERAPY

Patients who do not respond to thrombolytic therapy are at high risk and may be candidates for emergency rescue angioplasty or coronary artery bypass surgery. Therefore it is important to rapidly and noninvasively determine the presence of reperfusion.

Patients receiving thrombolytic therapy for acute MI have been studied[78-80] MI in hopes of identifying clinical and ECG markers of reperfusion and avoiding emergency coronary angiography. Of the patients who showed reperfusion on coronary angiography, 96% had relief of chest pain after 60 minutes. Early ECG signs of reperfusion are as follows:

- Transient increase in ST segment deviation (seen more often following thrombolytic therapy as opposed to primary PTCA)
- Normalization of the ST segment
- Terminal T wave inversion
- Accelerated idioventricular rhythm
- A twofold increase in premature ventricular complex (PVC)
- Transient increase in chest pain before ST normalization

ST Segment Resolution after Thrombolysis

Resolution of ST segment elevation after thrombolysis for acute MI has been shown to be directly related to clinical outcome and mortality rate,[80] and is most likely a direct consequence of restoration of myocardial blood flow. Patients with complete and stable (70% or more) resolution of ST segment elevation after short-term ischemia (less than 3 hours) have a better outcome and preservation of left ventricular function than patients with partial (30% to 70%) or no (less than 30%) ST segment resolution.[78] Patients with persistent ST elevation after reperfusion therapy may need additional interventions because they have more extensive myocardial damage and have a higher mortality rate.[80]

Note: Although early decrease in ST segment elevation identifies the success of thrombolytic therapy for acute MI, frequently this decrease is preceded by a transient elevation above the level noted at the start of thrombolytic treatment.

The extent of ST segment resolution after reperfusion for acute MI conveys useful early information to guide the physician regarding prognosis and follow-up[81]:

1. Excellent survival rate. Complete ST segment resolution identifies such patients; however, there is a slightly higher probability of nonfatal reinfarction, suggesting that a predischarge stress test may identify patients who would benefit from early angiography and revascularization.
2. Increasing risk of death over long term. Partial ST segment resolution identifies such patients, suggesting that they may benefit from vigorous adjunctive pharmacotherapy.
3. Poor prognosis. Lack of ST segment resolution indicates lack of reperfusion and identifies patients who may benefit from immediate coronary angiography and rescue PTCA.

Reperfusion Arrhythmias

Increase in the number of PVCs: In most patients with reperfusion arrhythmias, an increase in the number of PVCs occurs before other arrhythmias.

Accelerated idioventricular rhythm (AIVR): During acute MI the AIVR has been shown to be a sign of reperfusion (spontaneous or as a result of thrombolytic therapy), especially when it occurs early in the course of the infarction (within 6 hours). Approximately half of the patients with reperfusion have an AIVR when the ECG is recorded continuously after thrombolytic therapy. This finding is of practical clinical importance in that it may help in the recognition of both spontaneous and thrombolytic-induced reperfusion in the absence of coronary angiography. In general, antiarrhythmic treatment is not needed.

Q Waves

Successful reperfusion with thrombolytic therapy may accelerate the evolving ECG picture of infarction. Therefore rapid resolution of ST segment elevation is followed by rapid development of pathologic Q wave and loss of R wave amplitude.

T Wave Inversion

Terminal T wave inversion after thrombolytic therapy (within 24 hours) is a very specific (94%) sign of successful, effective reperfusion, although it lacks the sensitivity of ST segment normalization.[78]

COMPLICATIONS OF MI

Severe mitral regurgitation: May occur shortly after MI because of papillary muscle rupture or dysfunction.

This usually presents with acute pulmonary edema or cardiogenic shock.

Acute ventricular septal rupture: Often occurs at the posterobasal septum in inferior MI and at the apical septum in anterior MI and is associated with the appearance of a loud systolic murmur and frequently cardiogenic shock.

Acute free wall rupture: May present with acute bradycardia, asystolic cardiac arrest, or electrical-mechanical dissociation.

Ventricular aneurysm: A common complication of MI, a ventricular aneurysm is a dilation of the infarct region without disruption of the myocardial wall. It may predispose to ventricular arrhythmias and/or clots and embolic events.

Pseudoaneurysm: Another complication of MI, a pseudoaneurysm is a rupture of the myocardium with full thickness penetration through the wall with the rupture being contained by the pericardium.

Ventricular thrombus: May occur in the regions of infarction, even in the absence of thrombus formation and can be the cause of stroke.

Pericarditis and pericardial effusion: May be seen in the days after acute MI. Rarely this may lead to cardiac compression and tamponade.

DIFFERENTIAL DIAGNOSES OF ACUTE MI

The clinical presentation of acute MI may be mimicked by the following five relatively common clinical conditions, which always should be considered in the differential diagnosis of acute MI. They are acute pulmonary embolism, acute pericarditis, aortic dissection, pancreatitis, and cholecystitis. In addition a newly described syndrome, mimicking more acute MI, transient left ventricular apical ballooning without coronary artery stenosis, is also discussed. In addition, the ECG abnormalities that may mimic or mask acute MI are listed on Box 24-3..

BOX 24-3. Conditions Capable of Masking or Mimicking Acute Myocardial Infarction on Electrocardiogram

- Left ventricular hypertrophy
- Right ventricular hypertrophy
- Left bundle branch block
- Right bundle branch block
- Ventricular pacing
- Left anterior fascicular block
- Left posterior fascicular block
- Ventricular preexcitation
- Low voltage

Acute Pulmonary Embolism

Acute massive pulmonary embolism (see Chapter 28) involving the main pulmonary arteries may simulate acute MI, especially because both conditions may present with chest pain, shortness of breath, and hypotension and may be associated with a fall in cardiac output, abnormal Q waves, ST segment elevation, and T wave changes and modest troponin elevation. For example, right axis deviation with Q waves and T wave changes in the inferior leads mimics inferior MI. Although an RBBB pattern and ST segment elevation in lead V_1 causes one to suspect pulmonary embolism, especially if there is also a positive T wave in that lead, this pattern is also seen when RBBB is associated with acute anteroseptal infarction, acute pericarditis, and the early repolarization pattern, and it occurs in posterior wall MI. In acute pulmonary embolism the following differences help in the diagnosis, although none is truly specific:

1. The acute respiratory distress is more pronounced than would be expected in MI, unless the acute MI is accompanied by pulmonary edema.
2. The ECG, although abnormal, is not consistent with that usually seen in MI. For example, both inferior wall and anterior MI may be suggested in one 12-lead ECG; that is, Q waves may be seen in leads III and aV_F, but not in lead II, and these may be associated with changes in lead V_1.
3. The chest x-ray does not show pulmonary congestion, although there is severe dyspnea and hypoxemia.
4. The diagnostic usefulness of the ECG is enhanced when combined with emergency echocardiography. The diagnosis is established by computer tomographic angiography.

Acute Pericarditis

The signs and symptoms of pericarditis can mimic those of acute MI in that there may be chest pain, and there is ST segment elevation. The diagnosis of pericarditis is based on the following:

1. Characteristic chest pain that is sharp, pleuritic, worse on inspiration or with recumbency, and relieved by leaning forward,
2. No response to nitroglycerin, or
3. Pericardial friction rub heard along the left lower sternal border or the left precordium

ECG changes classically occur in four stages, with some cases that do not include all four stages:

Stage I: Diffuse concave ST segment elevation during the first few days of pericardial inflammation, lasting up to 2 weeks. The appearance of the ST segment elevation of pericarditis differs from the usually convex appearance of acute MI.

Stage II: Return of ST segments to baseline and flattening of the T wave lasts from days to several weeks.

Stage III: Inversion of the T waves begins at the end of the second or third week.

Stage IV: Gradual resolution of the T wave that may last up to 3 months.

Other helpful clues are the absence of Q waves, the absence of reciprocal changes, and the fact that the ST segment elevation does not localize into right or left coronary artery distribution.

The echocardiogram is the most helpful in making the differential diagnosis because frequently there is pericardial effusion as a result of pericarditis.

Aortic Dissection

The character of the pain may differ from that of acute MI, as follows:

- Frequently there is posterior transmission.
- Pain may be pulsatile, rhythmic, synchronized with systole.
- There is no response to nitroglycerin.
- The ECG may be normal or there may be ST segment changes, especially if there is hypertension and left ventricular hypertrophy.
- There may be ECG changes associated with pericarditis if the dissection involves the aortic root and there is pericardial hemorrhage.

The diagnosis is suspected on chest x-ray films and confirmed by computed tomographic scan, transesophageal echocardiography or magnetic resonance imaging. Aortography is rarely needed for diagnosis.

Myocarditis

The clinical presentation of myocarditis can mimic that of acute MI. Sarda et al[82] showed that among 45 patients who presented with symptoms of acute MI but had a normal coronary angiogram, 40% of them had myocarditis. The diagnosis is made by exclusion of acute MI, the clinical course of the patient, and if needed, endomyocardial biopsy.

Pancreatitis and Cholecystitis

Pancreatitis[83] and cholecystitis can present a clinical picture mimicking acute MI with chest pain. The differential diagnosis is made with abdominal ultrasound and determination of appropriate blood tests.

Transient Left Ventricular Apical Ballooning Without Coronary Artery Stenosis

Recently a new syndrome has been described by Tsuchihashi et al[84] that mimics acute MI. It is characterized by transient left ventricular apical ballooning without coronary stenosis. These patients present with chest discomfort and ECG changes mimicking myocardial ischemia or infarction and have elevated CK. Some patients present with pulmonary edema, cardiogenic shock, or ventricular fibrillation. There is no obstructive coronary artery disease and most patients have complete recovery quite rapidly. This is a newly described syndrome and our understanding of the pathophysiology and clinical course remains quite incomplete.

SUMMARY

The speedy diagnosis, identification of high-risk patients, and effective management of acute MI are extremely important in view of the potential benefits of early reperfusion via thrombolytic therapy or primary PTCA with the potential for myocardial salvage and reduction of mortality.

ST segment elevation is the sign of acute myocardial occlusion and myocardial injury; the higher the elevation and the more leads involved, the more extensive the injury. If occlusion persists, the injury evolves into acute MI. The key to locating the infarct is understanding the coronary circulation, the surfaces of the heart, and their reflecting leads. Briefly, leads V_1 to V_4 reflect anterior MI; when this finding is combined with ST segment elevation in leads I, aV_L, and V_5 to V_6, there is extensive anterolateral wall infarction. High-risk patients are recognized when RBBB or hemiblock appear. Leads II, III, and aV_F reflect inferior MI. High-risk patients are recognized when there is ST segment elevation of 1 mm or more in lead V_{4R}. In selected patients emergency echocardiography is useful in the diagnosis, evaluation, and determination of possible complications in acute MI.

REFERENCES

1. Wellens HJJ: Acute myocardial infarction and left bundle-branch block—can we lift the veil? *N Engl J Med* 334:528-529, 1996.
2. Albert JS, Thygesen K, Antman E, Bassand JP: Myocardial infarction redefined—a consensus document of the joint European Society of Cardiology/American College of Cardiology Committee for the redefinition of myocardial infarction, *J Am Coll Cardiol* 36:959-969, 2000.

3. Turnstall-Pedoe H: Comment on the ESC/ACC redefinition of myocardial infarction by a consensus dissenter, *Eur Heart J* 22:613-615, 2001; *J Am Coll Cardiol* 37:1472-1474, 2001.
4. Richards AM, Lainchbury JG, Nicholls MG: Unsatisfactory redefinition of myocardial infarction, *Lancet* 357:1635-1636, 2001.
5. Mulvihill NT, Foley JB, Murphy R et al: Evidence of prolonged inflammation in unstable angina and non-Q wave myocardial infarction, *J Am Coll Cardiol* 36:1210-1216, 2000.
6. Frink RJ, James TN: Normal blood supply to the human His bundle and proximal bundle branches, *Circulation* 47:8, 1973.
7. Pardee HEB: An electrocardiographic sign of coronary artery obstruction, *Arch Intern Med* 26:244, 1920.
8. Estes NAM III, Link MS, Homound M et al: ECG findings in active patients. Differentiating the benign from the serious. In Thompson PD, editor: *Exercise and sports cardiology series. The physician and sports medicine* 29:1-14, 2001.
9. Panju AA, Hemmelgarn BR, Guyatt GH et al: Is this patient having a myocardial infarction? *JAMA* 280:1256-1263, 1998.
10. Barrabés JA, Figueras J, Moure C et al: Prognostic significance of ST segment depression in lateral leads I, aV_L, V_5 and V_6 on the admission electrocardiogram in patients with a first acute myocardial infarction without ST segment elevation, *J Am Coll Cardiol* 35:1813-1819, 2000.
11. Atie J, Brugada P, Smeets JLRM et al: Clinical presentation and prognosis of left main coronary disease in the 1990s, *Eur Heart J* 12:495, 1991.
12. Sevilla DC, Wagner NB, Anderson WD et al: Sensitivity of a set of myocardial infarction screening criteria in patients with anatomically documented single and multiple infarcts, *Am J Cardiol* 66:792-795, 1990.
13. Hathaway WR, Peterson ED, Wagner GS et al: Prognostic significance of the initial electrocardiogram in patients with acute myocardial infarction. GUSTO-I Investigators. Global utilization of streptokinase and t-PA for occluded coronary arteries, *JAMA* 279:387-391, 1998.
14. Caceres L, Cooke D, Zalenski R et al: Myocardial infarction with an initially normal electrocardiogram—angiographic findings, *Clin Cardiol* 18:563-568, 1995.
15. Morrow DA, Antman EM, Charlesworth A et al: TIMI risk score for ST elevation myocardial infarction. A convenient, bedside, clinical score for risk assessment at presentation, *Circulation* 102:2031-2037, 2000.
16. Conti CR: Determining prognosis after acute myocardial infarction, *Clin Cardiol* 24:97-98, 2001.
17. Killip T, Kimball JT: Treatment of myocardial infarction in the coronary care unit. A two year experience with 250 patients, *Am J Cardiol* 20:457, 1967.
18. Birnbaum Y, Kloner RA, Sclarovsky S et al: Distortion of the terminal portion of the QRS on the admission electrocardiogram in acute myocardial infarction and correlation with infarct size and long-term prognosis (Thrombolysis in Myocardial Infarction 4 Trial), *Am J Cardiol* 78:396-403, 1996.
19. Tamura A, Nagase K, Watanabe T et al: Relationship between terminal QRS distortion on the admission electrocardiogram and the time course of left ventricular wall motion in anterior wall acute myocardial infarction, *Jpn Circ J* 65:63-66, 2001.
20. Fisch C: Electrocardiography and vectorcardiography. In Braunwald E, editor: *Heart disease,* ed 4, Philadelphia, 1992, WB Saunders.
21. Engelen DJ, Gorgels AP, Cheriex EC et al: Value of the electrocardiogram in localizing the occlusion site in the left anterior descending coronary artery in acute anterior myocardial infarction, *J Am Coll Cardiol* 34:389-395, 1999.
22. Kosuge M, Kimura K, Ishikawa T et al: Electrocardiographic criteria for predicting total occlusion of the proximal left anterior descending coronary artery in anterior wall acute myocardial infarction, *Clin Cardiol* 24:33-38, 2001.
23. Arbane M, Goy JJ: Prediction of the site of total occlusion in the left anterior descending coronary artery using admission electrocardiogram in anterior wall acute myocardial infarction, *Am J Cardiol* 85:487-491, A10, 2000.
24. Ben Gal T, Herz I, Solodky A: Acute anterior wall myocardial infarction entailing ST- segment elevation in lead V1: electrocardiographic and angiographic correlations, *Clin Cardiol* 21:399-404, 1998.
25. Birnbaum Y, Chetrit A, Sclarovsky S et al: Abnormal Q waves on the admission electrocardiogram of patients with first acute myocardial infarction: prognostic implications, *Clin Cardiol* 20:477-481, 1997.
26. de Gevigney G, Ecochard R, Rabilloud M et al: Worsening of heart failure during hospital course of an unselected cohort of 2507 patients with myocardial infarction is a factor of poor prognosis: the PRIMA study, *Eur J Heart Fail* 3:233-241, 2001.
27. Sakata K, Yoshino H, Houshaku H et al: Myocardial damage and left ventricular dysfunction in patients with and without persistent negative T waves after Q wave anterior myocardial infarction, *Am J Cardiol* 87:510-515, 2001.
28. Gunnarsson G, Eriksson P, Dellborg M: Bundle branch block and acute myocardial infarction. Treatment and outcome, *Scand Cardiovasc J* 34:575-579, 2000.
29. Lie KI, Wellens HJJ, Schuilenburg RM: Bundle branch block and acute myocardial infarction. In Wellens HJJ, Lie KI, Janse MJ, editors: *The conduction system of the heart,* Philadelphia, 1976, Lea & Febiger, pp 662-672.
30. Li SF, Walden PL, Marcilla O et al: Electrocardiographic diagnosis of myocardial infarction in patients with left bundle branch block, *Ann Emerg Med* 36:561-565, 2000.
31. Ryan TJ, Anderson JL, Antman EM et al: ACC/AHA guidelines for the management of patients with acute myocardial infarction: executive summary, *Circulation* 94:2341-2350, 1996.
32. Shlipak MG, Go AS, Frederick PD et al: Treatment and outcomes of left bundle-branch block patients with myocardial infarction who present without chest pain. National Registry of Myocardial Infarction 2 Investigators, *J Am Coll Cardiol* 36:706-712, 2000.
33. Wackers FJT, Lie KI, David G et al: Assessment of the value of electrocardiographic signs for myocardial infarction in left bundle branch block. In Wellens HJJ, Kulbertus HE, editors: *What's new in electrocardiography,* The Hague, The Netherlands, 1981, Martinus Nijhoff. pp 37-57.
34. Sgarbossa EB, Pinski SL, Barbagelata A et al: Electrocardiographic diagnosis of evolving acute myocardial infarction in the presence of left bundle-branch block, *N Engl J Med* 334:481-487, 1996.
35. Chauhan VS, Tang AS: Dynamic changes of QT interval and QT dispersion in non-Q-wave and Q-wave myocardial infarction, *J Electrocardiol* 34:109-117, 2001.
36. Furman MI, Dauerman HL, Goldberg RJ et al: Twenty-two year (1975 to 1997) trends in the incidence, in-hospital and long-term case fatality rates from initial Q-wave and non-Q-wave myocardial infarction: a multi-hospital, community-wide perspective, *J Am Coll Cardiol* 37:1571-1580, 2001.
37. Maeda S, Imai G, Kuboki K et al: Pathologic implications of restored positive T waves and persistent negative T waves after Q wave myocardial infarction, *J Am Coll Cardiol* 28:1514-1518, 1996.
38. Dacanay S, Kennedy, Uretz E et al: Morphological and quantitative angiographic analyses of progression of coronary stenoses: a comparison of Q-wave and non-Q-wave myocardial infarction, *Circulation* 90:1739, 1994.

39. Haim M, Hod H, Reisin L et al: Comparison of short- and long-term prognosis in patients with anterior wall versus inferior or lateral wall non-Q-wave acute myocardial infarction. Secondary Prevention Reinfarction Israeli Nifedipine Trial (SPRINT) Study Group, *Am J Cardiol* 79:717-721, 1997.
40. Tsuka Y, Sugiura T, Hatada K et al: Clinical characteristics of ST-segment elevation in lead V_6 in patients with Q-wave acute inferior wall myocardial infarction, *Coron Artery Dis* 10:465-469, 1999.
41. Berger PB, Ruocco NA, Ryan TJ et al: Incidence and prognostic implications of heart block complicating inferior myocardial infarction treated with thrombolytic therapy: results from TIMI II, *J Am Coll Cardiol* 20:533-536, 1992.
42. Laham CL, Hammill SC, Gibbons RJ: New criteria for the diagnosis of healed inferior wall myocardial infarction in patients with left bundle branch block, *Am J Cardiol* 79:19-22, 1997.
43. Erhardt LR, Sjögren A, Wahlberg I: Single right-sided precordial lead in the diagnosis of right ventricular involvement in inferior myocardial infarction, *Am Heart J* 91:571, 1976.
44. Braat SH, Brugada P, de Zwaan C et al: Value of electrocardiogram in diagnosing right ventricular involvement in patients with an acute inferior wall myocardial infarction, *Br Heart J* 49:368, 1983.
45. Klein HO, Tordjman T, Ninio R et al: The early recognition of right ventricular infarction: diagnostic accuracy of the electrocardiographic V_{4R} lead, *Circulation* 67:558, 1983.
46. Braat SH, Brugada P, den Dulk K et al: Value of lead V_{4R} for recognition of the infarct coronary artery in acute inferior myocardial infarction, *Am J Cardiol* 53:1538, 1984.
47. Horan LG, Flowers NC: Right ventricular infarction: specific requirements of management, *Am Fam Physician* 60:1727-1734, 1999.
48. Haji SA, Movahed Assad: Right ventricular infarction—diagnosis and treatment, *Clin Cardiol* 23:473-482, 2000.
49. Pasternak RC, Braunwald E, Sobel BE: Acute myocardial infarction. In Braunwald E, editor: *Heart disease,* Philadelphia, 1992, WB Saunders.
50. Porter A, Herz I, Strasberg B: Isolated right ventricular infarction presenting as anterior wall myocardial infarction on electrocardiography, *Clin Cardiol* 20:971-973, 1997.
51. Hurst JW: Comments about the electrocardiographic signs of right ventricular infarction, *Clin Cardiol* 21:289-291, 1998.
52. Wartman WB, Hellerstein HK: The incidence of heart disease in 2,000 consecutive autopsies, *Ann Intern Med* 28:41-65, 1948.
53. Isner JM, Roberts WC: Right ventricular infarction complicating left ventricular infarction secondary to coronary artery disease: frequency, location, associated findings and significance from analysis of 236 necropsy patients with acute or healed myocardial infarction, *Am J Cardiol* 42:885-894, 1978.
54. Braat SH, de Zwaan C, Brugada P et al: Right ventricular involvement with acute inferior wall myocardial infarction identifies high risk of developing atrioventricular nodal conduction disturbances, *Am Heart J* 107:1183-1187, 1984.
55. Zehender M: Right ventricular infarction as an independent predictor of prognosis after acute inferior myocardial infarction, *N Eng J Med* 328:981-988, 1993.
56. Flowers NC, Horan LG, Wylds AC: Relation of peri-infarction block to ventricular late potentials in patients with inferior wall myocardial infarction, *Am J Cardiol* 66:568-575, 1990.
57. Santolin CJ, Mukerji V, Alpert MA et al: Signal-averaged electrocardiographic detection of terminal QRS deflection suggesting late potentials, *South Med J* 84:1402-1404, 1991.
58. First SR, Bayley RH, Bedford DR: Peri-infarction block: electrocardiographic abnormality occasionally resembling bundle branch block and local ventricular block of other types, *Circulation* 2:31-38, 1950.
59. Rosenbaum MB, Elizari MV, Lazzari JO: *The hemiblocks: new concepts of intraventricular conduction based on human anatomical, physiological and clinical studies,* Oldsmar, Fla, 1970, Tampa Tracings.
60. Scherlag BJ, Gunn CG, Berbari EJ, Lazzara R: Peri-infarction (1950)–late potentials (1980): their relationship, significance and diagnostic implications, *Am J Cardiol* 55:839, 1985.
61. Casas RE, Marriott HJL, Glancy DL: Value of leads V_7-V_9 in diagnosing posterior wall acute myocardial infarction and other causes of tall R waves in V_1-V_2, *Am J Cardiol* 80:508-509, 1997.
62. Matetzky S, Freimark D, Feinberg MS et al: Acute myocardial infarction with isolated ST-segment elevation posterior chest leads V_7-V_9. "Hidden" ST-segment elevations revealing acute posterior infarction, *J Am Coll Cardiol* 34:748-743, 1999.
63. A Report of the American College of Cardiology/American Heart Association Task Force on Practice Guidelines (Committee on Management of Acute Myocardial Infarction): 1999 Update: ACC/AHA guidelines for the management of patients with acute myocardial infarction, *J Am Col Cardiol* 34:886-889, 1999.
64. The Gusto Investigators: An international randomized trial comparing four thrombolytic strategies for acute myocardial infarction, *N Engl J Med* 329:673, 1993.
65. Cannon CP, Sayah AJ, Walls RM: Prehospital thrombolysis: an idea whose time has come, *Clin Cardiol* 22(suppl IV):10-19, 1999.
66. Braunwald E: Optimizing thrombolytic therapy of acute myocardial infarction, *Circulation* 82:1510, 1990.
67. Cannon CP: The evolution of superaggressive management of AMI. Available online at http://www.chestpainonline.org/html/hottop 0922.htm. Accessed 2001.
68. Armstrong MD, Collen D: Fibrinolysis for acute myocardial infarction. Current status and new horizons for pharmacological reperfusion, Part I, *Circulation* 103:2862-2866, 2001.
69. Morrison LJ, Verbeek PR, McDonald AC et al: Mortality and prehospital thrombolysis for acute myocardial infarction: a meta-analysis, *JAMA* 283:2686-2692, 2000.
70. Ljosland M, Weydahl PG, Stumberg S: Prehospital ECG reduces the delay of thrombolysis in acute myocardial infarction, *Tidsskr Nor Laegeforen* 120:2247-2249, 2000.
71. Lamfers EJ, Hooghoudt TE, Uppelschoten A et al: Effect of prehospital thrombolysis on aborting acute myocardial infarction, *Am J Cardiol* 84:928-930, A6-7, 1999.
72. ACC/AHA Task Force Report: Guidelines for the early management of patients with acute myocardial infarction: a report of the American College of Cardiology/American Heart Association Task Force on assessment of diagnostic and therapeutic cardiovascular procedures, *J Am Coll Cardiol* 16:249, 1990.
73. Bär FW, Vermeer F, de Zwaan C et al: Value of admission electrocardiogram in predicting outcome of thrombolytic therapy in acute myocardial infarction, *Am J Cardiol* 59:6, 1987.
74. Clemmensen P, Grande P, Saunamäki K et al: Effect of intravenous streptokinase on the relation between initial ST predicted size and final QRS estimated size of acute myocardial infarction, *J Am Coll Cardiol* 16:12-52-1257, 1990.
75. The Global Use of Strategies to Open Occluded Coronary Arteries in Acute Coronary Syndromes (GUSTO IIb) Angioplasty Substudy Investigators: A clinical trial comparing primary coronary angioplasty with tissue plasminogen activator for acute myocardial infarction, *N Engl J Med* 336:1621-1628, 1997.
76. The GUSTO V Investigators: Reperfusion therapy for acute myocardial infarction with fibrinolytic therapy of combination reduced fibrinolytic therapy and platelet glycoprotein IIb/IIIa inhibition: the GUSTO V randomised trial, *Lancet* 357:1905, 2001.

77. The Clopidogrel in Unstable Angina to Prevent Recurrent Events Trial Investigators: Effects of clopidogrel in addition to aspirin in patients with acute coronary syndromes without ST-segment elevation, *N Engl J Med* 345:494-502, 2001.
78. Wehrens XHT, Doevendans PA, Ophuis TJO, Wellens HJJ: A comparison of electrocardiographic changes during reperfusion of acute myocardial infarction by thrombolysis or percutaneous transluminal coronary angioplasty, *Am Heart J* 139:430-436, 2000.
79. Vaturi M; Birnbaum Y: The use of the electrocardiogram to identify epicardial coronary and tissue reperfusion in acute myocardial infarction, *J Thromb Thrombolysis* 10:137-147, 2000.
80. van't Hof AW, Liem A, de Boer MJ et al: Clinical value of 12-lead electrocardiogram after successful reperfusion therapy for acute myocardial infarction. Zwolle Myocardial infarction Study Group, *Lancet* 350:615-619, 1997.
81. Schröder R, Dissmann R, Brüggemann T et al: Extent of early ST segment elevation resolution: a simple but strong predictor of outcome in patients with acute myocardial infarction, *J Am Coll Cardiol* 24:384-388, 1994.
82. Sarda L, Colin P, Boccara F et al: Myocarditis in patients with clinical presentation of myocardial infarction and normal coronary angiograms, *J Am Coll Cardiol* 37:786-792, 2001.
83. Hung SC, Chiang CE, Chen JD et al: Pseudo-myocardial infarction, *Circulation* 101:2989-2990, 2000.
84. Tsuchihashi K, Ueshima K, Uchida T et al: Transient left ventricular apical ballooning without coronary artery stenosis: a novel heart syndrome mimicking acute myocardial infarction, *J Am Coll Cardiol* 38:11-18, 2001.

CHAPTER 25

Congenital Long QT Syndrome

The congenital long QT (LQT) syndrome is a group of inherited disorders affecting cardiac repolarization and often resulting in a prolonged QT interval and T wave abnormalities. It is estimated that congenital LQT syndrome causes as many as 3,000 sudden deaths in children and young adults per year in the United States alone.[1] As with the acquired form of LQT syndrome, the congenital form may cause torsades de pointes (TdP), ventricular fibrillation, and sudden death. Unlike the acquired form, the congenital form may be precipitated by a variety of circumstances such as exercise, emotion, rest, or sudden arousal, depending on the affected gene. In most adults with congenital LQT syndrome, TdP is preceded by a pause (pause-dependent) that exacerbates the already prolonged QT interval. In children, who often have a more severe form of the disease, the onset of TdP is typically not pause-dependent.[2]

GENETICS

Gene mutations that cause congenital LQT syndromes have been identified on chromosomes 3, 4, 7, 11, and 21. The most common mutations occur in genes that form channels for potassium currents. Five mutant genes have thus far been identified and linked to LQT syndrome in different families. More than 180 different mutations of these five known genes have been described, with almost every family studied manifesting a different mutation. Surely, many more mutations await discovery.[1]

Four of these genes encode potassium channels (LQT1, LQT2, LQT5, and LQT6) and one gene encodes sodium channels (LQT3). The gene for chromosome 4-linked LQT (LQT4) is still unknown. Table 25-1 lists the genes causing LQT syndrome and TdP.

ECG RECOGNITION

QTc: In contrast with acquired LQT syndrome, the congenital form does not always live up to its name in that the QTc interval may be normal.[3] In fact, an overlap exists in QTc between normal individuals and those with congenital LQT syndrome. Thus, in nonsymptomatic members of a family with congenital LQT syndrome, measurement of the QTc may not be diagnostic and congenital LQT syndrome cannot be excluded on the basis of a normal QTc interval.

The range of QTc intervals in congenital LQT syndrome is from 0.41 second to more than 0.60 second.

TABLE 25-1 Genes Causing Torsades de Pointes

Phenotype Symbol	Gene Symbol	Ion Channel	Protein	T Wave
LQT1	KvLQT1 (KCNQ1)	I_{Ks}	KvLQT1	Broad-based
LQT2	HERG (KCNH2)	I_{Kr}	HERG	Low amplitude
LQT3	SCN5A	I_{Na}	SCN5A	Late onset
LQT4	Unknown	Unknown	Unknown	
LQT5	KCNE1	I_{Ks}	minK	Broad-based
LQT6	Unknown	Unknown	Unknown	Low amplitude

From Keating MT, Sanguinetti MC: Familial cardiac arrhythmias. In Scriver CR, Beaudet AL, Sly WS et al, editors: *The metabolic & molecular bases of inherited disease,* ed 8, New York, 2001, McGraw-Hill. Vol III, pp 5203-5222.

There is a wide QTc distribution in gene carriers with the LQT1, LQT2, and LQT3 genotypes. In LQT1 and LQT2 the QTc averages 0.49 second. In LQT3 this value may be longer, with a mean of 0.51 second. It has been shown that correcting the QT interval for heart rate may mask repolarization abnormalities in high-risk patients. The shape of the T wave may be an additional helpful diagnostic clue.

T wave morphology: The characteristic electrocardiogram (ECG) patterns seen in three distinct forms of LQT syndrome are show in Fig. 25-1. Note the variety of T wave morphology. Bifid T waves are sometimes seen. Fig. 25-2 depicts the bifid T wave and the U wave, and Fig. 25-3 shows a variety of bifid T waves; some more obvious than others.

TdP: The life-threatening ventricular tachycardia known as TdP is described and illustrated in Chapter 26. It is generally agreed that TdP is initiated by triggered activity because of an early afterdepolarization from a focal subendocardial site. A reentrant mechanism has been suggested for the maintenance of TdP.[4]

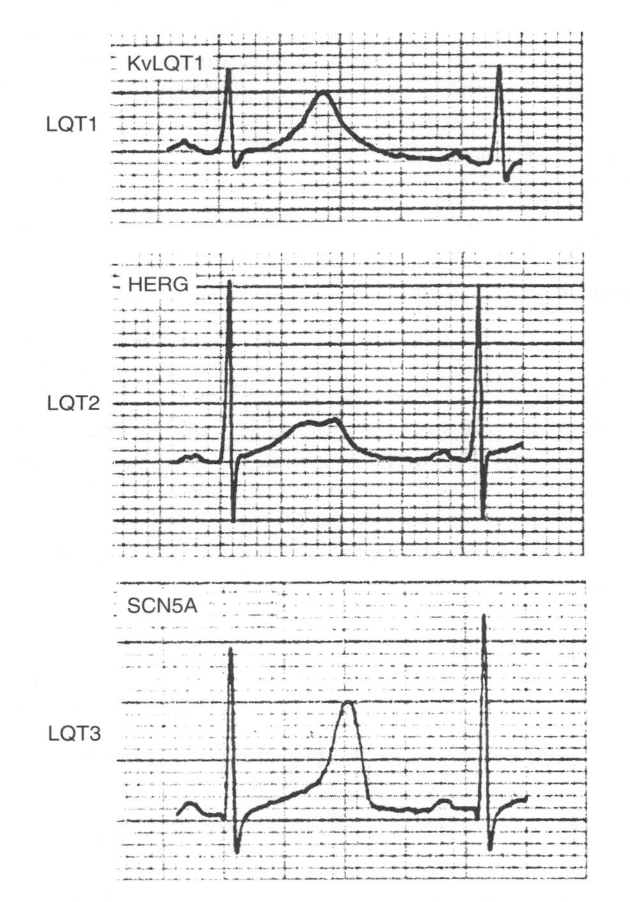

FIG. 25-1. Characteristic ECG patterns in three distinct forms of long QT syndrome: LQT1, LQT2, and LQT3, resulting from mutations in KvLQT1, HERG, and SCN5A, respectively. (From Keating MT, Sanguinetti MC: Familial cardiac arrhythmias. In Scriver CR, Beaudet AL, Sly WS, Valle D, editors: *The metabolic & molecular bases of inherited disease,* ed 8, New York, 2001, McGraw-Hill. Vol III, pp 5203-5222.)

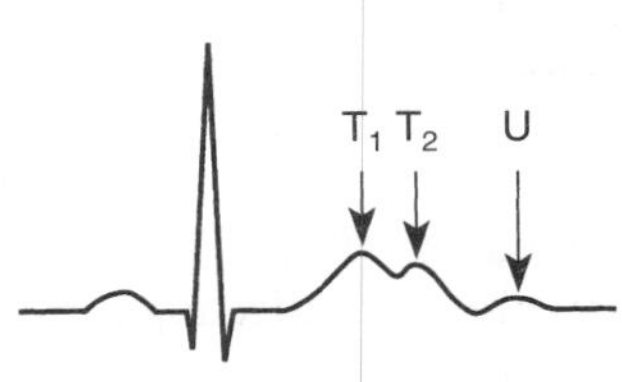

FIG. 25-2. Schematic depiction of an ECG complex showing the primary T wave *(T_1)*, a T wave hump *(T_2)*, and the U wave *(U)*. (From Lehmann MH, Suzuki F, Fromm BS et al: *J Am Coll Cardiol* 24:746, 1994.)

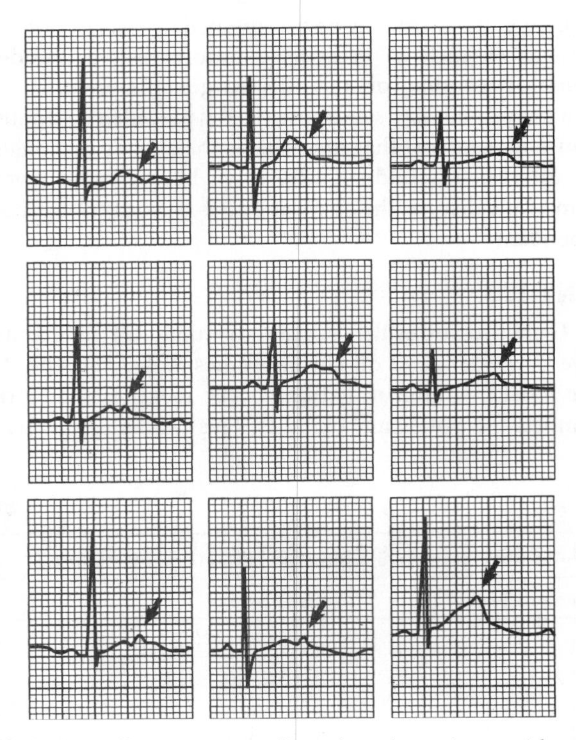

FIG. 25-3. Differing T wave distortions in patients with congenital long QT syndrome. Some T waves are bifid with a cleft; others are simply deformed by a bump on the T wave. (From Lehmann MH, Suzuki F, Fromm BS et al: *J Am Coll Cardiol* 24:746, 1994.)

The classical tracing from the original description of TdP by Dessertenne[5] is displayed in Fig. 25-4. Note the undulating QRS heights. The heart rate may range from 200 to 250 beats/min.

Fig. 25-5 is an example of TdP in a 19-year-old girl who had recurrent stress-induced syncope for 12 years. The sinus rhythm seen in the 12-lead ECG is rather bizarre looking because of the combination of a long QTc (550 ms) and T wave alternans, making the rhythm appear to be ventricular bigeminy. The intracardiac electrogram seen in Fig. 25-6 sorts it all out. The high right atrial electrogram demonstrates a regular sinus rhythm. The electrogram from the right ventricular apex and right ventricular outflow tract demonstrate sinus conducted beats. Of interest is the recording of the monophasic action potential showing alternating repolarization times. For this reason, every other QT interval is markedly prolonged (best seen in lead V_1), causing the next sinus conducted beat (with a shorter QT) to be superimposed on the preceding T wave.

MECHANISM

LQT syndromes are associated with a disruption of the flow of ions across the cardiac cell membranes during repolarization. A brief description of the normal cardiac electrical cycle (the action potential) places these ionic disruptions in perspective. The ventricular action potential (Fig. 25-7) has already been discussed in Chapter 2. Briefly, it consists of a resting phase (phase 4), depolarization of the membrane to threshold potential, rapid depolarization when the fast Na^+ channels and Ca^{2+} channels open (phase 0), a rapid brief beginning of repolarization in ventricular cells (phase 1), the plateau phase of repolarization (phase 2), and late rapid repolarization (phase 3).

The Na^+ Current

Normal. The initial rapid depolarization of most healthy cardiac cells during phase 0 of the action potential is mainly the result of a huge influx of Na^+ into the cell, depicted in the left panel of Fig. 25-8. The fast Na^+ channels open when the transmembrane voltage reaches a threshold potential and inactivate (close) rapidly (in <1 ms) not to open again until repolarization is completed, the cell has rested, and threshold voltage is again met.

Enhanced. Mutation of the gene that encodes the Na^+ channel (SCN5A) causes a channel malfunction; instead of

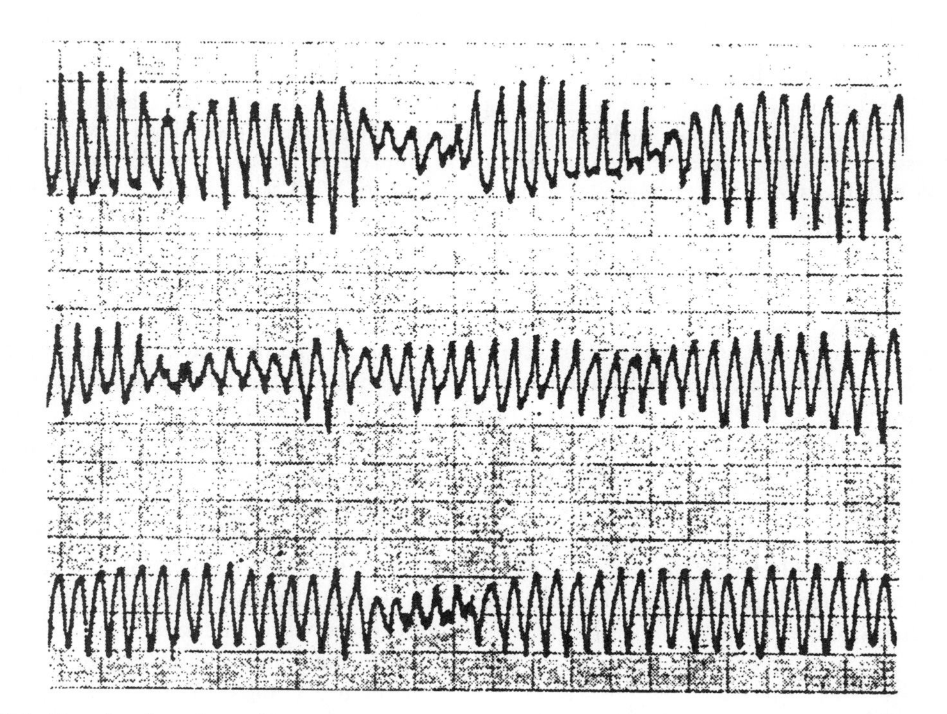

FIG. 25-4. Torsades de pointes. (From Dessertenne F: La tachycardie ventriculaire a deux foyers opposés variables, *Arch Mal Coeur* 59:263-272, 1966.)

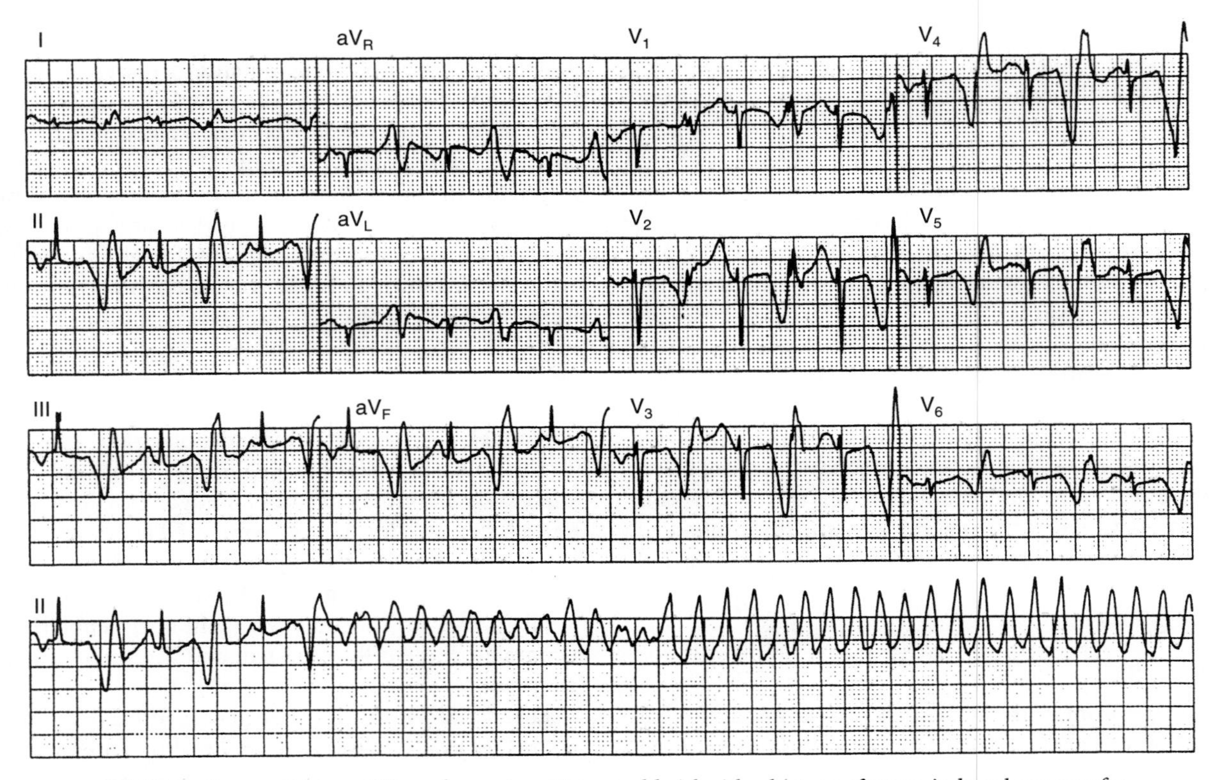

FIG. 25-5. Congenital long QT syndrome in a 19-year-old girl with a history of stress-induced syncope for 12 years. The QTc in her resting ECG was 550 ms. Torsades de pointes appears in the lead II rhythm strip. The confusing features of this bizarre-looking 12-lead ECG are the T wave alternans and the alternating QT intervals, which together hide the P waves (sinus tachycardia). The onset of torsades de pointes is seen in the lead II rhythm strip. The sinus rhythm in the 12 leads is best evaluated in leads V_1 or V_2, where the two distinct alternating T waves can be seen along with their QRS complexes. Note that one QT is longer than the other and that a QRS complex is superimposed on the end of the preceding T wave, creating the impression of an interpolated ventricular bigeminal rhythm. (From Liu YB, Chen WJ, Lee YT: Apparent ventricular bigeminy in the congenital long QT syndrome: What is the mechanism? *J Cardiovasc Electrophysiol* 11:371-372, 2000.)

inactivating and remaining closed, small Na^+ currents continue to enter the cell during phase 2 of the action potential. The normal inactivation of the fast Na^+ channel is depicted in the left panel of Fig. 25-8. Compare this figure with the one seen in the right panel of the same figure. You will note that during the plateau of the action potential Na^+ continues to enter the cell prolonging the repolarization process. These events, reflected in the surface ECG by a prolonged QT interval, result in one form of congenital LQT syndrome called *LQT3*.

The K^+ Currents

Normal. he plateau of the action potential (phase 2) is followed by repolarization of the cell in a timely manner (phase 3). The normal K^+ currents mainly responsible for the repolarization process are depicted in the left panel of Fig. 25-8. These are known as the cardiac *delayed rectifier K+ currents (IK);* they are normally active during phase 2 and 3 of atrial and ventricular myocardial cells and control the duration of repolarization and QT interval.

The term *delayed* is a relative term used to distinguish I_K from the rapidly activating Na^+ current during phase 0. In electrical terminology a rectifier permits a current to flow in only one direction, as if pressure were preventing flow in the opposite direction; in cellular electrical terminology it is applied in the same way, although not in the strict sense of the word. Although many K^+ channels are inwardly rectifying, preventing excessive loss of this impor-

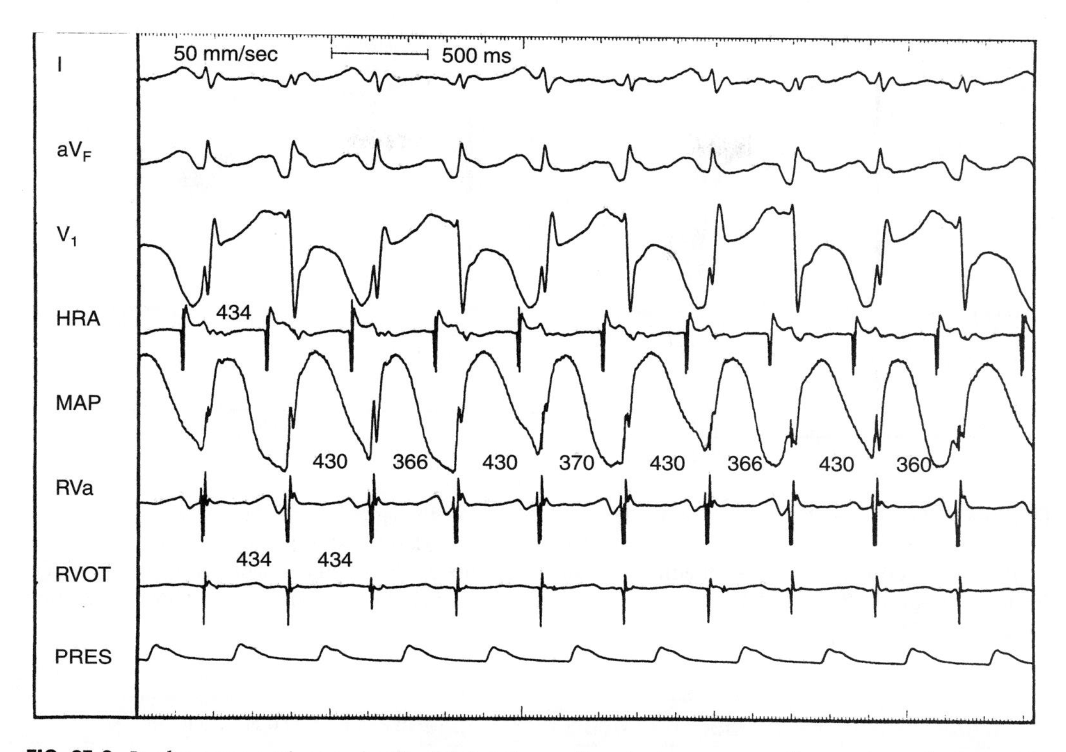

FIG. 25-6. In the same patient as in Fig. 25-5, intracardiac electrograms confirm a sinus rhythm with conducted beats to the ventricles and alternating lengths of repolarization time to explain the T wave alternans seen on the surface ECG. Look in the high right atrial *(HRA)* recording for the sinus rhythm and in the right ventricular apex *(RVa)* and outflow tract *(RVOT)* recordings for the ventricular responses. The alternating changes in action potential duration can be seen in the monophasic action potential recording *(MAP)*. *PRES,* Pressure recording. (From Liu YB, Chen WJ, Lee YT: Apparent ventricular bigeminy in the congenital long QT syndrome: What is the mechanism? *J Cardiovasc Electrophysiol* 11:371-372, 2000.)

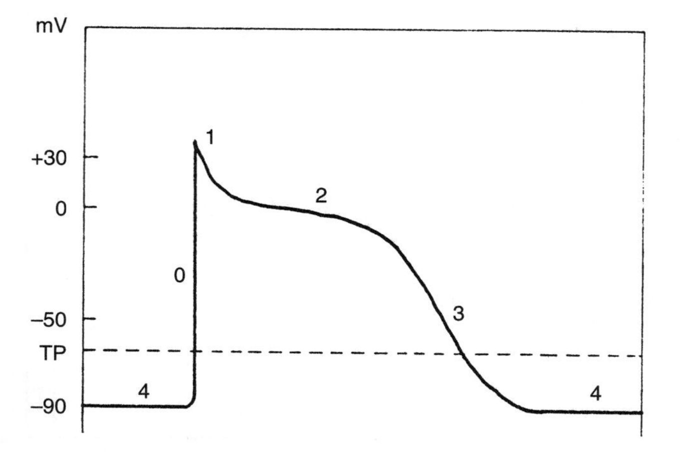

FIG. 25-7. The normal ventricular action potential. *TP,* Threshold potential.

tant intracellular ion, there are also small outward K^+ currents that activate during the plateau phase of the action potential and "fine tune" the duration of repolarization. It is this outward flow of K^+ that can be reduced by mutation of the genes that encode the K^+ channels (congenital LQT syndrome) and blocked by certain drugs, cardiac and noncardiac (acquired LQT syndrome). In addition to the drugs listed in Box 26-1, p. 386, those listed in Box 25-1 should also be avoided by patients with congenital long QT syndrome.[1]

Two components of I_K have important roles in the genesis of LQT syndromes because a rapidly activating component named I_{Kr} and a more slowly activating component named I_{Ks}. Each contribute uniquely to the action potential duration and QT interval.[6]

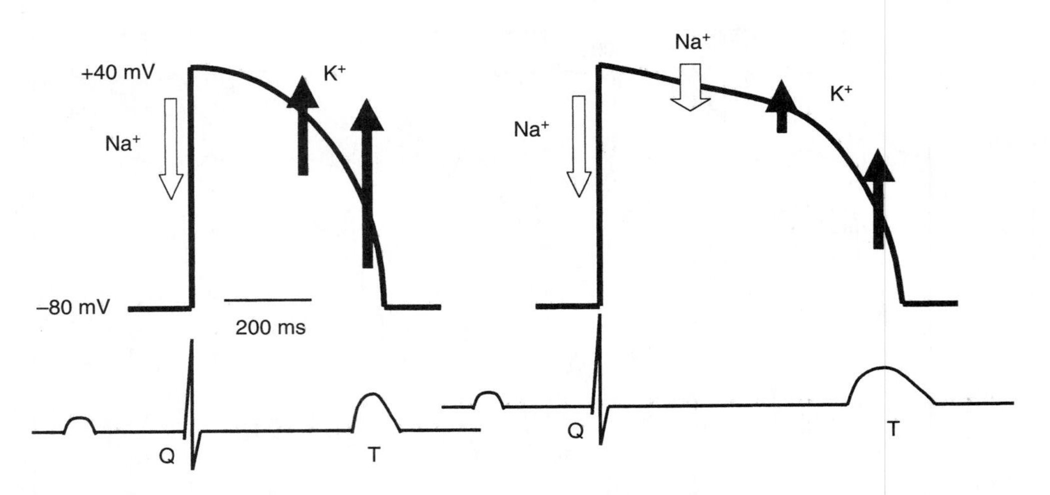

FIG. 25-8. The action potential seen on the left is normal. Note the large inward Na^+ current during phase 0 and two of the K^+ currents active during repolarization. The QT interval is normal. The action potential on the right is prolonged because of either an abnormal influx of Na^+ or an abnormal efflux of K^+, resulting in a prolonged QT interval. (Courtesy Michael C. Sanguinetti, PhD, Eccles Institute of Human Genetics, University of Utah, Salt Lake City, Utah.)

BOX 25-1. Additional Drugs to Be Avoided in Patients with Congenital Long QT Syndrome

ASTHMA/ALLERGY MEDICATIONS

- Ephedrine (adrenaline), Bronchaid, Epi, Epifin, Epinal, Epipen, Epitrate, Eppy/N, Medihaler, S-2, Isoproterenol (Isuprel, Medihaler-Iso)
- Epinephrine

DECONGESTANTS

- Phenyldrine, Propagest (Phindecon)
- Phenylpropanolamine (Acutrim, Dexatrim, Phenoxine, Pseudoephedrine)
- Phenylephrine (Neo-Synephrine) (Novafed, Pedia-Care Decongestant, Sudafed)

DRUGS TO PREVENT LOW BLOOD PRESSURE

- Midodrine (ProAmatine)
- Nor-epinephrine (Levophed)

ASTHMA MEDICATIONS

- Albuterol (Proventil, Ventolin, Ventolin Rotahaler or syrup, Volmax, Xopenex)
- Metaproterenol (Alupent, Metaprel, Metaproterenol)
- Salmeterol (Serevent)
- Terbutaline (Brethaire, Brethine, Brethine, Brethine-SC, Bricanyl)

DIET PILLS

- Fenfluramine (Pondimin)
- Phentermine (Adipex, Fastin, Ionamin, Obe-Nix, Obephen, Obermine Obestin, T-Diet)
- Sibutramine (Meridia)

DRUG TO PREVENT PRETERM LABOR

- Ritodrine (Yutopar)

From Vincent GM: Ventricular arrhythmias. Long QT syndrome, *Cardiol Clin* 18:309-325, 2000.

Note: The drugs presented in this table have the potential to stimulate the sympathetic nervous system and therefore would best be avoided by patients with congenital long QT syndrome. If these drugs must be given, careful monitoring of the heart rhythm is essential.

Reduced I_{Kr}. I_{Kr} can be reduced by either genetic mutations or drugs. Mutations of the genes HERG (human ether-a-go-go–related gene) and KCNE2 that encode the channel subunits for I_{Kr} result in congenital LQT syndromes named *LQT2* and *LQT6*, respectively.

The right panel in Fig. 25-8 illustrates the reduced outward flow of I_{Kr} that results in a prolonged QT interval.

Reduced I_{Ks}. I_{Ks} can be reduced because of mutations in two genes (KCNQ1 and KCNE1, also known as minK) that encode the subunits that coassemble to form I_{Ks} channels, resulting in congenital LQT syndromes named *LQT1* and *LQT5*, respectively.

SIGNS AND SYMPTOMS[7]

- Unexpected sudden death or cardiac arrest in an apparently healthy child or young adult, especially during exercise or emotional stress
- Sudden death during sleep, especially after the first year of life
- Syncope of sudden onset and without warning, during exercise, upon being startled by an alarm clock, when very excited (e.g., during an argument), causing a precipitous, hard, injury-producing fall to the ground
- Absence of major motor movements; there may be twitching or minor movements
- Labored breathing or apnea
- Absent pulse
- Once conscious, patient is instantly alert, orientated, and functional
- May feel tired; may have a headache

The features of neurally mediated syncope and seizures often differ as is demonstrated in Table 25-2.

EARLY DETECTION

In the Fetus

LQT syndrome should be in the differential diagnosis of the fetus with bradycardia and decreased heart rate variability in the absence of distress. Early diagnosis allows for preventive care in the infant and identification of family members at risk.[8] In the presence of unexplained fetal tachyarrhythmia, LQT syndrome should be considered a possible cause. The presence of atrioventricular dissociation, which can be detected with ultrasound, may be useful in prenatal diagnosis of LQT syndrome.[9]

In the Neonate

Early detection and treatment of congenital LQT syndrome in the neonate are mandatory to prevent TdP and sudden death.[10] The ECG may give some clues such as the following:

- Persistent QT prolongation
- Bizarre T waves
- Intermittent episodes of T wave alternans
- TdP not preceded by a pause (most episodes of congenital TdP in the older child and young adult are pause-dependent)[2]

LQT SYNDROME TYPE 1

In 1991 Keating et al[11] mapped the chromosomal location of the first congenital LQT syndrome gene. Because this was the first gene to be named, the syndrome produced by mutations in this gene was called long QT type 1 (LQT1).

Dominant Mutations

In 1996 Wang et al[12] discovered the gene associated with the LQT1 locus that encodes the pore-forming subunit of a K^+ channel. This gene was named KvLQT1 (now called KCNQ1), reflecting the ion channel (Kv), the long QT, and its place in the history of discovery (first). Since then, approximately 80 mutations of the KvLQT1 gene have been identified.[13]

When four KvLQT1 subunits are united with another subunit called *minK*, it forms channels that conduct the slow delayed rectifier K^+ current (I_{Ks}), as demonstrated in Fig. 25-9. Disruption of the function of this channel and its K^+ current results in prolonged cardiac repolarization (QT interval). However, individuals with a mutation of the KvLQT1 gene are often not plagued with TdP unless another factor that also prolongs the QT interval is intro-

TABLE 25-2 Characteristic Symptoms and Signs in the Differential Diagnosis of Long QTS

Condition	Prevention	Appearance at Onset	Motor Activity	Breathing	Unconscious	Afterwards
Long QT	No warning	Normal	None, flaccid	Gasping	30 sec–3 min	Alert, 1-2 min
Neurally mediated syncope	Dizziness, fainting	Pale, sweating	None, flaccid	Normal	Seconds	Alert, 1-2 min
Seizure	Aura	Glazed, confused	Stiff, jerking	Impaired	Minutes	Disoriented

duced, such as enhanced autonomic tone, hypokalemia, hypomagnesemia, sinus pauses, or potassium channel-blocking drugs.[13,14] Such drugs (cardiac and noncardiac) block the repolarizing channels of another K^+ current, the rapid delayed rectifier K^+ current, known as I_{Kr}. The channels for I_{Kr} are formed when four HERG subunits are united with another subunit called *?MiRP1*, as demonstrated in Fig. 25-10.

Recessive Mutations

The syndrome associated with the autosomal recessive form of LQT was first recognized by Jervell and Lange-Nielson in 1957 (Fig. 25-11).[15] They reported a family with four deaf children, QT interval prolongation, and sudden cardiac death in three of the four affected children. It is now known that the channels for I_{Ks}, the slow, delayed rectifer K^+ current, also conduct K^+ into the

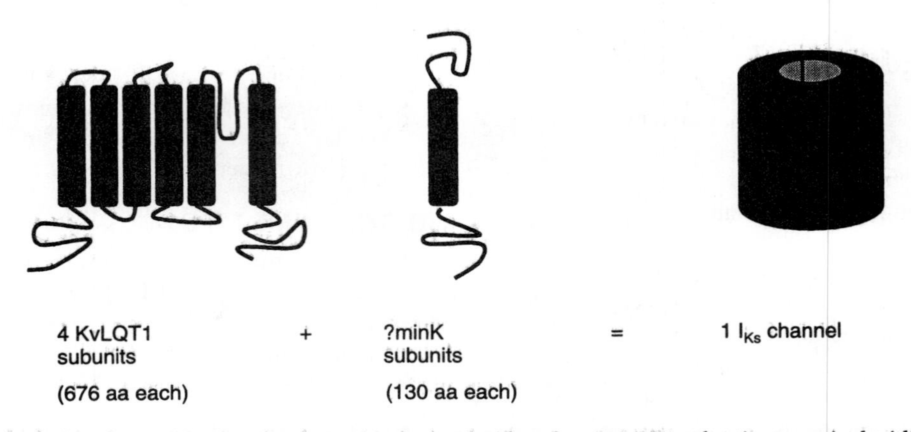

FIG. 25-9. The formation of an I_{Ks} channel is depicted. When four KvLQT1 subunits are united with another subunit called *?minK*, it forms channels that conduct the slow delayed rectifier K^+ current (I_{Ks}). Mutation of the KvLQT1 gene results in disruption of the function of this channel and its K^+ current, prolonging repolarization and the QT interval. *aa*, Amino acids. (Courtesy Michael C. Sanguinetti, PhD, Eccles Institute of Human Genetics, University of Utah, Salt Lake City, Utah.)

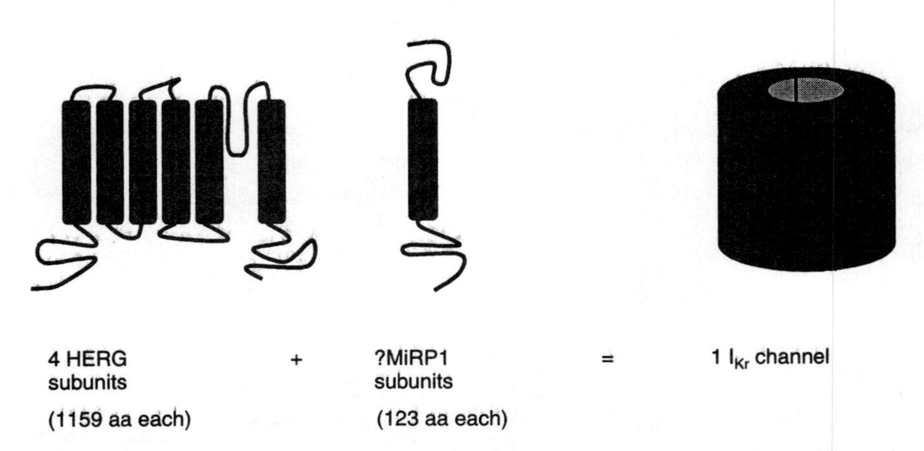

FIG. 25-10. The formation of an I_{Kr} channel is depicted. The channels for I_{Kr} are formed when four HERG subunits are united with another subunit called *?MiRP1*. Potassium channel-blocking drugs (cardiac and noncardiac) block the channels for I_{Kr}, prolonging the QT interval, especially in individuals with a mutation of the KvLQT1 gene. *aa*, Amino acids. (Courtesy Michael C. Sanguinetti, PhD, Eccles Institute of Human Genetics, University of Utah, Salt Lake City, Utah.)

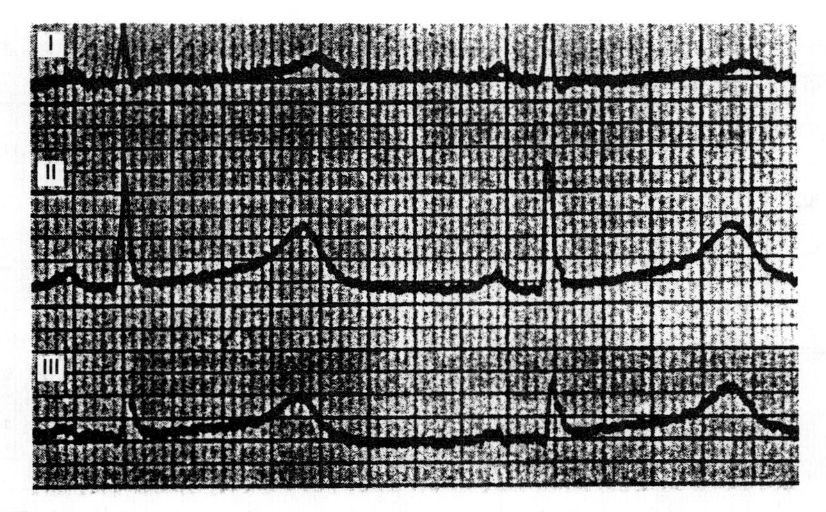

FIG. 25-11. The ECG of the first patient to be described with congenital long QT syndrome and deafness. (From Jervell A, Lange-Neilsen F: Congenital deaf-mutism, functional heart disease with prolongation of the QT interval, and sudden death, *Am Heart J* 54:59-68, 1957.)

inner ear, creating a potassium-rich endolymph fluid. Recessive mutations of the KvLQT1 or minK gene eliminates IKs, compromising the production of inner ear fluid and causing a degeneration of the organ of Corti. The individual will have neural deafness and more severe arrhythmias than seen in patients with the dominant mutation.[13]

ECG Patterns in LQT1

The QTc interval is 480 ms. The T wave is normal. ST-T wave patterns have been described[16] for the genotypes of congenital LQT1:

- Infantile pattern (2 months to 2 years, sometimes up to 5 years):
  - Normal pediatric ECG of sinus tachycardia and right ventricular predominance
  - ST segment short and ill-defined diagonal line to the T wave upslope
  - Bifid T waves common with second component highest
  - Steep T wave downslope
  - Broad-based, peaked, and asymmetrical T wave
  - QT borderline to obviously prolonged (QTc 490 ± 40 ms)
- Broad-based T wave pattern:
  - Single, smooth T wave in most leads
  - No distinct T wave onset
  - QT normal to obviously prolonged (QTc 490 ± 40 ms)
- Normal-appearing T wave pattern:
  - Normal-looking T wave
  - QT normal to obviously prolonged (QTc 460 ± 40 ms)
- Late-onset normal-appearing T wave:
  - Normal-looking T wave
  - Prolonged ST segment
  - QTc 490 ± 40 ms

Fig. 25-12 displays a typical ECG from a patient with LQT1.

The patient whose ECG is shown in Fig. 25-13 was a 20-year-old woman with a history of recurrent syncope and no hearing defect. She did not survive the episode of TdP seen in the bottom tracing.

LQT SYNDROME TYPE 2

LQT2 involves the mutation of HERG, a cardiac potassium channel gene, which encodes the I_{Kr} channel most commonly blocked by many structurally diverse drugs in the acquired LQT syndrome. More than 81 mutations of the HERG gene have thus far been identified (46% of the known LQT syndrome gene mutations).[1] In a few cases the QT intervals have only slightly or borderline prolongation.

ECG Patterns in LQT2[16]

Low-amplitude bifid T waves are the ECG hallmark of LQT2. It may be difficult at times to distinguish a bifid T wave from a T-U. Careful examination of all 12 leads usually helps.

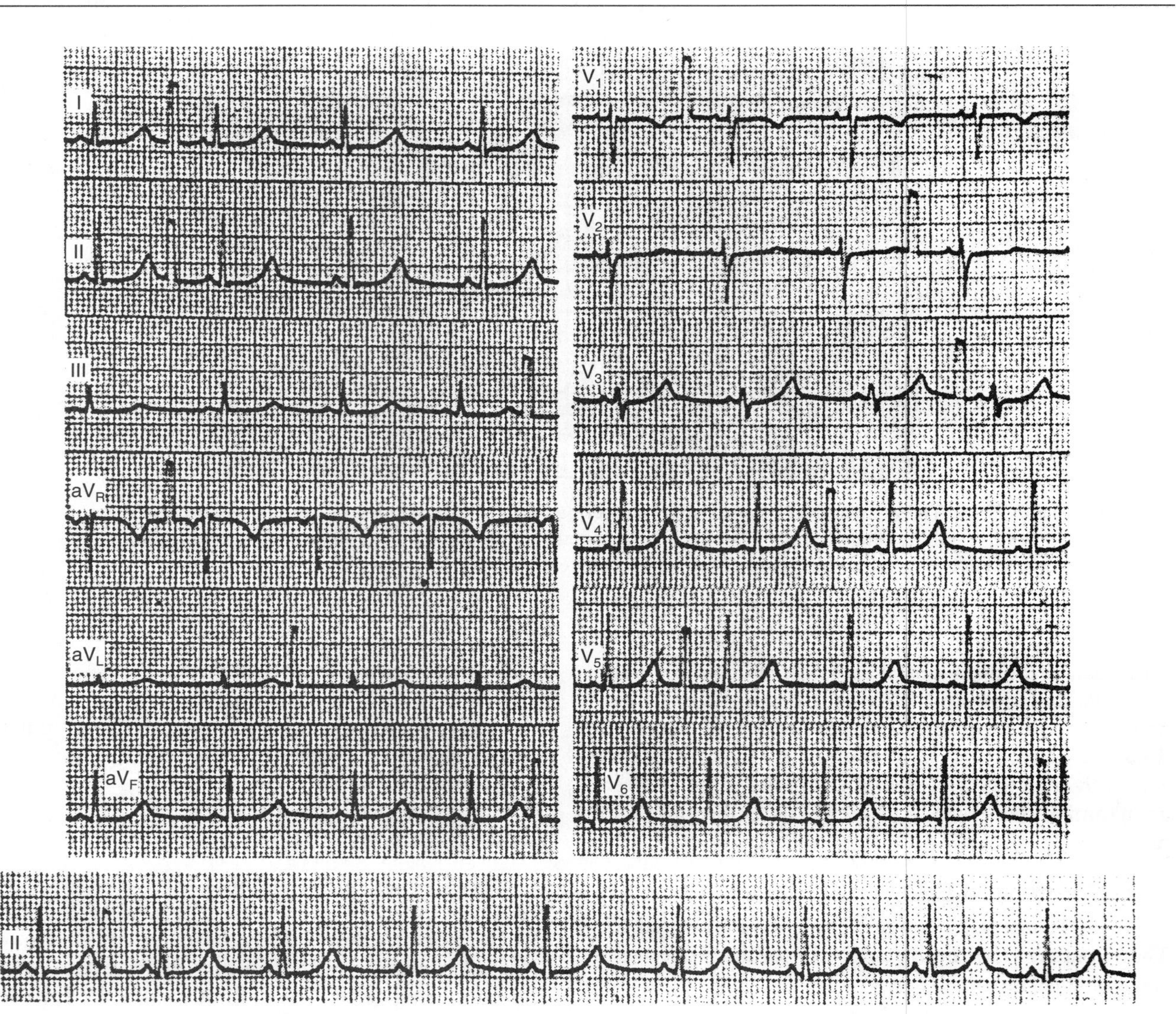

FIG. 25-12. An ECG from a patient with KvLQT1 long QT syndrome. The QTc is 0.48 second. The T wave is normal. This is a typical ECG for many patients with the K^+ channel genotypes. The degree of QT prolongation is about average for these patients. (From Vincent GM: The long QT syndrome. In Parmley WW, Chatterjee K, editors: *Cardiology physiology, pharmacology, diagnosis,* Philadelphia, 2002, Lippincott-Raven Publishers.)

- Four main types of bifid T waves are as follows:
  1. Obvious
  2. Subtle with the second component at the top of the T
  3. Subtle with the second component on the T downslope
  4. Low amplitude and widely split
- QT interval normal to markedly prolonged (QTc) 470 ± 30 ms)
- Onset of TdP often the classic "startle" response to auditory stimuli, which appears relatively specific for mutations in HERG[17]

LQT SYNDROME TYPE 3

LQT3 involves mutation of the cardiac voltage-dependent Na^+ channel gene, SCN5A. At least 13 mutations of this gene have been identified (6% of the known LQT syndrome gene mutations).[1] In these individuals, most events of TdP occur at night.

Mutations of the LQT3 gene cause a malfunction of the

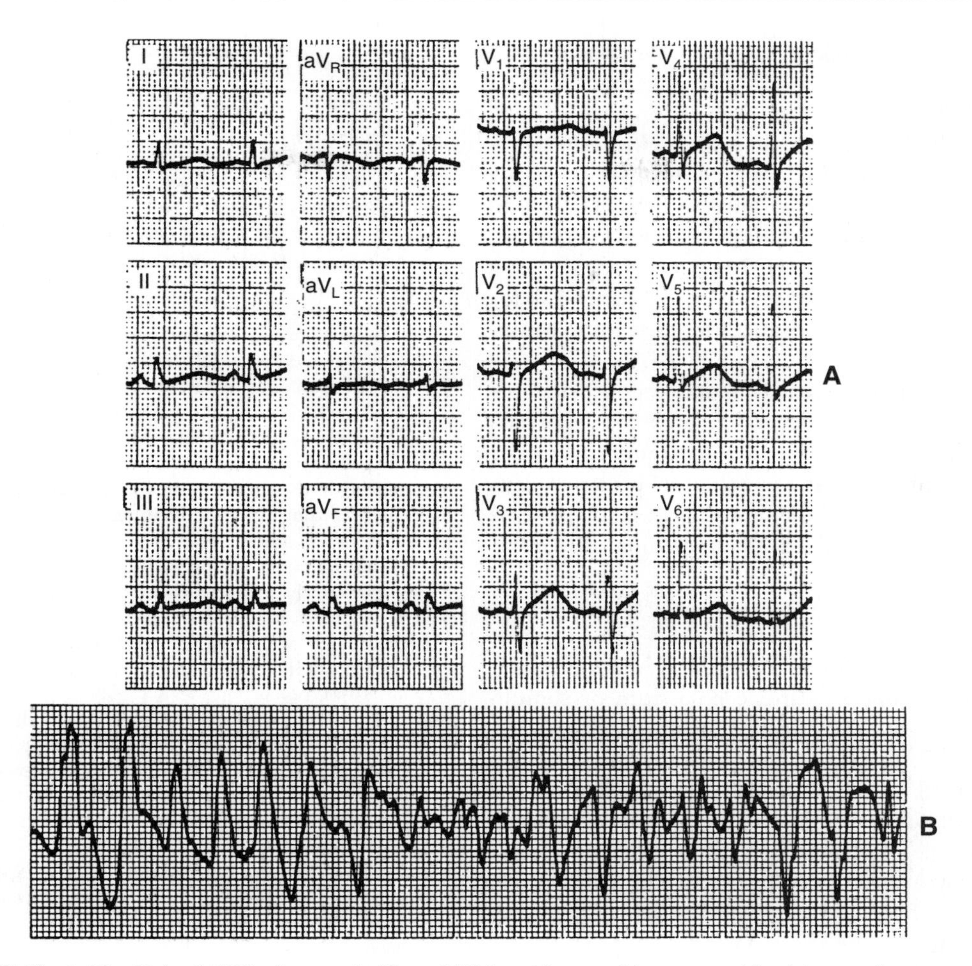

FIG. 25-13. **A**, The 12-lead ECG of congenital long QTS in a 20-year-old woman with a history of recurrent syncope. Her QTc was 0.61 second. She had no hearing defects. **B**, Torsades de pointes in the same patient. The patient died on the same day the 12-lead ECG was obtained. (From Chou TC: *Electrocardiography in clinical practice; adult and pediatric*, Philadelphia, 1996, WB Saunders. Fig. 26-23, p 566.)

fast Na^+ channels. Instead of remaining closed after rapid depolarization, they reopen to allow a small late Na^+ current to enter the cell during the plateau phase of the action potential, upsetting the intricate balance of ionic currents that control the length of repolarization. When Na^+ enters the cell inappropriately (or when K^+ cannot leave the cell as it should), the onset of phase 3 repolarization is delayed, and the QT interval is prolonged. Early after-depolarizations develop, and these may trigger TdP.

ECG Patterns in LQT3[16]

The typical ECG patterns of LQT3

- Late onset, peaked, biphasic T waves with the following:
  - Long ST segment
  - Distinct T wave onset and offset
  - Steep T wave downslope
  - QT interval often markedly prolonged (QTc 530 ± 40 ms)
- Asymmetric peaked T waves with the following:
  - Steep downslope
  - QTc 470 ± 30 ms

TREATMENT

Prevention of sudden death for patients with congenital LQT syndrome requires life-long therapy. Although beta blockers remain the mainstay of therapy, this may not be sufficient for cardiac arrest survivors and for those with LQT3.

Other future treatment options may be genotype

specific drugs and pacemakers, especially for patients with LQT2 or LQT3.

Although the antiarrhythmic effect of gene-specific drugs has yet to be established, they do significantly shorten the QT interval. Potassium channel openers do so for patients with inadequate potassium outflow (LQT1 and LQT2 genotypes) or sodium channel blockers for patients with excessive sodium inflow (LQT3).[18]

Cardiac pacemakers may prove to be beneficial for patients with LQT2 or LQT3 and for those with pause-dependent TdP.

A review of practical recommendations on programming pacemakers for pause-dependent arrhythmias, which differs from the standard pacemaker programming, can be found in the references.[19] Implantable defibrillators with dual-chamber pacing capability are indicated for patients at high risk for arrhythmic death, including all cardiac arrest survivors.

SUMMARY

Congenital LQT syndrome is caused by mutations in at least five genes coding for cardiac potassium or sodium channels that regulate the duration of ventricular action potentials (QT interval). If outward K^+ channels are reduced or inward Na^+ channels enhanced, the repolarization process can be prolonged, producing early afterdepolarizations capable of triggering TdP, a potentially lethal ventricular tachycardia. TdP be precipitated by a variety of circumstances such as exercise, emotion, rest, or sudden arousal, depending on the affected gene.

REFERENCES

1. Vincent GM: Long QT syndrome, *Cardiol Clin* 18:309-325, 2000.
2. Viskin S, Fish R, Zeltser D et al: Arrhythmias in the congenital long QT syndrome: How often is torsade de pointes pause dependent? *Heart* 83:661-666, 2000.
3. Roden DM: Torsade de pointes, *Clin Cardiol* 16:683, 1993.
4. Antzelevitch C, Yan GX, Shimizu W et al: Electrical heterogeneity, the ECG, and cardiac arrhythmias. In Zipes DP, Jalife J, editors: *Cardiac electrophysiology from cell to bedside,* ed 3, Philadelphia, 2000, WB Saunders.
5. Dessertenne F: La tachycardie ventriculaire a deux foyers opposés variables, *Arch Mal Coeur* 59:263-272, 1966.
6. Sanguinetti MC, Tristani-Firouzi M: Delayed and inward rectifier potassium channels. In Zipes DP, Jalife J, editors: *Cardiac electrophysiology from cell to bedside,* ed 3, Philadelphia 2000, WB Saunders.
7. Vincent GM: The long QT syndrome. In Parmley WW, Chatterjee K, editors: *Cardiology physiology, pharmacology, diagnosis,* Philadelphia, 2002, Lippincott-Raven Publishers.
8. Donofrio MT, Gullquist SD, O'Connell NG et al: Fetal presentation of congenital long QT syndrome, *Pediatr Cardiol* 20:441-444, 1999.
9. Ohkuchi A, Shiraishi H, Minakami H et al: Fetus with long QT syndrome manifested by tachyarrhythmia: a case report, *Prenat Diagn* 19:990-992, 1999.
10. Mache CJ, Beitzke A, Haidvogl M Jr et al: Perinatal manifestations of idiopathic long QT syndrome, *Pediatr Cardiol* 17:118-121, 1996.
11. Keating M, Atkinson D, Dunn C et al: Linkage of a cardiac arrhythmia, the long QT syndrome, and the Harvey ras-I gene, *Science* 252:704-706, 1991.
12. Wang Q, Curran ME, Splawski I et al: Positional cloning of a novel potassium channel gene: KVLQT1 mutations cause cardiac arrhythmias, *Nat Genet* 12:17-23, 1996.
13. Sanguinetti MC: Long QT syndrome: ionic basis and arrhythmia mechanism in long QT syndrome type 1, *J Cardiovasc Electrophysiol* 11:710-712, 2000.
14. Napolitano C, Schwartz PJ, Brown AM et al: Evidence for a cardiac ion channel mutation underlying drug-induced QT prolongation and life-threatening arrhythmias, *J Cardiovasc Electrophysiol* 11:691, 2000.
15. Jervell A, Lang-Nielsen F: Congenital deaf-mutism, function heart disease with prolongation of the LQ-T interval and sudden death, *Am Heart J* 54:59-68, 1957.
16. Zhang L, Timothy KW, Vincent GM et al: Spectrum of ST-T-wave patterns and repolarization parameters in congenital long-QT syndrome: ECG findings identify genotypes, *Circulation* 102:2849-2855, 2000.
17. Wilde AA, Jongbloed RJ, Doevendans PA et al: Auditory stimuli as a trigger for arrhythmic events differentiate HERG-related (LQQTS2) patients from KVLQT1-related patients (LQTS1), *J Am Coll Cardiol* 33:327-332, 1999.
18. Viskin S, Fish R: Prevention of ventricular arrhythmias in the congenital long QT syndrome, *Curr Cardiol Rep* 2:492-497, 2000.
19. Viskin S: Cardiac pacing in the long QT syndrome: review of available data and practical recommendations, *J Cardiovasc Electrophysiol* 11:593-600, 2000.

CHAPTER 26

Torsades de Pointes in the Acquired Long QT Syndrome

Torsade(s) de pointes (TdP) is a life-threatening polymorphic ventricular tachycardia (VT) of more than 170 beats/min with a unique undulating QRS pattern. It occurs against a background of prolonged QT intervals, ventricular ectopic beats, T and U wave abnormalities, and pauses. Its subjective symptoms are recurrent episodes of dizziness and syncope. The etiology of TdP (acquired or congenital) determines its classification under long QT syndrome (LQTS). Acquired LQTS is caused by QT prolonging drugs, heart block, cardiac, cerebral disease or electrolyte imbalance; congenital LQTS is the result of gene mutations (Chapter 25). The acquired form typically affects older individuals and is most often associated with specific pharmacologic agents, whereas the congenital form may be recognized in the child and rarely in the fetus.[1]

The term *torsade(s) de pointes* is a descriptive French term meaning "twisting of the points" that was applied to this unique pattern of VT when, in 1966, it was first distinguished from other VTs.[2] *Pointes,* of course, refers to the QRS peaks. However, there is disagreement regarding the French term for twisting. Should it be *torsade or torsades*? Some believe that the singular form *(torsade)* refers to a single salvo of tachycardia. The plural form *(torsades)* refers to more than one episode.[3]

ELECTROCARDIOGRAM SIGNS WARNING OF TdP

Typical warning signs seen in all but the sudden-onset type of TdP are one or more of the following, some of which can be seen in Figs. 26-1 to 26-3:

- Progressive lengthening of the QTc interval to more than 0.44 second during sinus rhythm, the hallmark of TdP and an important way to differentiate it from ischemia-related polymorphic VT
- Appearance of bizarre-looking T waves with giant U waves in the sinus complex after each postextrasystolic pause
- T wave alternans
- Onset of ventricular extrasystoles
- Short-long-short sequences and salvos of VT (classical and cascade type, described in the following section)
- Significant heart rate (HR) increase in the minute before the onset of TdP

ONSET OF TdP

The onset of TdP often is a classical short-long-short sequence beginning with a single ectopic beat followed by a pause. Fig. 26-4 is an example, although in this case the TdP is triggered by a pair of premature ventricular complexes (PVCs) (the first one a fusion beat). The onset may also be sudden; that is, not preceded by PVCs and pauses.

In patients with LQTS, a short-long-short sequence creates a myocardial milieu (inhomogeneity of refractoriness) favoring initiation and maintenance of TdP.[4] The tachycardia typically arises after the peak of the T wave in the cycle after the pause.

QUINIDINE-INDUCED TdP

In quinidine-induced TdP the QT intervals are quite long and may exceed 0.60 second, as in Figs. 26-4 and 26-5. This may be the case even with low quinidine plasma concentrations and absence of marked QRS prolongation. Other characteristic features of quinidine-related TdP are hypokalemia (K <4 mEq/L) and usually abrupt slowing of the HR just before the initiation of TdP.[5,6]

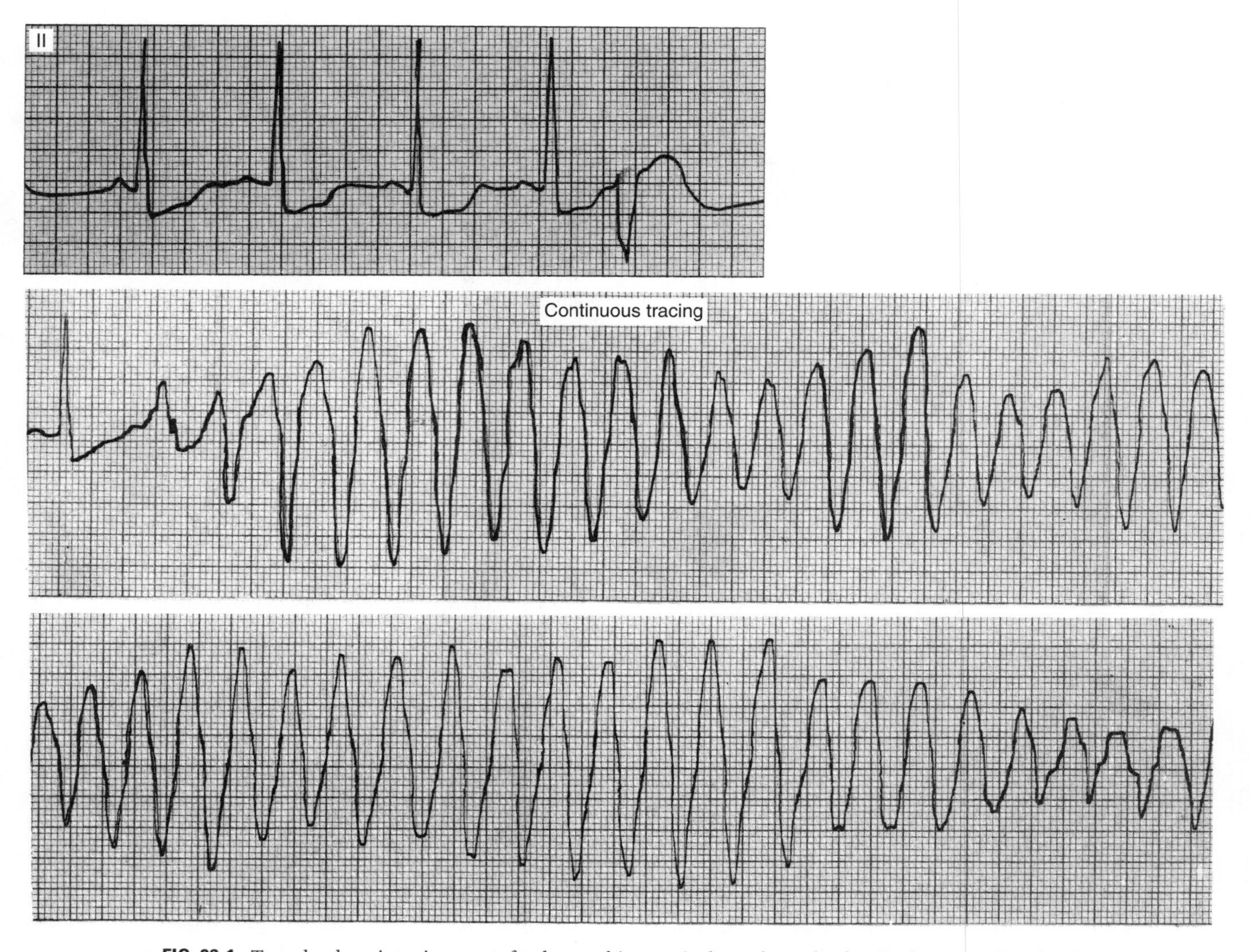

FIG. 26-1. Torsades de pointes is a type of polymorphic ventricular tachycardia that is often paroxysmal and that occurs in the setting of a long QT interval, which is commonly secondary to therapy with quinidine or quinidine-like drugs (procainamide and disopyramide) but which may also be the result of hypokalemia and complete heart block. This tracing is from a patient who had been receiving procainamide (500 mg four times a day, orally).

CORRECTED QT INTERVAL

The QT interval normally accommodates HR, lengthening with bradycardia and shortening with tachycardia. In order to correct the QT for HR (QTc) the square root of the RR interval is divided into the QT interval.

Rule of Thumb

For decades, clinicians have been using a "rule of thumb" to quickly determine if a QT interval is normal. This undocumented rule states that at a HR of 60 to 100 beats/min the normal QT does not exceed half the RR interval.[7] This shorthand rule was mathematically validated in 1998 by Phoon,[8] who plotted it against Bazett formula, the Framingham Heart Study's linear correction, and Fridericia's cube root prediction. The validated "rule of thumb" is essentially the same as the long-standing empirical one; the only change has been the heart rates at which it can be used. Thus the normal QTc is less than half the RR interval when the HR is more than 70 beats/min.

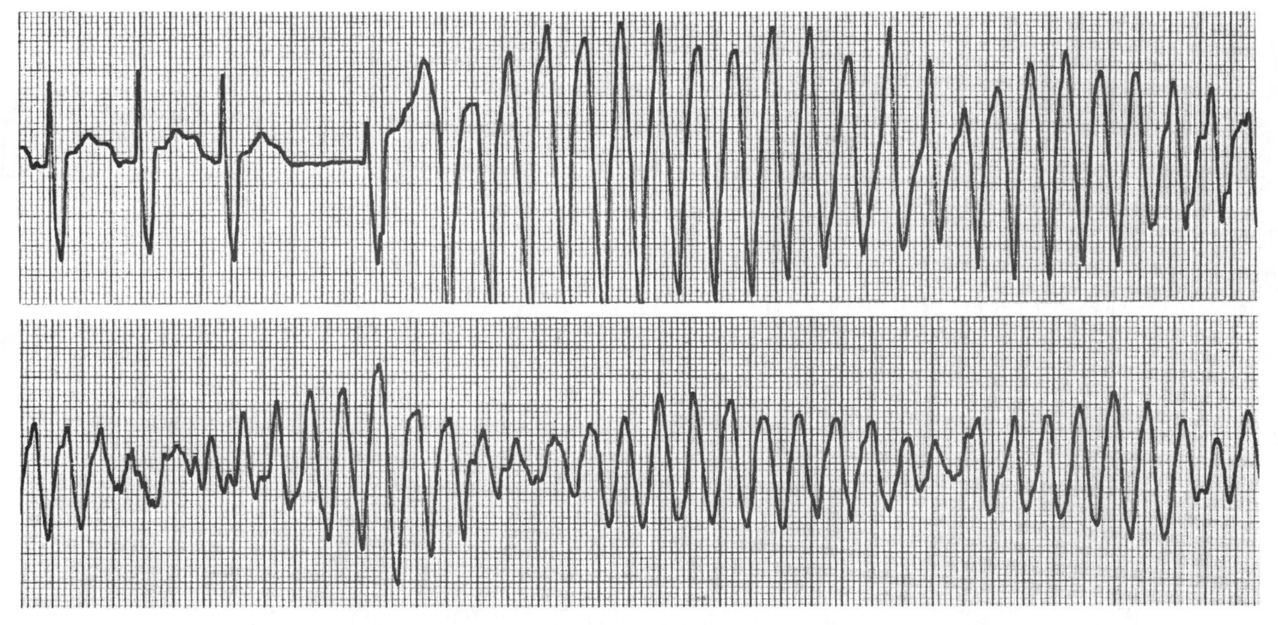

FIG. 26-2. A prolonged episode of torsades de pointes (continuous tracing) follows sinus tachycardia, an unexplained pause, and an ectopic beat. Note during sinus rhythm the prolonged QT interval, the distorted T wave during sinus rhythm, and the giant T wave in the beat after the pause. (From the late Dr. Alan Lindsay collection, Salt Lake City, Utah.)

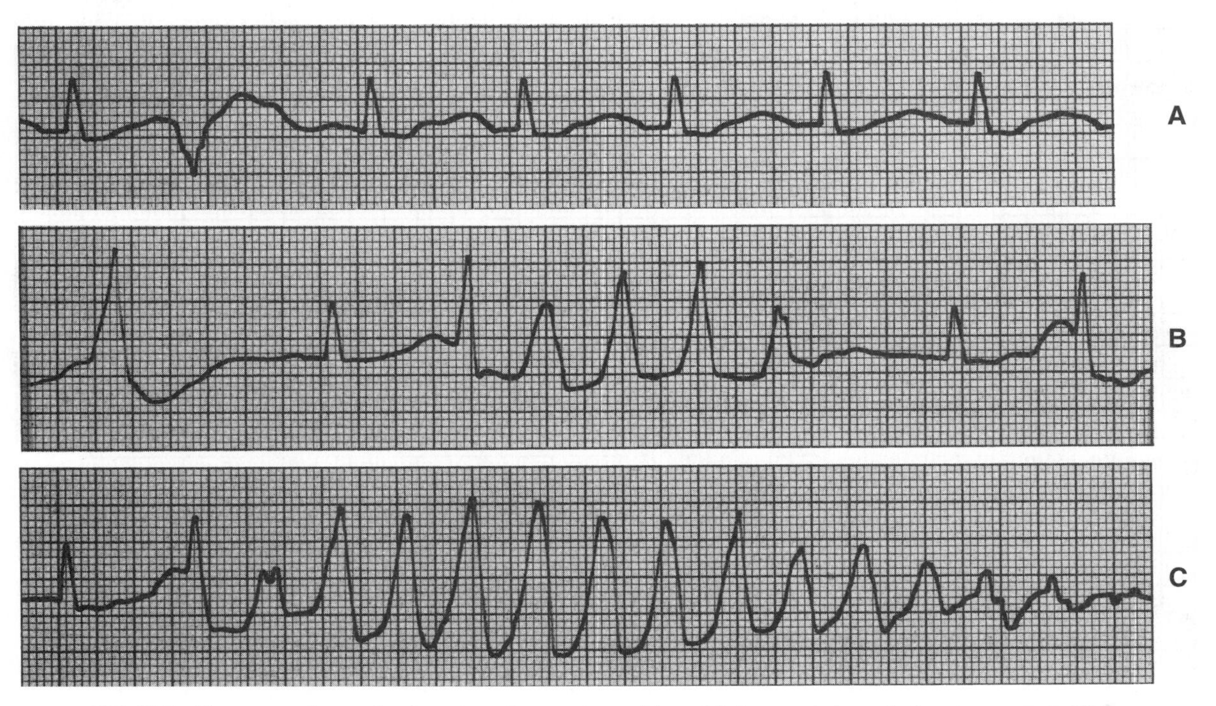

FIG. 26-3. The onset of torsades de pointes in a patient with multiple ectopic beats before its onset. **A,** Note the prolonged QT and the appearance of a premature ventricular complex (PVC) after the first beat. **B,** There are PVCs at the beginning and end of the tracing flanking a short run of ventricular tachycardia. **C,** The stage is finally set for the first episode of torsades de pointes.

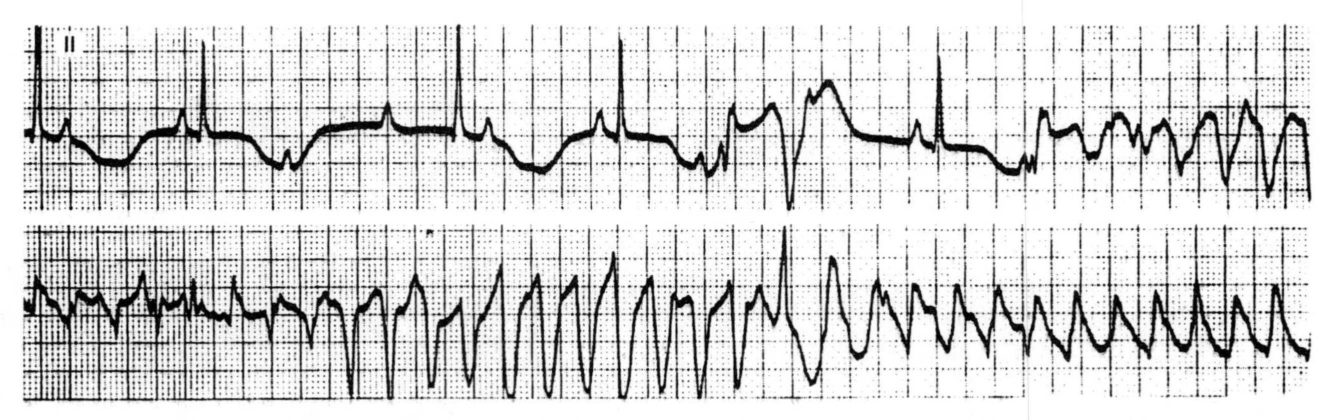

FIG. 26-4. Drug-induced torsades de pointes. The QT interval is 0.84 second. The high-grade AV block causes pauses in the rhythm, which compound the risk for torsades de pointes. (From Schamroth L: *Electrocardiographic excursions*, 1975, Blackwell Scientific Publications, Oxford.)

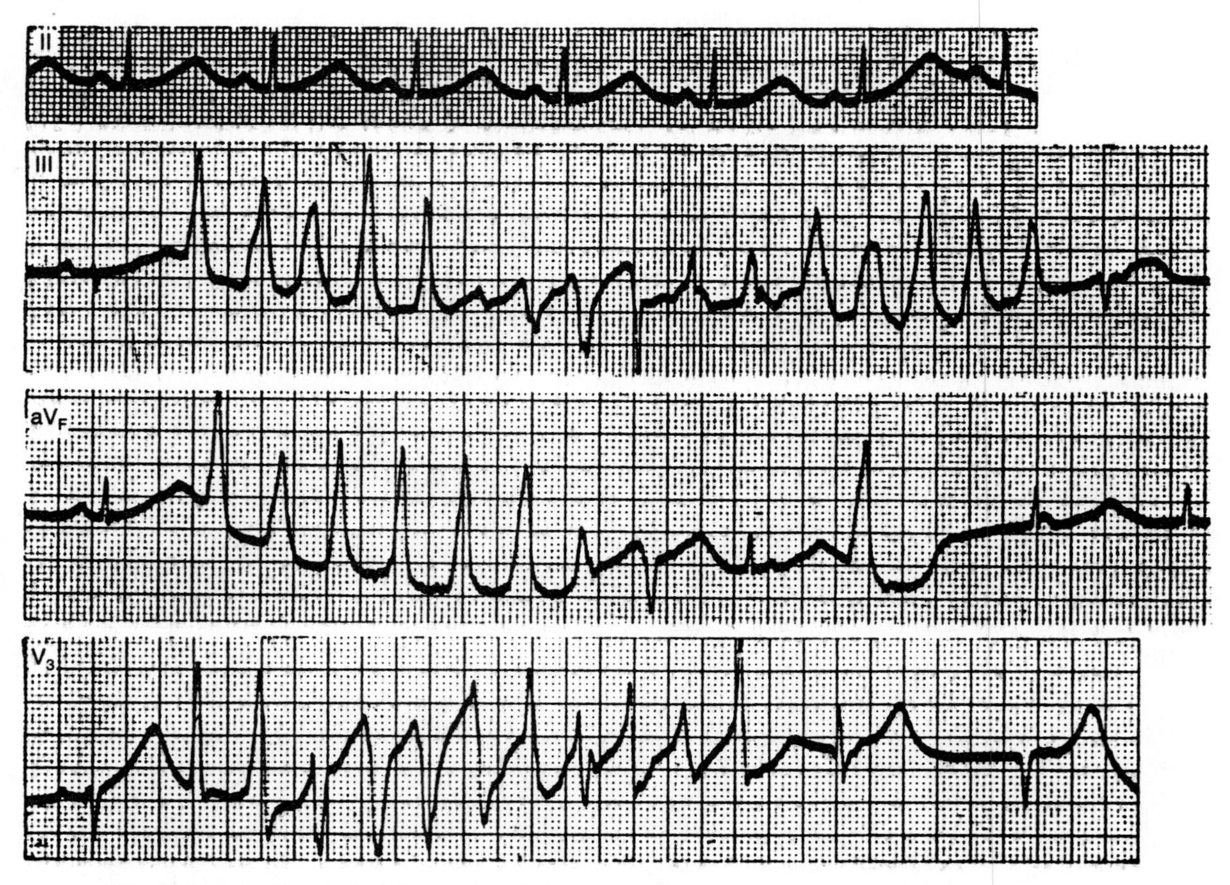

FIG. 26-5. Quinidine-induced torsades de pointes. The QT interval exceeds 0.60 second. (From Goldman MJ: *Principles of clinical electrocardiography*, ed 10, Los Altos, Calif, 1979, Lange Medical Publications.)

MECHANISMS

Acquired LQTS, as with congenital LQTS is caused by abnormal ventricular repolarization and has many features similar to congenital LQTS, but typically affects older individuals and is often associated with specific pharmacologic agents. A growing number of cardiac and noncardiac drugs have been found to block K^+ channels, prolonging the QT interval and causing TdP when administered alone, with another drug that also blocks K^+ channels, or to an individual whose K^+ or Na^+ channels are already genetically blocked (congenital LQTS). Potassium is the main ion in control of the duration of the action potential; its channels make fine adjustments in the speed with which K^+ leaves the cell, accommodating slow and fast HR by providing the shorter QT interval needed during tachycardia and the longer one needed during bradycardia.

Early Afterdepolarizations

Early afterdepolarizations are oscillations in the membrane potential toward the end of repolarization (phase 3 of the action potential). They are the result of a prolonged repolarization time, as reflected in the lengthening of the QT interval. The actual afterdepolarizations are not seen on the ECG.

The action potential can be prolonged by activation of inward currents carried by positive ions (sodium and calcium currents) or by blocking outward currents carried by potassium ions (various potassium currents), such as would occur in both acquired and congenital LQTS.

Fig. 26-6 shows normal (control panel) and abnormal action potentials followed by sudden onset TdP. The arrows point to the early afterdepolarizations elicited in animal experiments after administration of an antiarrhythmic drug that prolongs repolarization. When all conditions are met, the early afterdepolarization produces a triggered beat and the onset of TdP, as is evident in this tracing. Conditions can be met after pauses and during bradycardia, inducing reactivation of the L-type (slow) calcium current, an inward flux of Ca^{2+} into the cell. If this depolarizing Ca^{2+} current reaches a critical potential, it triggers TdP.[9,10]

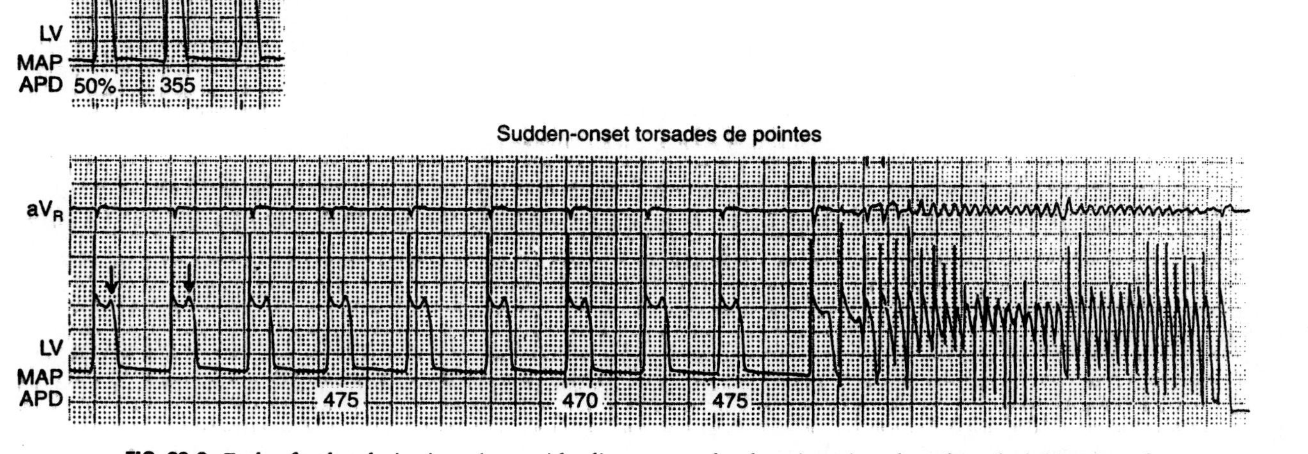

FIG. 26-6. Early afterdepolarizations *(arrows)* leading to torsades de pointes in a dog after administration of a class III antiarrhythmic drug. The tracing shows surface ECG lead AV_R with the coinciding endocardially recorded action potentials. The three action potentials on the left were recorded before administration of the drug. After administration, the action potential duration increases and the oscillation (early afterdepolarization) during its plateau appears. (From Vos MA, Gorenek B, Verduyn SC et al: Observations on the onset of torsades de pointes arrhythmias in the acquired long QT syndrome, *Cardiovasc Res* 48:421-429, 2000.)

Dispersion of Repolarization

Prolongation of the QT interval of itself is not necessarily a harbinger of TdP. Some antiarrhythmic drugs are, in fact, chosen precisely for this property. A prolonged action potential will generate an early afterdepolarization, but it is the dispersion of repolarization (unequal refractory periods within the ventricles) that tips the balance toward the initiation and support of TdP. Other factors may also prevent a QT prolonging drug from resulting in TdP. Amiodarone, for example, prolongs the QT interval, but has a very low incidence of TdP,[11] probably because it is a calcium channel blocker and, therefore, suppresses early afterdepolarizations and because it does not increase dispersion of refractoriness.[12]

BOX 26-1. Drugs That Prolong the QT Interval or Induce Torsades de Pointes

Acrivastine* (Semprex-D)
Ajmaline
Almokalant
Amantadine (Symmetrel)
Amiodarone (Cordarone)
Amitriptyline (Elavil, Endep, Etrafon, Limbitrol, Triavil)
Amoxapine (Asendin)
Ampicillin (Omnipen, Polycillin, Principen)
Amrinone (Inocor)
Aprindine
Astemizole† (Hismanal)
Azimilide
Bepridil (Vasocor)
Bretylium (Bretylate, Bretylol)
Budipine
Cetirizine* (Zyrtec)
Chloral hydrate
Chloroquine (Aralen)
Chlorpromazine (Largatil, Thorazine)
Cisapride‡ (Propulsid)
Citalopram (Celexa)
Clarithromycin (Biaxin)
Clemastine (Tavist)
Clofilium
Clomipramine (Anafranil)
Co-trimoxazole (Bactrim, Septra, SMX-TMP)
Desipramine (Norpramin)
Diphenhydramine (Benadryl)
Disopyramide (Norpace)
Dofetilide (Tikosyn)
Doxepin (Sinequan, Zonalon)
Droperidol (Inapsine)
Ebastine (Ebastel)
Erythrocin (Erythrostatin, Ilotycin, PCE, Staticin)
Erythromycin (Akne-Mycin, EES, E-Mycin, EryDerm, Erygel, Ery-tab, Eryc, EryPed, fexofenadine* [Allegra])
Flecainide (Tambocor)
Fludrocortisone (Florinef)
Fluphenazine (Permitil, Prolixin)
Gatifloxacin
Grepafloxacin
Halofantrine (Halfan)
Haloperidol (Haldol)
Hydroxyzine (Atarax, Atazine, Dovaril, Hypam, Vistacot, Vistaril, Vistawin)
Ibutilide (Corvert)
Imidazole (Lotrimin)
Imipramine (Tofranil)
Indapamide (Lozol)
Ipecac
Itraconazole (Sporanox)
Ketanserin (Aseranox, Ketensin, Perketan, Serepress, Sufrexal)
Ketoconazole (Nizoral)
Lipoflazine
Lithium
Loratadine* (Claritin)
Maprotiline (Ludiomil)
Mefloquine (Larium)
Mesoridazine (Serentil)
Milrinone (Primacor)
Mizolastine* (Mistamine)
Moricizine (Ethmozine)
N-acetyl-procainamide
Nortriptyline (Pamelor)
Papaverine, intracoronary
Pentamidine (NebuPent, Pentacarinat, Pentam)
Pericycline
Perphenazine (Trilafon)
Phenothiazines (Chlorpromazine, Compazine, Mellaril, Permitil, Prolixin, Serentil, Stelazine, Thorazine, Trilafon, Vesprin)
Pimozide (Orap)
Prenylamine† (Prenylamine)
Probucol (Lorelco)
Procainamide (Procan, Procanbid, Pronestyl)
Prochlorperazine (Compazine)
Propafenone (Rythmol)
Protriptyline (Vivacil)
Quetiapine (Seroquel)
Quinidine (Cardioquin, Duraquin, Quinaglute, Quinidex)
Quinine
Risperidone (Risperdal)
Sematilide
Sertindole† (Serdolect)
Sotalol (Betapace)
d,l-Sotalol, d-sotalol
Sparfloxacin
Spiramycin
Sultopride (Cloridrato)
Tamoxifen (Nolvadex)
Terfenadine‡ (Seldane)
Terodiline†
Thioridazine (Mellaril)
Thiothixene (Navane)
Timiperone
Trifluoperazine (Stelazine)
Trimethoprim sulfamethoxazole (Bactrim, Septra)
Troleandomycin (Tao)
Vasopressin (Pitressin)
Zimeldine (Zelmid)

Data from Vincent GM: Ventricular arrhythmias. Long QT syndrome, *Cardiol Clin* 18:309-325, 2000; Viskin S: Torsades de pointes, *Curr Treatment Options Cardiovasc Med* 1:187-195, 1999; Yap YG, Camm J: Risk of torsades de pointes with non-cardiac drugs, *BMJ* 320:1158-1159, 2000.
*New nonsedating antihistamine; effect on I_{Kr} needs confirmation.
†Off the market.
‡Off the market in some countries.

Multiple ectopic beats with their associated short-long-short sequences add to the ventricular milieu necessary to trigger TdP by creating differing action potential durations (repolarizations times) between cell layers and cell types.

Cardiac M Cells

The M cells constitute a layer of myocardium between the epicardium and endocardium in which the action potential duration is normally longer than that of more superficial cells. Weaker potassium currents in the M cells cause them to be more profoundly affected by bradycardia and drugs that prolong repolarization than the other myocardial layers. For this reason, the M cells may contribute to the arrhythmogenic environment required to initiate and sustain the reentry mechanism of TdP. The M cells have also been shown in experimental studies to be the last to repolarize, an event that is reflected by the end of the T wave, in which the abnormal U wave preceding TdP appears. The T wave alternans (alternating T wave amplitude or shape) that is sometimes seen as a warning sign of impending TdP is the result of side-by-side alternations in action potential durations within the layer of M cells.[12,13]

TdP IN WOMEN

The duration of the QT interval is affected by a number of factors, including gender. The longer QTc interval in women makes them more vulnerable than men to the effects of drugs that prolong ventricular repolarization (Box 26-1), accounting for as much as 70% of the occurrence of TdP.

Drici et al[14] observed a female predominance in Food and Drug Administration reports of erythromycin-associated cardiac arrhythmias. This greater propensity in women toward drug-induced TdP is also demonstrated by the fact that quinidine causes greater QT prolongation in women than in men at equivalent serum concentrations,[15] as does d,l-sotalol.[16]

Mechanisms

A gender difference in the duration of the QT interval is seen during adolescence when the QTc interval shortens in males, especially during bradycardia. Even in some forms of congenital LQTS (see Chapter 25) men exhibit shorter QTc intervals than both women and children.[17,18] Sex hormones have been implicated as possible mediators in this gender disparity,[19] although one study found that estrogen is not a factor because the prolongation of repolarization in women taking d,l-sotalol was independent of age, extending from pre- to postmenopause.[20]

Another possible reason for the longer QT interval in women and the difference in vulnerability to TdP may be that Purkinje fibers in women tend to have longer ventricular repolarization times.[21]

The variability of ventricular recovery time may also be a factor. Although women have longer QT intervals than men, they have less variability of ventricular recovery, possibly contributing to their increased risk of drug-induced TdP.[22]

CAUSES

The drugs that prolong the QT interval or induce TdP include antiarrhythmics, such as quinidine; nonsedating antihistamines, such as terfenadine (Seldane); and antipsychotic drugs, such as chlorpromazine (Thorazine, Largatil). Box 26-1 is an alphabetic list of cardiac and noncardiac drugs capable of causing QT prolongation and TdP. Some drugs that cause QT prolongation are more likely to do so when coadministered with other QT-prolonging drugs or metabolic inhibitors. Others cause TdP on their own, such as the class IA and class III antiarrhythmics. Conditions that may prolong the QT interval are listed in Box 26-2.

BOX 26-2. Conditions That May Prolong the QT Interval

Bradycardia
Cardiac hypertrophy
Cirrhosis
Congestive cardiac failure
Diabetes mellitus
Female gender
Hyperaldosteronism
Hyperparathyroidism
Hypocalcemia
Hypokalemia
Hypomagnesemia
Hypothyroidism
Intracranial trauma
Liquid protein diets
Liver diseases
Mitral valve prolapse
Myocardial ischemia
Myocarditis
Pheochromocytoma
Renal diseases
Right neck dissection or hematoma
Stroke
Subarachnoid hemorrhage
Thalamic hematoma

PUBLIC HEALTH RISK WITH NONCARDIAC DRUGS

The mechanism for QT prolongation of certain noncardiac drugs is the same as that of some of the antiarrhythmic drugs; they block the rapid component of the delayed rectifier potassium channel[23] and other positive outward currents. A significant public health risk continues to develop as more noncardiac drugs with QT prolonging effects become available. Many physicians are unaware of this expanding list and the dangerous potential to cause TdP. For example, tricyclic antidepressants are associated with a significant clinical risk of arrhythmia and death because of prolonged QT interval and TdP, especially because of overdose and in patients with pre-existing heart disease. Research is investigating the possibility that QTc prolongation associated with tricyclic antidepressants or other antipsychotic drugs may be mitigated by modulating serum potassium concentrations.[24]

SYMPTOMS

Often the patient is not aware of palpitations, but if the attack is prolonged, there are episodes of dizziness, syncope, and rarely, sudden death, probably from a deterioration of TdP into ventricular fibrillation. When syncope is the presenting symptom, patients are sometimes misdiagnosed as epileptic. Before we were aware of the mechanism and electrocardiogram (ECG) identification of TdP, the term *quinidine syncope* was used to describe these symptoms.[25]

Possible outcomes include the following:

1. Slowing and then spontaneous conversion
2. Conversion and then a new attack
3. Ventricular standstill
4. Ventricular fibrillation

CYTOCHROME P-450 3A4 INHIBITORS

The cytochrome P-450 system is a group of enzymes, found mainly in the liver and small bowel mucosa, that controls the concentrations of many endogenous substances and drugs by a number of metabolic processes. Because of its dual locations, inhibition of cytochrome P-450 3A4 (CYP 3A4) exerts its effect both before the drug enters the system (at the level of the small bowel mucosa) and during its metabolism in the liver. Clinically important CYP 3A4 inhibitors are listed in Box 26-3.

BOX 26-3. Cytochrome P-450 3A4 Inhibitors

Clarithromycin (Biaxin)
Cyclosporine (Neoral)
Danazol (Danocrine)
Delavirdine (Rescriptor)
Diltiazem (Cardizem)
Erythromycin (E-Mycin)
Ethinyl Estradiol
Fluconazole (Diflucan; weak inhibitor)
Fluvoxamine (Luvox)
Grapefruit and grapefruit juice* (active only in the small bowel mucosa)
Imidazole (Lotrimin)
Indinavir (Crixivan)
Isoniazid (INH)
Itraconazole (Sporanox)
Ketoconazole (Nizoral)
Methylprednisone
Metronidazole (Flagyl)
Mibefradil (Posicor)
Miconazole (Monistat)
Nefazodone (Serzone)
Nelfinavir (Viracept)
Nicardipine (Cardene)
Norethindrone
Norfloxacin (Norflex)
Oxiconazole (Oxistat)
Prednisone (Deltasone, Liquid Pred, Metocorten, Orasone, Panasol, Prednicen-M)
Quinine
Red wine†
Ritonavir (Norvir)
Saquinavir (Invirase)
Troleandomycin (TAO)
Verapamil (Calan)
Zafirlukast (Accolate)

*Bailey DG, Dresser GK, Kreeft JH et al: Grapefruit-felodipine interaction: effect of unprocessed fruit and probable active ingredients, *Clin Pharmacol Ther* 68:468-477, 2000.

†Chan WK, Delucchi AB: Resveratrol, a red wine constituent, is a mechanism-based inactivator of cytochrome P450 3A4, *Life Sci* 67:3103-3112, 2000.

Clinical Impact of CYP 3A4 Inhibitors

TdP can occur when CYP 3A4 inhibitors are coadministered with terfenadine (Seldane), astemizole (Hismanal), cisapride (Propulsid), or pimozide (Orap).

Grapefruit may cause TdP when taken with clinical doses of terfenadine.[26] Among other drugs known to be affected by grapefruit juice are calcium channel blockers[27,28]; tranquilizers[29]; the statins[30,31]; the antidepressant, sertraline (Zoloft)[32,33]; and ritodrine (Yutopar; for preterm labor).

Additionally, the metabolism of amiodarone is dramatically impaired by grapefruit, which completely inhibits the production of amiodarone's major metabolite, N-desethylamiodarone, for at least 3 days after ingestion of the fruit or its juice (processed or fresh).[34,35] The effects of grapefruit juice on amiodarone are reflected on the ECG by a decrease in PR and QTc intervals.[36]

PRECAUTIONS

Camm et al[12] have published measures to prevent the adverse effects of QT-prolonging drugs in clinical practice:

- Do not exceed the recommended dose
- Restrict the dose in patients with risk factors such as organic heart disease, particularly congestive heart failure, metabolic abnormalities (hypokalemia and hypomagnesemia), bradycardia, and female gender
- Avoid concomitant administration of drugs that inhibit drug metabolism or excretion, prolong the QT, or produce hypokalemia
- Check potassium level regularly when the patient is taking potassium-wasting diuretics
- If the patient develops TdP, stop the offending drug and correct electrolyte abnormalities
- When prescribing a QT-prolonging drug, warn the patient of the problems associated with its use
- Provide a card listing risk factors, including other drugs that prolong the QT interval
- Provide the patient with precautions and contraindications for coprescriptions

EMERGENCY RESPONSE

TdP that degenerates into ventricular fibrillation requires immediate direct current shock, using the "unsynchronized" mode, for termination. In the synchronized mode normally used for cardioversion the cardioverter may not recognize the QRS complexes and fail to fire. Otherwise, the following measures are taken for the emergency treatment of TdP[37,38]:

1. Continuous ECG monitoring. The presence of a long QT interval or U wave in the basic rhythm is documented.
2. All agents or conditions that may be potentially responsible for TdP and QT prolongation are immediately discontinued or corrected (Boxes 26-1 and 26-2).
3. When the QT is prolonged for any reason, intravenous (IV) potassium is given by slow infusion to raise the level to high normal (>4.5 mEq/L).[39] When extracellular potassium is increased so is the efflux of potassium ions from the cells, accelerating repolarization and shortening the QT interval.[40]
4. Prompt suppression of TdP in acquired and congenital LQTS[41] can be achieved with IV injection of magnesium (which is suggested even in normomagnesemia)[42] and potassium supplements. Tzivoni et al[43] were the first to demonstrate the lifesaving effects of magnesium in cases of TdP. Magnesium is contraindicated when there is renal failure; loss of deep tendon reflex; a serum magnesium level above 5 mEq/L; a drop in systolic blood pressure below 80 mm of mercury; or a heart rate below 60 beats/min.
5. If IV magnesium is unsuccessful, overdrive ventricular pacing or isoproterenol may be necessary as a means to increase the basic heart rate and thus shorten the QT interval. Temporary rapid ventricular pacing suppresses the VT and may be lifesaving.[44] Additionally, the TdP may remain abated after pacing is discontinued.[45] Isoproterenol is contraindicated in patients with TdP because of congenital LQTS and VT that is not pause-dependent, including polymorphic VT in the setting of coronary ischemia,[46] and the rarely seen catecholamine-sensitive idiopathic polymorphic VT.[47]
6. Alleviate fear and stress, recognized triggers for both congenital and acquired TdP.[48,49]
7. Direct current cardioversion is usually transiently effective in terminating TdP. When the arrhythmia is caused by high doses of class IA agents, repeated cardioversions may be necessary.

The class IA (quinidine, procainamide, and disopyramide) drug-induced TdP usually appears soon after the initial administration of the drug, while the patient is still in the hospital. In this setting the problem is recognized early, and treatment is straightforward.

POLYMORPHIC VT WITHOUT QT PROLONGATION

Most of the patients with polymorphic VT without QT prolongation have coronary artery disease. Akhtar[50] described two subgroups, one associated with chronic coronary artery disease and the other with acute myocardial ischemia caused by critical coronary artery stenosis.

Fig. 26-7 shows a polymorphic VT without QT prolongation with stable coronary artery disease and prior myocardial damage but with no evidence of acute ischemia. Treatment options are similar to those for sustained monomorphic VT in association with chronic coronary artery disease.[50]

Fig. 26-8 shows a polymorphic VT in a patient and acute ischemia caused by an occluding bypass graft. This type of VT is often, but not always, accompanied or preceded by angina or ischemic ECG changes, and it responds well to beta blockers and myocardial revascularization.

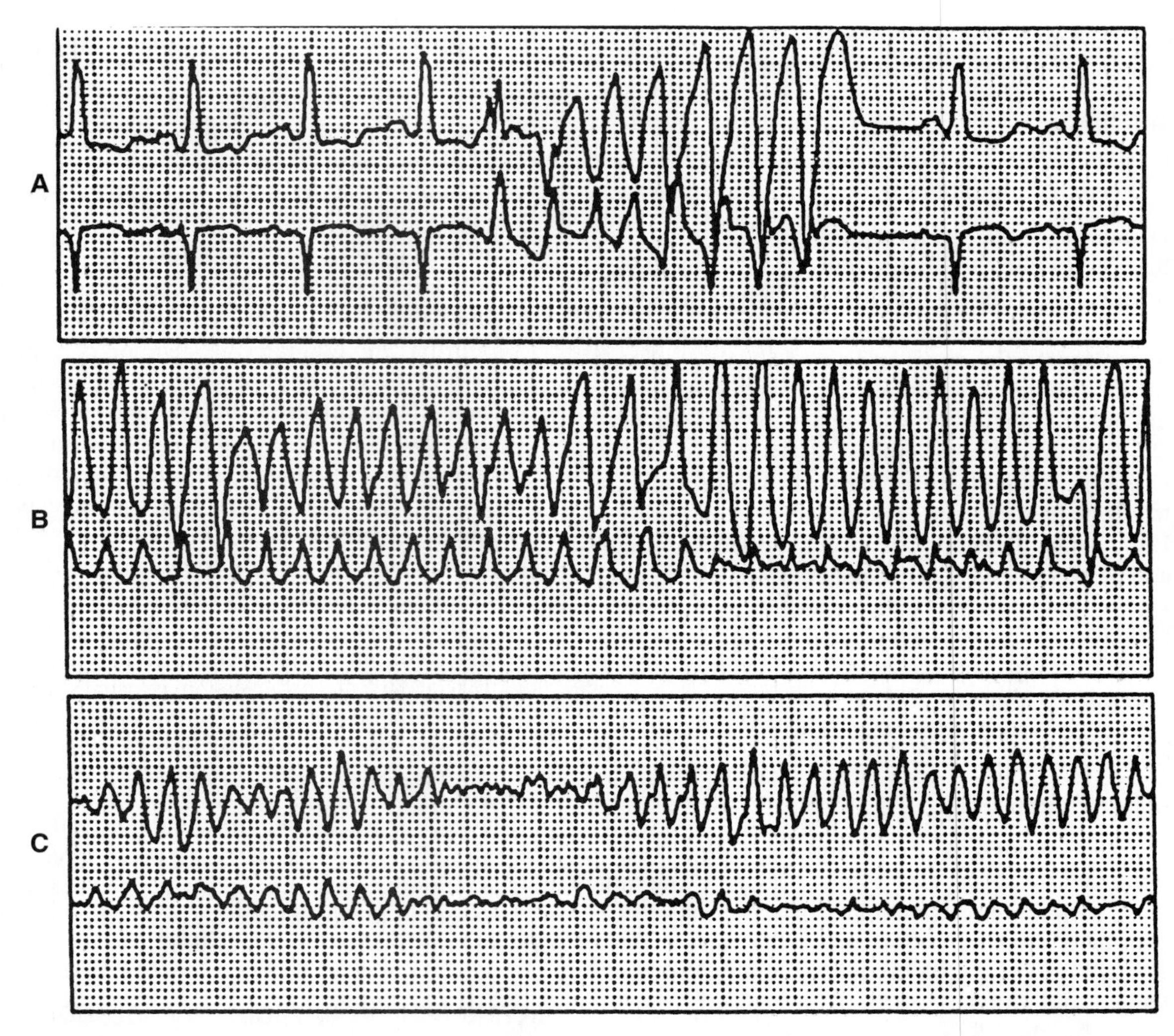

FIG. 26-7. Polymorphic ventricular tachycardia with a normal QT interval in a patient with chronic coronary artery disease. **A**, Spontaneous episode of polymorphic ventricular tachycardia. **B**, Sustained episode leading to ventricular fibrillation. **C**, Patient had coronary artery disease but continued to have such episodes after myocardial revascularization and beta blockade. Class I agents readily controlled this arrhythmia. (From Akhtar M: *Circulation* 82:1561, 1990.)

SUMMARY

Acquired TdP is a distinctive life-threatening paroxysmal polymorphic VT that, in most cases, occurs against a background of prolonged QT intervals, ventricular ectopic beats, and pauses. It may be caused by QT prolonging drugs, heart block, or electrolyte imbalance. When the QT interval reaches a critical duration oscillations appear during the plateau or beginning of phase 3 of the action potential. The oscillations are called early afterdepolarizations to distinguish them from the delayed afterdepolarizations that appear during digitalis toxicity. The pause that follows a PVC may further prolong the QT interval and cause the early afterdepolarization to reach threshold potential for the slow calcium channels, triggering the onset of TdP. Emergency treatment consists of discontinuing the offensive drug(s), and giving IV magnesium and potassium.

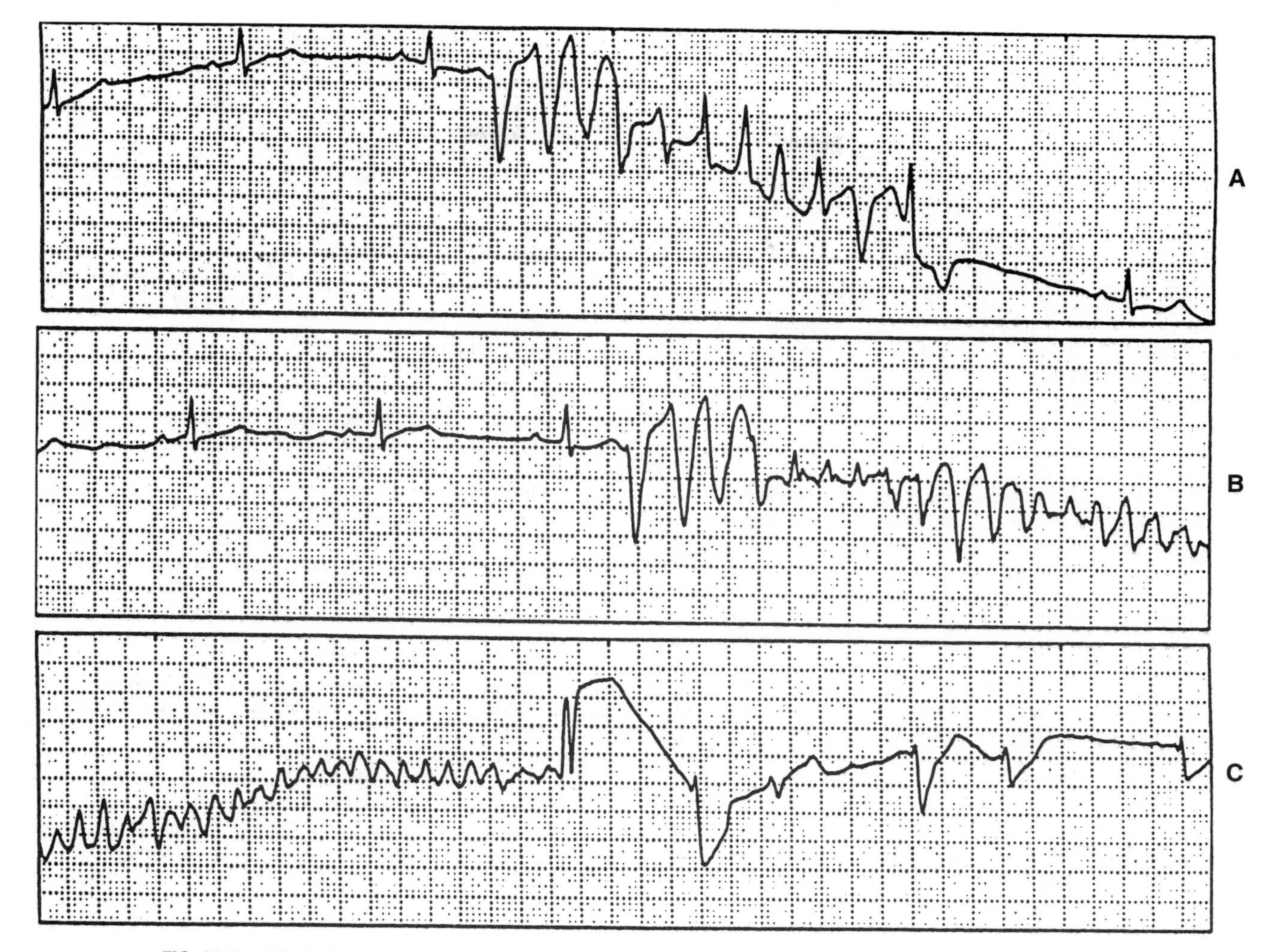

FIG. 26-8. Polymorphic ventricular tachycardia with a normal QT interval in a patient with acute myocardial ischemia. **A**, Nonsustained polymorphic ventricular tachycardia. **B**, Another episode that leads to rapid degeneration into ventricular fibrillation, followed by **C**, defibrillation. (From Akhtar M: *Circulation* 82:1561, 1990.)

REFERENCES

1. Ohkuchi A, Shiraishi H, Minakami H et al: Fetus with long QT syndrome manifested by tachyarrhythmia: a case report, *Prenat Diagn* 19:990-992, 1999.
2. Dessertenne F: La tachycardie ventriculaire à deux foyers opposés variables [Ventricular tachycardia with two variable opposing foci], *Arch Mal Coeur Vaiss* 59:263-272, 1966.
3. Coumel P, Leclercq JF, Dessertenne F: Torsades de pointes. In Josephson ME, Wellens HJJ, editors: *Tachycardia, mechanisms, diagnosis, treatment,* Philadelphia, 1984, Lea & Febiger.
4. Kay GN, Plumb VJ, Arciniegas JG et al: Torsades de pointes: the long-short initiating sequence and other clinical features: observations in 32 patients, *J Am Coll Cardiol* 2:806-817, 1983.
5. Roden DM, Thompson KA, Hoffman BF et al: Clinical features and basic mechanisms of quinidine-induced arrhythmias, *J Am Coll Cardiol* 8(1, Suppl A):73A, 1986.
6. Denes P, Gabster A, Huang SK: Clinical, electrocardiographic and followup observations in patients having ventricular fibrillation during Holter monitoring, *Amer J Cardiol* 48:9-16, 1981.
7. Marriott HJL: *Practical electrocardiography,* Baltimore, 1983, Williams & Wilkins.
8. Phoon CKL: Mathematic validation of a shorthand rule for calculating QT_c, *Amer J Cardiol* 82:400, 1998.
9. Volders PG, Vos MA, Szabo B et al: Progress in the understanding of cardiac early afterdepolarizations and torsades de pointes: time to revise current concepts, *Cardiovasc Res* 46:376-392, 2000.
10. Viswanathan PC, Rudy Y: Pause induced early afterdepolarizations in the long QT syndrome: a simulation study, *Cardiovasc Res* 42:530-542, 1999.
11. Singh B: Amiodarone: pharmacological, electrophysiological, and clinical profile of an unusual antiarrhythmic compound. In Singh BN, Wellens HJJ, Hiraoka M, editors: *Electropharmacological control of*

cardiac arrhythmias, Mount Kisco, NY, 1994, Futura Publishing, pp 497-522.
12. Camm AJ, Janse MJ, Roden DM et al: Congenital and acquired long QT syndrome, *Eur Heart J* 21:1232-1237, 2000.
13. Shimizu W, Antzelevitch C: Cellular and ionic basis for T-wave alternans under long-QT conditions, *Circulation* 99:1499-1507, 1999.
14. Drici MD, Knollmann BC, Wang WX et al: Cardiac actions of erythromycin. Influence of female sex, *JAMA* 280:1774-1776, 1998.
15. Benton RE, Sale M, Flockhart DA et al: Greater quinidine-induced QTc interval prolongation in women, *Clin Pharmacol Ther* 67:413-418, 2000.
16. Lehmann MH, Hardy S, Archibald D et al: JTc prolongation with d, l-sotalol in women versus men, *Am J Cardiol* 83:354-359, 1999.
17. Lehmann MH, Timothy KW, Frankovich D et al: Age-gender influence on the rate-corrected QT interval and the QT-heart rate relation in families with genotypically characterized long QT syndrome, *J Am Coll Cardiol* 29:93-99, 1997.
18. Pearl W: Effects of gender, age and heart rate on QT intervals in children, *Pediatr Cardiol* 17:135-136, 1996.
19. Drici MD, Burklow TR, Vedanandam H et al: Sex hormones prolong the QT interval and downregulate potassium channel expression in the rabbit heart, *Circulation* 94:1471-1474, 1996.
20. Lehmann MH, Hardy S, Archibald D et al: Sex difference in risk of torsades de pointes with d,l-sotalol, *Circulation* 94:253-254, 1996.
21. Lu HR, Marien R, Saels A et al: Are there sex-specific differences in ventricular repolarization or in drug-induced early afterdepolarizations in isolated rabbit Purkinje fibers? *J Cardiovasc Pharmacol* 36:132-139, 2000.
22. Costeas C, Bedi AK, Tolat A et al: Effects of aging and gender on QT dispersion in an overtly healthy population, *Pacing Clin Electrophysiol* 23:1121-1126, 2000.
23. Yap YG, Camm J: Risk of torsades de pointes with non-cardiac drugs. Doctors need to be aware that many drugs can cause QT prolongation, *BMJ* 320:1158-1159, 2000.
24. Hancox JC, WitchelHJ: Psychotropic drugs [letter], HERG, and the heart, *Lancet* 356:428, 2000.
25. Selzer A, Wray HW: Quinidine syncope. Paroxysmal ventricular fibrillation occurring during treatment of atrial arrhythmias, *Circulation* 30:17-26, 1964.
26. Dresser GK, Spence JD, Bailey DG: Pharmacokinetic-pharmacodynamic consequences and clinical relevance of cytochrome P450 3A4 inhibition, *Clin Pharmacokinet* 38:41-57, 2000.
27. Dresser GK, Bailey DG, Carruthers SG: Grapefruit juice–felodipine interaction in the elderly, *Clin Pharmacol Ther* 68:28-34, 2000.
28. Takanaga H, Ohnishi A, Matsuo H et al: Pharmacokinetic analysis of felodipine-grapefruit juice interaction based on an irreversible enzyme inhibition model, *Br J Clin Pharmacol* 49:49-58, 2000.
29. Lilja JJ, Kivisto KT, Backman JT et al: Effect of grapefruit juice dose on grapefruit juice-triazolam interaction: repeated consumption prolongs triazolam half-life, *Eur J Clin Pharmacol* 56:411-415, 2000.
30. Lilja JJ, Kivisto KT, Neuvonen PJ: Duration of effect of grapefruit juice on the pharmacokinetics of the CYP3A4 substrate simvastatin, *Clin Pharmacol Ther* 68:384-390, 2000.
31. Kantola T, Kivisto KT, Neuvonen PJ: Grapefruit juice greatly increases serum concentrations of lovastatin and lovastatin acid, *Clin Pharmacol Ther* 63:397-402, 1998.
32. Lee AJ, Chan WK, Harralson AF et al: The effects of grapefruit juice on sertraline metabolism: an in vitro and in vivo study, *Clin Ther* 21:1890-1899, 1999.
33. Kivisto KT, Lilja JJ, Backman JT et al: Repeated consumption of grapefruit juice considerably increases plasma concentrations of cisapride, *Clin Pharmacol Ther* 66:448-453, 1999.
34. Bailey DG, Dresser GK, Kreeft JH et al: Grapefruit-felodipine interaction: effect of unprocessed fruit and probable active ingredients, *Clin Pharmacol Ther* 68:468-477, 2000.
35. Takanaga H, Ohnishi A, Murakami H et al: Relationship between time after intake of grapefruit juice and the effect on pharmacokinetics and pharmacodynamics of nisoldipine in healthy subjects, *Clin Pharmacol Ther* 67:201-214, 2000.
36. Libersa CC, Brique SA, Motte KB et al: Dramatic inhibition of amiodarone metabolism induced by grapefruit juice, *Br J Clin Pharmacol* 49:373-378, 2000.
37. Haverkamp W, Shenasa M, Borggrefe M et al: Torsade de pointes. In Zipes DP, Jalife J, editors: *Cardiac electrophysiology from cell to bedside,* ed 2, Philadelphia, 1995, WB Saunders.
38. Wellens HJJ, Conover M: *The ECG in emergency decision making,* Philadelphia, 1992, WB Saunders.
39. Choy A, Lang C, Chomsky D et al: Normalization of acquired QT prolongation in humans by intravenous potassium, *Circulation* 97:2149-2154, 1997.
40. Yang T, Roden D: Extracellular potassium modulation of drug block of IK_r: implications for torsades de pointes and reverse use-dependence, *Circulation* 93:407-411, 1996.
41. Igawa O, Fujimoto Y, Kotake H et al: Treatment of torsade de pointes with intravenous magnesium in idiopathic long QT syndrome, *Jpn Circ J* 55:1057, 1991.
42. Iseri LT, Chung P, Tobis J: Magnesium therapy for intractable ventricular tachyarrhythmias in normomagnesemic patients, *West J Med* 138:823, 1983.
43. Tzivoni D, Banai S, Schuger C et al: Treatment of torsades de pointes with magnesium sulfate, *Circulation* 77:1395-1402, 1988.
44. Viskin S: Torsades de pointes, *Curr Treat Options Cardiovasc Med* 1:187-195, 1999.
45. Jackman WM, Friday KJ, Anderson JL et al: The long QT syndromes: a critical review, new clinical observations and a unifying hypothesis, *Prog Cardiovasc Dis* 31:115, 1988.
46. Wolfe CL, Nibbley C, Bhandari A et al: Polymorphous ventricular tachycardia associated with acute myocardial infarction, *Circulation* 84:1543-1551, 1991.
47. Leenhardt A, Lucent V, Denjoy I et al: Catecholaminergic polymorphic ventricular tachycardia in children. A 7-year follow-up of 21 patients. *Circulation* 91:1512-1519, 1995.
48. Schwartz PJ, Periti M, Malliani A: The long Q-T syndrome, *Am Heart J* 89:378-390, 1975.
49. Locati EH, Maison-Blanche P, Dejode P et al: Spontaneous sequences of onset of torsades de pointes in patients with acquired prolonged repolarization: quantitative analysis of Holter recordings, *J Am Coll Cardiol* 25:1564-1575, 1995.
50. Akhtar M: The clinical spectrum of ventricular tachycardia, *Circulation* 82:1561, 1990.

CHAPTER 27

Brugada Syndrome

In 1992[1] Brugada and Brugada described eight patients without structural heart disease, including three children, who had a history of aborted sudden cardiac death resulting from ventricular fibrillation (VF), right bundle branch block (RBBB), and a unique type of ST segment elevation in the right precordial leads (V_1 to V_3). Recognition of this electrocardiographic (ECG) pattern is important because it permits early identification and treatment of those at risk for sudden death.

ECG DIAGNOSIS

Figs. 27-1 and 27-2 are examples of Brugada syndrome during sinus rhythm. The following ECG signs of overt Brugada syndrome are limited to the right precordial leads V_1, V_2, and V_3:

- Exaggerated J wave
- Elevated J wave/ST segment dips (saddleback shape) into a positive T wave in least vulnerable of individuals, or into a negative T wave in the most vulnerable of individuals
- RBBB-like ECG pattern, possibly the combination of the J wave and the elevated to rapidly downsloping ST segment[2]
- Increase in the frequency of closely coupled premature ventricular complexes (PVCs) preceding the onset of ventricular tachycardia (VT)/VF[3]
- Left axis deviation is occasionally present[4]

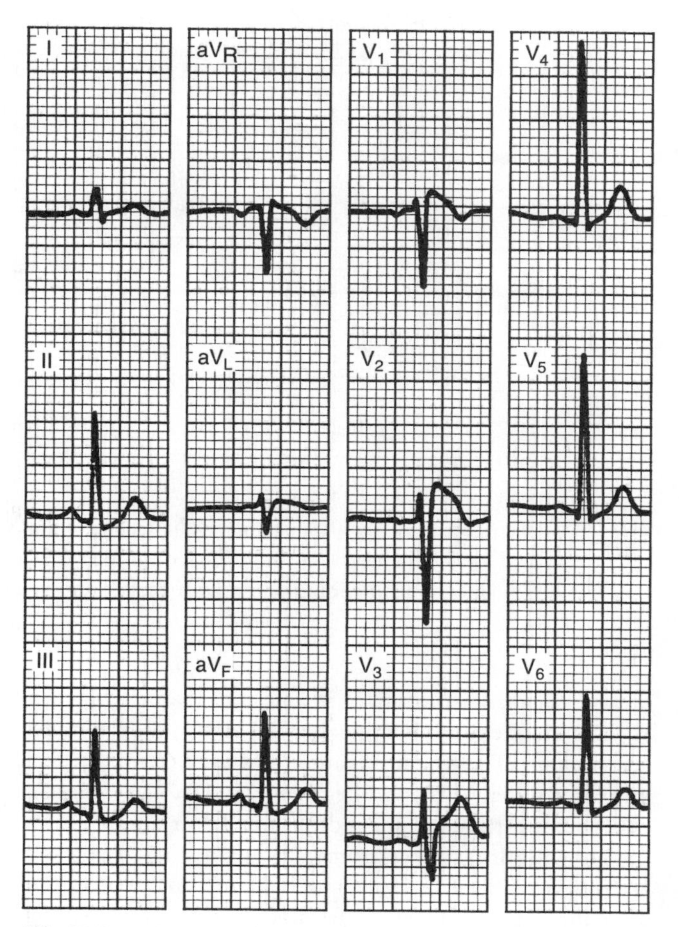

FIG. 27-1. Brugada syndrome in a 39-year-old patient. Note the typical coved ST segment elevation in V_1 and V_2. This patient previously experienced two unexplained episodes of syncope. (From Hermida JS, Lemoine JL, Aoun FB et al: Prevalence of the Brugada syndrome in an apparently healthy population, *Am J Cardiol* 86:91-94, 2000.)

Unmasking Concealed and Intermittent Forms

In cases of overt Brugada syndrome, the diagnosis is apparent to the informed observer. However, the concealed and intermittent forms are often not diagnosed, increasing the risk of sudden death.[5]

When the ECG signs of Brugada syndrome are not

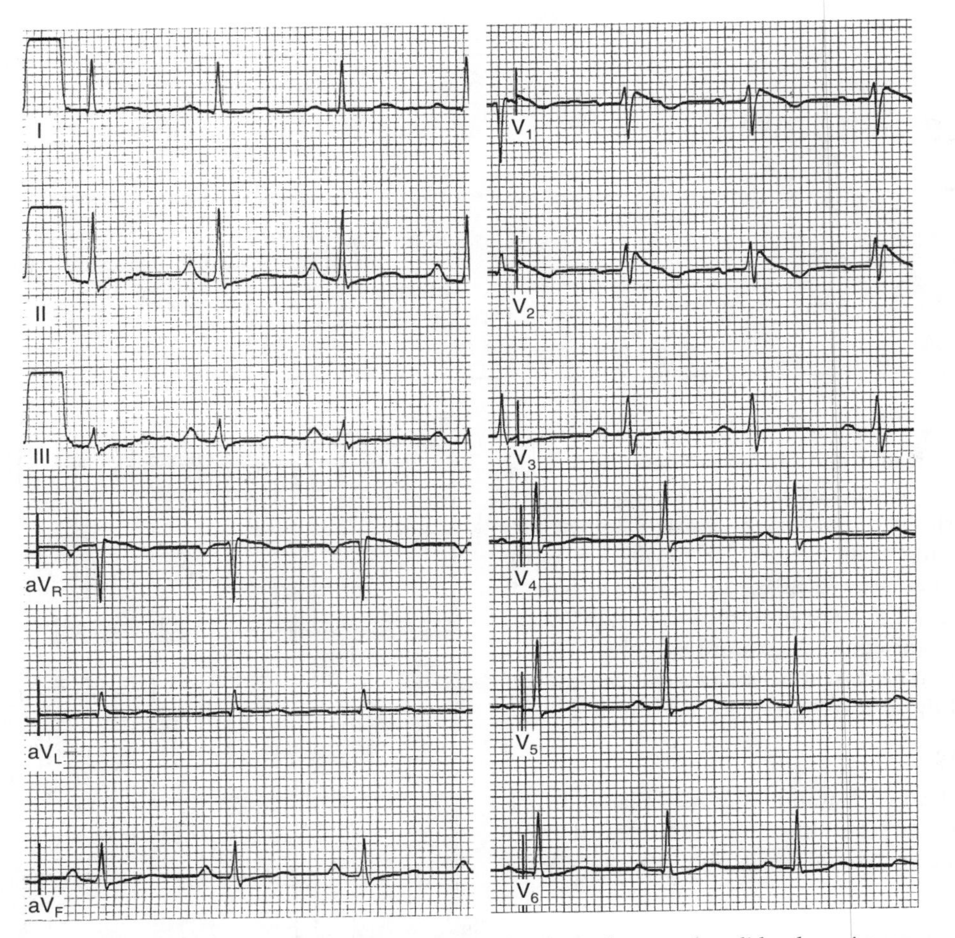

FIG. 27-2. Brugada syndrome. Note in leads V_1 and V_2 the elevated J wave that slides down into a negative T wave. The ECG is from a 37-year-old man who was admitted to the emergency department with complaints of palpitations and presyncope. (Courtesy Ara M. Tilkian, MD, Mission Hills, Calif.)

apparent, administration of a calcium channel blocker, such as intravenous ajmaline, flecainide, or procainamide, accentuates ST segment elevation and unmasks concealed and intermittent forms of the disease. In Fig. 27-3 Shimizu et al[6] demonstrate the effect of flecainide on the ECG of a patient with Brugada syndrome. It is interesting to note the transition of the ECG to a more threatening appearance after the administration of flecainide (a calcium channel blocker). The elevated J wave (*arrow*), saddleback ST segment, and positive T wave seen in lead V_2 of Fig. 27-3, *A*, are transformed *(B)* into a more elevated J wave and ST segment (*arrow*), and negative T wave because of the flecainide. Note in *B* that the ST segment in the second beat of the right precordial leads plunges into a negative T wave followed immediately by closely coupled PVCs. The cellular mechanism is illustrated in Fig. 27-6.

When the ECG signs are overt, beta-adrenergic stimulation (exercise, intravenous isuprel) normalizes the ECG,[7] whereas beta blockade may exaggerate the J wave.[8]

DIFFERENTIAL DIAGNOSIS

The diagnosis of Brugada syndrome is pursued after excluding the more common causes of sudden unexplained death (i.e., structural or coronary heart disease).[4] The same ECG pattern described by the Brugada brothers is seen in patients with arrhythmogenic right ventricular (RV) cardiomyopathy or dysplasia, acute RV ischemia, infiltrative cardiomyopathy, tricyclic drug overdose,[9-11] anteroseptal myocardial infarction,[12] Chagas disease (a tropical disease), myotonic dystrophy (Steinert disease),[13] and mediastinal tumors.[14]

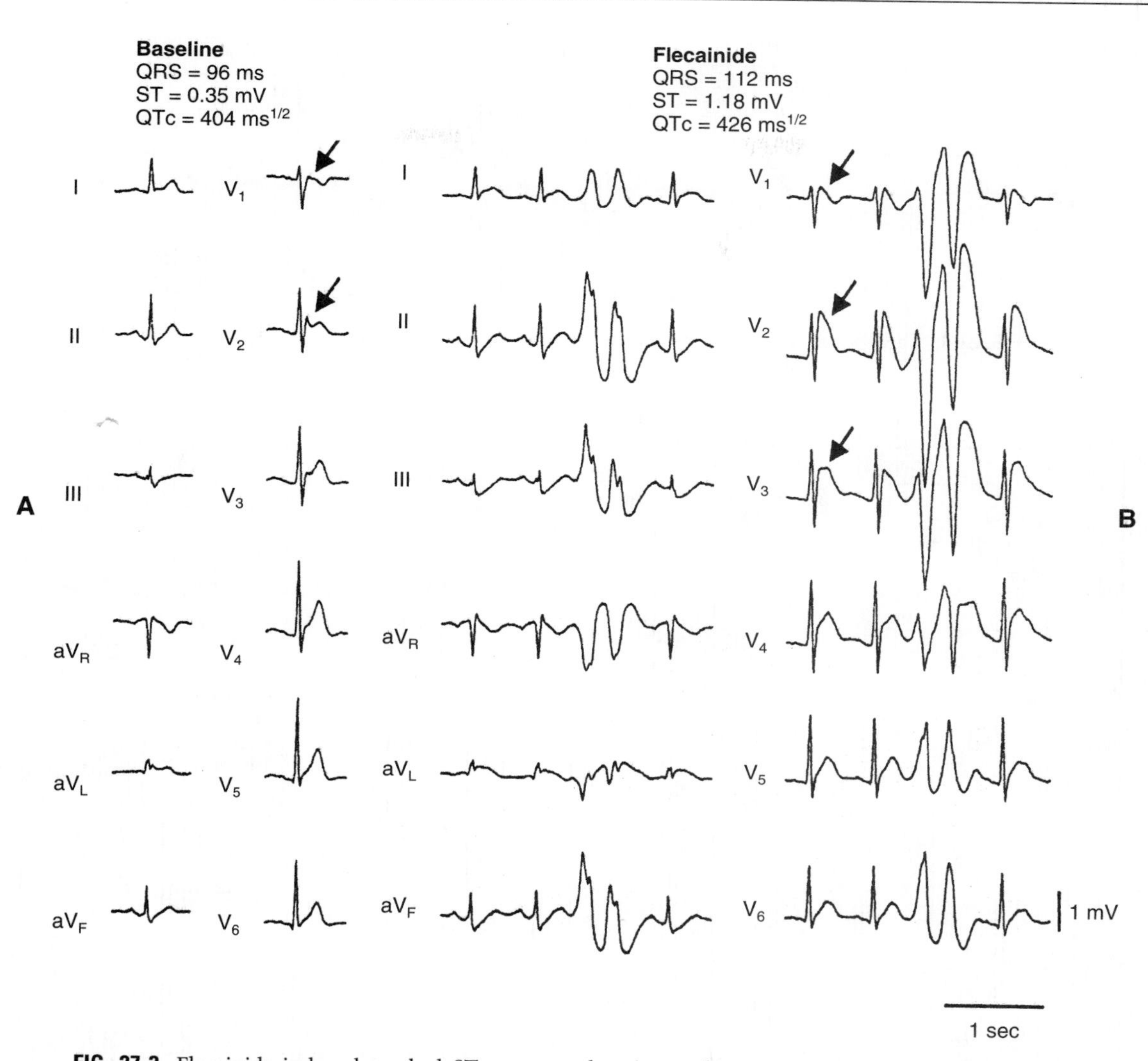

FIG. 27-3. Flecainide-induced marked ST segment elevation and premature ventricular complexes in a patient with Brugada syndrome. Coved and saddleback-type ST segment elevation (0.35 mV) was seen in leads V_1 and V_2; the QRS duration was normal under baseline conditions (**A**, *arrows*). Flecainide-induced ventricular couplets followed marked ST segment elevation (1.18 mV) without a major increase in QRS duration (112 ms) (**B**, *arrows*). The premature ventricular complexes displayed a left bundle branch block–like pattern with normal axis, suggesting a right ventricular outflow tract focus. (From Shimizu W, Antzelevitch C, Suyama K et al: Effect of sodium channel blockers on ST segment, QRS duration, and corrected QT interval in patients with Brugada syndrome, *J Cardiovasc Electrophysiol* 11[12]:1320-1329, 2000.)

MECHANISMS

The ECG signs of Brugada syndrome are seen in the right chest leads V_1 to V_3 because of the predominance of transient outward current in the right ventricular epicardium.[15]

The J point and J wave: The J point is the precise place at which the QRS and the ST segment meet (Fig. 27-4). When the J point is elevated it is called a *J wave*, also known as the *Osborn wave*.[16] It is a diagnostic sign in hypothermia and hypercalcemia. Fig. 27-5, *A* and *B*, are examples of the ECG seen in hypothermia. An elevation of the J point occurs when there is a difference in electrical potential between the ven-

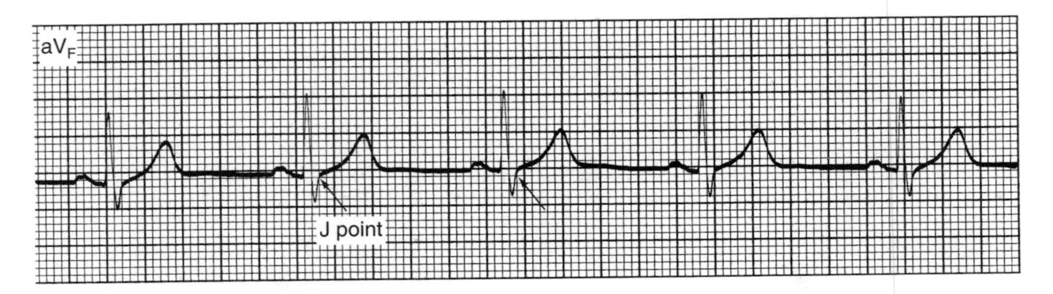

FIG. 27-4. The J point *(arrows)* is the spot where the QRS ends and the ST segment begins.

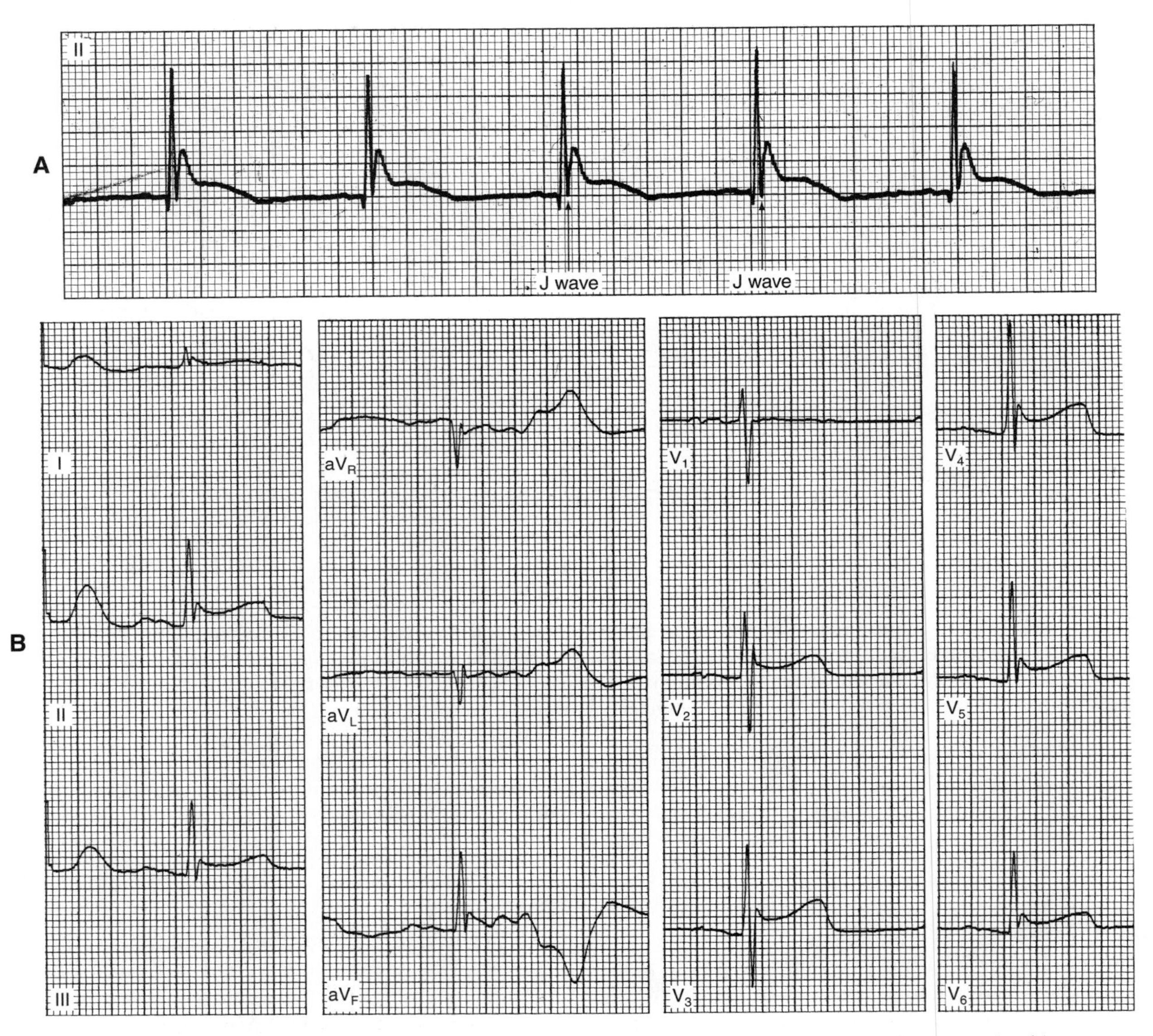

FIG. 27-5. The J wave of hypothermia. **A**, Note the J wave *(arrows)* and elevated ST segment in this hypothermic patient. **B**, J waves are seen in leads V_2 through V_6 in a hypothermic patient in Hawaii with a core temperature of 87.1° F. The hypothermia was secondary to hypothyroidism and hypoadrenalism associated with a hypothalamic cyst. (Courtesy M. Miller, RN, Oahu, Hawaii.)

tricular epicardium and endocardium, causing a current to flow between the two at the completion of the QRS complex.

Cellular Electrophysiology

In Fig. 27-6, Antzelevitch[2] schematically illustrates the cellular mechanisms thought to occur in the myocardium of patients with Brugada syndrome, providing a comparison with the normal and the early repolarization syndrome along with the resultant ECGs as seen in V_2.

Normal. In Fig. 27-6, *A*, the normal simultaneous action potentials from the three ventricular myocardial layers (epicardium, endocardium, and M layer between them) have slightly differing times of onset and termination, although there is no voltage gradient between them during the plateau (phase 2) of the action potential, thus an isoelectric ST segment and no J wave (the action potential is described on pp. 9-10). The epicardium normally repolarizes first, followed by the endocardium and M layer. Note that during the final phase of repolarization (phase 3) there is normally a voltage gradient, causing a current to flow. It is this normally occurring current that creates the positive T wave.

Early repolarization syndrome. In Fig. 27-6, *B*, which is an illustration of the cellular mechanism of the early repolarization syndrome, there is a distinct difference in the shapes of the two action potentials. The epicardial cells develop a sharp spike and dome not seen in the endocardium. The resultant small voltage gradient at the end of the depolarization process (phase 0) and beginning of repolarization (phase 1) causes a current to flow between the two myocardial layers. This is reflected in a small J wave, perceived as an ST segment elevation.

Bianco and colleagues[17] compared the ECGs of 155 male athletes to 50 sedentary men. They concluded from their study that early repolarization is almost always the rule in athletes. The ECG in early repolarization syndrome is, however, significantly different from that of Brugada syndrome. In athletes, the maximum ST elevation is not as high nor is the QRS duration as long as in patients with

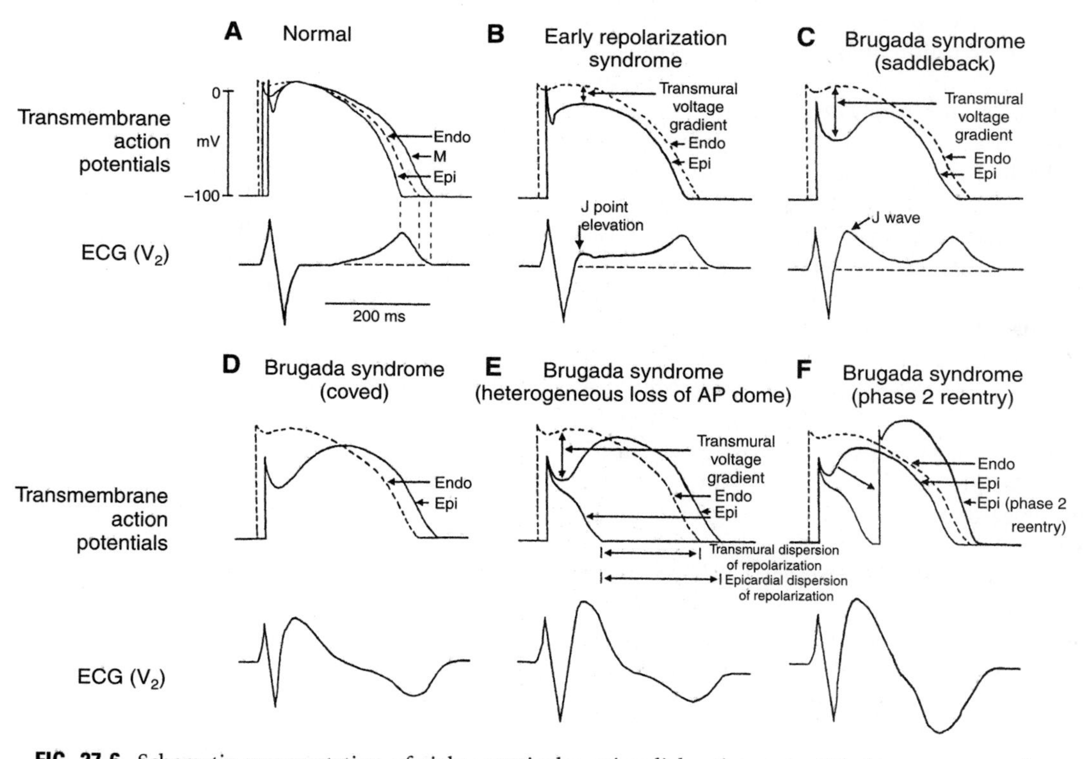

FIG. 27-6. Schematic representation of right ventricular epicardial action potential changes proposed to underlie the ECG manifestation of early repolarization syndrome (**B**) and Brugada syndrome (**C-F**). The normal is shown for comparison (**A**). Note in Brugada syndrome (**C-F**), as the difference between the endocardial *(Endo)* and epicardial *(Epi)* action potentials becomes progressively more marked, the J wave in the ECG becomes progressively higher. Please see text for explanation. (From Antzelevitch C: The Brugada syndrome: ionic basis and arrhythmia mechanisms, *J Cardiovasc Electrophysiol* 12:268-272, 2001.)

Brugada syndrome. This fact can be appreciated when comparing Fig. 27-6, *B* and *C*.

Brugada syndrome with a saddleback ST segment. When the disturbance of current flow is more profound due to mutation of a gene controlling Na^+ channels (Brugada syndrome), as in Fig. 27-6, *C*, the amplitude of phase 0 is lower resulting in a slowing of conduction velocity and accentuation of the action potential notch in epicardium, creating a marked voltage gradient in RV cells. The resultant current flow produces a tall J wave in right precordial leads. The repolarization sequence is still in its proper order with the epicardium repolarizing before the endocardium, reflected in a positive T wave and a "saddleback" look to the ST segment.

Brugada syndrome with a coved ST segment. The difference between the two voltages of RV epicardium and endocardium during phase 1 of the action potential is quite marked in Fig. 27-6, *D*, causing a current flow that is reflected in the large J wave deflection in right precordial leads. Additionally, the repolarization sequence is no longer in its proper order. The time it takes for the epicardium to repolarize now exceeds that of the endocardium, causing a reversal in the direction of current flow during phase 3 of the action potential. This is reflected on the ECG by a slightly coved ST segment and a negative T wave. The tall J wave and steeply downsloping ST segment into a negative T wave, typical of Brugada syndrome, may account for the RBBB appearance on the ECG, because, according to Brugada et al,[18] RBBB may be absent.

Brugada syndrome with loss of the action potential dome in some epicardial cells and not in others. In Fig. 27-6, *E*, there are two epicardial action potentials, one with and one without its dome. This situation represents relatively large differences in repolarization times within the epicardial layer and presents a window of opportunity for extra beats to be generated. When there is a difference in electrical potential between adjacent areas of the heart, a current will flow, thus the potential for an extra beat. Note that some areas of the epicardium are excitable (the brief action potential) whereas others are still refractory.

Brugada syndrome with phase 2 reentry. In Fig. 27-6, *F*, the scene is set for the generation of a very early PVC. Note that it is now possible for current to flow during phase 2 of the action potential from areas of the RV epicardium that still have an action potential with a spike and dome configuration to adjacent epicardial areas that have lost their dome and have therefore repolarized very early. Current flow during phase 2 of one epicardial cell to adjacent excitable epicardial tissue is represented by an arrow. The J wave is tall and a steeply falling ST segment dives into a negative T-QS combination that heralds the onset of VT/VF.

Phase 2 reentry. The distressing cellular milieu represented in Fig. 27-6, *F*, is capable of initiating and supporting a reentrant VT; the mechanism is called *phase 2 reentry* because it is generated from the voltage difference that exists between cells that are still negotiating phase 2 of the action potential and adjacent cells that are already repolarized and excitable. The resultant PVC that develops in the RV epicardial layer propagates to the endocardium away from the precordial leads, producing a QS complex that is simultaneous with the T wave and is therefore obscured by it. This PVC lines up with the second epicardial action potential seen in *F*.

CAUSE

As with the LQT3 syndrome discussed on p. 378, Brugada syndrome is an inherited arrhythmogenic syndrome caused by mutation of the cardiac voltage-dependent calcium channel gene, SCN5A, thus far the only gene linked to Brugada syndrome. At least 13 mutations of this gene have been identified.[19] So far, three of them have been linked to the Brugada syndrome.[20] Mutations of the SCN5A gene result in a reduction of the inward Na^+ current, possibly leaving unopposed the transient outward current (I_{to}). This current contributes to the notch of phase 1 of the action potential (J point on the ECG) and when unopposed creates a J wave.

LINK TO LQT3

Bezzina et al[21] describe a large SCN5A-linked family with ECG features of both LQT3 and Brugada syndrome, with some family members dying suddenly during the night, and suggest that both syndromes may be caused by the same mutation.

Priori et al[22] found that the typical manifestations of LQT syndrome (i.e., prolonged QT interval) and Brugada syndrome (ST segment elevation in V_1 through V_3) may coexist in a single individual, raising the question of the actual difference between the two conditions. A point in question is the use of flecainide to unmask concealed Brugada syndrome. Thirteen individuals from seven LQT3 families were given flecainide using the protocol for unmasking Brugada syndrome. Although the desired effect (QT interval shortening) occurred in all but 1 patient, the disturbing effect of ST segment elevation was observed in V_1 through V_3 in 6 of the 13 patients, demonstrating a link between LQT3 and Brugada syndrome.

INCIDENCE

The incidence of the disease is difficult to estimate, but it causes 4 to 10 sudden deaths per 10,000 inhabitants per year in areas such as Thailand and Laos. In these countries, the disease represents the most frequent cause of death in young adults. Up to 50% of the yearly sudden deaths in patients with a normal heart are caused by this syndrome.[15] Most of the reported cases of Brugada syndrome have been young men (8:1 ratio of males to females)[2] of Southeast Asian and Japanese origin, with an average age of 40 years (range, 22 to 65 years). In these geographic areas, the disease is thought to represent the most frequent cause of sudden death in young adults.

In Charlotte, North Carolina, over a 2-year period, Monroe and Littman[23] prospectively evaluated ECGs from 12,000 unselected, noncardiac patients. They found 52 patients with ECG patterns consistent with Brugada syndrome.

SYMPTOMS AND CLINICAL IMPLICATIONS

Symptoms are rarely subjective until the unexpected and tragic terminal event. Some individuals may report palpitations and syncope, prompting an ECG, or the diagnosis may be made from an ECG during a routine physical examination or because of a family history of sudden death or survival from cardiac arrest.

In Thailand, the Philippines, and Japan there are many word-of-mouth reports of young men in apparently good health thrashing with agonal respirations and then dying suddenly in their beds. Those who were resuscitated were found to have inducible polymorphic VT/VF in the electrophysiologic laboratory.[24]

Cardiac arrest because of VF is usually caused by coronary artery disease, cardiomyopathy, or other cardiac structural abnormalities.[25] However, about 10% to 20% of patients dying suddenly or resuscitated from VF do not have demonstrable heart disease; their episode is labeled "idiopathic ventricular fibrillation." Of those who survive, 40% to 60% are said to have Brugada syndrome.[26]

Of 27 Thai men studied, 16 were found to have an ECG pattern consistent with what we now know as Brugada syndrome; 11 had normal ECGs. On follow-up, the 16 men with the abnormal ECGs were found to have a greater risk of dying suddenly than those with the normal ECGs.[27]

TREATMENT

When treated with antiarrhythmic drugs such as amiodarone and beta blockers, sudden death is not prevented in those with or without symptoms; mortality is approximately 10% per year. The group IC antiarrhythmic drugs (e.g., flecainide, propafenone) have the potential to increase risk.[4]

The pivotal parameter in Brugada syndrome is a prominent I_{to}, the transient outward current that contributes to the notch of phase 1 of the ventricular action potential. Antzelevitch[2] has suggested that quinidine may be effective in blocking I_{to} and that beta-adrenergic agents (isoproterenol) and anticholinergic agents may also be efficacious. Others have reported clinical success with quinidine, but not with procainamide.[28-30]

The implantable defibrillator is the only proven effective treatment to prevent sudden death in patients with Brugada syndrome.[31] This having been said, a dilemma still exists regarding the management of young, apparently healthy individuals with an ECG suggestive of Brugada syndrome who have never manifested a symptom of the disease. In one study,[1] during follow-up of 22 such patients, 6 (27%) had VF.

SUMMARY

Brugada syndrome consists of syncopal episodes or sudden death in individuals with a structurally normal heart and a characteristic ECG. When overt, it is characterized by an exaggerated J wave that is perceived as an elevated ST segment in V_1 through V_3 and an RBBB-like ECG pattern. The disease is genetically determined with an autosomal dominant pattern of transmission resulting in the mutation of the gene, SCN5A, which forms channels for Na^+. This is the same gene mutation responsible for congenital LQT3 syndrome discussed in Chapter 12; cases of the two conditions coexisting have been reported. Three different mutations have been identified in one individual and two families afflicted with the disease.

The cellular mechanism responsible for the unique ECG pattern of Brugada syndrome is the genetically engineered reduction in the Na^+ current at the beginning of repolarization, leaving the transient outward current (I_{to}) unopposed. The result is a marked abbreviation of the epicardial action potential at some right ventricular sites. This combination causes a transmural voltage gradient and, at its worst, a voltage gradient between adjacent epicardial cells, setting the stage for phase 2 reentry capable of initiating closely coupled PVCs and supporting polymorphic VT, terminating in VF. There is no cure. Treatment is the implantable defibrillator, although the possibility of a pharmacologic therapy is being explored.

Although the diagnosis of overt Brugada syndrome is easily made by means of the ECG, it can be missed in concealed and intermittent forms. In suspicious cases, the ECG can be modulated by changes in autonomic balance and the administration of antiarrhythmic drugs. Beta-adrenergic stimulation normalizes the ECG, whereas intravenous ajmaline, flecainide, or procainamide accentuate the elevated J wave and are capable of unmasking the concealed and intermittent forms.

Antiarrhythmic drugs such as amiodarone and beta

blockers do not prevent sudden death in symptomatic or asymptomatic individuals. Gene therapy may offer a cure in future years. Implantation of an automatic cardioverter-defibrillator is the only currently proven effective therapy.[15]

REFERENCES

1. Brugada P, Brugada J: Right bundle branch block, persistent ST segment elevation and sudden cardiac death: a distinct clinical and electrocardiographic syndrome: a multicenter report, *J Am Coll Cardiol* 20:1391-1396, 1992.
2. Antzelevitch C: The Brugada syndrome: ionic basis and arrhythmia mechanisms, *J Cardiovasc Electrophysiol* 12:268-272, 2001.
3. Kakishita M, Kurita T, Matsuo K et al: Mode of onset of ventricular fibrillation in patients with Brugada syndrome detected by implantable cardioverter defibrillator therapy, *J Am Coll Cardiol* 36:1646-1653, 2000.
4. Alings M, Wilde A: "Brugada" syndrome: clinical data and suggested pathophysiological mechanism, *Circulation* 99:666-673, 1999.
5. Hermida JS, Lemoine JL, Aoun FB et al: Prevalence of the Brugada syndrome in an apparently healthy population, *Am J Cardiol* 86:91-94, 2000.
6. Shimizu W, Antzelevitch C, Suyama K et al: Effect of sodium channel blockers on ST segment, QRS duration, and corrected QT interval in patients with Brugada syndrome, *J Cardiovasc Electrophysiol* 11:1320-1329, 2000.
7. Brugada J, Brugada P, Brugada R: The syndrome of right bundle branch block ST segment elevation in V1 to V3 and sudden deathÑthe Brugada syndrome, *Europace* 1:156-166, 1999.
8. Kasanuki H, Ohnishi S, Ohtuka M et al: Idiopathic ventricular fibrillation induced with vagal activity in patients without obvious heart disease, *Circulation* 95:2277-2285, 1997.
9. Scheinman MM: Is the Brugada syndrome a distinct clinical entity? *J Cardiovasc Electrophysiol* 8:332-336, 1997.
10. Tada H, Sticherling C, Oral H et al: Brugada syndrome mimicked by tricyclic antidepressant overdose, *J Cardiovasc Electrophysiol* 12:275, 2001.
11. Rouleau F, Asfar P, Boulet S et al: Transient ST segment elevation in right precordial leads induced by psychotropic drugs: relationship to the Brugada syndrome, *J Cardiovasc Electrophysiol* 12:61-65, 2001.
12. Grace AA: Brugada syndrome, *Lancet* 354:445-446, 1999.
13. Antzelevitch C, Brugada P, Brugada J et al: Clinical approaches to tachyarrhythmias. In Camm AJ, editor: *The Brugada syndrome*, New York 1999, Futura Publishing, p 73.
14. Tarín N, Farré J, Rubio JM et al: Brugada-like electrocardiographic pattern in a patient with a mediastinal tumor, *PACE* 22:1264-1266, 1999.
15. Brugada P, Terradellas I: Brugada syndrome: from cell to bedside, *J Electrocardiol* 34:319, 2001.
16. Osborn JJ: Experimental hypothermia: respiratory and blood pH changes in relation to cardiac function, *Am J Physiol* 175:389-398, 1953.
17. Bianco M, Bria S, Gianfelici A et al: Does early repolarization in the athlete have analogies with the Brugada syndrome? *Eur Heart J* 22:504-510, 2001.
18. Brugada J, Brugada P: Further characterisation of the syndrome of the right bundle branch block, ST elevation, and sudden cardiac death, *J Cardiovasc Electrophysiol* 8:325-331, 1997.
19. Vincent GM: Long QT syndrome, *Cardiol Clin* 18:309-325, 2000.
20. Chen Q, Kirsch GE, Zhang D et al: Genetic basis and molecular mechanism for idiopathic ventricular fibrillation, *Nature* 392:293-296, 1998.
21. Bezzina C, Veldkamp MW, van den Berg MP et al: A single Na^+ channel mutation causing both long-QT Brugada syndromes, *Circ Res* 85:1206-1213, 1999.
22. Priori SG, Napolitano C, Schwartz PJ et al: The elusive link between LQT3 and Brugada syndrome: the role of flecainide challenge, *Circulation* 102:945-947, 2000.
23. Monroe MH, Littmann L: Two-year case collection of the Brugada syndrome electrocardiogram pattern at a large teaching hospital, *Clin Cardiol* 23:849-851, 2000.
24. Veerakul G, Nademanee K: What is the sudden death syndrome in Southeast Asian males? *Cardiol Rev* 8:90-95, 2000.
25. Zipes DP, Wellens HJJ: Sudden cardiac death, *Circulation* 98:2334-2351, 1998.
26. Butler JM: Brugada syndrome—the missed epidemic, *J Accid Emerg Med* 17:426-428, 2000.
27. Nademanee K, Veerakul G, Nimmannit S et al: Arrhythmogenic marker for the sudden unexplained death syndrome in Thai men, *Circulation* 96:2595-2600, 1997.
28. Belhassen B, Viskin S, Fish R et al: Effects of electrophysiologic-guided therapy with class IA antiarrhythmic drugs on the long-term outcome of patients with idiopathic ventricular fibrillation with or without the Brugada syndrome, *J Cardiovasc Electrophysiol* 10:1301-1312, 1999.
29. Yan GX, Antzelevitch C: Cellular basis for the Brugada syndrome and other mechanisms of arrhythmogenesis associated with ST-segment elevation, *Circulation* 100:1660-1666, 1999.
30. Suzuki H, Torigoe K, Numata O et al: Infant case with a malignant form of Brugada syndrome, *J Cardiovasc Electrophysiol* 11:1277-1280, 2000.
31. Brugada P, Brugada R, Brugada J: The Brugada syndrome, *Curr Cardiol Rep* 2:507-514, 2000.

CHAPTER 28

Acute Pulmonary Embolism

Acute pulmonary embolism is underdiagnosed in most clinical settings and is the most often missed diagnosis in cases of sudden death within the hospital. It accounts for hundreds of thousands of hospitalizations annually in the United States.[1] Weinberg[2] has described the following inscription on a tombstone in Bermuda:

> In memory of Richard Sutherland Dale. Eldest son of Commodore Richard Dale of Philadelphia in the US of America and midshipman in the US Navy. He departed this life at St. Georges, Bermuda on the 22nd day of Feb AD 1815 age 20 years 1 mo 17 da. He lost his right leg in an engagement between the US Frigate President and a squadron of his Brittanic Majesty's ship of war on the 15 da of Jan AD 1815. His confinement caused severe complaint in his back which in a short time terminated his life.

More than 185 years later, pulmonary embolism is all too often a cause of unexpected death.

VALUE OF THE ELECTROCARDIOGRAM

As a result of the increasing accuracy in diagnosing acute pulmonary embolism by isotopic ventilation-perfusion scintigraphy and pulmonary arterial angiography, the electrocardiogram (ECG) changes associated with acute cor pulmonale are being abandoned as a diagnostic tool for this life-threatening disease.[3] Not only does the ECG help exclude acute myocardial infarction (MI), but it is also useful for identifying a patient with a large pulmonary embolism and the ECG signs of right heart strain.[4] Although the ECG signs of acute pulmonary embolism are not diagnostic, certain signs should raise a high degree of suspicion. The Wellens group studied 49 consecutive patients who came to medical attention with acute symptoms and with subsequently proven pulmonary embolism.[4] The 12-lead ECG was reviewed in a blinded fashion to identify the ECG features of right ventricular overload. On the basis of the admission ECG alone a diagnosis of pulmonary embolism was suspected in 76% of patients. With the evaluation of serial tracings the diagnosis could be suspected in 82% of cases. Therefore it is imperative that emergency and critical care personnel be familiar with the ECG signs that warn of the possibility of acute pulmonary embolism and be prepared to institute emergency intervention.

Speed is of the utmost importance. Serial 12-lead ECG tracings are necessary. Although most ECG features of pulmonary embolism lack specificity and sensitivity, especially when prior cardiopulmonary disease is present, certain ECG findings may heighten the initial clinical suspicion.[5]

COMMON ECG FINDINGS IN THE ACUTE PHASE

In a study by the Wellens group[4] pulmonary embolism was considered probable when three or more of the following abnormalities were present. These ECG signs are transient, and serial recordings are necessary.

1. Incomplete or complete right bundle branch block (RBBB), which may be associated with ST segment elevation and positive T waves in lead V_1
2. S waves in leads I and aV_L of more than 1.5 mm
3. A shift in the transitional zone in the precordial leads to V_5
4. Q waves in leads III and aV_F, but not in lead II
5. Right axis deviation (more than 90 degrees); or an indeterminate axis (–90 to +180 degrees)
6. Low-voltage QRS complex (less than 5 mm) in the limb leads

7. T wave inversion in III and aV_F or V_1 to V_4 (subacute phase)

Other ECG Findings

Rhythm: Sinus tachycardia, atrial fibrillation, atrial flutter, premature atrial complexes (right atrial, positive in lead I), premature ventricular complexes (PVCs) (right ventricular, negative in V_1), ventricular fibrillation.

P waves: A shift in the P axis to the right, P-pulmonale (tall P waves [more than 2.5 mm]) leads II, III, and aV_F.

ST-T: ST elevation in V_1, aV_R, and III.

The ECG in Fig. 28-1 was taken the day of the acute event. Sinus tachycardia and the emergence of an incomplete RBBB pattern (terminal r wave is beginning to appear) in lead V_1 can be seen. There is also ST segment elevation in leads V_1 and aV_R, and clockwise rotation of the heart. The transitional zone is between V_4 and V_5, whereas the normal location is V_3 to V_4. The tall P wave in lead II (P-pulmonale) is another reflection of the acute dilation of the right side of the heart.

Fig. 28-2 is from the same patient as in Fig. 28-1, 2 days later. The height of the P wave in leads II, III, and aV_F has decreased.

Right chest leads. In addition to the 12-lead ECG, Chia et al[6] found ST segment elevation and a qs or qr pattern

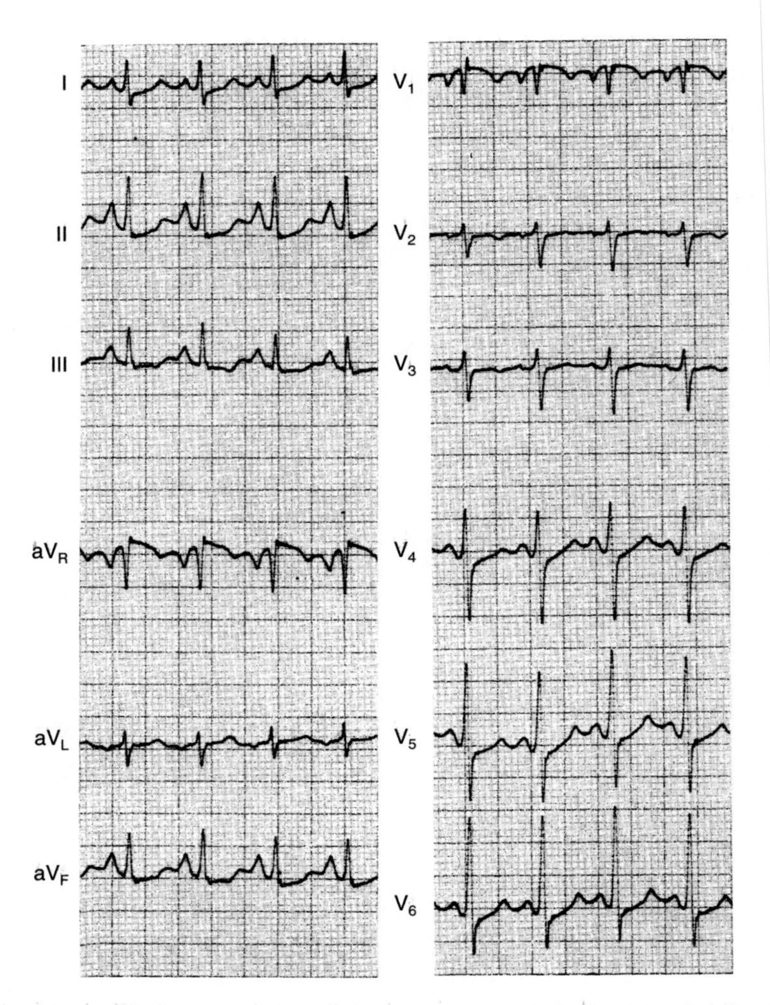

FIG. 28-1. A 12-lead ECG from a patient with acute pulmonary embolism recorded the day of the acute event. Note the sinus tachycardia; prominent P waves in leads II, III, and aV_F; S wave in lead I; incomplete RBBB (V_1); and ST segment elevation in leads V_1 and aV_R. (Courtesy Hein J.J. Wellens, MD, Maastricht, The Netherlands.)

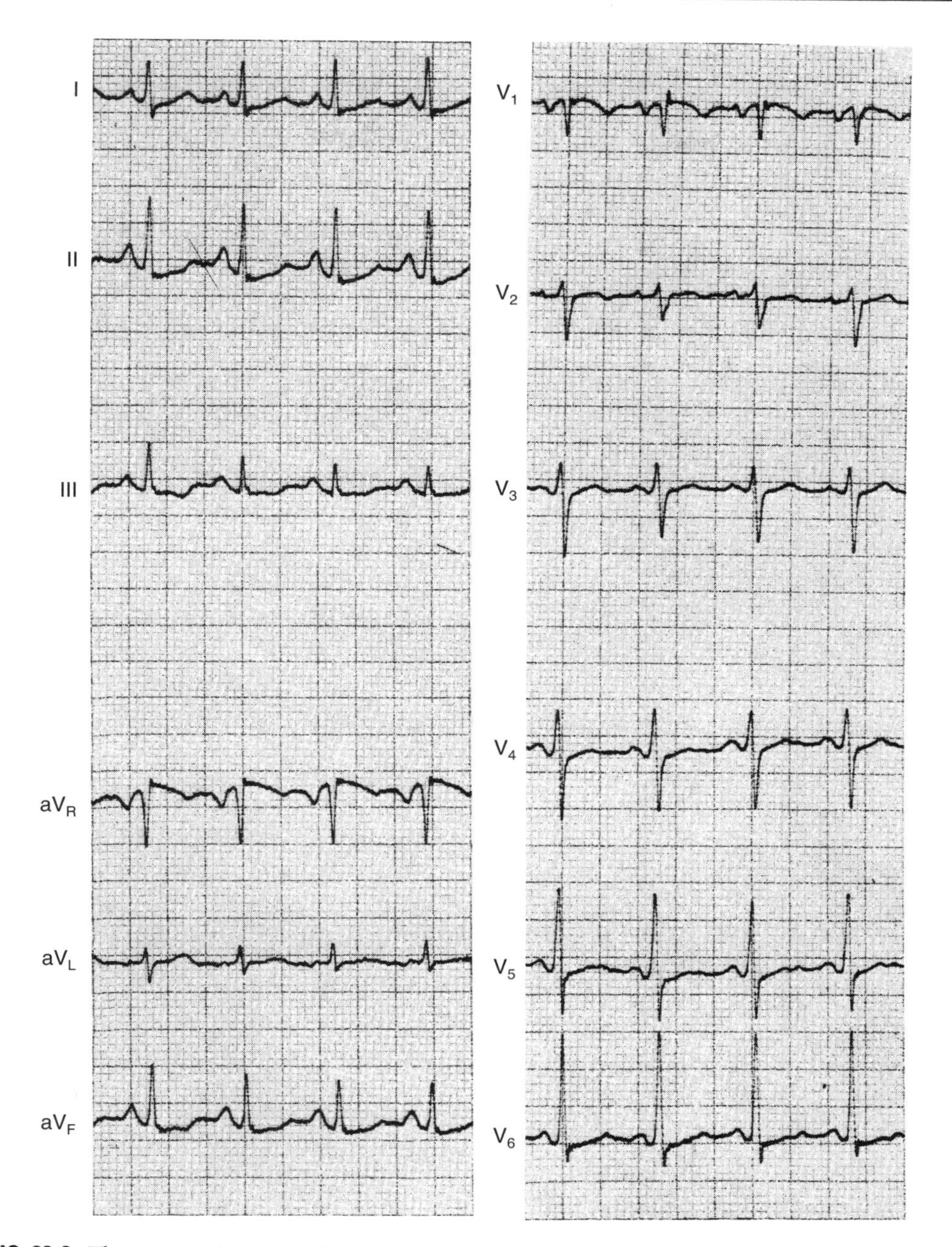

FIG. 28-2. The same patient as in Fig. 28-1, 2 days later. The same abnormalities are present, but the height of the P wave in leads II, III, and aV_F has markedly decreased. (Courtesy Hein J.J. Wellens, MD, Maastricht, The Netherlands.)

(with prominent q waves) in one to three of the right chest leads V_{4R}, V_{5R}, and V_{6R} to be useful in the ECG recognition of acute pulmonary embolism.

ECHOCARDIOGRAPHY

The diagnostic accuracy of the ECG is enhanced when combined with two-dimensional Doppler echocardiography. Tricuspid valve regurgitation and increased right ventricular end-diastolic diameter was revealed in all cases studied by the Wellens group.[4]

Echocardiography visualizes the right side of the heart and central vessels, in particular, the pulmonary arteries, providing a rapid, practical, and sensitive technique for the recognition of right ventricular overload following pulmonary embolism. It is also useful for risk stratification in that patients with right ventricular dysfunction are at increased risk for recurrent pulmonary embolism.[1]

Echocardiographic diagnosis is primarily based on indirect signs such as right ventricular dilation and hypokinesis, bowing of the interventricular septum into the left ventricle, tricuspid regurgitation, and preserved left ventricular function. Echocardiography also helps to exclude ventricular septal rupture, aortic dissection, and pericardial tamponade.[7]

PLASMA D-DIMER ENZYME-LINKED IMMUNOSORBENT ASSAY

Enzyme-linked immunosorbent assay (ELISA)–-determined plasma D-dimer is a blood test for pulmonary embolism screening. Some natural fibrinolysis takes place after acute pulmonary embolism in the body's attempt to break down the clot. The product of this break down is D-dimers, which can be assayed by monoclonal antibodies in commercially available kits.

CHEST X-RAY

Chest x-ray helps to exclude lobar pneumonia, pneumothorax, and acute MI, although pulmonary embolism may exist along with these disorders. More than half of the patients with pulmonary embolism have an abnormal chest film. Importantly, a near normal film in a patient with severe respiratory distress is highly suggestive of massive pulmonary embolism.[1]

VENTILATION-PERFUSION LUNG SCANNING

Ventilation-perfusion (V-Q) lung scanning is a principal diagnostic test. The V-Q scan is most useful if it is clearly normal or demonstrates a high probability of pulmonary embolism. The diagnosis of pulmonary embolism, however, is not excluded if the scan is of intermediate or low probability when the clinical suspicion is strong. Such cases are usually followed by selective pulmonary angiography.

PATHOPHYSIOLOGY

Fig. 28-3 is a pulmonary angiogram showing a large, acute pulmonary embolus. An understanding of the dynamic syndromes of pulmonary embolism as the severity of the condition increases from mild (pulmonary infarction syndrome), to moderate (isolated dyspnea syndrome), to severe (circulatory collapse) is helpful in the differential diagnosis.[8]

The processes involved in acute pulmonary embolism are dynamic. Immediately after sudden obstruction of a central or peripheral pulmonary artery, endogenous fibrinolysis begins to break down some of the fibrin clot to D-dimers (hence the use of the plasma D-dimer test) and improve pulmonary circulation. In the absence of cardiopulmonary disease, thrombi may lyse in a few days, but massive thrombi may cause death within minutes or hours.[9] The emergency nature of this condition cannot be overemphasized. One third of patients with acute pulmonary embolism die within 1 or 2 hours; the diagnosis in about 70% of them is unsuspected.[10] Most patients who survive long enough for a diagnosis to be made have the syndrome of pulmonary infarction (pleuritic pain or hemoptysis).

Massive obstruction of the main pulmonary trunk is reflected in a newly emerged RBBB pattern in V_1.[11] Significant obstruction results in the following pathophysiologic conditions:

- Acute pulmonary hypertension
- Right-side dilation
- Clockwise cardiac rotation

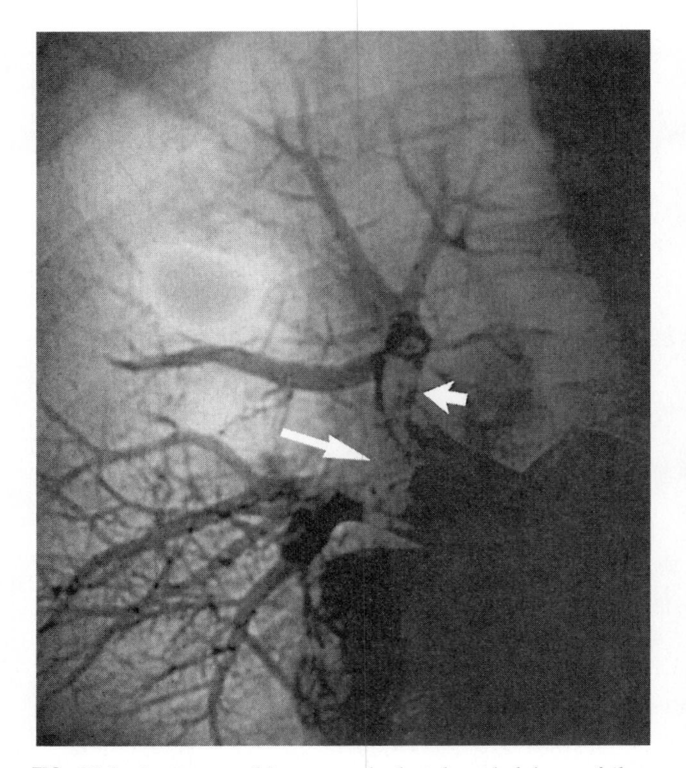

FIG. 28-3. A 77-year-old woman had right-sided heart failure despite 3 days of full-dose heparin. Therefore she underwent right heart catheterization and pulmonary angiography. Her pulmonary arterial pressure was 55/30 mm Hg. Seen on her baseline angiogram were large right middle and right upper lobe pulmonary emboli *(arrows).*

- Right ventricular failure
- Pulmonary infarction
- Marked V-Q disturbance
- Acute lowering of the cardiac output

RISK FACTORS

Common histories in patients with pulmonary embolism are hypertension, diabetes mellitus, obesity, atrial fibrillation, and hyperlipidemia. Patients in an especially high-risk group are those undergoing orthopedic surgery or gynecologic surgery for cancer and immobilized medical patients in whom pulmonary embolism may occur postoperatively as late as 1 month.

Other risk factors include the hypercoagulation state of occult cancer, use of oral contraceptives, the postpartum period, and especially the period after cesarean section.[7] Pulmonary embolism is the most common medical cause of maternal mortality associated with live births in the United States; the risk is much greater during the first 6 postpartum weeks than during the pregnancy itself.

Genetic Link

For patients with a family history of venous thrombosis or for young patients with venous thrombosis, Goldhaber[7] suggested that testing for a specific inherited hypercoagulable state may be justified. In a prospective evaluation of 218 men, the presence of the G20210A mutation in the prothrombin gene was associated with a significantly increased risk of recurrent venous thromboembolism, particularly among those who coinherited factor V Leiden.[12]

SIGNS AND SYMPTOMS

The three most common presenting symptoms of a life-threatening pulmonary embolism are dyspnea, syncope, or cyanosis. Pleuritic pain may signify a small embolism in the distal pulmonary tree. In patients with prior cardiopulmonary disease the most common sign is tachypnea; the most frequent symptom is dyspnea.

Physical findings are related to acute right ventricular volume overload, right ventricular failure, and the increase in pulmonary artery pressure. Other symptoms include hepatomegaly, palpable right ventricular impulse, increase in jugular venous *A* wave, increase in jugular venous distention, and palpable pulmonary artery pulsation.

The heart sounds that may be heard are tricuspid regurgitation, audible right ventricular fourth heart sound, third heart sound, narrow splitting of second heart sound with an exaggerated pulmonic second sound, and a pulmonary ejection murmur.

Sudden, unexplained shortness of breath in a patient who is a likely candidate for pulmonary embolism (recent surgery, debilitation, immobilized) is a finding that leads to a diagnosis.

DIFFERENTIAL DIAGNOSIS

The ECG patterns in acute pulmonary embolism often resemble those of acute MI. Abnormal Q waves, ST segment elevation, and T wave inversions that may occur in the inferior leads are similar to those of inferior wall MI, whereas the ST segment elevation in lead V_1 and the RBBB may mimic anterior wall infarction.

Helpful clues include the following:

1. The observation of ECG signs of apparent MI in both inferior and anterior wall leads should alert the examiner to the possibility of acute pulmonary embolism. Plus, the pattern in the 12-lead ECG, although abnormal, is not really typical of MI. For example, Q waves may appear in III and aV_F, but not in II, along with a QR in V_1.
2. Acute dyspnea is usually much more pronounced in acute pulmonary embolism than in acute MI. In spite of the severe dyspnea, the chest x-ray does not show pulmonary congestion.

TREATMENT[13]

1. Oxygen
2. Analgesics
3. Full-dose heparin; the major side effects of heparin are bleeding and thrombocytopenia (commonly heparin-induced platelet aggregation)
4. Intravenous thrombolytic therapy
5. Emergency pulmonary thromboendarterectomy (rarely necessary but is lifesaving in patients with acute massive pulmonary embolism who do not respond to or who have absolute contraindications to thrombolytic therapy); also considered a potential cure for patients with chronic pulmonary hypertension that is the result of undiagnosed or inadequately treated prior pulmonary embolism[14]

PREVENTION

- Avoid venous stasis by early mobilization and ambulation when possible
- External compression of the legs for patients on complete bed rest

Intensive preventive action is required for patients undergoing orthopedic or gynecologic cancer surgery and for immobilized medical patients. Goldhaber[1] advises adjusted-dose warfarin for total hip replacement.

Antithrombin agents may be shown to be even more effective.[15,16]

Graduated compression elastic stockings should be considered first-line prophylaxis in all hospitalized patients except those with peripheral arterial occlusive disease whose condition may be worsened by vascular compression. In patients at moderate to high risk the stockings may be used in combination with intermittent inflation of air-filled cuffs (pneumatic compression boots). The compression stockings serve to oppose perioperative venodilation, and the compression boots prevent venous stasis in the legs and may stimulate endogenous fibrinolysis.

SUMMARY

The common ECG findings in the acute phase of pulmonary embolism are the result of right ventricular failure and acute dilation of the right atria and right ventricle. Arrhythmias that occur in acute pulmonary embolism are sinus tachycardia, atrial fibrillation, atrial flutter, and right-sided premature atrial complexes and PVCs. ECG changes reflecting the acutely dilated right side of the heart are RBBB, P pulmonale, right axis shifts of the P wave and QRS complex, elevated ST segments in leads V_1 and aV_R, clockwise rotation of the heart, and an S_1, Q_3, T_3 pattern. The preceding changes, which begin abruptly, require serial ECG tracings and are confirmed with Doppler echocardiography. Speed in diagnosing and treating acute pulmonary embolism is important because of the high mortality in untreated cases.

REFERENCES

1. Goldhaber SZ, Braunwald E: Pulmonary embolism. In Braunwald E, editor: *Heart disease,* ed 5, Philadelphia, 1997, WB Saunders.
2. Weinberg SL: President's page: pulmonary embolism—diagnosis on a tombstone, *J Am Coll Cardiol* 22:328, 1993.
3. Hubloue I, Schoors D, Diltoer M et al: Early electrocardiographic signs in acute massive pulmonary embolism, *Eur J Emerg Med* 3:199-204, 1996.
4. Sreeram N, Cheriex EC, Smeets JL et al: Value of the 12-lead electrocardiogram at hospital admission in the diagnosis of pulmonary embolism, *Am J Cardiol* 73:298-303, 1994.
5. Vranckx P, Ector H, Heidbuchel H: A case of extensive pulmonary embolism presenting as an acute myocardial infarction—notes on its possible pathophysiology, *Eur J Emerg Med* 5:253-158, 1998.
6. Chia BL, Tan HC, Lim YT: Right sided chest lead electrocardiographic abnormalities in acute pulmonary embolism, *Int J Cardiol* 61:43-46, 1997.
7. Goldhaber SZ: Recognition and management of pulmonary embolism, *Heart Dis Stroke* 3:142, 1993.
8. Stein PD, Henry JW: Clinical characteristics of patients with acute pulmonary embolism stratified according to their presenting syndromes, *Chest* 112:974-979, 1997.
9. Pulmonary embolism. In *Merck Manual*, Whitehouse Station, NJ, 2001, Merck & Co.
10. Stein PD, Henry JW: Prevalence of acute pulmonary embolism among patients in a general hospital and at autopsy, *Chest* 108:978-981, 1995.
11. Petrov DB: Appearance of right bundle branch block in electrocardiograms of patients with pulmonary embolism as a marker for obstruction of the main pulmonary trunk, *J Electrocardiol* 34:185-188, 2001.
12. Miles JS, Miletich JP, Goldhaber SZ et al: G20210A mutation in the prothrombin gene and the risk of recurrent venous thromboembolism, *J Am Coll Cardiol* 37:215-218, 2001.
13. Wellens HJJ, Conover M: *The ECG in emergency decision making,* Philadelphia, 1992, WB Saunders.
14. Okubo S, Yoshioka T, Nakanishi N, et al: Acute fatal pulmonary embolism: its prevention, diagnosis and treatment, *Respir Circ* 38:375, 1990.
15. Turpie AG: Pentasaccharide Org31540/SR90107A clinical trials update: lessons for practice, *Am Heart J* 142(2 Suppl):S9-S15, 2001.
16. Eriksson BI: New therapeutic options in deep vein thrombosis prophylaxis, *Semin Hematol* 37(3 Suppl 5):7-9, 2000.

CHAPTER 29

Chamber Hypertrophy and Enlargement

ELECTROCARDIOGRAM SENSITIVITY AND SPECIFICITY

The electrocardiogram (ECG) diagnosis of right or left ventricular hypertrophy (LVH) has a low sensitivity (approximately 50%) but a high specificity (more than 90%). Thus approximately half of the individuals with ventricular hypertrophy cannot be recognized by the ECG. However, ventricular hypertrophy is most probably present if the ECG criteria are met.[1] Echocardiographic studies indicate that the ECG does not differentiate among concentric hypertrophy, eccentric hypertrophy, and dilation without hypertrophy, although the sensitivity of the ECG is greater in individuals with severe hypertrophy.[2]

CAUSES OF VENTRICULAR HYPERTROPHY

Increased metabolic demands or increased workload in the adult causes enlargement and structural alteration of myocardial cells and hyperplasia of nonmuscular cardiac components. Causes of cardiac hypertrophy are pressure and volume overload and neurohumoral factors. The two types of overload are compared with each other and with the normal heart in Fig. 29-1.

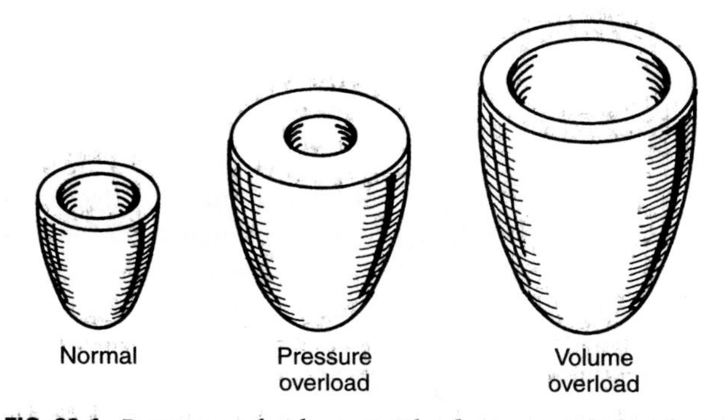

FIG. 29-1. Pressure and volume overload are compared with each other and with the normal heart. (Modified from Oparil S: *J Am Coll Cardiol* 5:57B, 1985.)

Pressure Overload or Systolic Overload

When the heart is forced to pump against increased resistance, as in aortic stenosis or systemic hypertension, the resultant increased cardiac work causes *concentric hypertrophy*, in which the ventricular wall thickens in relation to the ventricular cavity (Fig. 29-1). Systolic overload is characterized by increased QRS voltage, depressed ST segment, and inverted T waves in left precordial leads.

Volume Overload or Diastolic Overload

An increased end-diastolic wall stress caused by increased volume, as in valvular regurgitation and congestive heart failure, may cause the left ventricular chamber to stretch or dilate, leading to *eccentric hypertrophy;* that is, the left ventricular wall thickness remains normal relative to the increase in the radius of the left ventricle (chamber dilation), as seen in Fig. 29-1. In this situation systolic pressure remains unchanged. Diastolic overload is characterized by tall late R waves in V_5 and V_6.

LEFT VENTRICULAR HYPERTROPHY

The ECG diagnosis of LVH is based on the increase of QRS voltage generated from the increased muscle mass of the left ventricle.

Estes Scoring System

The box on p. 408 illustrates the Estes criteria for the diagnosis of LVH. The standard ECG is a poor screening test for the detection of LVH in individuals with essential hypertension.

Cornell Voltage Criteria

The Cornell voltage criteria has a sensitivity of 22% and specificity of 95%.

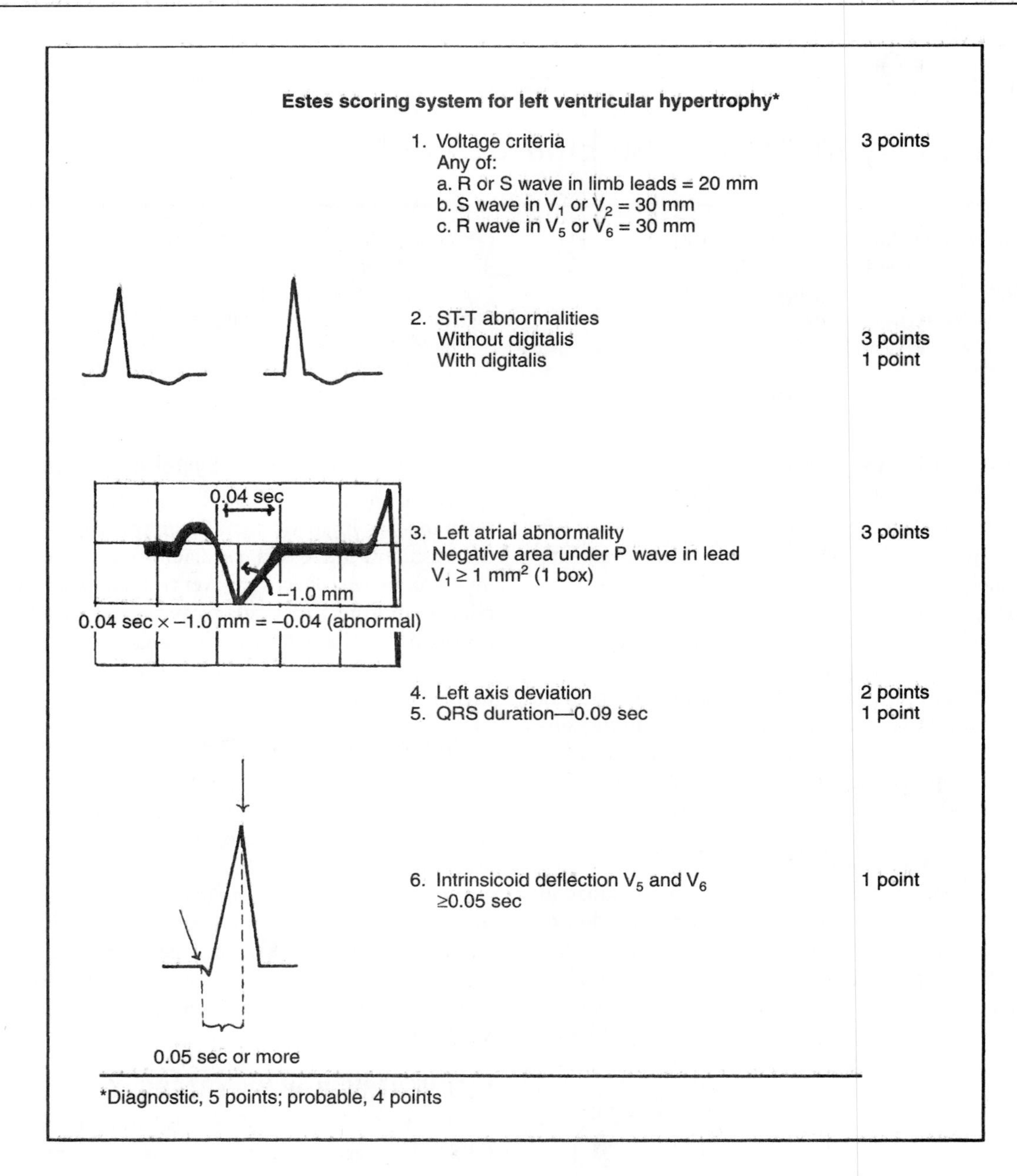

- S in V_3 + R in aVL >24 mm (men)
- S in V_3 + R in aVL >20 mm (women)

Limb Lead Voltage Criteria

- R in aV_L ≥11 mm or
- If left axis deviation: R in aV_L ≥13 mm plus S in III ≥15 mm

Chest Lead Voltage Criteria

- S in V_1 plus R in V_5 or V_6 ≥35 mm

The 12-lead ECG in Fig. 29-2 represents LVH. Note the increased voltage of the QRS; the late intrinsicoid deflection in lead V_6; left axis deviation; and the broad, deep, negative component to the P wave in lead V_1 (left atrial enlargement).

QRS amplitude. When LVH can be recognized on the ECG there are tall R waves in left precordial leads and deep S waves in right precordial leads.

Limitations. QRS voltage varies with age, sex, and race. It is greater in adolescents and young adults than in older

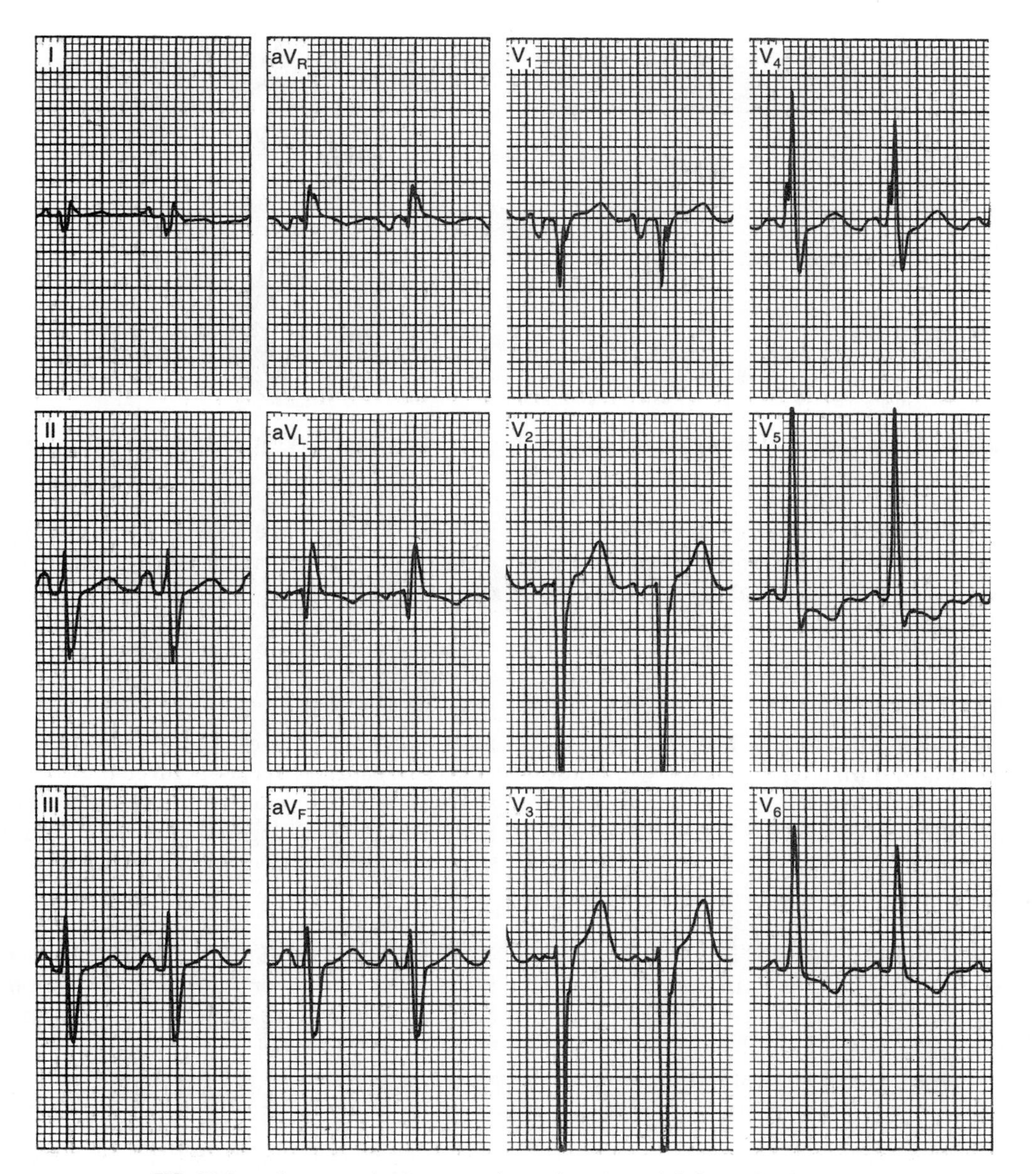

FIG. 29-2. Left ventricular hypertrophy and strain with left atrial enlargement.

individuals, in men than in women, and in blacks than in whites. The QRS voltage also depends on the mean frontal plane QRS axis, being greater in the lead whose axis is parallel with the mean current flow; is greater in individuals with a thin chest wall and is less in obese individuals, who may have LVH with normal QRS amplitude; and is less when there is lung disease, pericardial effusion, coronary artery disease, secondary myocardial disease (amyloidosis, scleroderma heart disease), or coexistent severe right ventricular hypertrophy.

In addition, there is day-to-day variability of voltage measurements, and young black individuals appear to have much higher voltages with normal ventricles than whites of the same age. However, despite its limitations, the ECG remains a valuable tool for the detection of hypertensive target organ damage and is recommended as an essential test in the office evaluation of the hypertensive patient.[3,4] Fig. 29-3 compares the normal QRS complex in leads V_1 and V_6 with that of LVH.

Intrinsicoid Deflection

The extra thickness of the left ventricle prolongs the QRS and the ventricular activation time and delays the intrinsicoid deflection. In lead V_6 the intrinsicoid deflec-

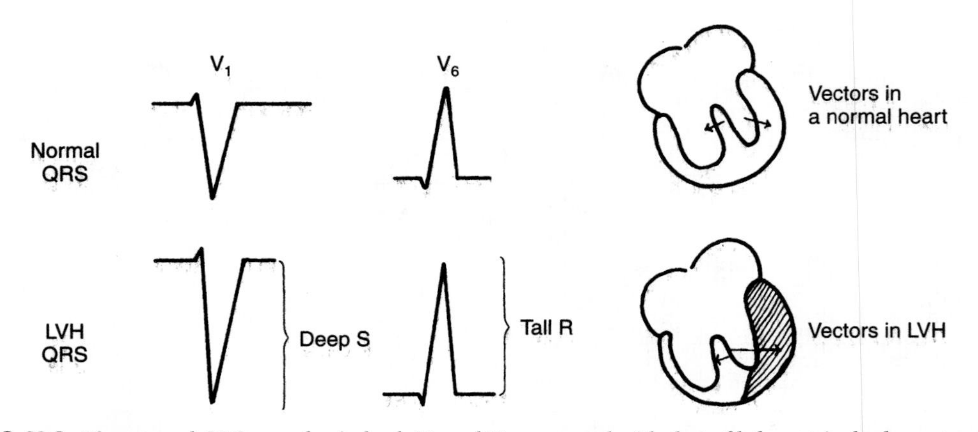

FIG. 29-3. The normal QRS complex in leads V_1 and V_6 compared with that of left ventricular hypertrophy.

tion is delayed in LVH to 0.05 second or more (Fig. 29-4), probably as a result of the extra time it takes to activate the hypertrophied ventricle. Although this delay in the intrinsicoid deflection is not specific, it occurs in 35% to 90% of cases.

Widened QRS/T Angle

A sensitive method for interpreting T waves is to compare the forces generated during repolarization with those of depolarization. To make this evaluation it is necessary to know the axis of both the QRS and the T wave. The angle between them is normally narrow, usually not more than 45 degrees in the frontal plane or 60 degrees in the horizontal plane.

The methods for plotting the QRS axis in the frontal plane have already been discussed in Chapter 4. The T wave axis is plotted in the same way. In Fig. 29-5 lead III has the T wave with zero net enclosed area; thus its axis is perpendicular to the axis of lead III and parallel to the axis of lead aV_R. Therefore the T axis is 30 degrees, the QRS axis is 60 degrees, and the angle between them is 30 degrees (normal).

Left Ventricular Strain Pattern

The left ventricular strain pattern denotes the pattern seen when the QRS/T angle widens because the ST segment and T wave are opposite in direction to that of the QRS. This pattern does not occur in uncomplicated hypertrophy but is associated with myocardial ischemia. The term itself is misleading in that the ECG records only electrical activity, not hemodynamic changes.

Mechanism

The increased QRS voltage is the result not only of the exaggerated leftward and posterior forces in the ventricle, but also because the thickened left ventricle is in close contact with the chest wall.

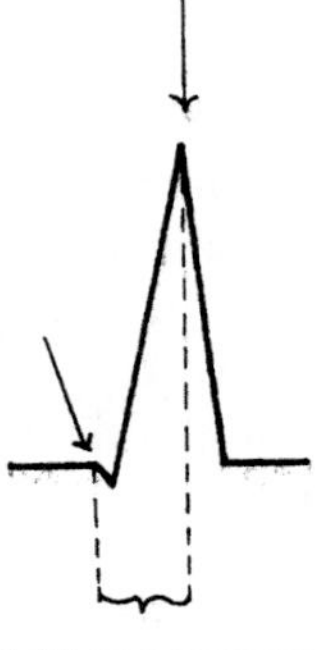

FIG. 29-4. The intrinsicoid deflection in lead V_6 in left ventricular hypertrophy.

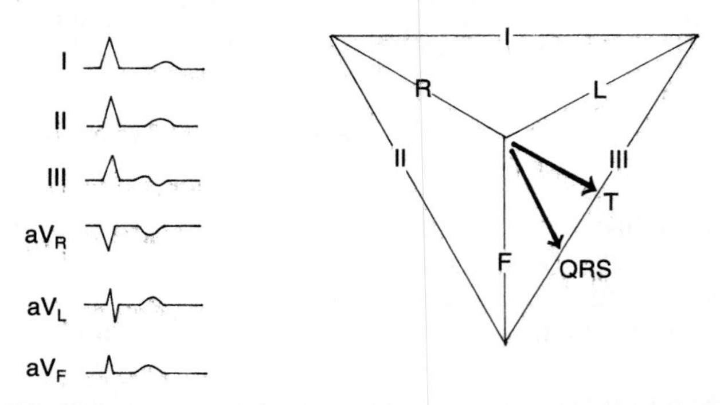

FIG. 29-5. QRS/T angle. The QRS axis is +60 degrees. In the example given, the T wave axis is +30 degrees, and the angle between them is 30 degrees. The T wave axis is plotted exactly the same as the QRS axis as described in Chapter 4. Look for the isoelectric T wave (lead III). The T axis is perpendicular to that lead axis and parallel with the lead axis of aV_R at +30 degrees.

Causes and Risks

Hypertension. LVH is causally related to high blood pressure. Its presence in hypertensive patients points to hypertensive target organ damage. When there is ECG evidence of LVH, there is an associated increased risk for a number of cardiovascular diseases, including myocardial infarction (MI), stroke, and congestive heart failure, especially in hypertensive patients.[5,6]

Arrhythmias. LVH is accompanied by specific changes in ventricular electrophysiology, which are potentially arrhythmogenic. The incidence of supraventricular and ventricular arrhythmias in patients with arterial hypertension is up to 96% and is about 10 times higher than in normotensives. Moreover, as QRS voltage or repolarization abnormalities increase, so does the risk. Likewise, as the voltage or repolarization abnormalities decline, so does the risk, suggesting that regression of the ECG signs of LVH is associated with improved prognosis.[7]

Differential Diagnosis

True LVH versus pseudo LVH. When high QRS voltage is encountered in adults younger than 40 years of age, the differential diagnosis between true LVH and pseudo LVH can be made by evaluating the QRS-T angle. In the early stages of true LVH the T wave in V_1 is upright and taller than the upright T wave in V_6 (T-V_1 >T-V_6). In the pseudo LVH seen in young adults, even though the ECG satisfies the voltage criteria for LVH, the T wave is inverted in V_1, as it would be in normal subjects.[8]

Wolff-Parkinson-White syndrome. In Wolff-Parkinson-White syndrome (see Chapter 21), the sequence of ventricular activation is altered and, depending on the anatomic site of the accessory conduction pathway, may result in pseudo ventricular hypertrophy and pseudo myocardial infarction ECG patterns. When the accessory pathway is on the right side, the depolarization current travels toward V_5 and V_6, amplifying the R waves and simulating LVH. When the accessory pathway is on the left side, the depolarization current travels toward V_1, amplifying the R waves and simulating right ventricular hypertrophy.[9]

Acute coronary ischemia. The altered morphologies of the ST segment or the T wave associated with LVH resemble features seen in acute ischemic heart disease.[10]

Voltage Discordance in Dilated Cardiomyopathy

A useful ECG sign of dilated cardiomyopathy is "voltage discordance"[8]; that is, low QRS voltage in the limb leads with good or preserved QRS voltage in the precordial leads as shown in Fig. 29-6.

RIGHT VENTRICULAR HYPERTROPHY

In mild cases of right ventricular hypertrophy (RVH), no ECG signs are seen. In severe RVH, such as would be seen in pulmonary stenosis and pulmonary hypertension, ST depression and T wave inversion are usually seen in right precordial leads.

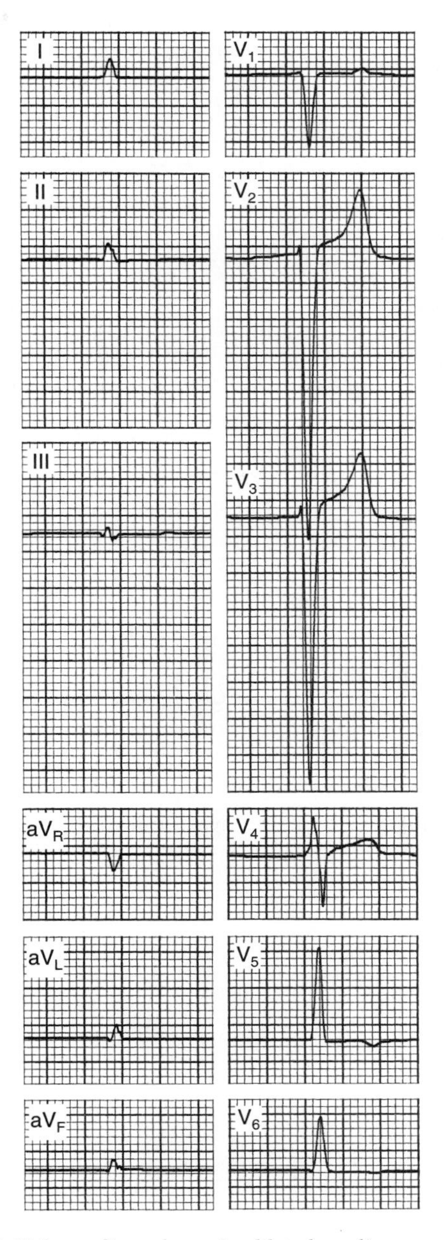

FIG. 29-6. Voltage discordance in dilated cardiomyopathy. Note the low voltage in the limb leads compared to the enhanced voltage in V_2 and V_3. (Courtesy G. Veerender Reddy, MD, Wilmington, Del.)

ECG Recognition[1]

General ECG signs:

- Right axis deviation of more than 90 degrees
- Tall R waves in the right precordial leads, V_1 being the most sensitive because of its proximity to the right ventricle

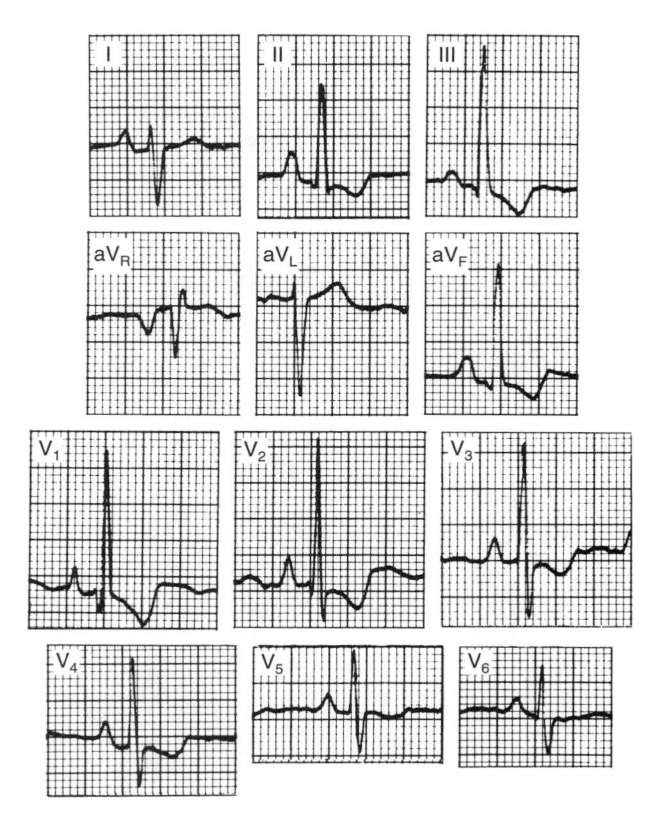

FIG. 29-7. Right ventricular hypertrophy with right atrial enlargement.

- Q waves sometimes precede the tall R waves in right precordial leads, in which case there is frequently right atrial hypertrophy and tricuspid regurgitation (tall, peaked P waves in leads II, III, aV_F, and, occasionally, V_1; Fig. 29-7)
- Deep S waves in the left precordial leads
- Slight increase in QRS duration
- Secondary ST-T abnormalities in the precordial and inferior leads in the form of wide QRS/T angle (the T wave is opposite in polarity to the QRS)
- Evidence of right atrial enlargement

When QRS duration is less than 0.12 second, one or more of the following will occur:

- Right axis >90 degrees associated with etiology for RVH
- R in aV_R ≥5 mm, or
- R in aV_R >Q in aV_R

Any one of the following in V_1:

- R/S ratio >1 with a negative T wave
- qR pattern (also seen in right bundle branch block (RBBB) with and without anteroseptal MI)
- R >6 mm, or
- S <2 mm, or
- rSR′ with R′ >10 mm

Note: An incomplete RBBB (rSR′ in V_1) pattern may signify RVH, dilation or overload of the right ventricle, but it is most frequently the result of other factors. It is seen in mitral valve disease with pulmonary hypertension and atrial septal defect and disappears following corrective surgery.

Fig. 29-8 compares the patterns seen in leads V_1 and V_6 in the normal heart with those of marked RVH. The patterns present a mirror image of the patterns seen in LVH.

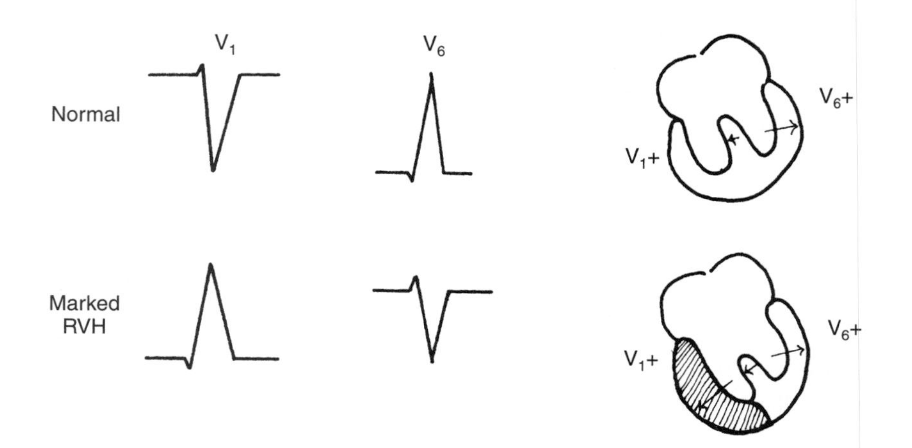

FIG. 29-8. The normal QRS complex compared with that in right ventricular hypertrophy *(RVH)*.

In healthy individuals a narrow rSr′ pattern with a small terminal r wave is found in 2.4% of individuals. In such a case, the amplitude of the r′ wave seldom is more than 5 mm, as well as being less than the R wave and the S wave. Recorded at a lower interspace, this finding disappears.

Other Chest Lead Criteria

- R in V_1 plus S in V_5 or V_6 10 mm
- R/S ratio in V_5 or V_6 <1
- R in V_5 or V_6 <5 mm
- S in V_5 or V_6 >7 mm

Secondary ST depression and T wave inversion may be seen in right precordial leads and is listed as supporting criteria.[11]

Mechanism

An increase in muscle mass in the right ventricle modifies its normal anterior and rightward forces in proportion to the degree of hypertrophy. Because the left ventricular walls are normally much thicker than those of the right ventricle, severe right ventricular hypertrophy must be present for the right ventricular forces to dominate and manifest on the ECG.

Causes

RVH is associated with conditions that cause the right ventricular mass to begin competing with the left ventricle, such as congenital pulmonary stenosis, tetralogy of Fallot, and primary pulmonary hypertension. Systolic overload occurs in pulmonary hypertension or pulmonary stenosis, resulting in right axis deviation and increased voltage in right precordial leads. Diastolic overload occurs in atrial septal defect causing right axis deviation with an rSr′ pattern in V_1 with little or no increase in QRS duration.

BIVENTRICULAR HYPERTROPHY

Biventricular hypertrophy is frequently present in *Eisenmenger's syndrome* (ventricular septal defect or patent ductus arteriosus and pulmonary hypertension). Right ventricular hypertrophy caused by pulmonary hypertension may be associated with and may obscure the ECG pattern of established LVH. When there is hypertrophy of both ventricles, the ECG may actually be normal because of the partial cancellation of electrical forces, making this diagnosis particularly difficult. The patient whose ECG is displayed in Fig. 29-9 had bilateral disease and probable biventricular hypertrophy.

ECG Recognition

- R/S ratio in V_5 or V_6 <1
- S in V_5 or V_6 >6 mm

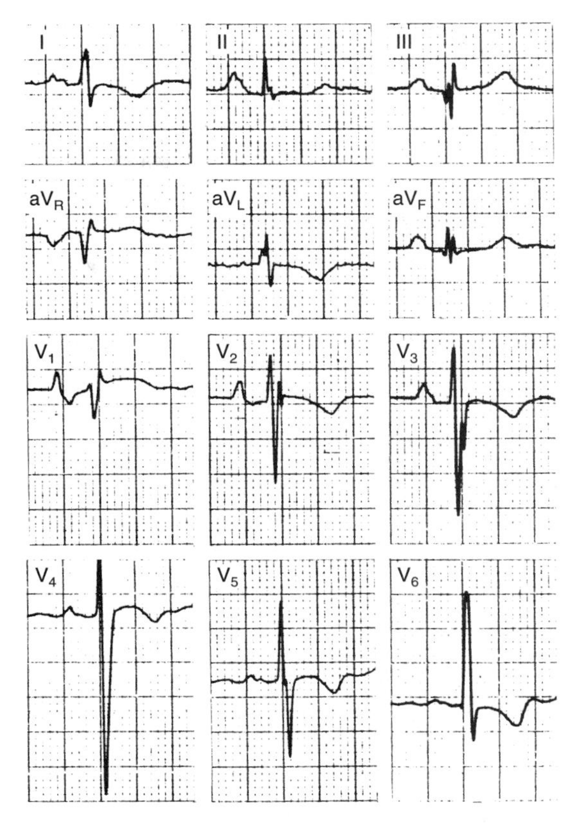

FIG. 29-9. A 12-lead ECG from a patient with hypertension. The notched, upright P wave in leads I, II, and V_4 to V_6 and the deep, broad terminal trough in lead V_1 are evident. (Courtesy Ara G. Tilkian, MD, Van Nuys, Calif.)

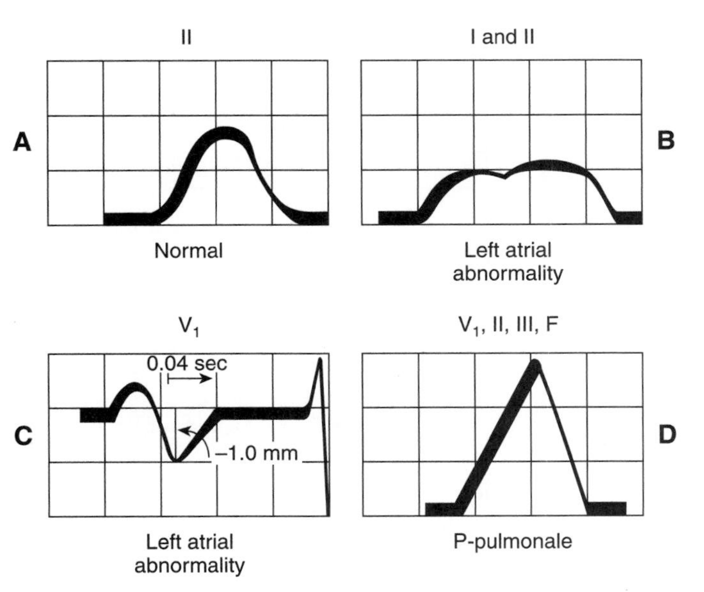

FIG. 29-10. **A-D,** The normal P wave compared with the P wave in left atrial abnormality and P-pulmonale.

- Right axis deviation of >90 degrees
- Signs of LVH and RVH
- Signs of LVH and right axis deviation or right atrial enlargement
- A shift to the left of the transitional zone in the precordial leads (a less reliable sign)

NORMAL P WAVE

- Less than 3 mm high and less than 0.12 second wide (Fig. 29-10, *A*)
- Upright in the left precordial leads and in leads I and II
- Usually diphasic in the right precordial leads
- P axis is about +60 degrees in the frontal plane
- Initial and terminal components corresponding to right (anterior) and left (posterior) atrial forces

LEFT ATRIAL ENLARGEMENT

The pattern associated with left atrial enlargement reflects a conduction abnormality within the atria, not actual hypertrophy or dilation. The ECG pattern of left atrial abnormality is often present in hypertension and may transiently occur in pulmonary edema.

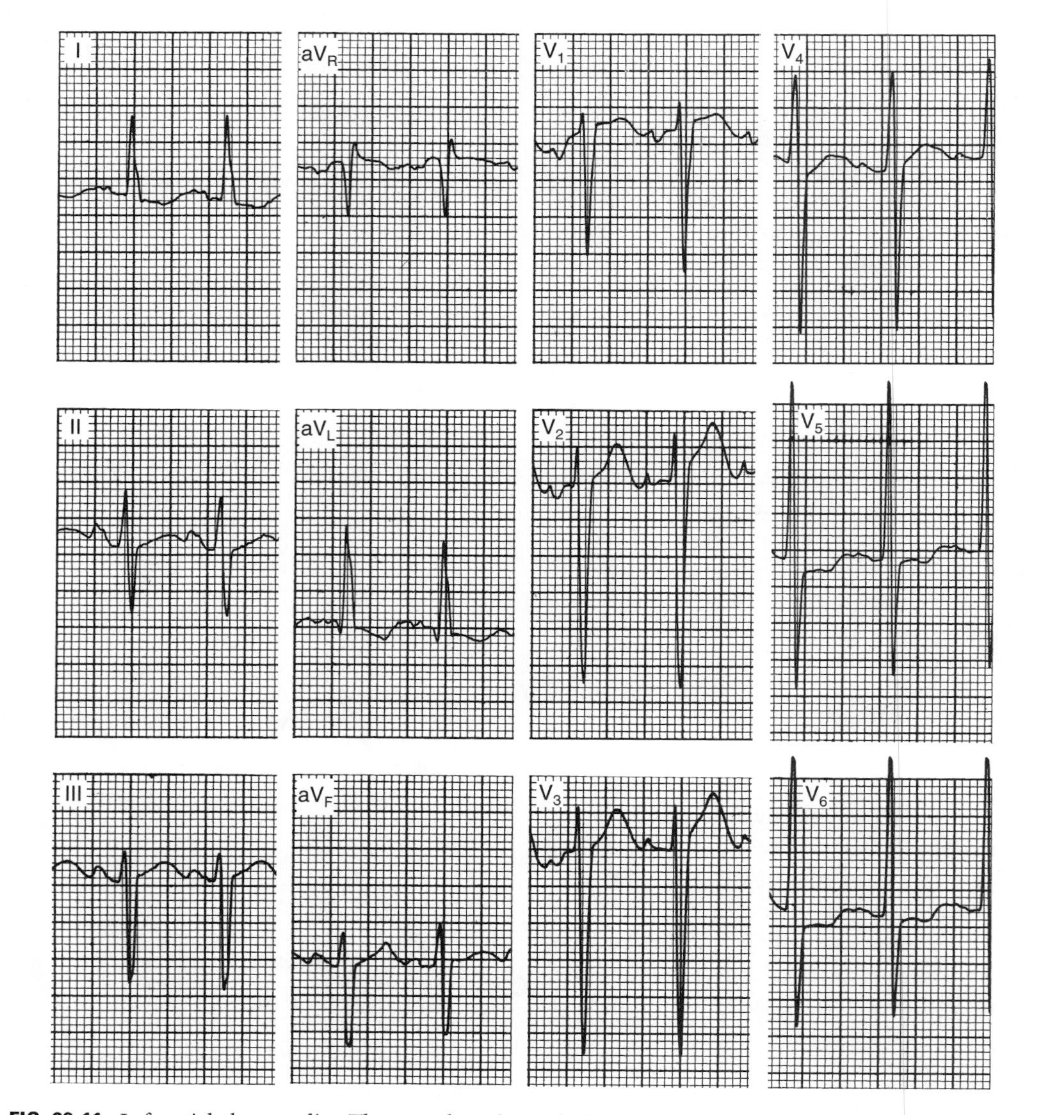

FIG. 29-11. Left atrial abnormality. There are broad, notched P waves in leads I, II, V_5, and V_6. The P wave in lead V_1 has a broad terminal trough. (Courtesy Ara G. Tilkian, MD, Van Nuys, Calif.)

ECG Recognition (Sensitivity 40%; Specificity 90%)

- Prolonged P wave duration (>0.12 second; usually in lead II)
- Notched upright P wave in leads I, II, and V_4 to V_6 with the interpeak duration of 0.04 second
- A deep, broad terminal trough in lead V_1 of ≥0.04 second; depth ≥1 mm

Left atrial abnormality causes the initial and terminal components of the P wave to separate, widening the P wave to 0.12 second or more. Thus on the ECG the P wave is upright and notched in leads I, II, and V_4 to V_6 (Fig. 29-10, *B*). It may be either positive or negative in leads III and aV_F. In lead V_1 the wide separation between the two components of the P wave is most noticeable, producing an initial upright component followed by an inverted component (Fig. 29-10, *C*). Left atrial abnormality is often accompanied by RVH.

Fig. 29-11 is a 12-lead ECG from a patient with hypertension. The notched, upright P wave in leads I, II, and V_4 to V_6 and the deep, broad terminal trough in lead V_1 can be seen.

RIGHT ATRIAL ABNORMALITY

The so-called P pulmonale pattern is associated with lung disease, pulmonary embolus, and other causes of pulmonary hypertension. When associated with lung disease the ECG changes may result from increased sympathetic stimulation (causing increased P amplitude) and low position of the diaphragm (causing the P axis to be rightward) associated with diffuse lung disease. The P pulmonale pattern aids in the evaluation of the severity of chronic obstructive lung disease (rightward P axis shift). The right axis deviation of the P wave is the best ECG change in evaluating the severity of chronic obstructive lung disease.

ECG Recognition

Chronic obstructive lung disease; P pulmonale. If the ECG changes are stable, consider the clinical presentation for lung disease and exposures to pulmonary irritants and toxins.

In patients with chronic obstructive lung dis ease the lungs are overaerated and provide an insulating effect. This effect, along with the change in the spatial orientation of the heart, causes these ECG changes.

- Tall, peaked P waves in leads II, III, and aV_F; amplitude increases with the severity of the disease (Fig. 29-10, *D*)
- Low R wave amplitude (less than 0.5 mV in lead V_6 as the disease becomes more severe)
- Wide, slurred S waves in leads I, II, III, and V_4 to V_6 that are caused by the late QRS vector being oriented superiorly and to the right (with more severe disease, the R:S ratio is equal to or less than 1 in lead V_6)
- Right axis deviation and a dominant S wave in precordial leads (the most reliable signs of RVH in chronic lung disease)[3]
- P axis to the right of +70 degrees

Fig. 29-12 is an ECG from a patient with chronic obstructive lung disease. Note the typical P pulmonale pattern.

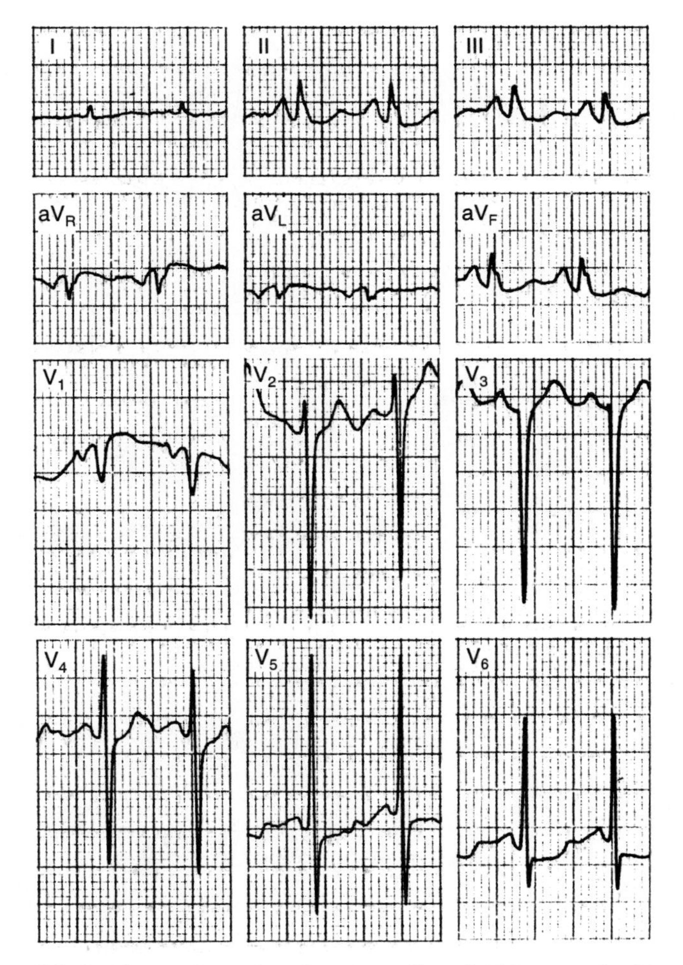

FIG. 29-12. P pulmonale. There are tall, peaked P waves in the inferior leads, and the P axis is rightward. (Courtesy Ara G. Tilkian, MD, Van Nuys, Calif.)

Acute pulmonary embolism. If the ECG changes are new, consider the clinical presentation for acute pulmonary embolism (sinus tachycardia, pleuritic chest pain, immobilization). The ECG signs are discussed in Chapter 28 and reviewed here:

- Incomplete or complete RBBB, which may be associated with ST segment elevation and positive T waves in lead V_1
- S waves in leads I and aV_L of more than 1.5 mm
- A shift in the transitional zone in the precordial leads to V_5
- Q waves in leads III and aV_F, but not in lead II
- Right-axis deviation (more than 90 degrees); or an indeterminate axis (–90 to ±180 degrees)
- Low-voltage QRS complex (less than 5 mm) in the limb leads
- T wave inversion in III and aV_F or V_1 to V_4 (subacute phase)
- Sinus tachycardia, atrial fibrillation, atrial flutter; premature atrial complexes (right atrial, positive in lead I), premature ventricular complexes (right ventricular, negative in V_1), ventricular fibrillation
- A shift in the P axis to the right
- P pulmonale (tall P waves [more than 2.5 mm]) leads II, III, and aV_F
- ST elevation in V_1, aV_R, and III

The ECG in Fig. 29-13 was taken the day of the acute

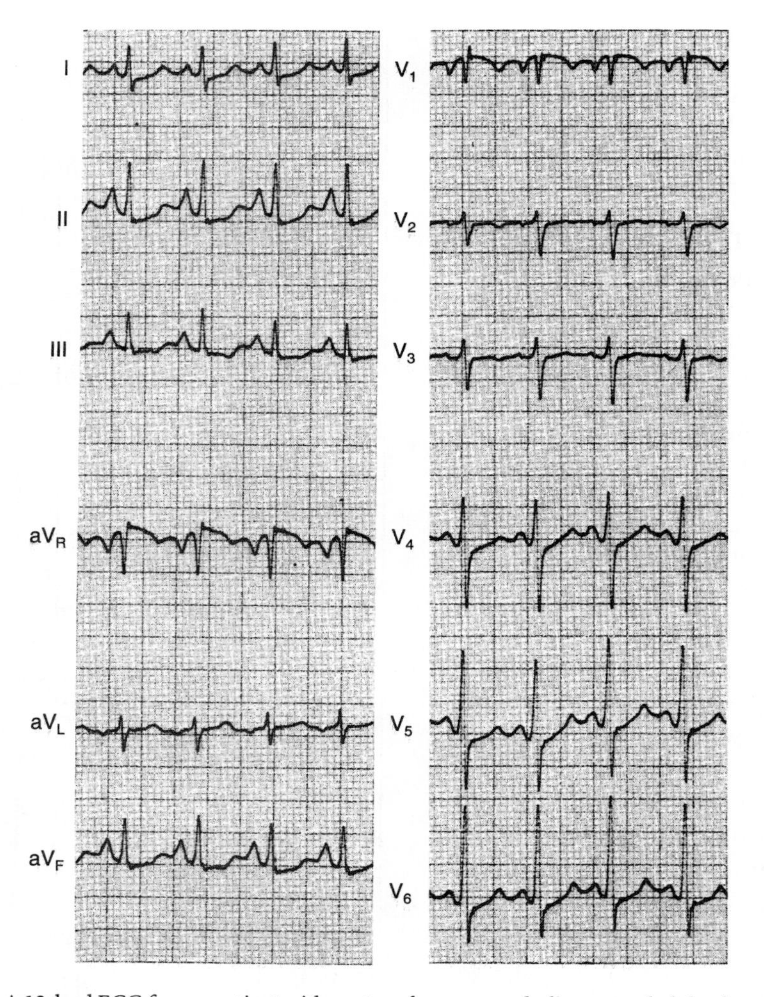

FIG. 29-13. A 12-lead ECG from a patient with acute pulmonary embolism recorded the day of the acute event. Note the sinus tachycardia; prominent P waves in leads II, III, and aV_F; S wave in lead I; incomplete RBBB (V_1); and ST segment elevation in leads V_1 and aV_R. (Courtesy Hein J.J. Wellens, MD, Maastricht, The Netherlands.)

event. Sinus tachycardia and the emergence of an incomplete RBBB pattern (terminal r wave is beginning to appear) in lead V_1 can be seen. There is also ST segment elevation in leads V_1 and aV_R and clockwise rotation of the heart. The transitional zone is between V_4 and V_5, whereas the normal location is V_3 to V_4. The tall P wave in lead II (P pulmonale) is another reflection of the acute dilation of the right side of the heart.

Emphysema. In emphysema the following ECG changes are noted:

- Low voltage
- QRS axis: posterior and superior
- P wave axis: to the right of +60 degrees in the frontal plane
- Associated right ventricular hypertrophy: rSR′ pattern in right precordial leads, a slurred S wave in left precordial leads, and a prominent R wave in lead aV_R

RIGHT ATRIAL HYPERTROPHY

In right atrial hypertrophy the major P vector is directed anteriorly. Right atrial hypertrophy results from congenital heart disease, tricuspid valve disease, and pulmonary hypertension.

ECG Recognition

- Tall, wide P waves in the limb leads and right precordial leads
- Often associated with RVH

Fig. 29-14 is the ECG of a patient with right atrial hypertrophy caused by tricuspid valve disease (or

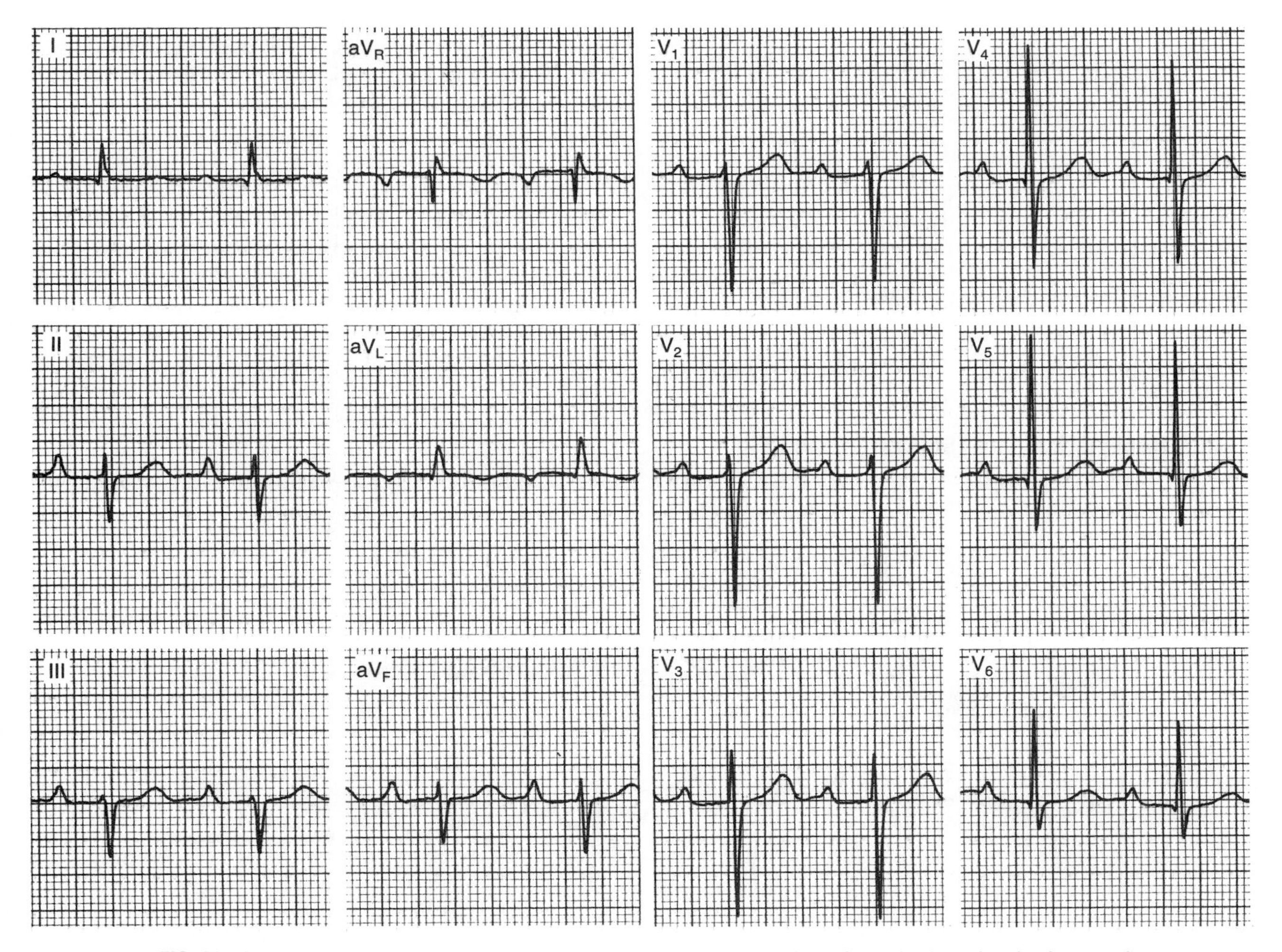

FIG. 29-14. Right atrial hypertrophy. There are tall, wide P waves in the inferior leads and in leads V_4 and V_5. (Courtesy Ara G. Tilkian, MD, Van Nuys, Calif.)

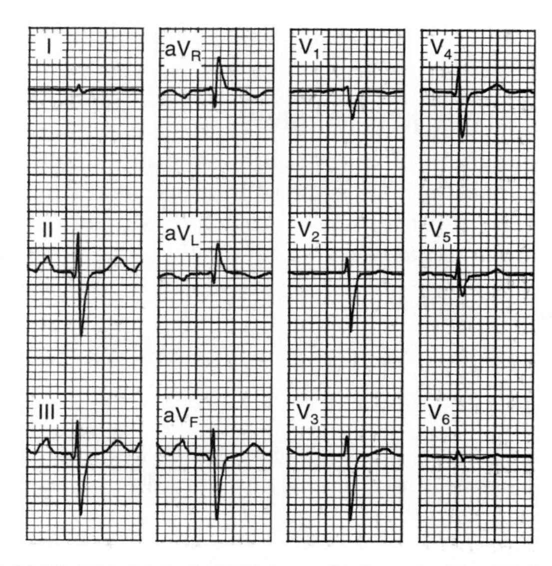

FIG. 29-15. This 12-lead ECG shows the "standard lead I sign" of emphysema. Note the isoelectric P, QRS, and T in lead I. (Courtesy G.V. Reddy, MD, Wilmington, Del.)

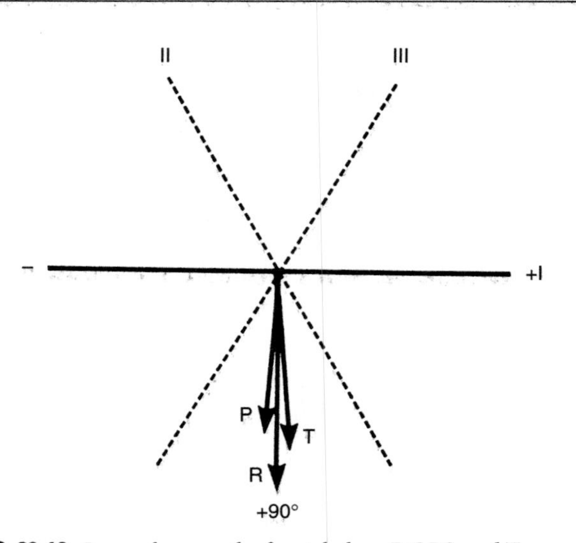

FIG. 29-16. In emphysema the frontal plane P, QRS, and T axes are all commonly directed at or about +90 degrees or perpendicular to the axis of lead I. (From Schamroth L: *Electrocardiographic excursions*, Oxford, 1975, Blackwell Scientific Publications.)

pulmonary hypertension). The tall, wide P waves in the inferior leads and right precordial leads are evident.

CHRONIC COR PULMONALE—EMPHYSEMA

Chronic cor pulmonale is secondary to intrinsic pulmonary disease, such as emphysema (rather than secondary to left ventricular failure).

ECG Recognition: The "Standard Lead I Sign"

- **Lead I:** The ECG in Fig. 29-15 shows the classic, almost pathognomonic "standard lead I sign" of emphysema (i.e., very low QRS voltage with isoelectric P, QRS, and T). This occurs because in emphysema the frontal plane P, QRS, and T axes are all commonly directed at or about +90 degrees or perpendicular to the axis of lead I (Fig. 29-16).[12,13]
- **P pulmonale:** Tall, peaked P waves are seen in leads I, II, II, and aV_F.
- **P axis:** The frontal plane P axis is usually directed at +90 degrees.
- **PR segment:** Sloping, as seen in Fig. 29-17, caused by the atrial repolarization wave (Ta wave).

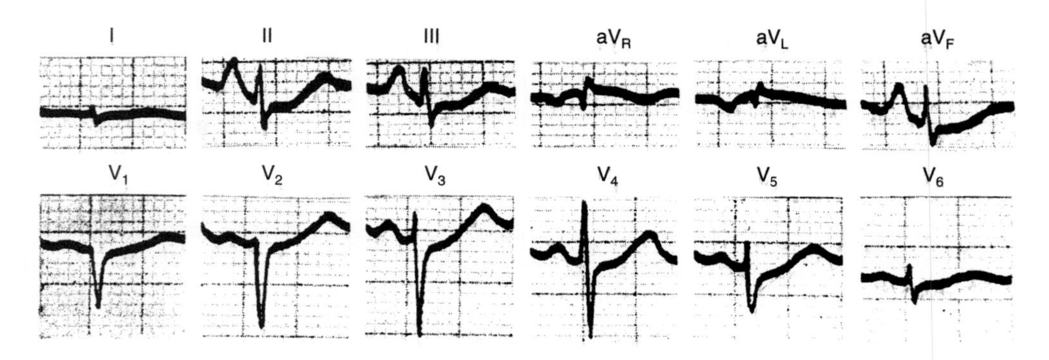

FIG. 29-17. A 12-lead ECG with the typical features of emphysema. Note the isoelectric P, QRS, and T in lead I and the sloping PR segment in leads II, III, and aV_F. The patient was a 54-year-old man who had smoked 40 cigarettes a day for at least 30 years. (From Schamroth L: *An introduction to electrocardiography*, ed 5, Oxford, 1976, Blackwell Scientific Publications.)

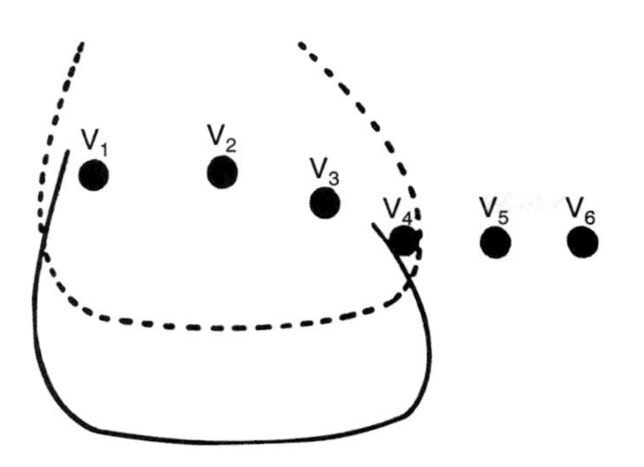

FIG. 29-18. Diagram illustrating the effect of the downward displacement of the heart in emphysema (i.e., the precordial electrodes become oriented to the upper or basal regions of the heart). (From Schamroth L: *An introduction to electrocardiography,* ed 5, Oxford, 1976, Blackwell Scientific Publications.)

- **QRS and T:** Generally low voltage, especially in the frontal plane leads and leads V_5 and V_6.

Mechanism

The ECG signs of chronic cor pulmonale are caused by right ventricular dominance, downward displacement of the diaphragm and heart (Fig. 29-18), and the voluminous lungs resulting in poor electrical transmission to the surface leads.

SUMMARY

Cardiac hypertrophy results from an increase in myocardial muscle mass, usually from valvular stenosis or hypertension. Atrial dilatation is the response of the thin-walled atria to volume overload and pressure overload. Ventricular dilatation is the response of the ventricle to volume (diastolic) overload. Ventricular hypertrophy is the response of the ventricle to pressure (systolic) overload. Cardiac enlargement includes dilatation and hypertrophy, which frequently occur together and are an expression of the heart's compensation to maximize cardiac output under stress.

REFERENCES

1. Yanowitz FG: *Left ventricular hypertrophy,* Salt Lake City, Utah, 2001, The Alan E Lindsay ECG Learning Center in Cyberspace, Lesson VIII.
2. Norman JE Jr, Levy D, Campbell G et al: Improved detection of echocardiographic left ventricular hypertrophy using a new electrocardiographic algorithm, *J Am Coll Cardiol* 21:1680, 1993.
3. Frohlich ED, Apstein C, Chobanian AV et al: The heart in hypertension, *N Engl J Med* 327:998, 1992.
4. The fifth report of the Joint National Committee on Detection, Evaluation, and Treatment of High Blood Pressure, *Arch Intern Med* 153:154, 1993.
5. Vakili BA, Okin PM, Devereux RB: Prognostic implications of left ventricular hypertrophy, *Am Heart J* 141:334-341, 2001.
6. Wachtell K, Rokkedal J, Bella JN: Effect of electrocardiographic left ventricular hypertrophy on left ventricular systolic function in systemic hypertension (The LIFE Study). Losartan Intervention for Endpoint, *Am J Cardiol* 87:54-60, 2001.
7. Perings C, Hennersdorf M, Vester EG et al: [Arrhythmia risk in left ventricular hypertrophy], *Kardiol* 89(Suppl 3):36-43, 2000.
8. Reddy GV: Personal communication, December 2001.
9. Khan IA, Shaw IS: Pseudo ventricular hypertrophy and pseudo myocardial infarction in Wolff-Parkinson-White syndrome, *Am J Emerg Med* 18:807-809, 2000.
10. Brady WJ: Electrocardiographic left ventricular hypertrophy in chest pain patients: differentiation from acute coronary ischemic events, *Am J Emerg Med* 16:692-696, 199.
11. Chou TC, Knilans TK: *Electrocardiography in clinical practice, adult and pediatric,* ed 4, Philadelphia, 1996, WB Saunders.
12. Schamroth L: *Electrocardiographic excursions,* Oxford, 1975, Blackwell Scientific Publishers.
13. Schamroth L: *An introduction to electrocardiography,* ed 5, Oxford, 1976, Blackwell Scientific Publishers.

CHAPTER 30

Expert ECG Evaluation: The Diagnostic Leads

THE BEGINNINGS OF IN-HOSPITAL CARDIAC MONITORING

Single-lead electrocardiogram (ECG) monitoring was initially introduced into hospitals in the early 1960s because of the discovery that lidocaine suppressed premature ventricular contractions and ventricular tachycardia (VT). With new hope for improving the outcome of patients with acute myocardial infarction (MI), hospitals across the country began establishing a special room for monitoring these patients and called it the *coronary care unit* (CCU). For the first time nurses were expected to make a diagnosis in response to the ECG signal seen on a simple, unprocessed oscilloscope (a light that immediately faded as it wrote). They were further expected to administer intravenous lidocaine immediately when indicated and appropriately cardiovert or defibrillate, acting upon standing orders. These unprecedented expectations of nurses spawned the need for inservice education. Before this time only the physician or laboratory technician entered a vein and the diagnosis of arrhythmias was unquestionably the physician's domain.

During this infant period of ECG monitoring, the only lead used was lead II. The simple justification for this choice, strangely enough, was that the P wave was bigger in that lead, even though recognition of ventricular ectopy and not the P wave was the objective of early CCUs. Realizing this, Dr. Henry Marriott modified the abandoned bipolar CL lead by placing the positive chest (C) electrode in the V_1 position and, for patient comfort, moved the negative left arm electrode (L)to the left upper chest, giving us MCL_1 (modified CL in the V_1 position), a bipolar lead simulating the unipolar V_1 and the best lead in which to distinguish aberrancy from ectopy.[1]

TABLE 30-1 Best Monitoring Leads

Digitalis Intoxication II and/or V_1	PSVT I, II, III, V_1, and V_6	Unstable Angina V_2 or V_3 Without Pain	VT V_1, V_2, and V_6	High-Risk MI Inferior V_{4R}; Anterior V_1, I, and II
II: P in atrial tachycardia If no conduction or atrial fibrillation: V_1 J F	CMT P AVNRT II P V_1 P	Critical proximal LAD stenosis (Wellens syndrome) 12-lead with pain ST ↑ V_1 and aV_R ST ↓ 8 other leads Left main or three-vessel coronary artery disease	**V_1 positive complex** V_1 V_1 need V_6 R: S < 1 **V_1 negative complex** V_1 and V_2	**Inferior** V_{4R} Proximal RCA occlusion RV MI **Anterior** or

AVNRT, Atrioventricular nodal reentry tachycardia; *CMT,* circus movement tachycardia; *LAD,* left anterior descending (coronary artery); *MI,* myocardial infarction; *PSVT,* premature supraventricular tachycardia; *RCA,* right coronary artery; *RV,* right ventricular; *VT,* ventricular tachycardia.

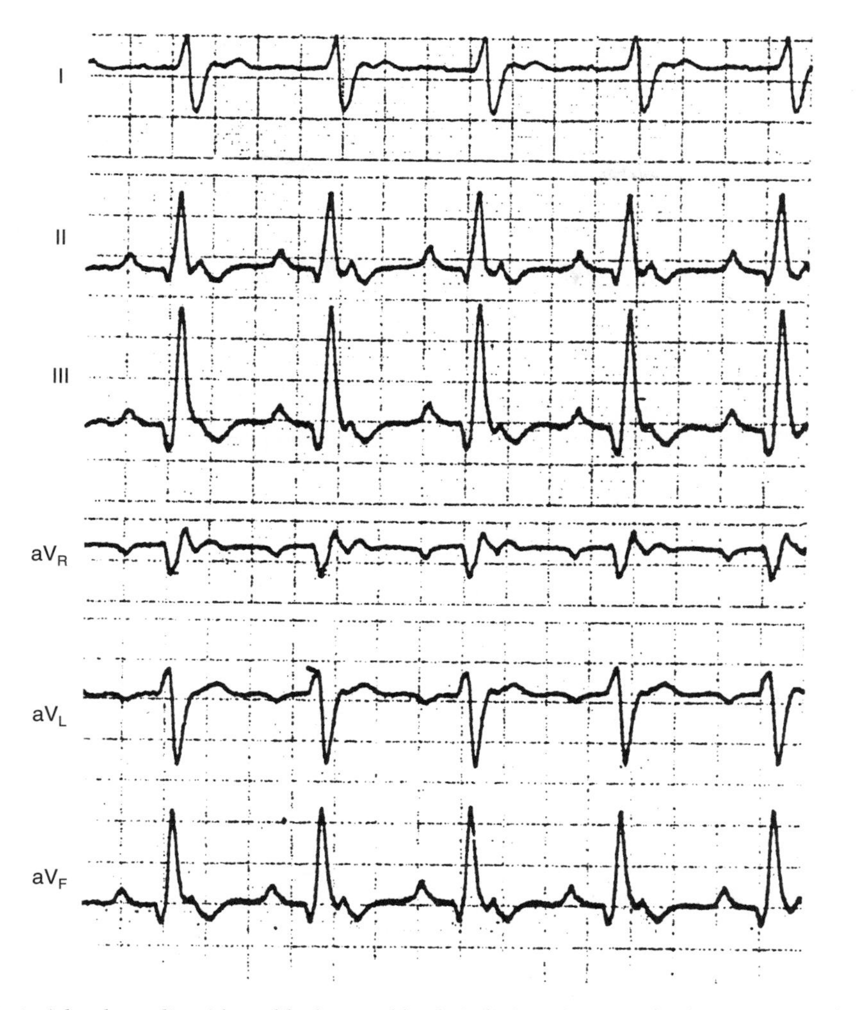

FIG. 30-1. Atrial tachycardia with 2:1 block caused by digitalis intoxication. The diagnosis is made in lead II because of the positive P wave, as well as the ventriculophasic PP intervals. The focus in this clinical setting is close to the sinus node, producing P′ waves that are positive in lead II and similar in appearance to sinus P waves. (Courtesy Hein J.J. Wellens, MD, The Netherlands.)

Today, multiple leads are used in many areas within the hospital and in emergency mobile units not only to recognize ventricular ectopy but also to do the following:

- Recognize the onset of ischemia
- Diagnose drug toxicity
- Diagnose congenital and acquired long QT syndrome
- Identify the culprit artery in acute MI
- Evaluate the risk and the amount of myocardium affected in MI
- Locate the accessory pathways
- Identify critical proximal left anterior descending (LAD) coronary stenosis in patients with unstable angina and thus avoid myocardial damage

The ideal monitoring protocol would be to monitor in all 12 leads continuously. However, because this is not possible with the equipment available in most hospitals in the United States, this chapter will supply you with the minimal ECG lead requirements for monitoring patients in the acute settings of digitalis intoxication, paroxysmal supraventricular tachycardia (PSVT), broad QRS tachycardia, unstable angina, and acute MI. Table 30-1 is a summary of the best monitoring leads and the ECG patterns seen in them.

DIGITALIS INTOXICATION

Best Leads: II and V_1

Lead II. Use lead II initially to look for P waves that resemble sinus P waves during atrial tachycardia. In Fig. 30-1 the ectopic P waves in this atrial tachycardia closely resemble sinus P waves; as would be expected in digitalis toxicity (p. 201).

Lead V_1 or MCL_1. If there is no conduction, you will need lead V_1 (or MCL_1) to determine whether the ventricular rhythm is junctional (rS pattern) or fascicular VT (rSR′ pattern). Chapter 15 discusses mechanism, ECG recognition, and treatment of digitalis intoxication. In cases of fascicular VT there will also be axis deviation, which can be determined by looking at leads I and II (right axis: I negative, II positive; left axis: I positive, II negative).

Best Diagnostic Leads in Fig. 30-2

Step 1. Look in lead II for P waves and atrioventricular (AV) conduction. The absence of P waves and the regular

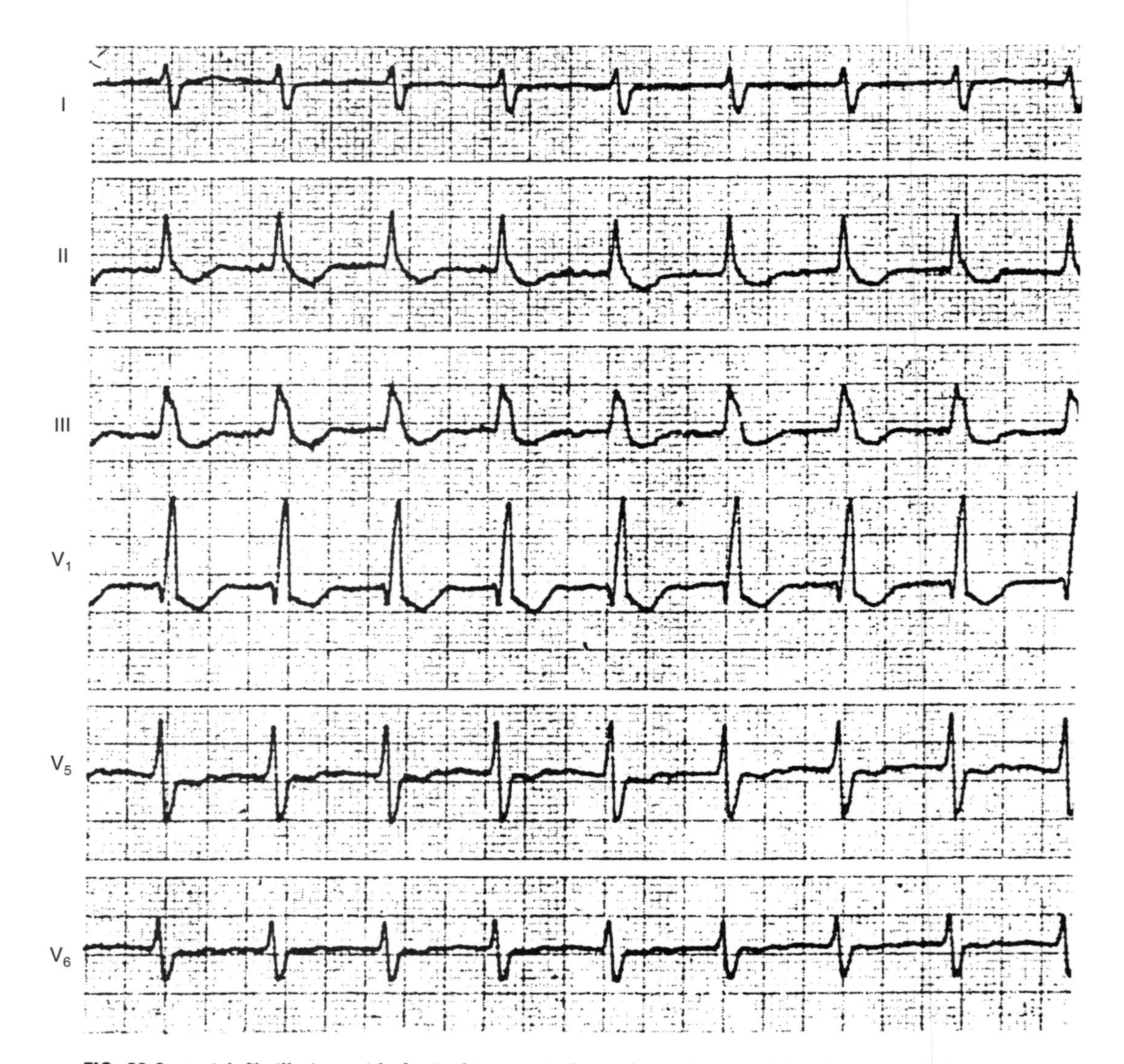

FIG. 30-2. Atrial fibrillation with fascicular ventricular tachycardia caused by digitalis intoxication. The diagnosis of atrial fibrillation is made in lead II (no P waves); absence of atrioventricular conduction is also noted in this lead (regular ventricular response). Lead V_1 shows a fascicular ventricular tachycardia (rSR′ pattern). Leads I and II show right axis deviation, indicating a left anterior fascicular focus (see Chapter 17). (Courtesy Hein J.J. Wellens, MD, The Netherlands.)

ventricular rhythm indicate atrial fibrillation with no conduction to the ventricles (AV dissociation).

Step 2. The ventricular rhythm must now be identified by evaluating the QRS morphology in V_1; an rS would indicate a junctional tachycardia, whereas an rSR′ would indicate a fascicular rhythm. The digitalis effect on the ST segment is noted (sagging ST segment). The diagnosis is atrial fibrillation with fascicular VT, and an emergency response is called for. The digitalis is discontinued and a hemodynamic assessment will determine the course of action.

Step 3. No further ECG analysis is necessary for the emergency care of this patient.

PAROXYSMAL SUPRAVENTRICULAR TACHYCARDIA

Best Leads: I, II, III, V_1, and V_6

In patients admitted for evaluation of PSVT the ability to monitor the patient on leads I, II, III, and V_1 is most efficacious because P waves are not seen in all leads. If only a single lead is available for monitoring, it can be any one of the four mentioned. However, keep in mind that the purpose of the patient's presence in your unit is to record the PSVT at least in the important leads. Everyone on the unit must be alert to this responsibility and ready to hook up additional leads when indicated. Often, patients with PSVT have been symptomatic for many years without ever having the rhythm recorded and a diagnosis made. It is extremely helpful to the electrophysiologist to have a record of the clinical arrhythmia. After you are successful in recording the problem arrhythmia, look in the leads mentioned for the ECG signs of AV nodal reentry tachycardia (P′ wave buried or distorting the end of the QRS) and circus movement tachycardia using an accessory pathway (P′ wave immediately following the QRS; if QRS alternans is present it is a helpful clue because it is most common in this type of PSVT).

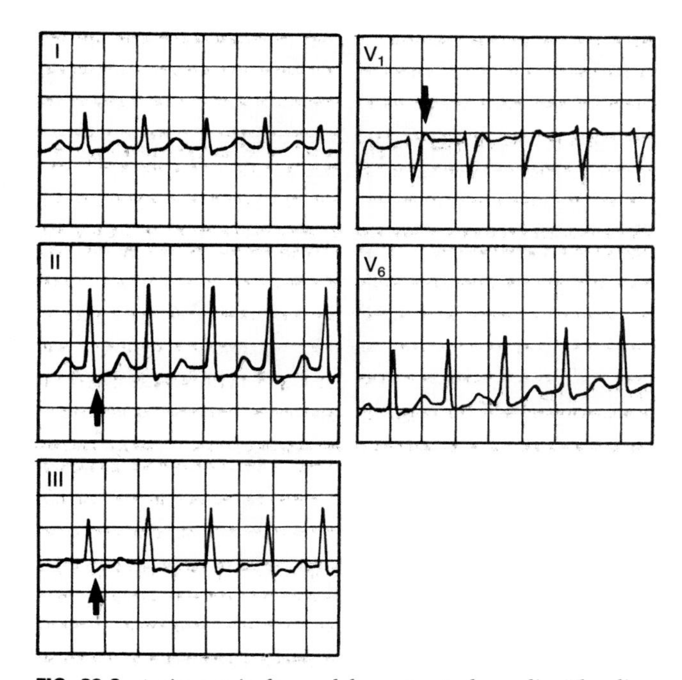

FIG. 30-3. Atrioventricular nodal reentry tachycardia. The diagnosis is made because the P′ wave is seen distorting the terminal QRS forces in leads V_1 (pseudo-r) and leads II, III, and V_6 (pseudo-S) *(arrows).*

Best Diagnostic Leads in Fig. 30-3

Step 1. Because AV nodal reentry tachycardia is the most common cause of PSVT, look in the five leads recorded for a P′ distorting the end of the QRS. This is seen in all leads. It is half-buried in the QRS, so you are only seeing the end of it. In leads I, II, III, and V_6 it is a pseudo–s wave *(arrows)*. In V_1 it is a pseudo–r wave *(arrow)*, diagnostic of AV nodal reentry tachycardia.

Best Diagnostic Leads in Fig. 30-4

Step 1. Using the same approach, in all leads available the end of the QRS is found to be without distortion. However, upon examining the ST segment, a P′ wave is seen in leads I, II, and III immediately after the QRS. In circus movement tachycardia using an accessory

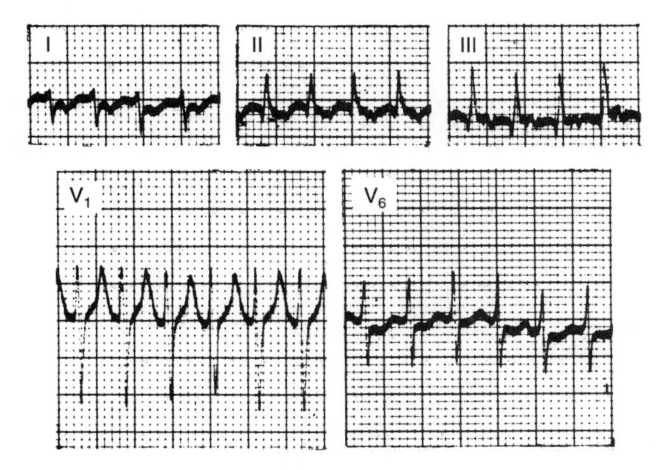

FIG. 30-4. Circus movement tachycardia. The diagnosis is made quickly because the P′ waves follow the QRS complexes and are separate from them. The P′ waves are clearly seen in the limb leads. In this case, a negative P′ wave in lead I is diagnostic of a left-sided accessory pathway. (From Marriott HJL, Conover M: *Advanced concepts in arrhythmias,* ed 2, St Louis, 1989, Mosby.)

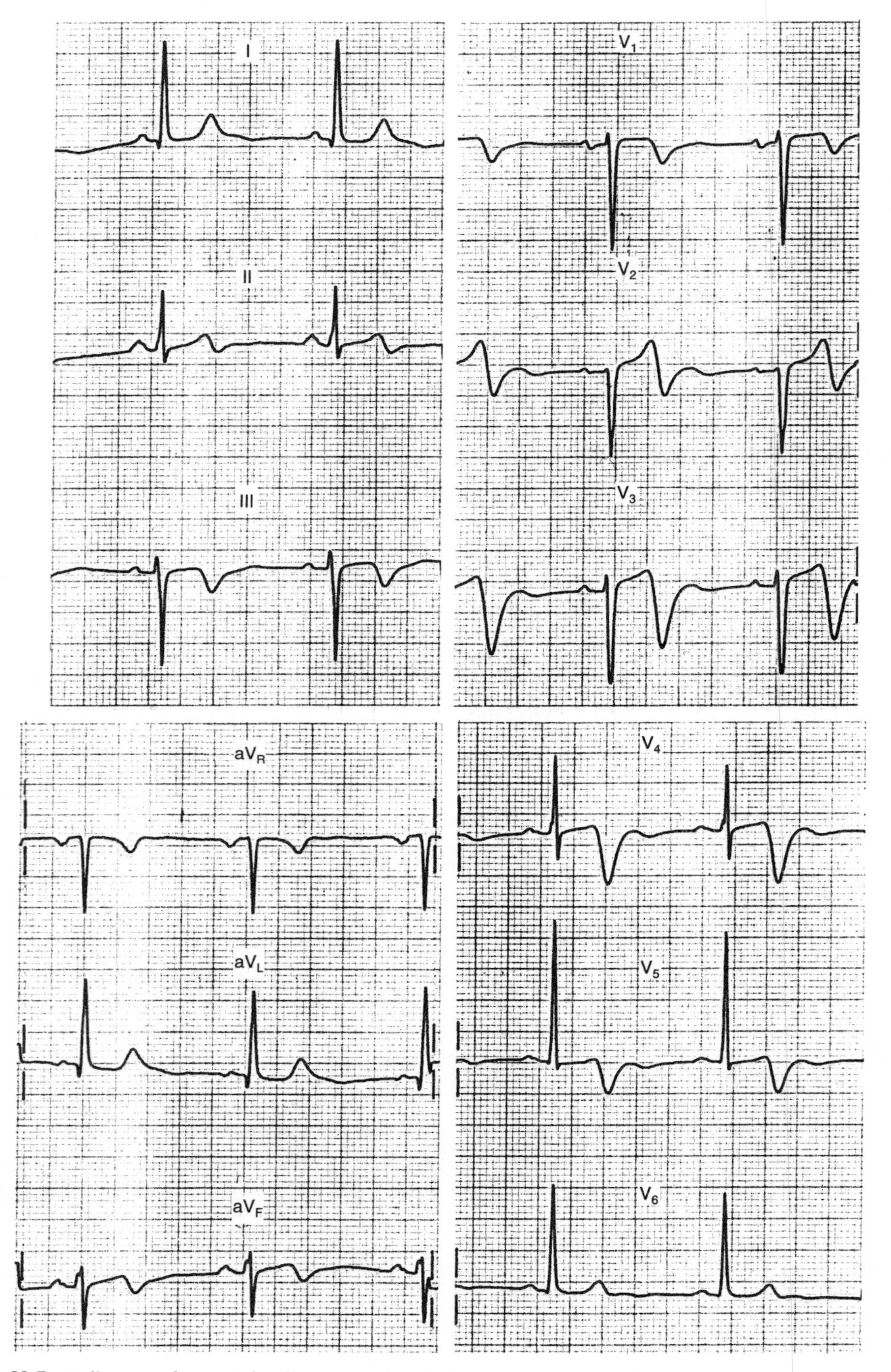

FIG. 30-5. Wellens syndrome. The diagnosis of critical proximal left anterior descending coronary artery stenosis is made because of the presence of unstable angina, along with the typical ST-T changes in leads V_2 and V_3, as described in Chapter 22 and noted here. When the patient is without pain, there is progressive deep, symmetric inversion of the T wave with little or no ST segment elevation or elevation in creatine kinase level and there is no loss of precordial R waves. (Courtesy Jerilyn Briten, RN, Nampa, Idaho.)

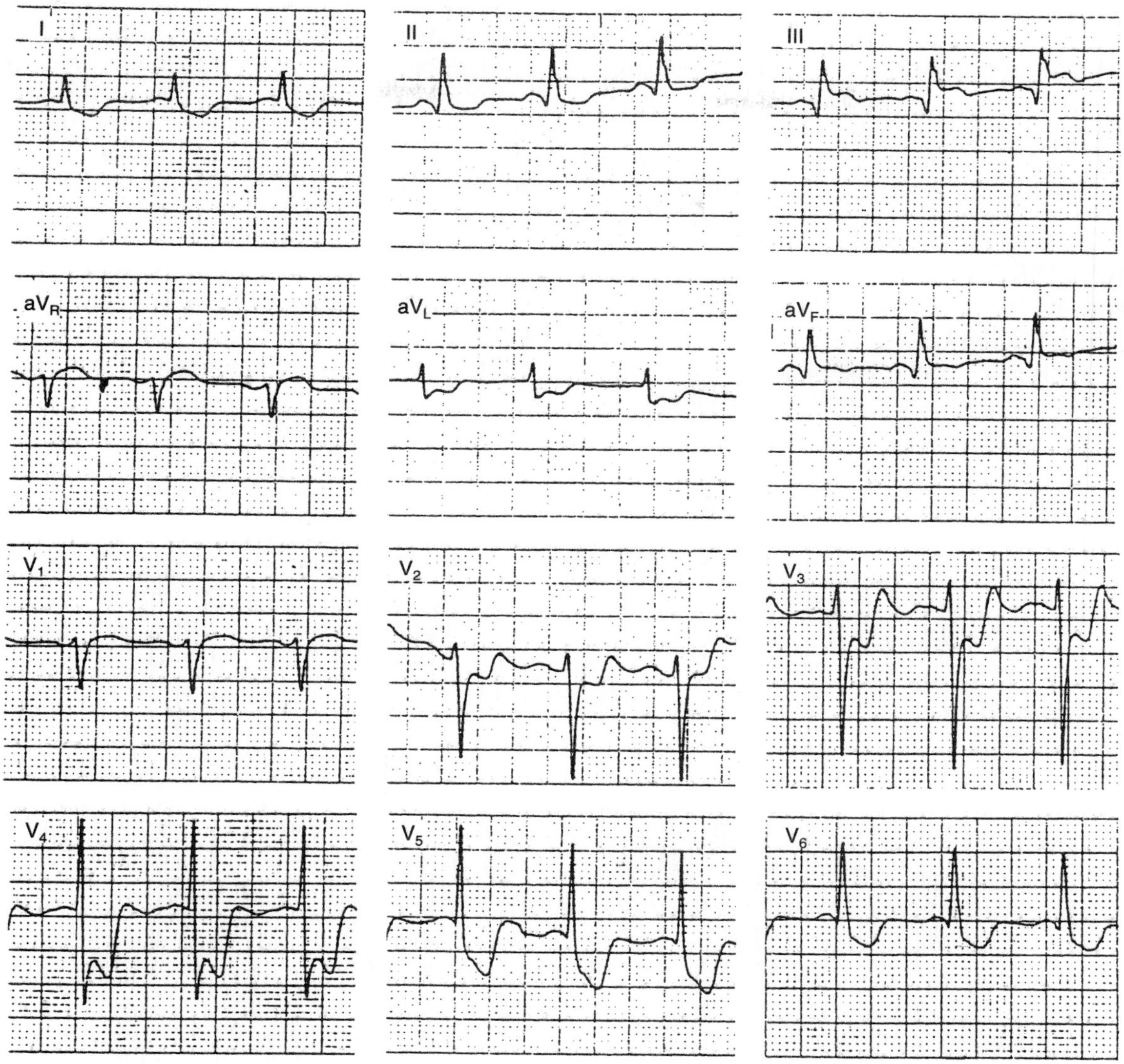
I
II
III
aVR
aVL
aVF
V1
V2
V3
V4
V5
V6

FIG. 30-6. The ECG pattern in left main stem disease. The diagnosis is made because of the presence of unstable angina, the ST elevation in leads V_1 and aV_R, and the ST depression in the remainder of the precordial leads and in I, II, and aV_L. (From Wellens HJJ, Conover M: *The ECG in emergency decision making,* Philadelphia, 1992, WB Saunders.)

pathway the P′ wave is separate from the QRS 100% of the time.

Step 2. Although no further examination is necessary to make the diagnosis, additional information can be obtained by evaluating the polarity of the P′ wave in lead I. It is negative, an indication of a left lateral accessory pathway. The QRS axis is right because the patient is only 3 weeks old.

UNSTABLE ANGINA

Diagnostic Leads: V_2 and V_3 Without Pain, All 12 Leads During Pain

For patients with unstable angina, leads V_2 and V_3 are minimal requirements to assess for Wellens syndrome (see Chapter 22). When the patient is without pain (Fig. 30-5) the indication of critical proximal LAD coronary artery stenosis is progressive, deep, symmetric T wave inversion in leads V_2 and V_3. Although the T wave inversion is not necessarily limited to these two leads, they are the diagnostic leads. This typical T wave inversion in patients with unstable angina is a sign of reperfusion in the pain-free periods.

During pain a 12-lead ECG is required to assess for left main or three-vessel coronary artery disease (Fig. 30-6). The diagnosis is made because of the ST elevation in leads V_1 and aV_R and the ST depression in the remainder of the precordial leads and leads I, II, and aV_L.

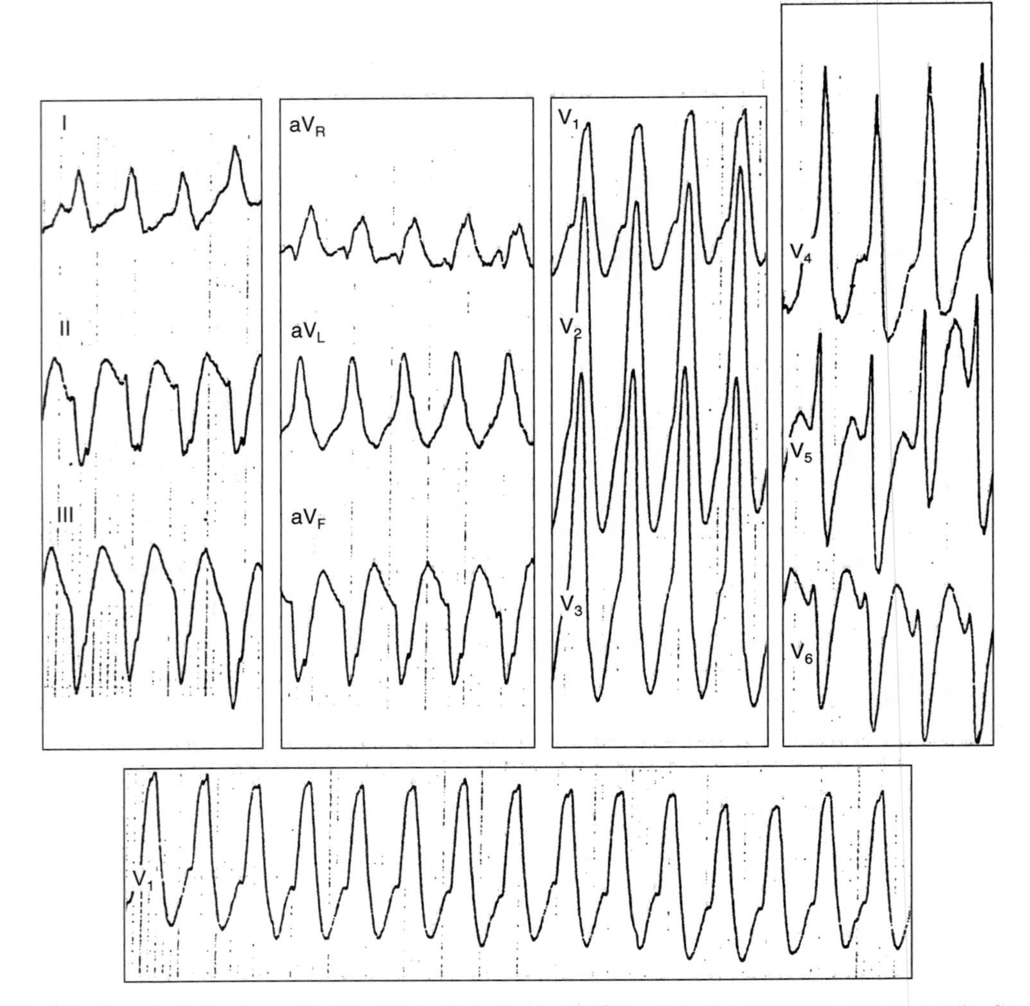

FIG. 30-7. Ventricular tachycardia. The diagnosis is made quickly because the QRS in lead V_1 is a monophasic R wave. Other clues are the deep S wave in V_6, QRS duration greater than 0.14 second, left axis deviation, and signs of atrioventricular dissociation in lead I.

BROAD QRS TACHYCARDIA

Best Leads: V_1, V_2, and V_6

The recording of lead V_1 is mandatory in broad QRS tachycardia. If V_1 looks like VT, it is VT unless there is an accessory pathway. If V_1 looks like supraventricular tachycardia (SVT) and is negative, you must also see V_2. If V_1 and V_2 have inconclusive patterns, lead V_6 is also necessary.

Best Lead in Fig. 30-7

Step 1. Look at V_1 and note that the ventricular complex is positive. Therefore a monophasic, biphasic, or taller left rabbit ear configuration would indicate VT. The ventricular complex in V_1 is a monophasic R wave—VT. No further evaluation is necessary in this emergency setting. The left axis deviation supports VT but is not diagnostic.

Best Lead in Fig. 30-8

Step 1. Look at V_1 and note that the ventricular complex is negative. Therefore V_1 and V_2 are evaluated for a broad R, slurred S downstroke, and delayed S nadir. There is a slurred S downstroke in V_1 and in V_2 there is a broad R and delayed S nadir. This is VT and no further evaluation is necessary in this emergency setting. The diagnostic sign of AV dissociation is noted (i.e., independent P waves in almost every lead).

Best Lead in Fig. 30-9

Step 1. Look at V_1 and note that the ventricular complex is negative. Therefore V_1 and V_2 are evaluated for a broad R, slurred S downstroke, and delayed S nadir, none of which are found. The downstroke of the QS wave is swift and clean and the nadir early. There is no q wave in V_6. This is supraventricular tachycardia with left bundle branch block aberration.

Chapter 14 discusses aberration versus ectopy and will help to make you aware of the tachycardias that do not follow the rules. That is, the SVTs that look like VTs use an accessory pathway to activate the ventricles. The VTs that look like SVTs are fascicular VT, idiopathic VT, and bundle branch reentry VT.

HIGH-RISK MI

Inferior MI High-Risk Assessment: Lead V_{4R}; Anterior MI High-Risk Assessment: Leads I, II, and V_1

The diagnosis of acute MI and the decisions regarding thrombolysis are made from the 12-lead ECG and lead V_{4R}.

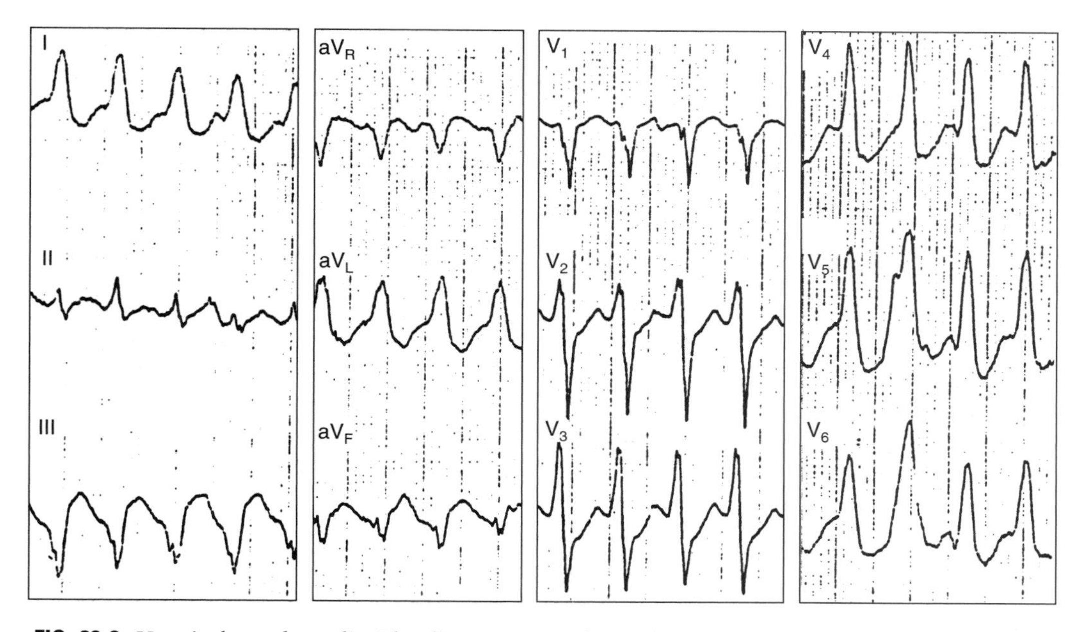

FIG. 30-8. Ventricular tachycardia. The diagnosis is made quickly because of the broad R wave, slurred S downstroke in lead V_1, broad R wave in lead V_2, and delayed S nadir in leads V_1 and V_2. Other clues are signs of atrioventricular dissociation in many leads, a fusion beat (lead II), and QRS duration greater than 0.14 second. It was only necessary, however, to spot the slurred downstroke in lead V_1 to make the diagnosis.

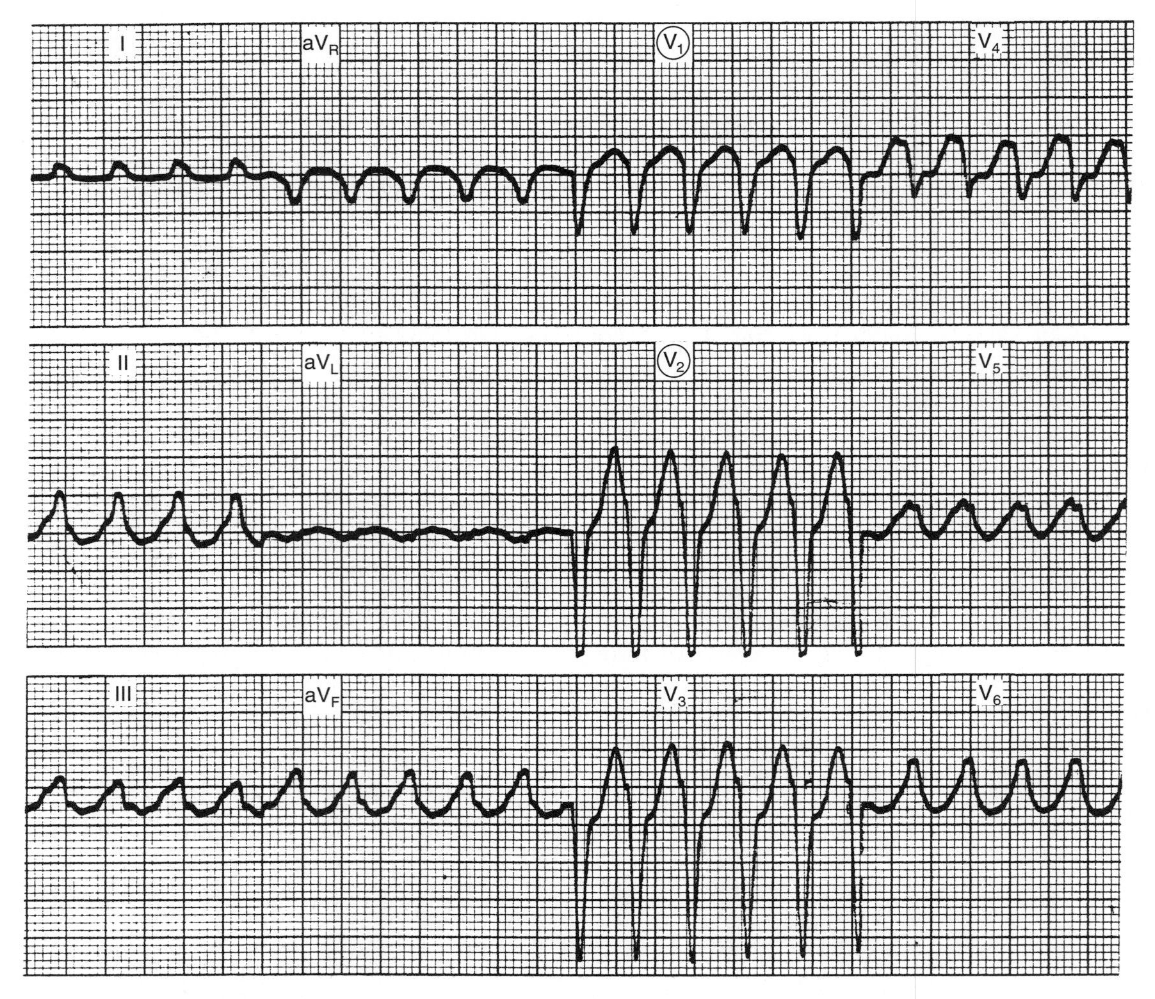

FIG. 30-9. Supraventricular tachycardia. The diagnosis is made because in leads V_1 and V_2 the S wave has a clean, swift downstroke. Both leads are necessary for this diagnosis because in some cases lead V_1 can look like supraventricular tachycardia, but V_2 will confirm that the condition is ventricular tachycardia.

Best Lead in Fig. 30-10

High-risk patients with acute inferior wall infarction are of course identified by the height of the ST segment. However, risk can also be evaluated in lead V_{4R}. Note the elevated ST segment in that lead indicating proximal right coronary artery occlusion, right ventricular infarction, the chances of developing high-grade AV block, and the need for aggressive therapy. The culprit right coronary artery is also identified because the ST segment elevation in lead III is higher than it is in lead II. The opposite configuration would indicate a circumflex occlusion (ST in II higher than ST in III).

Best Lead in Fig. 30-11

High-risk patients with acute anterior wall infarction have a proximal LAD occlusion and develop bundle branch block and hemiblock. Leads V_1, I, and II are necessary to access the intraventricular conduction system. Bundle branch block with anterior MI can be diagnosed in lead V_1 because of the QR pattern. The left anterior hemiblock is recognized in leads I and II because of the left axis deviation.

SUMMARY

This chapter emphasized the importance of monitoring each patient as an individual according to his or her

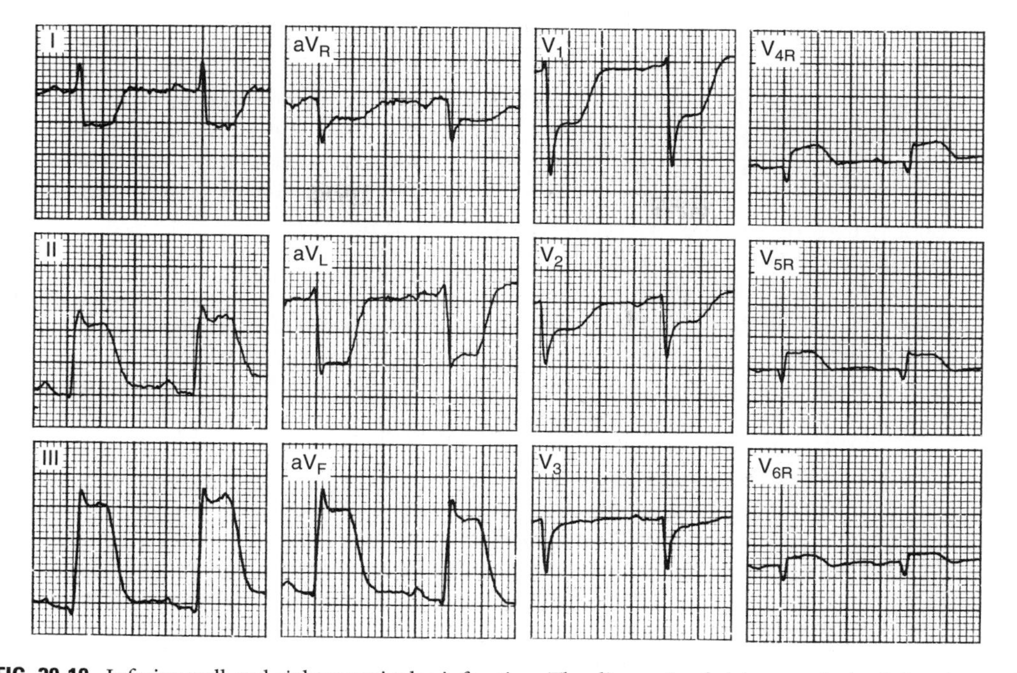

FIG. 30-10. Inferior wall and right ventricular infarction. The diagnosis of right ventricular infarction and high risk in a patient is made because of the elevated ST segment in lead V_{4R} (see Chapter 24).

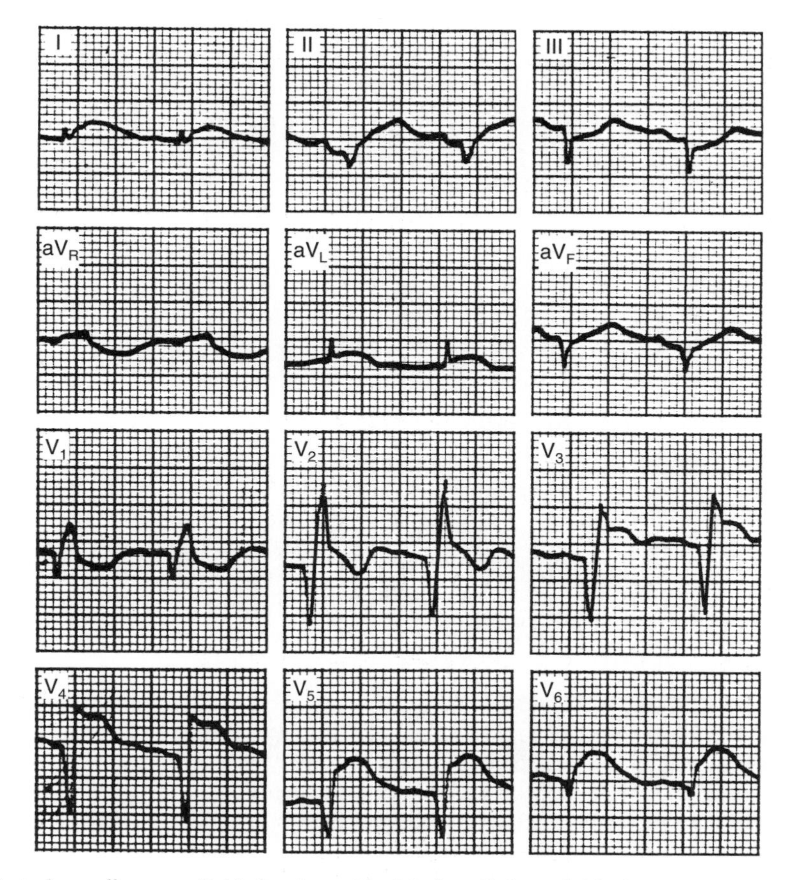

FIG. 30-11. Anterior wall myocardial infarction with right bundle branch block (V_1) and left anterior hemiblock (leads I and II) identify a high-risk patient. (Courtesy Peg McKnight, RN, Las Vegas, Nev.)

clinical situation. A designated single monitoring lead for a critical care unit is not logical and may even place the patient in jeopardy. A case in point is that of the patient with unstable angina. To monitor such a patient on lead II or V_1 denies that patient an early diagnosis of critical proximal stenosis of the anterior descending left coronary artery and may even be the cause of that patient losing cardiac muscle. Patients who are taking digoxin can easily slip into toxicity, especially the elderly, if the staff members are not aware of and practicing correct monitoring techniques. When a patient is admitted for PSVT, he or she is there for one purpose only—that the arrhythmia may be recorded in enough of the best possible leads so that a diagnosis can be made.

REFERENCE

1. Sandler JA, Marriott HJL: The differential morphology of anomalous ventricular complexes of RBBB type in lead V1; ventricular ectopy versus aberration, *Circulation* 31:551, 1965.

CHAPTER 31

In-Hospital Cardiac Monitoring

Mary G. Adams-Hamoda, RN, PhD • Michele M. Pelter, RN, PhD

There are two basic types of in-hospital monitoring strategies: hardwired bedside and telemetry. Typically the emergency department and critical care units monitor patients with bedside monitors that are wired with 3, 5, or 10 wires (Fig. 31-1).

As patients require less intensive nursing care, such as in transitional units, telemetry is often invoked as the choice of monitoring.[1] Through radio transmission, patients are no longer attached to a monitor but rather have the freedom to ambulate through their respective units (Fig. 31-2). With the current advancements in computers, most electrocardiographic (ECG) monitors are extremely sophisticated. Computer algorithms have the capacity to monitor both arrhythmias and myocardial ischemia.

Today, in-hospital cardiac monitoring is used to evaluate patients for arrhythmias and myocardial ischemia. Specifically, in-hospital cardiac monitoring is used to assess patients for life-threatening arrhythmias, symptomatic arrhythmias requiring intervention, and determine the success of both pharmacologic and invasive cardiac interventions. Because of the abrupt and transient nature of these conditions in-hospital cardiac monitoring must be maintained continuously so that immediate action can be taken to interrupt arrhythmias and halt the progression of myocardial ischemia into infarction.

CURRENT RECOMMENDATIONS FOR IN-HOSPITAL CARDIAC MONITORING

In light of the expanded use of cardiac monitoring, recommended guidelines have been developed for arrhythmia[2] and ischemia monitoring,[3] with the intent of

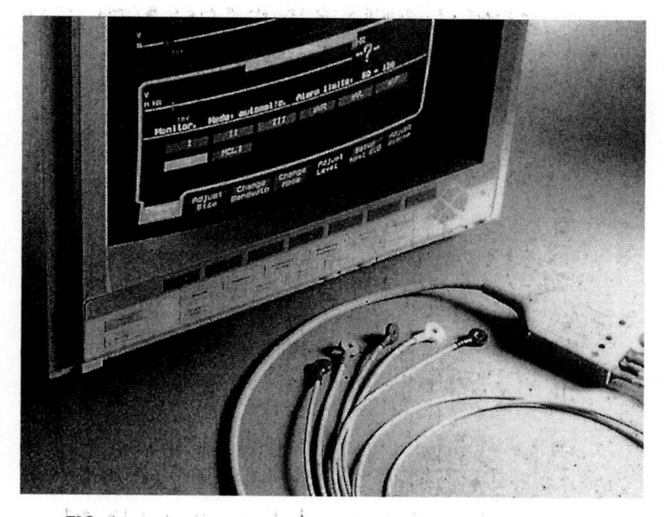

FIG. 31-1. Typical critical care bedside monitoring unit.

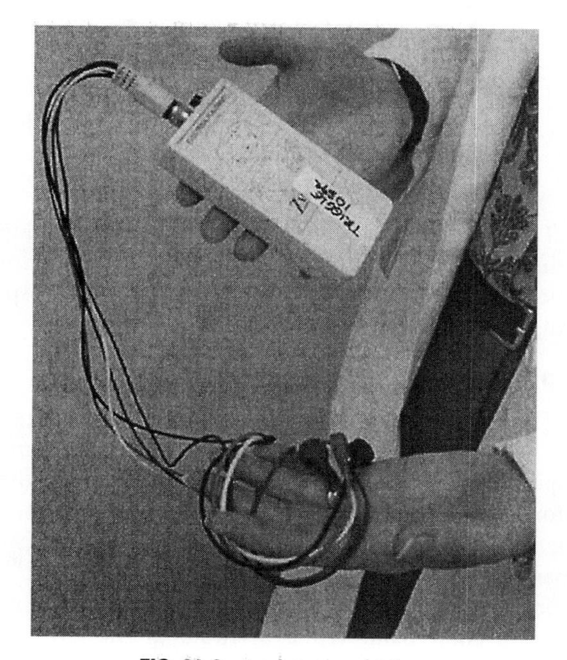

FIG. 31-2. A telemetry device.

assisting clinicians apply and use this technology in the hospital setting. The following section of this chapter will review the current guidelines for cardiac monitoring and offer clinical examples of the use of cardiac monitoring in select situations.

Cardiac Monitoring

The current recommendations for in-hospital cardiac monitoring were developed for the American College of Cardiology by the Emergency Cardiac Care (ACC-ECC) Committee.[2] The following are general guidelines that should be considered for in-hospital cardiac monitoring in all hospital settings:

1. There must be adequate human surveillance of the cardiac monitors 24 hours a day by medical, nursing, or paramedic personnel (monitor watchers) who are trained and qualified in ECG recognition of clinically significant cardiac rhythm disturbances.
2. Appropriately trained physicians and nurses must be responsible for decisions regarding the use of cardiac monitoring in each hospital clinical area using cardiac monitoring. These individuals must determine the following: (a) the specific degree of monitoring surveillance that is appropriate for each clinical area, (b) the minimal qualifications and training for the personnel assigned to watch the monitors, (c) the specific protocols and procedures for responding to arrhythmias, and (d) the unit-specific standards for initiation and discontinuation of cardiac monitoring.
3. Adequate numbers of physicians and nurses must be present or immediately available to treat life-threatening arrhythmias and myocardial ischemia.

The following rating system (Box 31-1) was developed by the ACC-ECC Committee to classify the more common clinical conditions for the application of in-hospital cardiac monitoring.

Patient Scenario

The following scenario is an example of how the guidelines might be useful when deciding how to implement in-hospital cardiac monitoring. A 72-year-old man with a history of hypertension, elevated cholesterol, diabetes, and a significant smoking history presented to the emergency department declaring, "I am having a heart attack." He reports that while he was walking, he developed acute nonradiating chest pain. While in route to the emergency department, his systolic blood pressure was 70 mm Hg, thus a dopamine drip and transcutaneous pacing was initiated. Figure 31-3 shows his presenting 12-lead ECG. Given the patient's history and presenting 12-lead ECG and using the ACC-ECG Guidelines, what class of monitoring does this patient require?

Given that the patient's presenting 12-lead ECG shows third-degree heart block with possible accelerated fascicular rhythm at 48 beats/min, class I monitoring would be recommended per the ACC-ECC guidelines. Importantly, cardiac monitoring is indicated in most if not all patients in class I. Specifically, in this example, the patient had essentially been at risk for cardiac arrest because of symptomatic third-degree heart block.

Myocardial Ischemia

The following guidelines were developed by the ST-Segment Monitoring Practice Guideline International Working Group that was composed of key physician and nurse scientists who were identified as leaders in the field of ST segment monitoring for detection of myocardial ischemia.[3] The general equipment requirements for ST segment monitoring include the following:

1. Installation of ST segment software into the bedside monitor, which is capable of providing computerized ST segment measurements, full disclosure of stored information, and ST "trends"
2. Capability to monitor all 12 ECG leads because the sensitivity of ischemia detection is substantially lowered when only 1, 2, or 3 ECG leads are available

Table 31-1 lists the patients who should have ST monitoring, its potential benefits, and the recommended time frames for monitoring during hospitalization.

Patient Scenario

The following patient scenario is an example of how the above guidelines might be useful when implementing in-hospital cardiac monitoring for detection of myocardial ischemia. A 78-year-old male patient presented to the emergency department with complaints of chest pain at rest. The patient had no prior history of acute coronary syndromes.

However, given the nature of his chest pain (rest angina) and the presence of coronary risk factors, which included diabetes and smoking, the patient was admitted to the telemetry unit with the diagnosis of chest pain to rule out MI. According to the ST segment guidelines, this patient might benefit from ST segment monitoring (chest pain that prompts a visit to the emergency department), and V_2 or V_3 should be evaluated for progressive sym-

BOX 31-1. ACC-ECC Committee Rating System for In-Hospital Cardiac Monitoring

Class I: Cardiac monitoring is indicated in most, if not all, patients in this group.

1. During first 72 hours in patients with suspected, and subsequently proven acute myocardial infarction (MI). This period should be extended for patients with clinically important complications (i.e., significant arrhythmias, conduction defects, silent ischemia, cardiac failure, or shock).
2. Patients with acute MI, as evidenced by clinical or electrocardiogram criteria, or both.
3. During and in the early convalescence (72 hours) after cardiac surgery, to include patients who receive an automated internal cardiac defibrillator (ICD). This period should be extended for patients with clinically important complications (i.e., significant arrhythmias, conduction defects, silent ischemia, cardiac failure, or shock).
4. Patients who have been resuscitated from cardiac arrest or in those patients at risk for cardiac arrest (i.e., Mobitz type II heart block, third degree heart block, new-onset, high-degree heart block, runs of sustained ventricular tachycardia, or new onset intraventricular conduction defects [fascicular, bundle branch block]).
5. Critically ill medical or surgical patients requiring care in an intensive care unit.
6. During the acute hospital phase in patients with drug toxicity with drugs known or suspected of having cardiac toxicity (e.g., tricyclic antidepressants, phenothiazines, digitalis, antiarrhythmic drugs).
7. During the acute phase of myocarditis.
8. During the initiation and loading of type I or type III antiarrhythmic drugs for potential life-threatening arrhythmias.
9. Immediately after percutaneous coronary interventions in patients with complications as a result of the procedure (i.e., coronary artery dissection or thrombosis).
10. Patients with unstable angina.
11. Patients with high-risk coronary lesions (e.g., left main coronary artery disease or its equivalent).
12. Patients treated for arrhythmias by catheter ablation.

Class II: Cardiac monitoring may be of benefit in some patients but is not essential in all.

1. Patients with acute MI after day 3, particularly those at higher risk for ventricular arrhythmias (i.e., anterior MI, conduction defects).
2. Patients with potentially lethal arrhythmias for several days after initial control of the arrhythmia.
3. Patients with underlying conditions who are deemed at risk for cardiac arrest, respiratory arrest, or development of hypotension.
4. Patients with non–life-threatening arrhythmias (e.g., atrial fibrillation) who are at risk for proarrhythmic effects of type I or type III antiarrhythmic agents.
5. Patients with symptomatic paroxysmal tachycardia or bradycardia.
6. During the acute phase of pericarditis.
7. Patients with unexplained syncope or other neurologic signs or symptoms that might be due to arrhythmias.
8. Immediately after percutaneous coronary intervention.
9. During the first 48 to 72 hours after insertion of permanent pacemaker.
10. Patients in stable condition after cardiac surgery.

Class III: Cardiac monitoring is not indicated because the patient's risk of a serious arrhythmia or the therapeutic benefit is low.

1. Postoperative patients at low risk (i.e., young patients after relatively simple surgeries).
2. Obstetric patients, unless such patients develop cardiac conditions defined in class I or II.
3. Patients with terminal illnesses who are not candidates for treatment of arrhythmias that may be detected.
4. Patients undergoing routine, uncomplicated coronary angiography.
5. Patients with chronic, stable atrial fibrillation.
6. Patients with stable asymptomatic premature ventricular contractions or nonsustained ventricular tachycardia who are hospitalized for conditions other than cardiac or hemodynamic compromise.
7. Patients with underlying cardiac diseases who have been stabilized and who have had no arrhythmias on 3 consecutive days during monitoring.

metric T wave inversion for Wellens syndrome. Fig. 31-4 presents three ECGs obtained during continuous 12-lead monitoring. This patient, who was initially admitted with unstable angina and a normal troponin I level, subsequently "ruled-in" for MI with positive troponin I level, which is not surprising given the ST segment deviation observed during ECG monitoring. ST segment monitoring proved invaluable in this scenario because the

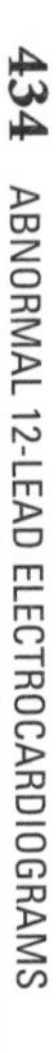

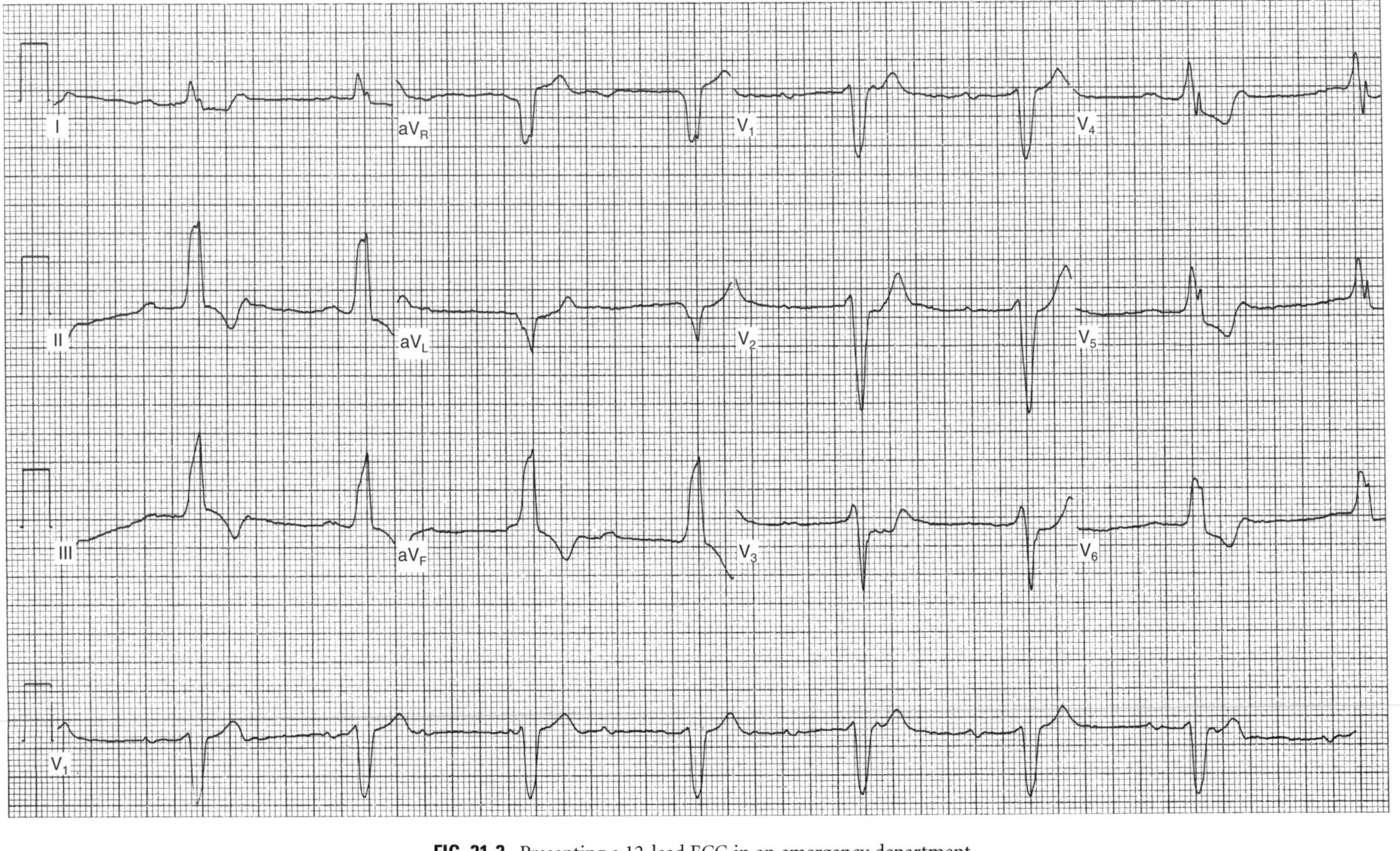

FIG. 31-3. Presenting a 12-lead ECG in an emergency department.

TABLE 31-1 ST Monitoring Patients, Goals, and Time Frames

Patients	Goals	Time Frame for Monitoring
HIGHEST PRIORITY PATIENTS		
Patients with either ST elevation or non–ST elevation acute MI	Assess patency of infarct-related artery Assess how much myocardium is at risk Detect recurrent ischemia and extension of acute MI Distinguish cardiac from noncardiac chest pain Assess readiness for early mobilization and possible discharge from hospital	24-48 hr
Patients with unstable angina	Assess efficacy of antianginal regiments Detect clinically silent ischemia Confirm ischemia in patients with atypical symptoms or in patients with the inability to communicate symptoms	24-48 hr
PATIENTS WHO MAY BENEFIT FROM ST SEGMENT MONITORING		
Patients presenting with chest pain that prompts a visit to the emergency department	Detect ischemia in patients with nondiagnostic ECG in whom ST segment elevation develops Monitor in V_2 or V_3 for critical proximal LAD stenosis (see Chapter 22)	8-12 hr
After percutaneous coronary interventions	Detect abrupt reocclusion Distinguish ischemic from nonischemic coronary vessel "stretch" chest pain Detect clinically silent reocclusion in cardiac transplant patients with reduced sensory discrimination	6-12 hr
Patient with coronary vasospasm	Confirm diagnosis by observing transient ST segment elevation Assess efficacy of therapy with calcium channel blockers	24-48 hr
After coronary artery bypass graft surgery	Distinguish incisional from ischemic chest pain Assess graft patency or reocclusion Determine whether postoperative cardiac arrhythmias have an ischemic origin	24-48 hr
Patients undergoing noncardiac surgery	Detect ischemia in patients at risk for cardiac complications (e.g., patients with left ventricular hypertrophy, coronary or vascular disease, or other cardiac risk factors)	24-48 hr

MI, Myocardial infarction; *ECG,* electrocardiogram.

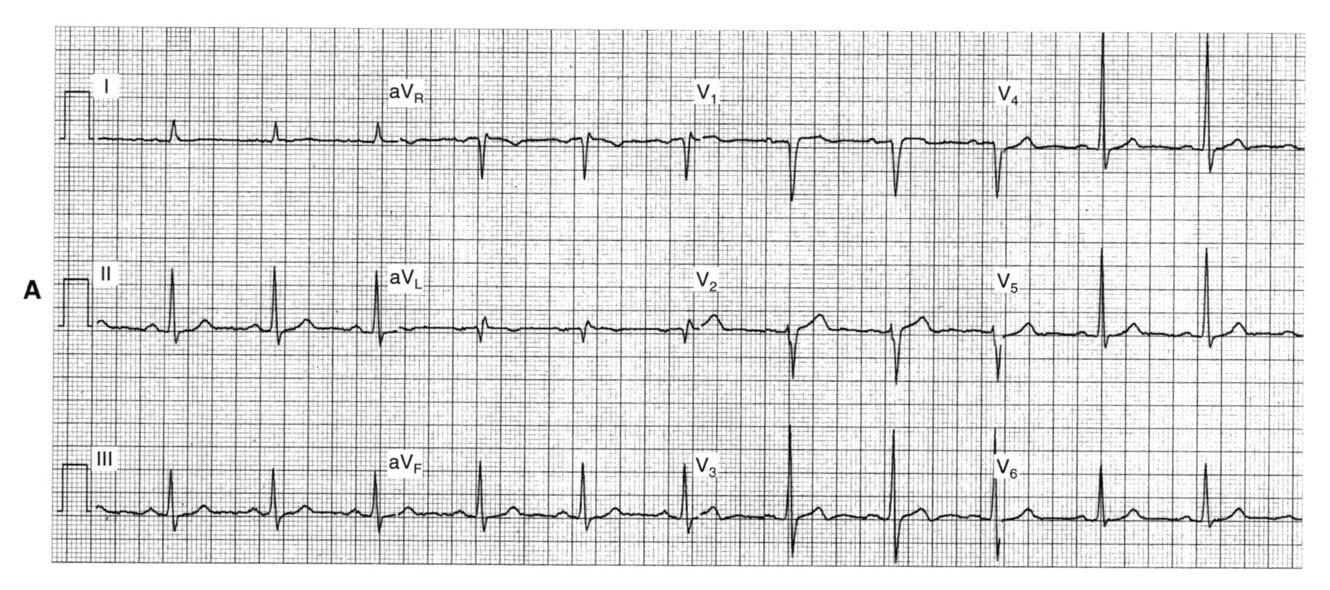

FIG. 31-4. A, 6:40 AM: Baseline 12-lead ECG.

Continued

ischemia was transient and the patient did not complain of chest pain during the ischemic event. The patient's angiogram later revealed a nearly 100% occluded left anterior descending coronary artery, which was treated with a coronary stent.

RECOMMENDED IN-HOSPITAL CARDIAC MONITORING LEADS

Use of all 12 ECG leads is ideal for in-hospital cardiac monitoring. This is essential for applying diagnostic criteria for distinguishing among arrhythmias. In addition, all 12 ECG leads are necessary for accurate detection and characterization of myocardial ischemia. However, when all 12 ECG leads are not available clinicians must choose the best 1- or 2-lead combination offered by the bedside ECG monitor.

Best Leads for Detection of Myocardial Ischemia

The goal of ST segment monitoring is detection ongoing or transient myocardial ischemia. Because ischemia is regional rather than global, all 12 ECG leads are necessary for accurate detection of ischemia. However,

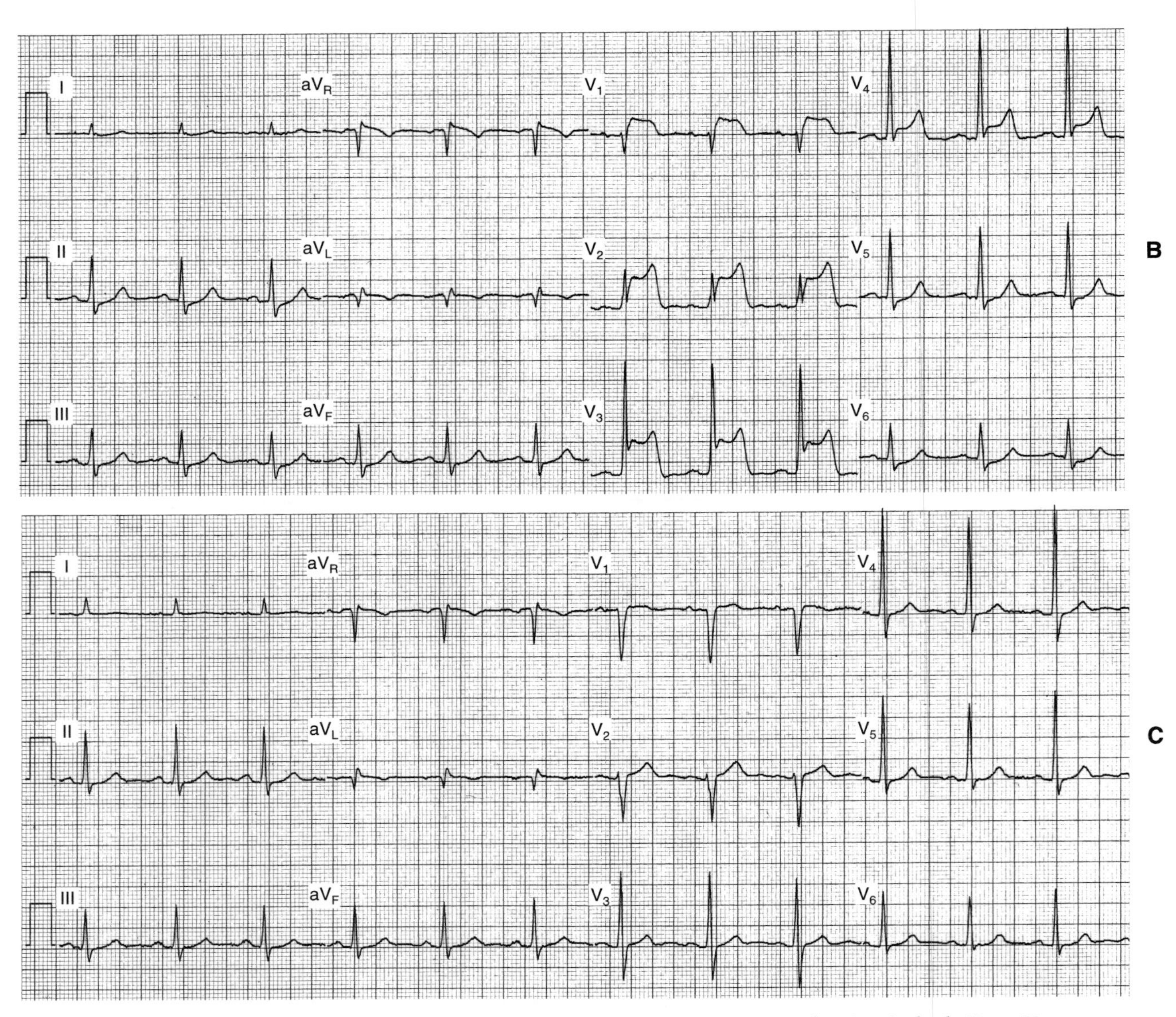

FIG. 31-4, cont'd. **B,** 7:00 AM: ST "event" 12-lead ECG. Note ST segment elevation in leads V_1 to V_4. Importantly, the patient did not complain of chest pain during this ischemic event. **C,** 7:30 AM: Return to baseline ST segment level. Note that ST segment elevation in leads V_1 to V_4 has returned to baseline level.

12-lead ECG monitoring is often not available, hence clinicians must chose the best one or two lead combination. To select the best lead thoughtful consideration regarding the myocardial zone at risk for ischemia should be considered. For instance, lead III is the best single lead for detecting ischemia in the inferior myocardial zone. This would be applicable to patients with acute coronary syndromes involving the right coronary artery. Whereas leads V_2 and V_3 are best for detecting ischemia in the anterior or posterior myocardial zone (Fig. 31-5). This would be applicable to patients with acute coronary syndrome involving the left anterior descending or the circumflex coronary artery.[4-6] Therefore, the best ECG lead combination for ischemia monitoring is lead III and V_2, or V_3.

LIMITATIONS OF ISCHEMIA MONITORING

Realistically, many significant forces hamper excellence in cardiac monitoring. Patton and Funk[7] surveyed 192 critical care nurses across America regarding the use of ST segment monitoring in coronary care units. The

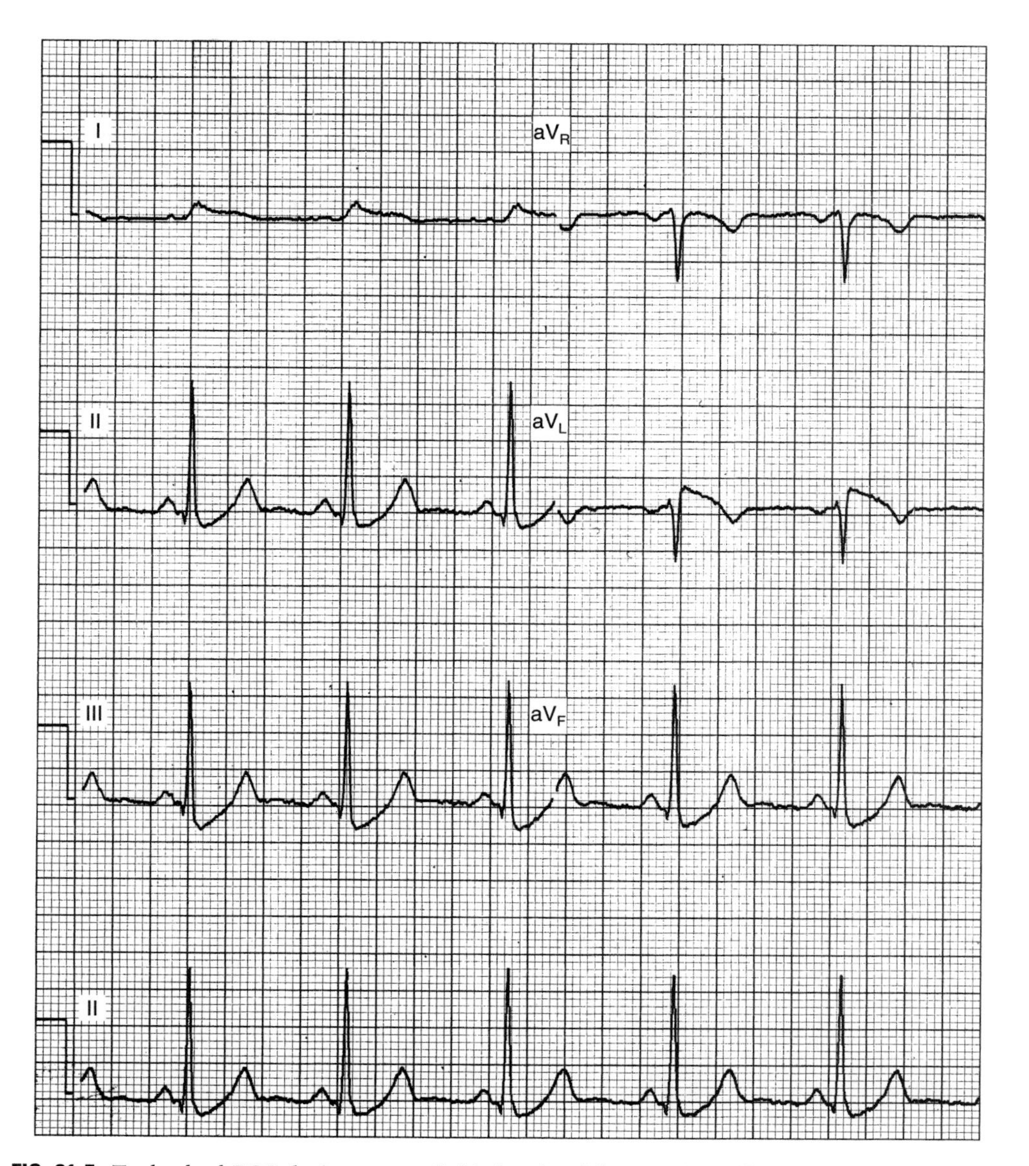

FIG. 31-5. Twelve-lead ECG during myocardial ischemia of the anterior wall. Lead V_4 shows the most ST segment deviation, whereas lead II remains insensitive.

Continued

study found that fewer than half of the nurses reported that ST segment monitoring was used in their respective critical care units. Of the nurses who did not use ST segment monitoring, the reason given most frequently was lack of interest on the part of the physician. Other common responses were lack of equipment or software, lack of staff expertise and too many false alarms. Not surprisingly, it is difficult for an engaged nurse to spend valuable time evaluating a physiologic parameter such as the ST segment because the physician may not use this information in clinical decision-making. Also, it is less than optimal for the same nurse to be inundated by false alarms. All of these forces make it difficult to ascend to excellence in cardiac monitoring.

Technical Problems

Of note, continuous in-hospital cardiac monitoring has the potential to produce substantial amounts of invalid data because of technical problems inherent in the recording and analysis of ECGs continuously recorded.

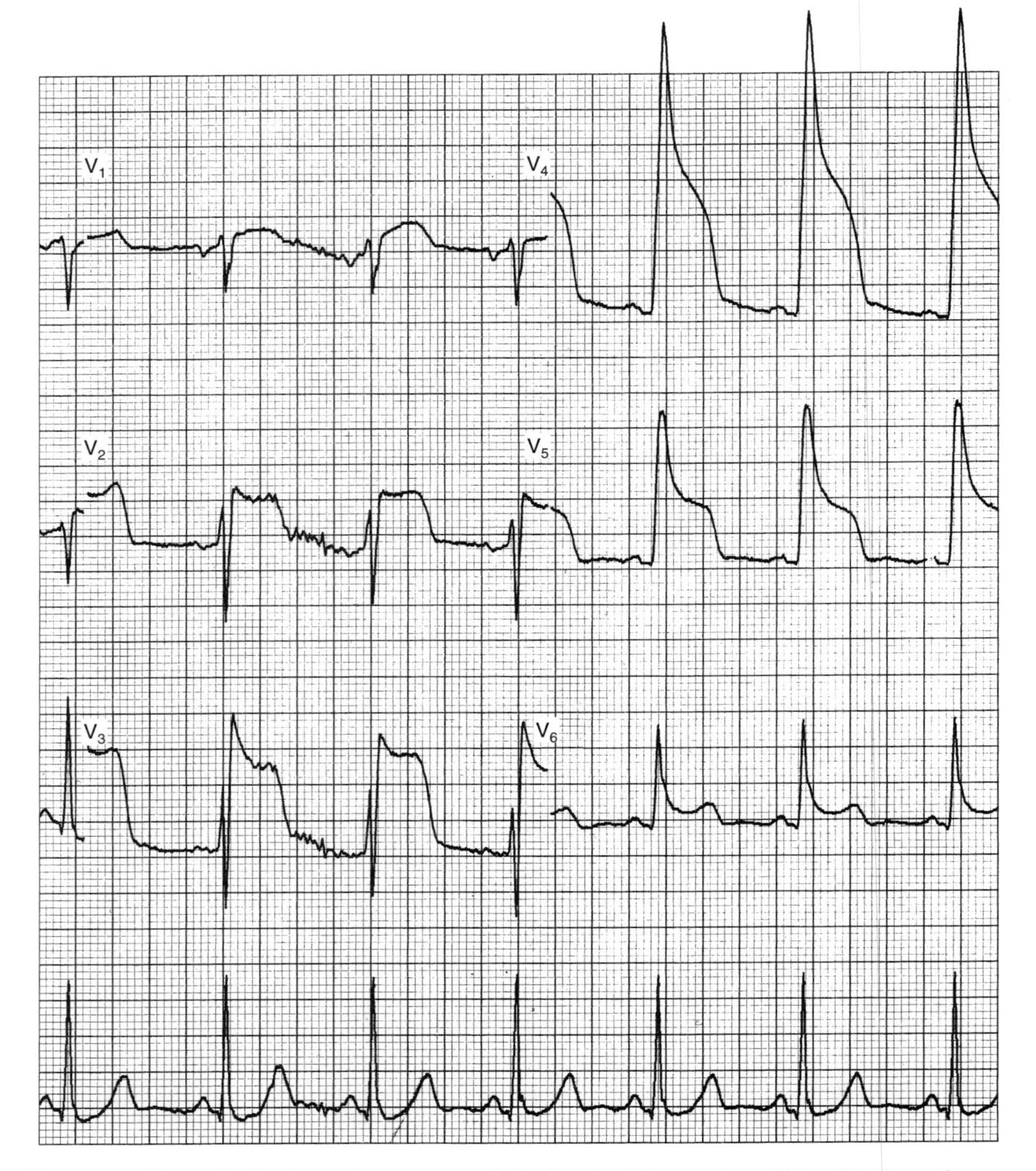

FIG. 31-5, cont'd. Twelve-lead ECG during myocardial ischemia of the anterior wall. Lead V_4 shows the most ST segment deviation, whereas lead II remains insensitive.

Thus interpretation of in-hospital cardiac rhythms, even when limited to arrhythmia and ischemia detection, is in certain respects more demanding than interpreting a standard 12-lead ECG. This is primarily because of noise interference from numerous sources that plague cardiac monitoring and that are essentially avoided with the standard 12-lead ECG, which is recorded while the patient is resting quietly in a supine position. Thus to some extent education, training, experience, and cognitive and technical skills are necessary for competent in-hospital ECG interpretation.

With prolonged monitoring, many patients manifest arrhythmias while monitored in the hospital that are not correlated with poor outcomes. These increase with patient age, cardiovascular disease, and the duration of monitoring. Conversely, arrhythmias that have prognostic importance for future cardiac events need to be recognized and reported promptly. Although in-hospital cardiac monitoring is noninvasive, inexpensive and with little risk, inappropriate interpretation and failure to correlate ECG findings with clinical assessment may result in serious iatrogenic complications. For example, interpretation of ST segment changes as ischemia in the absence of any supporting clinical signs or symptoms might result in an invasive cardiac catheterization.[8] In many cases, up to 40% of acute coronary syndrome patients have one or more false-positive alarms due to nonischemic conditions.[9] Therefore, it is important when reporting the significance of findings to appreciate the wide range of normal to avoid unnecessary interventions.

Computer Interpretation

Overall, the ECG is an important keystone for the care of patients with both cardiac and noncardiac disease. In recent years, computers have becomes an integral part of some ECG systems. Although computer programs provide accurate information regarding the heart rate, intervals, and electrical axis, all computer ECG interpretations-particularly interpretations of rhythm disturbances, ischemia or infarction-require careful overreading. Before an ECG can have proper diagnostic accuracy and clinical usefulness, the clinician is required to compare it with previous tracings and, particularly, to integrate clinical data that provides a differential diagnosis. Importantly, an incorrect ECG diagnosis can have significant undesirable medical and legal consequences.

False Alarms

As computer technology strives to improve algorithm sensitivity, specificity is often compromise, which can generate numerous false alarms. Fig. 31-6 shows a typical intensive care unit inundated by ECG tracings spieled out by the central algorithms monitor.

Recently, while continuously monitoring for myocardial ischemia, researchers reported the frequency and type of false-positive events.[9] Of 292 patients, 117 (40%) had one or more false-positive events for a total of 506 false-positive events. Specifically, the 506 false-positive events included 167 (36%) because of body positional change, 132 (26%) because of sudden increase in QRS complex/ST segment voltage, 96 (19%) because of transient arrhythmia or pacing, 80 (16%) because heart rate change in steeply sloped ST segment contours, 26 (5%) because of a noisy signal, and 5 (1%) because of lead misplacement. In addition, certain patient groups may not be candidates for currently available ST segment monitoring technology.[3]

Patients who should not have ST segment monitoring including those with (1) intermittent right bundle branch block (RBBB) or left bundle branch block (LBBB), (2) permanent LBBB, (3) ventricular pacemaker, (4) excessively noisy signal because of restlessness or confusion, or (5) wound dressing over the precordium. Figs. 31-7 and 31-8 illustrate why ST segment monitoring may not be appropriate in some patients.

Fig. 31-8 illustrates false-positive ST segment changes because of a heart rate change in a patient with permanent LBBB. The left ECG complex shows a QRS complex in lead V_1 of a patient with LBBB, illustrating the typical secondary repolarization abnormality of the ST segment,

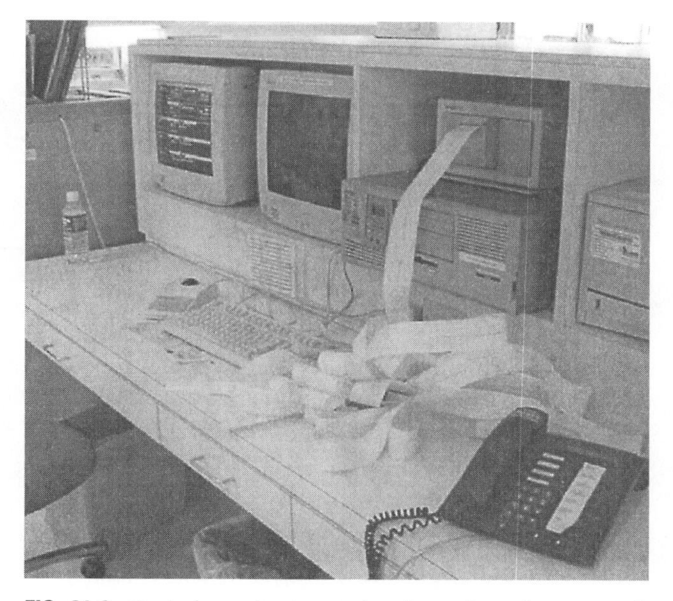

FIG. 31-6. Central monitoring station in an intensive care unit with numerous ECG tracing generated from patient alarms.

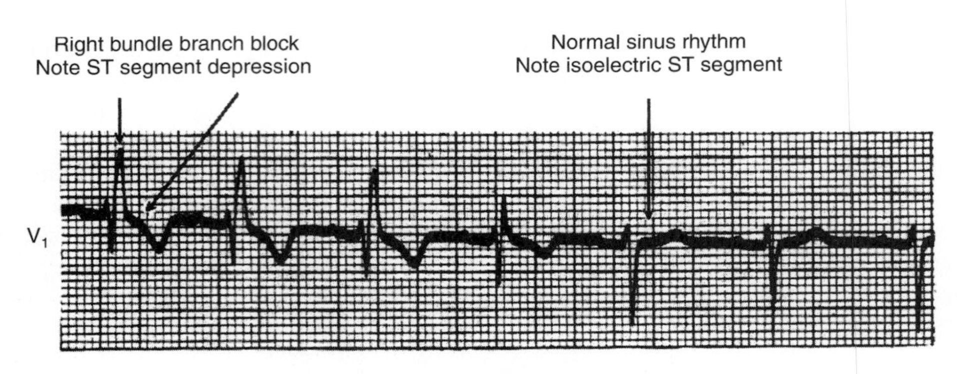

FIG. 31-7. Intermittent RBBB alters the ST segment.

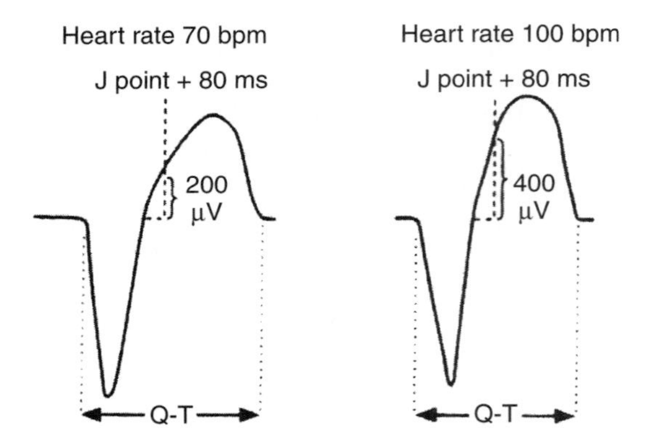

FIG. 31-8. Permanent LBBB with a heart rate change dramatically alters the ST segment measurement point.

which results in 200 μV of ST segment elevation, measured 80 ms past the J point. The right panel shows the ST segment changes that occur when the patient's heart rate increased from 70 to 100 beats/min, the QT interval shortened and the T wave fused with the ST segment, changing the contour of the ST segment. As a result, the J point plus 80 ms measurement point falls closer to the apex of the T wave, measuring 400 μV of ST segment elevation.

REDUCED LEAD CONFIGURATIONS

Use of all 12 ECG leads is the current recommendation for in-hospital ischemia cardiac monitoring.[3] However, the feasibility of maintaining 12-lead ECG monitoring continuously is extremely challenging. For example, multifunction pads (defibrillation or pacer) compete with precordial lead placement. In addition, precordial lead placement

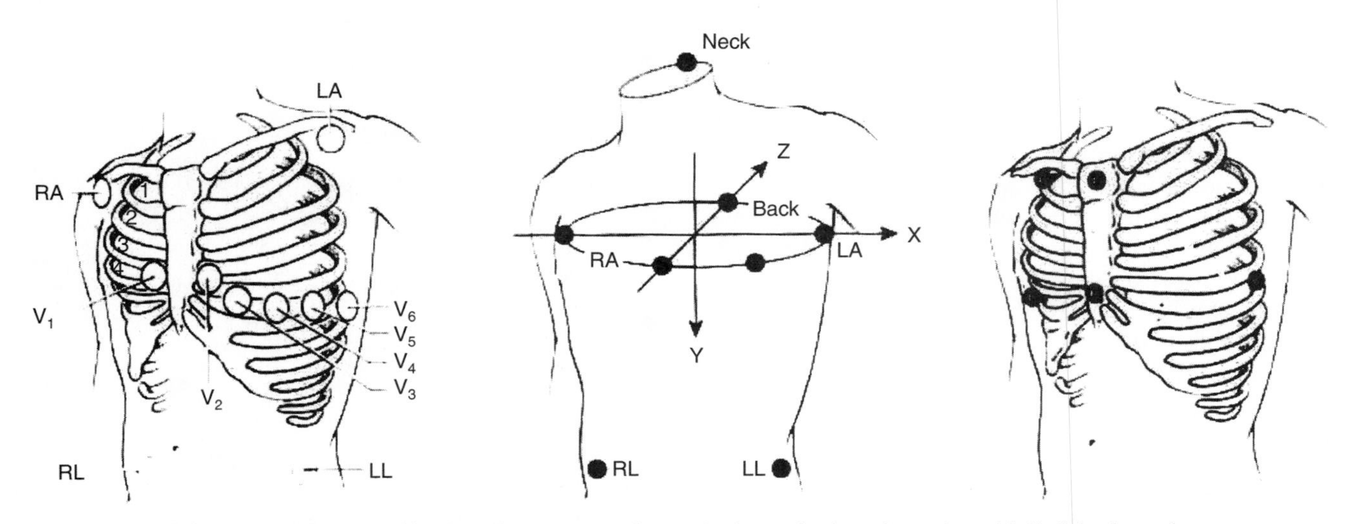

FIG. 31-9. Three reduced lead configurations. *Left,* Standard ECG lead configuration with limb leads on the body torso. *Middle,* Frank vectorcardiographic lead configuration with eight electrodes. *Right,* EASI lead configuration using five electrodes.

makes it difficult to perform routine procedures including echocardiography, chest x-ray, and emergency procedures such as defibrillation and cardiopulmonary resuscitation. Thus to meet the current recommendation of 12-lead monitoring, there have been efforts to develop reduced lead configurations that allow 12-lead ECG monitoring with fewer than 10 lead wires.

Frank Vectorcardiographic Configuration

The Frank vectorcardiographic lead configuration requires eight electrodes to record three channels of ECG information (X, Y, and Z orthogonal leads).[10] Information from the three orthogonal leads can then be transformed into a familiar 12-lead ECG format. The Frank lead configuration includes electrodes on the patient's back as well as an electrode under the right axilla so that this system may be more sensitive than the standard ECG for detecting posterior wall myocardial ischemia (Fig. 31-9). Practical limitations of the Frank lead configuration for continuous in-hospital ECG monitoring are the two posterior electrodes on the neck and back. Specifically, these electrodes can compromise skin integrity in immobile patients and are often uncomfortable for the patient to lie on.

EASI Configuration

A second reduced lead configuration was developed in 1988 by Dower et al.[11] The mathematically derived a 12-lead ECG uses three electrodes from the original Frank vectorcardiographic lead configuration, including electrodes E (lower sternum), A (left axilla), S (manubrium), and I (right axilla). A fifth electrode serves as a ground electrode and can be placed in any convenient location. An important advantage of the EASI lead configuration is the lead placement on the torso that allows access to the precordium (Fig. 31-9).

Two reduced lead configurations are the Frank vectorcardiographic and EASI, both of which are comparable with the standard 12-lead ECG for detection of arrhythmias and ischemia.[12,13] However, clinicians should be cautious when comparing serial ECGs recorded with two different lead configurations in a given patient because there may be subtle difference between the tracings. There are current investigations under way developing additional reduced lead configurations for in-hospital cardiac monitoring.

STRATEGIES TO IMPROVE IN-HOSPITAL CARDIAC MONITORING

The following section contains strategies to improve the accuracy and clinical usefulness of in-hospital cardiac monitoring.

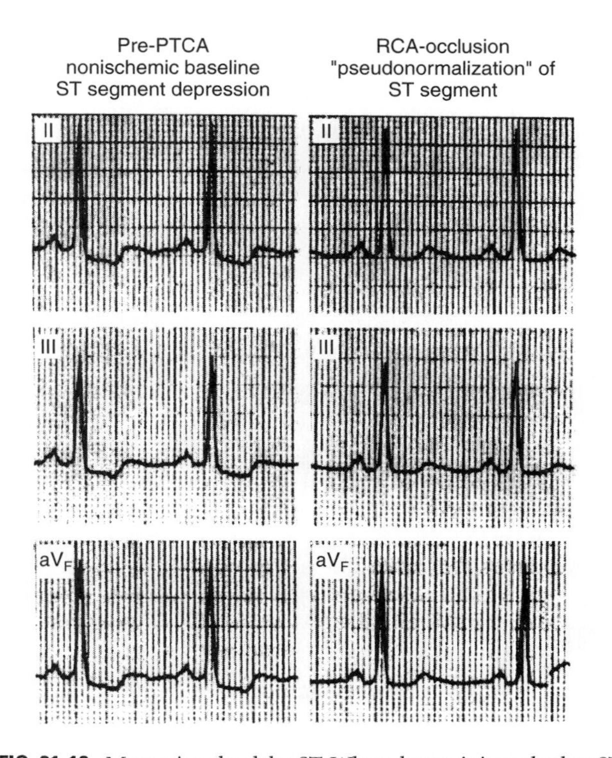

FIG. 31-10. Measuring the delta ST. When determining whether ST segment changes are because of myocardial ischemia, it is critical to establish the patient's baseline ST segment level, which may be deviated because of coronary artery disease, left ventricular hypertrophy, or drug therapy such as digitalis. This example illustrates this point. The *left panel* shows baseline ST segment depression pattern in leads II, III, and aV_F in a patient with left ventricular hypertrophy. The *right panel* shows the ST segment changes (elevation) that occurred during percutaneous coronary intervention. This is an example of "pseudonormalization" of the ST segment in a patient with left ventricular hypertrophy. (From Drew BJ, Wung SF, Adams MG et al: *J Electrocardiol* 30[Suppl]:157-165, 1998.)

Proper and Consistent ECG Electrode and Lead Wire Placement

- Mark chest electrode sites with indelible ink when monitoring is initiated so that electrodes can be replaced to the exact location during ECG monitoring.
- Assess electrode placement and lead wire attachment frequently during monitoring to ensure correct placement.

Individualize Alarm Parameters

- Assess patient's baseline ECG (heart rate, ST segment deviation, frequency of premature complexes).
- Individualize alarm parameters to minimize false-positive alarms. For example, if the patient's baseline heart rate is 55 beats/min the lower alarm threshold

should be set at 50 beats/min and not 60 beats/min to reduce the number of alarms.

Selection of J Point Measurement for Ischemia Monitoring

- Most ST segment software offers a choice of either J point +60 ms or J point +80 ms.
- The current recommendation is to use the J point +60 ms measurement point because this measurement point is less likely to coincide with the upslope of the T wave.

Measure "Delta ST"

- Establish the patient's baseline ST segment level, and then assess changes in the ST segment from this ST segment level. Importantly, in most patients with coronary artery disease the non-ischemic baseline ST level may *not* be isoelectric (i.e., flat) compared to the PR segment, but rather deviated (elevated or depressed) due to prior MI, medications (i.e., digitalis), or repolarization abnormalities (i.e., left ventricular hypertrophy) (Fig. 31-10).

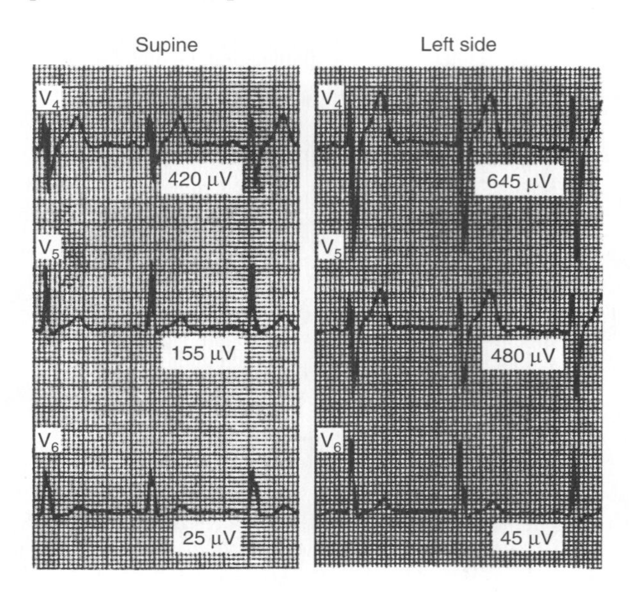

FIG. 31-11. This illustrates both ST segment and QRS changes because of shifts in body position. The *left panel* shows computer-generated microvolt values at the J point plus 80 ms measurement point in leads V_4 to V_6 while the patient was supine. The *right panel* shows the ST segment and QRS changes that occurred when a patient was turned to the left side-lying position. Specifically, ST segment elevation occurred, as much as 325 µV in lead V_5. In this same lead the QRS complex changed from predominantly upright to a predominantly downward complex. In addition, the kQRS complex became taller in the left side-lying position compared to the supine position in leads V_1 and V_6. (From Drew BJ, Wung SF, Adams MG et al: *J Electrocardiol* 30[Suppl]:157-165, 1998.)

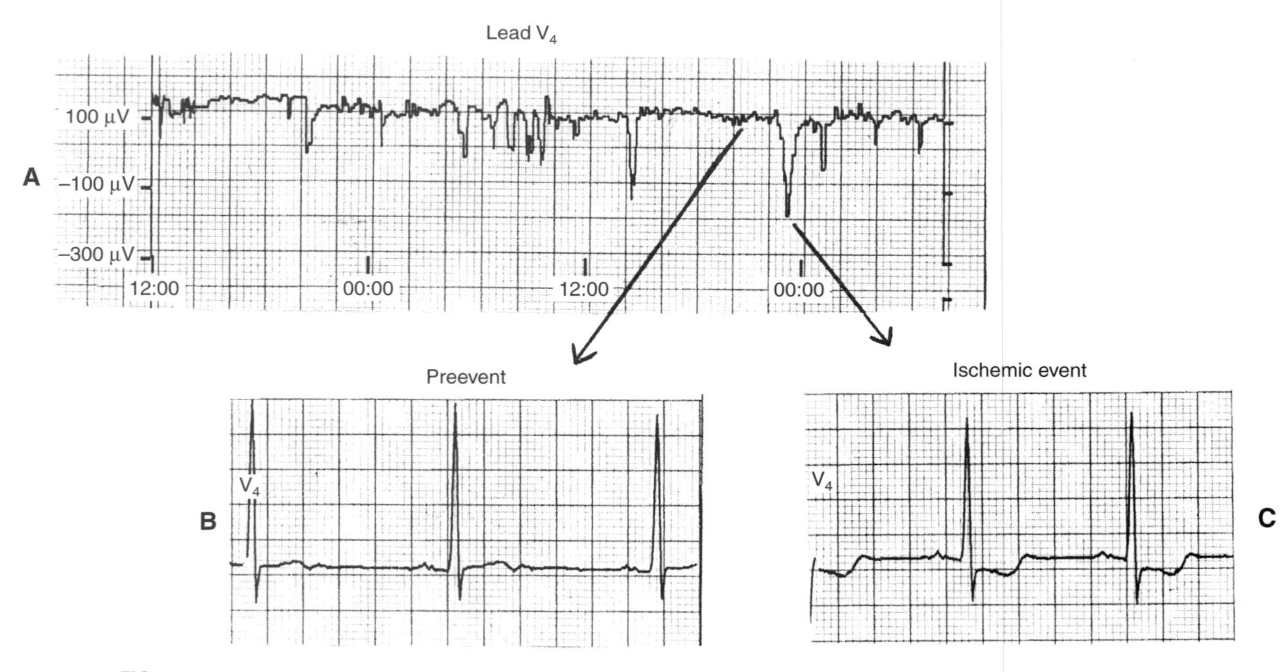

FIG. 31-12. A, A 48-hour ST trend in lead V_4, with the time interval along the x-axis and ST magnitude in microvolts along the y-axis. **B,** ST level before the ischemic event. **C,** ST level (depression) during an ischemic event. Because myocardial ischemia is transient and often clinically silent, evaluation of the ST trend is helpful for evaluating the presence or absence of myocardial ischemia over time.

Set ST alarms at 100 to 200 μV above the patient's baseline ST level. Many conditions in addition to myocardial ischemia cause transient ST segment deviations in patients including changes in body position, transient arrhythmias, pacing, noisy signal, and even lead misplacement (Fig. 31-11).

Use ST "trend" when available as a feature of the software program. This allows for quick assessment of the ST segments over time (Fig. 31-12).

SUMMARY

Accurate cardiac monitoring requires expertise in both arrhythmia and ischemia interpretation. Clinical guidelines have been developed with the intent to assist clinicians apply and use this technology in the hospital setting. An understanding of a patient's clinical situation and history should be considered when implementing in-hospital cardiac monitoring. Finally, careful consideration of the functions and limitations of current bedside monitoring devices can improve the quality of ECG data and aid clinicians with interpretation.

REFERENCES

1. Pelter MM, Adams MG, Drew BJ: Association of transient myocardial ischemia with adverse in-hospital outcomes for angina patients treated in a telemetry unit or a coronary care unit, *Am J Crit Care* 11(4):318-325, 2002.
2. Jaffe AS, Atkins JM, Field JM et al: Recommended guidelines for in-hospital cardiac monitoring of adults for detection of arrhythmias, *Am Coll Cardiol* 18:1431-1433, 1991.
3. Drew BJ, Krucoff MW: Multilead ST-segment monitoring in patients with acute coronary syndromes: a consensus statement for healthcare professionals. ST-Segment Monitoring Practice Guideline International Working Group, *Am J Crit Care* 8(6):372-386, 1999.
4. Drew BJ, Tisdale LA: ST segment monitoring for coronary artery reocclusion following thrombolytic therapy and coronary angioplasty: identification of optimal bedside monitoring leads, *Am J Crit Care* 2(4):280-292, 1993.
5. Mizutani M, Freedman SB, Barns E et al: ST monitoring for myocardial ischemia during and after coronary angioplasty, *Am J Cardiol* 66:389-393, 1990.
6. Wellens HJJ, Bar FW, Lie KI: The value of the electrocardiogram in the differential diagnosis of a tachycardia with a widened QRS complex, *Am J Med* 64:27-33, 1978.
7. Patton JA, Funk M: Survey of use of ST-segment monitoring in patients with acute coronary syndromes, *Am J Crit Care* 10(1):23-32, 2001.
8. Drew BJ, Adams MG. Clinical consequences of ST-segment changes caused by body position mimicking transient myocardial ischemia: hazards of ST-segment monitoring? *J Electrocardiol* 34(3):261-264, 2001.
9. Drew BJ, Wung SF, Adams MG et al: Bedside diagnosis of myocardial ischemia with ST-segment monitoring technology: measurement issues for real-time clinical decision making and trial design, *J Electrocardiol* 30(Suppl):157-165, 1998.
10. Frank E: An accurate, clinically practical system for spacial vectorcardiography, *Circulation* 13:737-349, 1956.
11. Dower G, Yakkush A, Nazzal S et al: Deriving the 12-lead electrocardiogram from four (EASI) electrodes, *J Electrocardiol* 21:S182-S187, 1988.
12. Dellborg M, Riha M, Swedberg K: Dynamic QRS-complex and ST-segment monitoring in acute myocardial infarction during recombinant tissue-type plasminogen activator therapy, *Am J Cardiol* 67:343-349, 1991.
13. Drew BJ, Pelter MM, Wung SF et al: Accuracy of the EASI 12-lead electrocardiogram compared to the standard 12-lead electrocardiogram for diagnosing multiple cardiac abnormalities, *J Electrocardiol* 32(Suppl):38-47, 1999.

PART IV

SPECIAL DIAGNOSTIC AND THERAPEUTIC PROCEDURES

CHAPTER 32

Signal-Averaged ECG and Fast Fourier Transform Analysis

Edward L. Conover

Patients surviving acute myocardial infarction (MI) may be at risk for development of life-threatening arrhythmias. In patients with a history of MI, certain low-level, high-frequency electrocardiographic (ECG) signals have been observed and correlated with increased risk of developing spontaneous arrhythmias.[1-4] These distinctive signals, called *ventricular late potentials (VLPs)*, are high-frequency, low-amplitude events that occur late in and are continuous with the QRS complex. They apparently arise from delayed, disorganized activity in areas of the myocardium at the interface of fibrous scar tissue and normal tissue.[5,6] Because these late potentials are a very low-level phenomenon, special techniques and equipment have been developed to record them.

Techniques such as the signal-averaged ECG (SAECG) are being used both to evaluate late potentials and as a tool for other noninvasive studies, such as His bundle activity,[7] evaluation of the effect of surgical repair on congenital heart disease,[8] determination of left ventricular mass,[9] and effects of thrombolysis.[10-12]

LEAD PLACEMENT: ORTHOGONAL X, Y, AND Z LEADS

The two types of averaging processes used clinically are temporal and spatial, the most common being temporal. The orthogonal x, y, and z lead placement for temporal SAECG has been shown to be best for detecting ventricular late potentials. This lead configuration is shown in Fig. 32-1 and is described here.

Horizontal Leads

The horizontal leads are x– and x+ and are located at the midaxillary lines in the fourth intercostal space.

Vertical Leads

The vertical leads are y– and y+ and are located at the suprasternal notch (y–) and the anterior superior iliac crest (y+).

Anterior/Posterior Leads

The anterior/posterior leads are z– and z+. They are located anteriorly (z–) in the ECG V_2 position (left sternal border; fourth intercostal space) and directly opposite posteriorly (z+), as shown in Fig. 32-1.

CLINICAL IMPLICATIONS[13]

Early Post–Acute MI

Although it is true that the abnormal SAECG recorded immediately after MI is associated with early ventricular tachycardia (VT) and ventricular fibrillation (VF), often these events occur before hospitalization. In addition to this, there are very real technical difficulties of early recording on admission or in the coronary care unit.

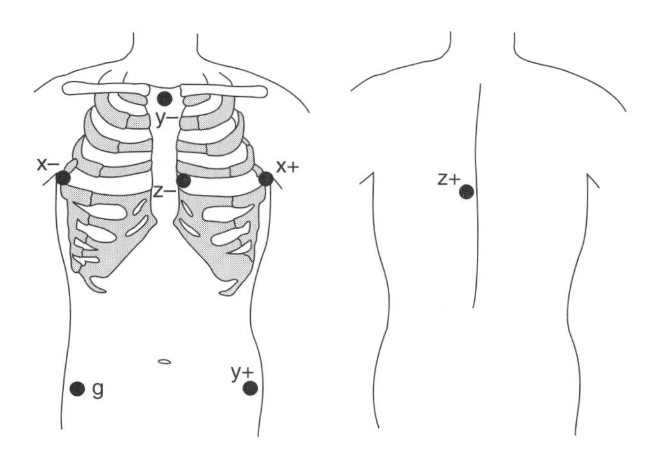

FIG. 32-1. Lead placement for the orthogonal x, y, and z leads used for temporal signal averaging.

Risk Stratification

During the weeks and months after MI, patients continue to be at risk for VT and VF because of the disruption of the normal architecture of the myocardium. Thus risk stratification must be performed early enough to identify patients in danger of sudden death. Patients with normal SAECG results have a significant advantage in survival than do patients in whom delayed potentials are detected on the SAECG.[14]

SAECG in Combination with Other Tests

Technology is evolving that will permit simultaneous recording of multiple indicators of high risk such as ventricular arrhythmias, heart rate variability, SAECG, and QT dispersion.

Unsustained VT, coronary artery disease, and left ventricular dysfunction. Gomes et al[15] found the SAECG to be a powerful predictor of poor outcomes in patients with unsustained VT, coronary artery disease, and left ventricular dysfunction. The combination of an abnormal SAECG and a reduced ejection fraction may be useful in selecting high-risk patients for intervention.

Predictor of atrial fibrillation after coronary artery bypass graft. The predictors of atrial fibrillation after surgery are left atrial enlargement on standard 12 lead ECG, right coronary artery lesion, and SAECG P wave duration. Among these predictors, Aytemir et al[16] found that the SAECG P wave duration was the best predictor.

PROBLEMS IN ANALYZING SMALL ECG SIGNALS

Although it is a demanding task to present the ECG of the electrical cardiac cycle in a noise-free manner, it is a much greater challenge to record and analyze microvolt-level ECG signals. The recording of the electrical cardiac cycle can be interfered with by noise from skeletal muscle movement, amplifier and instrumentation noise, power frequency and its harmonics, and tissue electrode interface. The small signals of late potentials are largely masked by larger, low-frequency signals (e.g., the ST segment) and noise.

Tissue-electrode artifacts can be minimized by lightly sanding the skin with fine sandpaper (no. 220), wiping with alcohol, and using silver–silver chloride electrodes. Shielding and twisting of input cables reduce power frequency noise, and investigations requiring extremely low noise levels enclose the patient and equipment in a Faraday cage. Muscle noise can be reduced by the use of muscle relaxants or spatial-averaging techniques.[17]

Further reduction of noise requires the use of sophisticated techniques that have been developed to separate the low-amplitude, high-frequency signals from the noise and low-frequency signals. These techniques are based on enhancing the characteristics of the signals that are desired while repressing the undesired ones.

SIGNAL AVERAGING

The objective of signal averaging is reduction of the noise that contaminates the ECG. Signal averaging can be accomplished by using either spatial averaging or temporal averaging: both have unique advantages and disadvantages and are used according to the situation. Both techniques are based on the assumption that the noise is random, whereas the signal of interest is coherent and repetitive. Consequently, when several inputs representing the same event are added together, the coherent signal will be reinforced and the noise will cancel itself. The degree of noise reduction obtained is proportional to the square root of the number of inputs averaged. The key lies in obtaining multiple inputs representing the ECG and maintaining coherence. Spatial averaging averages multiple electrodes over a single complex. Ensemble averaging uses a single vector electrode set over multiple complexes.

Spatial Averaging

Spatial averaging uses from 4 to 16 electrodes to obtain the necessary multiple inputs.[18] These inputs are then averaged to provide the noise reduction. The noise reduction available from the use of spatial averaging is restricted by the practical limit on the number of electrodes that can be placed, the possibility that closely spaced electrodes will respond to a common noise source and not cancel effectively, and the theoretical limit of a twofold to fourfold reduction in noise.

The advantage of spatial averaging is the ability to provide a signal-averaged ECG from a single beat, thereby allowing beat-to-beat analysis of transient events and complex arrhythmias.[17]

Temporal Averaging (Signal Averaging)

Temporal averaging, as applied to cardiology, is commonly referred to as *signal averaging*, and this term will be used hereafter. Other terms for temporal averaging are *ensemble averaging* and *serial averaging.* Most studies use temporal averaging as opposed to spatial averaging because of a greater noise reduction afforded by the collection of a larger number of complexes.

The multiple inputs necessary for signal averaging are gathered from standard orthogonal bipolar X, Y, and Z leads over a series of ECG cycles. Because the average can be taken over a large number of beats (typically 100 or more), the noise can theoretically be reduced by a factor of 10 or greater. The tacit assumptions underlying signal averaging are that the waveform is repetitive and can be captured without losing beat-to-beat synchronization.

Signal averaging is a computer-based process whereby each electrode lead input is amplified, its voltage measured or sampled at intervals of 1 ms or less, and each sample converted into a digital number with at least a 12-bit precision.[15] The ECG is thereby converted from an analog voltage waveform into a series of digital numbers that are, in essence, a computer-readable ECG of 100 or more QRS complexes. The digital QRS complexes are then aligned and averaged by a computer with a recognition template to reject ectopic or excessively noisy beats.

Fundamental to signal averaging is the establishment of a starting or fiducial point (usually a point on a fast-moving portion of the QRS) to use in aligning each of the series of QRS complexes. If the fiducial point is unstable (jitter) or the portion of the waveform of interest does not have a stable time relationship to the starting point, the waveform will be smoothed and high-frequency components lost.[19] To ensure that analysis uses valid data, the equipment often provides outputs to advise the user of the correlation coefficient and jitter. This signal-averaged data can be presented and analyzed in either the time domain or the frequency domain, or both.

TIME DOMAIN ANALYSIS OF THE SIGNAL-AVERAGED ECG

Time domain analysis, also referred to as high-pass filtering, presents the ECG as a function of time. After the individual lead signals have been signal-averaged, they are filtered and then combined to form the composite SAECG. Filtering removes the large, low-frequency components that would obscure the low-level, high-frequency late potentials. The following types of filters are commonly used in processing SAECG signals:

1. High-pass filters, which emphasize the high frequencies and minimize the low frequencies
2. Band-pass filters, which emphasize the midrange and high frequencies, minimizing both the low frequencies and the very high frequencies

Typically, the high-pass filters reject frequencies below 25 to 40 Hz, whereas the band-pass filters reject frequencies below 25 to 40 Hz and above 250 Hz.[17,20-24] The work of Vatterott et al[21] and El-Sherif et al[17] investigates the use of different filter frequency bounds. Most recent systems use a 40 Hz high-pass filter.[25] Generally a bidirectional four-pole Butterworth filter is used to minimize ringing and artifacts. After the X, Y, and Z leads have been signal-averaged and filtered, the vector magnitudes are combined $(X^2 + Y^2 + Z^2)^{1/2}$ to form the composite SAECG. Studies also have been made evaluating the filtered X, Y, and Z leads.[10,17]

Interpreting the Time Domain Signal-Averaged ECG

A typical filtered SAECG for a normal subject is shown in Fig. 32-2. Because very high gain is required to display the late potentials, the main portion of the complex exceeds the vertical range and is cut off or clipped. Investigation of late potentials centers around the magnitude and duration of the signals generated by the delayed depolarization of a portion of the myocardium. The areas of interest in the SAECG are the following:

1. Duration of the filtered QRS complex (QRSD), which is indicative of how long the completion of the QRS is delayed by late potentials[20]
2. Amount of energy in the late potentials as given by the root mean square (RMS) voltage in the terminal 40 ms of the QRS complex (RMS40)[20]
3. Duration of the late potentials as indicated by the duration of the low-amplitude signals of less than 40 μV in the terminal QRS region (LAS40)[20,21]

The preceding values either can be read from the SAECG itself or can be derived by the computer system.

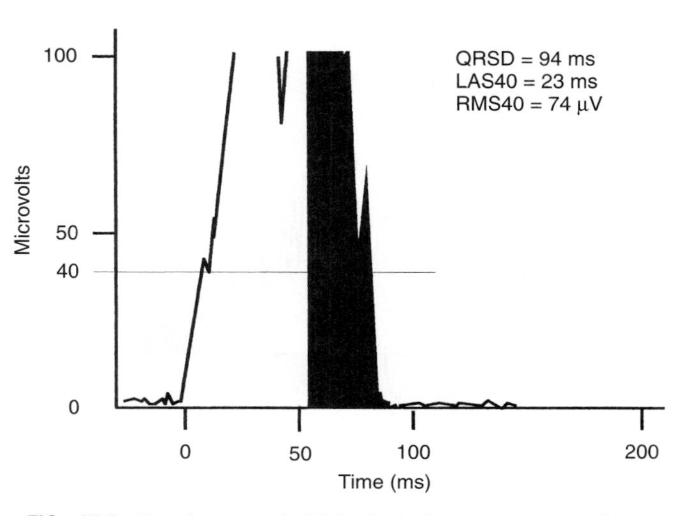

FIG. 32-2. Signal-averaged ECG depicting a normal subject. *QRSD,* The duration of the high-frequency QRS; *LAS40,* the duration of low-amplitude signals of less than 40 μV; *RMS40,* the root mean square voltage of the last 40 ms of the complex *(shaded area).*

In Fig. 32-2 the time base starts at the onset of the filtered QRS, and the QRSD is 94 ms. The shaded portion defines the final 40 ms of the complex. RMS40 is computed from this portion of the complex. The duration of the low-amplitude signals (LAS40) is the interval from the intersection of the 40-μV line and falling edge of the QRS to the termination of the filtered QRS complex.

Defining a late potential and scoring an SAECG as normal or abnormal are highly dependent on technique. Although a consensus among investigators has yet to emerge, representative criteria for 40 Hz filtering are that late potentials exist when the filtered QRS complex is longer than 114 to 120 ms, when there is less than 20 μV RMS of signal in the terminal 40 ms of the filtered QRS, or when the terminal portion of the filtered QRS remains below 40 μV for longer than 38 ms.[1,6,20,26] Different criteria are used to enhance sensitivity or specificity, usually one at the expense of the other.[27] The criteria are altered if bundle branch block is present, and frequency domain analysis may be preferred.[28,29] Fig. 32-3 depicts an abnormal SAECG with late potentials present.

FREQUENCY DOMAIN ANALYSIS OF THE SAECG

Analysis of the SAECG using the frequency domain offers a different way of displaying the ECG, one in which it mathematically is broken into its component frequencies, allowing the contributions of the individual frequencies to be examined.

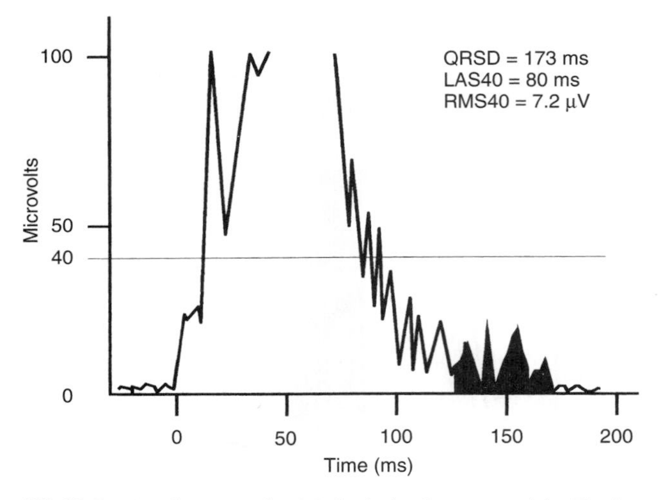

FIG. 32-3. Signal-averaged ECG depicting late potentials. The late potentials cause the duration QRSD to be lengthened; a substantial portion of the increase is caused by the slowly decaying low-level signals in LAS40. The energy level in RMS40 is now composed of low-level signals and contains much less energy. *QRSD,* The duration of the high-frequency QRS; *LAS40,* the duration of low-amplitude signals less than 40 μV; *RMS40,* the root mean square voltage of the last 40 ms of the complex *(shaded area).*

Any continuous time domain waveform, for example, an idealized ECG, is composed of a series of sinusoidal components. This series consists of a fundamental frequency and a series of harmonics whose frequencies are integer multiples of the fundamental. The process usually used to accomplish the transformation from the time domain to the frequency domain is the fast Fourier transform (FFT). Frequency domain analysis plots the amplitude of the fundamental and its harmonics against frequency. The resulting display of information offers new insights into the SAECG.

In the same manner that a rainbow spreads the component color spectrum of sunlight across the sky, a frequency domain ECG spreads the constituent frequencies along the horizontal axis. Frequency domain plots are often referred to as *spectral plots* and are the spectrum of the time domain waveform. As would be expected, there is a certain mirror relationship between the time domain and the frequency domain.

Frequency Domain

In the time domain ECG, events happening at different times are easy to discern. But events containing different frequencies occurring at the same time are very difficult to distinguish. The time domain SAECG attempts to compensate for this shortcoming through the use of filters, which tend to eliminate the undesired frequencies. These filters introduce artifacts that must be understood in reading the SAECG. In the frequency domain SAECG, events containing different frequencies occurring at the same time are easily discriminated; however, those of the same frequency but happening at different times pose a problem. Just as a filter is used in the time domain to reject signals occurring at unwanted frequencies, a "window" is used in the frequency domain to reject part of the waveform that occurs at unwanted times and select those occurring in the desired time slot. Fig. 32-4 depicts an arbitrary waveform, a unity data window, and the portion of the waveform selected by the window. Because the filter introduces some distortion in the time domain, so does the window in the frequency domain.

Methodology

Frequency analysis is performed using the signal-averaged inputs derived from Frank X, Y, and Z leads, although other corrected or uncorrected leads are used. Sampling rates of 1 kHz or greater are typically used. To eliminate filtering artifacts, the inputs are either unfiltered or filtered only to remove extremely low (less than 0.5 Hz) and

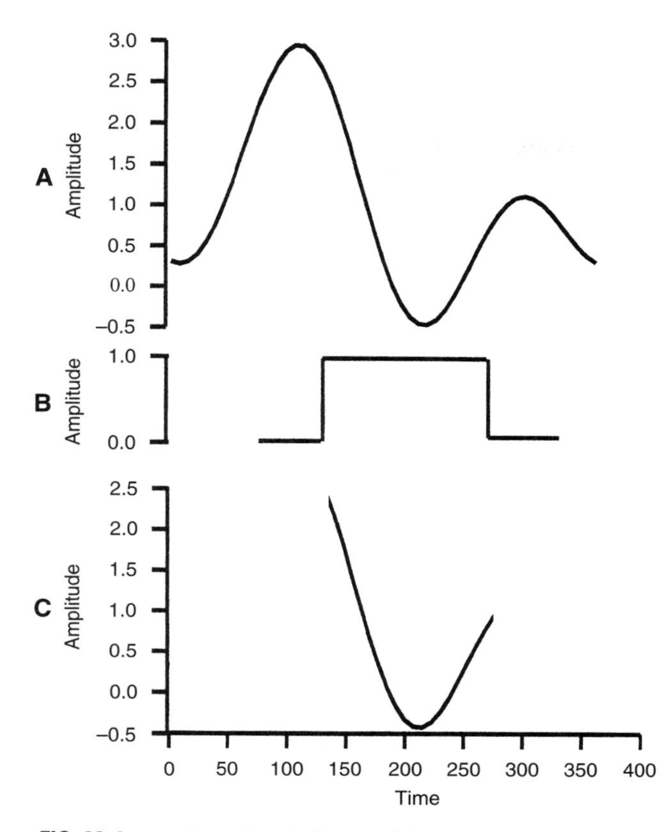

FIG. 32-4. A unity gain window used for selecting a section of a waveform. **A,** An arbitrary waveform. **B,** A unity data window positioned to select a segment of the top waveform in A. **C,** The selected result. The window can be lengthened or shortened and moved horizontally to select the desired portion of the waveform.

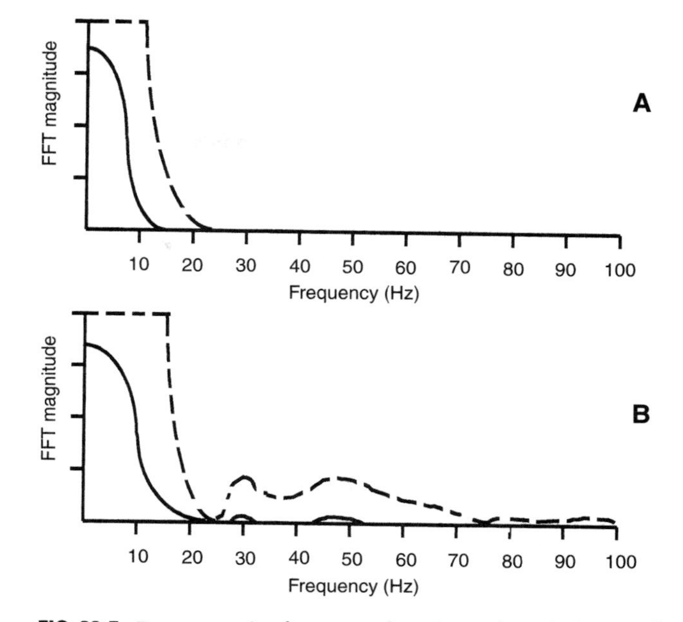

FIG. 32-5. Representative frequency domain tracings. **A,** A normal subject. **B,** The presence of high-frequency potentials is demonstrated. The dashed curve is a magnification ×10 of the solid curve. Evaluation of the fast Fourier transform (FFT) of an ECG is based on the areas or ratio of areas under the curve for different frequency ranges and the frequency and magnitude of peaks.

extremely high (greater than 450 Hz) frequencies. Existing as an array of numbers in a computer, the ECG can be displayed, scaled, and manipulated. By positioning the cursor window over the desired part of the waveform, the operator can make spectral plots of the entire QRS complex or any part of it. The terminal 40 ms of the QRS complex and the ST segment are of greatest interest. After the window is positioned and its length set, either manually or under computer control, the computer calculates the FFT and displays the frequency domain tracing. Because the degree of late potential activity is indicated by the energy in the high-frequency components, the frequency domain tracing often shows the magnitude squared (power is proportional to the square of the voltage), giving the power spectrum. Fig. 32-5 shows a representative FFT tracing.

One of the basic assumptions made in using the FFT on a portion of any waveform is that the signal is continuous; that is, the start point and end point of the signal are at the same level. If this is not the case, false frequency responses will be produced in the FFT. To reduce these errors, window-shaping functions such as Blackman-Harris are used to smooth the data to zero at the boundaries and reduce the false side lobes. Fig. 32-6 depicts the use of a shaped window to reduce edge discontinuities.

Shaped windows can reduce the high frequencies in the ECG and, if the sloped edge of the window is positioned over the late potentials, severely attenuate them. The spectral resolution is related solely to the reciprocal of the length of the window. A window length of 100 ms provides a frequency resolution of 1/0.100 second or 10 Hz. The fundamental will be 10 Hz, and the harmonics will be 20, 30, and 40 Hz and so forth. Longer windows provide greater resolution and vice versa. But it must be kept in mind that short windows, in addition to having poorer resolution, attenuate more of the signal with the sloped sides of the window. Each point in the FFT algorithm accepts one point (a point being one sample) of the ECG complex. A commonly used FFT is one of 512 points, which accommodates up to a 512-ms window at a 1-kHz sample rate. However, the windows chosen are usually much shorter,

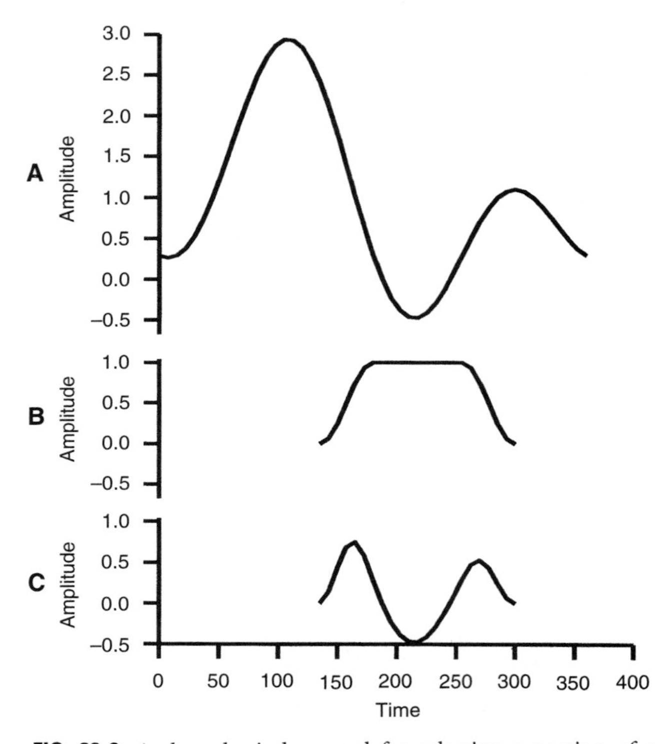

FIG. 32-6. A shaped window used for selecting a portion of a waveform. **A,** The same waveform as shown in Fig. 32-3. **B,** A shaped window (the slope of the sides is exaggerated for illustration; each slope usually is only about 10% of the total window length). **C,** The result of a sample-by-sample multiplication of the waveform A by the window. Portions of A that fall under the sloped sides are severely attenuated.

and the remaining unfilled points are filled with zeros. The selection of the length and position of the window can have a great effect on the results of tests on the same data. In a patient with anterior wall MI and recurrent VT Kelen et al[30] have shown that a small change in the boundary of the analyzed segment, in the order of 10 ms, can result in changes in the area ratio of several hundred percent. Some researchers have conducted FFT analysis over the entire cardiac cycle.[31]

Interpreting the Frequency Domain SAECG

The interpretation of the frequency domain SAECG is highly subject to technique. However, a common thread runs through the evaluation criteria, in that they evaluate the amount of high-frequency energy present, usually by means of an area ratio. This is the ratio of area of the high-frequency portion of the spectrum divided by the total area of the spectrum. The definition of what the high-frequency spectrum comprises varies according to the individual researcher.[32] Pierce et al[22] used the ratio of the area between 60 and 120 Hz to that of 0 to 120 Hz, whereas Cain et al[33] relied on the ratio of the region of 20 to 50 Hz to the area of 10 to 50 Hz. The area ratio of the 40- to 120-Hz to the 0- to 120-Hz regions was used by Kinoshita et al.[34] In addition to the area ratios, some researchers also consider the frequency peaks.[33]

The Fourier transform analysis is a powerful tool, and the implications of its usefulness are still evolving. Research in the field is moving rapidly, but repeatable criteria for distinguishing risk are still emerging.[35] The use of the FFT requires that the researcher, and eventually the clinician, be aware of the limitations of this technique.

OTHER ANALYTIC METHODS

The analytic methods previously described have been combined in various configurations to improve screening accuracy. Among these methods are the following:

1. **Spectral temporal mapping.** This mapping method displays both time and frequency information in a three-dimensional plot. The plot is generated by dividing the ST segment into 20 to 30 segments. Each of the segments is of the same length (typically 80 ms) but starts a few milliseconds later than the previous segment. By stepping the window through each of these segments, the frequency components of each segment are computed using the FFT. The data are then displayed as a three-dimensional surface map with amplitude on the vertical axis, frequency on the horizontal axis, and time on the Z axis.[36,37]
2. **Large electrode arrays.** Studies have been made using ensemble-averaging techniques on body map arrays of electrodes.[38,39] In these studies 28 to 87 body leads were used to gather ECG data. The data were then signal-averaged to reduce noise and evaluated. Tests in dogs have shown that the results of the body map array SAECG correlate more closely to the epicardial measurements than do the results of the standard three-lead SAECG.[40]
3. **Multivariate analysis.** Multivariate analysis statistically combines several factors that may affect the accuracy of determining risk factors. The factors combined are time domain SAECG, frequency domain SAECG, age, infarct location, number of diseased coronary vessels, left ventricular ejection fraction, infarct-related coronary artery patency, treatment received, delay between admission and

SAECG recording, and delay between admission and coronary angiography.[37,41-43]

SUMMARY

Sophisticated techniques from the radar and communication disciplines such as signal-averaging, digital filtering, and the FFT are being applied to the analysis of the ECG. These tools allow the researcher and diagnostician to examine portions of the ECG that were previously obscured by noise and artifacts. As the subject of the bulk of the clinical studies, the time domain signal-averaged ECG has emerged as an important tool in the evaluation of late potentials. Although the techniques and standards are still evolving, the time domain and frequency domain SAECGs alone or in combination with other tests and factors provide noninvasive tests to identify those MI patients at risk of sustained VT or sudden death.[44-46]

REFERENCES

1. Simson MB: Signal-averaged electrocardiography. In Zipes DP, Jalife J, editors: *Cardiac electrophysiology from cell to bedside,* ed 2, Philadelphia, 1995, WB Saunders.
2. Steinberg JS, Regan A, Sciacca RR et al: Predicting arrhythmic events after acute myocardial infarction using the signal-averaged electrocardiogram, *Am J Cardiol* 69:13, 1992.
3. Simson MB: Noninvasive identification of patients at risk for sudden cardiac death, *Circulation* 85(Suppl 1):1, 1992.
4. Lindsay BD, Ambos HD, Schechtman KB et al: Noninvasive detection of patients with ischemic and nonischemic heart disease prone to ventricular fibrillation, *J Am Coll Cardiol* 16:1656, 1990.
5. Klein H, Karp RB, Kouchoukos NT et al: Intraoperative electrophysiologic mapping of the ventricles during sinus rhythm in patients with previous myocardial infarction: identification of the electrophysiologic substrate of ventricular arrhythmias, *Circulation* 66:847, 1982.
6. Simson MB, Untereker WJ, Spielman SR et al: The relationship between late potentials on the body surface and directly recorded fragmented electrograms in patients with ventricular tachycardia, *Am J Cardiol* 51:659, 1983.
7. Hombach V: The high-resolution electrocardiogram: clinical aspects. In El-Sherif N, Samet P, editors: *Cardiac pacing and electrophysiology,* ed 3, Philadelphia, 1991, WB Saunders.
8. Stelling JA, Danford DA, Kugler JD et al: Late potentials and inducible ventricular tachycardia in surgically repaired congenital heart disease, *Circulation* 82:1690, 1990.
9. Vacek JL, Wilson DB, Botteron GW et al: Techniques for the determination of left ventricular mass by signal-averaged electrocardiography, *Am Heart J* 120:958, 1990.
10. Leor MD, Hod H, Rotstein Z et al: Effects of thrombolysis on the 12-lead signal-averaged ECG in the early postinfarction period, *Am Heart J* 120:495, 1990.
11. Zimmermann M, Adamec R, Ciaroni S: Reduction in the frequency of ventricular late potentials after acute myocardial infarction by early thrombolytic therapy, *Am J Cardiol* 67:697, 1991.
12. Moreno FLL, Karagounis L, Marshall H et al: Thrombolysis-related early patency reduces ECG late potentials after acute myocardial infarction, *Am Heart J* 124:557, 1992.
13. Berbari EJ, Steinberg JS: A practical guide to the use of the high-resolution electrocardiogram, Armonk, NY, 2000, Futura Publishing .
14. Kuchar DL, Thorburn CW, Sammel N: Late potentials detected after myocardial infarction: natural history and prognostic significance. Circulation 74:1280-1289, 1986.
15. Gomes JA, Cain ME, Buxton AE et al: Prediction of long-term outcomes by signal-averaged electrocardiography in patients with unsustained ventricular tachycardia, coronary artery disease, and left ventricular dysfunction, *Circulation* 104:436-441, 2001.
16. Aytemir K, Aksoyek S, Ozer N et al: Atrial fibrillation after coronary artery bypass surgery: P wave signal averaged ECG, clinical and angiographic variables in risk assessment, *Int J Cardiol* 69:49-56, 1999.
17. El-Sherif N, Restivo M, Craelius W et al: The high-resolution electrocardiogram: technical and basic aspects. In El-Sherif N, Samet P, editors: *Cardiac pacing and electrophysiology,* ed 3, Philadelphia, 1991, WB Saunders.
18. Flowers NC, Shvartsman V, Kennelly BM et al: Surface recording of His- Purkinje activity on an every-beat basis without digital averaging, *Circulation* 63:948, 1981.
19. Ros HH, Koeleman ASM, Akker TJ: The technique of signal averaging and its practical application in the separation of atrial and His-Purkinje activity. In Hombach V, Hilger HH, editors: *Signal averaging technique in clinical cardiology,* New York, 1981, FK Schattauer Verlag.
20. Breithardt G, Cain ME, El-Sherif N et al: Standards for analysis of ventricular late potentials using high-resolution or signal-averaged electrocardiography: a statement by a task force committee of the European Society of Cardiology, the American Heart Association, and the American College of Cardiology, *J Am Coll Cardiol* 17:999, 1991.
21. Vatterott PF, Vailey KR, Hammill SC: Improving the predictive ability of the signal-averaged electrocardiogram with a linear logistic model incorporating clinical variables, *Circulation* 81:797, 1990.
22. Pierce DL, Easley AR, Windle JR et al: Fast Fourier transformation of the entire low amplitude late QRS potential to predict ventricular tachycardia, *J Am Coll Cardiol* 14:1731, 1989.
23. Nalos PC, Gang ES, Mandel WJ et al: Utility of the signal-averaged electrocardiogram in patients presenting with sustained ventricular tachycardia or fibrillation while on an antiarrhythmic drug, *Am Heart J* 115:108, 1988.
24. El-Sherif N, Ursell SN, Bekheit S et al: Prognostic significance of the signal-averaged ECG depends on the time of recording in the postinfarction period, *Am Heart J* 118:256, 1989.
25. Cain ME, Anderson JL, Arnsdorf MF: ACC Expert consensus document. Signal-averaged electrocardiography, *J Am Coll Cardiol* 27:238-249, 1996.
26. Hood MA, Pogwizd SM, Peirick J et al: Contribution of myocardium responsible for ventricular tachycardia to abnormalities detected by analysis of signal-averaged ECGs, *Circulation* 86:1888, 1992.
27. Lander P, Barbari EJ, Rajagopalan CV: Critical analysis of the signal-averaged electrocardiogram, *Circulation* 87:105, 1993.
28. Buckingham TA, Lingle A, Greenwalt T et al: Power law analysis of the signal-averaged electrocardiogram for identification of patients with ventricular tachycardia: effect of bundle branch block, *Am Heart J* 124:1220, 1992.
29. Fontaine JM, Rao R, Henkin R: Study of the influence of left bundle branch block on the signal-averaged electrocardiogram: a qualitative and quantitative analysis, *Am Heart J* 121:494, 1991.
30. Kelen GJ, Henkin R, Fontaine JM et al: Effects of analyzed signal duration and phase on the results of fast Fourier transform analysis of the surface electrocardiogram in subjects with and without late potentials, *Am J Cardiol* 60:1282, 1987.

31. Cain ME, Ambos HD, Markham J et al: Diagnostic implications of spectral and temporal analysis of the entire cardiac cycle in patients with ventricular tachycardia, *Circulation* 83:1637, 1991.
32. Malik M, Kulakowski P, Poloniecki J et al: Frequency versus time domain analysis of signal-averaged electrocardiograms. I. Reproducibility of the results, *J Am Coll Cardiol* 20:127, 1992.
33. Cain ME, Lindsay BD, Arthur RM et al: Noninvasive detection of patients prone to life-threatening ventricular arrhythmias by frequency analysis of electrocardiographic signals. In Zipes DP, Jalife J, editors: *Cardiac electrophysiology,* Philadelphia, 1990, WB Saunders.
34. Kinoshita O, Kamakura S, Ohe T et al: Spectral analysis of signal-averaged electrocardiograms in patients with idiopathic ventricular tachycardia of left ventricular origin, *Circulation* 85:2054, 1992.
35. Engel TR, Pierce DL, Patil KD: Reproducibility of the signal-averaged electrocardiogram, *Am Heart J* 122:1652, 1991.
36. McClements BM, Adgey AAJ: Value of signal-averaged electrocardiography, radionuclide ventriculography, Holter monitoring and clinical variables for prediction of arrhythmic events in the survivors of acute myocardial infarction in the thrombolytic era, *J Am Coll Cardiol* 21:1419, 1993.
37. Steinberg JS, Prystowsky E, Freedman RA: Use of the signal-averaged electrocardiogram for predicting inducible ventricular-tachycardia in patients with unexplained syncope: relation to clinical variables in a multivariate analysis, *J Am Coll Cardiol* 23:99, 1994.
38. Ho DSW, Denniss RA, Uther JB: Signal-averaged electrocardiogram: improved identification of patients with ventricular tachycardia using a 28-lead optimal array, *Circulation* 87:857, 1993.
39. Shibata T, Kubota I, Ikeda K et al: Body surface mapping of high-frequency components in the terminal portion during QRS complex for the prediction of ventricular tachycardia in patients with previous myocardial infarction, *Circulation* 82:2084, 1990.
40. Freedman RA, Fuller MS, Greenberg GM et al: Detection and localization of prolonged epicardial electrograms with 64-lead body surface signal-averaged electrocardiography, *Circulation* 84:871, 1991.
41. Shin HH, Sagar KB, Stepniakowski K et al: Increased prevalence of abnormal signal-averaged electrocardiograms in older patients who have hypertension with low diastolic blood pressure, *Am Heart J* 125:1698, 1993.
42. De Chillou C, Sadoul N, Briançon S et al: Factors determining the occurrence of late potentials on the signal-averaged electrocardiogram after a first myocardial infarction: a multivariate analysis, *J Am Coll Cardiol* 18:1638, 1991.
43. Nogami A, Iesaka Y, Akiyama J et al: Combined use of time and frequency domain variables in signal-averaged ECG as a predictor of inducible sustained monomorphic ventricular tachycardia in myocardial infarction, *Circulation* 86:780, 1992.
44. Elami A, Merin G, Flugelman MY: Usefulness of late potentials on the immediate postoperative signal-averaged electrocardiogram in predicting ventricular tachyarrhythmias early after isolated coronary artery bypass grafting, *Am J Cardiol* 74:33, 1994.
45. Turitto G, Ahuja RK, Caref EB et al: Risk stratification for arrhythmic events in patients with nonischemic dilated cardiomyopathy and nonsustained ventricular tachycardia: role of programmed ventricular stimulation and the signal-averaged electrocardiogram, *J Am Coll Cardiol* 24:1523, 1994.
46. Guidera SA, Steinbert JS: The signal-averaged P wave duration: a rapid and noninvasive marker of risk of atrial fibrillation, *J Am Coll Cardiol* 21:1645, 1993.

CHAPTER 33

Electrical Stimulation Therapies

John R. Buysman, PhD

All cardiac contraction sequences in some part involve the mechanisms of cellular automaticity, conduction by specialized fibers, and cell-to-cell conduction. These mechanisms result from ion currents along, between, in, and through cardiac cell membranes. Because ion currents and cell membrane permeabilities can be affected by electrical effects; cardiac rhythms and contraction sequences can be artificially created, modified, or terminated by the application of electrical pulses. Many electrical cardiac therapeutic devices use electrical pulses to control arrhythmias and to resynchronize contractions to improve cardiac performance.

ORGANIZATION OF ARRHYTHMIAS WITH RESPECT TO ELECTRICAL THERAPIES

Table 33-1 organizes the known arrhythmogenic mechanisms (atrioventricular [AV] conduction failure, abnormal automaticity, triggered activity, and reentry) in a manner that facilitates visualizing how they are treated by electrical therapies. The normal electrical activity of the heart and arrhythmogenic mechanisms have already been discussed in Chapters 2 and 3.

GOALS OF ELECTRICAL THERAPIES

Because ventricular pumping is crucial for life, the most important therapeutic goal is to preserve, restore, or create useful ventricular rhythms. Atrial rhythms are not immediately critical to life if the ventricular rhythm is supported. However, useful atrial rhythms that provide rate variability to support various activities and that provide AV synchrony are highly important to cardiac performance factors affecting quality of life, and can affect ultimate longevity. In certain patients, especially heart failure patients in whom the left and right ventricles are not coordinated, resynchronization of the ventricles, and sometimes the atria, is important to maintain or improve cardiac performance. The latter is becoming known *as cardiac resynchronization therapy*.

ELECTRICAL THERAPIES FOR BRADYCARDIA

General Pacing Concepts

The most common way to treat bradyarrhythmias is to use electrical devices that apply tiny electrical stimuli to the atrial or ventricular muscle mass, or both, at a desired rate and sequence to cause these muscle masses to depolarize at that rate and sequence. Each atrial stimulus instantly produces a single atrial depolarization, and each ventricular stimulus instantly produces a single ventricular depolarization. These devices are called *pacemakers* because they set the pace of the heart; the stimuli are called *paces*.

The electrical pulses (stimuli) are produced by the pacemaker's electronic unit called the *pulse generator* and are conveyed to the atrial or ventricular muscle mass via insulated wires called *leads*. At the cardiac end of each lead there is an exposed contact called the *electrode*, which touches the heart and conveys the stimulus into the cardiac cells nearby. The stimulus needs only to be applied to a small cluster of cells in each mass because the depolarization there will spread throughout the muscle mass by cell-to-cell conduction.

Pacemakers are available as external devices for temporary applications, or as implantable devices for permanent applications. In this chapter the implantable types are discussed, but the principles are also applicable to the external type (Fig. 33-1).

Some patients who require implantable devices for tachycardia therapies also require pacing for bradycardia, thus full bradycardia pacemaker capabilities are included

TABLE 33-1 **Relationship of Common Arrhythmias to Basic Arrhythmic Mechanisms**

General Problem	Specific Problem	Typical Problem Location	Corresponding Rhythm	Systemic Result
AV conduction failure	Delayed conduction	AV node	First-degree block	Sinus rate
	One-sided block	Branch(es) of Purkinje system	Bundle branch block	Sinus rate
	Intermittent or complete block	AV node, bundle of His, or Purkinje system	Second- or third-degree block	Bradycardia
Abnormal cellular electrophysiology	Automaticity: too slow	Atria (SA node)	Sinus bradycardia	Bradycardia
	Automaticity: too fast	Atria	Atrial tachycardia	Tachycardia
		AV node, junction	Junctional tachycardia	Tachycardia
		Ventricle	Ventricular tachycardia	Tachycardia
	Triggered activity	Atria	Atrial tachycardia	Tachycardia
		Ventricle	Ventricular tachycardia	Tachycardia
Reentry	Small-loop reentry in a single mass	Atria	Atrial tachycardia	Tachycardia
		AV junction	Junctional PSVT	Tachycardia
		Ventricle	Ventricular tachycardia	Tachycardia
	Large-loop reentry in a single mass	Atria	Atrial flutter	Tachycardia
		Ventricle	Ventricular flutter	Tachycardia
	Meandering or multiloop reentry in a single mass	Atria	Atrial fibrillation	Tachycardia
		Ventricle	Ventricular fibrillation	Tachycardia
	Atrioventricular loop	Atria and ventricle	AV reciprocation PSVT	Tachycardia

Bradycardia reduces cardiac performance, resulting in loss of blood pressure. Mild bradycardia can cause dizziness and fainting. Profound bradycardia will cause death.

Extremely fast tachycardias may reduce cardiac performance, resulting in loss of blood pressure and pulselessness. Dizziness, fainting, and sometimes death can occur. Ventricular flutter and ventricular fibrillation cause a total loss of ventricular function, resulting in no blood pressure and pulselessness. Fainting occurs within 7 to 15 seconds, and death will occur within a few minutes if untreated.

AV, Atrioventricular; *PSVT*, paroxysmal supraventricular tachycardia.

in nearly all implantable devices for tachycardia therapies. Their pacing functions are identical except for certain features where bradycardia functions would be in conflict with antitachyarrhythmia therapies. In this chapter discussion centers on pacemakers, but almost all discussions also apply to the bradycardia features in antitachyarrhythmia devices.

Both pacemakers and antitachyarrhythmia devices may include, or be adapted to, cardiac resynchronization therapies.

General types of pacemakers. In all bradycardias, ventricular rate must be restored. Thus nearly all pacemaker systems are capable of *directly* pacing the ventricular muscle. Only in patients with *proven reliable conduction* may pacing be applied only to the atrial muscle.

Atrial pacemakers function solely by stimulating the atria, and *ventricular pacemakers* stimulate only the ventricles; *atrioventricular (AV) pacemakers* can stimulate both the atria and the ventricles. The two former types are *single-chamber pacemakers,* and the latter type is a *dual-chamber pacemaker. Dual* refers to an atrial chamber and a ventricular chamber; it does not connote "left" or "right." The term *chamber* extends to include the whole atrial muscle or the whole ventricular muscle, as applicable. Pacemakers and antitachyarrhythmia devices with cardiac resynchronization therapies that pace the right and left atria or the right and left ventricles have been introduced. These are noted by adding the terms *biatrial* or *biventricular.*

In pacemakers and implantable cardioverter defibrillators (ICDs), all functions are automatically controlled by a microcomputer inside the pulse generator according to the instructions programmed into it. The instruction parameters can be reprogrammed at any time by using an external programmer, a custom portable computer matching the brand of pacemaker or ICD being programmed. During reprogramming, the pulse generator and programmer

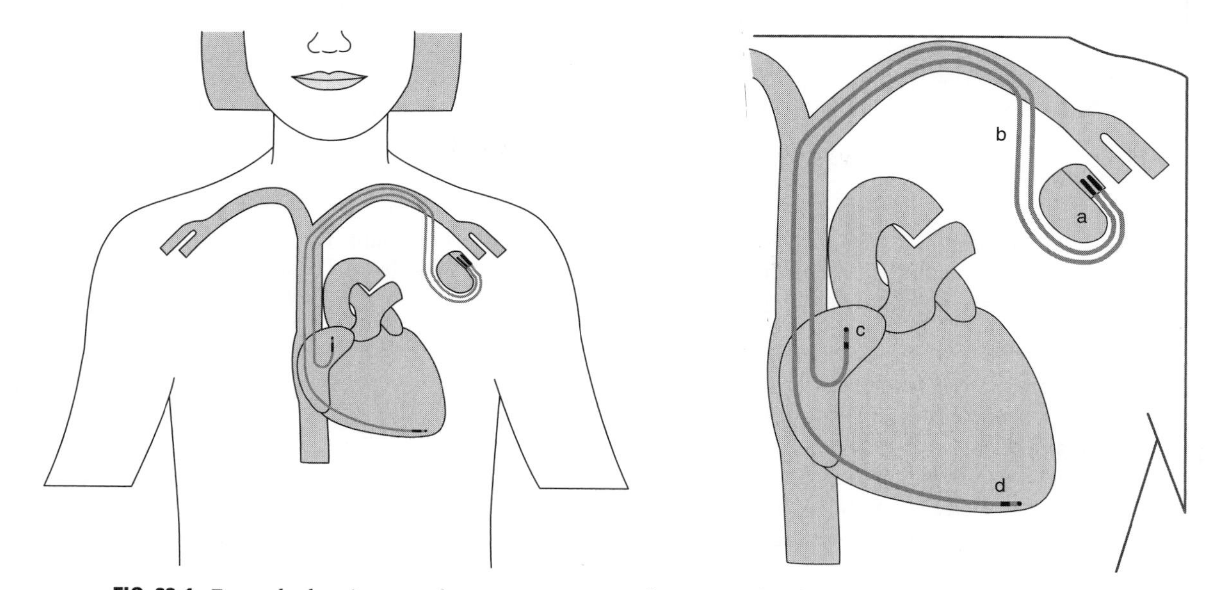

FIG. 33-1. Example showing use of a permanent pacemaker to treat bradyarrhythmia. An implantable pulse generator *(a)* produces tiny electric pulses, which are conveyed to the heart by leads *(b)*. Most systems employ two leads as shown here, one to pace and sense the atria and another to pace and sense the ventricle. At the tip of each lead (*c* and *d*) an electrode delivers the pulses to adjacent cardiac cells and depolarizes them. Depolarization then spreads by cell-to-cell conduction through the atrial and ventricular masses. In this sketch the atrial lead *(c)* is in the appendage of the atria.

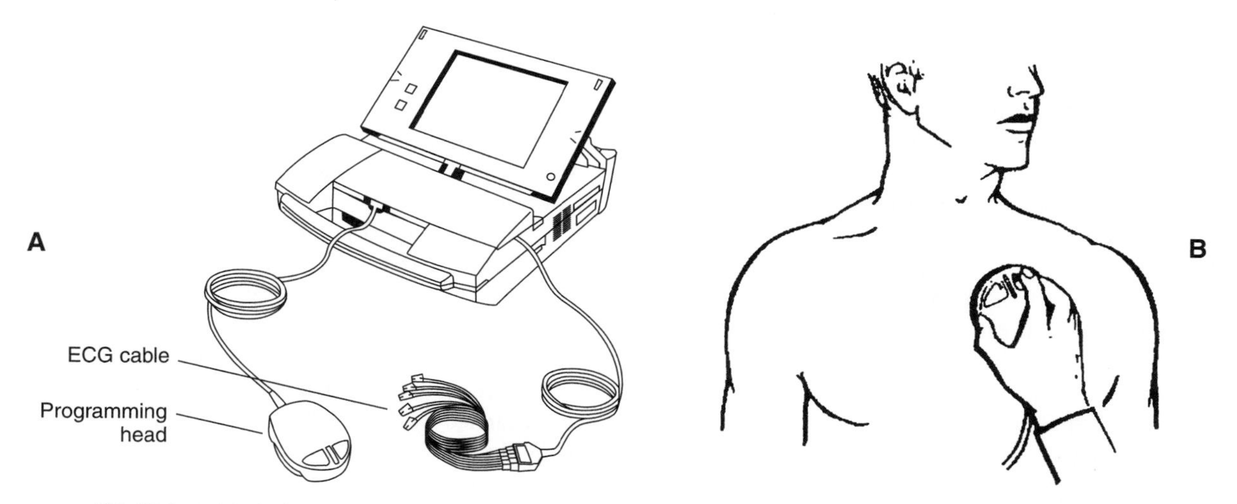

FIG. 33-2. A, Typical programmer. **B,** Programming head is placed over the generator that is in the patient, providing a radio magnetic link to receive data from the generator and to program new commands and parameters into the generator. (Courtesy Medtronic, Inc, Minneapolis, Minn.)

communicate using short-range radio magnetic telemetry signals that are usually exchanged through a "programming head," an external accessory placed over the generator area (Fig. 33-2).

Stimulus artifacts on the electrocardiogram. When the electrical stimulus is delivered, a small fraction of the stimulus voltage appears at the surface of the body and is usually recorded on the electrocardiogram (ECG) as a *stimulus artifact.* The size of the artifact is often not displayed uniformly on some ECG monitors and recorders,

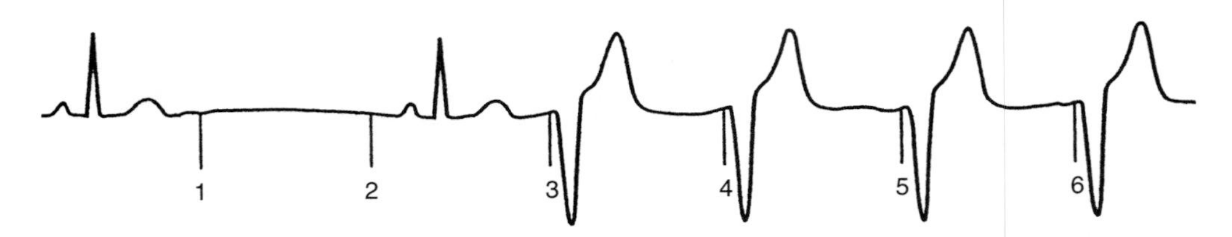

FIG. 33-3. Noncapture and capture (ventricular). Pacing stimuli *1* and *2* had insufficient strength to capture the ventricle. In the time between stimuli *2* and *3*, the pacing output was changed to a stronger setting. Stimuli *3* to *6* captured consistently.

and sometimes artifacts may be barely visible. Some other monitors employ a "pacemaker detect" feature that detects and replaces the real artifact with a standardized artifact mark that looks like a paced artifact. Standard artifacts all appear the same length. Occasionally, interference can be detected and marked as a pacing artifact, causing confusion.

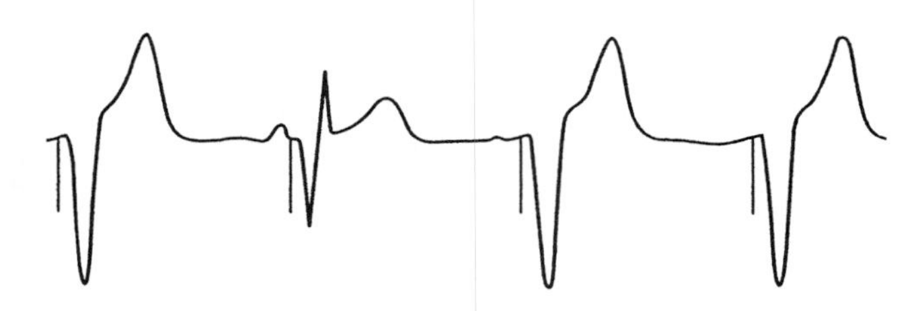

FIG. 33-4. Paced fusion (second complex). A pacing stimulus occurs immediately after the P wave and begins depolarizing the ventricles. The ECG complex begins showing the paced depolarization. Note the initial similarity to other paced depolarizations. Then normal conduction enters the Purkinje fibers, quickly completing depolarization of the ventricles and dominating the rest of the ECG complex. Repolarization is also affected, yielding a different T wave.

Stimulation Concepts

Mechanism of stimulation. When a pacing pulse appears at the electrode, an electrical field radiates from the electrode, penetrates the excitable cells, overwhelms the natural electrical potential of these cells and alters their membrane permeabilities, which in turn allows rapid influx of sodium, which produces depolarization. The depolarization then spreads by cell-to-cell conduction throughout the entire mass of cardiac tissue, *capturing* the mass and causing the mass to contract. Capture can be recognized as a depolarization observed immediately after the stimulus artifact (Fig. 33-3). The stimulus must be large enough to initiate rapid depolarization; that is, the stimulus must exceed a *threshold.*

Paced fusion. If a native depolarization enters the ventricles about the same moment a ventricular pace is delivered, two depolarization patterns develop simultaneously, one from the native depolarization and the other from the pace-initiated depolarization. Although these are two distinctly separate processes, the ECG records their combined voltages as a *paced fusion* beat (Fig. 33-4). A premature ventricular contraction (PVC) and paced beat can also fuse. In biventricular systems, the depolarizations from the two pacing sites fuse. An analogous process can occur in the atria.

Sensing Concepts

Reasons for sensing. Pacemakers must coordinate pacing with the natural depolarizations occurring in the heart. For example, pacing into refractory tissue (such as premature atrial contractions, PVCs, and conducted depolarizations) serves no purpose, and pacing into relative refractory tissue in rare cases may be arrhythmogenic, so must be avoided; that is, unwanted paces must be *inhibited.* Also, AV pacemakers must coordinate ventricular pacing to follow natural atrial activity, so as to mimic natural AV synchrony. To meet the preceding needs, pacemakers *sense* natural depolarizations and use the sensed information to control their timing functions.

Mechanism of sensing. When a depolarization occurs in cardiac muscle, ion movements during the depolarization process create a small voltage in the tissue. This voltage is carried by the lead into the pulse generator, where it is amplified and sent to various circuits to control the pacing functions.

Sensing involves voltages close to the electrode only; thus sensing is unrelated to the size of the surface complex, but it does occur within the time of the surface complex.

Undersensing and oversensing. Normal depolarizations repetitively follow the same path, thus are sensed uniformly beat after beat. Ectopic depolarizations vary; thus on rare occasions they may be unsensed by a normally operating pacemaker.

When a depolarization is not sensed, it is said to be

undersensed. When interference is sensed as if it were a depolarization, it is said to be *oversensed.*

Competitive pacing. The sensing feature can be switched off during certain standard pacemaker tests. With sensing switched off, pacing is not inhibited by native beats. Pacing in the presence of native beats may result in *competitive pacing,* causing some fused beats. If a native depolarization has already passed the electrode by the time the stimulus is delivered, the stimulus will have no effect because the tissue contacting the electrode is already depolarized. This occurrence is sometimes called *pseudofusion.* Similarly, an atrial stimulus occurring just after a P wave or a ventricular stimulus occurring during an ST segment will have no effect because the respective tissue is refractory. Later, a stimulus may start another depolarization if the tissue at the electrode has already repolarized, but if parts of the respective mass are still refractory, an abnormal cell-to-cell conduction will result (Fig. 33-5).

General Pacemaker Timing

Pacemakers control the timing of their stimuli by continuously monitoring the *sequence* and *timing* between depolarizations occurring in the heart, both natural and paced, and by checking these against desired sequences and time limit intervals electronically stored in the pulse generator. Whenever a natural depolarization fails to occur within an expected time, the pacemaker sends a stimulus to the delinquent muscle mass to produce a depolarization there.

Intercycle timing. A pacemaker uses an event from one cardiac cycle to set the time limit for the appearance of the next cycle. If the next cycle occurs naturally before the time limit expires, the existing time limit is canceled and immediately reset for the next cycle. But if the next cycle fails to occur by the end of the time limit, the pacemaker instantly initiates a new cycle by pacing.

Cardiac cycles contain an atrial event and a ventricular event, or at least a ventricular event. An "event" is either a natural depolarization or a pace that initiates a depolarization. If the pacemaker uses the atrial event of one cycle to set the time limit for the appearance of the atrial event of the next cycle, the pacemaker employs AA intercycle timing. If the pacemaker uses the ventricular event of one cycle to set the time limit for the atrial event of the next cycle, it employs VA intercycle timing. Likewise, if the ventricular event sets the limit for the start of the next ventricular event, it is VV intercycle timing. Because a historical naming quirk, VA timing is often called VV timing.

In atrioventricular timing schemes, PVCs occurring between cycles cancel the present time limit and typically initiate a VA intercycle time limit.

Recently, with the introduction of biatrial and biventricular pacing, the terms *AA* and *VV* are also being used to indicate the interatrial (right-left) and interventricular (right-left) intervals, which is confusing and requires interpretation from context.

Timing mechanisms. Pacing is described in terms of *rate,* but pacemakers operate with time *intervals* expressed in milliseconds. A basic pacing rate in pulses per minute (cycles per minute) can be converted to a basic pacing interval by the following formula:

$$\text{Interval (milliseconds/cycle)} = \frac{\text{60,000 (milliseconds/minute)}}{\text{Rate (cycles/minute)}}$$

Timing mechanisms are best understood from examples.

Single-chamber pacemakers. Single-chamber AA intercycle timing is illustrated by conventional atrial pacing in

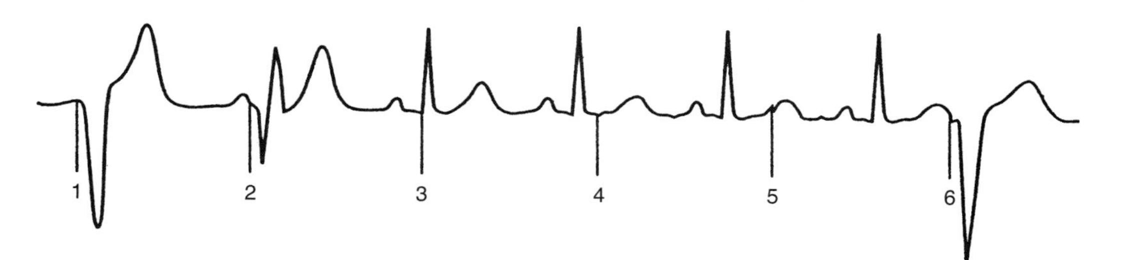

FIG. 33-5. Competitive pacing (ventricular example). When the sensing function is turned off, stimuli occur without regard to native depolarizations. Pace *1* results in a normal paced depolarization. Pace *2* is a fusion similar to that in Fig. 33-4. Pace *3* is fusion, but normal conduction is so far ahead that the complex appears normal; only a slight variation in the T wave is noticeable. Paces *4* and *5* fire into refractory muscle and hence do nothing. Pace *6* occurs after the muscle adjacent to the electrode has repolarized; thus it captures. However, the morphologic appearance shows that the depolarization pattern was altered by remaining refractory muscle.

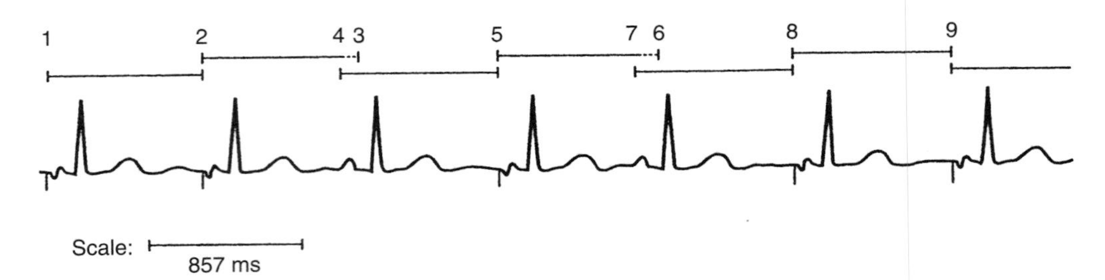

FIG. 33-6. Example of AA intercycle timing in a basic atrial pacemaker. The basic rate is programmed to 70 pulses/min, corresponding to an AA interval of 857 ms. A pace event at *1* sets a time limit that will expire 857 ms later at *2.* When the time reaches *2,* the atria are paced and the time limit is reset for another 857 ms to expire at *3.* Before the time reaches *3,* however, a native atrial depolarization occurs and is sensed at *4.* This event cancels the existing time limit and resets a new time limit for 857 ms to expire at *5.* When the time reaches *5,* a pace occurs and the limit is reset again for *6.* At *7* a native depolarization is sensed, which cancels *6* and resets the time limit for *8,* and so forth.

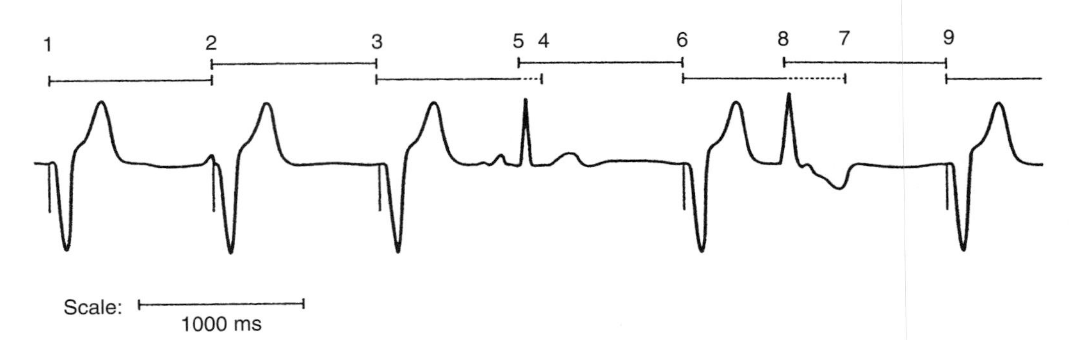

FIG. 33-7. Illustration of VV intercycle timing in a basic ventricular pacemaker. The basic rate is programmed to 60 pulses/min, corresponding to a VV interval of 1000 ms. A pace at *1* sets a time limit to expire at *2.* When *2* is reached, a pace occurs, and the limit is reset to expire at *3.* At *3* a pace occurs, and the limit is reset to expire at *4.* However, a ventricular sense occurs at *5,* which resets the time limit to expire at *6,* where a pace occurs and resets the limit for *7.* However, at *8* a premature ventricular contraction is sensed, canceling the pace for *7* and resetting the limit to *9.*

Fig. 33-6, and single-chamber VV intercycle timing is illustrated by conventional ventricular pacing in Fig. 33-7.

Dual-chamber pacemakers. Atrioventricular pacemakers have an additional time limit, the AV interval, which ensures that each atrial beat is followed by a ventricular beat within a specified time interval, the *AV interval.* In nearly all applications each atrial event sets the time limit for the next ventricular depolarization, and if a ventricular depolarization does not occur before the end of the limit, the limit expires and a ventricular pace is immediately delivered.

Dual-chamber pacing with AA intercycle timing is shown in Fig. 33-8, and dual-chamber VA intercycle timing in Fig. 33-9. Remember, a PVC is a special event that resets the atrial time limit to a value equal to AA minus AV.

Special pacing sequences. In addition to basic pacing functions, many pacemakers produce special pacing sequences in special circumstances. These sequences are often flagged by computerized hospital ECG monitors, ambulatory monitors, and automatic event recorders. Reviewers of ECGs who encounter an unknown sequence that presents no risk to the patient should contact the pacemaker manufacturer for information before assuming there is a problem. Of course, if a sequence presents risk, immediate attention must be given. Two common examples are noted below.

Ventricular safety pacing. AV pacemakers must assure that atrial paces can not be sensed by the ventricular lead (crosstalk) because this would inhibit ventricular pacing, which could be fatal in patients with heart block. Thus during and just after an atrial pace, the ventricular sensing function is electronically blanked for about 30 ms to allow

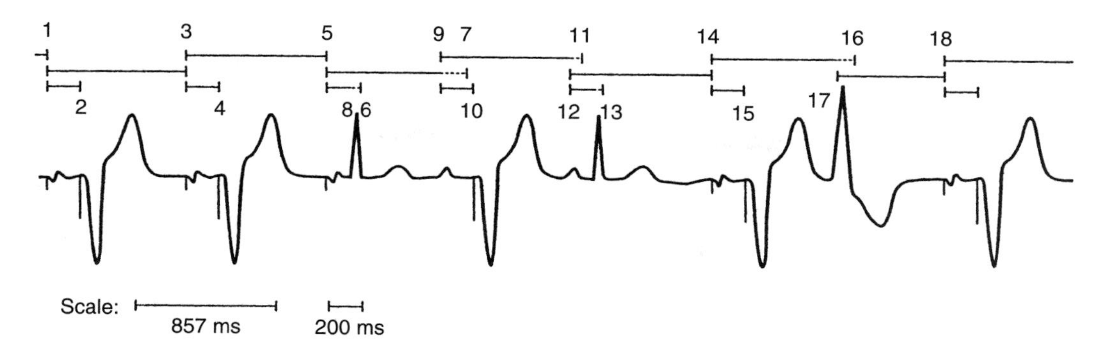

FIG. 33-8. Example of AA intercycle timing in a basic atrioventricular (AV) pacemaker capable of pacing and sensing both the atria and ventricles. The basic rate is programmed to 70 pulses/min, and the AV interval to 200 ms, corresponding to an AA interval of 857 ms and a special VA interval of 657 ms after premature ventricular complexes (PVCs). The atrial pace at *1* sets a time limit of 200 ms ending at *2* for the appearance of a ventricular event, and a limit of 857 ms ending at *3* for the next atrial event. At *2* a ventricular pace is delivered. At *3* an atrial pace is delivered, and both time limits are reset for a ventricular event by *4* and an atrial event by *5*. At *4* a ventricular pace is delivered. At *5* an atrial pace is delivered, and both time limits are reset for a ventricular event by *6* and an atrial event by *7*. At *8* a ventricular event is sensed, which cancels the time limit for *6*. At *9* an atrial sense occurs and sets the time limit for a ventricular event by *10* and an atrial event by *11*. A ventricular pace occurs at *10*. An atrial sense occurs at *12*, which cancels the time limit for *11* and resets the time limits for a ventricular event by *13* and an atrial event by *14*. A natural ventricular depolarization occurs just before *13*, which cancels the limit for *13* but leaves the limit for an atrial event by *14*. An atrial pace occurs at *14*, setting a limit for a ventricular event at *15* and an atrial event at *16*. A ventricular pace occurs at *15*. The PVC occurring at *17* cancels the atrial event time limit for *16* and resets it for 657 ms later for *18*. At *18* an atrial pace is delivered.

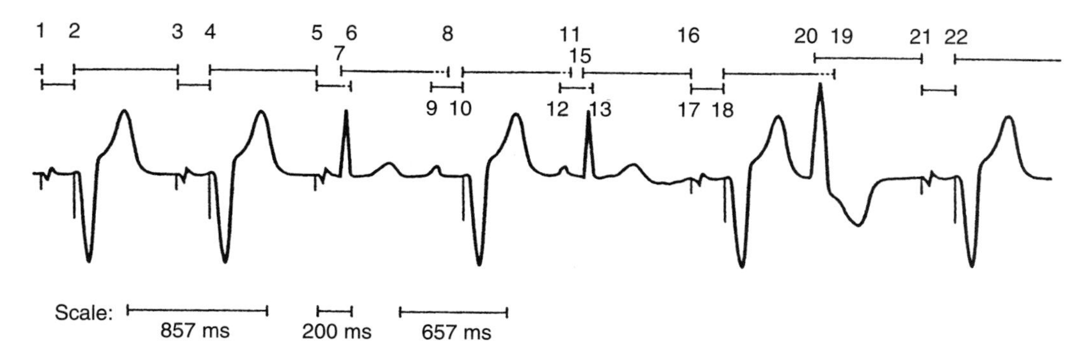

FIG. 33-9. Illustration of VA intercycle timing in a basic atrioventricular (AV) pacemaker capable of pacing and sensing both the atria and ventricles. The basic rate is programmed to 70 pulses/min and the AV interval to 200 ms, corresponding to an AA interval of 857 ms and a VA interval of 657 ms. The atrial pace at *1* sets a time limit of 200 ms, ending at *2* for the appearance of a ventricular event. At *2* a ventricular pace is delivered, and a time limit of 657 ms is set for the appearance of the next atrial event at 3. At *3* an atrial pace is delivered, and the time limit for a ventricular event is set for 4. At *4* a ventricular pace occurs, and the time limit for the next atrial event is immediately set to *5*. At *5* an atrial pace is delivered, and the time limit for a ventricular event is set for *6*. At *7* a ventricular sense occurs, canceling *6* and resetting for an atrial event by *8*. At *9* an atrial sense occurs and sets the time limit for a ventricular event by *10*. At *10* a ventricular pace occurs, and the time limit is set for an atrial event by *11*. An atrial sense occurs at *12*, which cancels *11*, and sets the time limit for a ventricular event by *13*. A ventricular depolarization occurs at *15* and sets the time limit for the next atrial event at 16, and so forth. A premature ventricular complex appears at *20*, canceling *19* and resetting the time limit for the next atrial event at *21*.

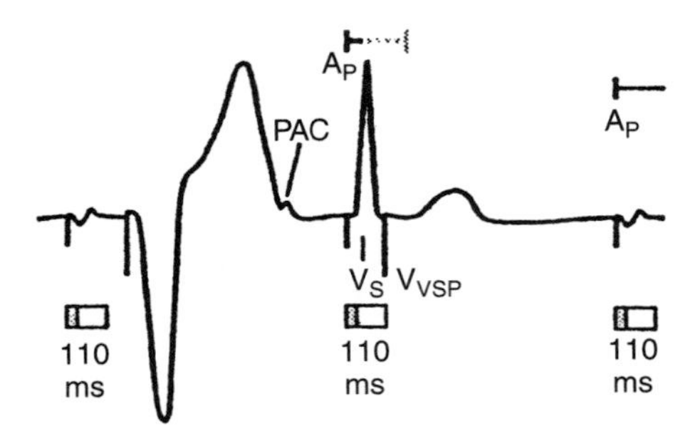

FIG. 33-10. Sketch illustrating ventricular safety pacing. During and after each atrial pace, ventricular sensing was blanked *(shading)*. After the blanking, any ventricular sense up to 110 ms would produce a committed ventricular safety pace. In the second cycle, a premature atrial complex was undersensed and thus an atrial pace occurred. Because of natural conduction from the premature atrial depolarization, a ventricular depolarization occurred and was sensed just after the blanking and produced a committed ventricular pace before the T wave. This was a normal pacemaker response. (It is very rare that a ventricular depolarization as received by the cardiac electrode will fit inside the blanking time, but if that occurs it is unsensed, and a full atrioventricular interval follows, and then the ventricle is paced. Although undesirable, this is not a device malfunction.)

pacing polarization potentials to dissipate. For added safety in the event that some potentials linger and are sensed, any ventricular sense event shortly after the blanking will initiate a committed (can not be inhibited) ventricular pace 110 ms after the atrial pace, to assure a ventricular beat. This short time (110 ms) is used so that if a random junctional, PVC, or conducted depolarization (from an undersensed atrial beat) might occur and be sensed during this moment, the ventricular pace will occur before the t wave. This feature is called *ventricular safety pacing*. It does not occur for atrial sensed events (Fig. 33-10).

Automatic determination of pacing thresholds. Some pacemakers automatically determine pacing thresholds, usually at preprogrammed times, by using special pacing sequences that appear in the ECG. These devices insert test paces of various sizes, sense for evoked potentials signifying capture, and note which paces did or did not capture.

Because some test paces will not capture, a backup pace of large size is delivered 110 ms later to assure a ventricular beat. This interval is deliberately short so that the backup pace will not be delivered into the t wave of any ventricular event (Fig. 33-11, *A* and *B*).

Magnet mode timing. Nearly all pacemakers and antitachyarrhythmia devices contain a magnetic switch that, when activated by a magnet, produces a special operation of the device, usually for testing.

In pacemakers. When a pacemaker is inhibited by natural depolarizations, there is no pacing to observe, thus all pacemaker functions can not be tested. To allow testing, magnet mode produces constant pacing at a *magnet rate*, which may be the same as the basic rate or may be a special rate. To indicate the beginning of a magnet mode, some pacemakers pace at an accelerated rate for about three to seven cycles and then go to the magnet rate. In AV pacemakers the AV interval is typically shortened during the accelerated cycles so that in patients who at present have AV conduction, ventricular capture can be evaluated before AV conduction occurs.

In antitachyarrhythmia devices. Magnet operations in antitachyarrhythmia devices vary with brands. They mostly concern tachycardia issues and have few of the magnet mode features of pacemakers.

Elective replacement indicators. Pacemakers and ICDs

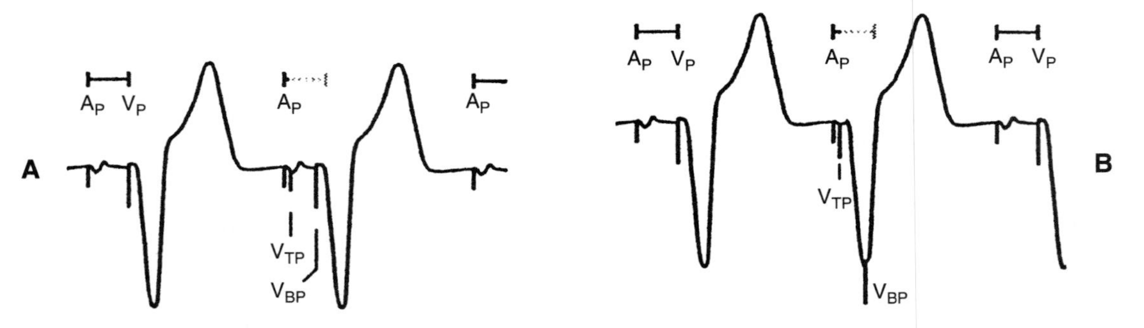

FIG. 33-11. Sketch illustrating a typical automatic ventricular threshold measurement sequence. **A,** The pacemaker inserted a ventricular test pace (V_{TP}) early in the cycle far ahead of any natural conduction and then monitored for a special signal signifying capture. There was no capture from this test pace. The backup pace (V_{BP}) provided capture. **B,** In a later cycle, a test pace of larger size captured and the backup pace occurred during tissue refractoriness, having no effect.

are powered by chemical batteries that will eventually have their energy consumed, requiring that the generator be replaced. Special circuits in the generator monitor the battery status and report it to the programmer during each check-up, giving advanced warning of the elective replacement time (ERT).

Occasionally patients are "lost to follow-up"; thus to attract the attention of the patient or general health care personnel, most pacemakers at ERT switch to a special rate called the *elective replacement indicator* (ERI) (65 ppm is common). Most dual-chamber pacemakers, to conserve remaining energy, convert to ventricular pacing only. Most ICDs do not undergo a pacing change upon ERT, but use some other method to attract attention; for example, one manufacturer's ICD, upon ERT, emits a 30-second audio tone every 24 hours.

Reviewers of ECGs should be alert to these special rates, and when seen, inquire about ERT status.

Advanced Pacing Therapies for Bradycardias

The details of newer pacing therapies for bradycardia are voluminous, thus are presented separately in Chapter 34.

ELECTRICAL THERAPIES FOR TACHYARRHYTHMIAS RESULTING FROM CELLULAR ABNORMALITIES

Electrical therapies used to treat tachycardias resulting from rapid repetitive cellular depolarizations (hyperautomaticity or trigger activity) are mainly electrical therapies of prevention because electrical therapies for the termination of these tachycardias are crude and incidental.

Prevention

Some tachycardias are initiated by transient bradycardia. Pacing to prevent the bradycardia helps prevent these tachycardias.

Some drug therapies that control tachycardia may produce bradycardia, which renders the therapy impractical. Pacing can prevent the bradycardia, allowing the drug therapy to be used. However, *pacing can mask signs of impending drug-induced ventricular proarrhythmia; thus caution is required* in this application.

Excitable tissue that is mildly unstable can sometimes be stabilized by pacing the tissue at a cycle length less than its natural cycle length. This is known as *overdrive suppression.*

A natural mixing of short and long natural cycle lengths appears to be associated with the formation of arrhythmias. Certain special programs can monitor for short cycles and then pace-shorten the following few cycles. This is believed to be stabilizing; various implementations are called *rate stabilization* or *rate regularization.*

In many patients ablation of the offending cells can provide a lifelong cure and may be preferable to electrical stimulation therapies.

In rare cases of nontreatable atrial tachycardia and fast AV conduction, ablation of the AV node can block the conduction, and ventricular pacing must then be used to support the ventricular rate.

Termination

In emergencies of last resort, tachycardias of cellular origin can sometimes be terminated with high-energy electrical shocks from a defibrillator. Although the mechanism is not defibrillation, it appears that the shock can stun or upset the offending cells, altering their behavior for better or for worse. This use of massive force certainly lacks therapeutic eloquence and specificity, but it is sometimes successful.

ELECTRICAL THERAPIES FOR TACHYARRHYTHMIAS RESULTING FROM REENTRANT LOOPS

Prevention

All the previously described preventive methods that calm excitable tissues can also be applied to prevent reentrant tachycardia. If all the loop pathways can be located and are accessible, ablations of the pathways may be curative and thus preferable to electrical stimulation therapies.

Termination

For any loop to continue to propagate, there must be nonrefractory tissue available so that the depolarizing wave front can advance into it. The key electrical termination therapies all work by artificially initiating depolarization of the tissue ahead of the advancing offending wave front so that when the offending wave front encounters the depolarized tissue, it will stop. After the tissues repolarize, it is hoped that a more normal depolarization pattern will spontaneously appear. The artificially initiated depolarization must not initiate any new loops, otherwise the original offending loop will just be replaced by a new offending loop.

Two therapeutic strategies are employed to depolarize nonrefractory tissue just ahead of the offending wave front: the application of a high-energy electric shock that instantly depolarizes all the nonrefractory tissue, or the application of a special series of pacing pulses which are critically timed to progressively redepolarize increasing amounts of the nonrefractory tissue over several heart cycles.

These therapeutic capabilities and conventional dual-chamber pacing modalities are combined in modern implantable devices called *ICDs*, an old name that understates the multiple capabilities of these newer devices.

In most applications the ICD generator (containing the electronic circuits and the batteries) is implanted in the front left shoulder. Electrical connections to the heart occur via transvenously placed leads, which at their cardiac end bear one or two small electrodes for sensing and pacing and one or two large electrodes for high-energy shocks. The metallic container of the generator also serves as a large electrode (Fig. 33-12).

For atrial sensing and pacing, the pair of small electrodes in the atria is used. For ventricular sensing and pacing, the pair of small electrodes in the ventricle is used. For tachycardia detection and classification, various combinations of all the electrodes can be used. For high-energy shocking, typically energy is applied to the large electrode in the right ventricle, and the electrodes of the superior vena cava and generator case are used to complete the circuit.

Principles of high-energy shock therapies. High-energy shock therapies were initially based on the concept that if all the cells in the heart could be depolarized simultaneously, there would be no nonrefractory tissue available to propagate the offending wave front; hence the arrhythmia would terminate.

Because an artificially applied electrical potential can disturb the cell membranes of excitable cells, causing them to depolarize, a large electrical shock applied to the entire heart can depolarize the entire heart. Depolarization of the entire heart was initially accomplished by externally applying large electrodes (paddles) onto the patient's chest and then delivering through them an enormous electrical shock from a bulky electrical apparatus. Although such devices could terminate all reentry tachycardia, they were mostly used to terminate fibrillation and so became known as defibrillators.

It later became apparent that it is not necessary to depolarize the entire heart; depolarizing just enough mass to prevent the wave front from spreading is all that is needed. This concept is known as the *critical mass hypothesis.*

With ICDs, when a rapid tachycardia occurs, the depolarization wave fronts repetitively pass by the sensing electrodes at short time intervals. As each wave passes, it produces in the sensing electrodes a small electrical signal that is conducted by the leads to the electronic unit. The electronics analyze the signals, and when the analysis indicates a sustained tachycardia, the device delivers a high-

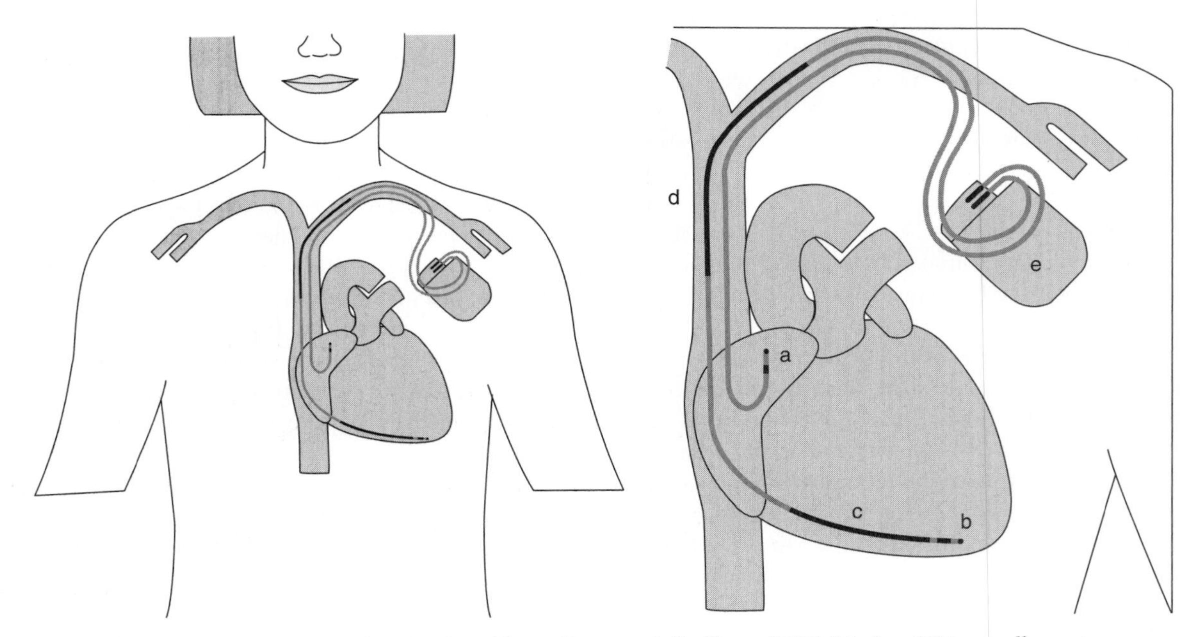

FIG. 33-12. Sketch of a modern implantable cardioverter defibrillator (ICD). Modern ICDs usually use transvenously placed leads, one in the atria *(a)* and one in the ventricle *(b)*. A pair of two small electrodes at the tip of each lead provides pacing and sensing for each lead. The high-voltage shock is delivered between a flexible electrode (approximately 5 cm long) in the ventricle *(c)* and a similar electrode in the superior vena cava *(d)* plus the metal containment of the electronic device *(e)*, which serves as an additional electrode.

energy shock. The shock may be as much as 750 volts and lasts for 5 to 8 ms.*

Cardioversion. During a tachycardia, at any time, part of the mass is depolarized (reverse-polarized and refractory) and part is nonrefractory (polarized). To terminate the tachycardia, it is necessary only to artificially depolarize the nonrefractory locations because the rest is already depolarized. Of course, at any location the states of depolarization and nonrefractoriness are constantly varying, so this is not easy to do selectively. However, if the depolarization pattern is a well-organized single-loop tachycardia, at any particular moment in each cycle a single location is nonrefractory whereas the rest of the mass is refractory. A smaller shock applied to a portion of the heart and synchronized to strike just at the moment when that portion is nonrefractory can depolarize that portion and prevent reentry into it and terminate the tachycardia. The concept of synchronizing a shock to the offending rhythm is called *cardioversion.*†

In contrast, if the depolarization pattern is chaotic and has multiple loops, the locations of nonrefractory regions at any instant are unpredictable, so cardioversion is usually not successful and large shocks are required.

In rare instances cardioversion may initiate new loops and cause fibrillation. Therefore cardioversion should be implemented only by devices that also have high-energy shock capabilities, so that if fibrillation should occur, a high-energy shock can be immediately delivered to terminate the fibrillation.

Principles of antitachyarrhythmia pacing therapies. Antitachycardia pacing (ATP) is based on the concept that in a single-loop tachycardia, any given location in the loop becomes momentarily nonrefractory as the loop rotates. If this location during this moment can be depolarized by pacing, then the looping depolarization cannot enter it and the looping will terminate.

To apply this therapy, in the tissue mass of interest, pacing pulses are applied for several seconds at a rate faster than the tachycardia rate, with the intention that the paced depolarizations will eventually invade the tachycardia loop and terminate it. This is known as burst-type antitachycardia pacing.

Typically, the wave of depolarization created by the first pace does not travel far toward the loop before it is blocked by a depolarization radiating from the loop; however, the paced depolarization blocks the depolarization that is radiating from the loop, thus preventing it from resetting the pacing site. Both areas repolarize and then the second pace quickly occurs. Because the pacing rate is faster than the tachycardia rate, the depolarization from this pace starts sooner so travels farther toward the loop before it is blocked by another depolarization radiating from the loop. This sequence repeats several times, and each successive paced depolarization travels a little farther toward the loop than the previous one, blocking the depolarizations from the loop progressively closer and closer to the loop. In time, a paced depolarization invades a location in the path of the loop during the moment when that location is nonrefractory, blocking the loop and terminating the loop. The timing is critical because the invading depolarization must collide with the leading edge of the looping depolarization to terminate the loop, yet not start a new loop where the terminating loop is repolarizing (Fig. 33-13).

When the loop terminates, only the depolarizations from the burst pacing remain. Because this rhythm is not looping, when the burst pacing stops, a natural or lower rate paced rhythm begins immediately. This is casually called a *type I break.*

Often depolarizations from the burst do not successfully enter the loop but instead only distort the loop. After the burst ends, the distorted loop may revert to the original form and the therapy then fails. More often, the distorted loop continues for several cycles and then spontaneously terminates, accomplishing the desired goal. This is casually called a *type II break* (Figs. 33-14 and 33-15).

Sometimes the burst may initiate fibrillation. This is not uncommon in atrial applications, and atrial fibrillation of this cause usually spontaneously terminates in a few seconds to several minutes, accomplishing the desired goal. In ventricular applications initiation of fibrillation in the ventricle is infrequent; however, ventricular fibrillation virtually never terminates spontaneously and is fatal if not immediately terminated by other means. Thus burst pacing in the ventricle may never be used unless high-energy shocks are available for ventricular defibrillation (see the section on Tiered Therapies and Fig. 33-16).

To improve the chance of termination, modern devices for burst pacing employ a variety of burst-pacing sequences. These devices monitor the natural heart intervals, analyze them, and then automatically select prepro-

*High-energy shocks are customarily measured in joules (J). External defibrillators deliver up to 360 J to the chest; about 10% to 20% of this amount reaches the heart. Automatic ICDs typically deliver directly to the heart 10 to 35 J for defibrillation and 0.1 to 10 J for cardioversion. All these shocks are painful, but fortunately they are very brief. By comparison, pacing stimuli are typically 0.000005 to 0.000025 J and are imperceptible.

†The term *cardioversion* has had several definitions over many years, including (1) any method used to terminate a tachycardia, (2) any method using electrical shocks to terminate a tachycardia, (3) a method for terminating atrial flutter or fibrillation in which the shock is synchronized to occur during a ventricular depolarization (it is assumed that this method is less likely to trigger a ventricular arrhythmia), and (4) a method for synchronizing a shock to a regular tachycardia to terminate the tachycardia.

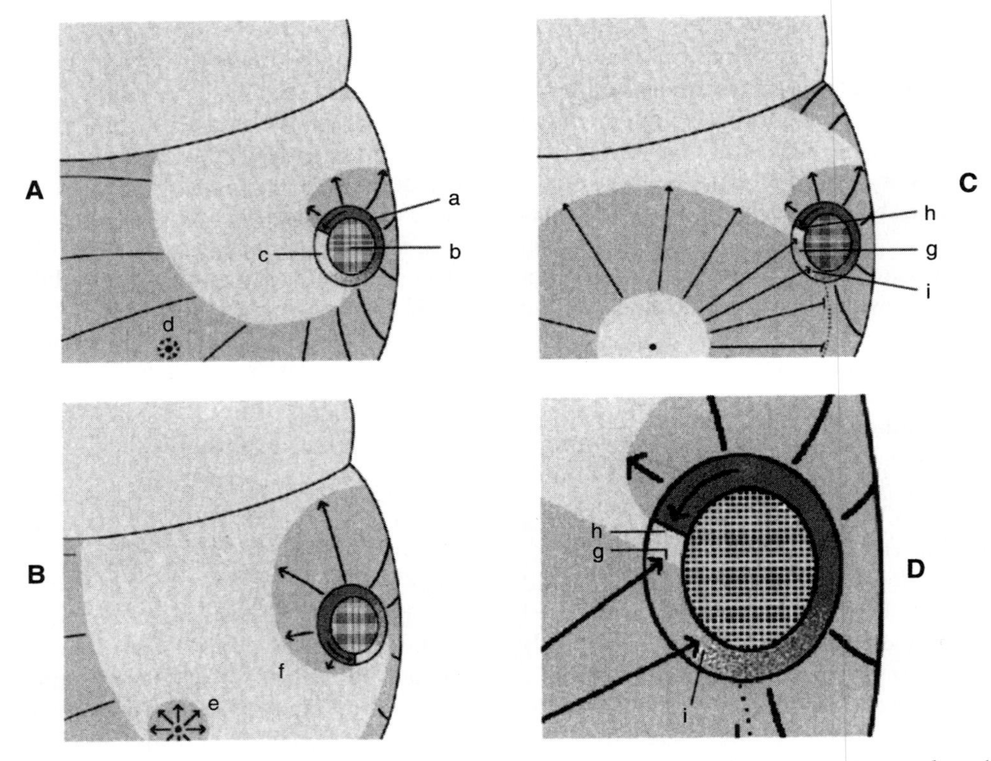

FIG. 33-13. Conceptualized termination of a single-loop reentry by antitachycardia pacing. **A,** Reentry loop *(a)* circles an anatomic obstacle *(b)*. There is a region of repolarized tissue *(c)* that rotates as part of the loop. Stimuli are introduced through an electrode at a site *(d)*. In this sketch the stimulus is unable to stimulate the tissue because the tissue is refractory *(medium shading)*. **B,** Several cycles later a stimulus occurs when the tissue is nonrefractory *(light shading)* and initiates a new depolarization radiating outward *(e)* from the electrode site. This depolarization will collide with the depolarization *(f)* coming from the loop. This collision blocks the depolarization that is coming from the loop from reaching the pacing site and resetting the site; thus the pacing site will respond to the next pacing stimulus. Because the pacing rate is faster than the looping rate, this step will repeat again and again and the paced depolarizations will gain additional distance toward the loop with each succeeding cycle. **C,** Eventually, paced depolarizations reach the loop. After several more cycles the loop becomes nonrefractory at the location where the paced depolarization arrives (shown here and in enlargement, **D**), and the paced depolarization will enter the loop. **D,** The paced depolarization *(g)* will collide with the looping depolarization *(h)* and terminate the loop. It is hoped that the paced depolarization will react favorably with repolarizing tissue *(i)* of the loop so that another loop is not started in the same path.

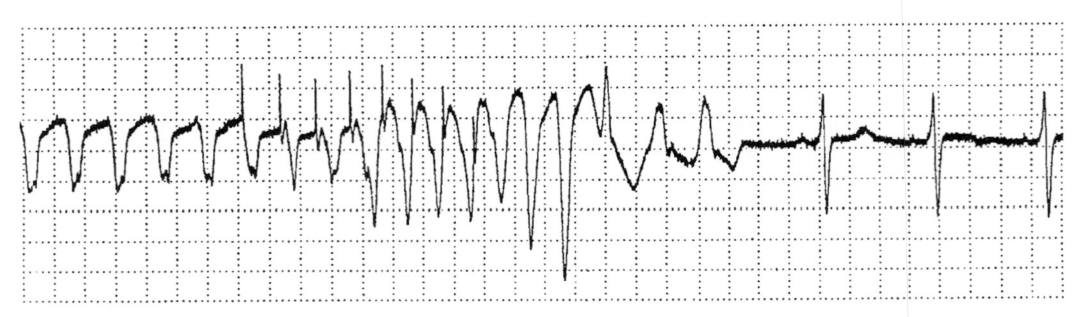

FIG. 33-14. Ventricular tachycardia terminated by antitachycardia pacing. A burst of eight pacing pulses was initially synchronized with the tachycardia and then decreased in interval with each successive pace. The paces modified the reentry path. Although modified reentry continued after the last pace, the modified rhythm was not self-sustaining and terminated after several more cycles.

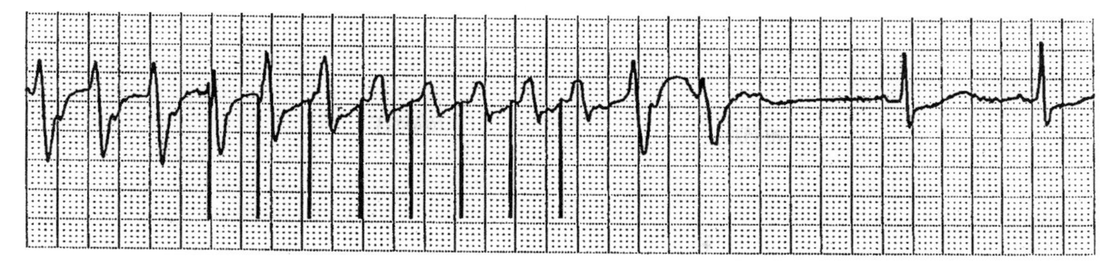

FIG. 33-15. Ventricular tachycardia terminated by antitachycardia pacing. A burst of eight paces modified the tachycardia; changes over the first five paces are evident. After the last pace the tachycardia seemed to reappear, but it was distorted too much to reestablish itself and so it terminated.

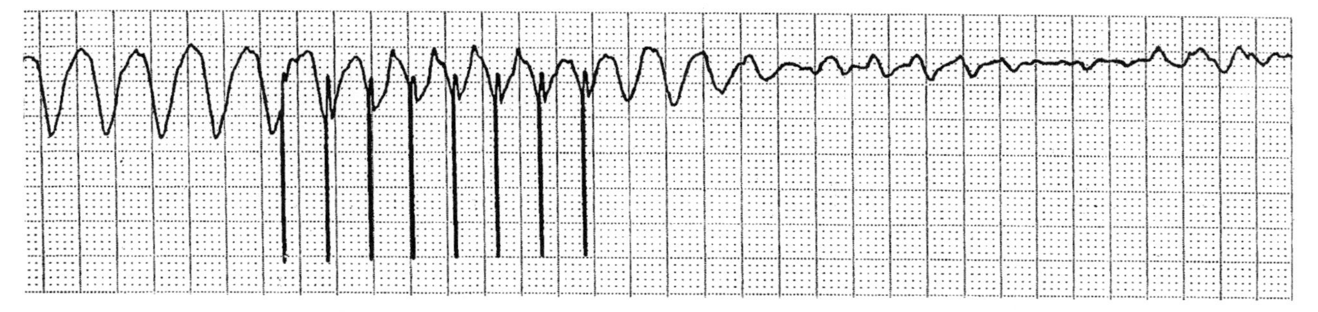

FIG. 33-16. Ventricular tachycardia accelerated by failed antitachycardia pacing. Laboratory demonstration showing a burst of eight paces, which modified the tachycardia into a reentry loop that converted to ventricular fibrillation. The importance of having backup ventricular defibrillation available whenever antitachycardia pacing is used in the ventricle is clear.

grammed burst sequences best suited to terminate the tachycardia. After each burst is applied the result is assessed. If the burst failed to terminate the tachycardia, another burst of the same or different design is tried. Some devices automatically select their first burst rate as a preprogrammed percentage above the tachycardia rate, some select an increment or decrement rate, and some set the number of paces in the burst or the duration of the burst.

Antitachycardia pacing is quite successful for terminating single-loop tachycardia that has a regular pathway, but it is much less satisfactory for multiloop or chaotic tachycardias. Ventricular fibrillation can almost never be terminated by antitachycardia pacing.

Fifty-hertz burst pacing in the atria. For some atrial tachyarrhythmia, constantly restimulating the atria for a second or two terminates the arrhythmia. This is easily done by applying 50 Hz or similarly pulsed stimuli for a second or two.

The mechanism is not totally understood, but it appears that this raises the complexity of the looping pathways to the extent that the loops are not self-supporting.

Reviewers of ECGs will see, where the therapy is applied, what looks like AC interference for about 0.5 to 3.0 seconds. ECGs recorded on monitors with the pacemaker detect feature will show continuous repetition of pacemaker markers.

This therapy must not be used in the ventricle because it will induce ventricular fibrillation that will not self-terminate. The atrial lead must be firmly anchored in the atria and pretested to ensure it cannot pace the ventricle.

Special case: atrioventricular reciprocating tachycardia. Many of the previously described preventive and termination methods are applicable to AV reciprocating tachycardia, but these methods are seldom used to treat this arrhythmia because most patients with this arrhythmia now receive a permanent cure by ablation.

Conventional AV pacemakers can also be easily used to block AV reciprocation. If the AV interval is programmed to a short value such as 70 ms, ventricular depolarization is forced to follow atrial depolarization so quickly that the ascending retrograde depolarization arrives at the atria while the atria are still refractory; thus the retrograde is blocked.

Types of Devices for Treating Tachyarrhythmias

ICDs with tiered electrical therapies. Modern ICDs can provide high-energy shocks, synchronized cardioversion, automated antitachycardia pacing, and conventional pacing, as needed.

The full range of automatic antitachycardia therapies and conventional pacing for bradycardia offer substantial advantages over any one therapy alone. For example, the conventional pacing can provide preventive benefits. Antitachycardia pacing can be used for single-loop reentrant tachycardia. High-energy shocks can be used for cardioversion, defibrillation, and termination of more resistant tachycardia. In addition, conventional pacing can prevent pauses after any tachycardia termination. Antitachycardia pacing and cardioversion can be employed in the ventricle if a high-energy shock is programmed to terminate ventricular flutter or ventricular fibrillation, if such should occur (Figs. 33-17 and 33-18).

Serious arrhythmias such as fibrillation sometimes evolve naturally from simple arrhythmias. With multifunction devices the prevention of simple arrhythmias by pacing, or their termination by antitachycardia pacing, helps prevent the emergence of serious arrhythmia, and in turn helps prevent the need for subsequent high-energy shocks. This benefit is highly significant in the ventricle because avoiding ventricular fibrillation is always desirable. In addition, conventional pacing and antitachycardia pacing is painless, whereas high-energy shocks for cardioversion and defibrillation are very painful, although quick.

Generally, devices are programmed to respond to

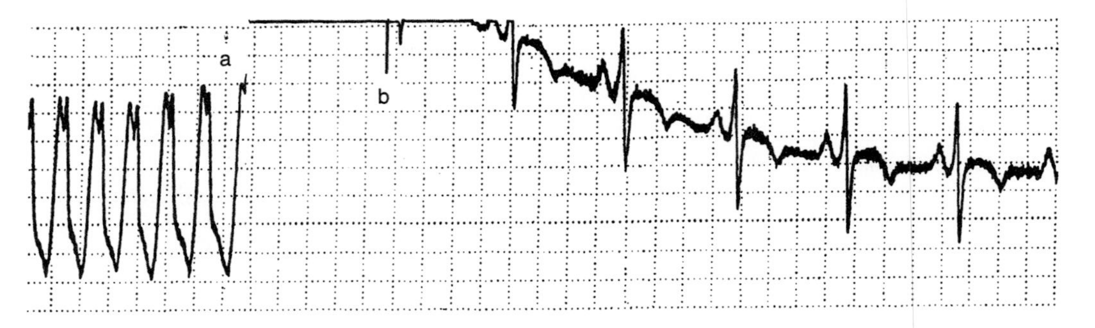

FIG. 33-17. Ventricular tachycardia terminated by cardioversion. A synchronized, low-energy shock of 0.2 J was applied to the ventricle *(a)* and terminated the tachycardia. This internal cardiac defibrillator also began backup pacing 1000 ms after the shock as can be partially seen off the upper edge of the paper *(b)*. Thereafter the native rate was faster than the pacing rate, so sensing inhibited pacing.

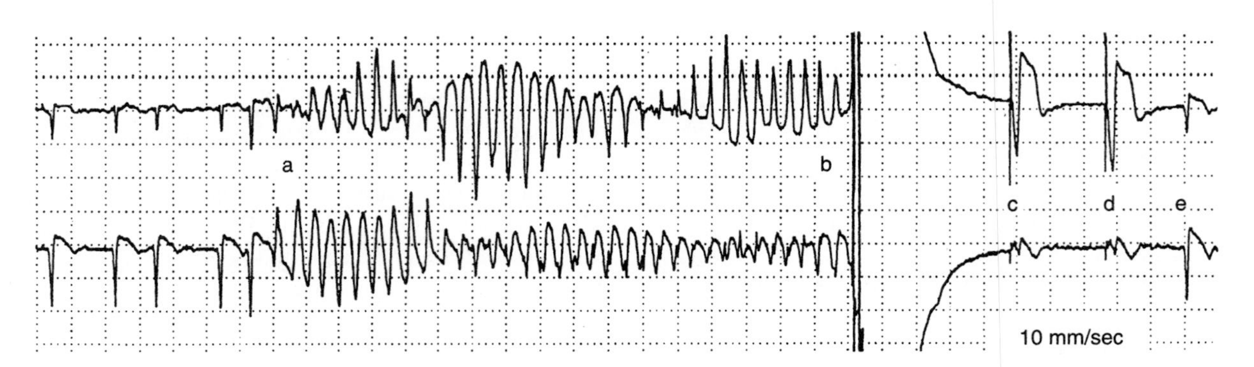

FIG. 33-18. Ventricular fibrillation terminated by high-energy shock. Tape-recorded episode of spontaneous ventricular fibrillation *(a)*. The internal cardiac defibrillator detected the rhythm and delivered a high-energy shock *(b)*, which terminated the ventricular fibrillation. When a natural rhythm did not return, backup pacing occurred (*c* and *d*) until a natural rhythm was sensed *(e)*.

simple tachyarrhythmias in a stepwise manner, automatically trying the pacing termination routines first and then increasing in aggressiveness until success is achieved. This is known as *tiered electrical therapy.* Generally these devices are also programmed to respond immediately to ventricular flutters and ventricular fibrillation by delivering an immediate high-energy shock, bypassing less aggressive tiers.

ICDs with additional atrial antitachyarrhythmia features. High-energy shocks to the ventricle usually produce sufficient collateral energy in the atria to terminate atrial reentry tachycardias. This is especially true if one of the high energy electrodes is placed in the superior vena cava, which draws current through the atria. There are special ICDs that exploit this effect. In addition to the tiered therapy features, these ICDs employ special features which detect and classify atrial tachyarrhythmias and apply atrial ATP therapies. If these are unsuccessful, high-energy cardioversion shocks can be delivered. In this application, shocks are synchronized to occur upon a ventricular event, to prevent initiating a ventricular arrhythmia (see previous footnote, p. 465).

Shocks for atrial purposes may be automatic or elective. For example, in one device, elective options allow selection of the hours of the day when shocks are allowed, or the patient can enable a shock manually by using an external activator, a little accessory device that can be held over the ICD to interrogate the ICD for present arrhythmia status, and if desired, allow a shock. In the rare event of a ventricular tachyarrhythmia starting during any of the atrial therapies, atrial therapies are stopped and ventricular therapies are applied.

Pacemakers with atrial antitachyarrhythmia features. AV pacemakers are also available with special antitachycardia therapies. These therapies are only used for atrial applications and in patients without accessory conduction paths. (Because antitachyarrhythmia pacing can occasionally induce fibrillation, ventricular applications cannot be safely performed without ventricular high-energy backup protection. Accessory conduction could carry accelerated atrial arrhythmia to the ventricle.)

These pacemakers are frequently used along with drug therapies and have extensive diagnostic capabilities to help guide drug management. For example, these pacemakers have built-in computer programs that constantly analyze the patient's rhythm and store significant information which can be read from the pacemaker when interrogated by an external receiver or programmer. The pacemakers also record and store internal ECGs of pertinent events for study upon interrogation.

Standard pacemakers. Standard pacemakers produced by some manufacturers for treating bradycardia can *in the*

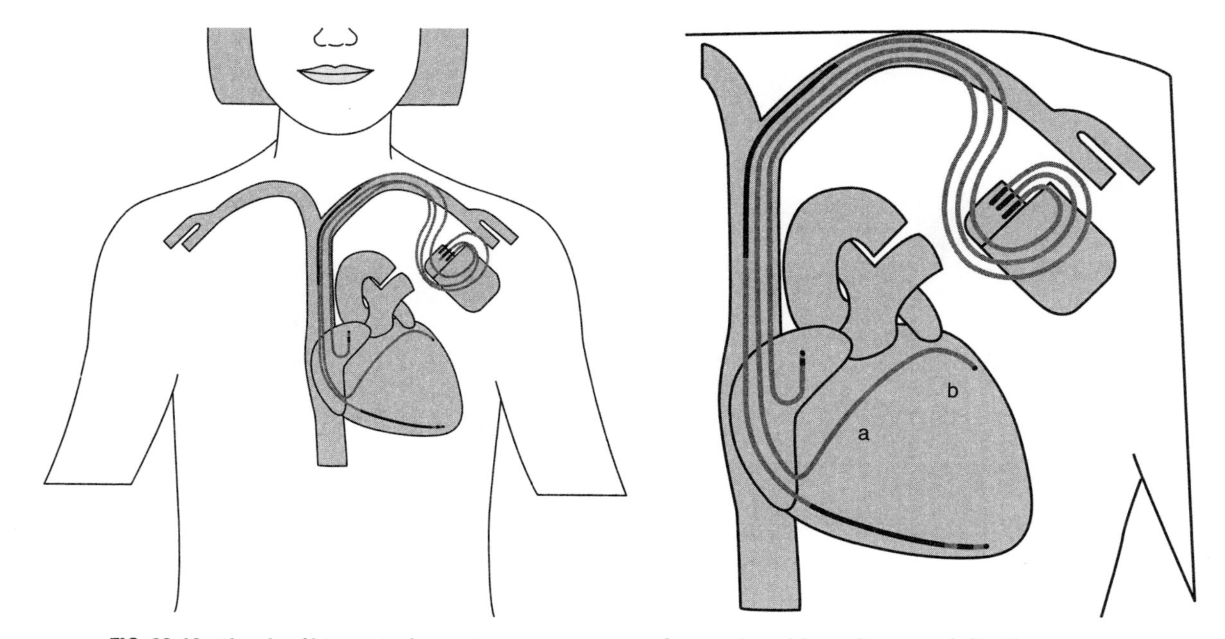

FIG. 33-19. Sketch of biventricular pacing system as part of an implantable cardioverter defibrillator system. A second ventricular pacing electrode was transvenously introduced and retrogradely passed through the coronary sinus *(a)* into a ventricular cardiac vein on the left ventricle *(b)*. Pacing occurs through the wall of the vein.

hospital setting be noninvasively linked to programmers to perform complex elective antitachycardia pacing routines in either the atria or ventricles. Certain noninvasive electrophysiologic studies can be conducted in this manner also.

ELECTRICAL THERAPIES FOR MAINTAINING OR RESTORING CARDIAC CONTRACTION SYNCHRONY

Until recently, for bradycardia applications with either pacemakers or ICDs, no particular attention was given to where in the atria or ventricle the pacing stimuli were delivered. Recently it has been shown that in some patients, especially heart failure patients, the efficiency of ventricular contractions can depend on the timing of the right and left ventricles and the location where stimulation occurs. It has also been shown that in heart failure patients with bundle branch block and normal heart rates, pacing to resynchronize the ventricles can be beneficial.

For resynchronization of the ventricles, using either a pacemaker or an ICD, the pacing system is similar to that described before except that there is an additional lead for pacing the left ventricle. An example showing a typical arrangement for an ICD is in Fig. 33-19.

Less commonly, resynchronization of the atria is employed, with an additional lead in the coronary sinus and curved upward for pacing the left atria.

The details of cardiac resynchronization are presented in Chapter 34.

ECGs FROM IMPLANTED ELECTRODE LOCATIONS

ECGs from Implantable Event Recorders (Implantable Loop Recorders)

Implantable event recorders are used to identify or rule out rhythm disturbances. They are implanted subcutaneously, usually in the upper left chest (Fig. 33-20). They constantly record the ECG, retaining the most recent minutes of recording. Upon automatic detection of a bradycardia or tachycardia or upon a patient command (using a tiny external transmitter), the most recent several minutes of ECG are stored for later retrieval using a programmer.

The recordings are for rhythm analysis only, so there are no standards for placement; recordings may be in any vector, and may even be upside-down from conventional recordings. Because the electrode spacings are short, the QRS voltages are typically about a fifth of standard recordings; thus the recordings are additionally amplified about five times for viewing. The higher amplification increases the appearance of muscle noise when patients are active. The frequency response is limited and introduces some variations in the amplitude compared to standard ECGs. An example is shown in Fig. 33-21.

Reviewers of ECGs must be adept at recognizing ECG

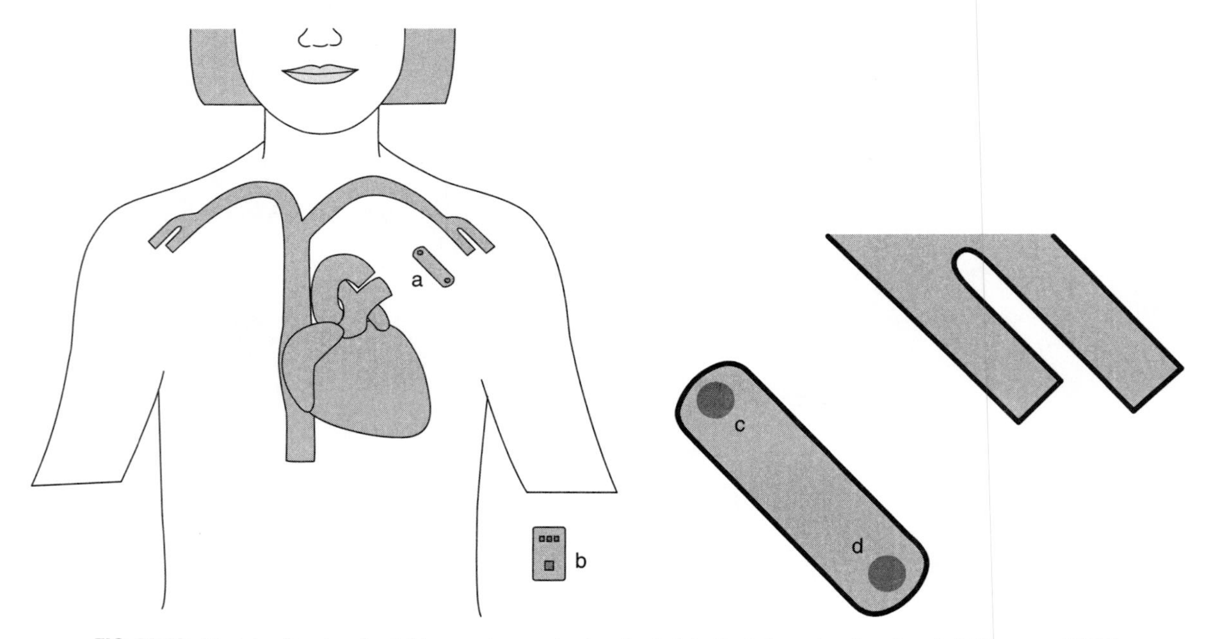

FIG. 33-20. Sketch of an implantable event recorder implanted in the left pectoral region *(a)*. Storage of ECG segments can be automatically or electively activated by using a remote transmitter *(b)*. The ECG is recorded through two electrodes 5 cm apart (*c* and *d*).

features in unusual vectors and in the presence of myopotentials.

ECGs from Pacemakers and ICDs

Dual-chamber pacemakers and ICDs have the distinct advantage of being able to record from the atria and ventricle separately and be relatively free from interferences. The frequency response of the ECGs is optimized for rhythm analysis and is not intended for analysis of ischemia or hypertrophy.

Reviewers of conventional ECGs for patients with existing pacemakers and ICDs will find the adjunctive use of intracardiac recordings, pacemaker markers, and patient activity record helpful when interpreting ECGs.

Although ambulatory monitors and event recorders are helpful in diagnosing arrhythmias, they do not always catch the event. Second, for very fast tachycardias, the mechanisms often remain ambiguous, usually because atrial activity is obscured by ventricular signals, myopotentials, and motion artifacts. Differentiating atrial causes from ventricular causes is critical to therapeutic strategies.

Many newer pacemakers and ICDs continuously monitor and analyze intracardiac ECGs, store analytical data, and store selected ECG segments and sense/pace markers for later retrieval. In addition they record the patient's activity level. Upon retrieval, analytical data are presented in charts, tables, and graphs, and the ECGs and markers as tracings.

Pacemakers and ICDs can record cardiac signals from between a pair of atrial cardiac electrodes, a pair of ven-

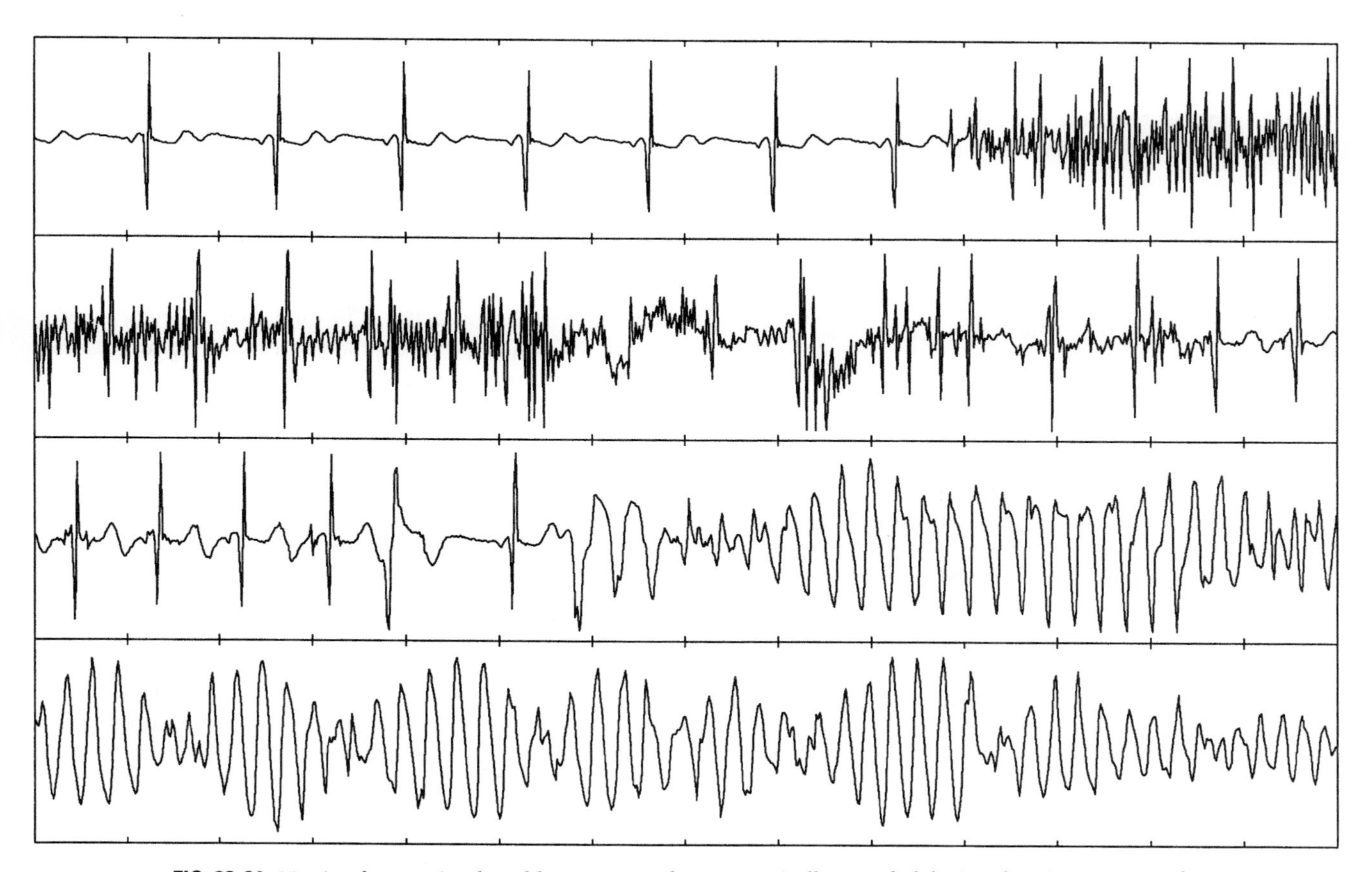

FIG. 33-21. Tracing from an implantable event recorder automatically recorded during sleep in a young male with recurrent sudden-onset syncope and negative neuro, cardiac, and drug provocation tests for long QT interval. This continuous recording begins with a heart rate of 44 beats/min and prolonged QT interval. The muscle activity recorded at the end of the first panel is followed by an acceleration in heart rate to 65 beats/min. The third panel nicely shows torsades de pointes and its classical beginning (i.e., a "short-long-short" sequence created by an ectopic beat followed by a pause). Fortunately, the arrhythmia self-terminated, and the patient is now protected from this potentially lethal event by a dual-chamber ICD. (Courtesy Robert S. Fishel, MD, West Palm Beach, Fla.)

tricular cardiac electrodes, an atrial cardiac electrode and the pulse generator, or a ventricular cardiac electrode and the generator (exact combinations and number of recordable channels depend on generator brand, model, and leads).

Cardiac signals at a distance from the heart. All cardiac cells, when they depolarize, radiate an electric potential that diminishes with distance. For locations more than several centimeters from the heart, the signal from each cell is extremely small, but the combined signals from millions of synchronized cells produce potentials of about 1 to 2 mV. The atrial and ventricular signals combine with each other. Electrodes in the superior vena cava and the generator record this signal.

Cardiac signals at the heart. An electrode in contact with the heart also records signals from the whole heart, but when the cells near the electrode depolarize, because of closeness their potential is not significantly diminished, so they contribute considerable potential to the electrode; the amount depends on the number of local cells (wall thickness), fiber orientation, depolarization direction, and other local factors. For the brief moment when atrial depolarization passes the atrial electrode, the potential there may reach as much as 6 mV (1 to 4 is typical). The ventricle is thicker and for the brief moment when the ventricular depolarization passes the ventricular electrode, the potential there may reach as much as 25 mV (8 to 15 is typical).

The choice of electrode sizes and locations (tip, ring, high voltage electrode, and generator case), the recording frequency response, the data sample rate, and other factors markedly determine the morphology of the waveforms displayed. In general, the waveforms are fast (20 to 40 ms in duration) because they are dominated by the local depolarization. The morphology also has a polarity reversal (similar to an intrinsicoid deflection) as the wave front passes the electrode (Fig. 33-22). Although there are no standards, different morphologies in the same recording indicate depolarizations from different origins. For example, in the atrial ECG, the morphology of a sinus beat is usually different from that of a retrograde beat.

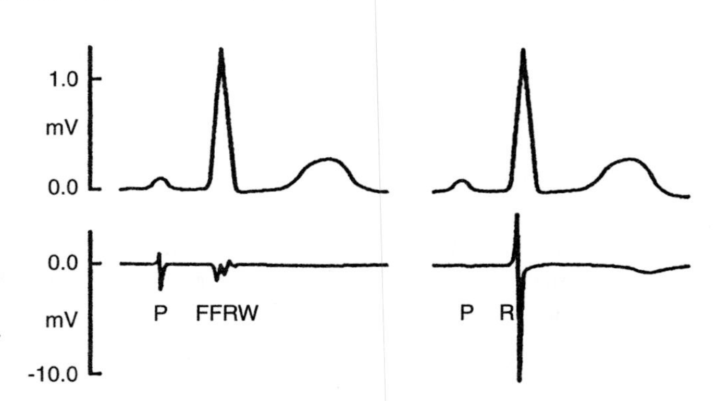

FIG. 33-22. Sketch of typical atrial electrogram (*lower left*) and ventricular electrogram (*lower right*). Note the scale is tenfold greater in the lower recordings. The main atrial and ventricular deflections are casually called "P" and "R" waves as in the surface ECG. Sometimes the ventricular depolarization contributes some signal to the atrial recording, and this is called a *far-field R wave (FFRW)*. Rarely does the atrial depolarization contribute measurable signal to the ventricular recording.

SUMMARY

In this chapter, only those features that are likely to be encountered in general cardiac care have been discussed, and only as an overview. In recent years there has been a rapid expansion of features in implantable devices. Major areas not discussed involve arrhythmia detections, differential rhythm classifications, therapeutic selections, internal patient monitoring, data collection, diagnostics, feature interactions, device self-monitoring, and outcome reporting.

As a result of the increasing complexity, management of arrhythmias and cardiac resynchronization by devices has become a specialty.

ACKNOWLEDGMENT

Thank you to Walter Olson, PhD, Sam Pollack, Steve Subera, and Rick Grooms of Medtronic, Inc.; and to Robert S. Fishel, MD, West Palm Beach, Fla, for sample ECGs. Appreciation is expressed to Medtronic Customer Services members and Ronald Stuedemann, director, for their support.

CHAPTER 34

Pacemaker Therapies for Bradyarrhythmias

John R. Buysman, PhD

GOALS OF PACING

Historically, pacing was intended to save the life of the patient, but in the last 20 years most new developments were made to improve the quality of life and extend the life of the patient. Indeed, recently pacing is being used to improve cardiac efficiencies in patients with naturally normal heart rates, a nontraditional application.

The principal goals for improving quality of life are as follows:

- To support normal arterial pressures and cardiac output for a wide range of varying activities
- Not to raise venous pressures (as some older pacing methods do)
- Not to stress the atria in ways predisposing to earlier onset of atrial disease (as some older pacing methods do)

Achievement of these goals came largely from two strategies:

- Constant adjustment of heart rate (HR) to match the activity of the patient
- Ensuring constant atrioventricular (AV) synchrony

In addition, for selected patients, resynchronization of the right-left heart timing has maintained or improved cardiac efficiencies.

Cardiovascular Regulation in Health

Cardiac output and pressure regulation. The vast array of blood vessels, capillaries, and organs can be reduced to the simplified circulatory diagram in Fig. 34-1.

In normal health, pressure in the systemic arteries pushes blood through the millions of capillaries in the tis-

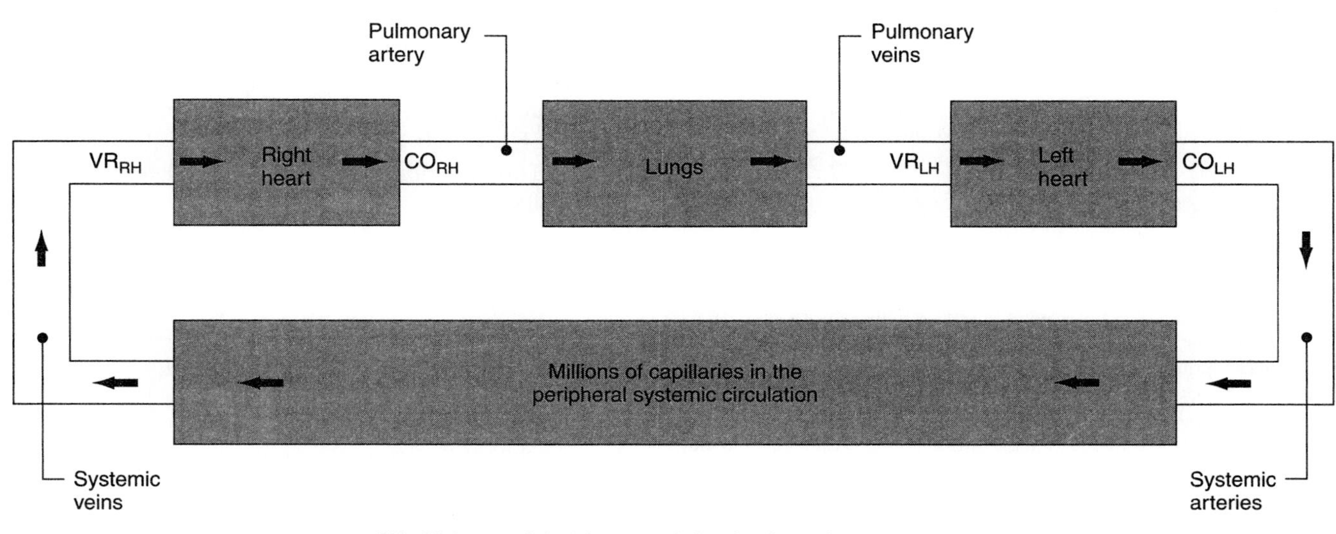

FIG. 34-1. Simplified functional sketch of circulatory system.

sues throughout the body. Each capillary opens and closes to allow through just the amount of blood it needs to service its local area. The arterial pressure has only a small effect on the capillary flow, provided the pressure is adequate to support the flow desired.

Blood leaving the capillaries combines into the systemic veins and returns to the heart. Thus it is the combined flow through the millions of capillaries that sets the total flow rate at which blood is returned to the heart. This flow is called the *systemic venous return* or the *venous return to the right heart.*

The heart can pump blood out of its ventricles forcefully; however, it has almost no ability to draw blood into itself to refill. The right ventricle is filled mostly by the systemic venous pressure, which although small, during cardiac diastole pushes blood through the right atria into the right ventricle. During late ventricular diastole, the atrial contraction swishes additional blood into the ventricle.

The amount of filling that occurs for each beat depends upon a balance between the systemic venous pressure (which forces filling) and the stretch characteristics of the right ventricle (which resists filling).

When the ventricular contraction occurs, blood is pumped out of the right ventricle into the pulmonary artery until a balance with the pulmonary arterial pressure occurs or ventricular systole ends, in either case leaving some blood still in the ventricle. The amount pumped out is called the *right heart stroke volume,* and it is approximately equal to the volume which was added to the ventricle during filling.

Over a short period, such as a minute, the balance between systemic venous pressure and right ventricular (RV) stretch properties adjusts such that the average stroke volume of the right heart (SV_{RH}) becomes equal to the systemic venous return to the right heart (VR_{RH}) divided by the HR.

The heart rate and right stroke volume determine the amount of blood pumped out by the right ventricle. Over a minute, the SV_{RH} times the HR equals the *cardiac output of the right heart* (CO_{RH}). Thus the systemic venous return determines right heart cardiac output.*

$$\frac{VR_{RH}}{HR} = SV_{RH} \text{ and } SV_{RH} \times HR = CO_{RH}$$

Right heart cardiac output fills the pulmonary arteries to produce the pulmonary arterial pressure needed to push blood through the lung capillaries. The lung capillaries have little self-regulating capabilities.

The combined flow through the lung capillaries provides the total flow rate at which blood is returned to the left atria. This flow is called the *pulmonary venous return* or the *venous return to the left heart.* The mechanisms for the left heart are the same as those for the right heart. The left ventricle is filled by pulmonary venous pressure plus some additional filling during atrial systole.

The amount of filling depends upon a balance between the pulmonary venous pressure and the stretch characteristics of the left ventricle. When the ventricular contraction occurs, blood is pumped out until a balance with the systemic arterial pressure occurs or ventricular systole ends, in either case leaving some blood still in the ventricle. The amount pumped out is called the *left heart stroke volume,* and it is approximately equal to the volume which was added to the left ventricle during filling. Over a short period the balance between pulmonary venous pressure and left ventricular (LV) stretch properties adjusts such that the average stroke volume of the left heart (SV_{LH}) becomes equal to the pulmonary venous return to the left heart (VR_{LH}) divided by the HR.

The HR and SV_{LH} determine the amount of blood pumped out by the left ventricle. Over a minute, the SV_{LH} times the HR equals the cardiac output of the left heart (CO_{LH}). Thus pulmonary venous return determines left heart cardiac output.

$$\frac{VR_{LH}}{HR} = SV_{LH} \text{ and } SV_{LH} \times HR = CO_{LH}$$

CO_{LH} fills the systemic arteries to produce the systemic arterial pressure needed to push blood through the peripheral capillaries.

Over several seconds, the pulmonary venous pressure adjusts such that the left heart pumps the same amount as what the right heart pumps. In summary, the systemic capillary flow sets the venous return to the right heart, which sets the right cardiac output, which sets the left cardiac

*The basis of this relationship can be seen by example. Assume to begin that the flow through the capillaries is constant and that the right heart cardiac output is equal to the total flow through the capillaries. If the HR was then increased, the cardiac output would become greater than the total flow through the capillaries, thus the veins would begin to empty, which would decrease venous pressure, which would decrease the degree of ventricular filling, which would decrease the stroke volume, which would decrease cardiac output. This would continue until the cardiac output was again equal to the total flow through the capillaries. A decrease in rate would bring about opposite changes, but end with the same result—that is that the cardiac output becomes the same as the incoming venous return. Consider another example, if the total flow through the capillaries were to increase, the venous pressure would increase, which would increase RV filling, which would increase stroke volume, which would increase cardiac output. This would continue until the cardiac output became equal to the total flow through the capillaries. A decrease in total flow though the capillaries would bring about the opposite changes, with the cardiac output becoming equal to the total flow through the capillaries. Thus cardiac output automatically adjusts to match the venous return.

output. Because over a short time, the right and left stroke volumes are equal, and the right and left cardiac outputs are equal, in casual discussions left and right distinctions are often not stated.

Response to changing activity. During activity, blood flow through the systemic capillaries in the tissues increases, which in turn increases the rate of blood return to the heart. In normal health the heart accommodates this return because there is an increase in heart rate and stroke volume.

HR mechanisms. The HR is normally increased by two mechanisms:

1. Activity produces a rise in sympathetic tone and catecholamine release, which increases heart rate.
2. The increased return of blood to the heart distends the atria, which enhances sinoatrial node automaticity.

Stroke volume mechanisms. Stroke volume increases by several mechanisms:

- The increased return of venous blood increases the venous pressure, which fills the ventricles, filling them more fully.
- The increased sympathetic and catecholamine drive does the following:
    1. Tightens the veins and increases venous pressure, which fills the ventricles more fully
    2. Enhances cardiac relaxation allowing filling to proceed more easily during diastole
    3. Increases cardiac contractility, which helps the heart to contract tighter and thus empty to a greater extent at the end of each systole

Cardiovascular Regulation in Abnormal Rhythms

In many cardiac patients, some of the above natural mechanisms are blunted or absent.

Inadequate heart rate. In patients with mildly inadequate heart rate, the return of venous blood raises venous pressure in excess of normal until the pressure produces enough ventricular filling to increase stroke volume sufficiently to accommodate the returning blood flow. This excess of venous pressure can result in systemic and pulmonary congestion and can distend the atria predisposing over time to atrial disease. The increased filling produces an exaggerated stroke volume that can cause the contractile process to become less efficient.

If adequate filling can not be accomplished during exercise, cardiac output is limited and may not be able to support arterial pressure; indeed, in such a case if exercise is not immediately stopped, collapse will occur.

If heart rate is profoundly inadequate, cardiac output is not sufficient to support arterial pressure even at rest, and collapse and death will occur.

Inadequate AV synchronization

Heart blocks. In patients with first-, second-, or third-degree heart block, the atrial contribution to ventricular filling may be inefficient, sparse, or absent. In such cases, even if rate is adequate (natural or paced without synchronization), the venous pressure will rise to produce the needed filling without the atrial contribution. If the ventricle is difficult to fill, the rise in venous pressure may be significant, resulting in systemic and pulmonary venous congestion, and may distend the atria predisposing over time to atrial diseases. In second- and third-degree block, HR is usually inadequate (unpaced), and the rise in venous pressures to compensate for the loss of the atrial contribution is in addition to the rise because of the slow rate.

Junctional, ventricular escaped, or AV-unsynchronized ventricular paced rhythms. In patients with junctional, ventricular escaped, or AV-unsynchronized paced rhythms, the atrial contribution to ventricular filling is either randomly timed or consistently malsynchronized, the latter if retrograde conduction into the atria causes atrial contractions during ventricular contractions. The atria has less pressure capability than the ventricles, so it cannot transfer blood into the ventricles during this time; indeed, during atrial contractions blood is pumped backwards out of the atria. The atrial consequences are the same as for complete heart block.

Diminished contraction capability resulting from atrial or ventricular dyssynchrony

Intra-atrial conduction delays (atrial dyssynchrony). In patients with intra-atrial conduction delays, the timing of the atrial contributions to ventricular fillings may not be optimal.

Bundle branch blocks (BBB) (ventricular dyssynchrony). In patients with BBB, the timings of the ventricular contractions relative to their received atrial contributions may not be optimal for both ventricles. The right and left pressure rises may not produce a normal pressure differential across the septum, causing septal displacement. AV valve closure might be affected. These effects can lower the efficiency of pumping, which is significant for patients with heart failure.

PACING THERAPIES FOR CORRECTION OF HEART RATE AND AV SYNCHRONY

Correction of heart rate and AV synchrony by cardiac pacing employs overlapping strategies that are discussed together in the following section. Correction of right-left conduction delays employs additional strategies that are discussed separately in a later section.

Determination of Desired Heart Rate for Various Activities (Sensor Rate)

Basic concept. Although several technologies have been developed to manage heart rate, they all are based on a common concept, as illustrated in Fig. 34-2.

When the patient is at rest, only a minimum HR is needed. Thus all pacemakers have a programmable lower rate limit (LRL). When the patient is active, there is a certain rate appropriate for the activity. Thus the pacemaker must determine the patient's present amount of activity and determine the corresponding desired rate. At very high activity, very high rates might adversely limit diastolic time (during which ventricular filling occurs and coronary flow occurs), thus all pacemakers have a programmable upper rate limit (URL) to forbid an excessive pacing rate.

Sensors. Pacemakers determine the desired rate for a given activity through the use of "sensors" that measure the amount of activity the person is engaged in. The three most common sensors are the following.

Activity sensors. Physical activity produces accelerations and vibrations in the body. The more active the person, the more the accelerations and vibrations. Activity-measuring pacemakers use sensors inside the pacemaker that directly measure these accelerations and vibrations. The desired rate is calculated according to activity estimates based on the amount of accelerations and vibrations present.

Respiratory sensors. Physical activity increases respiration. The more active the person, the greater the respiratory response. Respiration-measuring pacemakers measure the respiratory volume rate (analogous to minute ventilation) of the person. The respiratory volumes are estimated by passing a tiny electric current (less than pacing currents) through the lung space between the pacemaker and a lead electrode in the heart. During breathing, the size of the lung space changes, which changes its electric resistance. The desired rate is calculated according to activity estimates based on these resistance changes that reflect the amount of the respiratory response.

Sympathetic tone sensor. Physical and emotional stress cause a natural increase in sympathetic tone, which in cardiac cells causes a slight shortening of the time from depolarization to repolarization. The more active the person, the shorter the depolarization-to-repolarization time. The most common sympathetic tone-measuring pacemakers measure this time as recorded from the electrodes of the pacing system. This is casually called a *QT sensor* because it mimics the Q-T interval of a surface electrocardiogram (ECG). The desired rate is calculated according to activity estimates based on the amount of QT shortening present, which reflects activity and stress.

Some pacemakers employ two different sensors to provide improved responses.

The desired rate determined from sensor measurements is called the *sensor rate*. To assist physicians in appropriately adjusting and refining sensor rate program settings, pacemakers record and store data in the pacemaker for retrieval and analysis at follow-ups. Sensor data, HR, pacing and sensing data, tachycardia episodes, trends, mode changes, and so on provide extensive information. Recently, built-in computer algorithms allow some pacemakers to automatically program sensor settings themselves as needed in accordance with general guidelines prescribed (via programming) by the physician.

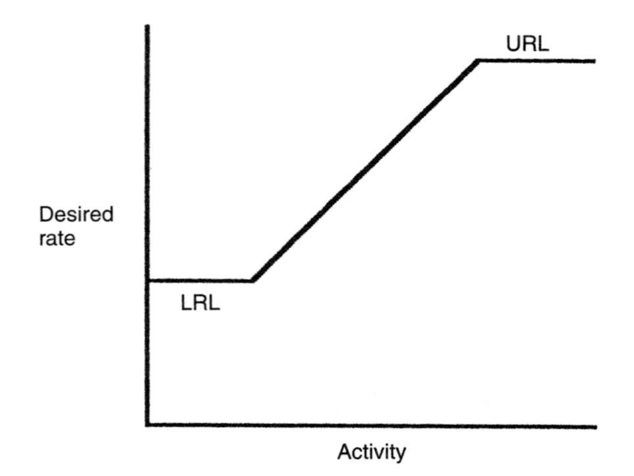

FIG. 34-2. Illustration showing that at minimum activity a basic rate is required, the lower rate limit *(LRL)*. At increased activity the desired HR is increased, and at high activity an upper rate limit *(URL)* is applied to the rate.

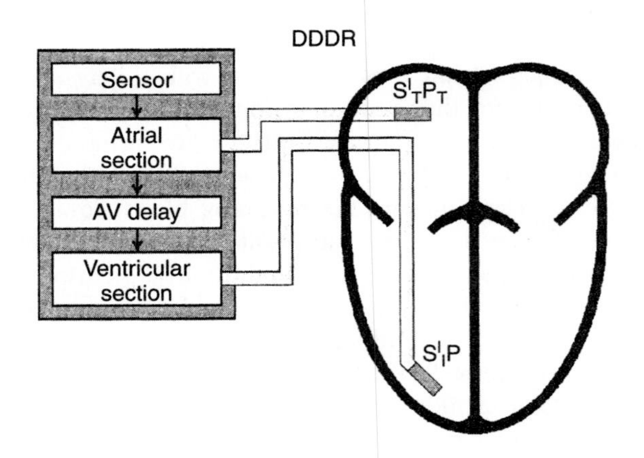

FIG. 34-3. Functional diagram of an atrioventricular pacemaker.

Implementing a Responsive HR and AV Synchrony

Various manufacturers use various methods, the most common is described here.

Most bradycardia patients have intermittently inadequate atrial rate responses to activity, and most have unreliable conduction. In these patients it is necessary to employ atrioventricular pacemakers with a sensor, operating in the DDDR mode.* The sensor continuously monitors the patient's activity to determine the desired rate at the present moment (Fig. 34-3).

The sensor continuously measures the activity of the patient and calculates the desired HR (sensor rate) for the activity.

The atrial section, upon the occurrence of an atrial event (sensed or paced), starts time limits for the appearance of the next ventricular event and the next atrial event. To start the ventricular time limit, the atrial event triggers the AV delay section, which operates the ventricular time limit.

The ventricular section monitors for any natural ventricular depolarization that might occur and be sensed before the ventricular time limit (AV delay) expires. If a natural ventricular depolarization is sensed, it inhibits (cancels) the impending ventricular pace. If not, when the time limit expires, the ventricle is immediately paced.

The atrial section monitors the atria for a natural depolarization signifying the start of the next cycle. If a natural atrial event is sensed, the time limit schedule for the next atrial pace will be inhibited. If no natural atrial event is sensed, when the atrial time limit expires, the atria will be paced. The atrial time limit is an interval corresponding to the sensor rate, so the pace is at the sensor rate. In either case, an atrial event starts the new cycle.

When natural atrial rate is greater than sensor rate. Many patients have normal naturally occurring atrial rates at times. It is preferable to use natural atrial contractions whenever possible, thus whenever the natural atrial rate is greater than the sensor rate, atrial pacing is by design inhibited and the natural atrial activity is *tracked*. Tracking also provides AV synchrony.

When a natural atrial event is sensed, the pacemaker establishes two time limits for future events: one to check for the appearance of the next natural ventricular event,

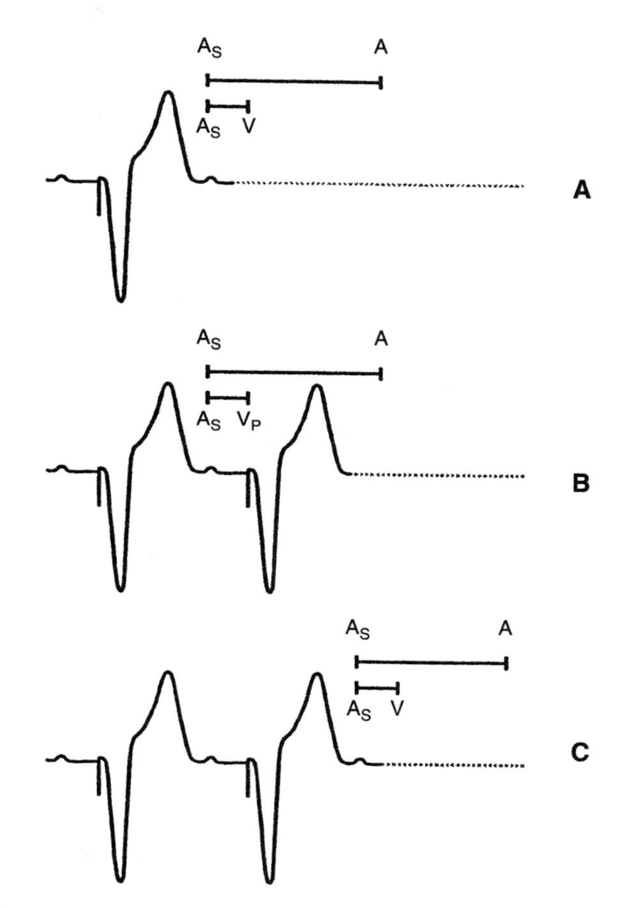

FIG. 34-4. Sketch illustrating tracking of a natural atrial rate when the natural atrial rate is greater than the sensor rate. **A,** Sensing of a natural atrial depolarization *(A_S)* started two time limits. The *upper bar* represents the time limit for the next atrial event *(A);* the *lower bar* represents that for the next ventricular event *(V).* The sensor constantly adjusts the A_SA time limit to be the interval equivalent of the sensor rate. The atrioventricular (A_SV) time limit is set to the AV interval. **B,** A natural ventricular event failed to occur before the ventricular time limit expired, so the ventricle was paced at the limit expiration and produced a ventricular beat. **C,** Because the natural atrial rate was adequate (greater than the sensor rate), the next atrial event occurred and was sensed before the existing atrial time limit expired; thus the scheduled potential atrial pace was inhibited and new time limits were immediately reestablished. Note that tracking produced a natural rate with pacemaker AV synchrony. The intervals are called AA, AV, and VA, respectively.

*Various combinations of pacing, sensing, and special features are called *modes*, and are typically named by a five-letter code, abbreviated here. The first letter designates where the device can pace: A, atria; V, ventricle; D, dual (both). The second letter designates where the device senses: A, atria; V, ventricle; D, dual (both). The third letter designates the action of sense(s): I, inhibit; T, trigger; D, dual (both). The fourth letter designates any special feature: R, Rate responsive. The fifth letter is for special antitachycardia features not discussed here. Most, but not all manufactures now use the letters S, D, and R in their model number to indicate S, single chamber (atria or ventricle); D, dual chamber; R, rate responsive—although this designation is not absolute.

and one to check for the appearance of the next natural atrial event. The time limit for the atria (atrial sense to future potential atrial pace) is automatically set to an interval that corresponds to the sensor rate, and varies beat-to-beat according to the sensor rate. The time limit for the ventricle is set to the AV interval (Fig. 34-4).

If natural conduction occurs before the ventricular time limit expires, sensing of the ventricular event will inhibit the ventricular pace because it is not needed. (Fig. 34-5).

When natural atrial rate would be less than sensor rate. There are times when the natural rate would be inadequate (natural rate would be less than the sensor rate) and so it is then necessary to pace the atria at the sensor rate. When an atrial pace occurs, the two time limits are established, with the AA interval set to the equivalent of the sensor rate, and the AV limit set to the AV interval (Fig. 34-6).

If natural AV conduction occurs before the ventricular time limit expires, sensing of the ventricular event will inhibit the ventricular pace because it is not needed (Fig. 34-7).

Prevailing rate. Note that whenever the natural atrial rate is higher than the sensor rate, the natural atrial rate is tracked and sets the HR. Whenever the natural atrial rate would be less than the sensor rate, atrial pacing occurs at the sensor rate and the sensor sets the HR. Whichever rate is higher prevails.*

In most methods, when a premature ventricular complex (PVC) occurs, the atrial time limit from the PVC is reset to an interval equal to the AA interval minus the AV interval.

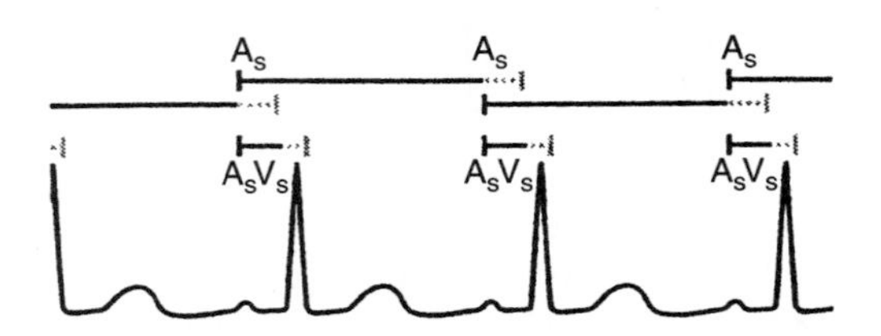

FIG. 34-5. In this example, a natural ventricular depolarization occurred and was sensed before each ventricular time limit expired. This inhibited the remainder of each ventricular time limit.

*In the examples shown, the cycle time limits are measured from atrial events, thus the method is called *AA timing.* Some manufacturers use timing schemes that set a ventricular time limit after each atrial event, and set an atrial time limit after each ventricular event. When troubleshooting pacemaker ECGs, it is important to know what method is used.

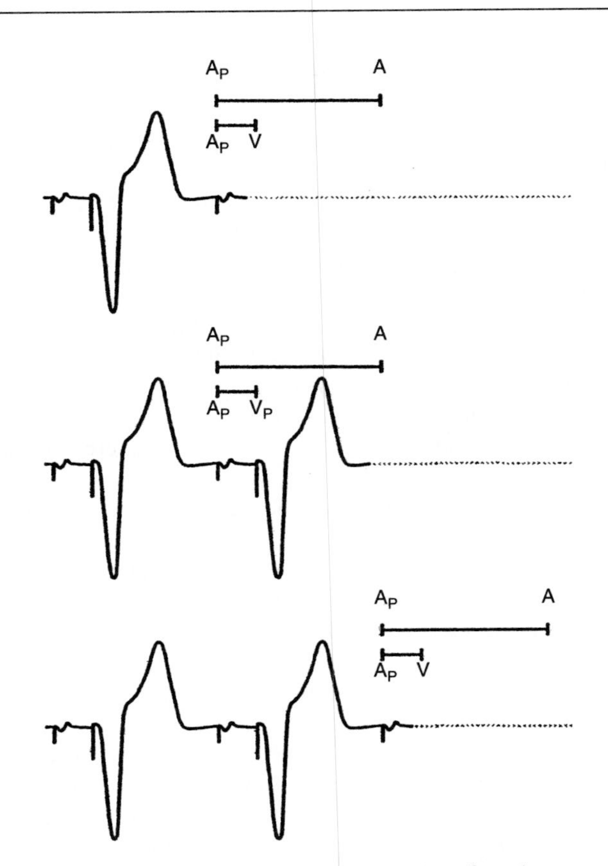

FIG. 34-6. Sketch illustrating sensor rate pacing when the natural atrial rate would be less than the sensor rate. **A,** Pacing of the atria starts two time limits. The *upper bar* represents a time limit for the next atrial event *(A), lower bar* for the next ventricular event *(V).* The sensor constantly adjusts the A_PA time limit to be the interval equivalent of the sensor rate. The atrioventricular (A_PV) time limit is set to the AV interval. **B,** A natural ventricular event failed to occur before the ventricular time limit expired, so the ventricle was paced at the limit expiration and produced a ventricular beat. **C,** Because the natural atrial rate is inadequate (would be less than the sensor rate), the atrial time limit expired and thus the atria was paced and new time limits were immediately reestablished. Note that this produced a sensor atrial paced rate with pacemaker AV synchrony.

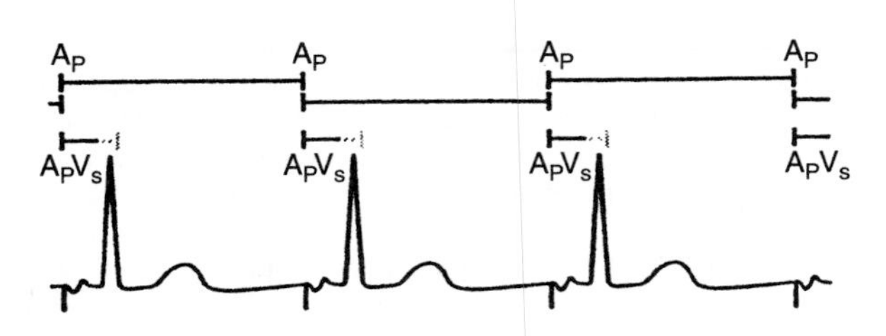

FIG. 34-7. A natural ventricular depolarization occurred and was sensed before each ventricular time limit expired. This inhibited the remainder of each ventricular time limit.

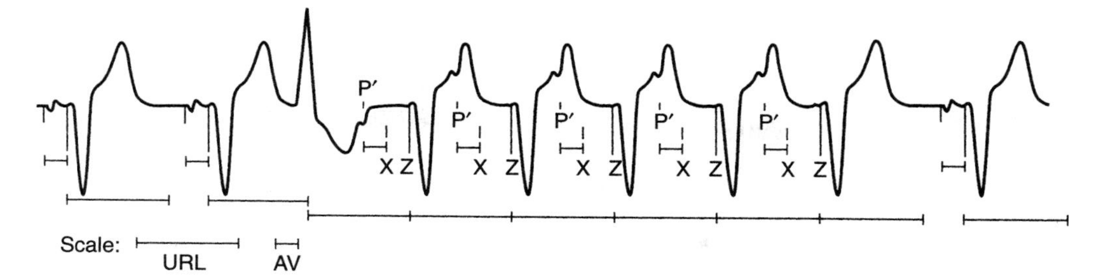

FIG. 34-8. Pacemaker-mediated tachycardia (PMT) caused by retrograde conductions. This pacemaker has a ventricular upper rate limit *(URL)*, which functions by delaying any ventricular pace that would otherwise cause the pacemaker to exceed the URL. After every ventricular event there is a limiting interval corresponding to the URL. Any ventricular pace that would occur within this interval is delayed until the interval expires. Every ventricular event, including the PVC, resets the URL interval. In the ECG the PVC conducts into the atria, producing a retrograde P wave at the first *P′* wave. This P wave is sensed and triggers an atrioventricular interval that expires at *X*. However, the ventricular pace is delayed until the URL interval completes at *Z*. The pace resets the URL interval again. The paced beat now conducts retrogradely to the atria. Because the preceding delay allowed the atria to repolarize, the atria accept the retrograde conduction and produce another retrograde P wave, and the cycle repeats. In the PMT shown, the retrograde mechanism fatigues and the PMT self-terminates.

Correction for Differences in AV Intervals

In the atria the conduction pattern of a natural beat is different from that of a paced beat. Thus there can be a difference in the mechanical AV timing between a sense-initiated AV interval (SAV) and a pace-initiated AV interval (PAV). In advanced pacemakers, these intervals can be independently programmed to compensate for these time differences.

Automatic Adjustment of AV Intervals According to Rate

In a healthy heart the PR interval naturally shortens in association with increases in rate. Advanced pacemakers can be programmed to similarly shorten their AV interval in response to rate increases. This is called *rate adaptive AV interval* and may be applied to the SAV or PAV.

Managing V-to-A Retrograde Conductions

In nearly all hearts with normal conduction, and even many with conduction disease, the AV conduction system is capable of conducting retrogradely from ventricle to atria. But because during normal rhythms the atria set the pace, the conduction is from atria to ventricle and the conduction system is rendered refractory to retrograde conductions. However, a premature ventricular event, such as a PVC or a mistimed ventricular pace, can produce VA retrograde conduction.

In modes that allow tracking of the atria, it is necessary to assure that atrial depolarizations caused by VA conduction are not tracked. If tracked, each atrial depolarization would cause a ventricular pace that would produce another retrograde conduction, and so on in a self-sustaining loop, causing a tachycardia known as a pacemaker-mediated tachycardia (PMT). An example of a PMT is shown in Fig. 34-8.

In this example the PMT is limited at the upper rate limit, but if very long AV intervals are present, the rate may be less than the URL.

To prevent tracking of retrograde beats after ventricular paced beats, an electronic atrial refractory period is initiated by the ventricular event.* Because it occurs after a ventricular event, this period is called a *postventricular atrial refractory period* (PVARP). It is programmed to be slightly longer than the time from the v-pace to the retrograded a-sense, so that the a-sense will not be responded to. With this condition, PMT can not occur. Because it cannot be known with certainty when a retrograde may occur, the PVARP is used after all ventricular events (Fig. 34-9).

*An electronic refractory period is a time during which sensed events are noted but not responded to in the usual manner. Refractory periods may contain a blanking period, during which all sensed events are totally ignored. In complex devices when multiple features are functioning simultaneously (such as bradycardia and tachycardia features), sensed events may be blanked in one feature yet be nonblanked refractory or sensed in another feature, and vice versa.

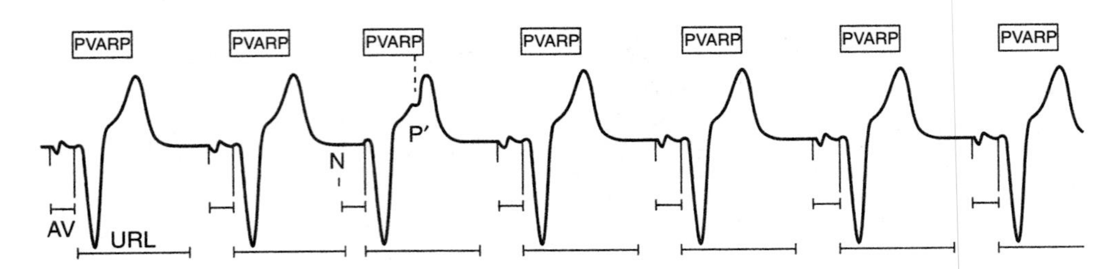

FIG. 34-9. Use of standard postventricular atrial refractory period *(PVARP)* to ignore retrograde conductions after paced beats. After the second complex a momentary intense interference (noise *[N]*) caused a false atrial sense that inhibited the next atrial pace and triggered a subsequent ventricular pace, the third complex. Because the atria had not been paced and had not depolarized intrinsically, a retrograde conduction from the paced beat initiated a retrograde P wave, *P′*. The PVARP covered this P′ wave, preventing tracking and pacemaker-mediated tachycardia. *URL*, Upper rate limit.

It is also desirable to not sense any atrial event after a PVC, thus most pacemakers insert a special PVARP after a PVC for one cycle. This PVARP is set long, usually 400 ms or more because a PVC may originate at a distant location and have a long retrograde conduction time. The pacemaker recognizes PVCs by noting the order of atrial and ventricular events; when a ventricular sense occurs after a preceding ventricular event, with no intervening atrial event, the ventricular sense is assumed to indicate a PVC (Fig. 34-10).

Other strategies are also used, though less commonly. For example, one method paces the atria whenever a PVC occurs. This causes the atria to depolarize so that a retrograde cannot enter the atria. Reviewers of ECGs who note pacemaker artifacts during PVCs should determine if this is the case or if some other explanation should be sought.

Managing Occasional Atrial Tachycardias

In modes that allow tracking of the atria, it is necessary to ensure that *occasional* atrial tachyarrhythmias, which can occur in these patients, are not fully tracked to the ventricle. Three methods are employed to prevent this:

- Limiting the time available for atrial sensing
- Directly limiting the ventricular pacing rate
- Switching temporarily to a nontracking mode with sensor rate during the tachyarrhythmias

The first two methods provide fixed safety limits, whereas the latter provides a desirable sensor-controlled rate.

Limiting the time available for atrial sensing. To limit the time available for atrial sensing, it is customary to program pacemakers to not track any atrial events detect-

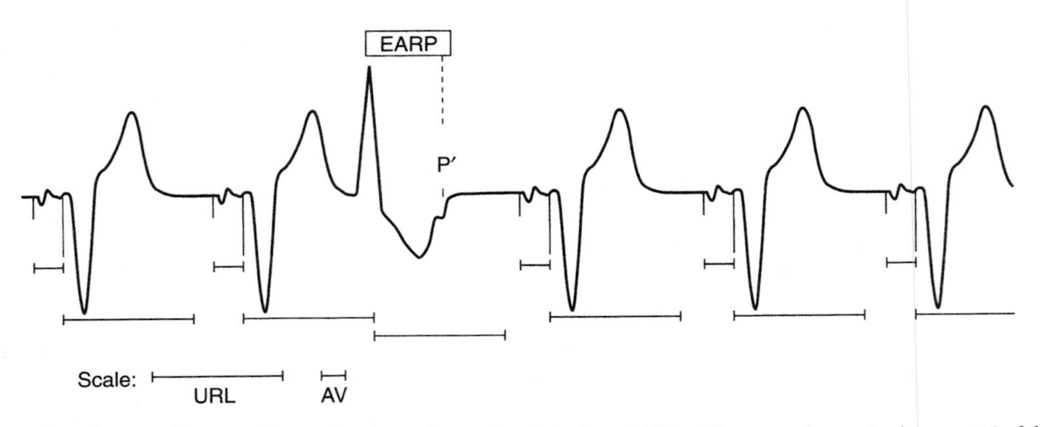

FIG. 34-10. Avoiding tracking of retrograde conductions from PVCs. The second ventricular event is followed by a sensed PVC, with no atrial event between. This sequence initiates an extended atrial refractory period *(EARP)*, which causes the retrograde P wave to be ignored.

ed soon after a ventricular event. This is accomplished by using the PVARP described earlier.

After a tracked atrial sense, no subsequent atrial events can be tracked until the SAV interval and the PVARP have completed. Thus the SAV + PVARP is the shortest atrial cycle length that can be tracked, and 60000/(SAV + PVARP) defines the corresponding rate, known as the maximum atrial tracking rate (MATR).

In patients with complete heart block, at atrial rates higher than the MATR, the ventricular rate will be half the atrial rate, a condition known as pacemaker 2:1 block (Fig. 34-11).

Directly limiting the ventricular pacing rate (to a rate less than the MATR). To directly limit the ventricular pacing rate, at each ventricular event, a time interval is set corresponding to the interval of the rate limit, usually the URL. Any ventricular pace called for during this interval is delayed until this interval has expired. If the natural atrial rate is regular and slightly above the ventricular rate limit, the ventricular paces and associated PVARPs are progressively delayed until a PVARP prevents an atrial sense from being tracked, causing a skipped tracking cycle. This effect is called pacemaker pseudo-Wenckebach (Fig. 34-12).

Suspending tracking and using sensor rate during an atrial tachycardia (mode switch). To switch to a nontracking sensor mode during an atrial tachycardia, one of several methods is used, depending upon the manufacturer. This concept is called *mode switch.* In the most common method, the atrial sensing rate is constantly monitored. If it exceeds a special given upper limit (the detection rate), tracking is temporarily suspended and the sensor rate is employed to control the pacing rate instead. When the atri-

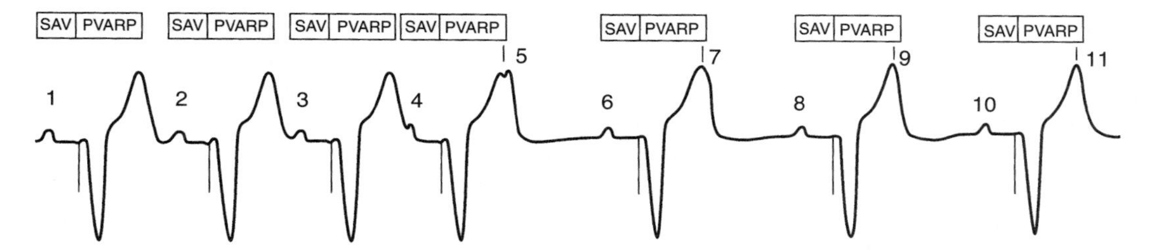

FIG. 34-11. Limitation of tracking rate caused by the total atrial refractory period (sense-initiated atrioventricular interval [*SAV*] + postventricular atrial refractory period *[PVARP]*). The trace illustrates a desirable, naturally increasing atrial tachycardia in a patient with complete heart block; the P waves are numbered. P waves *1* to *4* are tracked normally. As the length of the atrial cycle shortens, each new P wave becomes closer to the previous PVARP. When the atrial cycle length becomes even shorter *(5),* the atrial sense occurs in the previous PVARP and is ignored and a cycle is skipped. The next P wave *(6)* is sensed, but the one that follows *(7)* is ignored. Likewise, *8* is sensed and *9* is ignored, and so forth. When the atrial cycle length becomes less than the SAV + PVARP, every other P wave is sensed and 2:1 pacemaker block occurs.

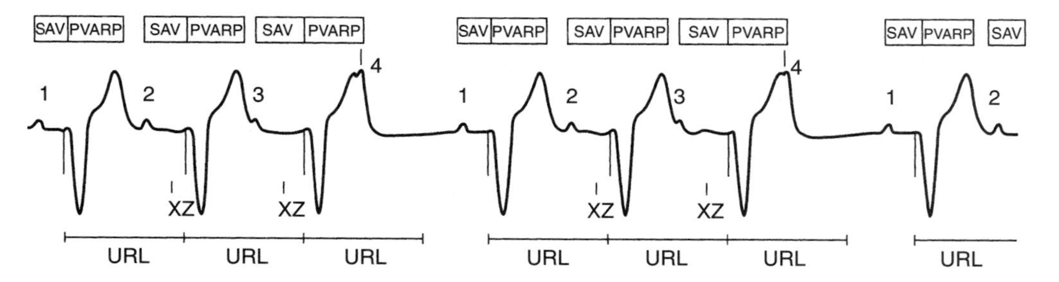

FIG. 34-12. Ventricular upper rate limit *(URL).* In this case the atrial rate is slightly faster than the URL but less than the maximum atrial tracking rate. The first P wave *(1)* is tracked normally. The second and third P waves (*2* and *3*) are tracked, but the URL delays their ventricular paces from *X* to *Z* in each case. The fourth P wave *(4)* occurs just before the end of the postventricular atrial refractory period *(PVARP)* and is ignored. On the next P wave the sequence repeats. In each sequence the first AV interval is in normal synchrony, the next few are lengthened, and the last is dropped: a Wenckebach-like rhythm. The ventricular rate within the sequence is at the URL, but because of dropped beats, the average rate is less than the URL.

al rate returns to below the detection rate, tracking is resumed.

Mode switch may take several seconds to activate, thus an appropriate rate setting for either the URL or MATR is still required (Fig. 34-13).

Alternate schemes are also used. For example, another system suspends tracking of any atrial sense that is more than a given percent higher in equivalent rate than the rate of previous cycles.

Managing Conflict Between Retrograde and Upper Rate Managements

If a long PVARP is required for retrograde protection, it may limit tracking of normally fast atrial rates during exercise, by establishing a restrictive MATR or pseudo Wenckebach (see Figs. 34-11 and 34-12). A new example readily illustrates management strategies. Consider a patient with complete heart block and a good atrial rhythm being exercised (Fig. 34-14, *A*). If the p-p cycle lengths become less than the sum of the SAV interval plus PVARP (the condition when the natural atrial rate is greater than the MATR), every other atrial sense will not be tracked and the ventricular rate will suddenly be half the atrial rate, which is physiologically stressing. Several strategies are used to prevent this large drop.

Sensor-driven override and fill-in. The sensor rate is adjusted to respond near the native atrial rate. When the sensor rate is above what would be the natural rate (Fig. 34-14, *B*), AV pacing occurs uniformly at the sensor rate regardless of tracking limitations. When the sensor rate is below the atrial rate (Fig. 34-14, *C*), the pacing rate will not drop below the sensor rate.

Rate-adaptive, sense-initiated AV intervals (RA-SAV). As can be seen in the MATR formula, MATR = 60000/(SAV + PVARP), shortening the SAV allows faster rates to be tracked. The rate-adaptive features of modern pacemakers can be programmed to automatically shorten the AV intervals when the native rate is fast. Typically both the sensed AV and the paced AV are shortened, so that transitions between them will be smooth.

Although RA-SAV raises the MATR considerably, at very high atrial rates, 2:1 block may still occur. Thus the sensor rate feature is still employed to prevent any large drop in rate (Fig. 34-14, *D*).

Reviewers of ECGs should be aware that AV intervals and the MATR may vary with rate.

Automatic control of PVARP. As can be seen in the MATR formula, shortening the PVARP allows faster rates to be tracked. In some patients increases in sympathetic mechanisms that raise the atrial rate also increase the speed of retrograde conductions, thus at high rates shorter PVARPs may be used in these patients. For patients who demonstrate this response, rate-adaptive features can be programmed to shorten the PVARP at fast rates.

Reviewers of ECGs should be aware that in some patients the PVARP and MATR may vary with rate.

Automatic PMT termination programs. For patients in whom PMT is unlikely, the PVARP is sometimes set short

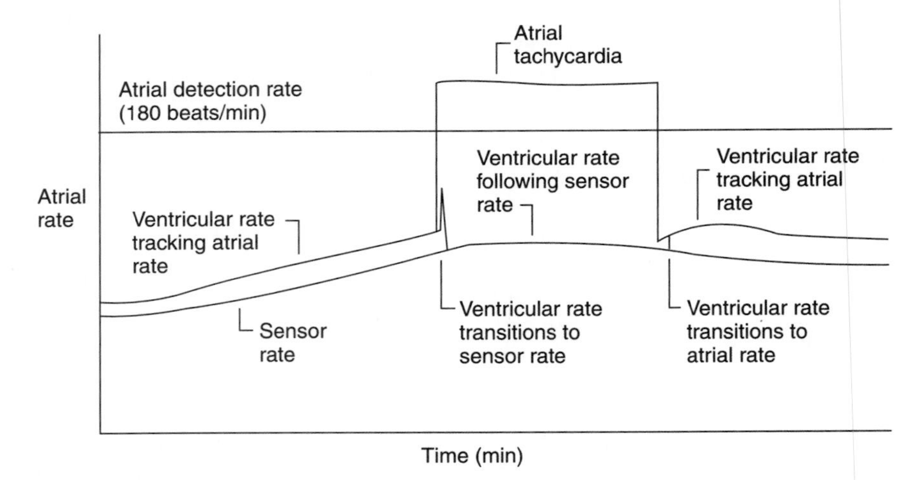

FIG. 34-13. Mode switch. In this example of a patient at moderate activity, the natural atrial rate is a little faster than the sensor rate, so ventricular pacing is initially tracking the atria. The pacemaker constantly monitors the atrial rate. When an atrial tachycardia suddenly appears, the atrial rate is above the atrial tachycardia detection rate (programmed here at 180 beats/min), so tracking is suspended and ventricular pacing assumes the sensor rate. After the tachycardia ends, normal tracking is resumed.

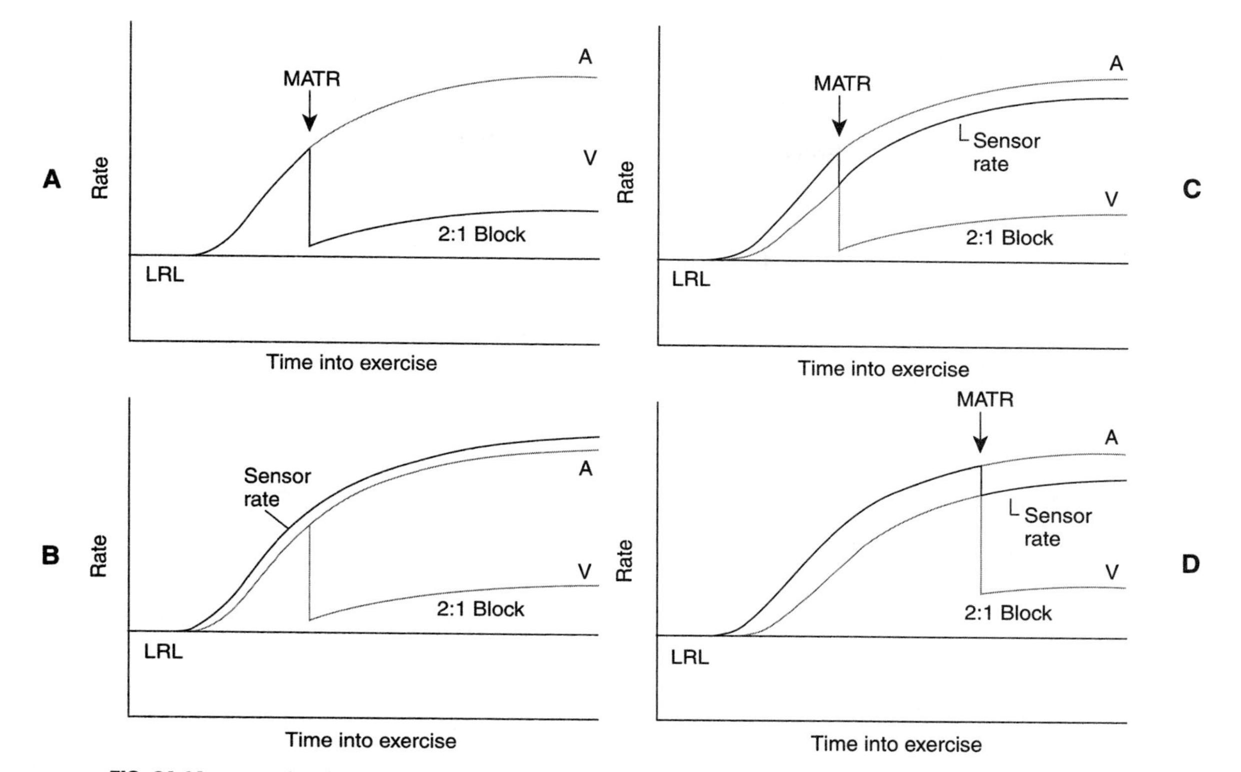

FIG. 34-14. Example of management of upper rate conflicts. **A,** A patient with a good atria and complete heart block undergoes maximal exercise. The atrial rate rises from the lower rate limit and after more than doubling ends at a high rate (A). When the atrial rate reached the maximum atrial tracking rate *(MATR),* alternating atrial depolarizations occurred during postventricular atrial refractory periods so were not tracked, causing the ventricle *(dark line)* to be paced at half the atrial rate. This illustrates the problem when no moderating features are employed. **B,** In this illustration the sensor was a little more aggressive than the natural atrial rate would have been, and both the atria and ventricle *(dark line)* were paced at the sensor rate. **C,** In this illustration the sensor was less aggressive than the natural atrial rate. When the atrial rate reached the MATR, the ventricular rate *(dark line)* dropped but the sensor prevented it from dropping below the sensor rate. **D,** In this illustration the rate-adaptive, sense-initiated AV interval (RA-SAV) shortened as the atrial rate increased, raising the MATR. The ventricular rate *(dark line)* tracked over a larger range before dropping to the sensor rate. When RA-SAV is used, most patients do not reach the MATR, but remain in 1:1 atrioventricular synchrony.

so not to restrict the MATR. Protection from PMT is then provided by a special program that monitors for PMT; when PMT is detected, the program inserts a single long PVARP to terminate the PMT. Various methods are used. For example, one method monitors for atrial senses within 400 ms after each ventricular pace. When eight such senses occur consecutively, a PMT is assumed and a single extended PVARP is applied to terminate it. A skipped beat will be seen on the ECG. Because very fast atrial rates during exercise may be mistaken for repetitive PMT by this method, termination PVARPs are only allowed to repeat every 90 seconds to avoid excessive skipped beats.

Reviewers of ECGs should be aware that various manufactures handle fast rates in various ways. If puzzling observations are seen that are not of urgent concern, contact the manufacturer before assuming a device malfunction. Of course, any dangerous situation should receive immediate attention.

Special Case: Proven Reliable Atrial Function

In a small percentage of patients, there is normal atrial function and unreliable conduction. A simpler pacing system is sometimes used. Because atrial pacing is not required, electrode contact with the atrial wall is not required, thus a single lead with two pairs of electrodes can be used. The atrial pair floats in the atria for atrial sensing, and the ventricular pair senses and paces conventionally.

Most previously discussed features are applicable except those for special circumstances desiring atrial paces (such as atrial pacing for atrial pauses after PSVTs), such paces are not available.

If the atrial rate becomes abnormally slow, below the lower rate limit, ventricular pacing occurs at the lower rate limit by default. This is the VDD mode (see footnote on p. 484 for explanation of letter code). Sensor rate may be used during mode switch operation.

Special Case: Proven Reliable AV Conduction

In a small percentage of patients there is intermittent atrial bradycardia and conduction that was proven by testing to be reliable and expected to be so for many years. In these patients it is only necessary to pace the atria with a responsive HR.

Because AV conduction might become unreliable over time, periodic testing of conduction (usually by temporarily pacing at high rates in a cardiac hospital environment) must be part of ongoing follow-up procedures.

The timing is similar to that described for AV pacemakers, except none of the ventricular features are present. An example is in the previous chapter (see Fig. 33-6).

Special Case: Atrial Fibrillation

Some patients have chronic atrial fibrillation with naturally poor conduction, or drug-depressed conduction. To ensure a good ventricular rate, the ventricle must be paced and sensed. It is fruitless to pace or sense the atria while they are fibrillating. Atrioventricular synchrony cannot be obtained, but a sensor can provide a responsive HR. This is the VVIR mode. An example of this mode (though not during atrial fibrillation) is given in Chapter 33 (see Fig. 33-7).

It is not uncommon to place DDDR-capable pacemakers in those patients who might respond to future pharmacologic conversion of their atrial fibrillation. With an implanted pacemaker present, some drug therapies for treating the atrial fibrillation that were impractical before because of drug-induced bradycardia after conversion may now be practical because if bradycardia happened to result it could be managed by the pacemaker. *Ventricular pacing may obscure warning signs of impending fatal ventricular arrhythmia; therefore, particular caution must be used with atrial drugs that have a ventricular proarrhythmic side effect.* If atrial conversion is likely, DDDR pacing is preferable. Conversion may be intermittent, thus a mode switch feature must be employed to automatically suspend tracking during atrial fibrillation.

Patients with older existing pacemakers that do not have mode switch features may be programmed to a non-tracking mode, usually DVIR or DDIR. The DVIR mode does not sense in the atria and may pace into the tachyarrhythmia, occasionally terminating it. The DDIR mode senses in the atria to inhibit atrial pacing, but these senses do not initiate an AV interval. In both, the ventricular pace occurs at a time corresponding to the sensor rate, and in both modes atrial *paces* trigger AV intervals.

Special Case: Maximizing Atrioventricular Synchrony When Using Ventricular Pacemakers

Many patients who would benefit from AV synchrony only have ventricular single-chamber pacemakers. Some of these patients have sinus rates between 60 and 75 beats/min with conduction much of the time, and only require pacing some of the time. For this select group of patients it may be desirable to permit sensing to rates as low as 60 beats/min because this inhibits pacing much of the time and allows the patient's heart to be in synchrony more of the time. However, when pacing is needed, this rate is too slow because synchrony is lost.

Many of these pacemakers have a feature that allows pacing at a faster rate yet sensing at a lesser rate, a feature called *rate hysteresis.* Whenever the rate drops below the sensing rate, pacing begins at the faster rate. Pacing continues at the faster rate until a natural depolarization is sensed above this faster rate; then the lower sensing rate is applied again (Fig. 34-15).

Retrograde conductions may somewhat reduce the effect of hysteresis by resetting the atria, making it a less frequent occurrence that a natural cycle is fast enough to overcome the pacing rate and reinitiate sensing at the lower rate. Some pacemakers with this feature introduce a lengthened cycle periodically during pacing to allow intrinsic cycles, if there are any, to appear. This concept is called *search hysteresis.*

PACING TO CORRECT FOR VENTRICULAR DYSSYNCHRONY RESULTING FROM CONDUCTION ABNORMALITIES

Preferable Use of Natural Conduction

There is general agreement that normal Purkinje conduction in the ventricle is preferable to either partial Purkinje conduction (as in BBB) or ventricular pacing. Abnormal conduction or single-focus ventricular pacing causes a time offset between the left and right heart that is believed to cause several adverse effects, such as an abnormal pressure differential across the septum, which results

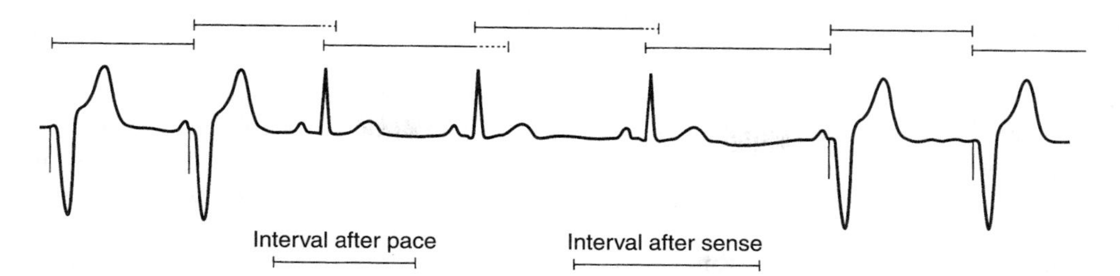

FIG. 34-15. Rate hysteresis. Pacing is occurring at the pacing rate *(shorter interval)*. Sensing of the third complex initiates sensing at the slower hysteresis rate *(longer interval)*. When the native rate becomes less than the hysteresis rate, pacing resumes at the pacing rate *(shorter interval)*.

in septal distortions, possible AV valve closure issues, contractile inefficiencies, and possibly over time a change in fiber organization (remodeling).

Long AV intervals. Historically, for patients with first-degree block or infrequent higher degree blocks, there has always been a notion that long AV intervals should be programmed to allow natural conduction to prevail as much as possible. In most patients this works satisfactorily, however, in some patients this is very problematic if natural AV conduction lengthens and ventricular pacing occurs, because long AV delays allow the atria to repolarize and conduct retrogradely, causing extraneous atrial beats that disrupt AV synchrony and may provoke arrhythmia.

Some pacemakers incorporate self-adjusting AV intervals intended to maximize native AV conduction when possible. Various manufacturers employ various schemes. For example, one device uses a medium AV interval for ventricular pacing and a longer AV for ventricular sensing; specifically, if a ventricular sense occurs while previously ventricular pacing, the device switches to the longer AV interval and continues at the long interval, but whenever conduction delays to beyond the longer AV interval, on the next cycle pacing resumes at the shorter AV. In another device, the AV interval readjusts within a range, but if the range is exceeded the device switches to a preprogrammed AV interval for several hours, and then resumes self-adjustment if operation within the range can again be accomplished.

Reviewers of ECGs may find variations in AV behavior. If this is of interest in the patient's evaluation, the pacemaker should be interrogated to determine which features are turned "on" and to what values parameters are programmed. ECGs that show ventricular pacing (as opposed to conduction) at long AV intervals should be scrutinized carefully for retrograde conduction and for potential loss of atrial capture because at medium-fast sensor rates the retrograded atrial beats may refractorize the atrial tissue to the next atrial pace. The use of long AV intervals requires study and periodic monitoring.

RV outflow tract pacing. In patients with heart failure, maximizing cardiac performance and efficiency is very important; therefore, in patients with ventricle-to-ventricle delays (QRS longer than 130 ms) new pacing strategies are being employed to reduce the delays. This has become known as ventricular resynchronization.

In patients in whom a block is located high in the conduction system and the lower portion is normal, it has been possible to place the ventricular pacing electrode high on the RV septum (RV outflow tract [RVOT]) and stimulate the conduction system well enough to provide simultaneous left and right Purkinje conductions. However, this method is limited to specific conduction situations, electrode positioning is very challenging, and high pacing voltages are required that severely shorten pacemaker battery longevity. In some cases RVOT pacing can provide some degree of resynchronization even if the conduction system is not engaged.

Reviewers of ECGs should note that results vary considerably, thus QRS morphologies also vary considerable from case to case. In the few cases where the Purkinje system is engaged well, the QRS presents a somewhat normal morphology.

Pacing to Synchronize the Ventricular Sequence

Pacing of delinquent chamber to match conducted chamber. In patients with BBB one side of the heart lags behind the other. In some cases it has been possible to pace the delinquent side and bring it into proper timing with the normally conducted side.

Lead placement is technically simple in patients with right-sided block who only need RV pacing, but unfortunately the majority of patients have a left-sided block. They require pacing of the left ventricle, which is technically challenging.

Although the timing of the paced chamber is electronically controlled, conduction to the other chamber varies somewhat. QRS morphologies display fusion and are highly variable and changeable because small time differences, left versus right, remarkably alter signal summations. Ideally, the overall QRS duration should be reduced from the unpaced QRS.

Pacing both left and right ventricles (biventricular pacing). An alternate approach has become more common. In this scheme, the right and left ventricles are separately paced. This has become known as *biventricular* pacing. Older devices pace the left and right simultaneously, whereas newer devices pace one chamber a little before or after the other, to adjust the timing to provide the best cardiac performance (Fig. 34-16).

Some patients with heart failure have no rate disturbances and only require pacing for resynchronization, but many also require protection against serious ventricular tachycardias. Thus resynchronization therapies are available as options in both pacemakers and implantable cardioverter defibrillators (ICDs) of certain models. An ICD with this option is sketched in Fig. 33-19.

Upon pacing of each electrode an artifact appears on the ECG. If the ventricular paces are simultaneous, only one artifact appears, but if they are not simultaneous, two appear. Some ECG monitors with "pacemaker detect" and transtelephonic monitors, may not be able to display the second pulse if the delay is very small.

A depolarization spreads outward from each electrode and the two wave fronts soon collide, and depolarization quickly completes. The surface ECG records the electrical summation of these depolarizations as a fusion beat with a shorter QRS duration (Fig. 34-17). The morphologies vary widely depending on the timing selected. Usually the AV intervals are programmed short such that the paced depolarizations complete before any intrinsic conduction enters the ventricle, but sometimes not if intrinsic conduction is helpful; if included, there is additional fusion.

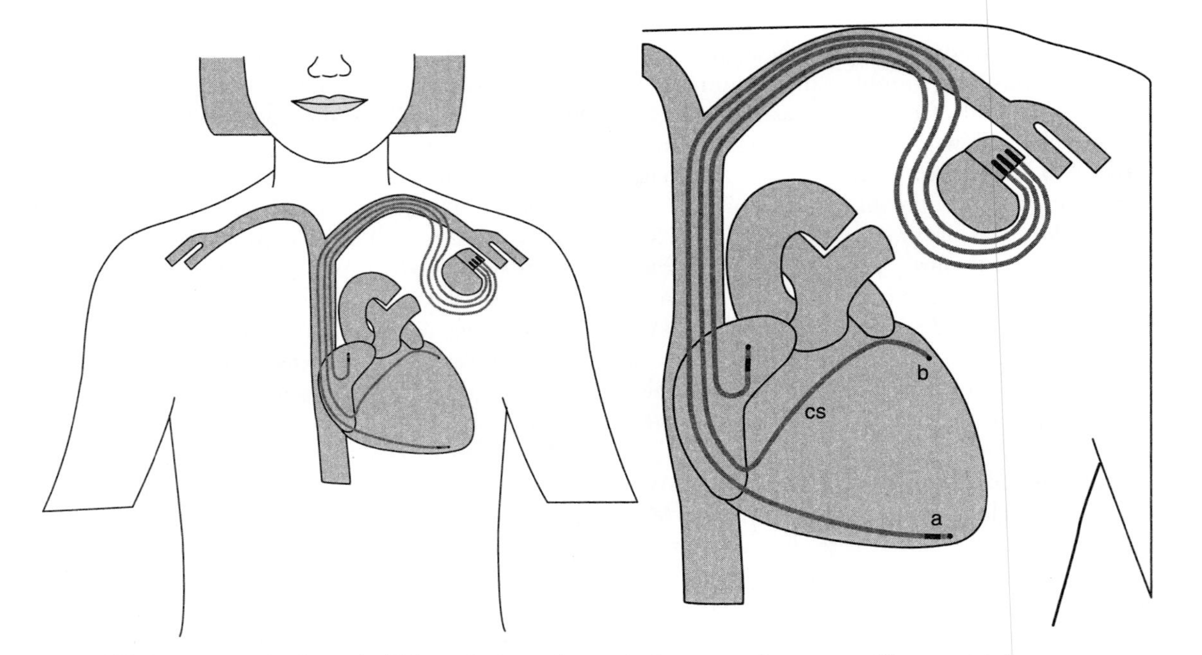

FIG. 34-16. Sketch of a typical biventricular atrioventricular pacemaker system. The ventricle has one pacing and sensing site in the RV apex *(a)* and another on the far LV *(b)*. Electrical access to the LV is usually made transvenously, but not into the left heart. (Leads may not be placed inside the left heart because tiny blood clots might form along the lead and disseminate systemically.) On the back side of the heart in the groove between the atria and ventricle, there is a tubular conduit called the coronary sinus *(cs)*. Some of the coronary veins, especially those from the left heart, drain into this sinus. The sinus in turn drains into the low right atria. To electrically access the LV, a pacing lead is advanced through the RA, leftward and upward through the coronary sinus, and into a coronary vein leading downward behind the LV. The electrode on the lead thus paces and senses the LV through the wall of the vein. Coronary vein access is technically difficult and not always accomplished, so on some such occasions, an epicardial electrode is placed on the LV epicardium via a minimally invasive thoracic approach.

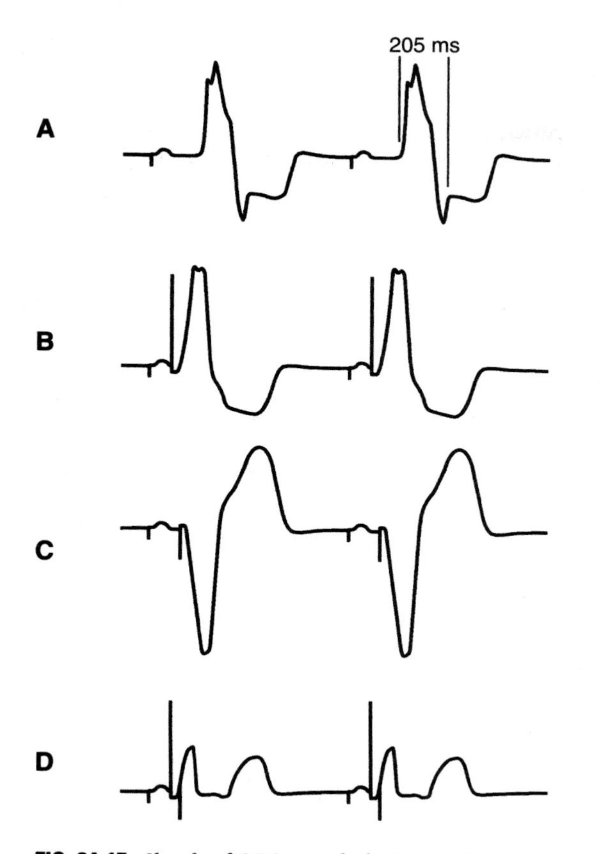

FIG. 34-17. Sketch of QRS morphologies in a biventricular pacing system. **A,** Delayed conduction (unpaced) results in a 205 ms ventricular depolarization. **B,** Pacing of left ventricle. **C,** Pacing of right ventricle. **D,** Biventricular pacing of ventricles. Note that in this case the left pacing site begins first and the QRS begins with that pattern. But as soon as the right pacing site begins, ECG fusion occurs producing a new morphology. Quite soon the depolarizations collide; note the abrupt completion of the complex.

In some pacemakers sensing can occur at either electrode, and in others just at one electrode. This can be a consideration in troubleshooting. For example, in normal operation, both electrodes pace and capture, refractorizing adjacent tissue, so no sensing occurs. However, if there is loss of capture at one electrode, depolarization from the capturing electrode can spread to the noncapturing electrode and be sensed there later (if the circuit for this electrode allows sensing).

ECG monitors in the intensive care or critical care units do not display the timing and internal ECG channels that can be transmitted to programmers by telemetry from pacemakers and ICDs. However, programmer printouts are often included in patient records and provide considerable understanding (Fig. 34-18).

On the left, biventricular pacing was occurring *(1-4)*. In the surface ECG note the abrupt termination of the QRS complex caused by the collision of the left and right wave fronts. Because both RV and LV electrodes captured, there was no conventional signal to be sensed at this time, thus the only timing event was the delivery of ventricular paces, as displayed on the marker channel *(VP)*.

In the atrial electrogram *(AEG; bottom tracing)* the large downward deflections are artifacts caused by the ventricular paces, which because of their high strength would have been recordable everywhere in the heart; each of these overwhelmed the internal ECG for about 40 ms. Apart from these artifacts, the atrial ECG shows atrial depolarizations *(8-11)* about 240 ms after each ventricular pace. Because of their consistency, these were almost surely caused by retrograde conductions from the ventricular beats. Note these are not visible on the surface ECG, yet clearly visible in the endogram, illustrating the insight gained from internal ECG recordings. The atrial deflections have a sharp appearance because the internal atrial electrodes recorded most strongly from their small region of contact with the heart wall, through which the depolarizations passed quickly.

Just after pace 3, a program command was sent. The cluster of pacing artifact markings seen there occurred because of the detection of the radio magnetic program commands from the programmer. These are often picked up by external ECG cables and trigger artifact markings; these are not true pacing artifacts. The internal ECG transmission was also suspended for this cycle.

The new program, which took effect just after pace 4, decreased the output such that the LV electrode lost capture. Capture *(5, 6)* continued at the RV electrode and depolarizations spread slowly to the LV electrode where they were sensed, as indicated by the marker channel *(VS)*, about 200 ms after the paces *(VP)*. In this particular case, the delay exceeded the electronic ventricular refractory period of the pacemaker (shortened for testing) and the pacemaker timing was reset, lowering the effective rate to 69 beats/min.

The atrial recording *(12)* shows an almost iso-electric signal, suggesting that at this slower rate the retrograde fused with a native atrial event. Several seconds later *(7)* several native cycles occurred. Note these internal p waves *(13, 14)* are different.

As ventricular depolarization *(7)* passed one electrode, it was sensed *(VS)* and set the electronic ventricular refractory period. As depolarization passed the other electrode about 130 ms later, it was sensed during the electronic refractory period and so marked *(VR)*. Senses during refractory periods do not affect the immediate timing.

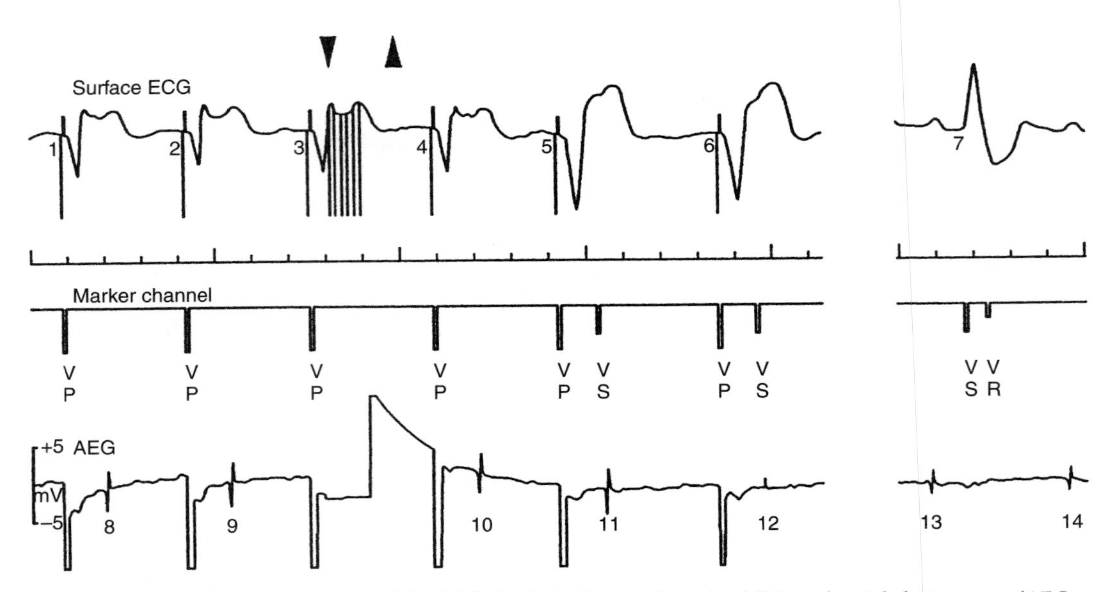

FIG. 34-18. Simultaneous tracings of the ECG *(top)*, timing markers *(middle)*, and atrial electrogram *(AEG; bottom)* are recorded during deliberate testing of a normal biventricular system that can sense from both left and right ventricles. Both ventricles were paced simultaneously, producing single-appearing pacing artifacts. In this test only the ventricular electrodes were programmed to pace and sense; the atrial electrodes were programmed to display the AEG, which was transmitted along with the timing marker to the programmer for display on the surface ECG. The marker channel marks when and where the pacemaker delivered paces and sensed; it does not discern capture or the nature of the signals that were sensed. See text for further explanation.

If the atrial sense marker had been programmed "on," the marker channel also would have marked those internal p waves, which would have been sensed.

SPECIAL FEATURES

Pacemaker Management of Vasovagal and Carotid Sinus Syndromes

These syndromes have two components: cardioinhibitory-induced bradycardia and low stroke volumes resulting from low venous pressures. Pacing can correct the bradycardia, and transiently pacing at a considerably elevated rate can increase cardiac output at small stroke volumes. AV pacing is always used because the atrial contraction aids ventricular filling. Several methods are used.

AV pacing with rate hysteresis. With this feature turned on, the pacing rate is faster than the sensing rate. For example, the pacing rate may be 80 beats/min and the sensing rate 50 beats/min. At the onset of a cardioinhibitory event the sinus rate may drop below 50 beats/min, initiating pacing at 80 beats/min. Later when the natural rate exceeds 80 beats/min, sensing resumes. Reviewers of ECGs can identify this feature by noting that the cycle preceding the first atrial pace is longer than the next paced cycle.

Rate-drop response pacing. This feature is designed specifically for treating cardioinhibitory bradycardias with low filling pressures. The pacemaker monitors a rate range just below the typical lower natural rates of the patient. When the atrial rate drops quickly through this range, a cardioinhibitory event is assumed and AV pacing is initiated at a fast rate. Pacing continues at the fast rate for several minutes and then decreases gradually until a reasonable natural rate is encountered. Reviewers of ECGs will note sudden drops in native atrial rate, followed by fast atrial-paced or AV-paced rates that reduce stepwise over several minutes.

Sleep Rates

Some pacemakers contain built-in clocks that can be programmed to permit lower rates during sleeping hours. A typical case might be where the rate declines gradually during a half hour in the late evening and increases gradually during a half hour in the early morning.

OBTAINING ASSISTANCE

Pacemakers of various brands and models may differ significantly from the preceding general descriptions. Most manufacturers have a 24-hour hotline staffed by experts who are familiar with their brand of pacemakers. These individuals can be quite helpful.

Index

F

G

H

I

J

K

L

S

Y